Principles and Techniques of Cutaneous Surgery

Principles and Techniques of Cutaneous Surgery

Gary P. Lask, M.D.

Clinical Professor of Medicine/Dermatology
University of California at Los Angeles
School of Medicine
Director of Dermatologic Surgery and Research
Harbor-UCLA Medical Center
Director, Dermatology Laser Center
University of California at Los Angeles Medical Center
Los Angeles, California

Ronald L. Moy, M.D.

Chief of Dermatologic Surgery
Veterans Administration–
West Los Angeles Medical Center;
Assistant Professor
Division of Dermatology
University of California at Los Angeles
Los Angeles, California

McGraw-Hill

New York   St. Louis   San Francisco   Auckland   Bogotá   Caracas   Lisbon   London   Madrid
Mexico City   Milan   Montreal   New Delhi   San Juan   Singapore   Sydney   Tokyo   Toronto

McGraw-Hill

A Division of The McGraw-Hill Companies

Principles and Techniques of Cutaneous Surgery

1 2 3 4 5 6 7 8 9 0   QPK QPK   9 8 7 6 5

ISBN 0-07-036471-0

This book was set in Times by Quebecor Printing/Kingsport. The editors were Michael Houston, Jamie Kircher, and Mariapaz Ramos Englis, and the production supervisor was Richard Ruzycka; the cover designer was Marsha Cohen/Parallelogram. The project was managed by David Marcus Green for Monotype Editorial Services. Quebecor Printing/Kingsport was printer and binder.

This book is printed on acid-free paper.

Library of Congress Cataloging-in-Publication Data

Principles and techniques of cutaneous surgery/[edited by] Gary Lask
and Ronald L. Moy.
    p.   cm.
  Includes bibliographical references and index.
  ISBN 0-07-036471-0
  1. Skin—Surgery. I. Lask, Gary P. (Gary Philip) II. Moy.
Ronald L.
  [DNLM: 1. Skin—surgery. 2. Skin Transplantation—methods.
3. Surgery, Plastic—methods.   WR 100 P957 1996]
RD520.P747 1996
617.4′77—dc20
DNLM/DLC
for Library of Congress   95-2894

Contents

PART I INTRODUCTION

1 Wound Healing • 1
Eric Bernstein / Alain Mauviel / John McGrath / Laura Bolten / Toby Frank / Jouni Uitto

2 Surgical Wound Dressings • 23
David S. Freitag

3 Surgical Anatomy • 35
Hubert Greenway

4 Sterilization of Equipment for Dermatologic Surgery • 47
Jack K. Sebben / Michael J. Fazio

5 Infection Control • 57
Mary E. Maloney

6 Local Anesthesia • 63
Seth L. Matarasso / Richard G. Glogau

7 Wound Closure Materials • 77
Jeffrey L. Melton / C. William Hanke

8 Instrumentations for Dermatologic Surgery • 85
Renuka Diwan

PART II EVALUATION AND MANAGEMENT OF THE SURGICAL PATIENT

9 Preoperative Evaluation of the Cutaneous Surgery Patient • 101
Barry Leshin / Timothy H. McCalmont

10 Perioperative Emergencies • 113
Rufus M. Thomas / Rex A. Amonette / John L. Buker

11 Postoperative and Ongoing Care Following Surgery • 125
Thomas H. King / Donald J. Grande

12 Medicological Issues for the Dermatologic Surgeon • 137
Abel Torres

PART III PROCEDURES AND TECHNICAL ASPECTS

13 Electrosurgery • 145
Daniel M. Siegel / David Kriegel

14 Cryosurgery • 153
Rodney P. R. Dawber

15 Cold Steel Surgery: The Ellipse • 165
Leonard H. Goldberg

16 Suturing Techniques • 171
George J. Hruza

17 Management of Excess Tissue: Dog-Ears, Cones, and Protrusions • 187
Daniel E. Gormley

18 The Elliptic Excision and Variations • 201
Peter B. Odland / Brian H. Kumasaka

19 Lines of Elective Incision on the Skin • 209
Gerald Bernstein

PART IV CHEMICAL DESTRUCTIVE TECHNIQUES

20 Surgical and Medical Treatment of Benign Cutaneous Lesions • 221
Harry M. Humeniuk / Gary P. Lask

21 Surgical Treatment of Malignant Lesions • 235
Christine M. Hayes / Duane C. Whitaker

22 Scar Revision • 249
David J. Leffell

v

23 Nails • 265
Bernard I. Raskin

24 Punch Graft • 283
David S. Orentreich

25 Full-Thickness Skin Grafts • 297
David E. Kent

26 Flap Surgery • 309
Roy C. Grekin

27 Lip Reconstruction • 329
Michael J. Fazio / John A. Zitelli

28 Reconstruction of the Forehead and Temple • 349
Glenn D. Goldstein / Jemshed A. Khan

29 Reconstruction of the Ear • 363
J. Ramsey Mellette, Jr.

30 Nasal Reconstruction • 381
Nicholas Telfer / Ronald L. Moy

31 Understanding Sclerotherapy • 403
David M. Duffy

32 Soft-Tissue Augmentation in the Practice of
Dermatology • 419
Arnold W. Klein / Gary D. Monheit / David M. Duffy

33 Microlipoinjection: Autologous Fat Grafting • 437
Richard G. Glogau / Seth L. Matarasso / Andrew C. Markey

34 Lasers in Dermatology • 445
Edward Glassberg / Kristin Walker / Gary P. Lask

**PART V   PROCEDURES AND TECHNICAL
ASPECTS**

35 Hair Replacement • 469
Walter P. Unger

36 Dermabrasion • 495
Stephen H. Mandy

37 Chemical Peel • 505
Lawrence S. Moy

38 Split-Thickness Skin Grafts • 519
John W. Skouge

39 Tumescent Liposuction with Local Anesthesia • 529
Jeffrey A. Klein

40 Scalp Reduction • 543
Paul T. Rose

41 Mohs Micrographic Surgery • 561
Paul O. Larson / Stephen N. Snow / Frederic E. Mohs

42 Ear Piercing Surgical and Repair of the Earlobe • 579
Deborah Atkin / Gary P. Lask

43 Blepharoplasty • 583
Sorin Eremia

44 Tissue Expansion • 605
*Windell Davis-Boutte / S. Rokhsan Taherpour / Ronald L.
Moy / Bernard Cohen / Gordon H. Sasaki*

Index • 619

Contributors

Rex A. Amonette, M.D. [10]
Clinical Professor of Dermatology, University of Tennessee, Memphis, Tennessee

Deborah H. Atkin, M.D. [42]
Resident in Dermatology, University of Arizona College of Medicine, Tucson, Arizona

Eric F. Bernstein, M.D. [1]
Assistant Professor, Department of Dermatology, Jefferson Medical College, Thomas Jefferson University, Philadelphia, Pennsylvania

Gerald Bernstein, M.D. [19]
Associate Professor, Department of Dermatology, University of Washington School of Medicine, Seattle, Washington

Laura L. Bolten, Ph.D. [1]
Worldwide Director of Scientific Affairs, Convatec, Bristol-Myers Squibb, Skillman, New Jersey; Adjunct Assistant Professor of Surgery, University of Medicine and Dentistry of New Jersey, Piscataway, New Jersey

Windell Davis-Boutte, M.D. [44]
Resident Physician, Emory Clinic, Atlanta, Georgia

John L. Buker, M.D. [10]
Assistant Clinical Professor of Dermatology, University of Tennessee, Memphis, Tennessee

Bernard Cohen, M.D. [44]
Clinical professor of Surgical Training
Department of Dermatology and Cutaneous Surgery
University of Miami School of Medicine
Miami, Florida

Rodney P. R. Dawber, M.D., F.R.C.P. [14]
Consultant Dermatologist, Clinical Senior Lecturer in Dermatology, Department of Dermatology, Churchill Hospital, Oxford University, Oxford, England

Renuka Diwan, M.D. [8]
Assistant Professor, Department of Dermatology, Case Western Reserve University, Cleveland, Ohio

David M. Duffy, M.D. [31, 32]
Assistant Clinical Professor of Medicine (Dermatology), University of California at Los Angeles; Associate Professor of Medicine (Dermatology), University of Southern California, Los Angeles, California

Sorin Eremia, M.D. [43]
Associate Clinical Professor of Medicine, School of Medicine; Director of Dermatology, University of California at Los Angeles, Los Angeles, California

Michael J. Fazio, M.D. [4, 27]
Clinical Assistant Professor of Dermatology, University of California, Davis, Sacramento, California

Toby Frank, M.D. [1]
Chief Resident, Dermatology Residency Training Program, Jefferson Medical College, Thomas Jefferson University, Philadelphia, Pennsylvania

David S. Freitag, M.D. [2]
Clinical Assistant Professor, Department of Dermatology, Howard University College of Medicine, Washington, DC

Edward Glassberg, M.D. [34]
Assistant Clinical Professor of Medicine (Dermatology), School of Medicine, University of California at Los Angeles; Associate-Director, Dermatologic Surgery and Research, Harbor-UCLA Medical Center, Torrance, California

Richard G. Glogau, M.D. [6, 33]
Clinical Professor of Dermatology, University of California, San Francisco, San Francisco, California

Leonard H. Goldberg, M.D. [15]
Professor of Clinical Dermatology, Chief, Dermatologic Surgery, Baylor College of Medicine, Texas Medical Center, Houston, Texas

Glenn D. Goldstein, M.D. [28]
Clinical Assistant Professor of Medicine, Kansas University Medical Center; Director Skin and Mohs Surgery Center, Baptist Medical Center, Kansas City, Missouri

Brackets refer to chapters written or co-written by contributors.

Daniel E. Gormley, M.D. [17]
Assistant Clinical Professor, Division of Dermatology, Center for Health Sciences, University of California, Los Angeles

Donald J. Grande, M.D. [11]
Assistant Professor of Medicine (Dermatology), University of Massachusetts Medical School, Worcester, Massachusetts

Hubert Greenway, M.D. [3]
Head, Mohs Surgery and Cutaneous Laser Unit, Director, Cutaneous Oncology Green Cancer Center, Scripps Clinic and Research Foundation; Assistant Clinical Professor, University of California San Diego, La Jolla, California

Roy C. Grekin, M.D. [26]
Associate Clinical Professor of Dermatology, Chief, Dermatologic and Mohs Surgery Unit, Department of Dermatology, University of California, San Francisco, San Francisco, California

C. William Hanke, M.D., F.A.C.P. [7]
Vice-Chairman and Professor of Dermatology, Professor of Pathology, Professor of Otolaryngology-Head and Neck Surgery, Indiana University School of Medicine, Indianapolis, Indiana

Christine M. Hayes, M.D. [21]
Assistant Professor of Dermatology, Tufts University School of Medicine; Director of Dermatologic Surgery, New England Medical Center, Boston, Massachusetts

George J. Hruza, M.D. [16]
Assistant Professor of Dermatology, Otolaryngology and Surgery, Washington University School of Medicine; Director Cutaneous Surgery Center, Barnes Hospital, St. Louis, Missouri

Harry M. Humeniuk, M.D. [20]
Assistant Clinical Professor, Medical College of Ohio, Department of Medicine, Division of Dermatology, Department of Pathology, Department of Otolaryngology

David E. Kent, M.D. [25]
Clinical Instructor Division of Dermatology, Department of Medicine, Medical College of Georgia, Augusta, Georgia; Clinical Assistant Professor Department of Medicine, Mercer University School of Medicine, Macon, Georgia

Jemshed A. Khan, M.D. [28]
Clinical Assistant Professor of Ophthalmology, Kansas University School of Medicine, Kansas City, Kansas; Director, Eyelid Plastic Surgery, Hunkeler Eye Center, Kansas City, Missouri

Thomas H. King, M.D. [11]
Chief, Dermatology Service, David Grant Medical Center; Assistant Clinical Professor of Dermatology, University of California, Davis, Sacramento, California

Arnold W. Klein, M.D. [32]
Associate Clinical Professor Dermatology/Medicine, Center for the Health Sciences, University of California at Los Angeles; Attending Physician, UCLA-Harbor General Hospital, Los Angeles, California

Jeffrey A. Klein, M.D. [39]
Capistrano Surgicenter, San Juan Capistrano, California

David Krieger, M.D. [13]
SUNY at Stony Brook, School of Medicine; Assistant Professor, Department of Dermatology; Chief of Dermatology, Northport Veterans Administration

Brian H. Kumasaka, M.D. [18]
Department of Dermatology, Virginia Mason Medical Center; Clinical Instructor, University of Washington, Seattle, Washington

Paul O. Larson, M.D. [41]
Associate Professor, Department of Surgery, Mohs Surgery Clinic, University of Wisconsin Hospital and Clinics, Madison, Wisconsin

Gary P. Lask, M.D. [20, 34, 42]
Clinical Professor of Medicine/Dermatology, School of Medicine, University of California at Los Angeles; Director of Dermatologic Surgery and Research, Harbor-UCLA Medical Center; Director, Dermatology Laser Center, University of California at Los Angeles Medical Center, Los Angeles, California

David J. Leffell, M.D. [22]
Associate Professor of Dermatology, Plastic Surgery and Otolaryngology, Yale University School of Medicine; Chief, Dermatologic Surgery, Yale-New Haven Hospital, New Haven, Connecticut

Barry Leshin, M.D. [9]
Associate Professor of Dermatology, Associate Professor of Otolaryngology, Director of Dermatologic Surgery, Wake Forest University Medical Center, Winston-Salem, NC

Mary E. Maloney, M.D. [5]
Associate Professor of Medicine, Director of Mohs Micrographic Surgery, Penn State University, College of Medicine, Hershey, Pennsylvania

Stephen H. Mandy, M.D. [36]
Clinical Professor of Dermatology, University of Miami; Director, Aspen Skin Clinic, Aspen, Colorado

Andrew C. Markey, M.D. [33]
St. John's Institute of Dermatology, St. Thomas Hospital, London, England

Seth L. Matarasso, M.D. [6, 33]
Assistant Clinical Professor of Dermatology, University of California School of Medicine, San Francisco, California

Alain Mauviel, Ph.D. [1]
Assistant Professor of Dermatology and Cutaneous Biology, Jefferson Medical College, Thomas Jefferson University, Philadelphia, Pennsylvania

Timothy H. McCalmont, M.D. [9]
Assistant Clinical Professor, Department of Pathology, Division of Dermatopathology, University of California at San Francisco, San Francisco, California

John McGrath, M.D. [1]
Post-doctoral Research Fellow, Department of Dermatology and
Cutaneous Biology, Jefferson Medical College, Thomas Jefferson
University, Philadelphia, Pennsylvania

J. Ramsey Mellette, Jr., M.D. [29]
Associate Professor of Dermatology; Director, Division of Mohs
Micrographic Surgery and Cutaneous Oncology, University of
Colorado Health Sciences Center, Denver, Colorado

Jeffrey L. Melton, M.D. [7]
Assistant Professor, Director of Dermatologic and Mohs Surgery,
Division of Dermatology, Loyola University of Chicago,
Maywood, Illinois

Frederic E. Mohs, M.D. [41]
Emeritus Clinical Professor, Department of Surgery, Mohs Surgery
Clinic, University of Wisconsin Hospital and Clinics, Madison,
Wisconsin

Gary D. Monheit, M.D. [32]
Assistant Professor, Department of Dermatology, University of
Alabama Medical Center, Birmingham, Alabama

Lawrence S. Moy, M.D. [37]
Private Practice, Manhattan Beach, California; Assistant Clinical
Professor of Medicine, School of Medicine University of California
at Los Angeles, Los Angeles, California

Ronald L. Moy, M.D. [30, 44]
Chief of Dermatologic Surgery, Veterans Administration–West Los
Angeles Medical Center; Assistant Professor, Division of
Dermatology, University of California at Los Angeles, Los
Angeles, California

Peter B. Odland, M.D. [18]
Assistant Professor of Medicine of Dermatology,University of
California at Los Angeles, Director of Dermatologic Surgery at the
Veterans Administration, West Los Angeles Medical Center, Los
Angeles, California

David S. Orentreich, M.D. [24]
Assistant Clinical Professor, Department of Dermatology, Mt. Sinai
School of Medicine; Assistant Attending, Department of
Dermatology, Mount Sinai Hospital, New York, New York

Bernard I. Raskin, M.D. [23]
Assistant Clinical Professor, Department of Medicine, Division of
Dermatology, University of California at Los Angeles, Los
Angeles, California

Paul T. Rose, M.D. [40]
Assistant Clinical Professor, Department of Dermatology,
University of South Florida; Director, Coastal Laser and
Dermatology Center, Tampa, Florida

Gordon H. Sasaki, M.D., F.A.C.S. [44]
Active Staff, Huntington Memorial Hospital, Pasadena, California

Jack K. Sebben, M.D. [4]
Associate Clinical Professor of Dermatology
University of California, Davis
Sacramento, California

Daniel M. Siegel, M.D. [13]
SUNY at Stony Brook, School of Medicine; Vice Chairman,
Department of Dermatology; Associate Professor of Dermatology;
Director, Division of Dermatologic Surgery

John W. Skouge, M.D. [38]
Assistant Professor, Johns Hopkins University, Baltimore,
Maryland

Stephen N. Snow, M.D. [41]
Associate Professor, Department of Surgery, Mohs Surgery Clinic,
University of Wisconsin Hospital and Clinics, Madison, Wisconsin

S. Rokhsan Taherpour, M.D. [44]
Resident Physician, County Hospital, University of Southern
California, Los Angeles, California

Nicholas R. Telfer, M.D., M.R.C.P. [30]
Consultant Dermatological Surgeon, University Department of
Dermatology, Manchester, England

Rufus M. Thomas, M.D. [10]
Private Practice, Clyde, North Carolina

Abel Torres, M.D., J.D. [12]
Associate Professor of Dermatology, Assistant Dean for Clinical
Education, Loma Linda University School of Medicine, Loma
Linda, California

Jouni Uitto, M.D., Ph.D. [1]
Professor of Dermatology, Professor of Biochemistry and
Molecular Biology, Chairman, Department of Dermatology,
Jefferson Medical College, Thomas Jefferson University,
Philadelphia, Pennsylvania

Walter P. Unger, M.D., F.R.C.P.(C.) [35]
Associate Professor of Medicine (Dermatology), University of
Toronto, Toronto, Canada

Kristin Walker, M.D. [34]
Dermatology Resident, LAC-USC Medical Center, Los Angeles,
California

Duane C. Whitaker, M.D. [21]
Professor, Director Dermatologic Surgery and Cutaneous Laser
Surgery, Department of Dermatology, University of Iowa Hospitals
and Clinics, Iowa City, Iowa

John A. Zitelli, M.D. [27]
Shadyside Medical Center, Pittsburgh, Pennsylvania

Preface

There has been tremendous growth in the area of cutaneous surgery over the last 15 years. This textbook has been written to teach the most current principles and techniques of cutaneous surgery, while maintaining a strong foothold in the basics necessary for optimal results. The authors recruited are some of the brightest and most innovative in the field, and the work illustrated herein represents the many changes and new procedures that now define cutaneous surgery. In addition, the text is based on the core curriculum developed by the American Society for Dermatologic Surgery and may offer a guideline for course of study by both cutaneous surgery residents and practicing dermatologic surgeons.

A variety of surgical techniques are required training during residency. Several advances have been made in recent years in the areas of hair restoration, laser surgery, liposuction, sclerotherapy and facial rejuvenation. Each of these areas is presented in the text by a renown surgeon specializing in the field, contains the necessary basic science, current discussion and illustrated procedures for a step by step approach. There is also new information on topics such as the basic science area of wound healing and cutaneous aging.

The initial impetus for the growth of dermatologic surgery was in large part thanks to Frederic Mohs. The Mohs micrographic surgery, with the advent of fresh tissue technique, is now recognized as the treatment of choice for certain cutaneous carcinomas and is documented to yield the highest cure rate with the least amount of tissue removed. Dermatologists are becoming more and more interested in reconstructive techniques that result from the removal of large tumors with Mohs micrographic surgery.

Dermatology has always been a leader in the area of hair restoration, from the early work of Orentrich to the more recent innovations of Unger and Stough resulting in smaller grafts with a more natural appearance.

The world of cutaneous laser surgery made dramatic advances in the last ten years due primarily to the innovative work of Rox Anderson and John Parrish of Harvard Medical School, with their development of the concept of selective photothermolysis. This theory resulted in the development of vascular- and pigment-specific lasers that can significantly diminish or remove a variety of vascular and pigment lesions including port-wine stains, tattoos, and nevus of Ota with minimal risk of scarring. These truly remarkable results have allowed lasers to fulfill some early promises they once held. Dermatologic surgery continues to be a driving and innovative force in the world of liposuction. With the development of the tumescent technique by Jeffrey Klein, the procedure can be performed under local anesthesia with minimal morbidity and better cosmetic results. The area of cosmetic dermatology continues to progress at a rapid rate and with the development of alpha-hydroxy acids by Van Scott, the demonstration of the usefulness of Retin-A on photo-aged skin, and the combination of a variety of peeling agents for facial rejuvenation. In the last several years, with the development of the North American Society of Phlebology, sclerotherapy has gone from a "simple technique for injection of spider veins of the legs" to a much more scientific overall approach to leg vein treatment.

Dermatologic Surgery continues to play a significant role in cutaneous surgery and at present has six societies using it as their primary and official journal. Perry Robins played an important roll in its development as the founding Editor-in-Chief and publisher. He was a founding member of the American Society for Dermatologic Surgery and the American College of Mohs Micrographic Surgery and Cutaneous Oncology, and had the first one-year surgery fellowship on which our present surgical fellowship program is based. He was also the founder of the International Society for Dermatologic Surgery. *Dermatology Surgery* has continued to play a significant role in the field thanks to the effort of the recent Editors-in-Chief William Hanke and, more recently, Leonard Dzubow.

We hope the textbook will continue to define cutaneous surgery and be helpful in teaching the basic as well as the newest concepts in cutaneous surgery.

Acknowledgments

We would like to thank our families for their consistent support; and of course, our staff for all their help.

We would also like to thank all those who have helped us achieve success in our careers.

I Introduction

Eric F. Bernstein   Laura L. Bolten
Alain Mauviel   Toby Frank
John A. McGrath   Jouni Uitto

1 Wound Healing

The discipline of surgery depends upon the proper healing of acute wounds inflicted to remove a variety of lesions from benign to malignant. The lesion to be removed may be acutely inflamed or infected or may be in a site which has received therapy such as radiation. Systemic therapies such as ionizing radiation, chemotherapeutic agents, or systemic retinoids may affect how healing will proceed. Also, the general health of the patients, including their nutritional status and disorders such as diabetes mellitus, contributes to patients' abilities to effectively heal a surgical wound.

A wound is a break in a contiguous body structure.[1] In the case of dermatologic surgery, the body structure in question is usually the skin. An *erosion* is defined as the focal loss of epidermis and does not penetrate into the dermis. An ulcer consists of the loss of both epidermis and dermis, while a fissure is merely an ulcer with sharp vertical walls.[1] Any variety of wounds may result from surgical procedures necessary to remove a constellation of lesions. Wounds may be closed with sutures or staples or left open to allow granulation, contraction, and eventually re-epithelializtion to take place. In the case of an open wound, a large degree of epidermal and dermal wound healing must take place to allow healing. However, a closed incision requires mostly dermal wound healing to take place, as only a minimal amount of epidermal regeneration is required to cover the defect. In all cases, wound strength is largely supplied by dermal collagen,[2–5] which regenerates with the help of a myriad of inflammatory cells, cytokines, and other dermal matrix components.

DERMAL EXTRACELLULAR MATRIX

The dermal matrix comprises the extracellular constituents of the dermis and includes collagens, elastic fibers, fibronectin, glycosaminoglycans, and proteoglycans. The fibrillar collagens form the bulk of the dermal matrix and are responsible for the ultimate strength of a healed wound.[2–4] Most of the extracellular matrix in the dermis is synthesized by dermal fibroblasts, which are influenced by a variety of factors, including inflammatory cells, cytokines, and even physical factors such as sunlight.

Collagen

Collagen is the main structural component of skin and is the most abundant extracellular matrix component of skin. The name collagen is derived from the Greek (*kolla,* glue; *genna,* to produce; *collagen,* glue former) because when boiled it produced glue.[6] Collagen types I and III form the bulk of the dermis, and their ratios in skin change following birth.[7,8] Other major types of collagen found in skin include collagen types IV, VII, and XVII, which constitute the basement membrane zone and anchoring fibrils of the dermal-epidermal junction. Other collagens found in substantial amounts in skin include collagens type V and VI.

The family of collagens is a closely related but genetically distinct group of extracellular matrix molecules. They are numbered in order of their discovery. Nineteen types of collagen have been described and named collagens I through XIX.[9,10] The protypical molecular configuration of collagen is the triple helix, which results due to the primary sequence of amino acids in the collagen α-chains. The collagenous, or triple-helical, portions of the collagen polypeptides contain a repeating sequence of three amino acids referred to as the *Gly-X-Y sequence. Gly* refers to glycine, and the *X* and *Y* positions are often the amino acids proline and hydroxyproline. Hydroxyproline requires ascorbic acid as a cofactor to stabilize the triple-helical conformation under normal physiologic conditions.[10]

Type I collagen

Type I collagen constitutes approximately 80 percent of the collagen in skin and is the major structural protein in the body.[11] Type I collagen consists of three polypeptide chains arranged in the typical α-helical configuration. Two of the chains are identical and labeled α1(I) chains, while the remaining chain is labeled α2(I). The entire primary sequence of these collagen chains has been found by sequencing the corresponding cDNAs.[12–14] The genomic DNA of type I collagen consists of approximately 50 coding regions, or exons, which are separated by intervening DNA sequences which do not code for amino acids composing the collagen chains, or introns. Type I collagen is produced in the dermis by fibroblasts, which may be induced to migrate to the site of a wound by a myriad of stimuli, including other matrix molecules or growth factors.

Collagen production involves a series of steps which occur within the fibroblast and in the extracellular space. To produce collagen, a messenger RNA precursor molecule is first transcribed from the DNA template containing sequences corresponding to both introns and exons. Posttranscriptional modification of the mRNA includes removal of introns by splicing (Fig. 1-1). In addition, capping of the 5′ and polyadenylation of the 3′ end of the mRNA molecule make it ready to serve as a template for translation of the preproα-chains from mRNA to a polypeptide. The procollagen molecules form a triple helix comprising two α1(I) and one α2(I) chains. They are secreted from fibroblasts into the extracellular space, and the nonhelical extensions on the N-terminal and C-terminal ends are removed by proteases. Collagen molecules then align into their fibrillar structure in a very specific way, with a banding pattern which has a periodicity upon examination by electron microscopy of approximately 68 nm (Figs. 1-2 and 1-3). Fibers are initially stabilized by noncovalent forces between collagen molecules or in some cases by disulfide bonds. Collagen fibers are further stabilized by the formation of cross-links produced by the deamination of lysyl and hydroxylysyl residues by lysyl oxidase, a copper-dependent enzyme.[15]

Type III collagen

Type III collagen has also been referred to as fetal collagen due to its abundance in fetal tissues.[16] It accounts for about half of the total collagen in fetal skin. Following birth, production of type I collagen exceeds that of type III collagen, with the resulting ratio of type I to type III collagen being approximately 6:1 in adult skin.[17] Type III collagen is composed of three identical α1(III) chains, arranged in the typical triple helix conformation. The distribution of type III collagen in skin is similar to that of type I collagen. Type III collagen is particularly abundant in extensible tissues, including the skin, gastrointestinal tract, and arterial blood vessels. In Ehlers-Danlos syndrome type IV, mutations are present in type III collagen. These patients have fragile skin and ruptures in the

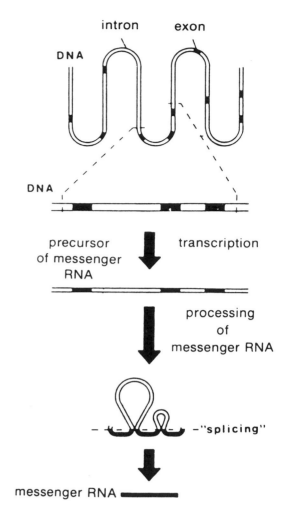

Figure 1-1.   Schematic representation of splicing. The information coding for amnio acid sequences resides in genomic DNA, which contains separate coding regions (exons) and intervening noncoding sequences (introns). The nucleotide sequences in DNA are transcribed to a precursor form of mRNA. The precursor molecule is then processed by several reactions, including splicing that removes the intron sequences. The processed mRNA can serve as a template for translation of polypeptides. (Reprinted with permission from Uitto J et al: Collagen: Its structure, function and pathology, in *Progress in Diseases of the Skin,* edited by R. Fleischmajer. New York, Grune & Stratton, 1981, pp 103–141.)

gastrointestinal tract and arteries, demonstrating the importance of type III collagen to the stability of these tissues.[9,18] Type III collagen has been shown to form thin fibrils which codistribute with type I collagen fibers in the dermis.[19] It may therefore play a role in development of dermal collagen fibers.

Type IV collagen

Type IV collagen is the major component of the basement membrane at the dermal-epidermal junction. It helps form the basement membrane zone of blood vessels in the dermis and elsewhere (Fig. 1-4). Type IV collagen is present mainly as a

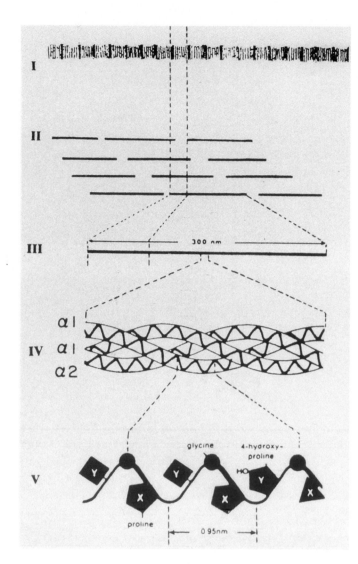

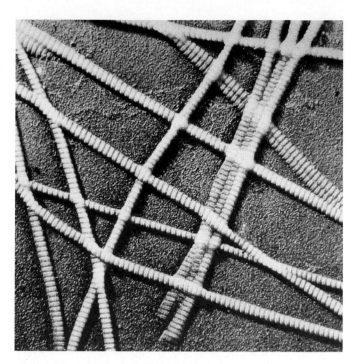

Figure 1-3. Electron micrograph of collagen fibers prepared from human dermis showing the regular banding pattern at an interval of 70 nm. Original magnification X45,000. (Reprinted with permission from Uitto J: Collagen, in *Dermatology in General Medicine,* 4th ed., edited by TB Fitzpatrick et al. New York, McGraw-Hill, 1993, pp 299–315.)

Figure 1-2. Schematic diagram representing the structure of type I collagen. The collagen fibers demonstrate a repeating periodicity evident upon electron microscopic examination and are composed of individual collagen molecules aligned in a quarter-stagger arrangement (II). Each type I collagen molecule is an approximately 300-nm-long rodlike structure (III) consisting of three individual polypeptides, called α chains, which are twisted around each other, forming a right-handed triple helix (IV). Each chain is composed of amino acids containing the collagenous repeating Gly-X-Y amino acid sequence (V), with the X position frequently occupied by a propyl residue and the Y position frequently occupied by a 4-hydroxy-propyl residue. (Reprinted with permission from Uitto J et al: Collagen: Its structure, function and pathology, in *Progress in Diseases of the Skin,* edited by R Fleischmajer New York, Grune & Stratton, 1981, pp 103–141.)

trimer composed of two α1(IV) chains and one α2(IV) chain. Unlike type I and type III collagens, which are fibrillar and make up the bulk of the dermis, type IV collagen has regions interrupted by noncollagenous segments lacking the typical Gly-X-Y repeating sequence. This may add flexibility to type

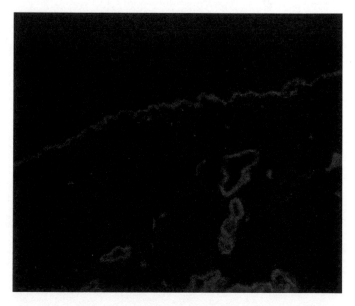

Figure 1-4. Immunofluorescent anti-type IV collagen labeling of normal skin. Positive staining is present along the dermal-epidermal junction and surrounding dermal blood vessels and nerves. Original magnification X160.

IV collagen and allow it to serve as a scaffold for incorporation of the numerous basement membrane components.[20]

Type VI collagen

Type VI collagen has a short, triple-helical segment with large amino- and carboxy-terminal globular domains. Type VI collagen is found in most tissues in the form of microfibrils.[21] It is a heterotrimer composed of three distinct polypeptide chains, $\alpha1(VI)$, $\alpha2(VI)$, $\alpha3(VI)$.[21] Because type VI collagen is located between dermal collagen fibers and has cell adhesion and collagen-binding properties, it has been suggested that type VI collagen is involved in adhesion between different connective tissue components. It is a major gene product of cultured skin fibroblasts.[22]

Type VII collagen

Type VII collagen is composed of 3 identical $\alpha1(VII)$ chains, which are much longer than those of the dermal fibrillar collagens, collagen types I and III.[23] The anchoring fibrils which extend from the basement membrane zone at the dermal-epidermal junction to the upper dermis are composed of type VII collagen (Fig. 1-5). Like type IV collagen, type VII collagen is thought to posess flexibility due to several interruptions in the Gly-X-Y collagen structure.[24] Anchoring fibrils extend from the lamina densa within the basement membrane zone to the papillary dermis. In the papillary dermis, some of the fibrils attach to anchoring plaques, while others form U-shapes in which the fiber entraps dermal collagen fibers and both ends of the type VII fibril are attached to the lamina densa.[24] The necessary role of anchoring fibrils is demonstrated by dystrophic epidermolysis bullosa (EB), a hereditary blistering disorder with mutations in type VII collagen. Patients with dystrophic EB develop blisters below the lamina densa, highlighting the importance of type VII collagen in maintaining integrity of the skin (Figs. 1-6a–b).

Other collagen types

Collagen types XII and XIV are part of a family of collagens known as FACIT or fibril associated collagens with inter-

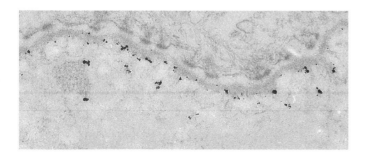

Figure 1-5. Immunogold electron microscopy labeling of type VII collagen in normal skin. Immunogold deposits are present at both ends of anchoring fibrils, within the lamina densa and in the upper papillary dermis. Original magnification X27,500.

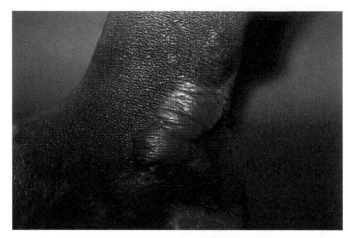

a

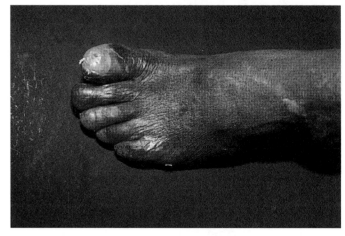

b

Figure 1-6. A patient with dystrophic epidermolysis bullosa. (*a*) Abnormal type VII collagen in the papillary dermis results in skin fragility with blister formation; (*b*) considerable scarring with loss of nails.

rupted triple helices.[25] They have been found to associate with type I collagen fibers of the dermis. Collagen types XII and XIV, along with type III and V collagens and the small proteoglycan, decorin, are thought to participate in regulation of collagen fiber diameter. Type XVII collagen, like type VII collagen, is a component of the basement membrane zone. The polypeptides of type XVII collagen are 180 kDa in size and contain a large noncollagenous amino-terminal end, with 15 collagenous domains on the carboxy-terminal end.[26,27] This collagen is the 180-kDa bullous pemphigoid antigen (BPAg2).[28]

Elastic Fibers

Although elastic fibers compose only 1 to 2 percent of the dry weight of non-sun-exposed skin,[29–31] they provide resilience and elasticity to skin. Elastic fibers are composed of amorphous elastin, as well as a fibrillar component, fibrillin. Elas-

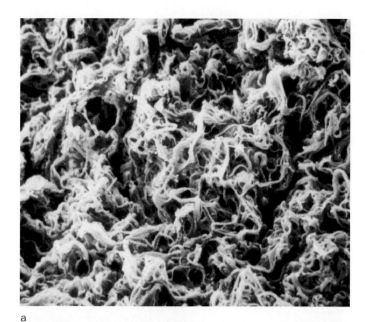

a

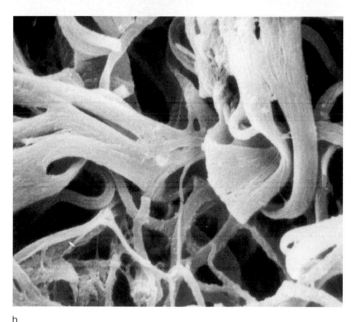

b

Figure 1-7. Scanning electron microscopy of elastic fibers in human skin. Original magnifications (*a*) X2000; (*b*) X5000. (Reprinted with permission from Uitto J, Christiano AM: Elastic fibers, in *Dermatology in General Medicine,* 4th ed., edited by TB Fitzpatrick et al. New York, McGraw-Hill, 1993, pp 339–349.)

tic fibers are significantly thinner than the dermal collagen fibers and are found parallel to collagen fibers in the reticular dermis. In the papillary dermis, a plexus of thin elastic fibers, termed *elaunin fibers,* runs parallel to the dermis. These elaunin fibers contain small amounts of cross-linked elastin. Other fibers, the oxytalan fibers, extend vertically from the papillary plexus of elaunin fibers to the dermal-epidermal junction and consist solely of fibrillin.

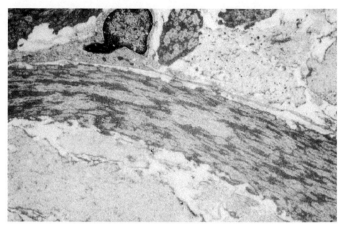

Figure 1-8. Transmission electron microscopy of elastic fibers in human skin reveals electron-lucent elastin and the electron-dense microfibril component of elastic fibers composed of fibrillin. Original magnification X16,000. (Reprinted with permission from Uitto J, Christiano AM: Elastic fibers, in *Dermatology in General Medicine,* 4th ed., edited by TB Fitzpatrick et al. New York, McGraw-Hill, 1993, pp 339–349.)

On examination by scanning electron microscopy, the elastic fiber network appears as a meshwork of fibers distributed among the collagen fibers (Figs. 1-7*a–b*). Transmission electron microscopy reveals elastic fibers to be composed of relatively electron-lucent elastin and an electron-dense fibrillar component composed of fibrillin (Fig. 1-8). Elastin is a polypeptide synthesized as a precursor, tropoelastin. The composition of elastin is characteristic. Elastin is rich in hydrophobic amino acids such as glycine, valine, proline, and alanine. Like collagen, about one-third of the amino acids in elastin are glycine residues. But unlike collagen, these residues are not distributed as every third amino acid in a Gly-X-Y distribution. Glycine residues in elastin are grouped with other hydrophobic amino acids. Unique to elastic fibers is the presence of the amino acid derivatives desmosine and its isoform, isodesmosine. Cross-links are formed between these desmosines using lysyl oxidase as a catalyst.[29] These desmosines are unique to elastic fibers among mammalian proteins and thus may be used to measure the amount of cross-linked elastic fibers present in skin.[30,31] One explanation for the elastic properties of elastin is the fact that when elastin is stretched, the hydrophobic domains are exposed to the aqueous extracellular milieu. Contraction then ensues by folding of elastin into its original conformation with the hydrophobic residues into the interior. This is expressed as elasticity in tissues like skin.[32] A massive accumulation of abnormal elastic fibers is seen in photodamaged skin in the upper portion of the dermis (Figs. 1-9*a–b*).

The fibrillins are a recently described group of proteins which constitute the fibrillar component of elastic fibers (Fig. 1-10).[33–35] It has been suggested that they function as a scaffold for the formation of elastic fibers. Their orientation may

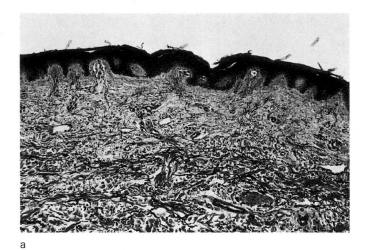

a

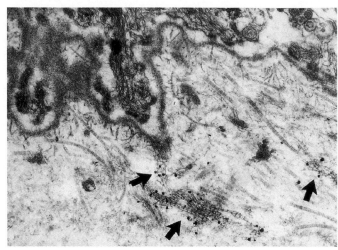

Figure 1-10.   Immunogold electron microscopy labeling of fibrillin within the papillary dermis. Labeling is present on lattice-like elastic dermal microfibrils (*arrows*) beneath the linear electron-dense lamina densa of the dermal-epidermal basement membrane zone. Larger dermal collagen fibers with the characteristic banding pattern are also seen. Original magnification X25,500.

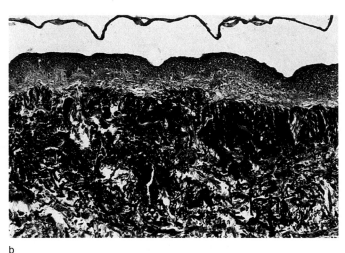

b

Figure 1-9.   (*a*) Staining for elastic fibers in non-sun-exposed skin; (*b*) photodamaged skin from the same individual reveals a massive accumulation of abnormal, clumped elastic fibers beneath a small uninvolved "grenz" zone. Elastic fibers stain black, while collagen stains red. Original magnification X100.

be such that elastic fibers of a specific diameter will be formed consistently. Abnormalities of fibrillin-1 have been associated with Marfan syndrome, which is a disease affecting highly elastic tissues, including the aorta and skin.[36] Alterations in fibrillin-2 have also been associated with a Marfan-like condition by genetic linkage analysis.[37] These disease-associated alterations in elastic fibers resulting from fibrillin abnormalities demonstrate the importance of fibrillin in proper elastic fiber formation.

Glycosaminoglycans and Proteoglycans

Glycosaminoglycans are polysaccharides composed of repeating disaccharide units. They are widely distributed in skin, although they constitute only a small fraction of the dry weight of the dermis. They do, however, bind a substantial amount of water to the dermis relative to their weight. With the exception of hyaluronic acid, which is quite widely dis-

tributed in skin, glycosaminoglycans are linked to a protein by the terminal-reducing sugar residue forming proteoglycans.[38,39] Proteoglycans have a variety of functions which include regulation of cellular interactions, cell movement within tissues, and basement membrane integrity. This explains their wide distribution on and between dermal matrix fibers, on cell surfaces, and within basement membranes.

Hyaluronic acid is the largest glycosaminoglycan and is composed of repeating D-glucuronic acid and N-acetylglucosamine residues. It does not contain sulfate, is in high concentrations in skin, and is not associated with a core protein.[40] Chondroitin sulfate is composed of alternating uronic acid and N-acetylgalactosamine residues. It is sulfated at the C4 or C6 of the N-acetylgalactosamine.[40] Unlike hyaluronic acid, chondroitin sulfate is attached to a core protein to form a proteoglycan. The heparan sulfates include the related compound heparin and are composed of alternating N-substituted glucosamine and a uronic acid.[40]

The small chondroitin sulfate (CS) proteoglycan, decorin, is widely distributed in normal dermis. It is the major proteoglycan produced by human fibroblasts in culture.[41] Its small size is attested to by the fact that only one chondroitin sulfate chain is attached to the core protein.[42] Immunohistochemical localization demonstrates ubiquitous decorin staining localized to dermal collagen fibers. Decorin has been shown to bind to specific regions on the collagen fiber.[43] Decorin affects collagen fiber formation and results in a specific lateral alignment of collagen fibrils in vitro.[44,45] It is thought to regulate assembly of collagen fibers and may have an effect on collagen fiber diameter.[46,47]

Versican is a very large CS proteoglycan present in significant amounts in the dermis. Versican mRNA is expressed by both fibroblasts and keratinocytes in vitro,[48] although im-

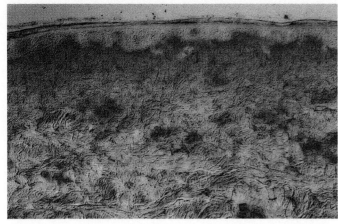

a

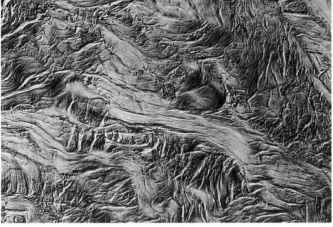

b

Figure 1-11. Immunohistochemical staining for versican (red) reveals a diffuse accumulation of versican immunostaining just below the dermal-epidermal basement membrane zone. Below this, a pattern identical to that seen when elastin or fibrillin antibodies are seen. Elastic fiber staining is evident between the much larger collagen fibers of the reticular dermis (blue). Original magnifications (*a*) X100; (*b*) X200. (Photographed using Nomarski optics.)

munohistochemical staining reveals significant versican staining only in the dermis (Figs. 1-11*a–b*). Versican has two epidermal growth factor-like repeats and a hyaluronic acid-binding domain.[45] Immunohistochemical staining has revealed that versican codistributes with elastin in the dermis.[48] Like decorin, versican associates with extracellular matrix fibers in the dermis, although the role of versican in elastic fiber formation remains to be discovered.

Fibronectin

Fibronectin is a glycoprotein with a variety of properties important to developing an environment to promote wound healing. Circulating fibronectin may be deposited in a wound from plasma, or it may be produced at the site of a wound by fibroblasts. Plasma and cellular fibronectin differ somewhat in their structure, although the clinical importance of these

differences remains to be elucidated.[49,50] Fibronectin contains an amino acid sequence, Arg-Gly-Asp-Ser (RGDS) sequence, which is the active portion of the fibronectin cell-binding domain.[49,51,52] Vitronectin, laminin, and thrombospondin are other cell adhesion proteins, which may play a role in wound healing.[49]

Extracellular matrix deposition and wound healing

After wounding occurs, hemostasis takes place with deposition of fibrin, which is the first matrix material deposited in a wound.[53] Glycosaminoglycans are also among the first extracellular matrix molecules deposited in a healing wound.[40] It is thought that fibrin and hyaluronic acid may create the initial matrix for cell migration and proliferation within wounded tissues.[54,55] As wound healing proceeds, hyaluronic acid deposition gives way to other glycosaminoglycans.[49,55] The active edges of a wound demonstrate significant amounts of hyaluronic acid, but newly deposited granulation tissue contains the more sulfated proteoglycans, such as chondroitin sulfate and dermatan sulfate.[56,57]

In addition to fibrin, fibronectin is deposited at the site of wounds from plasma.[58] Adding to the circulating fibronectin deposited at the site of wounds is fibronectin produced by cells at the site of injury. Fibronectin is a major matrix component of early wounds.[53,59–64] It is the first fibril secreted by fibroblasts at the site of a wound.[65] Fibronectin functions as a binding site for fibroblasts and other cells migrating to the site of a wound and as a scaffold for the deposition of collagen fibers. The initial provisional matrix is replaced by collagen. Type III collagen is the initial collagen to be deposited in a healing wound, followed by type I collagen.[66] Wound integrity and wound strength are provided by collagen, which is remodeled and strengthened by cross-links as healing continues.[67–69]

KERATINOCYTE MIGRATION

As dermal healing takes place, the dermal connective tissue requires epidermal overgrowth to protect the newly formed dermis. Keratinocytes must migrate from wound edges and epidermal appendages to form a protective barrier and maintain cutaneous integrity. Keratinocytes of the innermost (basal) layer of the epidermis possess several diverse behavioral characteristics that may be induced or influenced by contact with the extracellular matrix, including collagens and glycosaminoglycans. These different basal keratinocyte behavioral properties include attachment to the basement membrane zone, differentiation to form a multilayered epidermis, and migration to restore or maintain epithelialization.

Attachment to the subjacent basement membrane zone is secured by rivet-like structures known as *hemidesmosomes*. These cellular structures contain bullous pemphigoid antigens[70] and $\alpha6/\beta4$ integrin receptors[71] that have an adhesive interaction with various laminin molecules, including laminin-1 (EHS laminin), laminin-5 (nicein/kalinin), and laminin-6 (K-laminin),[72] within the lamina lucida of the cutaneous basement membrane zone.

This mechanism of focal cementing of basal keratinocytes to the extracellular matrix is temporarily lost when keratinocytes are required to migrate—for example, in wound healing. In such circumstances, the behavior of keratinocytes changes from adhesion to migration in an attempt to restore an intact epithelium.

The provisional matrix of wounds consists of both fibronectin and fibrin,[73] and fibronectin is of particular importance in promoting early keratinocyte migration.[73,74] More specifically, keratinocyte migration over fibronectin has been shown to be mediated by $\alpha 5/\beta 1$ integrins, with the important part of the fibronectin molecule being a 120 kDa cell-binding domain near the carboxy-terminal.[75,76]

Apart from fibronectin, other macromolecules may also influence keratinocyte migration. In vitro studies have demonstrated the promotion of keratinocyte migration by type I collagen (the main interstitial collagen of the dermis) and by type IV collagen (present in the lamina densa of the basement membrane zone).[77] Other molecules, including vitronectin[78] and thrombospondin,[79] may also promote keratinocyte migration. Albumin, type V collagen, and heparan sulfate proteoglycan seem to have no significant influence on this aspect of keratinocyte behavior.[77]

In contrast, however, keratinocyte migration is strongly inhibited by laminin (laminin-1).[77] This observation supports the concept that in anchored, nonmigrating basal keratinocytes there is a rich bed of laminin molecules beneath the keratinocytes that prevents keratinocyte migration. However, in wound healing, this "anchor" is removed as the new wound bed contains little laminin in the early stages of healing, and migration of keratinocytes over different, less adhesive, macromolecules is therefore allowed to proceed.

Thus, keratinocyte migration is an important and complex physiologic response in skin homeostasis and one which is greatly influenced by the nature of the surrounding extracellular matrix.

RESIDENT CELLS OF THE DERMIS

Fibroblasts belong to the family of connective-tissue cells and are responsible for the formation of most of the dermal extracellular matrix in normal skin and in a healing wound (Fig. 1-12). Fibroblasts migrate to the site of a wound in response to a variety of growth factors and extracellular matrix molecules, which result from the postwounding inflammatory response. Platelet aggregation at the site of injury not only results in hemostasis, but also causes the release of cytokines which cause fibroblast growth, migration, and activation. The alpha granules of platelets contain growth factors such as platelet-derived growth factor (PDGF),[80,81] epidermal growth factor (EGF),[82] and transforming growth factor-β (TGF-β).[83]

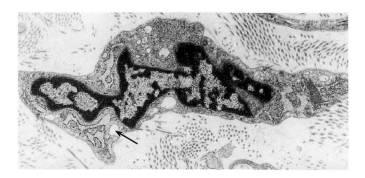

Figure 1-12. Transmission electron micrograph of a fibroblast within the dermis. There is dilation of the cisternae of the rough endoplasmic reticulum (*arrow*) indicative of active collagen synthesis. Original magnification X8000. (Courtesy of George F. Murphy, M.D., and Diana Whitaker Menezes.)

Mast cells are bone marrow-derived cells[84] which serve several functions in the dermis, including the release of vasoactive substances that may exert an effect on the healing response. They mostly reside around blood vessels in the dermis (Fig. 1-13).[85,86] Mast cells contain prominent granules with large amounts of heparin and histamine, stain metachromatically purple with the Giemsa stain,[87] and have a characteristic appearance on electron microscopy (Fig. 1-14). A variety of stimuli are capable of stimulating release of mast cell granules, including immune stimuli such as complement and interleukin 1 (IL-1) or nonimmune stimuli such as drugs or physical factors like heat or cold.[88,89] Substances released from mast cells include vasoactive mediators such as histamine and prostaglandins, chemotactic factors, enzymes, and proteoglycans such as heparin.[88,90] Mast cells are involved in a number of normal processes and pathological conditions

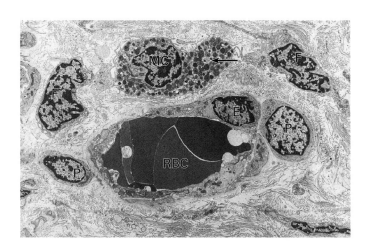

Figure 1-13. Transmission electron micrograph of a small blood vessel and surrounding cells. RBC = red blood cell, P = pericyte, E = blood vessel endothelial cell, MC = mast cell, F = fibroblast. Numerous secretory granules are present within the mast cell cytoplasm (*arrow*). Original magnification X3,000. (Courtesy of George F. Murphy, M.D., and Diana Whitaker Menezes)

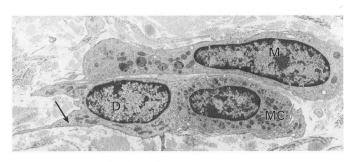

Figure 1-14. Transmission electron micrograph of resident cells within the dermis. In this field there is a dermal dendrocyte (D) with dendritic process (*arrow*), a macrophage (M), and a mast cell (MC) with characteristic granules. Original magnification X4000. (Courtesy of George F. Murphy, M.D., and Diana Whitaker Menezes).

and have been considered a cell necessary for normal wound healing to take place.[91–93] They have also been implicated in the pathogenesis of fibrotic disorders such as scleroderma.[88,94]

The dermal dendrocyte is a bone marrow-derived cell which stains positively with an antibody to clotting factor XIIIa.[95–97] Dermal dendrocytes are primarily located in the papillary dermis in the vicinity of blood vessels (Fig. 1-14).[97] They express monocyte-, macrophage-, and antigen-presenting cell markers and possess phagocytic capabilities.[97] They may be capable under a variety of conditions to function like macrophages[97–99] and antigen-presenting cells.[97,100,101] Dermal dendrocytes may be induced by interferon gamma (IFN-y) to express intercellular adhesion molecule 1 (ICAM-I), thus increasing their ability to interact with T-lymphocytes.[97] They are increased in a number of dermatologic disorders[102–104] and like mast cells possess numerous functions in health and disease states.

Macrophages are cells of bone marrow origin which develop from circulating monocytes (Fig. 1-14).[105] They function as phagocytes in the skin, manufacturing large quantities of lysosomal enzymes.[106] This is an important function in a healing wound, where injured tissue and bacteria need to be removed so that new extracellular matrix may be deposited. They play a pivotal role in wound repair[107,108] and promote angiogenesis in healing wounds.[109]

CYTOKINES

Pathway of Normal Wound Repair

Following tissue injury, normal wound repair takes place in an organized, sequential manner. After the initial fibrin clot formation, there is massive invasion of the injured tissue by mononuclear cells and granulocytes. These events are subsequently followed by angiogenesis, fibroblast proliferation, formation of granulation tissue, and matrix deposition. The

last phase of the healing process is maturation of the scar tissue, which involves contraction of the dermal collagen network in full-thickness wounds and squamous differentiation of the keratinocytes as part of the re-epithelialization process. Finally, wound closure is followed by tissue remodeling.[110]

The reparative phase of wound healing includes (1) neovascularization and (2) fibroblast activation to proliferate and to produce extracellular matrix components, leading to the formation of granulation tissue. This reparative phase is initiated in response to signals generated during the preceding inflammatory phase. This conclusion is based on observations that experimental wounds depleted of monocyte/macrophages by treatment with corticosteroids and anti-macrophage serum exhibit decreased fibroplasia and tissue granulation, and the rate of healing is significantly delayed.[111] These observations clearly demonstrate the fundamental role of infiltrating macrophages in tissue repair. The inflammatory cells then secrete cytokines and growth factors which exhibit potent chemotactic properties for fibroblasts and stimulate them to produce various extracellular matrix components.[112] Finally, after scar formation, remodeling occurs concomitantly with the production of new matrix proteins and the secretion of various degradative enzymes, including matrix metalloproteinases (MMPs). This remodeling step is essential for the realignment of fibrous elements along the tension lines in the skin, and it is carefully controlled by factors that cause the release, activation, or inhibition of various proteolytic enzymes, together with the synthesis and processing of matrix proteins. Also, during the remodeling period, progressive cross-linking of collagens takes place, resulting in increased tensile strength of the wound.

Effects of Cytokines on the Extracellular Matrix Gene Expression

The formation and repair of a functional extracellular matrix require coordinate expression of a number of genes, including those encoding for matrix proteins (such as the collagens, fibronectin, elastin, and the core proteins of various proteoglycans) and those encoding for regulatory enzymes, among them those involved in the posttranslational modification of collagen molecules, and various proteases.

Extensive in vitro studies have shown that a variety of inflammatory signals produced by circulation-derived cells in tissue are capable of modulating the metabolism of the extracellular matrix. Among the plethora of soluble factors released by monocytes macrophages are several with well-defined biologic functions: (1) proinflammatory cytokines, such as IL-1 and tumor necrosis factor-α (TNF-α); (2) growth factors, such as EGF, PDGF, and the acidic and basic fibroblast growth factors aFGF, bFGF); and (3) perhaps the most extensively studied growth factor, TGF-β.

Selected data on the effects of various growth factors on the extracellular matrix metabolism are presented in Table 1-1.

TABLE 1-1

Effects of Growth Factors on Extracellular Matrix Metabolism in vitro

Cytokine	Collagen	Fibronectin	Elastin	Proteoglycans	MMP-1 MMP-2	MMP-2 MMP-9	TIMP	Proliferation Migration	Angiogenesis
IL-1	+/−		+	+	+	+	+	+	
IL-4	+	+			−	−	=		
IL-6	=/+			+	+/−/=				+
IL-8	−								
TNF-α	−	−	−		+		+	+/−	
LT	−				+	+			
LR	−	−		+	+		=	=	
IFN-α/γ	−	+/−	−		+/−	−		−	
IGF-I	+							+	
EGF	−				+	+		+	
bFGF	−				+			+	+
PDGF								+	
TGF-β	+	+	+	+/−	+/−	+	+	+/−	+

* Effects include up-regulation (+), down-regulation (−), and no effect (=).
Source: Mauviel and Uitto.[112] Used by permission.

Mechanistic Interactions Between Growth Factor

The results of the experiments presented above were obtained in most cases using either highly purified or recombinant growth factors and cytokines usually tested under carefully controlled in vitro conditions. One should realize that these conditions do not necessarily reflect in vivo situations, where a variety of cytokines and growth factors are simultaneously present in the sites of inflammation and the healing wound. In fact, a number of in vitro studies have established that cytokines and growth factors interact with each other to modulate the production of extracellular matrix components by fibroblasts. For example, IL-1, TNF-α, IFN-γ, and leukoregulin (LR) have been shown to counteract the up-regulatory effect of TGF-β on type I collagen gene expression.[113–116] These antagonist effects may take place at the transcriptional level (TNF-α and LR)[113,116] or at the posttranscriptional level (IFN-γ),[113,115] and they may be additive or synergistic, as has been demonstrated for TNF-α and IFN-γ.[113,117] Interestingly, the authors have recently demonstrated that TGF-β and certain pro-inflammatory cytokines, such as TNF-α, IL-1, or LR, enhance fibroblast type VII collagen gene expression in an additive or synergistic manner.[118] These data suggest a potential role for these cytokines in inducing the formation of anchoring fibrils (type VII collagen) in tissue repair processes and demonstrate uncoordinate regulation of type I and type VII collagen genes.

Modulation of Degradative Events by Cytokines

The modulation of the expression of MMPs is another way for growth factors and cytokines to alter the net deposition of various extracellular matrix components in tissues.[119,120] MMPs compose a family of enzymes capable of degrading the macromolecules of the extracellular matrix. Three subclasses of MMPs, as defined by their specific substrates, have been delineated: collagenases, stromelysins, and gelatinases. The members within each MMP family share homologies at the levels of amino acid sequences and various structural domains. They are secreted as zymogens that require activation for proteolytic activity, and, once activated, they are inhibited by specific tissue inhibitors of metalloproteinases, the TIMPs. Transcriptional regulation of MMP-1 and MMP-3 (interstitial collagenase and stromelysin, respectively) gene expression by cytokines and growth factors involves oncogenes of the Fos and Jun families.[119,120] Specifically, c-Fos and c-Jun are required for the induction of collagenase gene expression by IL-1 and TNF-α, whereas it has recently been demonstrated that Jun B mediates TGF-β inhibition of collagenase gene expression in normal human fibroblasts in culture.[121] Therefore, characterization of the expression of oncogenes of the Fos and Jun families in pathological situations, such as in decubitus ulcers, may lead to fundamental insights into the transcriptional mechanisms leading to altered MMP gene expression in chronic wounds.

Cytokine Modulation of Cell Proliferation and Migration

The formation of granulation tissue results from both increased cellularity and the accumulation of extracellular matrix. The former event is controlled by different cytokines and growth factors which exhibit potent chemotactic activities on mesenchymal and epithelial cells, resulting in the migration and division of cells at the site of the wound.[122] These chemotactic agents eventually act indirectly to increase collagen biosynthesis by recruiting cells which synthesize extracellular matrix proteins and by inducing the proliferation of resident cells capable of synthesizing the matrix components.[123]

Regulation of Angiogenesis by Cytokines

Angiogenesis, the formation of new capillary blood vessels by a process of sprouting from preexisting vessels, is a key component of granulation tissue formation. After the initial breakdown of the basement membrane of the parent vessel, endothelial cells begin to migrate and form a capillary sprout. Further migration and endothelial cell replication allow the sprout to elongate, and eventually lead to formation of a mature capillary, once a lumen and a functional basement membrane have been formed. The migration and proliferation of capillary endothelial cells are probably triggered by growth factors released from the tissue adjacent to proliferating capillaries or from the endothelial cells.[124]

Relevance of In Vitro Observations to Wound Healing In Vivo

Immunocytochemistry and in situ hybridization techniques have provided tools to detect the expression of a number of cytokines and growth factors either in normal skin or following tissue injury. As discussed above, many of these growth factors can modulate cell proliferation, cell migration, and extracellular matrix deposition in vitro. These observations have then led to the conclusion that these growth factors may play an essential role in wound healing also in vivo.

To better understand the normal healing processes and the factors that impair healing, a variety of animal models have been developed to evaluate wound healing in vivo in a systematic and controlled setting. In this context, one should distinguish models of impaired wound healing, which mimic clinical examples of compromised healing of chronic wounds, such as bedsores and diabetic ulcers, as well as incisional wound models, which may reflect normal wound healing in patients undergoing surgery. Also, various approaches have been developed to study granulation tissue formation and the role of growth factors in this process. Among these models are (1) viscose sponges implanted into the dermis into which fibroblasts can migrate and produce extracellular matrix or (2) porous wound chambers releasing growth factors into the dermis. These experimental approaches have allowed investigation of various parameters of wound healing, such as the healing rate, the wound strength (which correlates with the type I collagen content in tissue), the formation of granu-

TABLE 1-2

Effects of Growth Factors on Experimental Wound Healing in vivo*

Cytokine	Granulation Tissue	Healing Rate	Tensile Strength	Proliferation Migration	Angiogenesis
IL-1	−			+	
IL-8					+
TNF-α	−	−	−		
IFN-γ	−				
IGF-I	+			+	
EGF	+	+	+	+/−	+
aFGF					+
bFGF	+	+		+	+
PDGF	+	+		+	
TGF-α					+
TGF-β	+	+	+	+	+

* Effects include up-regulation (+), down-regulation (−, and no effect (=).
Source: Mauviel and Uitto.[112] Used by permission.

TABLE 1-3

Clinical Studies Investigating the Use of Topical Growth Factors for Wound Healing

Wounds	Targeted Effects	Side Effects	Compound, Concentration, Vehicle	
			Active (N)	Control (N)
Blisters (suction)	No healing difference.	None	EGF µg/0.1 ml saline (5)	Saline 0.1 ml (5)
Diabetic Ulcers (some mixed etiology)	Questionable efficacy.	None	Partially purified autologous platelet derived factors	Buffered saline in gauze
Donor site Partial-thickness	Silver sulfadiazine with EGF accelerates rate of epidermal regeneration compared to control (25% and 50% by 1 day and 75% and 100% by 1.5 days) (a < 0.02)	None	SSD cream with EGF 10 µg/ml (12)	SSD cream (12)
Ulcers, Chronic	Homologous Platelet Derived Wound Healing Factor (HPDWHF) reduced ulcer area 94% vs 73% for placebo.	None	HPDWHF (7)	Placebo (6)
Ulcers, Mixed	HPDWHF 100% epithelization in 9.67 ± 4.9 weeks (a < 0.01)	None	HPDWHF plus SSD dressing: Decubitus (3) Diabetes (9) Arterial insufficiency (3) Venous stasis (2) Other (7)	Historic control, Saline plus SSD dressing: Decubitus (3) Diabetes (9) Arterial insufficiency (3) Venous stasis (2) Other (10)
Ulcers, Mixed	EGF healed 8/9 wounds in 34 days vs none healed for control.	None	EGF 10 µg/g Silvadene every 12 h (9)	Historic control: Silvadene and debridement 3 weeks–6 months (9)
Ulcers, Pressure	bFGF increased fibroblast and capillaries (a < 0.05) over control; > 70% wound closure with bFGF.	No toxicity, significant serum absorption, or antibody formation.	bFGF 1.0 µg/cm^2 (11) bFGF 5.0 µg/cm^2 (13) bFGF 10.0 µg/cm^2 (11)	Placebo (14)
Ulcers, Pressure	Patients treated with rPDGF-BB 1.0 µg/cm^2 wound demonstrated pronounced healing over placebo.	No toxic effect by rPDGF-BB	rPDGF at 1.0 µg/ml (4) rPDGF at 10.0 µg/ml (4) rPDGF at 100.0 µg/ml (5)	Placebo (7)
Venous Ulcers	Subjective increase in granulation and epithelization	None	Placental GF in saline in Geliperin Dry 26 µg protein/cm^2 gel (11)	Buffered saline without placental GF in gauze (7)
Venous Ulcers	No significant effect on healing (a = 0.01)	None	EGF 10 µg/ml water 2 × daily (17)	Water 2 × daily (18)

lation tissue, blood vessel formation, and the proliferation and migration of connective tissue cells.

A summary of the effects of cytokines and growth factors in the various experimental models of wound healing in vivo is given in Table 1-2 (previous page).

The essential conclusions from these studies are: (1) that

TGF-β appears as a potent pharmacologic agent that can accelerate normal wound healing; (2) that TGF-β, PDGF, βFGF, and EGF have the propensity to accelerate the healing of impaired wounds; and (3) that combinations of growth factors may induce synergistic effects on wound healing.

Clinical Trials of Growth Factors in Wound Healing

Clinical trials with crude preparations of growth factors isolated from cultured epithelial cells or from platelets have shown some efficacy in the repair of previously nonhealing cutaneous wounds. For example, in a preliminary study, a platelet-derived wound healing formula, consisting of platelet alpha granule lysate (growth factors) in a solution of platelet buffer obtained from patients' blood was applied topically to nonhealing ulcers.[125] Successful re-epithelialization was observed in 96 percent of the patients (48 of 50). This preliminary study has been followed with a placebo-controlled, double-blind crossover trial, which led to similar results.[126] Similar, but somewhat less clear-cut, data have been obtained with crude porcine and bovine preparations of platelet lysates.[127] Also, recent trials with recombinant (PDGF-BB) have shown some efficacy for the treatment of chronic pressure wounds.[128] Histologic observations of biopsies revealed an active wound healing response compared to placebo-treated patients, without disruption of the normal healing sequence. Other clinical trials investigating the use of topical growth factors for promoting healing are summarized in Table 1-3 (previous page).[129–137]

Although these clinical trials are preliminary, it is tempting to speculate that application of cytokines or growth factors, in optimal combinations, is a promising way to restore wound healing in chronic ulcers. Complete understanding of the molecular mechanisms mediating growth factor action is a prerequisite for the elaboration of more efficient growth factor-derived wound healing formulas.

THE INTEGRATED HEALING RESPONSE

The Wound Healing Process

Wounds disrupt normal anatomic structure and function.[138] Healing progresses differently for different depths of wounds, depending on the appendages remaining to repopulate the skin with vessels, nerves, hair follicles, and sweat glands (Fig. 1-15). As healing occurs, nature restores structure and function either imperfectly (repair) or perfectly (regeneration). Species, age, wound site, and depth of injury determine whether a given wound will regenerate or repair. Regeneration progresses through blastema formation to perfect reconstruction of the missing tissue.[139] Epidermis truly regenerates. A few mammals regenerate full-thickness wounds at special sites: fruit bat wings, rabbit ears, and deer antlers.[139] Phylogenetically "lower" species and perhaps very young or embryonic humans regenerate limbs, digits, or excised tissue.[140] Dermal wounds in humans do not normally regenerate. Therefore, cutaneous wound healing focuses on repair of normal tissues with what is usually an approximation of normal structures, where the clinician can make enormous differences in the healing outcome.[141,142]

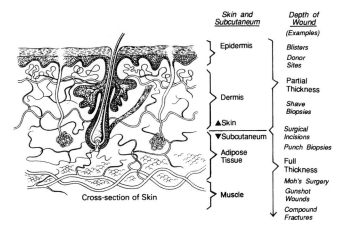

Figure 1-15. Layers of skin corresponding to different wound depths. (Reprinted with permission from Bolton L, van Rijswijk L. Wound dressings: meeting clinical and biological needs. *Dermatology Nursing* **3:**146–161, 1991.)

Repair occurs through a series of interactive phases (Fig. 1-16) progressing in an orderly and timely fashion (acute or normal repair), or, if any of the phases are prolonged, renewed, or disordered, the repair process is deemed chronic.[138] Variables that can delay repair are listed in Table 1-4.[143,144] In general, if there are potentially chronic wounds, such as pressure ulcers or leg ulcers, do not diminish these by 20 to 40

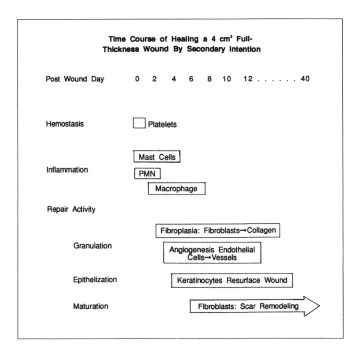

Figure 1-16. Typical course of secondary intention full-thickness healing for a 4 cm² wound with smooth, round edges. Events may be shortened if the wound is kept moist. (Reprinted with permission from Bolton L, van Rijswijk L. Wound dressings: meeting clinical and biological needs. *Dermatology Nursing* **3:**146–161, 1991

TABLE 1-4

Causes of Delayed Wound Healing

1. Reinjury due to trauma or pressure

   Ischemia

   Crushed vasculature

2. Vascular diseases

   Venous

      Edema due to reduced venous reflux

      Compromised lymphatic function

   Arterial

      Arteriosclerosis

      Drug abuse: e.g., nicotine, alcohol, etc.

3. Nutritional deficiency

   Water

   Vitamins, e.g., A, B_6, B_{12}, C, folate

   Minerals, e.g., zinc, iron, calcium

   Protein (kwashiorkor)

   Protein/Calories (marasmus)

4. Compromised immune system

   Immunosuppressive drugs

   HIV/AIDS

   Advanced age

   Radiation therapy

5. Metabolic disorders

   Diabetes

   Gout

   Porphyria (Cutanea Tarda)

   Impaired fibrin metabolism

6. Infections (local or systemic)

   Parasitic (e.g., elephantiasis)

   Bacterial (e.g., *S. aureus, P. aeruginosa*)

   Viral (e.g., herpes or HIV)

percent in the wound area during the first 2 to 4 weeks of treatment with a given modality; the cause of delay should be reassessed.[141,142,145] For example, occlusive wound dressings can aid debridement and provide an environment which optimizes repair only if the cause of tissue breakdown is alleviated.[143]

Once the wound is healed, maturation of the repaired tissue continues for months to years. Any resulting abnormal structures and functions are called *scar.* Scars can be normal, hypertrophic, or keloidal,[146] depending on the degree to which they surpass the skin's normal physical, biochemical, and physiological limits.

Biochemistry and Physiology of Wound Healing

To simplify descriptions of the healing process we divide it into the successive overlapping phases of healing (Fig. 1-16).

Nature often follows a much more erratic pattern, especially in chronic wounds which may be breaking down at one site or time and healing at another, depending on the microenvironment and the factors delaying healing, such as aging[147] or systemic steroids.[148] Local cells function both physiologically and biochemically to heal wounds, forming structures and releasing the following classes of molecules into the surrounding tissue:

- Growth factors or cytokines, which trigger or inhibit repair
- Matrix molecules, which form the structures of repair
- Ground substances, on which cells migrate

A nonexhaustive summary of components of wound healing is listed in Table 1-2.[149,150] The epithelial cells, fibroblasts, and endothelial cells are stimulated or inhibited by local growth factors and other cytokines. The latter two migrate on ground substance molecules and interact to build a collagen matrix through which new blood vessels course. This is red and appears granular because its surface is covered with capillary loops. The new granulation tissue fills and contracts the repairing wound as local fibroblasts contract within the matrix. The wound is usually considered healed once it is covered with epithelium, which migrates across the granulation tissue surface, proliferates, and differentiates to form the outer barrier layer, the stratum corneum. However, granulation tissue may continue to remodel for months or years after it is healed as the scar matures. This dynamic balance of collagen in the scar is mediated by enzymes and collagen release from local fibroblasts.

Measures of Healing and Scarring

If clinicians attempt to link the biochemistry and physiology of wound healing to clinical experience, they need to know which of these measures predict clinically valid healing outcomes. Table 1-6[142,143,145,148,151–165] lists clinical measures of healing which have face validity. These are generally viewed in medical practice as intrinsically important outcomes of wound repair.

Much work is needed to determine which of the biochemical and physiological parameters of wound healing listed in Table 1-5 have predictive validity for the outcomes in Table 1-6. Once this work is done, clinicians will be able to better test validated wound parameters and predict important clinical outcomes, such as a wound's potential to heal within a given time or the quality of healing.

OCCLUSIVE DRESSINGS AND WOUND HEALING

One of the fundamental questions in wound healing is whether the healing process benefits from dressing a wound or from leaving it exposed to the air. In an answer to this, extensive evidence has emerged to suggest that covering a wound in order to create a moist wound environment is the

TABLE 1-5

Cellular Physiology and Biochemistry of Wound Repair

Cell	Activities	Some Compounds Released	Functional Responses
Platelet	Aggregate, form plug, activate clotting cascade	Chemical transmitters Clotting factors PDGF, $TGF_{\alpha,\beta}$, arachidonic acid metabolites	Vasoconstriction Hemostasis/clotting time Chemotaxis, mitosis of fibroblasts, smooth muscle and epithelial cells
Polymorphonuclear neutrophil (PMN)	Diapedesis, chemotaxis Phagocytosis, ingest foreign matter	U-Plasminogen Activator Lysozymes Oxygen-free radicals	Lysis of fibrin Digestion of dead tissue Bacterial killing, phagocytosis
Mast cells	Migration, phagocytosis, granule release	Histamine Heparin Serotonin	Vasodilation Angiogenesis Vasoconstriction
Macrophages	Migration, chemotaxis Phagocytosis	Lysozymes PDGF, aFGF, bFGF, $TGF_{\alpha,\beta}$ EGF, $TGF\alpha$ IL-1,-2, MDGF, PDGF, TGF_{β}	Digestion of dead tissue Phagocytosis Angiogenesis Epithelization Fibroplasia
Fibroblast	Synthesize and extrude collagen; proliferate; release metalloproteases; contract; differentiate to quiescent state (apoptosis).	Procollagen converted outside cell to collagen; metalloproteases IGF-1	Granulation; remodeling IGF-1 stimulates fibroblast proliferation, collagen synthesis
Endothelial cell	Proliferate, migrate, bud to form vasculature	bFGF, PDGF, IGF-1, IL-1	Form vessel lumen; capillary budding
Smooth muscle cell	Proliferate, migrate, attach to blood vessels	IGF-1, PDGF	Vasoconstriction Vasodilation
Epithelial cell	Migrate, proliferate Differentiate to form stratum corneum	EDF, EGF, PDGF, IGF-1, IL-1, TGF_{α}	Epithelization, moisture and microbial barrier

better option. Specifically, dressings that have this property are referred to as *occlusive dressings*. Such dressings have been shown to accelerate the rate of re-epithelialization in acute wounds[166] and to improve the quality of granulation tissue in chronic wounds.[167] Other proven benefits of occlusive dressings include aiding debridement of necrotic wound material[168] and partial relief of pain in the wound site.

There are several different types of occlusive dressings: transparent polymer films, polymer foams, gels and hydrogels, hydrocolloids, and calcium alginates (Table 1-7).[169]

Polymer Films and Polymer Foams

Polymer film dressings consist of thin, nonabsorbent polyurethane (or similar polymer) material with adhesive material on one side. They are useful in treating superficial wounds, such as donor sites or abrasions. The films are permeable to moisture vapor and oxygen but impermeable to liquid and bacteria. The lack of absorbency means that polymer films are not the most suitable dressings for wounds with a heavy exudate. In contrast, polymer foams are suitable for exudative wounds or deep chronic wounds. These dressings are highly absorbent yet allow maintainance of a moist healing environment with permeability of oxygen and water vapor. Such dressings may be bulky, however, because a second light compression or elastic bandage is necesssary to keep the polymer foam attached to the wound.

Gels and Hydrogels

Hydrogels consist of cross-linked polymers (e.g., polyethylene oxide or polyacrylamides) that are extremely hydrophilic, often containing over 95% water. They have similar properties of vapor and oxygen permeability and absorbency to polymer foams and also require a secondary stabilizing dressing. Wounds such as superficial burns, donor sites, and some chronic ulcers may be treated by hydrogel dressings. The

TABLE 1-6

Clinically Validated Measures of Healing and Scarring

Clinical Outcome	Measures
Hemostasis	Clotting Time; Thrombin time; Prothrombin time
Inflammation	Pain, Quality of Life: Visual Analog Scale Erythema: Vascular perfusion, area, ordinal or ratio scales Edema: Ultrasound, Organ/extremity thickness, circumference (% normal) Warmth: Thermography, IR Thermometry (degree above normal) Myeloperoxidase (biochemical marker for neutrophils and macrophages)
Granulation	Fibrinolysis, necrotic tissue debridement: % area clean Angiogenesis: Laser Doppler Vascular Flow (LDVF), histology Matrix formation: Collagen, Hydroxyproline, protein, DNA, RNA Cell proliferation: thymidine incorporation Percent of wound covered with granulation tissue Wound Area, length, width or depth
Epithelization	Migration: histology, acridine orange stain, skin splitting Proliferation: thymidine uptake, mitotic counts Differentiation: % clinically healed, moisture vapor transmission rate (MVTR)
Maturation (Scar formation)	Scar length, width, area, depth, elevation, tracings, elasticity, organization Ordinal scales or visual analog scales for: suppleness, induration, pigment changes, retraction, pain, deformity, patient acceptance; degrees of range of motion; mm of pedunculation

semifluid nature of hydrogels allows good apposition of the dressing to the wound surface, and these dressings also have a high absorbent capacity for wound exudates. In addition, hydrogel dressings cool the skin surface for several hours after application, which may have beneficial effects on pain relief and reducing inflammation.

Hydrocolloid Dressings

Hydrocolloid dressings have different physical characteristics and properties compared to polymers and hydrogels. They comprise compounds containing elastomeric, adhesive, and gelling agents, for example, sodium carboxymethylcellulose. As such, these dressings form an impermeable barrier. Although some absorption of exudate is possible, this is not a major function of this type of dressing. The barrier nature of hydrocolloids is, however, extremely useful in preventing

TABLE 1-7

Trade Names of Dressings

Dressing	Company
Transparent Films	
Tegaderm Transparent Dressing	3M
Acu-Derm	Acme United Corporation
Transparent Adhesive	Baxter Healthcare
Hi/Moist Transparent	Catalina Biomedical
Vari/Moist Modifiable Transparent Dressing	Catalina Biomedical
Bioclusive Transparent Dressing	Johnson & Johnson
Polyskin II Transparent Dressing	Kendall Healthcare
Blister Film Transparent Dressing	Sherwood Medical
Opsite Wound Dressing	Smith & Nephew United
Transite Exudate Transfer Film	Smith & Nephew United
Uniflex Transparent Dressing	Smith & Nephew United
Visi Derm II by Medline	WTS
Foams	
Lyofoam	Acme United Corporation
Cutinova Plus Foam Gel Film	Beiersdorf Inc
Epi-Lock Synthetic Wound Dressing	Calgon Vestal
Mitraflex Dressing with Adhesive	Calgon Vestal
Allevyn Hydrophilic Polymer Dressing	Smith & Nephew United
Gels and Hydrogels	
Vigilon	Bard Home Health
Carrington Wound Dressing Gel	Carrington
Biolex Wound Gel	Catalina Biomedical
Nu-Gel	Johnson & Johnson
Intrasite Gel Hydrogel	Smith & Nephew United
Elasto-Gel	Southwest Tech
2nd Skin Dressing	Spenco
Clearsite by NDM	WTS
Hydrocolloids	
Tegasorb Ulcer Dressing	3M
Intact	Bard Home Health
Hydrapad	Baxter Healthcare
Cutinova Hydro	Beiersdorf Inc
Comfeel Ulcer Care Dressing	Coloplast Inc
Duoderm	Convatec
Restore Wound Care Dressing	Hollister Inc
J & J Ulcer Dressing	Johnson & Johnson
Ultec	Sherwood Medical
Intrasite Wound Dressing	Smith & Nephew United
Sween-A-Peel	Sween Corporation
Oraheslve	Convatec
Calcium Alginates	
Kaltostat Wound Dressing	Calgon Vestal
Sorbsan Absorbent Dressing	Dow B. Hickam, Inc
Algosteril	Johnson & Johnson

Reprinted with permission from Helfman T., Ovington L., Falanga V. Occlusive dressings and wound healing in Bernstein E. F. (guest editor), Clinics in Dermatology: Wound Healing, Elsevier Science Inc., New York, 1994 pp 121–127.

bacterial entry into the wound. Chronic wounds and burns are suitable for treatment with hydrocolloid dressings.

Calcium Alginates

Calcium alginate dressings consist of polysaccharide material derived from seaweed, usually in the form of nonwoven mats. They have similar properties to polymer foams with good permeability and absorbency. However, optimal results from calcium alginates depend on the dressing's absorbing some exudate from the wound and forming a gel. This gel is then able to provide the moist microenvironment conducive to wound healing. In addition, calcium alginate dressings may be useful in reducing malodor associated with chronic exudative wounds.

Occlusive Dressings and Tissue Repair

Occlusive dressings benefit both epidermal and dermal wound healing. In the epidermis, occlusive dressings may assist keratinocyte migration and prevent desiccation.[170] In the dermis, wounds beneath occlusive dressings show the earlier appearance of fibroblasts, new interstitial collagen, and new blood vessel growth.[170] In addition, the degree of new collagen synthesis is increased in wounds treated with occlusive dressings.[171] The inflammatory response in wound healing may also be modified. Occlusive dressing treatment accelerates the transition in acute wounds from neutrophils to macrophages and also dampens down the entire inflammatory phase of wound healing.[172,173]

Occlusive Dressings and Wound Bacteriology

Occlusive dressings of the hydrocolloid type have been shown to protect wounds from exogenous bacteria.[174] In contrast, other types of occlusive dressings may all result in an increased growth of commensal and pathogenic bacteria in occluded wounds.[175,176] However, this increased bacterial colonization does not correlate with an increased rate of infection.[177] On the contrary, in donor sites and chronic ulcers, occlusive dressings appear to be associated with a lower infection rate compared to nonocclusive dressings, such as cotton gauze.[177] Thus, occlusive dressings can be used on contaminated wounds unless signs of infection, such as cellulitis, are present.

Topical Agents and Occlusive Dressings

The beneficial effects on wound healing from occlusive dressings may be further enhanced, in some circumstances, by the addition of topical agents such as antibiotics. For example, silver sulfadiazine has been incorporated into a flexible, adhesive nylon sheet.[178] This antibiotic-occlusive dressing combination has proved useful in treating certain burn wounds.[179] Nevertheless, caution should always be applied

when considering the use of topical antibiotics to the skin, particularly in terms of the development of an allergic contact dermatitis that may have deleterious effects on wound healing. In a patch-test population, over 6 percent of individuals have been shown to have a positive reaction to the frequently used topical antibiotic neomycin.[180]

Thus, occlusive wound dressings appear to have numerous properties with beneficial effects on wound healing. In the future, it is likely that further developments will evolve both to help control the degree of wound exudate associated with certain wounds and to improve the permeability of some types of occlusive dressings. The incorporation of various drugs into occlusive dressings to act as drug-delivery systems is another development with considerable therapeutic potential.

REFERENCES

1. Mostow EN: Diagnosis and classification of chronic wounds. *Clin Dermatol* **12:**3–9, 1994
2. Gorodetsky R et al: Assay of radiation effects in mouse skin as expressed in wound healing. *Radiat Res* **115:**135–144, 1988
3. Hunt TK et al: Cellular control of repair, in *Soft and Hard Tissue Repair,* edited by TK Hunt et al. New York, Praeger, 1984, pp 3–19
4. Fleischmajer JS et al: Collagen fibrillogenesis in human skin. *Ann N Y Acad Sci* **460:**246–257, 1985
5. Bernstein EF et al: Transforming growth factor-β improves healing of radiation-impaired wounds. *J Invest Dermatol* **97:**430–434, 1991
6. Uitto J et al: Extracellular matrix of the skin: 50 years of progress. *J Invest Dermatol* **92:**61S–77S, 1989
7. Bauer EA, Uitto J. Collagen in cutaneous diseases. *Int J Dermatol* **18:**251–270, 1979
8. Weber L et al: Collagen type distribution and macromolecular organization of connective tissue in different layers of human skin. *J Invest Dermatol* **82:**156–160, 1984
9. Kivirikko KI: Collagens and their abnormalities in a wide spectrum of diseases. *Ann Med* **25:**113–126, 1993
10. Prockop DJ et al: Intracellular steps in the biosynthesis of collagen, in *Biochemistry of Collagen,* edited by GN Ramachandran, AJ Reddi. New York, Plenum, 1976, pp 163–273
11. Uitto J: Molecular pathology of collagen in cutaneous diseases, in *Advances in Dermatology.* St. Louis, Mo, Mosby-Year Book, 1990, pp 313–328
12. Kuivaniemi H et al: Structure of full-length cDNA clone for the pre pro-α2(I) chain of human type I procollagen. *Biochem J* **252:**633–640, 1988
13. Chu M-L et al: Characterization of three constituent chains of collagen type VI by peptide sequences and cDNA clones. *Eur J Biochem* **168:**309–317, 1987
14. Myers JC et al: Complete primary structure of the human a2

type V procollagen COOH-terminal pro-peptide. *J Biol Chem* **260**:2315–2320, 1985

15. Hämäläinen ER et al: Molecular cloning of human lysyl oxidase and assignment of the gene to chromosome 5q23.3-31.2. *Genomics* **11**:508–516, 1991

16. Epstein EH: α1(III)₃ Human skin collagen, release by pepsin digestion and preponderance in fetal skin. *J Biol Chem* **249**:3225–3231, 1974

17. Uitto J et al: Altered steady-state ration of type I/III procollagen mRNAs correlates with selectively increased type I procollagen biosynthesis in cultured keloid fibroblasts. *Proc Natl Acad Sci U S A* **82**:5935–5939, 1985

18. Kuivaniemi H et al: Mutations in collagen genes: Causes of rare and some common diseases in humans. *FASEB J* **5**:2052–2060, 1991

19. Fleischmajer R et al: Type I and type III collagen interactions during fibrillogenesis. *Ann N Y Acad Sci* **580**:161–175, 1990

20. Timpl R: Structure and biological activity of basement membrane proteins. *Eur J Biochem* **180**:487–502, 1989

21. Timpl R, Engel J: Type VI collagen, in *Structure and Function of Collagen Types,* edited by R Mayne, RE Burgeson. Orlando, Fla, Academic Press, 1987, pp 105–153

22. Olsen DR et al: Collagen gene expression by cultured human skin fibroblasts: Abundant steady-state levels of type VI procollagen mRNAs. *J Clin Invest* **83**:791–795, 1989

23. Burgeson RE: Type VII collagen, anchoring fibrils, and epidermolysis bullosa. *J Invest Dermatol* **101**:252–255, 1994

24. McGrath JA et al: Structural variations in achoring fibrils in dystrophic epidermolysis bullosa: Correlation with type VII collagen expression. *J Invest Dermatol* **100**:366–372, 1993

25. Shaw LM, Olsen BR: FACIT collagens: Diverse molecular bridges in extracellular matrices. *Trends Biochem Sci* **16**:191–194, 1991

26. Li K et al: Cloning of type XVII collagen: Complementary and genomic DNA sequences of mouse 180-kDa bullous pemphigoid antigen (BPAG2) predict an interrupted collagenous domain, a transmembrane segment, and unusual features in the 5′-end of the gene and the 3′-untranslated region of the mRNA. *J Biol Chem* **268**:8825–8834, 1993

27. Giudice GJ et al: Cloning and primary structural analysis of the bullous pemphigoid autoantigen, BP180. *J Invest Dermatol* **99**:243–250, 1992

28. Giudice GJ et al: Bullous pemphigoid and herpes gestationis autoantibodies recognize a common non-collagenous site on the BP180 ectodomain. *J Immunol* **151**:5742–5750, 1993

29. Uitto J: Biochemistry of the elastic fibers in normal connective tissues and its alterations in disease. *J Invest Dermatol* **72**:1–10, 1979

30. Uitto J et al: Elastic fibers in human skin: Quantitation of elastic fibers by computerized digital image analyses and determination of elastin by a radioimmunoassay of desmosine. *Lab Invest* **49**:499–505, 1984

31. Starcher BC: Determination of the elastin content of tissue by measuring desmosine and isodesmosine. *Anal Biochem* **79**:11–15, 1977

32. Gray WR et al: Molecular model for elastin structure and function. *Nature* **246**:461–466, 1973

33. Sakai LY et al: Fibrillin, a new 350-kDa glycoprotein, is a component of extracellular microfibrils. *J Cell Biol* **103**:2499–2509, 1986

34. Lee B et al: Linkage of Marfan syndrome and a phenotypically related disorder to two fibrillin genes. *Nature* **352**:330–334, 1991

35. Dietz HC et al: Marfan syndrome caused by a recurrent de novo missense mutation in the fibrillin gene. *Nature* **352**:337–339, 1991

36. Dietz HC et al: Four novel FBN1 mutations: Significance for mutant transcript level and EGF-like domain clacium binding in the pathogenesis of Marfan syndrome. *Genomics* **17**:468–475, 1993

37. Tsipuoras P et al: Genetic linkage of the Marfan syndrome, ectopia lentis, and congenital contractural arachnodactyly to the fibrillin genes on chromosome 15 and 5. *N Engl J Med* **326**:905–909, 1992

38. Comper WD, Laurent TC. Physiological function of connective tissue polysaccharides. *Physiol Rev* **58**:255–315, 1978

39. Pearce RH et al: Fractionation of rat cutaneous glycosaminoglycans using an anion-exchange resin. *Anal Biochem* **50**:63–72, 1972

40. Weitzhandler M, Bernfield MR: Proteoglycan glycoconjugates, in *Wound Healing: Beochemical and Clinical Aspects,* edited by IK Cohen et al. Philadelphia, Saunders, 1992, pp 195–208

41. Krusius T, Ruoslahti E: Primary structure of an extracellular matrix proteoglycan core protein deduced from cloned cDNA. *Proc Natl Acad Sci* U S A **83**:7683–7687, 1986

42. Vogel KG, Heingard D. Characterization of proteoglycans from adult bovine tendon. *J Biol Chem* **260**:9298–9306, 1985

43. Scott JE, Orford CR: Dermatan sulphate-rich proteoglycan associates with rat tail-tendon collagen at the d band in the gap region. *Biochem J* **197**:213–216, 1981

44. Vogel KG et al: Specific inhibition of type I and type II collagen fibrilogenesis by the small proteoglycan of tendon. *Biochem J* **223**:587–597, 1984

45. Uldbjerg N, Danielsen CC: A study of the interaction in vitro between type I collagen and a small dermatan sulphate proteoglycan. *Biochem J* **251**:643–648, 1988

46. Fleischmajer R et al: Decorin interacts with fibrillar collagen of embryonic and adult human skin. *J Struct Biol* **6**:82–90, 1991

47. Bianco P et al: Expression and localization of the two small proteoglycans biglycan and decorin in developing human skeletal and non-skeletal tissues. *J Histochem Cytochem* **38**:1549–1563, 1990

48. Zimmerman DR et al: Versican is expressed in the proliferating zone in the epidermis and in association with the elastic network of the dermis. *J Cell Biol* **124**:817–825, 1994

49. Grinnell F: Cell adhesion, in *Wound Healing: Biochemical and Clinical Aspects,* edited by IK Cohen et al. Philadelphia, Saunders, 1992, pp 209–222

50. Kornblihtt AR, Gutman A: Molecular biology of the extracellular matrix proteins. *Biol Rev* **63**:465–507, 1988

51. Pierschbache MD, Ruoslahti E: Cell attachment activity of fibronectin can be duplicated by small synthetic fragments of the molecule. *Nature* **309**:30–33, 1984

52. Yamada KM, Kennedy DW: Dualistic nature of adhesive protein function: Fibronectin and its biologically active peptide fragments can autoinhibit fibronectin function. *J Cell Biol* **99**:29–36, 1984

53. Whalen GF, Zetter BR: Angiogenesis, in *Wound Healing: Biochemical and Clinical Aspects,* edited by IK Cohen et al. Philadelphia, Saunders, 1992, pp 77–95

54. Weigel PH et al: A model for the role of hyaluronic acid and fibrin in the early events during the inflammatory response and wound healing. *J Theor Biol* **119**:219–234, 1986

55. Toole BP, Gross J: The extracellular matrix of the regenerating newt limb: Synthesis and removal of hyaluronate prior to differentiation. *Dev Biol* **25**:57–77, 1971

56. Alexander SA, Donoff RB: The glycosaminoglycans of open wounds. *J Surg Res* **29**:422–429, 1980

57. Bently JP: Rate of chondroitin sulfate formation in wound healing. *Ann Surg* **165**:186–190, 1967

58. Yamada KM: Fibronectin and other structural proteins, in *Cell Biology of the Extra Cellular Matrix,* edited by ED Hay. New York, Plenum, 1981, pp 95–114

59. Clark RAF et al: Fibronectin is produced by blood vessels in response to injury. *J Exp Med* **156**:646–651, 1982

60. Alitatlo K et al: Fibronectin is produced by human macrophages. *J Exp Med* **151**:602–613, 1980

61. Viljanto J et al: Fibronectin in early phases of wound healing in children. *Acta Chir Scand* **147**:7–13, 1981

62. Grinnell F et al: Distribution of fibronectin during wound healing in vivo. *J Invest Dermatol* **76**:181–189, 1981

63. Holund B et al: Fibronectin in experimental granulation tissue. *Acta Pathol Microbiol Immunol Scand* [A] **90**:159–165, 1982

64. Kurkinen M et al: Sequential appearance of fibronectin and collagen in experimental granulation tissue. *Lab Invest* **43**:47–51, 1980

65. McDonald JA et al: Role of fibronectin in collagen deposition: F′ab to the gelatin-binding domain of fibronectin inhibits both fibronectin and collagen organization in fibroblast extracellular matrix. *J Cell Biol* **92**:485–492, 1982

66. Jackson DS: Development of fibrosis: Cell proliferation and collagen biosynthesis. *Ann Rheum Dis* **36**(suppl):2–4, 1977

67. Gorodetsky R et al: Assay of radiation effects in mouse skin as expressed in wound healing. *Radiat Res* **115**:135–144, 1988

68. Hunt TK et al: Cellular control of repair, in *Soft and Hard Tissue Repair,* edited by TK Hunt et al. New York, Praeger, 1984, pp 3–19

69. Fleischmajer JS et al: Collagen fibrillogenesis in human skin. *Ann N Y Acad Sci* **460**:246–257, 1985

70. Stanley JR et al: Characterization of bullous pemphigoid antigen: A unique basement membrane protein of stratified squamous epithelia. *Cell* **24**:897–903, 1981

71. Sonnengerg A et al: Integrin a6/b4 complex is located in hemidesmosomes, suggesting a major role of epidermal cell-basement membrane adhesion. *J Cell Biol* **113**:907–917, 1991

72. Burgeson RE: A new nomenclature for laminins. *Matrix Biol* **14**:209–211, 1994

73. Clark RAF et al: Fibronectin and fibrin provide a provisional matrix for epidermal cell migration during wound re-epithelialization. *J Invest Dermatol* **79**:264–269, 1982

74. O'Keefe EJ et al: Spreading and enhanced motility of human keratinocytes on fibronectin. *J Invest Dermatol* **85**:125–130, 1985

75. Clark RAF: Fibronectin matrix deposition and fibronectin receptor expression in healing and normal skin. *J Invest Dermatol* **94**:128S–136S, 1990

76. Kim JP et al: Mechanism of human keratinocyte migration on fibronectin: Unique roles of RGD site and integrins. *J Cell Physiol* **151**:443–450, 1992

77. Woodley DT et al: Laminin inhibits human keratinocyte migration. *J Cell Physiol* **136**:140–146, 1988

78. Brown C et al: Fibronectin: Effects on keratinocyte motility and inhibition of collagen-induced motility. *J Invest Dermatol* **96**:724–728, 1991

79. Nickoloff BJ et al: Modulation of keratinocyte motility. *Am J Pathol* **132**:543–551, 1988

80. Morgan CJ, Pledger WJ: Fibroblast proliferation, in *Wound Healing: Biochemical and Clinical Aspects,* edited by IK Cohen et al. Philadelphia, Saunders, 1992, pp 63–76

81. Ross R et al: The biology of platelet-derived growth factor. *Cell* **46**:155–169, 1986

82. Oka Y, Orth DN: Human plasma epidermal growth factor/β-urogastrone is associated with blood platelets. *J Clin Invest* **72**:249–259, 1983

83. Assoian RK et al: Transforming growth factor-β in human platelets: Identification of a major storage site, purification and characterization. *J Biol Chem* **258**:7155–7160, 1983

84. Hatanaka K et al: Local development of mast cells from bone marrow-derived precursors in the skin of mice. *Blood* **53**:142–147, 1979

85. Enerback L: Mast cells in rat gastrointestinal mucosa: I. Effects of fixation. *Acta Pathol Microbiol Scand* **66**:289–302, 1966

86. Mikhail GR, Miller-Milinska A: Mast cell population in human skin. *J Invest Dermatol* **43**:249–254, 1964

87. Lever WF, Schaumberg-Lever G: *Histopathology of the Skin,* 7th ed. Philadelphia, Lippincott, 1990, p 62

88. Rothe MJ et al: The mast cell in health and disease. *J Am Acad Dermatol* **23**;615–624, 1990

89. Tharp MD: The mast cell and its role in human cutaneous diseases. *Prog Dermatol* **22**:1–14, 1987

90. Kerdel FA, Soter NA: The mast cell in mastocytosis and pediatric dermatologic disease. *Adv Dermatol* **4**:159–182, 1989

91. Wichmann B-E: The mast cell count during the process of wound healing: An experimental investigation on rats. *Acta Pathol Microbiol Scand [Suppl]* **108**:1–35, 1955

92. Boyd JF, Smith AN: The effect of histamine and a histamine releasing agent (compound 48/80) on wound healing. *J Pathol Bacteriol* **78**:379–388, 1959

93. Persinger MA et al: Mast cell numbers in incisional wounds in rat skin as a function of distance, time and treatment. *Br J Dermatol* **108**:179–187, 1983

94. Nishioka K et al: Mast cell numbers in diffuse scleroderma. *Arch Dermatol* **123**:205–208, 1987

95. Cerio R et al: Histiocytoma cutis: A tumour of dermal dendrocytes (dermal dendrocytoma). *Br J Dermatol* **120**:197–206, 1989

96. Cerio R et al: Identification of factor XIIIa in cutaneous tissue. *Histopathology* **13**:362–363, 1988

97. Cerio R et al: Characterization of factor XIIIa positive dermal dendritic cells in normal and inflamed skin. *Br J Dermatol* **121**:421–431, 1989

98. Cooper KD et al: Antigen-presenting IKM$_{5+}$ melanophages appear in human epidermis after ultraviolet radiation. *J Invest Dermatol* **86**:363–370, 1986

99. Cooper KD et al: Murine dermal cells in suspension contain T cell-activating antigen presenting cells. *J Invest Dermatol* **88**:482, 1987

100. James WD et al: Inflammatory acquired oral hyperpigmentation: Association with melanophages demonstrating phenotypic characteristics of antigen presenting cells and activated monocytes. *J Am Acad Dermatol* **16**:220–226, 1987

101. Shen HH et al: Functional subsets of human monocytes derived by monoclonal antibodies: A distinct subset of monocytes contains the cells capable of inducing the autologous mixed lymphocyte culture. *J Immunol* **130**:698–705, 1983

102. Nickoloff BJ, Griffiths CEM: Factor XIIIa expressing dermal dendrocytes are increased in AIDS associated Kaposi's sarcoma. *Science* **243**:1736–1737, 1989

103. Cerio R et al: A study of factor XIIIa and Mac 387 immunolabeling in normal and pathological skin. *Am J Dermatopathol* **12**:221–233, 1990

104. Nestle FO et al: Characterization of dermal dendritic cells in psoriasis. *J Clin Invest* **94**:202–209, 1994

105. Hirsh BC, Johnson WC: Concepts of granulomatous inflammation. *Int J Dermatol* **23**:90–100, 1984

106. Lever WF, Schaumberg-Lever G: *Histopathology of the Skin,* 7th ed. Philadelphia, Lippincott, 1990, pp 59–62

107. Leibovitch SJ, Ross R: The role of the macrophage in wound repair: A study with hydrocortisone and anti-macrophage serum. *Am J Pathol* **78**:71–100, 1975

108. Diegelman RF et al: The role of wound macrophages in wound repair: A review. *Plast Reconstr Surg* **68**:107–113, 1981

109. Hunt TK et al: Studies on inflammation and wound healing: Angiogenesis and collagen synthesis stimulated in vivo by resident and activated wound macrophages. *Surgery* **96**:48–54, 1984

110. Clark RAF: Overview and general considerations of wound repair, in *The Molecular and Cellular Biology of Wound Repair,* edited by RAF Clark, PM Henson. New York, Plenum, 1988, pp 3–33

111. Leibovich SJ, Ross R: The role of the macrophage in wound repair: A study with hydrocortisone and antimacrophage serum. *Am J Pathol* **78**:71–100, 1975

112. Mauviel A, Uitto J: The extracellular matrix in wound healing: Role of the cytokine network. *Wounds* **5**:137–152, 1993

113. Kähäri V-M et al: Tumor necrosis factor-α and interferon-γ suppress the activation of human type I collagen gene expression by transforming growth factor-β1: Evidence for two distinct mechanisms of inhibition at the transcriptional and post-transcriptional levels. *J Clin Invest* **86**:1489–1495, 1990

114. Heino J, Heinonen T: Interleukin-1β prevents the stimulatory effect of transforming growth factor-β on collagen gene expression in human skin fibroblasts. *Biochem J* **271**:827–830, 1990

115. Varga J et al: Interferon-γ reverses the stimulation of collagen but not fibronectin gene expression by transforming growth factor-β in normal human fibroblasts. *Eur J Clin Invest* **20**:487–493, 1990

116. Mauviel A et al: Leukoregulin down-regulates type I collagen mRNA levels and promoter activity, and counteracts the up-regulation elicited by transforming growth factor-β. *Biochem J* **284**:629, 1992

117. Scharffetter K et al: Synergistic effect of tumor necrosis factor-α and interferon-γ on collagen synthesis of human skin fibroblasts in vitro. *Exp Cell Res* **181**:409–419, 1989

118. Mauviel A et al: Differential cytokine regulation of type I and type VII collagen gene expression in human dermal fibroblasts. *J Biol Chem* **269**:25–28, 1994

119. Woessner JF Jr: Matrix metalloproteinases and their inhibitors in connective tissue remodeling. *FASEB J* **5**:2145–2154, 1991

120. Mauviel A: Cytokine regulation of metalloproteinase gene expression. *J Cell Biochem* **53**:288–297, 1993

121. Mauviel A et al: Transcriptional interactions of transforming growth factor-β with pro-inflammatory cytokines. *Current Biol* **3**:822–831, 1993

122. McKay IA, Leigh IM: Epidermal cytokines and their roles in cutaneous wound healing. *Br J Dermatol* **124**:513–518, 1991

123. Grinnell F: Wound repair, keratinocyte activation and integrin modulation. *J Cell Sci* **101**:1–5, 1992

124. Klagsbrun M, D'Amore PA: Regulators of angiogenesis. *Annu Rev Physiol* **53**:217–239, 1991

125. Knighton DR et al: Classification and treatment of chronic non-healing wounds; Successful treatment with autologous platelet-derived wound healing formula (PDWHF). *Ann Surg* **204**:322–330, 1986

126. Knighton DR et al: The use of platelet-derived wound healing formula in human clinical trials, in *Growth Factors and Other Aspects of Wound Healing: Biological and Clinical Implications,* edited by A Barbul et al. New York, Alan R Liss, 1988, pp 319–329

127. Carter DM et al: Clinical experience with crude preparations

of growth factors in healing of chronic wounds in human subjects, in *Growth Factors and Other Aspects of Wound Healing: Biological and Clinical Implications,* edited by A Barbul et al. New York, Alan R Liss, 1988, pp 303–317

128. Robson MC et al: Recombinant human platelet-derived growth factor-BB for the treatment of chronic pressure ulcers. *Lancet* **339:**23–24, 1992

129. Greaves MW: Lack of effect of topically applied epidermal growth on man in vivo. *Clin Exp Dermatol* **5:**1–13, 1986

130. Grunfeld C: Diabetic foot ulcers: Etiology, treatment and prevention. *Adv Intern Med* **37:**103–132, 1991

131. Brown GL et al: Enhancement of wound healing by topical treatment with epidermal growth factor. *N Engl J Med* **321:**76–79, 1989

132. Steed DL et al: Randomized prospective double-blinded trial in healing chronic diabetic foot ulcers: CT-102 activated platelet supernatant, topical versus placebo. *Diabetes Care* **15:**1598–1604, 1992

133. Atri SC et al: Use of homologous platelet factors in achieving total healing of recalcitrant skin ulcers. *Surgery* **108:**508–512, 1990

134. Brown GL et al: Stimulation of healing of chronic wounds by epidermal growth factor. *Plast Reconstr Surg* **88:**189–194, 1991

135. Robson MC et al: Recombinant human platelet-derived growth factor-BB for the treatment of chronic pressure ulcers. *Ann Plast Surg* **29:**193–201, 1992

136. Burgos H et al: Placental angiogenic and growth factors in the treatment of chronic varicose ulcers: Preliminary communication. *J R Soc Med* **82:**598–599, 1989

137. Falanga V et al: Topical use of human recombinant epidermal growth factor (h-EGF) in venous ulcers. *J Dermatol Surg Oncol* **18:**604–606, 1992

138. Lazarus GS et al: Definitions and guidelines for assessment of wounds and evaluation of healing. *Arch Dermatol* **130:**489–493, 1994

139. Goss RJ: Wound healing and antler regeneration, in *Epidermal Wound Healing,* edited by HI Maibach, DT Rovee. Chicago, Year Book, 1972, pp 219–228

140. Adzick NS, Longaker MT: Scarless wound healing in the fetus: The role of the extracellular matrix, in *Clinical and Experimental Approaches to Dermal and Epidermal Repair: Normal and Chronic Wounds,* edited by A Barbul et al. New York, Wiley-Liss, 1991, pp 177–192

141. van Rijswijk L, Multi-Center Leg Ulcer Study Group: Full-thickness leg ulcers: Patient demographics and predictors of healing. *J Fam Pract* **36:**625–632, 1993

142. van Rijswijk L: Full-thickness pressure ulcers: Patient and wound healing characteristics. *Decubitus* **6:**16–21, 1993

143. Bolton L, van Rijswijk L: Wound dressings: Meeting clinical and biological needs. *Dermatology Nursing,* **3:**146–161, 1991

144. Seiler WO, Stahelin HB: Identification of factors that impair wound healing: A possible approach to wound healing research. *Wounds* **6:**101–105, 1994

145. Margolis DJ et al: Planimetric rate of healing in venous ulcers of the leg treated with pressure bandage and hydrocolloid dressing. *J Am Acad Dermatol* **28:**418–421, 1993

146. Rockwell WB et al: Keloids and hypertrophic scars: A comprehensive review. *Plast Reconstr Surg* **84:**827–837, 1989

147. West MD: The cellular and molecular biology of skin aging. *Arch Dermatol* **130:**87–95, 1994

148. Buffoni F et al: Skin wound healing: Some biochemical parameters in guinea pigs. *J Pharm Pharmacol* **45:**784–790, 1993

149. Howell JM: Current and future trends in wound healing. *Emerg Med Clin North Am* **10:**655–663, 1992

150. Kiritsy CP, Lynch SE: Role of growth factors in cutaneous wound healing: A review. *Crit Rev Oral Biol Med* **4:**729–760, 1993

151. Reid TJ, Alving BM: A quantitative thrombin time for determining levels of hirudin and hirulog. *Thromb Haemost* **70:**608–616, 1993

152. Sanborn TA et al: A multicenter randomized trial comparing a percutaneous collagen hemostasis device with conventional manual compression after diagnostic angiography and angioplasty (with comments). *J Am Coll Cardiol* **22:**1273–1282, 1993

153. Ferrell BR et al: Quality of life as an outcome variable in the management of cancer pain. *Cancer* **63:**2321–2327, 1989

154. Choiniere M et al: Visual analogue thermometer: A valid and useful instrument for measuring pain in burned patients. *Burns* **20:**229–235, 1994

155. Lansdown ABG: Animal models for the study of skin irritants. *Curr Probl Dermatol* **7:**26–28, 1978

156. McCreesh AH, Steinberg M: Skin irritation testing in animals. *Advances in Modern Toxicology* **4:**193–210, 1977

157. Lundberg C, Arfors KE: Polymorphonucler leukocyte accumulation in inflammatory dermal sites as measured by 51-Cr-labelled cells and myeloperoxidase. *Inflammation* **7:**247–254, 1983

158. Lydon MJ et al: Dissolution of wound coagulum and promotion of granulation tissue under DuoDERM®. *Wounds* **1:**95–106, 1989

159. Field CK, Kerstein MD: Overview of wound healing in a moist environment. *Am J Surg* **167**(suppl):2S–6S, 1994

160. Falanga V, Eaglstein W: Wound healing: Practical aspects. *Progress in Dermatology* **22:**1–12, 1988

161. Surinchak JS et al: Skin wound healing determined by water loss. *J Surg Res* **38:**258–262, 1985

162. Christophers E: Kinetic aspects of epidermal healing, in *Epidermal Wound Healing,* edited by HI Maibach, DT Rovee. Chicago, Year Book, 1972, pp 53–69

163. Pirone LA et al: Wound healing under occlusion and non-occlusion in partial-thickness and full-thickness wounds in swine. *Wounds* **2:**74–81, 1990

164. Hein N et al: Facilitated wound healing using transparent film dressing following Mohs micrographic surgery. *Arch Dermatol* **124:**903–906, 1988

165. Michie DD, Hugill JV: Influence of occlusive and impregnated gauze dressings on incisional healing: A prospective, randomized controlled study. *Ann Plast Surg* **32:**57–64, 1993

166. Eaglstein WH, Mertz PM: New method for assessing epidermal wound healing: The effects of triamcinolone acetonide and polyethylene film occlusion. *J Invest Dermatol* **71:**382–384, 1978

167. Falanga V: Occlusive wound dressings: Why, when, which? *Arch Dermatol* **124:**872–877, 1988

168. Eaglstein WH et al: Occlusive dressings. *Am Fam Physician* **35:**211–216, 1987

169. Helfman T et al: Occlusive dressings and wound healing. *Clin Dermatol* **12:**121–127, 1994

170. Winter GD: Epidermal regeneration studied in the domestic pig, in *Epidermal Wound Healing,* edited by HI Maibach, DT Rovee. Chicago, Year Book, 1972, pp 71–112

171. Alvarex OM et al: The effect of occlusive dressings on collagen synthesis and re-epithelialization in superficial wounds. *J Surg Res* **35:**142–148, 1983

172. Dyson M et al: Comparison of the effects of moist and dry conditions on dermal repair. *J Invest Dermatol* **91:**434–439, 1988

173. Linsky CB et al: Effect of wound dressing on wound inflammation and scar tissue, in *The Surgical Wound,* edited by P Dineen. Philadelphia, Lea & Febiger, 1981, pp 191–206

174. Mertz PM et al: Occlusive wound dressings to prevent bacterial invasion and wound infection. *J Am Acad Dermatol* **12:**662–668, 1985

175. Mertz PM, Eaglstein WH: The effect of a semiocclusive dressing on the microbial population in superficial wounds. *Arch Surg* **119:**287–289, 1984

176. Marshall DA et al: Occlusive dressings: Does dressing type influence the growth of common bacterial pathogens? *Arch Surg* **125:**1136–1139, 1990

177. Hutchinson JJ: Prevalence of wound infection under occlusive dressings: A collective survey of reported research. *Wounds* **1:**123–133, 1989

178. Cruse CW, Daniels S: Minor burns: Treatment using a new drug delivery system with silver sulfadiazine. *South Med J* **9:**1135–1137, 1989

179. Gerding RL, et al: Outpatient management of partial-thickness burns: Biobrane versus 1% silver sulfadiazine. *Ann Emerg Med* **19:**121–124, 1990

180. Dupuis G, Benezra C: *Allergic Contact Dermatitis to Simple Chemicals: A Molecular Approach.* New York, Marcel Dekker, 1982.

David S. Freitag

2 Surgical Wound Dressings

Along with the upsurge in interest in dermatologic surgery procedures, a corresponding interest in wound healing and wound dressings has flourished. Dressing materials were developed subsequent to our growing knowledge of the needs of fresh wounds. The application of a particular dressing to a wound creates a specific subdressing environment.[1] The evolution from dry adhesive bandages to moist ones and finally to the development of synthetic occlusive materials constitutes the science of wound dressings which has become as integral to superior outcomes as proper surgical techniques. Reduced pain and infection rates, more rapid healing, and improved scar appearance are all products of this expanding knowledge. Yet patience, experience, technique, and common sense are also requisites for appropriate dressings.

A historical view of wound dressing innovation was recently published using both antiquated and modern examples.[2] For instance, the ancient Egyptians used a paste of beans and papyrus to dress burns. During the fourteenth century, people believed that pouring boiling oil into a gunshot wound would benefit the victim. Even within the last two decades, some have proposed the use of maggots to debride necrotic tissue from certain wounds. Though such methods would be castigated today, they were probably considered the superlative modalities of their time. Similarly, our newer occlusive materials will certainly be viewed as rudimentary by our colleagues in the twenty-first century.

The development of an optimal wound dressing has been actively pursued for centuries. Earlier dressings were used primarily to seal the open wound and to provide a visual barrier. This role has been extended, however, as our understanding of pathogens and wound healing developed. The reasons for applying dressings over open wounds have evolved to the optimal promotion of healing by preventing both the ingress of potential contaminants and the egress of bodily fluids.[1]

Before the 1960s, wounds were often left uncovered to encourage eschar formation. This was believed to curb bacterial proliferation by avoiding moisture accumulation and, therefore, promoting epithelialization.[2] In fact, more recent studies have concluded that a clean sutured wound left open to air following a 24 hour dressing is no more likely to become infected than one kept dressed until suture removal. These studies presented advantages to leaving wounds undressed, including easy wound inspection, cost containment, and patient hygiene; however, neither study mentions the speed with which they healed nor the postoperative appearance of the wounds after healing, and both studies were on general surgery patients, not wounds on smaller and simpler skin excisions.[3,4]

Occlusive dressings were rarely used until recently because many feared that the dressings created environments conducive to pathogen colonization, despite the demonstration that occluded wounds healed 50 percent faster than wounds left open to air.[5–7] Hutchinson surveyed nearly 70 reports encompassing many wound types and found the incidence of infection under occlusive dressings to be 2.6 percent compared to 7.1 percent found in wounds under traditional dressings.[8] *Clinical wound infection is probably more related to intraoperative tissue damage than to dressing type and subsequent bacterial load.* Additionally, occlusive dressings have been shown to permit surgical wounds to heal with a smaller, more agreeable scar.

Both dermal and epidermal wound healing improve under occlusive or semiocclusive dressing therapy. Occluded wounds develop less inflammation, a smaller area of fibrosis, and a more rapid return of the barrier function of the stratum corneum. Thus, wounds covered with occlusive dressings

TABLE 2-1

Characteristics Required for the Ideal Dressing

Handling of excess exudate

Removal of toxic substances

Maintenance of moist environment over wound

Gaseous exchange permitted*

Barrier to microorganisms

Thermal insulation provided

Freedom from particulate contaminants demonstrated

Removal without trauma to new tissue

Adheres well to a thin margin of surrounding skin

Does not adhere to the wound

Nontoxic and nonreactive

Conforms well to bodily contours and motion

Promotes patient comfort and is not bulky or conspicuous

Readily available and inexpensive

Long shelf life

Modified from Hutchinson and McGuckin[1]
*This may not be as important as previously thought.

usually have less pain, erythema, edema, and often a more cosmetically pleasing result.[7,9] The cosmetic appearance of the final scar may publicly reflect upon the skill and technique of the surgeon responsible. Because of this, choosing a dressing incorrectly may reap unwanted notoriety.

No surgical wound dressing exists that will suit the needs of every wound. Dermabrasion wounds or those healing by second intention ooze substantially and require maximum absorbency; sutured wounds are drier and require little absorbency. Each wound should be assessed individually for its healing requirements to determine the appropriate dressing.

Sometimes one must choose a dressing for reasons other than promoting faster healing. Often the choice depends upon the patient's circumstances. For example, a debilitated patient may be better off with a bulkier absorbent bandage which will remain in place for a week rather than a thinner nonabsorbent one which may need daily changing. In any case, a dressing created in the office should be both functional and aesthetically pleasing.[10]

Table 2-1 represents the properties deemed most desirable in an ideal dressing.

This chapter will attempt to review fundamental techniques and current materials for wound dressings in dermatologic surgery. Since the performance of a dressing depends on its basic structure and composition, traditional composite dressing materials and the newer occlusive or semiocclusive ones will be reviewed and contrasted. Examples of special situations and suggested dressings for certain locations will also be offered.

THE COMPOSITE DRESSING

The composite dressing is the traditional surgical covering and is normally composed of four layers: a *hydrating layer* of antibiotic ointment, a *contact layer,* an *absorbent layer,* and an outer *securing layer* of tape.[10] Each layer contributes some benefit to enhance the therapeutic value of the dressing. While this dressing has been the standard for years, the development and availability of synthetic occlusive dressings are making the composite dressing a second choice for many surgical wounds.

A layer of *antibacterial ointment* is useful to hydrate the wound bed and act as a short-term deterrent to bacterial growth. Generally, only a small amount is needed since the wound itself will create a certain amount of moisture in the form of serum exudate. Many types are readily available (Table 2-2).

The *contact layer* is placed adjacent to the wound. Only nonadhesive materials should be used to avoid damaging the healing wound upon removal. Either nonadhesive pads (e.g., Telfa, Release) or dressing materials impregnated with nonadhesive substances (e.g., Vaseline Petrolatum Gauze, Xeroform) will meet this requirement.

The *absorbent* third layer provides both pressure and absorbency. This layer is usually made of dry gauze or a cotton/rayon filler. By filling in a contour on the skin, the gauze adds pressure to the new wound which will aid in hemostasis during the critical first 24 hours. Its wicking action draws away excess exudate. This layer should extend past the margins of the contact layer.

The outer or *securing layer* affixes the dressing to the patient while holding the separate components in their proper places. It also provides mechanical support and distributes firm but comfortable pressure to the underlying surgical wound. In most cases, an appropriate surgical adhesive tape suits this function best. The use of a tactifier in conjunction

TABLE 2-2

Antibacterial Ointments

Brand Name	Active Antimicrobial Ingredients
Bacitracin	Bacitracin zinc
Polysporin	Bacitracin zinc, polymyxin B sulfate
Neosporin	Neomycin sulfate, bacitracin zinc, polymyxin B sulfate
Gentamicin	Gentamicin
Ilotycin	Erythromycin
Aquaphor Faster Healing Ointment	Bacitracin zinc, polymyxin B sulfate
Eucerin	
White petrolatum	

with surgical tape enhances adhesion which is especially helpful when one is applying pressure dressings.

A variety of surgical adhesive tapes are available. Most of these are hypoallergenic. Nonwoven rayon paper tape (e.g., Micropore, 3M, St. Paul, MN; Tender Skin, Kendall Co., Mansfield, MA) is most commonly used in dermatologic surgery. The tapes are usually offered in different sizes to accommodate various wound requirements, and some even incorporate pigments (i.e., flesh-toned). Paper tapes are lightweight and seldom cause irritation, thereby making them most useful in dressings requiring long-term application.

Other materials used for outer layers include roller gauze, tubular gauze, and elastic roller bandages. Tubular gauze is useful in dressing many areas such as the scalp, face, and fingers and can often be substituted for roller gauze. Specific uses for these outer layer materials will be discussed more fully below.

TACTIFIERS

Prior to securing a dressing, a final preparation of the wound and adjacent skin is warranted. Cleaning removes contaminants, dried blood, and skin oils which might reduce the adhesion of the bandage materials or tape. Skin may vary considerably in texture, perspiration, hair, and sebum secretions; wound types vary in size, location, and exudate. The use of adhesive compounds to augment the adhesion between dressings and skin has become standard practice in surgical wound management.

Mastisol (Ferndale Labs, Ferndale, Michigan) and compound tincture of benzoin USP are the two more commonly known liquid adhesives available. Mastisol is a straw-colored resinous liquid containing gum mastic, styrax liquid, methyl salicylate, and alcohol. Compound tincture of benzoin USP contains 10 percent benzoin, 2 percent aloe, 8 percent styrax, and 4 percent tolu balsum in alcohol. Although compound tincture of benzoin will enhance tape adhesion, Mastisol pro-

vides considerably more adhesive stability. Sensitization is a common problem with benzoin. Once sensitization to tincture of benzoin develops, cross-sensitization to Mastisol will often follow.[11,12]

Sensitization is rarely a problem with a silicon-based adhesive known as Dermistik (Medi-Flex, Overland Park, Kansas). Dispensed in a single-use applicator, this clear, colorless liquid has the distinct advantages of adhesion retention in the presence of moisture and a rapid drying time (5 to 10 s). The individual packaging, SEPP (sterile easy prepping product), contributes to both cost and ease of use without contamination.

Another hypoallergenic tactifier currently available is Skin-Prep (Smith & Nephew, Largo, Florida). This adhesive contains a citric acid which leaves a sticky film for adhesion and protection and alcohol which may degrease the skin somewhat. Table 2-3 lists some readily available spray and liquid tactifiers.

For best results, apply the liquid tactifier in a thin layer and allow it to dry before securing the dressing in place with tape. Mastisol and benzoin need 30 to 90 s to dry for optimal adhesiveness; the other listed products are quick drying and need only 5 to 10 s.[11,12] The wooden end of a cotton-tipped applicator is useful to efficiently apply liquid adhesives in a linear fashion, such as alongside suture lines. This method offers good control without waste, preventing contamination of the wound with the liquid. However, the cotton-tipped end proves more useful on more circular or concave sites like the ears or ala nasi. In any case, the liquid adhesives should be applied carefully and only to the normal intact skin.[11]

Other substances are produced specifically to eliminate residual adhesives following dressing changes. These are generally organic solvents which may also be used to degrease skin prior to applying liquid adhesives or tape. These products should also be prevented from entering the healing wound.

Adhesive removers may be obtained as individually packaged towelettes (e.g., Clinipad, Clinipad Corp., Guilford, Connecticut, or Adhesive Remover Pads, Moore Medical, New Britain, Connecticut) or as a liquid (e.g., Detachol, Ferndale Labs). Other substances, including acetone, isopropyl alcohol, or ether, can also be used to remove adhesives or degrease the skin; however, these substances are flammable.

T A B L E 2 - 3

Tactifiers

Product	Form	Source
Tincture of benzoin	Liquid	USP
Mastisol	Liquid	Ferndale Labs, Ferndale, MI
Dermistik	Liquid (SEPP)	Medi-Flex, Overland Park, KA
Derma-Prep	Liquid or spray	Mowbray, Inc, Waterloo, IA
JC-5 Tape Adherent	Spray	Aeroseptics, Erie, PA
Pedi-Pre-Tape	Spray	Pedinol, Farmingdale, NY
Pedi-Skin Adherent #2	Liquid	Pedinol, Farmingdale, NY
SkinPrep	Liquid	Smith & Nephew, Largo, FL

ADHESIVE BANDAGES

Adhesive bandages represent the most ubiquitous of wound dressings available. Found in homes and health care settings alike, these wound dressings come in a variety of shapes and sizes adaptable to many anatomic loci. All bandages are packaged as individually wrapped units composed of a thin contact layer with a pressure sensitive adhesive backing.[13]

The forerunner in this category is the plastic Band-Aid strip (Johnson & Johnson, New Brunswick, New Jersey).

More than 2 billion Band-Aid brand sheer strips are used annually in the United States. The author favors adhesive bandages which are fairly elastic (e.g., Coverlet, Beiersdorf, Co., Norwalk, CT). These often provide additional pressure to wounds and the elasticity is useful in adhering to curved surfaces.

OCCLUSIVE DRESSINGS

Occlusive dressings satisfy many of the criteria listed in Table 2-1 while also demonstrating the potential for faster and better healing.[1,7] Four basic types are now marketed. In general, they are all rather expensive and somewhat difficult to place and secure properly. However, the advantages they afford more than compensate for the expense and trouble incurred. Once occlusive dressings are introduced to a practice, the results as seen in improved healing, scar appearance, and patient comfort make them difficult to abandon.

The application of an occlusive dressing creates a specific subdressing environment.[1,14] Wounds exude a fluid medium rich in nutrients and chemicals which facilitate healing. Preventing the escape of this medium while excluding outside contamination is critical to the satisfactory functioning of the dressing.

Four general classes of occlusive dressings are available: films, foams, hydrogels, and hydrocolloids. They functionally differ in *adherence, absorbency, transparency,* and *vapor permeability* (Table 2-4). It is advantageous for materials to *adhere* to wounds so that another material such as tape is not needed to secure it. Adherence can also pose a problem if the fragile new epithelium sticks to the undersurface of the bandage and is stripped during dressing changes. *Absorbency* is that inherent quality of several dressing types to remove excess wound exudate. *Transparency* is one quality of some dressings that may be overrated. There is an occasional need to inspect a wound through a dressing several days following surgery. For the most part, however, all surgical wounds are left covered until the patient returns for suture removal or another dressing change. Transparency is an advantage in dressings but only a minor one. *Vapor permeability* is useful in allowing the evaporation of sweat from the skin, thereby avoiding maceration.

Moderate attention has been paid to the *gas permeability* of the newer surgical dressings. Falanga has noted that oxygen permeability "has not been an advantage either experimentally or clinically."[14] Varghese showed that wound exudate was uniformly hypoxic whether the dressing was oxygen permeable (OpSite) or not (DuoDerm).[15] Oxygen permeability is therefore not as important as some authors have previously surmised.

Films

These dressings, composed primarily of polyurethane (PUE), are permeable to water vapor but not to water.[6] They are, for the most part, adherent to the skin adjacent to the wound. Broad clinical use of occlusive dressings began with OpSite (Smith & Nephew), a thin, transparent, semiocclusive, somewhat elastic PUE coated unilaterally with a polyvinyl ethyl ether adhesive. OpSite permits the passage of water vapor through its membrane but prevents the egress of larger molecules (e.g., proteins, cytokines). Wound exudate collects below the membrane and prevents the adhesive bond directly above the wound bed. Because of its permeability to water vapor, PUE films permit the vaporization of sweat which helps to avoid maceration. These dressings are transparent thereby permitting inspection of the covered wound.[5,16–18]

Although best suited for split-thickness skin graft donor sites, PUE films may be used on any wound not overly contaminated. The author has successfully used a variety of the brands available on small sutured wounds or wounds allowed to heal secondarily following Mohs micrographic surgery. Split-thickness graft donor sites are notoriously painful and annoying; however, these dressings reduce this pain significantly while enhancing the rate of epithelialization.[17,19]

To the novice, most PUE films are difficult to apply as they may fold over and stick to themselves. Patience and practice will be rewarded since these dressings are superb for a variety of wounds. Apply the dressing after achieving hemostasis, cleaning the surrounding skin, and applying a tactifier. The edges must extend 1 to 2 cm beyond the wound and may be secured with tape to prevent the dressing from rolling and sticking to clothes. Placing gauze or a similar compressive dressing over the film can minimize the exudate in the first 24 to 48 h postoperatively. This also provides padding for patient comfort.[19] Excessive wound drainage will mandate dressing changes. This can sometimes be avoided by aspirating a portion of the exudate with a hypodermic needle and syringe and then covering the puncture site with another piece of PUE film.

Film dressings impregnated with antimicrobials are also available. Two of these, OpSite CH [chlorhexidine (Smith & Nephew)] and Tegaderm Plus [povidone-iodine (3M)], were recently compared along with their unimpregnated versions.[20]

TABLE 2-4

Characteristics of Synthetic Occlusive Dressings

	Adherent	Absorbent	Transparent	Vapor Permeable
Films	+	- *	+	+
Foams	Few	+	-	Partially
Hydrocolloids	+	+	-	-
Hydrogels	- †	+	+	+

*Except Omiderm (Omikron Scientific).
†Except ClearSite.

TABLE 2-5

Transparent Synthetic Films

Bioclusive	Johnson & Johnson
Ensure-It	Deseret
Omiderm	D.R. Laboratories
OpraFlex	Professional Medical
OpSite	Smith & Nephew
OpSite CH	Smith & Nephew
Polyskin II	Kendall
Tegaderm	3M
Tegaderm Plus	3M
Tegaderm Pouch	3M
Vari/moist	Catalina Biomedical
Visi Derm II	Medline Industries

Modified from Krasner.[26]

Impregnation appears to reduce the adhesive strength of these dressings. OpSite CH proved superior in suppressing bacterial proliferation. Regular (unimpregnated) Tegaderm demonstrated the least antimicrobial properties. (Table 2-5)

Special mention should be made of a particular film. The Omiderm membrane (Omikron Scientific, Ltd., Rehovot, Israel; distributed by D.R. Labs, San Francisco, California) was developed in 1982 at the Soreq Nuclear Research Center, Israel. An identical membrane is now also available as Jobskin (Jobst Institute, Inc., Toledo, Ohio). Omiderm is a PUE copolymer membrane created by grafting acrylamide and hydroxymethylmethacrylate to the material. The resulting membrane is flexible, transparent, and, unlike most other PUE films, extremely hydrophilic with the ability to absorb exudate up to 100 percent of its weight. Although relatively inelastic when dry, Omiderm becomes very elastic and comformable after absorbing moisture. Dressing removal causes neither pain nor tissue damage since adherence occurs via hydrophilia rather than adhesives. The components are not cytotoxic to fibroblasts or keratinocytes, unlike some adhesive-backed films that have demonstrated cytotoxicity in vitro.[6,21,22] Because of its meshed texture and the hydrophilic polymer included in its composition, this membrane has both a great permeability to water vapor and an ability to permit the diffusion of many drugs through the dressing.[6,21,23] These qualities may permit wound therapy without requiring dressing removal. For instance, antibiotic ointments may be applied directly to the membrane's outer surface and allowed to diffuse through to the wound.

Omiderm is the most vapor-permeable film dressing by a factor of five to ten. Thus, Omiderm clearly proves superior in preventing excessive fluid accumulation below the dressing which in turn may help avoid maceration.[6]

This membrane is useful as a wound covering over dermabrasions, partial and full-thickness dermal excisions, skin grafts and donor sites, curettage sites, and chronic wounds such as decubitus ulcers.[6,21,23–25] The membrane self-adheres to moist wound surfaces and will lose adhesiveness as healing progresses.

Raab describes the advantages of using Omiderm in facial dermabrasions.[21] Using the full face sheet rather than several smaller overlapping sheets, the surgeon can cut appropriate holes and trim the unit to size. Several extra centimeters are left around the perimeter to overcome any shrinkage or slippage sometimes occurring toward the latter stages of healing. The author suggests leaving the Omiderm in its package while this preparation takes place for easier handling. The resulting masklike dressing is thin, elastic, and conformable to the difficult anatomy of the face and therefore is more comfortable for the patient. Use of Mastisol around the normal skin periphery will help anchor the dressing unit in place. This dressing may be removed by day 6 or 7, after epithelialization has neared completion, and any residual areas not fully healed should be treated with frequent applications of an antibiotic ointment.[21]

Foam Surgical Dressings

Foam dressings are useful for open or exudative wounds. This class of covering is usually a bilaminate material consisting of an inner PUE foam pad and a larger outer semiocclusive film (e.g., polypropylene). The reticulated inner pad has a porous composition which helps absorb excess fluid while allowing collagen deposition. The formation of granulation tissue is stimulated.[27,28] Unfortunately, this is both an advantage and a disadvantage as occasionally the dressing may incorporate into the wound which is disrupted when the dressing is stripped away. Therefore, care must be taken not to allow foam dressings to stay in place more than 2 to 4 days without a change.

These dressings are not transparent, a disadvantage since their main use is in large, open wounds which would benefit from inspection prior to dressing changes. They are quite absorbent of fluids and somewhat permeable to water vapor. These qualities maintain a moist environment conducive to epidermal migration. Epigard (Ormed Corp., Santa Barbara, CA), Cutinova Plus (Beiersdorf), and Lyofoam (Acme United Corp., Fairfield, CT) are examples in this class which do not adhere to the wound and therefore need tape to secure them. Nu-Derm (Johnson & Johnson) and Lyofoam A are island dressings which differ in that their outer layer has an adhesive coating which allows for more secure placement.

Most of these dressings are larger (i.e., 6- by 6-cm or greater) pads. Large pads such as these are useful in chronic wounds such as venous ulcers. But only *larger* partial-thickness surgical wounds such as those following large Mohs micrographic surgery cases would require such ample dressings. These are sometimes well suited as temporary dressings to stimulate a granulated bed for an incipient skin graft. The author has not found a place for them in dressing sutured wounds.

Hydrogel Dressings

Though lacking mechanical strength, hydrogels have been used extensively as surgical wound dressings because they possess many of the aforementioned optimal properties. Most of the materials in this class are composed of polyethylene oxide suspended in water (up to 96 percent) on a lattice framework. The pads are generally packaged between two polyethylene sheets. The water vapor permeability of the dressing can be altered by removing either one or both of the films. The gel pad is placed directly on the wound and immediately begins absorbing wound exudate. The tremendous absorptive capabilities can be several times the weight of the pad. The pads are impermeable to bacteria, virtually transparent, and can nearly double the rate of wound epithelialization.[29]

Secondary dressings or tapes are required to secure most hydrogel dressings because the gel sheets offer only mild water adhesion. ClearSite (NDM Corp., Dayton, OH) is an exception since this material has an adhesive ring attached. The gel cushions against trauma and will not disrupt the healing wound during dressing changes. This flexible dressing conforms very well to wound beds and other irregular surfaces.[7,14] Its inherent absorptive quality favors its use on weeping or open wounds. The combination of soothing pain relief, superior absorption, and ease of removal during changes makes this dressing a top choice for dermabrasions. Chilling the dressing prior to application will enhance the analgesic properties.

Hydrogel pads are individually expensive which may be compounded by the need for frequent changing. Yet, like the other synthetic dressings, they maintain a moist wound bed which speeds epithelialization. A variety are available (Table 2-6).

A comparative study of several occlusive dressings (Vigilon, DuoDERM, and OpSite) demonstrated that Vigilon tends to create a better environment for *Staphylococcus aureus* proliferation than the others.[30] Another study showed Vigilon impregnated with povidone-iodine not only prevented wound infections but also sped healing when compared to controls using plain Vigilon.[31]

Hydrocolloids

Hydrocolloid surgical dressings (HCD) are synthetic occlusive wafers useful in lightly exudative wounds. Although usually comprised of two layers, several other forms do exist (see Table 2-7). The first layer consists of a hydrophilic polymer complex with a pressure-sensitive adhesive. The outer layer is a PUE or polypropylene film coating which is impermeable to water and water vapor. These pads require no secondary dressing as do many hydrogels or foam dressings.

T A B L E   2 - 6

Polyethylene Gels/Hydrogels

Biolex Wound Gel	Catalina Biomedical
Carrington Dermal Wound Gel	Carrington Laboratories
Elasto-Gel	Southwest Technologies
Geliperm (sheet & granular)	Fougera
IntraSite Gel	Smith & Nephew
Spand-Gel	Medi-Tech
Hydron Burn (Wound) Dressing	Bioderm Sciences
Second Skin	Spenco
Vigilon	Bard Home Health Care
Vigilon Plus	Bard Home Health Care
Cutinova Gel Film	Beiersdorf AG
Nu-Gel	Johnson & Johnson
ClearSite	NDM Corporation

Modified from Krasner.[26]

T A B L E   2 - 7

Hydrocolloids

Standard	
Comfeel	Kendall Healthcare
DuoDERM	ConvaTec
Hydropad	Baxter
Intact	Bard Home Health
IntraSite	Smith & Nephew
J & J Ulcer Dressing	Johnson & Johnson
Restore	Hollister
3M Tegasorb	3M
ULTEC	Sherwood Medical
Sween A-Peel	Sween
Paste	
Comfeel	Kendall Healthcare
DuoDERM	ConvaTec
Powder	
DuoDERM	ConvaTec
Special	
Actiderm	ConvaTec
Comfeel Pressure Rel.	Kendall Healthcare
Comfeel Transparent	Kendall Healthcare
DuoDERM CGF	ConvaTec
DuoDERM Extra-Thin	ConvaTec
Restore CX	Hollister

Modified from Krasner.[26]

They adhere well to irregular body surfaces and can be molded. Similar to other occlusive dressings, they reduce pain. Since they are usually opaque, they must be removed prior to wound inspection.

When in contact with wound exudate, the inner polymer complex liquefies into a gellike medium which speeds healing by providing an improved environment.[18,26,29,32,33] The pH of the exudate remains low, interfering with bacterial proliferation.[34] HCD may be the only dressings which effectively exclude heavy contamination by both gram-positive and gram-negative organisms.[30] In reviewing 70 papers, Hutchinson found infection rates of only 1.3 percent in wounds dressed with hydrocolloids. This was significantly lower than the other dressings, even other occlusive ones mentioned above.[1] Yet, since DuoDERM creates an oxygen-deficient environment below the dressing, it may allow anaerobic bacterial proliferation and should not be used as a dressing over known or suspected wound infections.[33]

DuoDERM (ConvaTec, Princeton, NJ) is a very popular hydrocolloid dressing which has found extensive use in the treatment of chronic ulcers, burns, minor abrasions, skin graft donor sites, and even skin biopsies.[18,35] For all the observed clinical advantages, no adverse histologic effects have been documented with this material.[36]

When applied, the dressing should extend several centimeters beyond the wound edge and thus provide an airtight seal. Since the outer layer is water impermeable, patients can bathe or shower without disrupting the dressing. Falanga warns that the only time a new dressing is needed is after the accumulation of wound fluid causes the gradual separation of the dressing from the wound.[14] Patients should be warned of the foul odor and purulent appearance of the liquefied hydrocolloid present during dressing changes.[32,33] This should not be mistaken for infection. The wound may be gently cleaned with normal saline before it is assessed.

MISCELLANEOUS DRESSINGS

Calcium Alginate

Alginates are naturally occurring polymers comprising an essential component in brown seaweed. Calcium alginate fabrics are useful in surgical wound dressings, especially in open or exudative ones. Sorbsan Topical Wound Dressing (Dow B. Hickam, Inc., Sugar Land, TX) and Algosteril (Johnson & Johnson) are sterile nonwoven pads which can absorb up to 20 times their weight in exudate.[37] The unique mechanism of the alginate permits only *vertical* wicking of exudate, even where the dressing extends beyond the wound, and thus avoids maceration of healthy tissue. Alginates have been shown to possess both hemostatic properties and an ability to be used on clinically infected wounds.[32,37,38] They are nontoxic, nonallergenic, and completely biodegradable and, therefore, cause little or no local tissue reaction.[38,39] This

dressing material requires moderate wound drainage to function properly. Because of this, the dressing cannot be used throughout the entire healing cycle. Furthermore, calcium alginate wound dressings require a secondary dressing placed over them as an outer covering. Either gauze or a PUE film dressing will serve this purpose.[37]

When in direct contact with a sodium-rich solution (e.g., saline or wound exudate), the calcium alginate pad forms a soft sodium alginate hydrogel. The exudate is drawn vertically into the outer dressing. The gel maintains a physiologically moist environment over the wound and thereby benefits healing. In addition, this hydrogel provides a nonadhesive interface with the wound bed, permits gaseous exchange, and provides a physical barrier against accidental contamination.[37,38]

Because the gel will not adhere to the wound bed, dressing changes are atraumatic. Residual gel can be rinsed using normal saline solution. Hence, the pain and wound disruption sometimes associated with other dressing materials may be avoided.

Calcium alginate pads should be changed when the secondary dressing becomes moist or begins leaking. Dressing changes become less frequent as wounds progress toward healing because of the decline in exudate production. When the wound stops draining, different dressing materials may be necessary for the remainder of the healing process. (Table 2-8)[32,37–39]

Biobrane

Biobrane (Winthrop Pharmaceuticals, New York, NY) is a trilaminate biosynthetic dressing composed of an ultrathin, semipermeable, silicone rubber membrane bonded to a flexible knitted nylon fabric with a loop structure providing both a larger surface area and an anchoring system for attachment to the wound base. The two layers are covalently bonded on both sides to a thin coating of porcine collagen peptides (type I collagen) which enhances wound adherence.[18,28] Biobrane is sold in large sheets (10 by 15 in) and may have some utility in covering large cutaneous burns. Its usefulness in dermatologic surgery may be limited to that of a temporary dressing over larger full-thickness open wounds prior to skin grafting. For dermabrasions and sutured wounds, the material offers no significant advantage over other readily available dressings yet is much more expensive.

TABLE 2-8

Calcium Alginate Pads

Sorbsan	Dow B. Hickham
Kaltostat	Calgon-Vestal Laboratories
Algosteril	Johnson & Johnson

OTHER INNOVATIONS IN WOUND DRESSING MANAGEMENT

In an editorial regarding wound dressings, Falanga pointed out that "the greatest benefit of occlusive dressings has been to bring about the realization that the wound and its microenvironment can be greatly modified by what covers them. The dressing is actually a pharmacologic agent, a drug with its own benefits and risks."[14] In the not-too-distant future, many dressings will possess the ability to influence the healing process selectively by modalities such as regulatory peptides, extracellular matrix materials, and other active agents. Eaglstein predicts that some future dressings may even deliver or modify laser or electric energy in improving the healing response.[7]

Dozens of growth factors have been recognized and are being synthesized. Although clinical use of growth factors and other multifunctional peptides is currently limited, evidence indicates that they play a significant role in homeostasis.[35,40,41] *Growth dressings* may be developed by impregnating currently available occlusive materials with slow-released growth factors which might stimulate specific patterns of healing.[14] Sawada et al. showed that survival of skin flaps in rats could be improved when dressed with silicone gel sheets impregnated with the drugs prostaglandin E_1, a potent vasodilator, and ofloxacin. Controls dressed with nothing, OpSite, or plain silicone sheeting had no increase in flap survival.[42]

Although the mechanism of action remains unknown, plain silicone gel has been demonstrated to be an effective modality in the prevention and treatment of hypertrophic scars.[43] Sawada and Sone postulate that the gel's impermeability to water is the cause, yet this mystery has not been fully explained.[44]

Fulton compared wound healing in facial dermabrasions by dressing half of each face with a hydrogel dressing (Second Skin) and the other half with the same dressing impregnated with aloe vera. The aloe vera-treated sides re-epithelialized 3 days faster and had a more rapid reduction in exudate than those covered with the hydrogel alone.[45] As our knowledge of wound healing expands, so do the horizons for manipulating surgical outcomes after the operative period.

DRESSING TECHNIQUES

Dressing techniques vary depending on wound types and modes used to create them. A slovenly applied dressing reflects negatively the professionalism of the entire medical staff. Moreover, such a dressing may prove therapeutically detrimental to the surgical wound itself. The dressing should be functional, comfortable, and aesthetically pleasing. Before leaving the office, the patient should be instructed (verbally and in writing) how to care for both the dressing and the underlying wound. Patients should also be provided with a point

of contact in case they experience dressing problems or require further information not previously understood or given.

When patients are seen in follow-up for suture removal of closed wounds, it is important to continue to support the wound and remove any tension from the developing scar. The longer the scar can heal without tension, the thinner it tends to be at maturity.[46] The author places supportive strips (e.g., Steri-Strip, 3M; Coverstrip II, Beiersdorf) across recently sutured wounds for 4 to 6 weeks following the procedure in an effort to reinforce such immature scars.[47] While the short follow-up visits require attention from the clinical office staff, a conspicuous scar on a patient is often a walking testimony to one's skill or lack thereof.

PRESSURE DRESSINGS

Pressure dressings are designed to maintain pressure over wounds in order to reduce exudate or maintain hemostasis. Since bleeding is most common in the first 24 h, the author finds it useful to apply pressure dressings of gauze and paper tape over film dressings for this period. The outer dressing can then be removed, exposing a much smaller or thinner film dressing which, if clean, is left in place until sutures are removed or until the dressing itself mandates a change.

Common sense is critical in applying pressure dressings. A key word is *pressure*—not strangulation. Excessive pressure will impede circulation and possibly result in tissue necrosis. Therefore, one must use caution when applying pressure dressings, especially in circumstances requiring the use of wrapping techniques over appendages.

Winton and Salasche published suggestions for dressing specific surgical wounds which remains an excellent reference for surgical or nursing staff alike. They note that "the design of a dressing for a difficult anatomic area may require considerable amounts of ingenuity and improvisation."[10] The following are tips for dressings of particular sites which may be added to their compendium.

Scalp

Dressings on the scalp are usually attached by wrapping successive layers of roller gauze around the head and securing it with tape. Before it is wrapped, the wound should be cleaned and dressed as any other local wound. Additional pressure may be exerted during the postoperative period by wrapping the head circumferentially. The gauze may be secured with tape at the forehead, preauricular, and postauricular regions. This dressing offers mild-to-moderate pressure depending on the elasticity of the roller gauze and the quantity of packing.

The *tennis headband* provides a simple means of applying mild-to-moderate pressure to a scalp wound. These bands are readily available and easy to apply. The author buys them by the dozen at a local sports store for less than a dollar each. At the author's office, they have taken the place of roller gauze

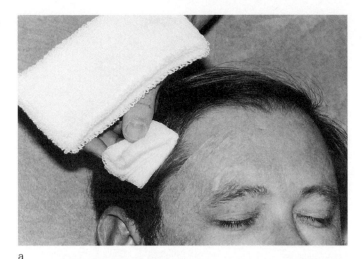

a

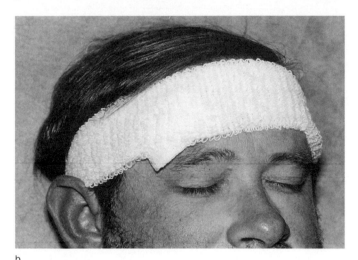

b

Figure 2-1 *(a, b)* Once a primary dressing is taped in place on the forehead and scalp, a piece of gauze may exert extra pressure under an elastic tennis headband to reduce edema, postoperative hemorrhage, and even orbital purpura—which is common from forehead wounds.

for head wounds. Size and elasticity of the headband, along with the packing material, will dictate the amount of pressure applied (Fig. 2-1*a–b*).

A third type of head dressing may be created by using no. 6 tubular gauze. Simply cut a 12- to 15-in piece of tube gauze and tie a knot at one end. Apply the dressing by drawing it over the patient's head like a stocking cap.[10] This dressing will exert mild-to-moderate pressure over wounds.

Care should be taken to prevent the ear from being pinned back with a circumferential-type scalp dressing. Chondrodynia can accompany such distortion. If pressure is exerted over the ear, a wedge of gauze or a dental roll should be placed in the postauricular sulcus.

The scalp can be dressed several different ways. Not all wounds will require a bulky dressing. Many times a simple application of collodion over small, nondraining wounds will

suffice. This "paint-on" dressing has been used for decades without producing the toxic side effects often associated with plastic spray dressings. Collodion is a viscous solution of nitrocellulose in ether and alcohol which forms a tacky semisynthetic covering when applied.

Ear

Dressing wounds on the ear can be extremely frustrating. Its irregular outer surface creates many problems. These problems are enhanced by the sebaceous nature of the pinna which makes adhesion more difficult.

For moderate-to-large wounds, or wounds requiring any amount of pressure, the addition of bulky dressing material to the dressing will help significantly. The bulky material will conform more easily to the irregular surfaces, thereby keeping the contact layer in place over the wound.

Ear wounds may offer the additional dilemma of exposed cartilage. Such wounds can develop chondritis if they become desiccated. Therefore, liberal applications of antibiotic ointment should be made. Moreover, because ear infections are associated more frequently with gram-negative microorganisms, a topical application of Garamycin, supplemented with an oral antibiotic if necessary, will enhance protection.

Before dressing wounds on the inner surface of the ear, particularly within the concha or tragal regions, one should place cotton gently into the external auditory meatus. This will help prevent the ingress of ointment and wound drainage which might lead to otitis media. Wounds on this surface may sometimes require more flexibility in the contact layer. Telfa or Release pads can be pulled apart so that only one surface is glossy. These function well on these rolling surfaces. The contact layer may be secured with cotton or "fluffed" gauze which is then taped in place over the dorsum of the ear (Fig. 2-2). Because the skin covering the ear is usually sebaceous, a tactifier will be beneficial.

As mentioned above, care should taken to prevent pinning back the ear by placing gauze in the postauricular sulcus.

Nose

The nose presents problems similar to those found in dressing an ear. This structure also presents concavities and convexities on its surfaces. The sebaceous nature of the nose will impede tape adhesion. Wounds on the nose may also expose cartilage.

Pressure dressings over the ala nasi are difficult since the alae will collapse. Sometimes the nose can be packed to provide counterpressure between the ala and the outer dressing. This may be achieved by simply inserting a piece of balled gauze into the nostril before securing the dressing down with tape (Fig. 2-3*a–b*).

In order to maintain pressure over wounds in the nasal sulcus, extra fluffed gauze must be placed to build up the dress-

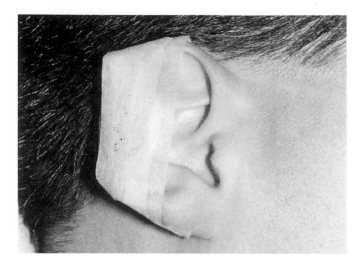

Figure 2-2 After placing a tactifier on the postauricular skin, fluffed gauze may be securely attached to the irregular anterior surface by taping over the edges of the ear.

ing to a level where tape across the nasal bridge to the adjacent cheek will still maintain pressure below.

Eyelids

Often, small wounds on the eyelids, canthi, or other periorbital structures may be allowed to heal with only a coating of ophthalmic antibiotic ointment. However, larger defects or full-thickness ones may leave the globe only partially covered, thereby necessitating an eye patch. Before placing the eye patch, apply some ophthalmic ointment below the conjunctiva to protect the globe. Eye patches should not be left in place for more than 24 h.[10]

Digits

Of greatest concern when dressing the digits is compromising the blood supply. Tubular gauze provides an efficient outer covering for wound dressings on the digits. The dressing under the tubular gauze may include a nonstick pad and tape; neither one of these materials should wrap tightly around the digit. The tubular gauze will provide adequate pressure without compromising vascular supply.

We often have patients elevate their hand for 24 to 48 h with a sling. Not only will this help reduce pain, but the forced inactivity of the extremity may serve to reduce swelling and bleeding as well.

Scrotum

Incisions on the scrotum are frequently followed by hematoma formation. To help prevent this malady, pressure must be applied firmly and evenly over the scrotal wound. This may seem somewhat difficult at first blush; however, a

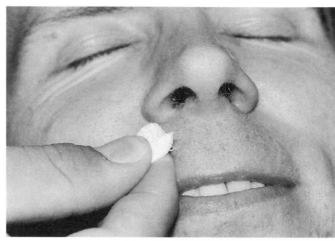

a

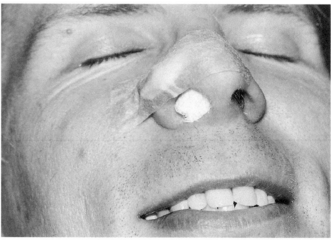

b

Figure 2-3 (a) A small piece of gauze is balled up and inserted just under the ala nasi. (b) A pressure bandage on an alar wound then has a counter-force to prevent excess bleeding during the critical first 24 hours.

simple modification to an ordinary athletic supporter creates an easy mode of applying effective pressure. The wound can be loosely dressed with ointment, contact layer, and gauze. The supporter acts as an outer covering to hold the dressing in place while applying rather uniform pressure. A hole may be cut near the top of the supporter so that the penis may be released and the supporter left in place without interfering with urination.

CONCLUSION

Dressing a surgical wound requires patience, skill, experience, and a good dose of common sense. A slovenly applied dressing not only reflects poorly on medical staff but, more importantly, may impede optimal healing. For better healing, wounds should be kept clean, moist, and covered. A dressing created in the office should be both functional and aesthetically pleasing. Often, this may be as simple as using flesh-colored tape and rounding off the corners to give the illusion of blending. Appropriate use of the newer dressing materials may lead to lower infection rates, reduced pain, faster healing, and a more pleasing scar. How a surgical wound heals may often reflect the skill and technique of the surgeon responsible. Knowing the materials available and applying them with common sense will serve to enhance such a reflection.

REFERENCES

1. Hutchinson JJ, McGuckin M: Occlusive dressings: A microbiologic and clinical review. *Am J Infect Control* **18**:257–268, 1990

2. Cuzzell JZ, Stotts NA: Trial and error yields to knowledge. *Am J Nurs* **90**:53–63, 1990

3. Longombe A: Postoperative dressings: Are they really necessary? *Trop Doct* **20**:41–42, 1990

4. Chrintz H et al: Need for surgical wound dressings. *Br J Surg* **76**:204–205, 1989

5. Gilchrist B, Hutchinson JJ: Does occlusion lead to infection? *Nursing Times* **86**:70–71, 1990

6. Limova M et al: Clinical experience with a new, nonadhesive film dressing. *Wounds* **2**:213–217, 1990

7. Eaglstein WH et al: Wound dressings: Current and future, in *Clinical and Experimental Approaches to Dermal and Epidermal Repair: Normal and Chronic Wounds.* New York, Wiley-Liss, 1991, pp 257–265

8. Hutchinson JJ: Prevalence of wound infection under occlusive dressings: A collective survey of reported research. *Wounds* **1**:123–133, 1989

9. Lynch WS: Wound healing, in *Skin Surgery,* edited by E Epstein, E Epstein Jr. Philadelphia, Saunders, 1987, pp 56–70

10. Winton GB, Salasche SJ: Wound dressings for dermatologic surgery. *J Am Acad Dermatol* **13**:1026–1044, 1985

11. Mikhail GR et al: The efficacy of adhesives in the application of wound dressings. *J Burn Care Rehabil* **10**:216–219, 1989

12. Rubio PA: Use of adhesive tape for primary closure of surgical skin wounds. *Int Surg* **75**:189–190, 1990

13. Norris P, Storrs FJ: Allergic contact dermatitis to adhesive bandages. *Dermatol Clin* **8**:147–152, 1990

14. Falanga V: Occlusive wound dressings: Why, when & which? *Arch Dermatol* **124**:872–877, 1988

15. Varghese MC et al: Local environment of chronic wounds under synthetic dressings. *Arch Dermatol* **122**:52–57, 1986

16. Poulsen TD: Polyurethane film (OpSite) vs. impregnated gauze (Jelonet) in the treatment of outpatient burns: A prospective randomized study. *Burns* **17**:59–61, 1991

17. Madden MR et al: Comparison of an occlusive and semi-occlusive dressing and the effect of the wound exudate upon keratinocyte proliferation. *J Trauma* **29**:924–931, 1989

18. Feldman DL et al: A prospective trial comparing Biobrane, DuoDERM and Xeroform for skin graft donor sites. *Surg Gynecol Obstet* **173**:1–5, 1991

19. Morris WT, Lamb AM: Painless split skin donor sites: A controlled double-blind trial of OpSite, scarlet red and bupivacaine. *Aust N Z J Surg* **60**:617–620, 1990

20. Wille JC, Blusse van Oud Alblas A: A comparison of four film-type dressings by their antimicrobial effect on the flora of the skin. *J Hosp Infect* **14**:153–158, 1989

21. Raab B: A new hydrophilic copolymer membrane for dermabrasions. *J Dermatol Surg Oncol* **17**:323–328, 1991

22. Behar D, Juszynski M: Omiderm, a new synthetic wound covering: Physical properties and drug permeability studies. *J Biomed Mater Res* **20**:731–738, 1986

23. Borenstein A et al: Transparent polyurethane (Omiderm) dressing for free flaps. *Ann Plast Surg* **26**:200, 1991

24. Golan J et al: Influence of a temporary synthetic skin substitute on capillary stasis in burns. *Eur J Plast Surg* **12**:201–204, 1989

25. Staso MA et al: Experience with Omiderm. A new burn dressing. *J Burn Care Rehabil* **12**:209–210, 1991

26. Krasner: Wound care products. *Ostomy/Wound Management* **33**:47–60, 1991

27. Roth RR, Winton GB: A synthetic skin substitute as a temporary dressing in Mohs surgery. *J Dermatol Surg Oncol* **15**:670–672, 1989

28. Zitelli JA: Synthetic skin. *Adv Dermatol* **4**:323–342, 1989

29. Corkhill PH et al: Synthetic hydrogels. *Biomaterials* **10**:3–10, 1989

30. Mertz PM et al: Occlusive wound dressings to prevent bacterial invasion and wound infection. *J Am Acad Dermatol* **12**:662–668, 1985

31. Mandy SH: Evaluation of a new povidone-iodine-impregnated polyethylene oxide gel occlusive dressing. *J Am Acad Dermatol* **13**:655–659, 1985

32. Alderman C: Supplement dressings. *Nursing Standard* **1**:49–54, 1989

33. Fowler E et al: Healing with hydrocolloid. *Am J Nurs* **91**:63–64, 1991

34. Sawada Y et al: Silicone gel including antimicrobial agent. *Br J Plast Surg* **43**:78–82, 1990

35. Nemeth AJ et al: Faster healing and less pain in skin biopsy sites treated with an occlusive dressing. *Arch Dermatol* **127**:1679–1683, 1991

36. Phillips TJ et al: Histologic evaluation of chronic human wounds treated with hydrocolloid and nonhydrocolloid dressings. *J Am Acad Dermatol* **30**:61–64, 1994

37. Motta GL: Calcium alginate topical wound dressings: A new dimension in the cost-effective treatment for exudating dermal wounds and pressure sores. *Ostomy/Wound Management* **25**:52–56, 1989

38. Tintle TE, Jeter KF: Early experience with a calcium alginate dressing. *Ostomy/Wound Management* **28**:74–81, 1990

39. Attwood AI: Calcium alginate dressing accelerates split skin graft donor site healing. *Br J Plast Surg* **42:**373–379, 1989

40. Rothe M, Falanga V: Growth factors: Their biology and promise in dermatologic disease and tissue repair. *Arch Dermatol* **125:**1390–1398, 1989

41. Lynch SE et al: Growth factors in wound healing. *J Clin Invest* **84:**640–646, 1989

42. Sawada Y et al: A new system of treating wounds by a continuous topical application of medication. *Br J Plast Surg* **43:**83–87, 1990

43. Ahn ST et al: Topical silicone gel for the prevention and treatment of hypertrophic scar. *Arch Surg* **126:**499–504, 1991

44. Sawada Y, Sone K: Treatment of scars and keloids with a cream containing silicone oil. *Br J Plast Surg* **43:**683–688, 1990

45. Fulton JE Jr: The stimulation of postdermabrasion wound healing with stabilized aloe vera gel-polyethylene oxide dressing. *J Dermatol Surg Oncol* **16:**460–467, 1990

46. Burgess LPA et al: Wound healing: Relationship of wound closing tension to scar width in rats. *Arch Otolaryngol Head Neck Surg* **116:**798–802, 1990

47. Moy RL, Quan MB: An evaluation of wound closure tapes. *J Dermatol Surg Oncol* **16:**721–723, 1990

Eric A. Breisch
Hubert T. Greenway

3 Superficial Anatomy of the Head and Neck

SURFACE ANATOMY OF THE FACE

The physician can easily identify certain bony prominences and foramina, providing quick reference points for important anatomic structures which enable the clinician to describe and localize cutaneous lesions on the face accurately.

The squamous portion of the frontal bone forms the foundation of the forehead. The superciliary arches located deep to the eyebrows form prominent ridges which unite medially forming in midline the glabella. The nasion, a craniometric point located just inferiorly to the glabella, is formed by the median articulation of the paired nasal bones with the frontal bone. On each side, approximately 2 cm laterally from the nasion along the superior margin of the orbit is the supraorbital notch or foramen, through which emerges the supraorbital nerve and artery. The lateral and inferior margins of the orbit are formed by the zygomatic bone with the malar portion forming the prominence of the cheek. The temporal process of the zygomatic bone joins the zygomatic process of the temporal bone to form the zygomatic arch. The maxillary bone forms the inferior and medial margins of the orbit, and located in the body of the maxilla approximately 5 mm below the inferior margin of the orbit is the infraorbital foramen, which transmits the infraorbital nerve and artery onto the face.

The tip of the chin is formed by the mental protuberance of the mandible. The body of the mandible lodges the lower dentition and presents an easily palpable sharp inferior margin. Lateral to the mental protuberance, the mental foramen is located midway in the height of the body of the mandible.

A vertical line drawn on the face, initiated at the supraorbital foramen and extended inferiorly to the inferior margin of the mandible, will intersect the infraorbital foramen 5 mm below the inferior margin of the orbit and the mental foramen midway in the height of the body of the mandible (Fig. 3-1). Note that in patients with dentures the position of the mental foramen is best located by measuring approximately 1 cm from the inferior margin of the mandible superiorly along the vertical line. This vertical line is a valuable reference line since it allows the clinician to identify quickly the surface anatomy of three foramina and their associated sensory nerves.

Posteriorly, the body of the mandible ends at the angle, and the mandible continues superiorly as the ramus. The ramus terminates as the condylar process, which is positioned directly anteriorly to the external auditory canal.

The mastoid process of the temporal bone is palpable just behind the auricular cartilage at the level of the external auditory meatus. The mastoid process of the adult protects the main trunk of the facial nerve as it exits the skull through the stylomastoid foramen. In children, pneumatization of the mastoid region does not begin until approximately 5 years of age, rendering the facial nerve at risk during superficial surgical procedures in this region of the neck.

The use of facial diagrams and a millimeter ruler allows the dermatologic surgeon to use the fixed bony prominences to assist in providing exact localization of cutaneous surface tumors and lesions.

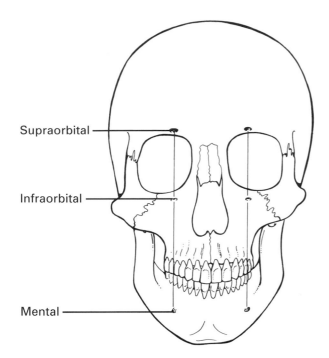

Figure 3-1.   Bony prominences and foramina. Note vertical line intersecting supraorbital, infraorbital, and mental foramina.

FACIAL MUSCULATURE

The mimetic muscles are all innervated by branches of the facial nerve and in general arise from the facial skeleton to insert into the skin. These muscles are grouped with regard to the region of the face: mouth, nose, periorbital, ear, and scalp (Fig. 3-2).

Mouth

The oral musculature arises from different regions on the face inserting into the skin and mucosa of the mouth. Generally these muscles can be divided into four groups:

1. The muscles of the lower lip (depressor group)
2. The muscles of the upper lip (elevator group)
3. The cheek bulk muscle (buccinator muscle)
4. The orbicularis oris (lip proper muscle)

The Muscles of the Lower Lip (Depressor Group)

The muscles of the lower lip are the depressor anguli oris, the depressor labii inferioris, and the mentalis.

The depressor anguli oris muscle, originates from the anterolateral aspect of the body of the mandible, inserts into the skin and mucosa at the labial commissure, and depresses the corner of the mouth.

The depressor labii inferioris muscle arises from the mandible deep to the depressor anguli oris muscle; it inserts into the skin and mucosa of the lower lip and depresses the lower lip.

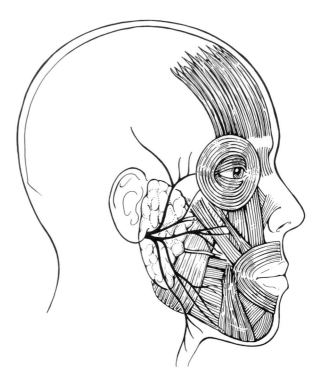

Figure 3-2.   Facial muscles with associated branches of the facial nerve and parotid gland and duct.

The mentalis muscle, arising from the body of the mandible medially to the depressor labii inferioris muscle, inserts into the skin overlying the tip of the chin, effecting protrusion of the lower lip and dimpling of the skin.

All of the lower lip muscles are innervated by the marginal mandibular branch of the facial nerve with secondary innervation from the buccal branches of the facial nerve.

The Muscles of Upper Lip (Elevator Group)

The upper lip consists of the risorius, zygomaticus major and minor, levator labii superioris, levator labii superioris alaeque nasi, and levator anguli oris muscles.

The risorius muscle originates from the parotid fascia, inserts into the skin and mucosa at the corner of the mouth, and pulls the labial commissure laterally, widening the mouth.

The zygomaticus major muscle, originating from the posterolateral aspect of the zygomatic bone, inserts into the skin and mucosa of the lateral upper lip and elevates the labial commissure.

The zygomaticus minor muscle arises just medially to the zygomaticus major muscle, inserts into the skin and mucosa of the upper lip, and elevates the upper lip.

The levator labii superioris muscle arises from the maxilla just above the infraorbital foramen and inserts into the skin and mucosa of the medial upper lip; it is an elevator of the upper lip.

The levator labii superioris alaeque nasi muscle arises from the medial margin of the orbit, first yields fibers into the ala of the nose, and then continues inferiorly to insert finally into the medial aspect of the skin and mucosa of the upper lip. This muscle is an elevator of the lip and dilates the nares.

The levator anguli oris muscle originates from the maxilla just below the infraorbital foramen and inserts into the skin and mucosa at the labial commissure; this muscle elevates the corners of the mouth.

The muscles associated with the upper lip are innervated by the buccal branches of the facial nerve with secondary innervation from the zygomatic branches of the facial nerve.

The Cheek Bulk Muscle (Buccinator Muscle)

The key muscle of the cheek is the buccinator muscle, arising from the posterolateral aspect of the maxilla, the medial aspect of the mandible near the last molar, and the pterygomandibular raphe; it inserts into the skin and mucosa of the labial commissure and the upper and lower lips. This muscle flattens the lips and cheeks against the teeth. The buccinator is innervated by the buccal branches of the facial nerve and is the only muscle of facial expression to receive its innervation from the superficial aspect.

The Orbicularis Oris (Lip Proper Muscle)

The core musculature of the lips is formed by the orbicularis oris muscle, which consists of concentrically arranged fibers circumscribing the mouth. These fibers provide a sphincteric function allowing pursing and protrusion of the lips. The orbicularis oris muscle is innervated by the buccal branches of the facial nerve.

Nose

The muscles of the nose are highly variable in their development and consist of the nasalis and depressor septi muscles.

The transverse portion of the nasalis muscle originates from the body of the maxilla and along with its associate from the opposite side inserts into an aponeurotic sling which passes over the bridge of the nose. A smaller alar portion of this muscle inserts into the lateral crus of the alar cartilage of the nose. The transverse portion of the nasalis compresses the nares, while the alar portion dilates the nares. The nasalis muscle is innervated by the buccal branches of the facial nerve.

The depressor septi muscle, arising from the incisive fossa of the maxilla, inserts into the columella and nasal septum; it narrows the nares. This muscle is innervated by the buccal branches of the facial nerve.

Periorbital

The muscles of the periorbital region include the orbicularis oculi, corrugator supercilii, and the procerus. The orbicularis ocili muscle is a concentrically arranged muscle which is typically divided into two parts: palpebral and orbital. The palpe-bral part is that portion of the muscle which covers the eyelid; it originates from the superior and inferior aspect of the medial palpebral ligament. Fibers pass laterally in both the upper and lower lids to interdigitate finally at the lateral aspect of the eyelid, thereby forming the lateral palpebral raphe. The orbital part of the orbicularis oris muscle originates from the medial palpebral ligament, the frontal process of the maxillary bone, and the nasal process of the frontal bone; its fibers extend out beyond the bony margins of the orbit in a series of concentric loops to insert into the overlying skin in the regions of the forehead, as well as the malar and infraorbital areas of the cheek. The palpebral part of this muscle acts to close the eyelid gently, while the orbital part is used for blinking and tight closure of the eyelid. The motor innervation of the orbicularis ocili muscle is from the temporal and zygomatic branches of the facial nerve. Paralysis of the these nerve branches leads to ectropion of the lid and inability to close the lids. Reconstruction of various defects in this area may involve local flaps containing not only skin and subcutaneous tissue, but also including underlying muscle (i.e., myocutaneous flap).

The corrugator supercilii muscle arises from the medial part of the superciliary ridge to insert into the skin of the eyebrow; it pulls the eyebrow medially. This muscle is innervated by the temporal branches of the facial nerve.

The procerus muscle originates from the superior aspect of the nasal bones to insert into the skin overlying the root of the nose; it pulls the medial aspect of the eyebrows inferiorly. The procerus muscle is innervated by the temporal branches of the facial nerve.

Ear

The anterior auricular muscle, the superior auricular muscle, and the posterior auricular muscle arise from the scalp and insert into the skin and auricle as their names suggest. Functionally, these muscles are of no clinical importance and are innervated by posterior and temporal branches of the facial nerve.

Scalp

The most important epicranial muscle of the scalp is the occipitofrontalis muscle. The small occipital belly arises from the mastoid process and superior nuchal line of the occipital bone to insert into the galea aponeurosis of the scalp; this muscle pulls the scalp posteriorly. The frontal belly arises from the anterior aspect of the galea aponeurosis and inserts into the skin of the forehead and eyebrows; it acts to pull the scalp anteriorly and elevates the eyebrows. The occipital belly is innervated by the posterior auricular branch of the facial nerve, and the frontal belly is innervated by the temporal branch of the facial nerve. Selecting or removing a portion of the temporal branch will result in lack of innervation of the frontalis muscle with possible drooping of the eyebrow and ptosis of the upper lid.

THE SUPERFICIAL MUSCULAR APONEUROTIC SYSTEM

The *superficial muscular aponeurotic system* (SMAS) is defined as the combination of the muscles of facial expression and the investing layer of superficial fascia. This fascial layer envelops the facial muscles more distinctly and definitively in certain areas, specifically the lower face, mid-face, and forehead regions.

The fascial component of SMAS originates in the neck as the superficial cervical fascia, envelops the platysma muscle, sweeps over the mandible, and invests the muscles of the face. The fascia is tightly bound to the mastoid process of the temporal bone, the deep fascia investing the sternocleidomastoid muscle, and the fascia of the parotid gland approximately 1 to 2 cm anterior to the tragus, with points of attachment to the periosteum of the zygomatic arch via fine fasciculi. The fascia is very thin within the temporal zone and is difficult to separate from the deep temporal fascia.

The fascia provides a functional network which binds nearly all of the muscles of facial expression together, allowing them to act in concert with one another, providing a mechanism for evenly distributing the pull of the muscles upon the overlying skin, and acting as a fire screen preventing the spread of infection from superficial to deep areas of the face.

THE PRIMARY RESTING SKIN TENSION LINES

The muscles of facial expression insert into the overlying skin, causing the skin to fold or crease in a predictable pattern. These creases are referred to as *resting skin tension lines* (RSTLs), and typically they occur perpendicular to the long axis of the underlying muscle (Fig. 3-3). Incisions made parallel to these lines produce a fine linear scar, while incisions made perpendicular to these lines will produce an irregular hypertrophic scar.

The position of RSTLs on the face is usually very predictable, although certain areas of the face seem to contradict the prediction formula for RSTLs (e.g., the periorbital region). However, since SMAS is very tenuous in the periorbital region, the muscle attachment to the overlying skin is very weak, thereby permitting RSTLs to be primarily influenced by gravity and muscles of the orbit. In order to best demonstrate the position of the RSTLs, the physician should ask the patient to perform a variety of exaggerated facial expressions which should help predict the position of the RSTLs.

The RSTLs of the forehead are oriented horizontally due to the frontalis muscle. In the region of the glabella, RSTLs can be found as vertical lines due to the corrugator supercilii muscle and transverse lines over the nasion due to the pull of the procerus muscle.

The periorbital regions demonstrate radial lines at the me-

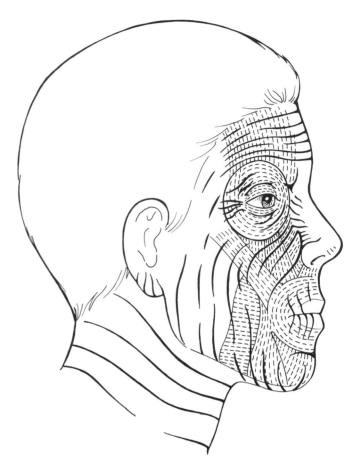

Figure 3-3. Primary resting skin tension lines of the face. Typically they occur perpendicularly to the long axis of the underlying muscles.

dial and lateral canthi due the orbicularis oris muscle. The RSTLs of the lids are horizontal due to the pull of gravity and the levator palpebrae superioris muscle of the orbit.

The skin of the nose demonstrates no predictable RSTLs.

The skin of the mid-face and perioral regions demonstrates the expected RSTLs. The pull of the orbicularis oris causes skin tension lines to radiate from the perimeter of the mouth. The zygomaticus muscles help accentuate the melolabial fold, while the risorius muscle helps create the vertical skin folds found over the cheek.

It should be remembered that some variation of the RSTLs will occur from one individual to the next. Secondary skin tension lines, which frequently occur perpendicular to RSTLs, can be due to aging of the skin, sun damage, altered states of hydration, or redundant folds of skin due to recent weight loss.

The placement of excision and/or closure lines within or parallel to RSTLs may provide a more favorable cosmetic result. However, on certain occasions, one may violate this principle in order to avoid or protect underlying critical anatomic structures (i.e., temporal branch of the facial nerve).

BLOOD SUPPLY OF THE FACE

The arteries supplying the face form a network derived from branches of the external carotid and the internal carotid arteries (Fig. 3-4).

The facial artery, a branch of the external carotid artery in the neck, grooves the submandibular gland to then hook upward around the mandible to reach the face. Palpable as it crosses the mandible at the anterior edge of the insertion of the masseter muscle, the facial artery passes superficially to the buccinator muscle and pursues a tortuous course toward the medial angle of the eye. The first branches arising from the facial artery are the inferior and superior labial arteries, which anastomose freely across the midline with their associates from the opposite side and weave sinuously through the muscle fibers of the orbicularis oris muscle. The facial artery continues as the angular artery, and, as it runs along the lateral margin of the nose toward the eye, it supplies the lateral nasal artery, which supplies most of the external nose.

Numerous anastomoses exist between the facial artery and branches of the maxillary and superficial temporal arteries: the inferior labial artery with the mental artery from the inferior alveolar artery over the chin, as well as small muscular branches of the facial with the buccal and infraorbital arteries derived from the maxillary artery.

The facial artery terminates at the medial aspect of the eye as the angular artery. The angular artery freely communicates with the supraorbital artery, the supratrochlear artery and dorsal nasal arteries which are each derived from the ophthalmic artery via the internal carotid artery.

The temporal region is supplied by the superficial temporal artery. The forehead receives the frontal branch of the superficial temporal artery and is reinforced by the supraorbital and supratrochlear arteries. The posterior scalp is supplied by the occipital and postauricular arteries derived from the external carotid artery. The remainder of the scalp is supplied via branches from the occipital, postauricular, superficial temporal, and supraorbital arteries.

The facial venous system parallels the arterial distribution. The temporal and lateral forehead regions drain into the superficial temporal vein, while the medial forehead drains into the supratrochlear and supraorbital veins which communicate with the ophthalmic venous system and the angular vein at the medial aspect of the eye. The angular vein descends along the lateral aspect of the nose and receives the venous drainage of the nose. The angular vein is joined by the superior and inferior labial veins to form the anterior facial vein. The anterior facial vein crosses the mandible just posteriorly to the facial artery to join the internal jugular vein. The temporal and parietal scalp, anterolateral ear, and posterior facial regions drain into the superficial temporal vein which joins the maxillary vein to form the retromandibular vein. The retromandibular vein passes through the parotid gland and bifurcates into an anterior and a posterior branch. The anterior branch joins the anterior facial vein, while the posterior division joins the posterior auricular vein to form the external jugular vein.

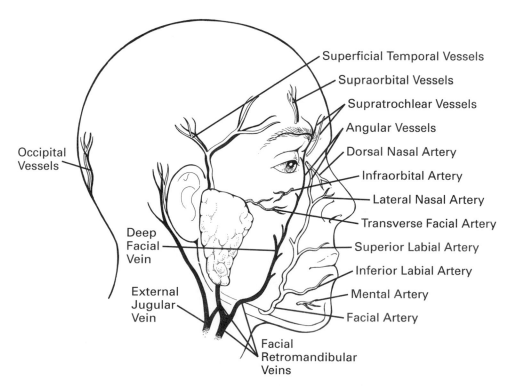

Figure 3-4. Vascular supply to the face. Both the external carotid and internal carotid systems contribute to facial vasculature.

LYMPHATICS OF THE HEAD

The lymphatic system of the scalp and face drains into regionally located lymph nodes found in close association with the primary venous pathways.

The occipital region drains into scattered occipital nodes found along the superior nuchal lines. The retroauricular nodes located over the mastoid process receive lymphatic drainage from the occipital, parietal, and temporal scalp as well as the posteromedial auricle (Fig. 3-5).

The forehead, temporal, and lateral canthal regions drain into preauricular or superficial parotid nodes. The medial eyelids, nose, cheek, and upper lips drain into the scattered facial nodes which parallel the facial vein.

The lips and mental region drain into submental and submandibular nodes located within the neck. The upper lips drain into the ipsilateral submandibular nodes; the lateral aspect of the lower lips drains into the ipsilateral submandibular nodes, while the medial aspect of the lower lips drains into ipsilateral and contralateral submental and submandibular lymph nodes. Squamous cell carcinomas of the skin of the head and neck which metastasize normally do so to the first echelon lymph nodes; thus, evaluation of those nodes is critical.

THE PAROTID GLAND

The parotid gland is positioned superficially to the masseter muscle, just anteriorly to the ear, and has a somewhat triangular configuration (Fig. 3-6). The superior pole of the parotid gland is located just anteriorly to the ear and immedi-

ately below the zygomatic arch; the inferior pole extends inferiorly, nearly to the angle of the mandible. The gland's posterior margin parallels the posterior edge of the ramus of the mandible, while its isthmus lies wedged between the external auditory canal and the ramus of the mandible; the anterior margin extends a variable distance anteriorly over the masseter muscle toward the buccal region of the cheek. The parotid duct emerges from the anterior border of the gland, turns medially at the anterior edge of the masseter, and then penetrates the buccinator muscle to empty into the buccal vestibule opposite the second upper molar. The duct is easily palpable at the anterior edge of the masseter at a point midway between the zygomatic arch and the labial commissure. At times, the duct may be injured when deep tumors are removed. Immediate repair is indicated if possible.

THE FACIAL NERVE

The facial nerve leaves the base of the skull via the stylomastoid foramen, coursing downward, laterally, and anteriorly. The first extracranial branch, the posterior auricular, passes posteriorly to supply the occipital belly of the occipitofrontalis muscle and the posterior auricular muscle. Continuing anteriorly, the facial nerve penetrates the deep surface of the parotid gland, which protects the nerve during its intraglandular course. Within the parotid gland, the facial nerve divides into five major branches (temporal, zygomatic, buccal, marginal mandibular, and cervical), which then leave the parotid gland and are named for the region of the face they supply (Fig. 3-7).

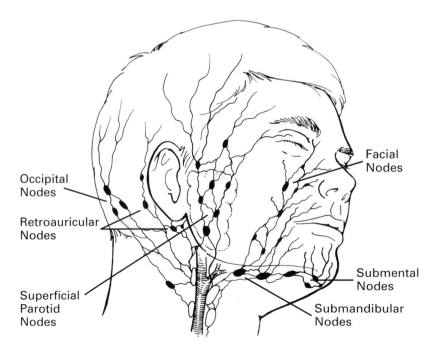

Figure 3-5. Lymphatics of the scalp and face. In the event of metastasis, most cutaneous squamous cell carcinomas of the face and scalp will spread initially to the draining lymph nodes.

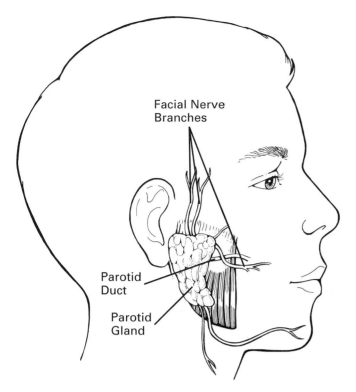

Figure 3-6. The parotid gland and duct. In many patients, the duct can be palpated at the anterior edge of the masseter muscle.

The extraparotid course of the facial nerve branches may be divided into safe and danger zones. The branches of the facial nerve have not arborized extensively within its danger zone, and cutting a nerve branch in this area may cause a motor deficit. The area outside the danger zone is called the "safe zone" because the facial nerve branches have extensively arborized, and cutting a small peripheral branch creates no significant motor deficits. The danger zone is delineated by a line drawn 1 cm above and parallel to the zygomatic arch, starting at the auricle and finishing at the lateral margin of the orbit. A vertical line is drawn from the lateral margin of the orbit inferiorly to the inferior margin of the mandible at the insertion of the masseter muscle; this is connected to a line curving 2 cm below the mandible to terminate at the angle of the mandible posteriorly. The area circumscribed by these boundaries on the posterior face is defined as the *danger zone* of the facial nerve (Fig. 3-8).

The temporal branches of the facial nerve leave the superior pole of the parotid gland and pass superficially to the zygomatic arch to supply the anterior and superior auricular muscles, the orbicularis oculi muscle, the frontal belly of the occipitofrontalis muscle, the corrugator supercilii muscle, and the procerus muscle. Damage to the nerve may cause drooping of the ipsilateral eyelid and inability to close the lid tightly. In dermatologic surgery, this branch of the facial nerve is the one most commonly injured.

The zygomatic branches of the facial nerve leave the anterosuperior aspect of the parotid gland and proceed toward

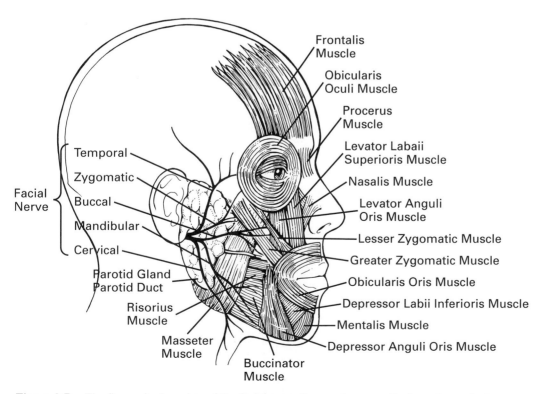

Figure 3-7. The five major branches of the facial nerve (temporal, zygomatic, buccal, marginal mandibular, and cervical).

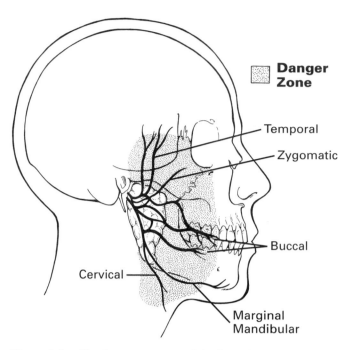

Figure 3-8. The danger zone area of the face where the branches of the facial nerve may be more at risk for damage during cutaneous and superficial surgical procedures (see text for boundaries).

the lateral angle of the eye. These branches supply the orbicularis oculi muscle and the zygomaticus major and minor muscles, with secondary innervation to the levators of the lip. Damage to this branch results in an ectropion of the lower eyelid, weakness in blinking, inability for tight closure of the eyelid, and moderate facial asymmetry when smiling. The use of an eye patch may be indicated.

The buccal branches emerge from the anterior border of the parotid gland and parallel the parotid duct, supplying the buccinator muscle, risorius muscle, orbicularis oris muscle, levators of the lip, depressor septi muscle, and nasalis muscle, with secondary innervation to the depressor anguli and depressor labii inferioris muscles. Injury to these branches results in weakness in the oral sphincter (unable to whistle or pucker lips) and facial asymmetry related to unopposed pull from the normal side.

The marginal mandibular branches of the facial nerve exit the inferior pole of the parotid gland to parallel the inferior margin of the mandible. In elderly patients, these nerve branches may descend 2 cm below the inferior margin of the mandible before they ascend back up onto the face at the insertion site of the masseter muscle into the mandible. The marginal mandibular branches continue forward, superficially to the facial artery and vein, finally to innervate the depressor anguli oris, depressor labii inferioris, and mentalis muscles. Damage to these branches causes facial asymmetry when talking or smiling. This branch may be more susceptible to damage toward the mid-face due to its lack of peripheral branches.

The cervical branches of the facial nerve emerge from the inferior pole of the parotid gland, descending behind the angle of the mandible into the neck to innervate the platysma muscle.

The use of local anesthetics may also cause temporary deinnervation of the various nerve branch or branches, with subsequent lack of muscle innervation and muscle drooping, asymmetry, and so forth. Depending on the type of anesthesia and duration of action (i.e., longer for long-acting local anesthetics such as Marcaine), this deficit may exist for several hours. Thus a patient with inability to close the eye due to local anesthetic action may require a temporary eye patch to protect the eye until the action of the local anesthetic has worn off.

SENSORY INNERVATION OF THE FACE AND SCALP

The sensory innervation to the skin of the face is primarily from the trigeminal nerve via its three divisions: ophthalmic, maxillary, and mandibular (Fig. 3-9).

Ophthalmic Division

The supraorbital and supratrochlear nerves supply the skin of the medial upper eyelid, forehead, and scalp as far superiorly as the crown. The infratrochlear nerve innervates skin over the medial upper eyelid and bridge of the nose. The lacrimal nerve supplies skin over the lateral upper eyelid.

The dorsal external nasal nerve is the terminal branch of the anterior ethmoidal nerve and supplies a strip of skin over the dorsum of the nose down to the tip.

Maxillary Division

The infraorbital nerve supplies the skin of the lower eyelids, lateral sides of the nose, upper lips, and buccal cheek.

The zygomatic nerve splits into zygomaticofacial and zygomaticotemporal nerves which supply skin over the malar region of the cheek and anterior temporal scalp region.

Mandibular Division

The mental nerve innervates the skin of the chin and lower lip extending laterally to the labial commissure.

The buccal nerve descends into the cheek between the temporalis and buccinator muscles, supplying the skin of the buccal cheek.

The auriculotemporal nerve passes posterior to the neck of the mandible to accompany the superficial temporal artery; it supplies the upper antero-lateral quadrant of the auricle, anterior half of the external auditory canal and tympanic membrane, and most of the temporal scalp region.

The use of nerve blocks (i.e., supraorbital, infraorbital, and

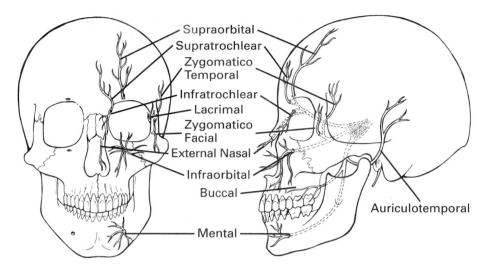

Figure 3-9.   Sensory innervation to the skin of the face via branches of the trigeminal nerve.

mental) may offer advantages in dermatologic surgery in many instances.

The Neck

Surface Anatomy of the Neck

Several landmarks are palpable in the neck and provide useful reference points (Fig. 3-10).

Approximately 2.5 to 3 cm below the chin, the body of the hyoid bone is identified in midline. Inferior to the hyoid bone, the prominence of the thyroid cartilage is palpated in midline.

Just below the thyroid cartilage, the anterior lamina of the cricoid cartilage is easily identified. The interspace between the thyroid and cricoid in midline is filled by the cricothyroid ligament and represents an important site for emergency access to the airway. Inferior to the cricoid are the prominent tracheal rings.

In the posterior neck, the superiormost reference point is the external occipital protuberance, palpable in midline on the occipital bone. When the patient's neck is flexed, the first palpable spinous process is the spinous process of the seventh cervical vertebra (vertebra prominens), demarcating the base of the neck.

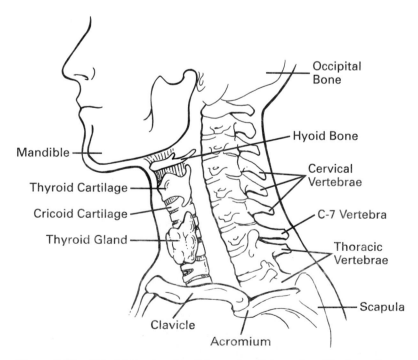

Figure 3-10.   Palpable landmarks of the neck which can be utilized as reference points.

Triangles of the Neck

The important landmarks of the *anterior triangle* (Fig. 3-11) of the neck are as follows: the mastoid process of the temporal bone, the tip of the chin, the midpoint of the manubrium, and the anterior border of the sternocleidomastoid muscle. The anterior triangle is further subdivided into four smaller triangles: the submandibular, the submental, the carotid, and the muscular.

The submandibular triangle is outlined by lines drawn from the mastoid process to the tip of the chin, to the lesser cornu of the hyoid bone, and back to the mastoid process. This triangle contains the submandibular gland, facial artery and vein, branches of the facial nerve (cervical and marginal mandibular), and lymph nodes.

The boundaries of the submental triangle are a line drawn from the tip of the chin to the middle of the hyoid bone, laterally to the lesser cornu of the hyoid, and back to the tip of the chin; it contains scattered lymph nodes.

The boundaries of the carotid triangle are identified by lines drawn from the mastoid process to the lesser cornu of the hyoid, from the hyoid to the junction of the lower one-third with the middle one-third of the anterior border of the sternocleidomastoid muscle, and back to the mastoid process. The major structures contained within the carotid triangle are the carotid arteries, the internal jugular vein, and associated lymph nodes. The muscular triangle, extending from the middle of the hyoid, inferiorly to the manubrium, along the anterior edge of the sternocleidomastoid muscle to its junction of the lower one-third with the middle one-third, back to the middle of the hyoid, contains the thyroid gland.

The *posterior triangle* of the neck, initiated at the mastoid process, is bounded posteriorly by the anterior edge of the trapezius muscle, anteriorly by the posterior border of the sternocleidomastoid muscle, and inferiorly along its base by the clavicle. An important superficial structure located within the posterior cervical triangle is the spinal accessory nerve, which emanates from the posterior border of the sternocleidomastoid muscle (Fig. 3-11) and traverses the triangle obliquely to penetrate the anterior edge of the trapezius muscle. The spinal accessory nerve is at risk for damage during its entire course through the posterior cervical triangle since it is covered only by the superficial cervical fascia and skin. The external jugular vein, formed near the angle of the mandible, descends vertically across the sternocleidomastoid muscle, finally emptying into the subclavian vein at the base of the posterior cervical triangle.

SUPERFICIAL CERVICAL MUSCULATURE

Overlying nearly the entire anterior triangle of the neck from the clavicle to the mandible, the paper-thin platysma muscle arises from the upper thoracic fascia to insert into the skin of the lower face and lower lateral lip. The platysma tenses the skin over the neck, pulls the lower lip downward and laterally, and is innervated by the cervical branches of the facial nerve. This muscle never shelters the accessory spinal nerve within

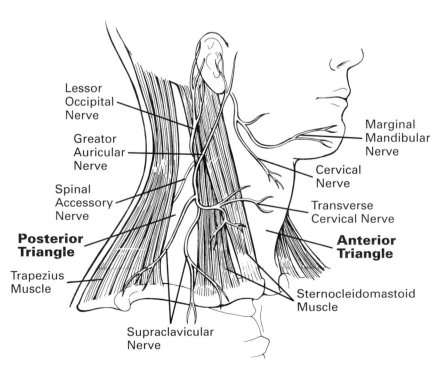

Figure 3-11. Anterior and posterior triangles of the neck with sternocleidomastoid muscle. Motor and sensory nerve supply.

the posterior cervical triangle and covers only the most inferior aspect of the posterior cervical triangle. The most important landmark within the neck is the sternocleidomastoid muscle, which extends obliquely across the neck from the clavicle and sternum, inserting into the mastoid process of the temporal bone and innervated by the spinal accessory nerve.

BLOOD SUPPLY OF THE NECK

The deeply positioned external carotid artery and thyrocervical trunk supply penetrating branches to the overlying skin and superficial structures located within the anterior and posterior cervical triangles.

The superficial veins of the neck consist of the anterior and external jugular venous systems. The anterior jugular vein, small and irregularly placed, located just deeply to the platysma muscle, originates within the submental triangle, descends toward the lower aspect of the muscular triangle, and passes posteriorly to the sternocleidomastoid muscle to terminate in the external jugular vein. The external jugular vein arises over the sternocleidomastoid muscle by the union of the postauricular vein and descends vertically to enter the subclavian vein within the posterior cervical triangle.

The superficial lymphatic system of the neck drains into the nodes of the superficial cervical lymphatic chain which parallels the external jugular vein. Scattered nodes located within the submental and submandibular triangles drain into the jugulodigastric node with direct drainage into the deep cervical lymphatic chain.

NERVES OF THE NECK

The most important motor nerve encountered in a superficial dissection of the neck is the spinal accessory nerve (Fig. 3-11). Emerging from approximately the junction of the upper and middle one-third of the posterior border of the sternocleidomastoid muscle, it passes inferiorly and obliquely across the posterior cervical triangle to innervate the trapezius muscle finally. The spinal accessory nerve is at risk for damage during its entire passage within the posterior cervical triangle because it is covered only by thin skin and a layer of fascia.

Another motor nerve which briefly traverses the neck is the main stem of the facial nerve. Emerging from the base of the skull through the stylomastoid foramen, the facial nerve quickly penetrates the posterior aspect of the parotid gland and splits into five terminal branches (temporal, zygomatic, buccal, marginal mandibular, and cervical). Only the cervical and marginal mandibular branches have important relationships in the neck. The cervical branches of the facial nerve exit the inferior pole of the parotid gland and descend below the angle of the mandible to innervate the platysma muscle. The marginal mandibular branch of the facial nerve normally parallels the inferior margin of the mandible, but in the elderly it frequently descends into the submandibular triangle of the neck before it ascends back up onto the face to supply the lower lip musculature.

The cutaneous sensory input is provided via branches of the cervical plexus (Fig. 3-11). These nerves emerge from the posterior edge of the sternocleidomastoid muscle at approximately its midpoint to supply the overlying skin of the anterior and posterior cervical triangles. The largest and most frequently injured of the cervical plexus branches is the greater auricular nerve; it crosses superficially to the sternocleidomastoid muscle to ascend directly toward the auricle, and supplies the skin overlying the upper half of the sternocleidomastoid muscle, posteromedial and anterolateral auricle, and the posteroinferior region of the face. The lesser occipital nerve passes along the posterior border of the sternocleidomastoid muscle supplying skin overlying the apex of the posterior cervical triangle, the posteromedial auricle, and occipital scalp. The transverse cervical nerves cross the superficial aspect of the sternocleidomastoid muscle horizontally, supplying the skin overlying the anterior cervical triangle. The supraclavicular nerves (medial, intermediate, and lateral), descend to supply the skin overlying the lower half of the posterior cervical triangle, upper chest, and lower one-third of the anterior cervical triangle.

Knowledge of the normal superficial anatomy of the head and neck is critical to proper tumor removal, reconstruction, and dermatologic surgery.

SUGGESTED READINGS

1. Breisch EA, Greenway HT: *Cutaneous Surgical Anatomy of the Head and Neck,* edited by RC Grekin. New York, N.Y., Churchill-Livingstone, 1992

2. Hollinshead WH: *Anatomy for Surgeons: The Head and Neck,* vol 1, 2d ed. Harper & Row, 1969

3. Williams PL, Warwick R (eds): *Gray's Anatomy,* 36th British ed. Philadelphia, Saunders, 1980

Jack E. Sebben and Michael J. Fazio

4 Sterilization of Equipment for Dermatologic Surgery

All surgical instruments and intraoperative equipment used for dermatologic surgical procedures must be completely sterile. Hospitals have infection control procedures to ensure the sterility of equipment. However, most cutaneous surgery is done in the outpatient setting, usually in the private office. In the office, it is the physician's responsibility to ensure adequacy of sterile technique. Individual practices may vary from levels of sterility approaching those of the hospital operating room environment down to very low levels where little sterile technique is observed. Previous surveys have shown a wide variation for infection control procedures in dermatologists' offices.[1] For the benefit of patients as well as medical personnel, surgical equipment must be handled properly and be subjected to a reliable, effective means of sterilization. This chapter will discuss proper handling and storage of surgical instruments as well as other items of equipment used in cutaneous surgery.

SURGICAL INSTRUMENTS

Instrument Construction

All instruments used for standard surgical procedures should be high quality. Well-constructed instruments are a pleasure to use and may facilitate the performance and efficiency of surgical procedures. The instruments will be subjected to repeated sterilization procedures, and high-quality instruments tolerate such treatments with minimal degradation. The instruments should be constructed of stainless steel whenever possible. Chromium-plated steel instruments are available at budget prices but do not hold up well with repeated use and sterilization. In addition, the chromium plating will eventually chip away and leave foreign material within wounds. Most metal surgical instruments are available either in a highly polished finish or what is referred to as a *luster* or *satin* finish. The luster-finished instruments tend to retain their original appearance longer than the highly polished varieties.[2] Most metal surgical instruments are available in a black finish to reduce the chance of reflections when used for laser surgery. However, many experienced laser surgeons find the black-finished instruments unnecessary.

The exceptions to the total stainless steel construction recommendation are needle-holders and scissors. Because the working surfaces are subjected to much wear and tear, a tungsten carbide insert is often desirable (Fig. 4-1). These inserts in needle-holders will wear much longer than the stainless steel surface. Tungsten carbide blade edges on scissors resist dulling. However, these tungsten carbide surfaces are fragile and can chip. If the instruments are immersed in sterilizing or holding solutions, they may be subject to degradation. In the past, there have been complaints that the tungsten carbide inserts separate from the body of the stainless steel instrument.

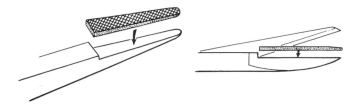

Figure 4-1 The useful longevity of needle-holders and scissors can greatly be increased by choosing those models with tungsten carbide inserts along the working surfaces. Needles-holders will retain their ability to securely grasp fine needles and suture material; scissors will resist dulling. Tungsten carbide inserts are excellent for small, medium, and large scissors. Extremely delicate scissors seldom benefit from these inserts because of the added thickness required.

This was a problem when the inserts were applied with epoxy bonding. Most manufacturers use silver solder for the bonding, and separation is not a problem.[3,4]

Instrument Cleaning

All foreign matter and organic debris should be removed from the instruments as soon as possible. If the instruments are subjected to sterilization with dried-on material, some microorganisms may be protected from the sterilization process. In addition, the dried material may be baked onto the instrument with heat sterilization and subsequently interfere with instrument operation.

The cleaning process will be facilitated if blood is not allowed to dry on the surfaces. The instruments should be placed in a basin of water for soaking immediately after they are taken from the operating room. The process may be facilitated if a small amount of neutral pH detergent is added to the soaking solution. A mechanical process is usually necessary to remove some of the debris. This may be accomplished by hand scrubbing with a brush. If hand scrubbing is performed, the technician should wear gloves to minimize injury and exposure to blood and tissue products.

Employee exposure is further minimized if an ultrasonic cleaner is used. It is also faster than manual scrubbing. The instruments are placed in an ultrasonic cleaner for approximately 5 min (Fig. 4-2). The ultrasonic energy is transferred to small, collapsing bubbles that implode adjacently to the instruments, acting like small depth charges to free the debris. On some instruments with tight joints or narrow openings, there may be some residual debris that may require cleaning with a small brush and then a second ultrasonic cycle.

It must be remembered that the ultrasonic cleaner is only a mechanical cleaning process and in no way destroys bacteria. All instruments must be considered to be as contaminated when they leave the ultrasonic cleaner as when they were initially placed inside. A neutral-based detergent is added to the ultrasonic cleaner to facilitate debris removal, but it has very little antibacterial activity. Therefore, the solution in the ultrasonic cleaner should be changed frequently. The detergent should only be a specially recommended neutral-based detergent. Acid or alkaline detergents or detergent antiseptics should never be placed in contact with surgical instruments because they may damage the surfaces and will often leave an orange or black discoloration, which appears after heat sterilization.[2,4] Once the ultrasonic cycle is completed, instruments should be rinsed under running water to remove the detergent solution.

After the cleaning procedure, the instruments should be dried before packing. Some instruments may become stiff after repeated use. If this occurs, the instruments may be dipped in instrument milk, which is a lubricant specially designed for surgical instruments. Ordinary household lubricants, including silicone and oil, should never be used. If an instrument becomes particularly stiff, the offending debris or corrosion may be removed by soaking the instrument overnight in a solution of 50 percent ammonia water and 50 percent isopropyl alcohol.[5]

Instrument Packing

Nonpacked Instruments

A few offices use nonpacked surgical instruments. The instruments are processed loose in an autoclave, and, after sterilization has been completed, they are placed in individual holding trays, either dry or in a disinfectant solution. This

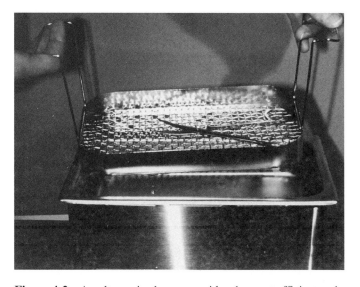

Figure 4-2 An ultrasonic cleaner provides the most efficient and safest means of instrument cleaning. The basket of instruments is immersed in the ultrasonic basin containing a neutral pH detergent. Ultrasonic waves remove debris from the instruments. The ultrasonic cleaner does not sterilize the instruments.

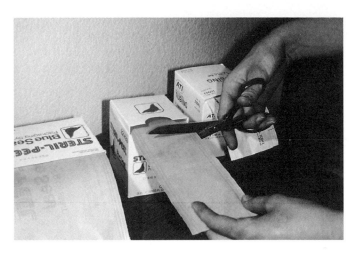

Figure 4-3 Sterile tubing is available in a variety of widths for packing surgical instruments prior to steam autoclaving. The appropriate length of tubing is cut with scissors, and the instruments are placed between the transparent plastic and the paper backing.

technique is not approved in any hospitals and is strongly discouraged. The instruments are constantly exposed to unseen contamination, especially if stored in trays of multiple instruments. If the instruments are placed in a disinfectant holding solution, contamination risks are increased, and surgical instruments tolerate constant moisture exposure poorly. In addition to being much safer, an accepted means of instrument packing usually involves less employee time.

Cloth Packing

Cloth packs are often used in hospitals, particularly for large surgical packs. Cloth packing is less convenient for the private office. The packing material is more expensive than paper materials and must be cleaned for repeated use. The cloth should be constructed of tightly woven cotton, and instruments should be wrapped in multiple layers. Even with multiple layers, the cloth material is a less effective contamination barrier than the modern disposable materials.[6]

Paper Packing Materials

Disposable paper drapes are available that are used in the same manner as the cloth packs. They are more convenient than the cloth packs but still require careful folding.

Paper/Transparent Pouches

The see-through pouches are the first choice for most offices. The instruments can be quickly packed in the pouches and they are easily sealed. The most economical form comes in long rolls of tubing in varying widths. Strips of tubing are cut off in the appropriate lengths, and the ends are sealed with autoclave tape after the instruments have been inserted (Figs. 4-3 and 4-4). It does take a little time to seal the end with autoclave tape or a heat sealer. Sometimes opening the pack by removing the autoclave tape can be a slow process. As a result, the most highly recommended forms are self-sealing pouches available in several sizes (Figs. 4-5 and 4-6). They are slightly more expensive than the tubing, but the instruments are easily packed and quickly opened at the time of surgery. These paper/transparent pouches also provide the maximum safe storage time of up to 1 year if handled and stored properly.[7]

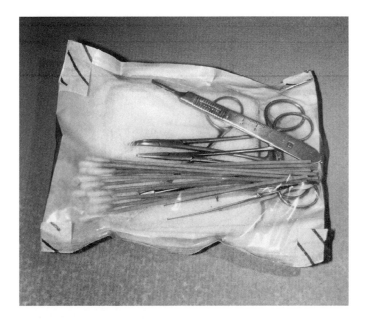

Figure 4-4 This surgical pack has been placed in surgical sterilizing tubing and the ends are sealed with autoclave tape. This is an economical means of packaging, but the packs open slowly because the autoclave tape must be carefully removed.

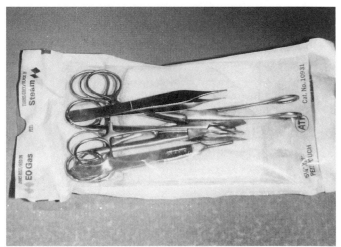

Figure 4-5 This surgical pack uses a self-sealing envelope which is more efficient than surgical tubing. Once the instruments are inserted, the ends self-seal quite quickly.

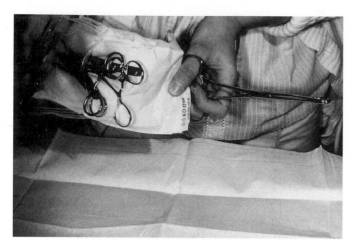

Figure 4-6   The self-seal packs peel open more efficiently than taped packs.

Additional Packing Considerations

When clamping-type instruments are packed for sterilization, they should be placed in the unlocked position. This includes needle-holders, hemostats, towel clamps, and any other instrument where two surfaces meet under tension. The tightly closed area may be protected from the sterilization process. In addition, for heat sterilization, the metal instrument under tension will be subjected to metal fatigue with heat exposure.

Sometimes instruments are placed in packs in bundles which are secured with rubber bands. Small pieces of surgical tubing are occasionally placed over delicate tips for protec-tion. The problem with either of these procedures is that the rubber band or tubing may protect bacteria from exposure to the sterilizing agent.[8]

Instrument Sterilization

After the instruments have been properly packed, they must be subjected to some form of sterilization (Table 4-1). The vegetative forms of bacteria and most viruses are easily de-stroyed with a wide variety of sterilization or disinfection techniques. The major concern is for bacterial spores which are very resistant to sterilization. Spores are even more resis-tant to chemical inactivation. Therefore, heat sterilization is most reliable and is highly recommended.[9]

Steam Autoclave

The basic steam autoclave is the most popular form of steril-ization in both hospitals and in private offices. It is a very simple and reliable modification of a pressure cooker. With appropriate temperatures, pressures, and exposure times, the steam heat will destroy all vegetative and spore forms of bac-teria. Most steam autoclaves use a pressure of two atmo-spheres with a temperature of 121° C. An exposure time of 15 min will destroy all bacteria, but the 15-min period does not start until the steam has reached all areas of the pack. There-fore, the manufacturer's recommended exposure times must be followed. The usual autoclave cycle takes 20 to 30 min de-pending upon the size. The steam autoclave works very well for metal instruments, cloth, paper, glassware, and heat-resis-tant plastics. The 100 percent humidity present during the

TABLE 4-1

Methods of Instrument Sterilization

Method	Active Agent	Exposure Time	Advantages	Disadvantages
Steam autoclave	Heat (121°C); water	20–30 min	Reliable; simple	Can't be used on material sensitive to moisture or moderate heat
Chemiclave	Heat (121°C); water; alcohol; acetone; ketone; formaldehyde	20–30 min	Minimal moisture; items dry at end of cycle	Can't be used on moderate heat-sensitive materials; must use special chemical solution
Dry heat	Heat (170°C)	60 min or more	No moisture; good for very sharp instruments; inexpensive	Very high heat eliminates use of cloth, paper, or plastic; must use special containers or foil for packing
Gas	Ethylene oxide	Hours	No heat or moisture; excellent for all heat- and moisture-sensitive instruments	Very long cycle; complex and expensive; toxic; use limited to hospitals
Chemical	Various solutions: glutaraldehyde; quaternary ammonium compounds; phenolic agents	Minutes for vegetative bacteria; many hours for spores	Inexpensive; no special equipment; no packing required	Unreliable; contamination-prone; short storage time

autoclave cycle may tend to dull some very sharp surgical instruments. If high-quality stainless steel instruments are used, the damage for sharp edges such as scissors will be insignificant. Scalpel blades as well as dermatome blades and hair transplant punches will receive some dulling, and alternative measures should be used.[10]

Chemiclave

A modified form of the steam autoclave which produces less humidity is available as the Chemiclave (MDT Corp., North Charleston, South Carolina). Over the years, it has been more popular in dental offices. The physical process is very similar to a steam autoclave but requires a chemical solution instead of distilled water. The solution contains methyl ethyl ketone, acetone, formaldehyde, and three alcohols. As a result, the humidity remains less than 15 percent, and the instruments are dry at the end of the autoclave cycle. There is less damage to moisture-sensitive instruments. The Chemiclave is very effective and reliable but does release some chemical vapors.[11]

Dry Heat Sterilization

Dry heat sterilization will effectively destroy microorganisms on any surgical materials that will withstand high heat exposure. Because no chemical or humidity is involved, the temperatures must be considerably higher than a steam autoclave, and the exposure times are longer. It is a very effective, economical way of sterilizing metal surgical instruments. The main problem is that the most commonly used packing materials will not withstand the high temperatures. After dry heat sterilization, the instruments must be placed in sterile metal or foil containers. Dry heat sterilization is a practical alternative to steam sterilization for very sharp metal instruments.[12]

Gas Sterilization

Gas sterilization involves the use of ethylene oxide, which is a mutagenic chemical that produces extremely effective sterilization for any materials that cannot be subjected to heat. Ethylene oxide is a toxic and flammable gas that requires a prolonged exposure time followed by an adequate period of aeration. Most gas sterilization procedures are performed in hospitals. There are small models of gas sterilizers that may be used in the medical office. There have been some studies that question the reliability of the smaller models, and there are concerns about toxic exposures within the office.[13–15]

Cold Sterilization

The use of liquid chemical agents for disinfection of surgical instruments is not truly complete sterilization. There are a number of germicide agents available as holding solutions for surgical instruments. Most contain a quaternary ammonium compound that is a relatively weak antiseptic that is prone to contamination. Phenol-based disinfectants are also available but are not considered effective for instrument sterilization.[16–18]

The only chemical agent considered somewhat reliable for cold sterilization is glutaraldehyde. Glutaraldehydes are weak disinfectants in the stable acidic state. In order to achieve maximum effectiveness, the pH must be raised to 8.5 with a buffering agent. The buffering agent will slowly polymerize, resulting in loss of effectiveness after a very few weeks. Cidex and Cidex-7 (Surgikos Co., Arlington, Texas), Glutarex (3M Co., St. Paul, Minnesota), and Acu-Sol (Acuderm, Inc., Fort Lauderdale, Florida) are popular glutaraldehyde preparations.[19,20]

Although glutaraldehyde preparations destroy the vegetative forms of bacteria within 10 min, highly increased exposure times are required for the eradication of spores. Glutaraldehyde is irritating to tissue and can stain or sensitize the skin. The solution should be removed from the instruments with sterile water prior to use.[21]

The major risk with cold sterilization is that there is no way of monitoring the effectiveness or absence of contamination in the solution. Cold sterilization is not approved by the Joint Commission on the Accreditation of Healthcare Organizations, the Centers for Disease Control (CDC), or the American College of Surgeons. It should not be used in the private office.[22]

Instrument Storage

The useful life of a sterile instrument pack will vary according to the packing material and how the pack is handled. Each pack should be dated at the time of sterilization. Cloth packs stored properly should only be considered sterile for a few weeks. Paper/transparent pouches are considered sterile up to 1 year if handled properly. Proper handling means that the instruments should never be exposed to any moisture or wet surfaces. They should be placed on a shelf or within a cabinet so that they are not subjected to repeated handling and moving.[7]

Surgical Tray Setup

The surgical instruments must be presented to the operating area in a manner that ensures their continued sterilization. In the outpatient setting, this is best accomplished by removing the instruments from the pack in a sterile manner and placing them upon a stand such as a Mayo table. The table should be covered with a sterile drape. If cloth packs are used, the pack may be unfolded in a manner so that the outer cover of the pack provides the initial drape for the table. With the more popular paper/transparent packs, the Mayo table should first be covered with a sterile disposable drape, preferably one that provides a moisture barrier. The more popular barrier drapes are triple layered. The two outer layers are paper, and the inner layer consists of a thin layer of polyethylene film providing a moisture barrier. If the moisture barrier is not present, moisture from solutions or blood may soak through the drape and allow the migration of bacteria from the underlying table.

As the surgical pack is opened, the instruments should fall gently onto the sterile drape so that the instruments are not damaged and so that they cannot puncture the drape and become contaminated. The instruments then are often arranged in a useful presentation on the drape with the aid of transfer forceps. Care should be taken to ensure that the tips of the transfer forceps are sterile.[3]

ELECTROSURGICAL EQUIPMENT

Electrosurgical Electrodes

It once was thought that the electrodes used for high-frequency electrosurgery were self-sterilizing. There is now ample evidence that this does not occur.[23,24] All electrodes used for sterile surgical procedures should be either disposable or sterilized between uses. Most metal electrodes can be resterilized. However, some contain insulating materials that may not tolerate heat sterilization. Popular choices for disposable electrodes include the Electrolase electrode (Birtcher Corp., Irvine, California), Acuderm needle electrodes (Acuderm), and metal-hubbed hypodermic needles used as electrodes when placed on special adapters (Figs. 4-7 and 4-8).

Electrosurgical Handles and Cords

Electrosurgical coaglation of blood vessels is often required for incisional surgical procedures. If the electrosurgical handle is introduced into the surgical field and used by personnel who are gloved and sterile, a technique must be used which prevents contamination. The easiest solution to the problem is

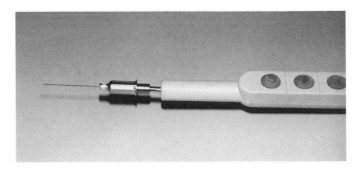

Figure 4-8 Metal-hubbed hypodermic needles can be used as electrodes. Some dermatologists use the same needle for anesthetic infiltration. The needle is then removed from the syringe and placed on a special adapter such as the Bernsco adapter shown above.

to use a sterile, disposable electrosurgical handle and cord. The varieties that contain a switching mechanism are often expensive and make their use cost prohibitive for the brief requirement during the course of minor surgical procedures (Fig. 4-9).[25] Nonswitching handles are available in sterile packs that are quite economic. An alternative is to sterilize reusable handles and cords. However, most models do not hold up well to steam heat sterilization, and gas sterilization is not readily available in most offices.[26] Instead of using a sterile electrosurgical handle and cord, many surgeons prefer to use a sterile cover over the instrument. Short, sterile covers for the handles are now available from Acuderm (Fig. 4-10) and Birtcher. Some surgeons will use a sterilized Penrose drain to cover the handle (Fig. 4-11). The drain should be at

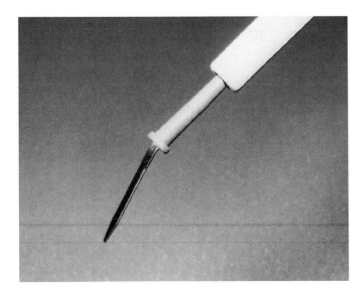

Figure 4-7 Because of concerns of cross-contamination, disposable electrosurgical electrodes have become quite popular. Shown above is the blunt model of the Birtcher Electrolase disposable electrode.

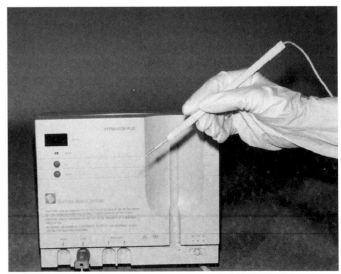

Figure 4-9 Sterile disposable handles and cords are available for attaching to various electrosurgical units which allow the surgeon to maintain sterility while performing electrosurgery in a sterile surgical field.

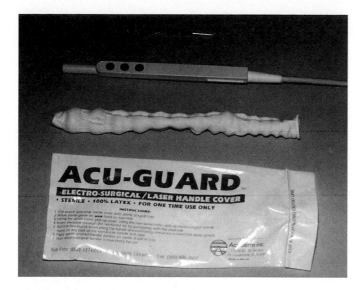

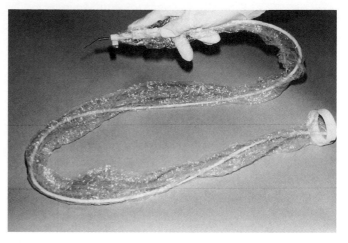

Figure 4-12   The Sani-Sleeve illustrated above is a protective sterile cover originally designed for laser handpieces but works very well for covering electrosurgical handles.

Figure 4-10   A variety of covers are available which may be placed over electrosurgical handles to maintain sterility and also to prevent cross-contamination between patients.

least 5/8-in diameter and 12 in long. A longer plastic cover is available as a Sani-Sleeve (Nieusma R&D, Inc., Lincoln, Nebraska), which will cover the electrode handle and a long length of cord. However, the Sani-Sleeve may be nearly as expensive as some disposable handles and cords (Fig. 4-12).

DERMABRASION EQUIPMENT

Dermabrasion Handpieces

Some portions of some dermabrasion handpieces are removable and can be sterilized with steam heat. The motor portion of most handles will not tolerate the exposure to heat and

moisture.[27] It is best to make arrangements with a local hospital so that the entire handpiece can be gas sterilized. A very acceptable alternative would be to use the above-mentioned Sani-Sleeve.

Dermabrasion Fraises and Brushes

Nearly all diamond fraises and wire brushes will tolerate most of the popular means of sterilization. For most offices, steam heat is most practical. Special attention should be paid to dried-on materials. They may require prolonged soaking and ultrasonic cleaning treatment in order to free all debris. Special abrasive blocks and pads are available for removing debris from diamond fraises.

Equipment Maintenance

Lubrication is essential for dermabrasion handpieces. Sterilization procedures will often remove the lubrication. Be sure to note the manufacturer's recommendations about maintenance of lubrication.

LASER EQUIPMENT

Laser light energy is delivered to the surgical site by means of either an articulating arm or a fiber optics pathway. Some of the smaller, more compact units may allow introduction of the entire laser-generating portion at the surgery site. Distal portions of the laser arm are sometimes removable and sterilizable. However, the most practical solution to laser use is to use a specially designed plastic laser cover or a Sani-Sleeve so that the laser delivery apparatus may be manipulated without fear of contamination.

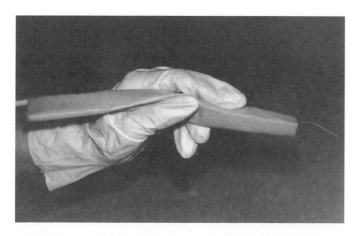

Figure 4-11   Twelve inches of a 5/8-in wide Penrose drain can be sterilized and placed over the electrosurgical handle to maintain sterility.

HUMAN IMMUNODEFICIENCY VIRUS AND HEPATITIS B VIRUS CROSS-CONTAMINATION RISKS

These viruses are easily inactivated by even the mildest forms of sterilization. Therefore, any adequate means of sterilization eliminates the risk of viral transfer on instruments. The main risks of cross-contamination occur in minor surgical procedures where strict sterility is not maintained. These include procedures such as simple biopsies or shave excisions where a full surgical tray is not used. Potentials for contamination occur when contaminated instruments are placed on nonsterile trays and countertops that may be adequately sterilized between procedures. Adequate measures must be taken so that there is a means to ensure that patient-to-patient contamination will not occur between procedures. Barrier drapes, disposable trays, or sterilized trays should be used for instruments, even for minor procedures, in order to ensure that cross-contamination will not occur (Fig. 4-13).[3,28]

The CDC has established universal precautions to prevent occupational HIV and hepatitis B virus (HBV) transmission.[29,30] These guidelines should be followed in hospitals and other health care facilities when workers are exposed to blood or other potentially infectious body fluids. Since there can be a long latency period prior to clinical symptoms of these viral diseases, all patients should be assumed to be infectious. Surgical personnel should be educated on the epidemiology of blood-borne infections (e.g., HIV and HBV), and a standard operating procedure should be defined. All surgical personnel should wear gloves, mask, eyewear, and protective clothing. Following these precautions will help minimize the risk of blood contact between the patient and the surgical staff.

During the surgical procedure, sharp instruments should not be passed between the surgeon and assistant. Also, needles should never be recapped or manipulated by hand. After the surgery, all syringes, needles, scalpel blades, and other sharp items should be disposed of in puncture-resistant containers. All nonsharp, disposable items are double bagged, marked with appropriate biohazard labels, and disposed of according to local regulations. If there has been any blood contamination of the surgical area, it should be cleaned immediately using an Environmental Protection Agency- (EPA) approved germicide or a 1:100 solution of sodium hypochlorite (household bleach). Proper cleaning, disinfecting, and sterilizing of surgical equipment are critically important in preventing transmission of blood-borne pathogens. Instruments suspected of HIV or HBV should be gently placed in 95 percent ethanol for 2 to 10 min for initial treatment of the viral particles.[31,32] Sodium hypochlorite is highly destructive to some surgical instruments and is not recommended for instrument decontamination. The instruments should then be cleansed and sterilized according to standard protocol as outlined above.

In the Mohs surgical unit, the tissue technician must also follow general precautions since a cryostat is a potential reservoir for HIV and HBV contaminants.[33] When working with tissue suspected of contamination, the technician should wear gloves and protective clothing while handling tissue. If fluid spattering is a concern, a face shield or a mask and protective eyeglasses should be worn. The mounting-medium dispenser should not be allowed to touch the tissue. Tissue sections are carefully placed on the slide and immersed in 10 percent formalin. The specimen is then processed in a normal fashion. The refrigeration in the cryostat is turned off, and the microtome knife is immersed in 95 percent alcohol for 15 min. The cryostat is cleaned with a sponge soaked in 95 percent ethanol, the knife is replaced, and refrigeration is resumed.

CONCLUSION

In the office surgical practice, it is the responsibility of the individual physician to ensure that the standards of a safe surgical environment are met. In addition to sterile surgical instruments, there are three other spheres of infection control that must be carefully established: (1) The surgical field must be maintained in a sterile manner, (2) the procedures must be performed in an operating room that is adequately equipped, and (3) the entire office environment must be maintained in a manner that minimizes the risks of infection exposure for both the patients and office personnel.

REFERENCES

1. Sebben JE: Survey of sterile technique in dermatologic surgeons. *J Am Acad Dermatol* **18**:1107–1114, 1988

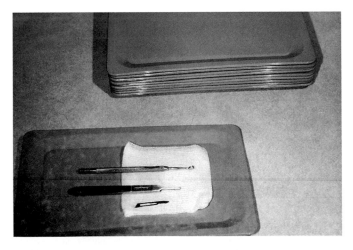

Figure 4-13   For minor procedures, such as biopsies, an entire surgical pack is seldom necessary. The physician should have some means of holding instruments. The plastic tray shown above can be sterilized, therefore preventing cross-contamination.

2. Kuhn R: Care and handling of surgical instruments, pt 2. *Med Product Sales* **13:**84–86, 1982

3. Sebben JE: Sterilization and care of surgical instruments and supplies. *J Am Acad Dermatol* **11:**381–392, 1984

4. Byrd DH, McElmurry M: Prevent spotting of surgical instruments. *AORN J* **17:**87, 1973

5. Sebben, JE: Sterile technique and the prevention of wound infection in office surgery, pt 1. *J Dermatol Surg Oncol* **14:**1364–1371, 1988

6. Laufman H et al: Scannine electron microscopy of moist bacterial strikethrough of surgical materials. *Surg Gynecol Obstet* **150:**165–170, 1980

7. Mallison GF, Standard PG: Safe storage times for sterile packs. *Hospitals* **48:**77–80, 1974

8. Schultz J: Back to basics in steam sterilization. *AORN J* **25:**67–68, 1977

9. Powell JF: Isolation of diplocolonic acid from spores of *Bacillus megaterium*. *Biochem J* **54:**210–211, 1953

10. Ernst RR: Sterilization by heat, in *Disinfection, Sterilization, and Preservation,* edited by SS Block. Philadelphia, Lea & Febiger, 1977, pp 481–521

11. Lyon TC, Devine MJ: Evaluation of a new model vapor sterilizer. *J Dent Res* **53:**213, 1974

12. Sykes G: *Disinfection and Sterilization.* London, E & FN Spon, 1958, p 288

13. Parisi AN, Young WE: Sterilization with ethylene oxide and other gases, *Disinfection, Sterilization, and Preservation,* edited by SS Block. 4th ed. Philadelphia, Lea & Febiger, 1991, pp 580–595

14. Schultz JR: Nurses' concerns with possible EO restrictions. *AORN J* **25:**1237–1238, 1977

15. Taguchi JT et al: Serious limitations of a portable ethylene oxide sterilizer. *Am J Med Sci* **245:**299–303, 1963

16. Spaulding EH et al: Chemical disinfection of medical and surgical material, in *Disinfection, Sterilization, and Preservation,* edited by SS Block. Philadelphia, Lea & Febiger, 1977, pp 654–684

17. Kaslow RA et al: Nosocomial pseudobacteremia: Positive blood culture due to contaminated benzalkonium chloride. *JAMA* **236:**2407–2409, 1976

18. Sebben JE: Protection from hepatitis B. *J Am Acad Dermatol* **11:**909–910, 1984

19. Scott EM et al: A review: Antimicrobial activity, uses and mechanism of action of glutaraldehyde. *J Appl Bacteriol* **48:**161–190, 1980

20. Pepper RE: Comparison of the activities and stabilities of alkaline glutaraldehyde sterilizing solutions. *Infect Control* **1:**90–92, 1980

21. Townsend TR et al: An efficacy evaluation of a synergized glutaraldehyde-phenate solution in disinfecting respiratory therapy equipment contaminated during patient use. *Infect Control* **3:**240–244, 1982

22. Sebben JE: Cold (tray) sterilization of hepatitis B virus. *J Am Acad Dermatol* **12:**718–719, 1985

23. Sherertz EF et al: Transfer of hepatitis B virus by contaminated reusable needle electrodes after electrodesiccation in simulated use. *J Am Acad Dermatol* **15:**1242–1246, 1986

24. Sebben JE: The hazards of electrosurgery (editorial). *J Am Acad Dermatol* **16:**869–872, 1987

25. Sebben JE: Blood vessel coagulation for incisional surgery. *J Dermatol Surg Oncol* **15:**1050–1053, 1989

26. Stoner JG et al: Penrose sleeve. *J Dermatol Surg Oncol* **9:**523–524, 1983

27. Young R, Walsh P: Sterilization of powered surgical instruments. *AORN J* **37:**945–953, 1983

28. Centers for Disease Control. Recommendations for prevention of HIV transmission in health care settings. *MMWR* **36:**1–18, 1987

29. Centers for Disease Control. Recommendations for prevention of HIV transmission in health care settings. *MMWR* **36**(suppl 25): 1987

30. Centers for Disease Control. Guidelines for prevention of transmission of HIV and HBV to health-care and public safety workers. *MMWR* **38**(suppl 6), 1989

31. Spire B et al: Inactivation of lymphadenopathy-associated virus by chemical disinfectants. *Lancet* **2:**899–901, 1984

32. Martin LS et al: Disinfection and inactivation of the human T lymphotropic virus type III/lymphadenopathy-associated virus. *J Infect Dis* **152**(2):400–403, 1985

33. Swisher BL, Ewing EP Jr.: Frozen Section Technique for Tissues Infected by the AIDS virus. *J. Histopathoc* **9:**29, 1986.

Mary E. Maloney

5 Infection Control

septic technique is a misnomer because it is impossible to render the patient or the environment sterile, as is implied by the term. The goal then is to decrease bacterial counts to as low a level as possible at the surgical site and to decrease or eliminate contamination from any other contact. This chapter is designed to identify potential sources of contamination and methods for avoidance of such contamination.

SKIN PREPARATION

The preparation of a surgical site is possibly the most important of all preoperative rituals. There exists what is termed *normal* or *resident flora,* and these bacteria are often credited with decreasing or holding down the numbers of pathogenic bacteria by competing for nutrients. These bacteria include Micrococcaceae (including *Staphylococcus epidermidis*), diphtheriods (including *Corynebacterium*), *Pityrosporum, Acinetobacter,* and *Propionibacterium.*[1] While each of these bacteria is considered to be of low "virulence," in sufficient numbers the bacteria may lead to wound infection, especially in the altered host.

Contaminating or *transient flora* include the organisms more commonly associated with wound infection. However, even some of these bacteria may be found "normally" in healthy patients. An example of this is *Staphylococcus aureus,* coagulase-positive, which can colonize the perineum or nose of 20 percent of healthy adults.[2] Such colonization can lead to infection with transfer of such bacteria to nonintact skin.

There are a number of conditions and medications which will alter the flora or rate of infection. Environmental conditions include a hot moist environment (which includes an occluded environment) and body location. Hospitalization itself increases colonization with pathogenic bacteria.[1] Diseases such as diabetes and HIV infection clearly affect host resistance. In one study, up to 76 percent of diabetic children were staphylococcus carriers as compared to 44 percent of nondiabetic children. The rate for staphylococcus carriers fell to 53 percent among insulin-dependent adult diabetics and 35 percent among non-insulin dependent diabetic adults, as compared to 34 percent among nondiabetic adults.[3] The need for insulin clearly affected this carrier state. Skin diseases such as the papulosquamous disorders, eczematous disorders, and bullous disorders may affect colonization. Medications may alter the resident or transient flora. These include antibiotics, retinoids, steroids, hormones, and immunosuppressive agents.

The list of conditions and medications affecting the flora or rate of infection is long, and surgeons need to be aware of the risk factors, especially should a wound infection occur. A low-risk patient with no known change in bacterial flora is not an excuse for inadequate surgical preparation. All patients must be approached as if wound infection is equally likely. This requires careful education of the entire surgical team.

SKIN PREPARATION AGENTS

In choosing an antiseptic skin-preparing agent, the surgeon wants one that has rapid onset of action, broad spectrum of action, prolonged action, and low skin irritation. There are a number of good, unrelated topical surgical preparatory agents available. The fact that these substances are unrelated allows alternatives, especially for the patient who develops an allergy.

Alcohols

Both ethyl and isopropyl alcohol are effective disinfectants when used in 70% to 90% concentrations. They act by denaturing proteins and thereby killing bacteria. While alcohol is very rapid in its onset of action, it must dry to be bactericidal. Studies do not outline the recommended method of applying alcohol,[4,5] but it does need to contact the skin fully and should be used after debris has been removed. A quick swipe followed by immediate initiation of surgery will not be sufficient. Alcohol may be superior to other agents in killing gram-negative bacteria, and it is virucidal for HIV and cytomegaloviruses.[6] It certainly compares favorably to other agents when used in an appropriate way.[4,5]

There are disadvantages to this inexpensive and generally effective antimicrobial agent. Alcohol is flammable and will ignite if cautery or laser equipment is used before the alcohol fully dries. This flammability also requires that alcohol not be stored in a location where it could be ignited by this equipment inadvertently. It is also not sporicidal and will kill only some of the fungi and viruses. It has no residual activity and does dry the skin with multiple applications.

Iodine and Iodophor

Iodine and iodophor act by releasing free iodine, which will penetrate the cell walls of microorganisms and lead to cell death. Release of free iodine and cellular uptake requires time, and several minutes of contact time are required for the antimicrobial activity to take place. Still this activity is considered to be relatively fast. Activity does not depend on the material's drying, and in fact drying ends the release of free iodine, ending any further activity. Because the activity of iodophor depends on continued release of iodine, wiping the solution from the skin preoperatively also ends its bactericidal activity. There is good activity against most bacteria.

There are disadvantages to this agent, as there are to all agents. Iodophor has some residual activity, but this is brief. The killing activity of this agent is neutralized by blood, or other organic material,[7] and is diminished if wiped away before the procedure is begun. This is a mechanical problem only for the surgeon who may find the tissue slippery or sticky with this preparatory agent in place. These agents are sensitizing in some individuals and are irritants to most. They are toxic to host cells as well as microorganisms and should not be used on open wounds.[8]

Chlorhexidine

Chlorhexidine is the newest agent for use as a topical antibacterial agent. It works by attacking the cell membranes, thereby causing cell death, and it has a rapid onset of action. One of the most important aspects of this agent is that it binds to the skin and maintains its activity for hours.[7] Activity of chlorhexidine is not decreased by the presence of alcohol, and there is a preparation which includes both alcohol and chlorhexidine. It is not degraded by organic materials and will not be systemically absorbed.

It can be ototoxic if instilled into the ear and can cause an irritant keratitis with corneal erosion and long-term corneal opacification if instilled into the eye. At very low concentration, chlorhexidine has been used as a disinfectant for soft contact lenses without any adverse effects. Ocular toxicity therefore appears to be related to concentration and contact time.[9] Complications of higher concentrations on preparatory agents with long exposure times can result in severe complications; thus, it is not worth the risk.

Other Agents

Hexachlorophene was for many years a popular topical antimicrobial. It is a chlorinated bisphenol which persists on the skin after application. Activity is additive with further applications. It is, however, absorbed percutaneously and can be demonstrated in the blood after a surgical scrub. In neonates, it will cross the blood-brain barrier, causing neurotoxicity. It has fallen to minor use after birth defects were found in fetuses whose pregnant mothers had used it for hand washing, and after toxicity in newborns led to the death of a number of infants.[10–12]

Benzalkonium chloride, a quaternium ammonium compound, has been used as an antiseptic. It is inactive against many of the gram-negative bacteria[13] but does have the benefit of being nonirritating to mucous membranes. It is easily contaminated in its container and can be a source of bacteria in those instances.

The final choice of skin antiseptic agent must depend on the location of the surgical site, the patient's sensitivities, the possible type of bacterial contamination, and the suspected length of the procedure. Several agents should be available to cover all situations.

SURGICAL SCRUBBING

Hand washing has reached art form in operating rooms, but it may be neglected when clinicians move from room to room to see patients in follow-up. Handling a contaminated wound of one patient may allow transfer of bacteria to another patient's wounds. Hands should be washed before handling a wound to prevent contamination of that patient and after handling the wound to prevent contamination of the next patient.

The method of hand washing and the antiseptic with which to wash has been much studied. Recommendations abound; however, knowledge of hand-washing methods and antiseptic preparations, in addition to common sense, is the best guide. Brief hand-washing with ordinary soap or even just tap water will remove recently acquired bacteria (i.e., bacteria acquired with a dressing change or a visit to the lavatory).[14] Preoperative hand-washing or scrubbing is very important in decreasing the bacterial load carried on the hands. The nail area carries up to 90 percent of organisms found on the hands.[15] Anything that mechanically improves cleaning of the nails will decrease the load of organisms. This includes keeping the nails short, avoiding artificial nails, and treating any periungual disorder that might harbor organisms. Jewelry also provides places where organisms may avoid removal, even with a good hand scrubbing. Rings and watches should be removed before hand-washing.

The goal of scrubbing is not only to remove all possible dirt, grease, and resident and transient bacteria,[16] but also to delay bacterial repopulation as long as possible. In this regard, an antiseptic solution that has prolonged activity is the best, depending on skin tolerance. Several studies have demonstrated the benefits of chlorhexidine over other agents. These benefits are probably related to the broad-spectrum activity of this agent as well as its prolonged activity.[13,19] It is important that whatever scrub is used does not cause a dermatitis that will harbor more organisms, creating a vicious circle.

The duration of the scrub has changed slowly over the years. A scrub of at least 7 min was originally recommended by Price in 1938.[17] This has now been shortened to a 2- to 4-min scrub. Some authors recommend a 4-min scrub before seeing the first patient, with subsequent 2-min scrubs,[18] while others feel a 2-min scrub is adequate, assuming attention is paid to the nail unit area.[20,21]

HAIR REMOVAL

Preoperative shaves were the standard for years; only more recently have practices changed. When razor shaving was compared to a depilatory or no hair removal, an infection rate of 5.6 percent was found in the razor group, while both the depilatory and no hair removal had an infection rate of 0.6 percent.[22] Another study showed that hair removal by clipping or shaving the evening before surgery or shaving the morning of surgery all had a significantly higher rate of wound infection compared to clipping hair the morning of surgery.[23]

Clearly, if hair removal is necessary, clipping the hair or using a depilatory just before surgery will be associated with the lowest postoperative infection rates. No hair removal was associated with just as low of an infection rate as depilatory use and can be recommended whenever possible.

GLOVES

Surgical gloves help protect the patient from bacterial contamination and protect the wearer from blood-borne diseases such as hepatitis B and HIV. Surgical gloves should never be viewed as a substitute for good hand washing.

Hand washing is imperative for decreasing microbial counts as described above. However, bacterial counts will increase again during the procedure due to the warm, moist environment. The longer the procedure, the greater will be the bacterial proliferation,[24] and therefore the greater the contamination will be if the glove is punctured.

The integrity of an unused glove is a very important consideration. Studies show that 1 to 3 percent of sterile gloves are not "intact" before the surgeon gloves.[25,26] This percentage may increase with the actual gloving procedure. Some defects may be easily noted, while others may not be visible but may still allow the movement of bacteria and fluids back and forth from patient and surgeon.

The failure rate of nonsterile gloves is significantly higher[26] and will depend in large part on the manufacturers and their level of quality control. Gloves that are difficult to put on may tear at that time, increasing risks of contamination.

The chance of glove perforation increases with the length of time required to complete the procedure.[27] Fingertips are the most likely site of perforation, probably because of the suturing needle, correlating nicely to the site of greatest bacterial growth. One should suspect a perforation, even if there is a small perceived prick that does not appear to have violated the integrity of the glove. Gloves should be changed for any suspected perforation, as cultures done on the inside of surgical gloves after the completion of a procedure have shown a significant incidence of S. aureus.[24] Despite the presence of bacteria on the surgeon's hands, perforation of the surgical glove has not been shown to lead to an increase in wound infection if appropriate action is taken when the perforation is noted.[28]

DRAPES

Drapes have multiple roles: they provide a sterile field on which the surgeon can work; instruments, gauze, and the sterile cautery handle can be placed on the drapes for convenient use; and sterilely gloved hands can be rested on them without contamination.

Drapes also prevent contamination of the prepared skin from surrounding skin or clothing. In this role, permeability is a factor. Drapes that are fluid-permeable can wick bacteria from underlying skin or clothing to the field itself.[29] Barriers that are impermeable will avoid that problem. Many surgeons prefer cotton towels because of their ease of use and their ready availability. If used, towels should be replaced as soon as they are contaminated by blood or fluids. Disposable drapes with a layer of plastic to prevent wicking of bacteria may be a better barrier. Some are very lightweight and move easily if not provided with an adhesive backing. If the drapes move out of the sterile field, their usefulness is greatly diminished.

Other benefits of drapes include protecting the patient's eyes from the bright operating lights when the patient is awake and surgery is being performed on the face. They may also keep the patient warm and in the outpatient setting protect the patient's clothing from surgical debris.

Overall, draping has not played a major role in causing or preventing wound infection,[5,28] although it will continue to be a part of the operative procedure.

UNIVERSAL PRECAUTIONS

There are two aspects of precautions aimed at control of blood-borne infections, especially HIV and hepatitis. The first is prevention of transmission from one patient to another, and the second is protection of the surgical team itself. The Centers for Disease Control and Prevention (CDC) couples these two issues under the single heading of "universal precautions."[30] A basic tenet of this is that all patients should be approached as if they were infected with HIV, hepatitis B, or other blood-borne pathogens. This means that universal precautions should be practiced for every patient.

Universal precautions as outlined by the CDC do not include contact with saliva, breast milk, urine, or feces unless these substances are grossly bloody.[31] Jackson and Lynch[32] expanded universal precautions in what they term "body substance isolation." In this set of recommendations, all contacts with fluids and mucous membranes fall within precaution recommendations.[32]

Many areas of precautions deserve special attention; each deserves monitoring by all staff. It is important for the surgeon to set the example of adherence to the guidelines and insist on compliance by the entire staff. Similarly, staff members must feel free to point out practices that do not meet the standards established. The entire team must work together in this important area.

Needle-sticks are clearly the most common risk that health care workers, especially surgical staffs, face.[33] Many surgeons find the recommendation for disposing all needles after use impractical; for example, local anesthetics may require supplementation throughout the procedure. Needle recapping is as dangerous (or possibly more dangerous) than leaving an uncapped needle on a tray. There are now several procedures for handling this problem. The first is a one-handed recapping technique. This is a safe and efficient method but requires some practice for dexterity. The cap is placed on the tray and the needle is threaded into the cap; the two are then tilted to "snap" the cap on fully and securely. There are several devices that can be placed on the sterile field into which uncapped needles may be placed. This leaves the needle in a safe location without the necessity for recapping. These devices can clutter the sterile tray. More recently, a sliding needle cap has been developed, allowing the cap to slide back to allow injection, and then it slides forward to cover the exposed needle when it is placed on the sterile tray. It should be an inviolate rule that no uncapped needle is left on the tray and that no needle is recapped with the two-handed method.

Eye protection has not been emphasized enough; this may be because it is an underestimated hazard.[34] Brearley and Buist[35] reported splashes on the glasses of the surgical team in 25 percent of procedures.[35] Many physicians still do not wear eye protection for surgical cases, and even fewer wear protection for simple procedures such as biopsies. It is not uncommon to get splash-back from local anesthesia injection through follicular structures or eroded skin.

Eye protection comes in many forms today. There are full plastic goggles, shields attached to masks, and more conventional glasses with the wraparound splash guards. Each member of the surgical team needs eye protection and should not be allowed at the operating table if protective eyewear is not in place.

Masks protect both patient and staff from droplet spread of disease. They also protect the nose and mouth from splashes of blood or other splash fluids (splashes of anesthesia from injection, etc.). Laser masks, with the ability to filter smaller particles, are necessary to protect the staff from smoke plumes.

Clothing should be specific for the operating room. This means that street clothes should not be worn. Such clothing not only can bring microorganisms into the surgical area, but can also become contaminated by blood or other fluids; therefore, street clothes can transfer contamination to other areas at work or at home. By the use of scrub suits, one eliminates the risk of clothing contamination adversely affecting the procedure. However, it does not prevent the shedding of bacteria from the surgical staff's skin. This shedding may occur from the open neck, sleeves, and pant legs or through the loose weave of the cloth itself.[36] To prevent any such contamination, a tight-weave, fluid-resistant gown must be worn. To date, there is no evidence that the use of such gowns affects infection rates for dermatologic surgery, and therefore scrub suits are appropriate for most dermatologic procedures.[37] However, if there is going to be extensive splashing such as with dermabrasion, gowning with fluid-resistant gowns is appropriate. Changing contaminated clothing should occur as soon as is practical and always before seeing another patient.

PROPHYLACTIC ANTIBIOTICS

The use of prophylactic antibiotics in selected patients is common. Use of such antibiotics must always be weighed against the risks of adverse reactions which include drug reactions, drug interactions, emergence of bacterial resistance, and even cost. There does not appear to be a role for antibiotic prophylaxis in uncomplicated cutaneous surgery on the otherwise completely healthy patient. Antibiotics should not be substituted for attention to sterile technique.

The risk of bacteremia with cutaneous surgery has been shown to be the greatest when the skin (or lesion to be removed) is ulcerated or clinically infected. The risk of bacteremia during skin surgery when the skin is intact and without clinical evidence of infection is exceedingly low.[38,39] The considerations for several subgroups of patients are not always clear cut. For example, total joint replacement can be complicated by late infection. The results of these late infections are costly and may be devastating. The mortality may reach 20 percent, and the permanent morbidity after a second prosthetic implanation may lead to joint fusion, an unstable joint, or even a chronic osteomyelitis.[40] The most common causative organisms are *S. aureus* and *S. epidermidis,* accounting for 50 percent of late infections of total hip replacements.[41] Patients with rheumatoid arthritis may have a risk as high as 4.2 times that of those patients whose joint was replaced for other reasons.[42]

Patients with valve replacement and known rheumatic heart disease are well recognized for being at risk of valvular infection following bacteremia. Complications of valvular infection are life threatening and clearly need to be prevented.

The question of who needs prophylaxis is not easy to answer. Patients at risk for seeded infections (those with total joint replacement, valve replacement, and rheumatic heart disease) should receive antimicrobial prophylaxis if there is surgery in a clearly contaminated or even an eroded tumor or if surgery will involve the mouth. Particular attention should be paid to identifying patients with a total joint replacement because of rheumatoid arthritis. They may be at higher risk of infection. Prophylaxis in other situations should be decided in conjunction with the patient's orthopedist, cardiologist, or general physician. Close communication is the key to good patient care.

The timing of antibiotic administration is key in its effectiveness as a prophylactic agent. The lowest incidence of surgical wound infections (0.6 percent) is seen when prophylaxis is administered preoperatively (0 to 2 h before the incision). Perioperative administration (within 3 h of the incision) yielded an incidence of 1.4 percent. Early preoperative (2 to 24 h before the incision) and postoperative (more than 3 h after the incision) administration had similar incidences of infection, 3.8 and 3.3 percent respectively.[43] When prophylaxis is chosen, it should be administered 0 to 2 h preoperatively and continued for 48 to 72 h.

OPERATING ROOM PROTOCOL

Operating room protocol should always be geared toward patient and staff protection (Table 5-1). The entire staff should stay attuned to new techniques and equipment and always be ready to try new methods. Everyone should be vigilant to adhering to protocol and changing that protocol when some aspect is not working. Constant attention is needed for both the patient's and the staff's sake.

Much of the protocol will be tailored to a specific office, procedure, or patient. The staff needs to be familiar with all of the variables and adjust them appropriately. For this reason, frequent staffing changes may be very disruptive and increase risks to all.

The basics of protocol are simple common sense coupled with a knowledge of aseptic technique. A patient history is imperative to identify any allergies, particularly allergies to antiseptics. The surgical site must be adequately exposed to allow access for an adequate preparation and the procedure itself. It is impossible to prepare a patient through a tiny "window" of clothing. The skin preparation must be performed

TABLE 5-1

Operating Room Protocol

Patient history to identify risks, medicines, allergies

Surgical site adequately exposed

Skin preparation performed

Sterile drape applied

Surgical team properly attired

Hand washing performed

Team gloved without contamination

Procedure performed without contamination or contaminated material discarded

Drapes disposed properly

Sharps discarded in appropriate containers

Gloves and other contaminated material disposed immediately and appropriately

Room appropriately cleaned before next patient

within a large enough field to allow tissue movement and undermining. It must also be performed before the area is draped, and the surgeon must not contaminate the site by touching it after the preparation has occurred. The surgical team must enter the surgical area properly attired, and good hand washing must be done by the entire team before gloves are donned. The procedure should be done without contamination, but, more importantly, if contamination occurs, corrective action should be taken immediately. A punctured glove should be replaced as should a wet drape. Blood-contaminated clothing should be changed as soon as possible. The surgical tray and field should both be kept clean of saturated gauze, dirty swabs, or other debris. As soon as the procedure is completed, drapes should be disposed of properly and the "sharps" placed in the appropriate containers. Gloves should be removed before any clean surface is touched. This means that soiled gloves should be removed, the dressing material gathered, and then the nurse should reglove to dress the wound. The only exception should be if the dressing material is already on the surgical tray. Lastly, the room should be appropriately cleaned before the next patient is brought to the room.

In the above outline for operating room protocol, there are many areas that require close attention, and reminders should be given to the staff involved. Protocol is such an important area that all staff should constantly monitor the procedures and look for possible sites of contamination.

REFERENCES

1. Roth RR, James WD: Microbiology of the skin: Resident flora ecology infection. *J Am Acad Dermatol* **20**:367–390, 1989

2. Emmerson AM: The role of the skin in nosocomial infection: A review. *J Chemother* **1**:12–18, 1989

3. Smith JA, O'Connor JJ: Nasal carriage of Staphylococcus aureus in diabetes mellitus. *Lancet* **2**:776–777, 1966

4. Davies J et al: Disinfection of the skin of the abdomen. *Br J Surg* **65**:855–858, 1978

5. Cruse PJE, Foord R: The epidemiology of wound infection. *Surg Clin North Am* **60**:27–40, 1980

6. Hobbs E: Surgical microbiology, antibiotic prophylaxis, and antiseptic technique, in *Cutaneous Surgery,* edited by Wheeland, R.G. Philadelphia, PA, WB Saunders Co., 1994, pp 64–75

7. Brown TR et al: A clinical evaluation of chlorhexidine gluconate spray as compared with iodophor scrub for preoperative skin preparation. *Surg Gynecol Obstet* **158**:363–366, 1984

8. Lineaweaver W et al: Topical antimicrobial toxicity. *Arch Surg* **120**:267–270, 1985

9. Nasser RE: The ocular danger of Hibiclens. *Plast Reconstr Surg* **89**:164–165, 1992

10. Check W: New study shows hexachlorophene is teratogenic in humans. *JAMA* **240**:513–514, 1978

11. Shuman RM et al: Neurotoxicity of hexachlorophene in the human: A clinicopathologic study of 46 premature infants, pt 2. *Arch Neurol* **342**:320–325, 1975

12. Powell H et al: Hexachlorophene myelinopathy in premature infants. *J Pediatr* **82**:976–981, 1973

13. Sebben JE: Sterile technique and the prevention of wound infection in office surgery, pt 2. *J Dermatol Surg Oncol* **15**:38–48, 1989

14. Sprunt K et al: Antibacterial effectiveness of routine hand washing. *Pediatrics* **52**:264–271, 1973

15. Maley MP: Extend handwashing to the forearms? *Am J Nurs* **89**:1437, 1989

16. Lowburg EJL: Skin disinfection. *J Clin Pathol* **14**:85–90, 1961

17. Price PB: The bacteriology of normal skin: A new quantitative test applied to a study of the bacterial flora and the disinfectant action of mechanical cleansing. *J Infect Dis* **63**:301–318, 1938

18. Aly R, Maibach HI: Comparative antibacterial efficacy of a 2-minute surgical scrub with chlorhexidine gluconate, povodine-iodine, and chloroxylenol sponge-brushes. *Am J Infect Control* **16**:173–177, 1988

19. Smylie HD et al: From pHisoHex to Hibiscrub. *Br Med J* **4**:586–589, 1973

20. O'Shaughnessy M et al: Optimum duration of surgical scrub time. *Br J Surg* **78**:685–686, 1991

21. Masterson BJ: Skin preparation. *Clin Obstet Gynecol* **31**:736–743, 1988

22. Seropian R, Reynolds BM: Wound infections after preoperative depilatory versus razor preparation. *Am J Surg* **121**:251–254, 1971

23. Alexander JW et al: The influence of hair removal methods on wound infection. *Arch Surg* **118**:347–352, 1983

24. Burke JF: Identification of the sources of staphylococcus contaminating the surgical wound during operation. *Ann Surg* **158**:898–904, 1963

25. Yangco BG, Yangco NF: What is leaky can be risky: A study of the integrity of hospital gloves. *Infect Control Hosp Epidemiol* **10**:553–556, 1989

26. Korniewicz DM et al: Integrity of vinyl and latex procedure gloves. *Nurs Res* **38**:144–146, 1989

27. Nakazawa M et al: Incidence of perforations on rubber gloves during ophthalmologic surgery. *Ophthalmic Surg* **15**:236–240, 1984

28. Sawyer RG, Pruett JL: Wound infections. *Surg Clin North Am* **74**:519–536, 1994

29. Whyte W: The role of clothing and drapes in the operating room. *J Hosp Infect* **11**:2–17, 1988

30. CDC. Update: Universal precautions for prevention of transmission of human immunodeficiency virus, hepatitis B virus, and other bloodborne pathogens in health-care settings. *MMWR* **37**:377–382, 387–388, 1988

31. Lynch P et al: Implementing and evaluating a system of generic infection precautions: Body substance isolation. *Am J Infect Control* **18**:1–12, 1990

32. Jackson M, Lynch P: An attempt to make an issue less murky: A comparison of four systems for infection prevention. *Infect Control Hosp Epidemiol* **12**:48–49, 1991

33. CDC. Update: Acquired immunodeficiency syndrome and human immunodeficiency virus infection among health-care workers. *MMWR* **37**:229–239, 1988

34. Vaughn RY et al: HIV and the dermatologic surgeon. *J Dermatol Surg Oncol* **16**:1107–1110, 1990

35. Brearley S, Buist L: Blood splashes: An underestimated hazard to surgeons. *Br Med J [Clin Res]* **299**:1315, 1989

36. Ritter MA, Marmion P: The exogenous sources and controls of microorganisms in the operating room. *Orthop Nurs* **7**:23–28, 1988

37. Bennet RG: Microbiologic considerations in cutaneous surgery, in *Fundamentals of Cutaneous Surgery.* St. Louis, Mo, Mosby, 1988, pp 136–178

38. Sabetta JB, Zitelli JA: The incidence of bacteremia during skin surgery. *Arch Dermatol* **123**:213–214, 1987

39. Zack L et al: The incidence of bacteremia after skin surgery. *J Infect Dis* **159**:148–149, 1989

40. Blackburn WD, Alarcon GS: Prosthetic joint infections. *Arthritis Rheum* **34**:110–117, 1991

41. Cioffi GA et al: Total joint replacement: A consideration for antimicrobial prophylaxis. *Oral Surg Oral Med Oral Pathol* **66**:124–129, 1988

42. Maderazo EG et al: Late infections of total joint prostheses: A review and recommendations for prevention. *Clin Orthop* **229**:131–142, 1988

43. Classen DC et al: The timing of prophylactic administration of antibiotics and the risk of surgical wound infection. *N Engl J Med* **326**:281–286, 1992

Seth L. Matarasso and Richard G. Glogau

6 Local Anesthesia

Cutaneous surgery is fast becoming routine in the practice and teaching of dermatology. Oncologic, reconstructive, and aesthetic surgery now supplement the ranks of simple procedures. However, prior to undertaking surgery, the obvious—anesthesia—must not be overlooked.

The word *anesthesia* was reputedly coined in 1846 by Oliver Wendell Holmes, who combined the Greek terms *without perception* to signify the absence of perception by the senses. Anesthesia thus is simply the loss of sensation, and local anesthesia is the temporary and circumscribed absence of pain without affecting vital functions.

While the selection and proper administration of anesthetic agents are important parts of dermatologic surgery, it is no longer sufficient to simply reduce the physical pain, but similarly the perception of pain must be addressed. Administration of anesthesia and discomfort and anxiety levels contribute to the patient's cooperation during the procedure and willingness to participate in future surgery. Toward this end, it is important to establish a good rapport, establish a trusting atmosphere, and ensure that the patient comprehends the procedure and has realistic expectations. The patient must then appreciate that whether surgery is medically indicated or elective, he or she must be psychologically prepared for the procedure in advance and realize that adequate anesthesia will be obtained. Assuring patients that the procedure will not commence until a satisfactory level of anesthesia has been achieved is important. As well, patients should be aware that the sensations of pulling and pressure will not be relieved with local anesthesia. Explaining this in simple language and occasionally showing the instrumentation will help to allay fears. Similarly, a nonthreatening environment, preoperative medication, and topical anesthetics are also useful in administering local anesthesia.

ENVIRONMENT

The patient's physical comfort is an important consideration when the physician administers local anesthesia. Head support, a semireclining position, flexed knees, and loosening or removal of constricting garments can contribute greatly to the patient's comfort. When one is operating on the face, direct lighting on the eyes can be uncomfortable and can be avoided by placing moistened gauze sponges on closed eyes. Music, preferably of the patient's choice, is also quite soothing and also masks operative noises like those made during suctioning, curettage, or procedures on bone. For procedures around the ear, cotton placed in the ear canal absorbs any drainage and dulls operative noises.

PREOPERATIVE MEDICATIONS

Patients with a high degree of anxiety or who are to undergo a lengthy procedure will often require ancillary preoperative medication. Although these agents are not intended to completely eliminate all pain, they are helpful in calming the patient sufficiently to allow for the smooth induction of local anesthesia. Given roughly 30 min prior to the procedure, preoperative medications should ideally decrease anxiety without making the patient unduly drowsy, relieve pain, and produce some degree of anesthesia. They should, however, not be used in lieu of patient-physician communication.

It is crucial to document the patient's medications, allergies, medical history, and a review of systems (inclusive of last menstrual period). The elderly, and patients with hepatorenal, thyroid, and central nervous system diseases, and those with anemia can be quite sensitive to low doses of medications. Conversely, patients who smoke, regularly take

TABLE 6-1

Preanesthetic Medications*

Hypnotics

    Barbiturates

        Phenobarbital/Luminal

    Antihistamines

        Diphenhydramine/Benadryl

        Hydroxyzines/Atarax or Vistaril

    Promethazine/Phenergan

Tranquilizers

    Benzodiazepines

        Diazepam/Valium

        Flurazepam/Dalmane

        Midazolam/Versed

        Chlordiazepoxide hydrochloride/Librium

        Alprazolam/Xanax

    Phenothiazines

        Prochlorperazine/Compazine

        Trifluoperazine/Stelazine

Narcotics

    Morphine

    Meperidine/Demerol

    Hydromorphone/Dilaudid

    Fentanyl/Sublimaze

* Drug dosing depends upon patient age, weight, sex, physical and psychological condition, and procedure to be performed.

sedatives, consume alcohol, or are extremely apprehensive often require higher doses. The choice of medication should not only be determined by the medical status of the patient but should also be determined by the type and duration of the procedure, the surgeon's degree of comfort in administering systemic medications, and the emergency and resuscitative equipment available. It is often wiser and safer to err conservatively and undermedicate with the flexibility for supplemental medication.

If the physician anticipates using preoperative anesthesia that may dull the sensorium, it is wise to have a responsible adult available for the patient's transportation and an area for postoperative recovery. Establishing intravenous access is generally not necessary; however, it is a good safety measure when narcotics and other powerful medications are to be administered.

There are three basic categories of preoperative medications (see Table 6-1). In general, the hypnotics produce drowsiness, the tranquilizers have a calming effect, and the narcotics relieve pain. [Naloxone (Narcan), a narcotic antagonist, should be readily available whenever narcotics are used parenterally.] There is occasionally overlap between groups and no clear-cut distinction between pharmacologic action.

INHALANTS

Physician-supervised inhalant analgesics such as Methoxyflurane and nitrous oxide are advantageous over other preoperative medications in their rapidity of action, short half-life, and potential for modulation. They are quite helpful in preparing patients for local anesthesia, especially when there is a fear of needles. Patients experience an intoxicated lethargic-like state and become less aware of their surroundings. There is less perception of pain and decreased anxiety, and yet patients are fully communicative and vital signs are preserved.

Methoxyflurane (Penthrane) is a fluorinated ether that is a colorless liquid with a pungent fruity odor. It is nonflammable and nonexplosive and volatile when exposed to air. Its preparation is simple: 2 to 3 mm of Penthrane saturates a felt wick within a lightweight cylindric hand-held analgizer. The patient intermittently inhales the fumes until feeling lightheaded. The analgizer can be periodically refilled until the degree of analgesia required is achieved (Fig. 6-1).

Methoxyflurane induces both gradual analgesia and, with discontinuation, a prompt return to baseline. Patients experi-

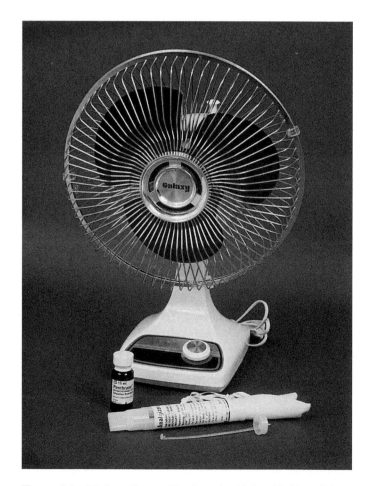

Figure 6-1 Methoxyflurane (Penthrane) with hand-held analgizer (Abbott Laboratories, Chicago, Illinois), portable fan, and tubing for disposal of vapors.

ence no hangover and are quickly capable of resuming normal daily activities. It is well tolerated and has a high margin of safety. Idiosyncratitic hepatic toxicity and dose-related nephrotoxicity have been reported; thus, patients with a history of hepatorenal dysfunction are not suitable candidates. Self-administration produces discontinuous anesthesia which lowers the probability of untoward problems—but it should not be delivered for more than 4 h, and the maximum dose for one session is 15 mL. Further, this agent can cause a loss of the gag reflex, and, with emesis, aspiration can occur. The solution and products exhaled by the patient can be noxious to the staff, and adequate ventilation is important.

Nitrous oxide (N_2O), first used in 1844 by Priestly, is still one of the most frequently administered anesthetic agents. It is an inert colorless inorganic gas with a fruity odor and is nonflammable and nonexplosive. The equipment, separate and clearly identified tanks for pure oxygen and nitrous oxide, tubing, and nasal masks, should be professionally installed and routinely monitored.

The patient accommodates to the mask by breathing pure oxygen. The physician gradually adds and increases the concentration of nitrous oxide. The recommended flow rates for nitrous oxide and oxygen are 1 to 2 L per min. The effects of nitrous oxide are a function of its concentration.

Because of its low blood gas solubility, nitrous oxide has a rapid onset and emergence. Usually after 3 to 4 min of breathing a nitrous oxide-oxygen mixture of 30 to 60 percent, the desired level of analgesia is produced. The physician can titrate the depth and duration of analgesia to the patient's pain threshold. Once analgesia is established, the flow rates are generally maintained. Large volumes (20 to 30 L) of nitrous oxide are taken up during the course of the procedure. At the conclusion, the patient should breathe 100 percent oxygen to flush out the nitrous oxide from the blood and lungs to prevent dizziness and light-headedness.

The use of nitrous oxide for outpatient surgery has not been associated with many problems, and most are readily reversible with lowering the concentration of nitrous oxide and administration of pure oxygen. Occasionally, patients become nauseated and vomit, but the risk of aspiration is minimal as the gag reflex is maintained. Irritability, restlessness, and hypermobility are evidence that the level of anesthesia is becoming too deep. It is a mild myocardial depressant and a cerebral vasodilator, and it can diffuse into air-containing cavities. The bowel can become distended, pneumothoraces and cerebral ventricular air pockets can become enlarged, and air emboli are possible. Patients with impaired respiratory response with pulmonary disease, or those who have taken sedatives or alcohol, or those who have a history of myocardial ischemia are contraindicated.

While the toxicity and safety of nitrous oxide are well documented, the occupational exposure risks have not been well defined. There is some evidence of nitrous oxide-induced neuropathy with numbness, tingling, and muscular weakness. Screening devices, scavenging masks, and properly maintained equipment reduce atmosphere pollution. As with any chemical or drug, pregnant women or women wishing to become pregnant should avoid exposure.

SURFACE ANESTHESIA

In either of its two forms, aerosol or topical, anesthesia of the superficial epithelium is important as a sole agent to remove isolated lesions and as an adjunct to decrease patient discomfort and anxiety prior to the physician's injecting a local anesthesia. From the surgeon's perspective, they are important as they do not distort tissue and resting skin tension lines and therefore allow for optimal surgical planning.

CRYOANESTHESIA

Cryoanesthesia has a similar mechanism of action as local anesthetics—it blocks pain fibers, then thermal fibers, and lastly tactile fibers. In its purest form, cryoanesthesia simply with the use of ice has been practiced for hundreds of years and is still a viable modality today. Ten seconds of ice applied with pressure will provide roughly 2 s of anesthesia.

The commercially available refrigerants (see Table 6-2) are still popular; however, there is increasing concern over their detrimental effects on the ozone layer. The sprays are directed toward the skin from a distance of 4 to 6 in until the skin frosts. The anesthetic effect will last 10 to 15 s after the frost disappears. When using any of these sprays, it is important that all those present shield both their eyes and avoid inhaling large quantities. Atrophic scarring, temporary sensory nerve damage, and pigmentation (hypo- and hyperpigmentation) have been reported when extreme cold has been used for lengthy periods of time.

It is not always necessary to use one of the commercial aerosol preparations. The same effect may be achieved with liquid nitrogen. Although its lower temperatures may cause more immediate and greater postoperative discomfort, paint-

T A B L E   6 - 2

Refrigerants

Ethyl chloride

Frigiderm [dichlorotetrafluoroethane (Freon 114)]

Fluoro Ethyl (25% ethyl chloride and 75% dichlorotetrafluoroethane)

CryOsthesia ($-30°C$ and $-60°C$)

Aerofreeze [dichlorodifluoromethane (Freon 12) and trichlorofluoromethane (Freon 11)]

CryoKwik

MediFrig [dichlorodifluoromethane (Freon 12)]

Liquid nitrogen

ing the area with a cotton swab as opposed to a spray may diminish these untoward effects.

TOPICAL ANESTHETICS

On intact skin, topical cream anesthetics diffuse slowly and penetrate to the papillary dermis, providing anesthesia to pinprick in roughly 3 h. With occlusive dressings or on an abraded surface with a denuded epithelial barrier, there is more effective penetration. However, care should be exercised when applying topical anesthesia to severely traumatized mucosa and over large areas where rapid systemic absorption can parallel intravenous dosing and precipitate toxicity. When mucosal surfaces are anesthetized, reflexes—both corneal and gag—can be impaired for up to 30 min. Patients should be observed until normal function returns.

Derived from the leaves of *Erythroxylon cocoa,* cocaine was the first topical anesthetic. It is the only local anesthetic with vasoconstrictive properties and is thus advantageous in vascular areas such as the mucous membranes of the nasal cavity. Cotton balls saturated with a 3% to 4% solution provide anesthesia in 2 to 5 min and last as long as 30 to 45 min. The maximal safe dose is 200 mg (10 mL of 2% solution). Due to its many potential systemic side effects, cocaine has largely been replaced with other agents for topical anesthetic.

Available in many forms and ranging from 5% to 20%, benzocaine is an effective anesthetic that provides anesthesia for several hours on mucosal surfaces. Despite a high incidence of contact sensitization, benzocaine is still commercially available as a 20% gel or aerosol and a 2.5% to 20% solution. Catacaine, an aerosol containing 14% benzocaine, 2% butylaminobenzoate, and 2% tetracaine, produces anesthesia of mucosal surfaces in 30 s.

Tetracaine 0.5% solution will provide anesthesia of the mucous membranes for up to 45 min. A mixture of tetracaine 0.5%, adrenaline 1:2000, and cocaine 11.8% in normal saline (TAC solution) provides both anesthesia and vasoconstrictive activity. Tetracaine does have potential toxicity (maximum dosage 50 mg) and cross-reacts with benzocaine.

Topical lidocaine has been used effectively as both a mucosal and cutaneous anesthetic. Available as a 2% jelly or viscous solution, 2.5% to 5% ointment, 4% nonviscous solution, and as a 10% aerosol, it can provide reliable topical anesthesia on mucosal surfaces within 15 to 30 min, with an approximate duration of action of 15 min. It is readily available, inexpensive, easy to apply, and safe. It has been recommended that the maximum dosage of 30 mL or 600 mg of 2% lidocaine jelly should not be exceeded in 12 h. If vasoconstriction is desired, lidocaine can be combined with phenylephrine (Neo-Synephrine), which is available as a 0.5% solution or jelly. Specially compounded 30% lidocaine in an acid mantle cream has been recommended for skin surfaces. This, however, can be unpredictable and often requires lengthy occlusion to ensure adequate penetration and successful anesthesia.

Lidocaine 2.5% has been combined with 2.5% prilocaine to form a eutectic mixture of local anesthetic (EMLA), an oil and water emulsion cream. It is optimally effective by degreasing the skin and applying the cream under occlusion for 30 to 60 min; it induces superficial cutaneous vasoconstriction and anesthesia to pinprick. EMLA cream has been found to be nontoxic and produces low plasma levels. It has recently been approved by the U.S. Food and Drug Administration, and is available from Astra Pharmaceutical (Oslo, Sweden).

OPHTHALMIC ANESTHETICS

Local anesthetics prepared for injection often produce a burning sensation when placed on the conjunctival surface. For this reason, ophthalmic preparations are specially recommended for topical anesthesia.

Proparacaine 0.5% hydrochloride (Ophthaine, Ophthetic) solution is useful for procedures around the eyes. One or two drops instilled into the conjunctival sac provide a momentary sting followed by rapid absorption and anesthesia that lasts up to 30 min. Manipulation around the eye, including insertion of a corneal shield, is greatly enhanced as the blink reflex is diminished. If one is not using a shield, it is important that extreme care be taken to avoid damage to the cornea. Other topical eye preparations include 0.5% tetracaine (Pontocaine) and 0.4% benoxinate (Dorsacaine).

IONTOPHORESIS

Iontophoresis, introducing ionized particles into the tissues through an electric current, has also been successfully employed as a method of achieving anesthesia without the pain of injection and distortion of tissues. However, iontophoresis of local anesthetics has not gained widespread popularity as it requires the purchase of a special current-controlled electrical system, is short lived, and is time consuming to perform.

LOCAL ANESTHETICS

For the majority of procedures in cutaneous surgery, local injectable anesthetics are ideal. They are a class of compounds that is inexpensive, readily available, requires minimal equipment, and is easy to administer. In addition, their effects are quickly felt, they are relatively free of side effects, and their lack of effect on the patient's sensorium makes them suitable for ambulatory procedures.

Mechanism of Action

Local anesthetic agents interfere with the ionic gradient of the nerve membrane by decreasing membrane permeability to sodium, thereby preventing the action potential from reaching the threshold level required for depolarization. This results in temporary blockage of electrical conduction in the nerve fiber. Proposed mechanisms of action include a specific receptor binding versus nonspecific membrane absorption. Diffusion of anesthetics across the axoplasm depends in part on the diameter of the nerve fiber. Thus small unmyelinated fibers carrying pain and temperature are readily blocked, and large myelinated fibers that carry sensations of touch, vibration, and pressure are least affected. Therefore, it is important to warn the patients that they may feel pressure and pull despite the lack of pain.

Structure and Classification of Local Anesthetics

The molecular structure of local anesthetics consists of a hydrophilic molecule (amine) linked to a hydrophobic aromatic residue by either an intermediate ester or an amide group (Fig. 6-2). The amine portion is responsible for the water solubility properties and in the charged cationic form binds with the nerve cell membrane receptors. The aromatic portion is lipophilic and is responsible for its interaction with the highly lipid nerve membrane. Increasing the lipid solubility of the anesthetic increases the anesthetic potency, and increasing the

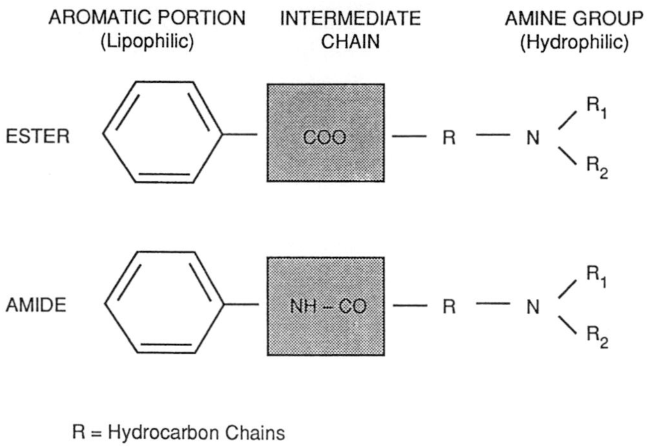

Figure 6-2 Basic structure of ester- and amide-type local anesthetics.

affinity for the protein receptors increases the duration. Therefore, an alteration in either end of the compound will change both the lipid solubility and protein-binding activity.

Local anesthetics are subdivided into ester and amide classes based upon the structural linkage of the intermediate chain (see Table 6-3). Ester-type local anesthetics have an es-

TABLE 6-3

Common Local Anesthetics

Generic (trade) name	Concentration available (%)	Potency	Approx. onset (min.)	Approx. duration (min.) W/O epi*	W epi†	Maximum dose (mg)
Esters **(plasma metabolism)**						
Cocaine	2–10 (topical)	High	Rapid	45	N/A	200
Procaine (Novocain)	0.5, 1.0, 2.0	Low	Rapid (5)	15–45	30–90	600–1000
Chloroprocaine (Nesacaine)	0.5, 1.0, 2.0	Mid	Rapid (5–6)	30–60	N/A	600–1000
Tetracaine (Pontocaine)	0.1, 0.25 (0.5 ophthalmic)	High	(7)	120–140	240–480	100
Amides **(hepatic metabolism)**						
Lidocaine (Xylocaine)	0.5, 1.0, 2.0 (2.0, 5.0 ophthalmic)	Intermed	Rapid (5)	30–120	60–400	300–500
Mepivacaine (Carbocaine)	1.0, 2.0	Intermed	Rapid (3–5)	30–120	60–400	300–500
Prilocaine (Citanest)	1.0, 2.0, 3.0	Intermed	Rapid (5–6)	30–120	60–400	600
Bupivacaine (Marcaine/Sensorcaine)	0.25, 0.5, 0.75	High	Mod (8)	120–140	240–480	150–250
Etidocaine (Duranest)	0.5, 1.0	High	Rapid (3–5)	200	240–360	300–400

* W/O epi = without epinephrine.

† W epi = with epinephrine.

ter linkage at the intermediate chain and share a similar metabolic fate. The anesthetic quality and potential toxicity of these agents have an inverse correlation to the rate of hydrolysis; those with slow hydrolysis exert longer duration and more potential toxicity. They are generally metabolized rapidly by plasma pseudocholinesterase to yield paraaminobenzoic acid (PABA) and diethyl-amino ethanol (DEAE) which are excreted by the kidneys. Patients who have a genetic deficiency in plasma pseudocholinesterase and thus an inability to degrade the anesthesia experience an elevation in blood levels and toxicity. Further, patients who have been sensitized to PABA may develop an allergic reaction to this group of anesthetics (see "Adverse Reactions" below). The most common ester-type local anesthetics include procaine, chloroprocaine, tetracaine, and cocaine.

Procaine (Novocain) was synthesized by Einhorn in 1905 and is the prototype for this group of agents. Although it has a rapid onset of action, it is rapidly hydrolyzed and therefore has a short duration and a high safety profile. It is contraindicated in patients who are allergic to PABA or procaine penicillin.

Chloroprocaine (Nesacaine) is slightly more potent than procaine. It, too, has a rapid onset of action, but, as it is the most rapidly hydrolyzed, it produces the shortest duration of action of the local anesthetics. It is used in patients who are quite ill and for very short surgical procedures. Blood levels do not rise significantly, making it also a drug of choice during pregnancy.

Tetracaine (Pontocaine) is hydrolyzed slowly and is the longest-acting ester compound and consequently has a high potential for toxicity.

Cocaine has its greatest utility as a topical surface anesthetic, particularly for procedures involving the mucosal surfaces of the nose or mouth. It is no longer available for internal use because of systemic side effects.

Amide anesthetics are metabolized by hepatic microsomal enzymes and have a longer duration of action. Patients with liver disease may have a reduced tolerance to this class of agents and are at an increased risk of systemic toxicity. Unlike the esters, the amides are generally not associated with allergic reactions and are considered safer than the ester-type anesthetics.

Lidocaine has a rapid onset and a long duration and has become the most common local anesthetic currently in use. It is effective both topically on mucous membranes (see "Topical Anesthetics" above) as well as in the injected form. The injectable form can be purchased in multiuse vials from 0.5% to 1% with or without epinephrine and up to 2% for nerve blocks.

It has been reported that mepivacaine (Carbocaine) has a more rapid onset and longer duration than lidocaine. However, the main advantages are its lower potential for toxicity and therefore the ability to use larger amounts of anesthesia.

Bupivacaine (Marcaine) is more potent and potentially more toxic than lidocaine. Due to a slower onset and longer duration, it is very useful both for nerve blocks (lasting up to 4 h) and when used adjunctively with other shorter acting injectable agents. Less free drug is available to cross the placenta and makes bupivacaine another drug of choice during pregnancy.

When compared to lidocaine, mepivacaine has a more rapid onset and longer duration and prilocaine slower onset and a longer duration. However, these differences are not great enough to warrant their widespread use.

Etidocaine (Duranest), introduced in 1973, is the newest amide local anesthetic. It has a short onset of action, and a longer duration, and is quite potent without a dramatic increase in toxicity. These advantages may prove ideal when a long procedure is planned and when epinephrine cannot be used.

Addition of Vasoconstriction and Neutralizing Agents

With the exception of cocaine, all local anesthetics produce vascular smooth muscle relaxation. This results in vasodilation which enhances the drug absorption and a concomitant decrease in amount of active drug at the site of injection. The addition of vasoconstrictors, usually epinephrine [alternatives are phenylephrine (Neo-Synephrine), levonordefrin (Neo-Cobefrin), and norepinephrine (Levophed)], restricts the anesthesia to the area in which it is placed and thus decreases absorption and toxicity while increasing duration of anesthesia. Since it slows the rate of systemic absorption and allows the body more time to metabolize the anesthesia, greater amounts of anesthesia can be injected when epinephrine is used.

Many local anesthetics are commercially available premixed with epinephrine usually at a concentration of 1:100,000 (1 mg/100 mL). Some practitioners, however, recommend freshly preparing the anesthesia with epinephrine as a higher pH is obtained, and there is less patient discomfort upon injection. For instance, combining 0.3 mL of 1:1000 epinephrine in a standard 30 mL lot of lidocaine will yield a concentration of 1:100,000. Increasing the concentration of epinephrine is not more advantageous and only increases the risk of tissue necrosis because of prolonged ischemia. Conversely, decreasing the concentration (1:200,000) appears to provide sufficient vasoconstriction for most dermatologic procedures.

The initial effect of vasoconstrictors is actually a brief vasodilation. Although the intradermal injection of lidocaine results in almost immediate anesthesia, the vasoconstrictor properties begin after a few minutes and are not at full effect until 15 min. Vasoconstriction is recognized clinically by the blanching of the overlying skin which at a later time may be followed by cyanosis. The blanching and anesthesia are not always congruent and pinprick tests should be made to ensure adequate anesthesia.

A stabilizer to prolong the shelf life is added to the stock solution of lidocaine, which slightly acidifies it (pH 3.3 to 5.5) and causes stinging on injection. The addition of 8.4% sodium bicarbonate in a ratio of 1 sodium bicarbonate/10 epinephrine 1:100,000 or 1 sodium bicarbonate/15 epinephrine 1:100,000 alkalizes the acidic pH to a natural physiologic 7.4 and attenuates the discomfort. Buffered solution can only be maintained with acceptable stability for 2 weeks if kept refrigerated.

Adverse Reactions

Local anesthetics are generally very safe drugs. Although it is rare for the dermatologist to encounter toxicity or adverse reactions, it is wise for the physician to be well versed in normal sequelae and complications and their respective treatments.

Reactions to anesthesia, like those to all drugs, may be classified as either localized or generalized. Local adverse reactions are usually temporary and attributable to injection technique. Ecchymosis and hematoma formation can occur if the patient has a bleeding diathesis, is taking anticoagulants, or there is a laceration of a blood vessel. In addition, once the effect of epinephrine has worn off, there is a further risk of bleeding, and meticulous hemostasis should be undertaken. Albeit rare, and usually associated with peripheral nerve blocks, laceration of the nerve can result in permanent nerve damage. (Loss of motor function and sensation due to diffusion of anesthesia is common and temporary.) Infection with abscess formation has been reported and is invariably due to improper sterile technique.

True allergic reactions to ester-type local anesthetics have occurred, but those attributed to amides are extremely rare. Many of the reactions occurring with the use of ester compounds have been attributed to the added preservatives (parabens). This group of local antibacterials is routinely added to multidose vials of anesthesia and cross-reacts with PABA, the major metabolite of the esters (single-dose vials are labeled "preservative free"). Most reactions occurring with the use of amide anesthetics are due to epinephrine side effects or to a vasovagal response. If a true allergic reaction is suspected, intradermal injections of saline or diphenhydramine (Benadryl) will often provide brief but excellent anesthesia for small procedures.

As with local adverse reactions, systemic toxicity is uncommon. Although local anesthetics are administered and have their greatest effect regionally, they are absorbed and can affect distant organ systems.

Toxic reactions usually can occur with low blood levels (allergic or idiosyncratic response); however, most occur when high blood levels are reached. High blood levels usually result from overdosage during lengthy procedures, rapid absorption upon injection into highly vascular areas over a short period of time, or inadvertent injection into a blood vessel. Elevated blood levels can also occur when metabolism of the anesthetic is impaired (hepatic or renal disease). The maximum amount of lidocaine that can be safely injected at one time for adults is 7.5 mg/kg, 500 mg total (50 mL) with epinephrine, and 4.5 mg/kg, 300 mg total (30 mL) without epinephrine.

The toxicity guidelines for lidocaine are expanded when discussing the tumescent or wet technique for liposuction surgery. An estimate of a safe lidocaine dose with this technique has been found to be 35 mg/kg, much higher than the recommended dose for lidocaine in "normal healthy adults." This higher safety profile is due to both the slow rate of absorption from relatively avascular subcutaneous adipose and the diluted concentration of the anesthesia (0.1% to 0.05% lidocaine and 1:1,000,000 epinephrine). (See Table 6-4.)

The central nervous and cardiovascular systems are particularly susceptible to the action of local anesthetics (see Table 6-5). The sequence of events related to the central nervous system after a progressive increase of local anesthetic agents is as follows: tingling sensation, dizziness or light-headedness, drowsiness, excitation, abnormal behavior, twitching, and tremors. Ultimately, in severe toxic reactions, colonic muscular contractions and convulsions occur.

The cardiovascular system is somewhat more resistant to the toxic effects of local anesthetics than the central nervous system. At high blood levels, most local anesthetics are direct myocardial depressants which, coupled with their intrinsic vasodilatory properties, can produce hypotension (more common in patients with preexisting conduction disturbances). Higher blood levels can lead to atrioventricular block, bradycardia, and ventricular arrhythmias. Most cardiovascular side effects are primarily caused by the stimulatory effects of epinephrine. The most common systemic adverse reaction from epinephrine is a mild transient tachycardia. With large amounts, this can progress to headache, palpitations, diaphoresis, anxiety, pallor, chest pain, and an increase in blood pressure. The maximum dosage of epinephrine should not exceed 1 mg (100 mL of 1:200,000) at any one time.

Epinephrine is a very helpful adjunct and is used extensively, but its powerful systemic effects should not be under-

T A B L E   6 - 4

Recipes for Anesthetic Solution for Tumescent Technique for Liposuction Surgery

	Illouz Formula*	Klein Formula†
Normal saline (0.9%)	900 cc's	1,000 cc's
Lidocaine	50 cc's (2%)	50 cc's (1%)
Epinephrine	1 cc (1:1000)	0.65 cc (1:1000)
Sodium bicarbonate	—	10.0 cc's (8.4%)
Hyaluronidase (Wydase)	6 cc's	—
Triamcinalone	—	0.25 cc's (40 mg/mL)

* 0.1% lidocaine, 1:1,000,000 epinephrine.
† 0.05% lidocaine, 1:1,000,000 epinephrine.

TABLE 6-5

Lidocaine Toxicity and Treatment

		Signs	Treatment
Central nervous system	Early 1–5 µg/mL*	Tinnitus; circumoral pallor; metallic taste; light-headedness; nausea; emesis; diplopia	Recognition, observation; symptomatic treatment; no further lidocaine
	Mid 5–12 µg/mL*	Nystagmus; slurred speech; hallucinations; muscle tremors; twitching; seizures	Diazepam; airway maintenance; observation
	Late 20–25 µg/mL*	Apnea; coma	Respiratory support
Cardiovascular system	High blood levels*	Myocardial depression; bradycardia; atrioventricular arrhythmias	Oxygen; vasopressors; cardiopulmonary resuscitation
Allergy		Pruritus; urticaria; angioedema; nausea	Antihistamines; epinephrine, 0.3 mL 1:1000 SQ; oxygen; airway maintenance
Psychogenic		Pallor; diaphoresis; hyperventilation; light-headedness; nausea; syncope	Trendelenburg position; cool compresses; observation

*Blood levels

Reprinted from Auletta MJ & Grekin RC. *Local Anesthesia For Dematologic Surgery,* NY, Churchill Livingston, 1991.

estimated. Absolute contraindications include compromised vasculature (severe cardiovascular disease, hypertension, and peripheral vascular disease), hyperthyroidism and pheochromocytoma.

Pregnant women as well as cutaneous areas supplied by an end artery that makes these areas avascular (digits, glans penis, nasal tip, and ear) are relative contraindications. Using epinephrine in patients taking beta blockers is also relatively contraindicated. Patients can experience a marked paradoxical hypertension followed by a reflex of bradycardia which can ultimately lead to cardiac arrest or hypertensive stroke. If vasoconstriction is considered necessary in a patient with a contraindication, a very dilute concentration of epinephrine should be used (1:300,000 or 1:400,000).

Equipment

Infection is not a common complication with local anesthesia, but its risk may be further minimized with routine precautions. With simple procedures, complete surgical preparation is unnecessary; however, cleaning the skin surface for a few seconds with alcohol (ethyl or isopropyl) or chlorhexidine gluconate (Hibiclens) will minimize nosocomial contamination. Similarly, gloves should always be worn to reduce the potential transmission of blood-borne diseases (hepatitis and immunodeficiency virus). Clean but not sterile gloves are acceptable, and latex gloves provide better tactile sensation. While a cap and gown are usually not necessary, eye protection (goggles) and a mask are physical barriers that prevent transmission of aerosolized blood-borne illnesses. Recapping

of needles is dangerous and is the most common cause of needle-stick injury. Needles and all sharp objects should be discarded immediately after use in a clearly visible and accessible puncture-proof container.

Disposable plastic Luer-Lok syringes have a prethreaded sheath that allows the needle hub to be securely screwed into the syringe which prevents inadvertent needle dislodgment with pressure. Narrow-barreled syringes are easy to manipulate and to inject with; however, size should depend upon the quantity of anesthetic that will be required (Fig. 6-3).

Small-gauge (no. 30) needles are less intimidating to the patient, less painful upon insertion, easier to handle, and force the operator to inject slowly and, therefore, less painfully (Table 6-6). However, the small diameter does not allow for aspiration of blood, and intravascular injection is a potential risk. Small-gauge needles (no. 32) are not useful for injection of local anesthetics because they are too flexible and cannot successfully penetrate the skin. Needles with a larger diameter (no. 18- to no. 25-gauge) are useful for initially drawing solution into the syringe, to inject large quantities of solution (after a small bleb of anesthesia has been raised), in areas of thick skin (scalp, palms, and soles), and when aspiration prior to injection is important.

Needle length should also be considered. Half-inch, 1-in, and spinal (3 in and longer) needles are available. The longer needles are useful for addressing both large areas and ring blocks. With these needles, one cutaneous needle puncture with subcutaneous threading and rotation can instill anesthesia in a large diameter. The larger needles are very fine and quite malleable. They tend to bend with thick skin, repeated

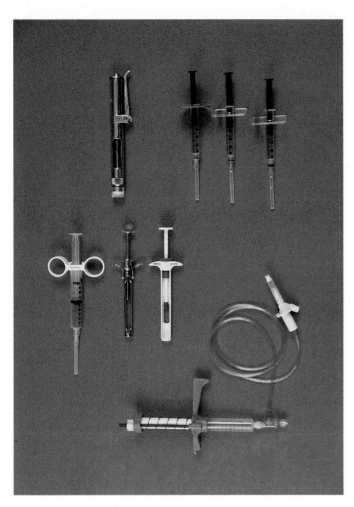

Figure 6-3   Syringes available for injection. Refilling syringe (McGhan), often connected to an intravenous bag containing local anesthetic solution, allows for anesthesia of large areas. Disposable cartridges and reusable plastic or metal syringes provide an alternate system for delivery of local anesthesia. Finger leverage plates slip over barrel of syringe to increase surface area and power of the plunger. Dermajets allow for administration of anesthesia without needles.

injections, or when changing directions upon infiltration. This can result in loss of control and—more importantly—needle breakage. The $^1/_2$-in length 30-gauge needle has become the workhorse in cutaneous surgery.

Technique of Injection of Local Anesthesia

Administration of local anesthesia can be accomplished topically or percutaneously through local infiltration, field (or ring) block, or nerve block. Topical and local infiltration anesthesia primarily affect nerve endings, the former by diffusion and the latter through an injection delivered either intradermally or into the subcutaneous fat. Nerve blocks require deposition of anesthesia close to a nerve trunk and thereby im-

TABLE 6-6

Hints for Minimizing Pain with Injectable Anesthesia

Patient comfort

   Preoperative sedation

   Atmosphere

   Topical anesthesia

Needle

   Small

   Sharp

   Patent

   Bevel up

   Without air

Anesthesia

   Buffered (with sodium bicarbonate)

   Epinephrine added freshly

   Warmed solution, (?)

Injection

   Pinch skin (counterirritation)

   Enter through pore at 90°

   Raise initial bleb (wheal)

   Inject slowly and steadily

   Minimize number of needle punctures (re-insert through anesthetized skin)

   Wait until anesthesia is effective (pinprick test)

   Supplement with long-acting agents

pede conduction of nervous impulses along the nerve. Field blocks occur when anesthesia is infiltrated more distally to a major nerve trunk but still proximally to the nerve ending (see Fig. 6-4).

Local infiltrative anesthesia is the most frequently used type in cutaneous surgery. It is easily administered and rapidly effective. Intradermal injection of anesthesia directly into the lesion produces almost immediate and, due to better localization, prolonged anesthesia. However, there is temporary tissue distortion of the surgical site. Conversely, introduction of anesthesia into the subcutaneous plane causes less tissue distortion and is therefore less painful; however, there is shorter duration due to subcutaneous diffusion and rapid absorption.

Circumferential or injection in a fan-shaped pattern around a lesion is a variation of infiltrative anesthesia and is called a *ring* or *field block*. Essentially, the operative field is encircled with walls of anesthesia, and the actual surgical site is preserved and not directly anesthetized. To obtain the optimal effect, anesthesia is injected in both the superficial and deep planes. Ring blocks are preferable to direct infiltration anesthesia when distortion of the anatomy is undesirable, to avoid

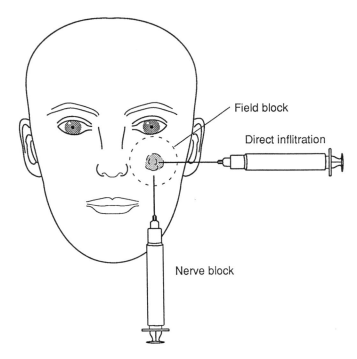

Figure 6-4 Three approaches to local anesthesia of a facial lesion: Field block places a wall of anesthesia around the lesion; direct infiltration affects the nerve endings; nerve blocks prevent conduction at the nerve trunk.

theoretic cancer cell implantation with neoplastic lesions, when addressing a large area that would normally require a large amount of anesthesia (scalp), and when anesthetizing tissue that is nondistensible (ears and nose).

Nerve blocks have a similar role as ring blocks—they, too, are useful when using large amounts of anesthesia, when tissue distortion is undesirable, and when direct infiltration would cause much patient discomfort. The most common nerve blocks in dermatologic surgery are on the face and digits, but they can also be used on the scalp, ear, penis, feet, and hands.

Nerve blocks can be achieved in two ways. Either a large volume of anesthesia is placed in the same fascial compartment as the nerve to be blocked, or the anesthesia is placed adjacently to the nerve as it exits the foramen; with either method, the anesthesia is injected in the subcutaneous plane. Due to this deep placement, there is less tissue distortion but also a delayed onset of action (3 to 10 min) and a more rapid absorption. As the duration is shorter and the vasoconstriction that occurs is in the immediate area of the nerve block, once adequate anesthesia has been achieved, supplemental vasoconstricting and long-acting agents can be added.

Peripheral nerve blocks are generally more difficult and riskier to perform as they require one's having knowledge of local neuroanatomy. Risks include inadvertent injection directly into the foramen, nerve laceration, loss of motor function, and, as blood vessels lie in close apposition to nerves, in-

travascular injection with subsequent toxicity and hematoma formation.

The easiest to learn is the digital nerve block. It is commonly used for procedures that involve the phalanges and nails. Digital innervation is supplied by two dorsal and two plantar nerves that run along the side of the digit, and, with two injections, these nerves can be blocked. The needle is first inserted at the web space, midway between the dorsal and plantar aspects, and anesthesia is deposited superficially and deeply down to bone. Without being removed, the needle is partially withdrawn and advanced along both the dorsal and plantar aspects of the digit. The procedure is repeated on the contralateral side of the finger. As necrosis can occur, epinephrine should be used cautiously when one is performing digital blocks. Reversible and controllable vasoconstriction can be better obtained with a tourniquet.

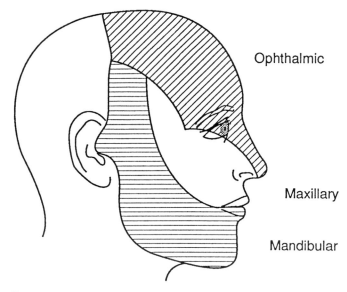

a

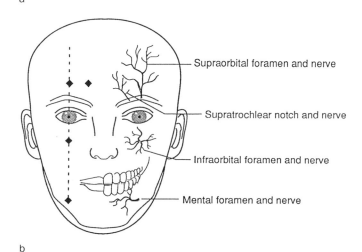

b

Figure 6-5 (*a*) Cutaneous sensory distribution supplied by the trigeminal nerve; (*b*) location of major branches of the trigeminal nerve as they exit their foramen.

To produce facial anesthesia requires a more precise knowledge of cutaneous innervation and anatomy. The sensory supply to the face is primarily through the trigeminal nerve (fifth cranial nerve) and its three branches: ophthalmic (V1), maxillary (V2), and mandibular (V3). These branches exit predictably through their respective foramen in the midpupillary line (around 2.5 cm from the midline). (See Figs. 6-5a–b.) By the accurate location of these sites, a large area of the face can be anesthetized with only a few milliliters of local anesthetic deposited around the nerve. Facial nerve blocks can be performed effectively by injecting bupivacaine or 0.5% to 1.0% lidocaine with or without epinephrine.

The supraorbital and supratrochlear nerves are terminal branches of the ophthalmic branch of the trigeminal nerve. The supraorbital nerve lies in the midpupillary line along the inferior ridge of the supraorbital ridge. It is blocked by depositing 1 to 2 mL of solution at the supraorbital notch. The supratrochlear nerve exits the orbit at about 1 cm lateral to the midline, along the upper medial corner of the orbit. It can be blocked by injection of anesthesia at the junction of the medial border of the upper rim of the orbit with the root of the nose. Blockade of these two nerves will anesthetize the skin of the forehead.

The maxillary branch of the trigeminal nerve exits the infraorbital foramen as the infraorbital nerve. The foramen is located in the midpupillary line, 1 cm inferior to the infraorbital ridge. Nerve blockade can be approached either percutaneously or intraorally. Once the bony landmarks are palpated, a 30-gauge needle is slowly advanced through the skin but not to the bone. The alternate approach to the infraorbital nerve is through the oral cavity. The foramen lies 1 cm (a 1-in needle

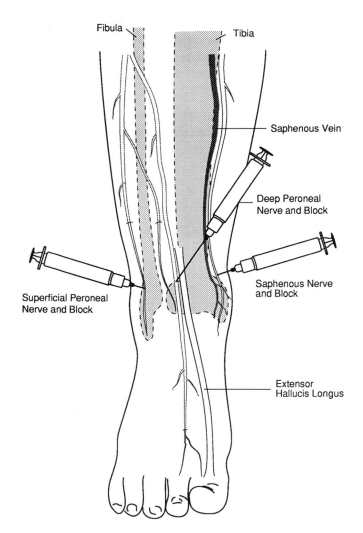

Figure 6-7 Anterior ankle block of superficial peroneal saphenous and deep peroneal nerves.

is therefore required) above the superior labial sulcus at the apex of the first bicuspid (premolar). With both approaches, 2 mL of solution deposited around the foramen will anesthetize the lower eyelid, part of the cheek, nasal side wall, and upper lip.

The mental nerve, a terminal branch of the mandibular division, leaves the mandible through the mental foramen in the midpupillary line and innervates the skin of the chin and lower lip. The anatomic position of the mental foramen varies with the age of the patient. In the adult, the foramen lies midway between the upper and lower edge of the mandibular bone below the second bicuspid and approximately 2.5 cm from the midline of the face.

As with the infraorbital nerve, the mental nerve can be approached either percutaneously or through the mucosa. With the intraoral approach to nerve blocks, topical anesthesia applied to the mucosa prior to the injection will decrease patient discomfort and anxiety.

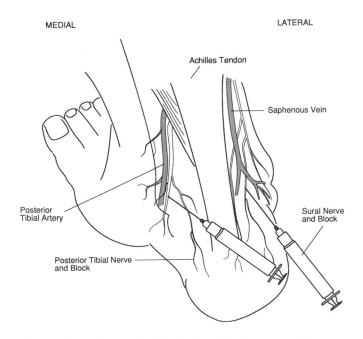

Figure 6-6 Posterior ankle block of sural and posterior tibial nerves.

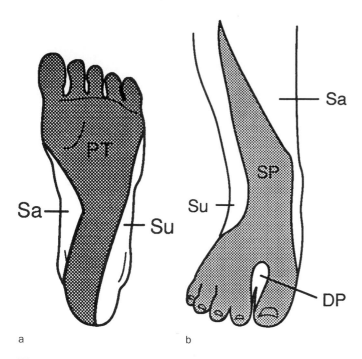

Figure 6-8 Cutaneous pattern of sensory innervation of the foot. (*a*) Plantar surface (Sa = saphenous nerve, PT = posterior tibial nerve, Su = sural nerve); (*b*) dorsal surface. (SP = superficial peroneal nerve, DP = deep peroneal nerve).

Other nerve blocks that are helpful in cutaneous surgery are wrist and ankle blocks. Infiltration of the ulnar and median nerves results in anesthesia of the volar surface of the hand. The ulnar nerve is located deeply to the pulsation of the ulnar artery and lies adjacently to the flexor carpi ulnaris tendon. The median nerve lies deeply to the large palmaris longus tendon, which can be visualized upon wrist flexion.

Ankle nerve blocks are more complicated but preclude painful injection into the foot. A block of the posteriorly located sural and posterior tibial nerves anesthetizes the plantar aspect (Fig. 6-6), and anterior blockage of the saphenous, superficial peroneal, and deep peroneal nerves anesthetizes the dorsum of the foot (Fig. 6-7).

The sural nerve innervates the posterior and lateral sole (Fig. 6-8*a*) and is blocked by depositing anesthesia where it becomes superficial, midway between the Achilles tendon and the lateral malleolus.

The posterior tibial nerve is medial to the Achilles tendon and immediately posterolateral to the pulsation of the posterior tibial artery. A needle directed toward the second toe is inserted at the level of the upper half of the medial malleolus, just posteriorly to the posterior tibial arterial pulse and medially to the Achilles tendon. (For both sural and posterior tibial nerve blocks, the patient should be prone.) Successful blockade will result in anesthesia of a large portion of the anterior aspect of the sole.

The superficial peroneal nerve innervates a major portion of the dorsum of the foot [except for the first web space (Fig.

6-8*b*)] and is blocked by injecting anesthesia midway between the lateral malleolus and the anterior tibial surface.

The saphenous nerve closely parallels the great saphenous vein and innervates the skin around the medial malleolus. This block is performed by injecting anesthesia medially to the saphenous vein (best visualized with the patient standing) and immediately above and anterior to the malleolus.

The deep peroneal nerve innervates the first web space, and local infiltration is generally adequate for this area.

Several points should be reiterated regarding peripheral nerve blocks. Injections should be made subcutaneously in the region surrounding the nerve trunk and should not enter bony foramens or the nerve itself. The diameter of cutaneous nerves is large; therefore, a 5-to-10-min delay occurs before optimal anesthesia is in effect. As nerves often lie in close proximity to arteries, it is important to aspirate prior to injection to avoid intravascular placement of anesthesia. Finally, nerve blocks do not produce effective vasoconstriction. To obtain adequate hemostasis, it is helpful to infiltrate the lines of incision and lines of dissection with an epinephrine-containing compound. However, epinephrine should not be used in patients with ischemic lesions of the foot and with advanced diabetes.

CONCLUSION

We have come a long way since the days when anesthesia consisted of a "shot of whiskey and a bullet to bite on." The who, what, where, when, why, and how of dermatologic surgery have been tremendously expanded with the pharmacologic advancement of local anesthesia. However, in a rush to expand our surgical horizons, we should not forget that local anesthetics are powerful medications, and their safety profile should be reviewed and tailored to each patient. It is of paramount importance that the surgeon be knowledgeable in the properties of anesthetics, including duration, onset, metabolism, and drug interactions. Recognition of local adverse reactions and systemic toxicity and their treatment is mandatory prior to beginning any procedure.

SUGGESTED READINGS

Abadir A: Use of local anesthetics in dermatology. *J Dermatol Surg Oncol* **1:**65–70, 1975

Alpert CC, Thomas JD: General anesthesia. *Clin Plast Surg* **12:**33–42, 1985

Arndt KA et al: Minimizing the pain of local anesthesia. *Plast Reconstr Surg* **72:**676–679, 1983

Ashinoff R, Geonemus RG: Effect of the topical anesthetic EMLA on efficacy of pulsed dye laser treatment of portwine stains. *J Dermatol Surg Oncol* **16:**1008–1011, 1990

Auletta MJ, Grekin RC: *Local Anesthesia for Dermatologic Surgery.* New York, Churchill Livingston, 1991

Bennett RG: *Fundamentals of Cutaneous Surgery.* St. Louis, Mosby, 1988

Bezzant JL et al: Painless cauterization of spider veins with the use of iontophoretic local anesthesia. *J Am Acad Dermatol* **19:**869–875, 1988

Cohen SJ, Roenigk RK: Nerve blocks for cutaneous surgery on the foot. *J Dermatol Surg Oncol* **17:**527–534, 1991

Courtiss EH: Tetracaine with epinephrine as an alternative to cocaine intranasally. *Plast Reconstr Surg* **806:**167, 1990

Covino BG: Local anesthesia. *N Engl J Med* **286:**1035–1042, 1972

Covino BG: Local anesthetic agents for peripheral nerve blocks. *Reg Anaes* **3:**33–37, 1980

Glinert RJ, Zachary CB: Local anesthetic allergy. *J Dermatol Surg Oncol* **17:**491–496, 1991

Goldberg MP: Induction of anesthetic in portions of the face by intranasal injection. *J Dermatol Surg Oncol* **5:**570–571, 1979

Gordon HL: The selection of drugs in office surgery. *Clin Plast Surg* **10:**278–284, 1983

Gormley DE: Local anesthesia: Pain control with proper injection technique. *J Dermatol Surg Oncol* **13:**35–36, 1987

Grekin RC, Auletta MS: Local anesthesia in dermatologic surgery. *J Am Acad Dermatol* **19:**599–614, 1988

Hutton KP et al: Regional anesthesia of the hand for dermatologic surgery. *J Dermatol Surg Oncol* **17:**881–888, 1991

Klein JA: Anesthesia for liposuction in dermatologic surgery. *J Dermatol Surg Oncol* **14:**1124–1132, 1988

Larson PO et al: Stability of buffered lidocaine with epinephrine used for local anesthesia. *J Dermatol Surg Oncol* **17:**411–414, 1991

Maloney JM: Local anesthesia obtained via iontophoresis as an aid to shave biopsy. *Arch Dermatol* **128:**331–332, 1992

Maloney JM et al: Plasma concentrations of lidocaine during hair transplantation. *J Dermatol Surg Oncol* **8:**950–954, 1982

Painge WR: Local anesthesia of the face. *J Dermatol Surg Oncol* **5:**311–315, 1979

Rardle HW et al: Know your anatomy: Local anesthesia for cutaneous lesions of the head and neck—practical applications of peripheral nerve blocks. *J Dermatol Surg Oncol* **18:**231–235, 1992

Robins P, Ashinoff R: Prolongation of anesthesia in Mohs micrographic surgery with 2% lidocaine jelly. *J Dermatol Surg Oncol* **17:**649–652, 1991

Salasche SJ et al: *Surgical Anatomy of the Skin.* Norwalk, Conn, Appleton & Lange, 1988

Sperling LC et al: Toward less painful anesthesia: Water, saline, and lidocaine. *J Dermatol Surg Oncol* **7:**730–731, 1981

Stegman SJ et al: *Basics of Dermatologic Surgery.* Chicago, Year Book, 1982

Stewart JH et al: Neutralized lidocaine with epinephrine for local anesthesia. *J Dermatol Surg Oncol* **15:**1081–1083, 1989

Swanson JG: Assessment of allergy to local anesthetic. *Ann Emerg Med* **12:**316–318, 1983

Swinehart JM: The ice-saline-xylocaine technique. *J Dermatol Surg Oncol* **18:**28–30, 1992

Jeffrey L. Melton and C. William Hanke

7 Wound Closure Materials

Important functions of sutures and other closure materials include ligation of vessels, approximation of structures, and obliteration of dead space. When healing by primary intention is elected, the final outcome depends not only upon the technique of the surgeon but also on the closure materials chosen. Only through a working knowledge of the mechanical properties of closure materials can the surgeon exploit their use to the fullest benefit of the patient.

Historically, a wide variety of materials have been used to close wounds. In recent decades, several new materials have become available, providing tremendous benefits to both the patient and the physician. The efficacy of suture materials has been greatly increased by development of synthetic materials in both absorbable and nonabsorbable types. Significant improvements have also led to increased use of closure tapes and strips. Stainless steel staples are another fairly recent development in wound closure. More recently, tissue glues have been developed, investigated, and used.

Several factors come into play when choosing the optimal materials for closing a particular wound; cosmesis and function are often foremost in these considerations. Anatomic site influences function and cosmesis of the area to be repaired. In facial wounds, cosmesis and patient acceptance are of obvious importance. Cosmesis is often less important on the scalp, particularly in females, and where androgenic alopecia is not anticipated. Rapidity of healing is also in part site-dependent, and thus surgical site has implications for choice of closure materials. Facial, scalp, and intraoral wounds do not often require prolonged artificial apposition, while truncal and extremity (particularly lower extremity) wounds may require substantial prolonged support. The size and geometry of the defect and type of repair also affect the degree of tension on the wound. These factors should be taken into account when choosing materials for closure.

Practicality, for both patient and physician, is important. Patient acceptance and compliance should be considered, particularly with respect to closure tapes or staples. Speed and ease of use can also be important considerations. The color of suture materials can be important in that more visible colors facilitate easier placement and removal.

The nature of implanted materials is important with respect to infectious and reactive processes. Although infection is not a common complication of cutaneous surgery, it can be a consideration in the choice of closure material.[1] For example, a host may have a chronic tendency toward staphylococcal carriage or have chronic inflammatory disease of the skin or neighboring tissues. All percutaneous closure materials represent foreign bodies. As such, all provoke some degree of host response. Thus, the number of sutures placed should not be excessive. The degree of response inherent in an individual material should be correlated with the anticipated healing time and length of support needed for the wound and the time of removal or degradation of the closure material.

SUTURE MATERIALS AND NEEDLES

Sutures

The primary differences among sutures relate to their configuration. Multifilament sutures are made of more than one strand of material, and the majority of these are of a braided configuration. In general, braided suture materials are more prone to infection than are monofilament sutures. Braided sutures also induce a greater degree of tissue reaction than do monofilament sutures. Advantages of braided sutures include ease of handling, low memory, and increased knot security. Ease of handling is inversely related to the memory of the suture. *Memory* is the tendency of the suture material to retain its original shape. *Knot security* is inversely related to memory and is the ability of a knot to hold under tension without slipping, stretching, or breaking.

A monofilament suture material is a single strand of material, usually round in transverse section. Monofilament sutures tend to have more memory, poorer handling characteristics, and less knot security than multifilament sutures. However, monofilament sutures in general have a decreased tendency of infection. Another advantage of monofilament sutures is ease of passage through tissue, including ease of removal. Although usually not an important consideration with interrupted sutures, a monofilament suture may be preferred for its ease of removal when running nonabsorbable sutures are used, particularly with subcuticular placement.

The second major characteristic of a suture material is its absorbability. Sutures are classified as absorbable or nonabsorbable in a relative sense, based on how rapidly tensile strength is lost after tissue implantation. The United States Pharmacopeia (USP) defines *nonabsorbable sutures* as those which retain the majority of their tensile strength at 60 days postimplantation. *Absorbable sutures* are defined as those which lose the majority of their tensile strength by 60 days. Thus, an absorbable suture may be present in tissue for a prolonged period albeit with a significantly reduced tensile strength. Contrariwise, a nonabsorbable suture can, in fact, completely absorb over a prolonged time period.

While the tensile strength of implanted sutures declines, tensile strength of the wound increases. During the first 4 to 6 days of wound healing, minimal wound strength is present.[2] At 2 weeks, wounds have 3 to 5 percent of their original strength; at 3 weeks, 20 percent; and at 1 month, 50 percent of their original strength. The rate of increase in wound tensile strength should be kept in mind when choosing a suture and when removing it. Sutures need not bear the tensile strength of normal, nonwounded skin. In fact, wounds will only strengthen to 80 percent of the original tensile strength regardless of length of healing. The breaking strength of nonwounded skin is far higher than that required for everyday activities and is probably only approached with significant blunt trauma. In general, buried absorbable sutures are relied upon for adequate wound support while wound tensile strength is inadequate. Superficial sutures are relied upon only for fine approximation of epidermal edges, since suture tracts and bridging scars result if percutaneous sutures are placed under tension or are left in place long enough for adequate wound strength to develop.[3]

A third major classification of suture materials is *natural* versus *synthetic*. The only natural sutures in general use in dermatologic surgery are silk and catgut. Advances in polymer chemistry have resulted in improved synthetic suture materials and thus in a relative decline in the use of natural materials.

The size of the suture material needs to be chosen regardless of what type is used. Because sutures act as foreign material, the caliber of the suture used should be the smallest which can hold the wound in apposition without breaking or cutting through the tissue.[4] The two factors which influence the volume of the tissue reaction sheath are the nature of the suture material and the size of the suture.[5,6] Suture sizes do not refer to a specific diameter but rather a range of diameters which corresponds to a specific tensile strength for the material in question. Thus, two 4–0 sutures of different materials may have somewhat different diameters. Suture sizes range from 11–0 to #3. The smallest suture is 11–0, with increasing diameter to 1–0. Sutures heavier than 1–0 are designated by a pound sign and a digit or simply a digit. These range from #1 to #3. Thus, a #1 suture is intermediate between 1–0 and #2. In cutaneous surgery, commonly used suture sizes range from 6–0 to 3–0. Finer sutures, such as 6–0, are frequently used on thin-skinned areas of low tension such as the eyelids. They are also well suited to affixing full- and split-thickness skin grafts. The 5–0 sutures are generally preferred on most other areas of the face. The 4–0 size is often selected for facial areas closed under some tension, such as the forehead, and for other body sites. Thick-skinned areas closed under tension, such as the scalp, back, and scapular areas, may require 3–0 or even 2–0 sutures to maintain wound integrity.

Absorbable Sutures

Catgut
Catgut (also referred to as *gut* or *surgical gut*) sutures have been used for hundreds of years. They are derived from the submucosa of the small intestine of sheep. As such, they are one of the few nonsynthetic suture materials in use. Even their use has declined due to the availability of improved synthetic materials. Plain catgut retains significant strength for only 4 to 5 days, with 60 percent of initial strength present at 7 days and essentially no strength remaining by the fourteenth day (Table 7-1). *Chromic gut* is catgut that has been treated with chromic salts. This delays absorption somewhat, although tensile strength beyond 14 days is minimal. A marked inflammatory phagocytic response accompanies the absorbtion of gut sutures.

A variant of catgut, called Fast Absorbing Gut (Ethicon, New Brunswick, NJ) degrades very quickly. Thus, it need not be removed. It can be useful where suture removal is difficult, without disrupting the wound, as in split-thickness grafts and in areas such as the eyelids.

Polyglycolic Acid
Polyglycolic acid (Dexon [Davis+Geck, Danbury, CT]) is a synthetic, absorbable, braided suture material which features high tensile strength, low reactivity, and slower and more predictable absorption compared to catgut.[7] The low reactivity is due to its degradation by enzymatic hydrolysis rather than phagocytic degradation (Fig. 7-1). Dexon was the first synthetic absorbable suture introduced in 1970. It was a significant advance since it was the first absorbable suture to maintain tensile strength for a prolonged period. Fifty percent of Dexon's tensile strength is present at 14 days after implantation, with complete degradation by 90 to 120 days.[8] The orig-

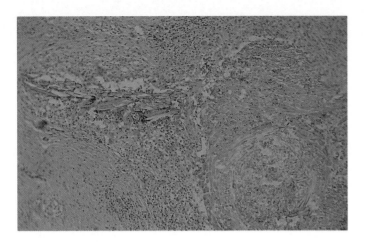

Figure 7-1 Dexon suture 30 days postimplantation. A mild lymphohistiocytic infiltrate is present (×100).

inal suture is still available, but it is now called Dexon S. Dexon is available only in a braided form. In order to improve its knot-tying qualities, a coating (Poloxamer 188) was added; this suture was called Dexon Plus. Due to the relatively disappointing performance of that coating, a polycaprolate coating is now used, and this suture is called Dexon II. Thus, the two Dexons currently available are Dexon S (uncoated) and Dexon II (coated). The suture strand is identical; the coating (which is also absorbed) is the only difference. The absorbable coating allows knots to slide down more smoothly, with less "chatter," as well as easier passage through tissue. The disadvantage of any such coating is some compromise in knot security. Both varieties of Dexon are available in two colors: "beige" (nearly white) and green.

Polyglactin 910
Polyglactin 910 [Vicryl (Ethicon)] is a synthetic, braided, absorbable polymer with many of the characteristics of Dexon.

It loses 50 percent of its tensile strength over 14 days, and resolves completely over 90 to 120 days.[8] Like Dexon, absorption of Vicryl is by enzymatic hydrolysis, with little inflammation. A coated Vicryl is also available. The coating, polyglactin 370, eases passage through tissue and knot tie-down. The coating is also absorbed. Vicryl is available as a white suture or dyed violet.

Polydioxanone
Polydioxanone [PDS (Ethicon)] is a more recently introduced synthetic absorbable suture. It is available only as a monofilament. PDS retains significant tensile strength longer than Dexon or Vicryl. It absorbs completely over 180 days with minimal tissue reaction. Fifty percent of original strength is present at 4 weeks and 25 percent at 6 weeks. Thus PDS is particularly useful where prolonged support is desired in an absorbable suture. Handling is somewhat better than other monofilament sutures but not as good as braided sutures. A newer version, PDS-2, was aimed at improving handling and knotting characteristics, but the difference was found to be minimal in one study.[9] PDS is available clear or dyed violet.

Polyglyconate
Polyglyconate [Maxon (Davis+Geck)] is the most recently developed synthetic absorbable suture. It is a copolymer of polytrimethylene carbonate and glycolide and has good tensile strength. The rate of loss of tensile strength with Maxon is similar to that of PDS, retaining approximately 50 percent of tensile strength for 21 to 28 days. Maxon has very good handling characteristics for a monofilament suture. In fact, Maxon is felt by some to have handling characteristics superior to Vicryl, which is a braided suture.[10] Maxon has relatively low memory and thus good knot security. As a monofilament, the suture passes through tissue easily. The suture is available in green or clear.

TABLE 7-1

Absorbable Suture Materials

Material	Tensile Strength Half-Life, Days	Tissue Reaction*	Configuration	Ease of Handling*	Knot Security*	Color†
Gut (fast absorbing)	2‡	2	Mono	1	1	N
Gut (plain)	4‡	4	Mono	1	1	N
Gut (chromic)	7‡	4	Mono	1	2	N
Dexon	14	2	Braided	3	4	G, W
Vicryl	14	2	Braided	3	4	V, W
PDS	28	2	Mono	2	3	C, V
Maxon	21–28	2	Mono	3	3	C, G

* 1 = lowest, 4 = highest.
† C = clear, G = green, N = natural, V = violet, W = white.
‡ Variable.

TABLE 7-2

Nonabsorbable Suture Materials

Material	Tissue Reaction*	Configuration	Ease of Handling*	Knot Security*	Color†
Silk	4	Braided	4	4	B, W
Nylon (mono)	1	Mono	2	2	B, C, G, K
Nylon (braided)	2	Braided	3	4	B, W
Polypropylene	1	Mono	1	1	B, C
Polybutester	1	Mono	2	3	B
Polyester (uncoated)	1	Braided	3	3	G, W
Polyester (coated)	2	Braided	4	2	B, G, W

* 1 = lowest, 4 = highest.

† B = blue, C = clear, G = green, K = black, W = white.

Nonabsorbable sutures

Silk

Silk is available as a braided suture. Although classified as a nonabsorbable suture, it is actually very slowly absorbed with significant tissue reaction. Due to the wicking action of a braided material which absorbs water, somewhat higher wound infection rates are associated with silk sutures (Table 7-2). Because of these disadvantages, and the advent of newer materials, silk sutures are now infrequently used in cutaneous surgery. The chief virtue of silk is its unsurpassed handling qualities. The softness of silk lends it to intraoral, and intertriginous use. Most silk sutures are now coated with silicone to ease passage through tissue.

Nylon

Nylon is a synthetic material which may be braided [Nurolon (Ethicon)] or monofilament. The monofilament sutures are much more commonly used. The braided suture has better handling characteristics but has a slightly higher incidence of wound infection. Nylon has low tissue reactivity and high tensile strength. Monofilament nylon is available in black, blue, green, or clear. Nurolon is available in black or white.

Polypropylene

Polypropylene (Prolene [Surgilene, Davis+Geck, Danbury, CT]) is a monofilament synthetic polymer with very low tissue reactivity. It is a good choice for temporary running sutures, particularly with running subcuticular placement, due to its ease of withdrawal. Polypropylene has a fairly high degree of memory. Therefore, it is somewhat more difficult to handle than other monofilament sutures and has poorer knot performance.[9] It is available clear or blue.

Polybutester

Polybutester (Novafil [Davis+Geck, Danbury, CT]) is available as a monofilament synthetic polymer. It is one of the newer such polymers introduced. For a monofilament nonabsorbable suture, it has above average handling qualities. It also has fairly high elasticity, allowing some stretching to occur during postoperative edema.

Polyester

Polyester is a synthetic polymer suture material. It comes only in a braided configuration and has handling characteristics similar to silk. As a braided suture, it has a slightly increased association with wound infection. It is available in several colors. The basic differences among polyester sutures are whether or not they are coated. The coatings decrease friction, thus improving handling while sacrificing knot security. Examples of polyester sutures include the uncoated Mersilene (Ethicon) and the coated Ethibond (Ethicon).

Others

Other nonabsorbable suture materials are available which are rarely used in cutaneous surgery. These include cotton and stainless steel sutures.

Future trends

Possible future developments in suture material will likely be aimed at producing monofilament sutures with improved handling characteristics because of the ease of tissue passage and decreased infection rate associated with monofilaments. Also, antimicrobial substances may be incorporated into the suture material or applied as coatings on the surface.[11]

Needles

Minimally traumatic cutaneous surgery is a prerequisite for obtaining the fastest healing, greatest patient comfort, minimal incidence of wound infection, and optimal cosmetic and functional results. Proper choice and use of needles is one of the keys to minimizing surgical trauma. The thickness of the needle is markedly greater than that of the suture and therefore defines the size of the path in which the suture lies. Mod-

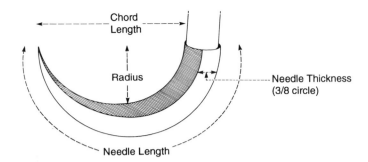

Figure 7-2 Measurements defining needle size.

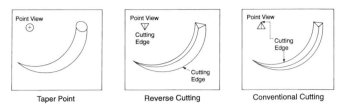

Figure 7-4 Needle points.

ern cutaneous surgery generally employs the use of swaged needles which come permanently affixed to the suture material rather than the older eyelet needles which were threaded by hand. Needles also figure prominently in the cost of disposable surgical materials. In fact, the most important factor in suture cost is the needle to which it is attached.

Needles used in cutaneous surgery are in the shape of a three-eighths or half circle. Measurements defining the size of the needle are the needle length, chord length, radius, and needle thickness (Fig. 7-2). The three parts of the needle are the point, body, and shank (Fig. 7-3). The soft shank, or swaged end, is hollow and accommodates the suture. As such, the needle bends easily if grabbed in this area. Thus, the needle should be grasped with the needle-holder at least one-fourth of the way toward the point from the swaged end to decrease the possibility of bending or breaking the needle. The swaged end affixes the needle to the suture permanently in all but the detachable types. These detachable needles are commonly referred to as *pop-offs* and are marketed under the names Control Release (Ethicon) and D-Tach (Davis+Geck). Detachable needles are not very commonly used in cutaneous surgery but can be useful in the deep closure of large wounds when interrupted suture technique is used. They allow rapid placement of many sutures.

The point of the needle may be of two basic types, cutting or tapered (Fig. 7-4). The tapered needle is round in cross section and has no cutting edge. Tapered needles are reserved for tissues in which a minimum of cutting and tearing is desired, such as subdermal structures. Thus, they can be useful for approximation of muscle, subcutaneous fat, and in suture ligature of vessels.

The cutting needle is the workhorse of cutaneous surgery. Two types are available, *cutting* (conventional cutting) and *reverse cutting*. Both are triangular in cross section, and each corner of the triangle is a cutting surface. The conventional cutting needle has its third cutting edge (point) of the triangle on the inside or concave side of the needle, while the reverse cutting needle has the third cutting edge on the outside or convex aspect of the needle (Fig. 7-4). The advantage of the reverse cutting needle is that it decreases the tendency of the suture to cut upward from the bottom of the wound or inward from the outer aspect of the suture tract. Consequently, the reverse cutting needle is generally preferred for cutaneous surgery.

Conventional cutting needles include the PC [precision cosmetic (Ethicon)] designation. Reverse cutting needles are designated FS, P, or PS in the Ethicon series; CE or PRE in the Davis+Geck series. The FS, P, and PS designations refer to "for skin," "plastic," and "plastic skin," respectively. In honing and sharpness, the PS is the finest, followed by the P, then the FS. In the Davis+Geck series, the reverse cutting needles are designated C (cutting) and PR (premium cutting). The PR is the more finely honed of the two. In Davis+Geck nomenclature, an E indicates a three-eighths-circle needle, whereas the lack of it indicates a half-circle needle. The sharpness of a needle is an important consideration, particularly in the finest cosmetic applications, since sharper needles induce less tissue trauma. In applications (or sites) of less cosmetic importance, the less finely honed needles may be preferred on the basis of lower cost, while the more finely honed needles may be reserved for precision cosmetic work.

SUTURELESS CLOSURE MATERIALS

Tissue Glues

Tissue glues have been used in cutaneous surgery for the past 30 years, although as a sole method of wound closure they have not met with wide acceptance. However, they have been successfully used in certain specialized applications discussed below. Two basic types of tissue glues have been used: *fibrin*

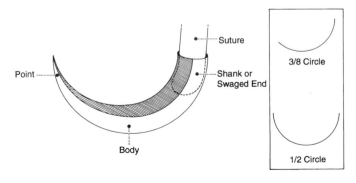

Figure 7-3 Needle components.

glues and *cyanoacrylate glues.* Perhaps continued research in biomaterials will result in refined tissue glues, leading to expanded applications and broader use.

Fibrin glues

The development of fibrin sealing began in the early 1970s and resulted from the observation of the adhesive and wound-healing properties of fibrin clots.[12] Since then, fibrin sealant, obtained from human plasma, has been used for tissue sealing, hemostasis, wound support, and promotion of wound healing. Because it is not a strong adhesive, it cannot be used to maintain significant tension. As a homologous material, fibrin glue is naturally degraded and does not interfere with wound healing. Since it is hemostatic, it may be useful in patients with disorders of hemostasis and in bloody procedures such as rhinophyma reduction.[13] Because of the combination of hemostatic and adhesive properties, it has been successfully used in the placement of skin grafts. In this application, it is particularly useful in concave areas and in other sites where grafts are difficult to affix and has resulted in significant reduction in blood loss and operative time to achieve hemostasis.[14]

However, despite stringent donor criteria, concern exists regarding transmission of HIV and hepatitis with the pooled fibrinogen preparation currently available. A single-donor fibrin glue has recently been developed and successfully used.[15] Perhaps newer techniques in molecular biology will result in an in vitro genetically produced product in the future.

Cyanoacrylate glues

Cyanoacrylate glues have been used since the 1960s for hemostasis, closure, reinforcement of wounds after suture removal, and in other specialized applications. The chief advantages cyanoacrylate glues offer are speed, strength of adhesion, and cost. Several different glues have been used. Differences in these materials include polymerization speed, polymerization temperature, histotoxicity, biodegradation rate, and wetting and spreading ability. These parameters relate primarily to the chain length of the molecule. Newer, longer alkyl chain derivatives, such as *N*-butyl cyanoacrylate (NBC) and isobutyl cyanoacrylate (IBC), cause a lesser tissue response while retaining the adhesive properties of the older methyl-2-cyanoacrylate (M2C).

In contrast to fibrin glues, adhesion of cyanoacrylate is strong enough for the approximation and closure of many wounds. Due to foreign-body reaction, however, the material may be expelled or sloughed when used for dermal closure. But superficial sutures can be reduced in number or eliminated by the coaptation of epidermal wound edges with cyanoacrylate droplets.

Cyanoacrylates may also be used for prolonged superficial wound support following suture removal, particularly in periorificial or moist sites where wound closure tapes are difficult to use. Cyanoacrylate glues have also been used in hair transplant donor graft placement to prevent up or down movement.[16] As with fibrin glues, perhaps the greatest application of cyanoacrylate glues is in skin grafting. Again, the primary benefit is greatly reduced operative time. However, in contrast to fibrin glues, the material causes too much tissue reaction to be used beneath grafts and is best used only on cornified surfaces to join the edges of grafts to each other or to the wound margin.

Wound Closure Tapes

Wound closure tapes have long been used in cutaneous surgery and have perhaps been more frequently used over the past two decades.[17] Tapes may be used to reinforce wounds after suture removal, to decrease tension on sutured wounds, and even for wound closure. Advantages associated with wound closure tapes include ease of application and removal, improved cosmesis by allowing earlier removal of nonabsorbable sutures, and prolonged wound support without percutaneous foreign bodies after such sutures are removed. In addition, a lesser tendency for wound infection is seen when tapes alone are used for wound closure. However, closure with tapes alone is efficacious only in wounds which can be closed under almost no tension. Certain body sites lend themselves poorly to the use of tapes, such as periorificial areas and moist or hairy areas. Another disadvantage of tapes is the frequent trapping of exudate which may interfere with superficial approximation of tissue.

Many types of tapes are presently available, including Steri-Strip (3M Medical-Surgical Division, St. Paul, MN), Suture Strip Plus (Genetic Laboratories, St. Paul, MN), Shurstrip (Shur Medical Corporation, Beaverton, OR), Coverstrip and Coverstrip II (Beirsdorf), Proxi-Strip (Ethicon), Clearon (Ethicon), Appose (Davis+Geck), and Op-Site Wound Closure (Smith & Nephew, Largo, FL).

The adhesiveness of most tapes is markedly increased by pretreating the skin with Mastisol or tincture of benzoin. In addition, any remaining skin surface lipid or soap-type surgical scrub should be removed before applying mastisol or benzoin. The tapes are applied after the latter agents are air dried. Mastisol has been found to have significantly greater adhesiveness than tincture of benzoin.[18] Tapes found to have significant adhesion without a pretreating agent were Proxi-Strip and Coverstrip II.[18]

A closure tape with increased elasticity has been introduced. It is said to decrease the tendency toward blistering at the distal aspects of rigid tapes.[19] Such blistering has not been a significant problem in the authors' experience.

Staples

Staples are frequently used for wound closure in general surgery and other surgical specialties. They are finding increased use in dermatologic surgery as well. All skin staplers currently in use utilize stainless steel staples. Inserted staples have an incomplete rectangular configuration, with a top cross-member parallel to the skin surface, bridging the wound; two vertical legs extending into skin; and two pointed tips directed toward the center of the wound. Squeezing the trigger on the stapler forces the staple into this configuration while one is inserting it into the skin.

The most impressive advantage of wound closure by stapling is considerable time savings. Typically, wounds can be stapled in one-fourth to one-half the time required for suture closure.[20] Consequently, staples are often considered for closing long wounds, particularly on the trunk and extremities. Since stapling offers good wound approximation while everting skin edges, cosmetic results can approach that of a well-sutured wound under certain conditions. In addition to approximating wounds, staples have also been used to affix split-thickness grafts and can even be used to affix the bolster.[21–23]

Although staples can work well on the face, many patients are uncomfortable with the idea of having staples in this location. Pain due to staples has been reported but has not been a significant complaint in the authors' experience. The largest single drawback to staples, after patient resistance, is cost. In 1995 prices, the cost per staple ranges from $.16 to $.80; the cost of the disposable staplers ranges from $3.80 to $35. If only a few staples are used and the unit is then discarded, the cost per staple is even higher. Some suggest that the units can be gas sterilized (after cleaning) and reused.[24]

Removal of the staples requires the use of a staple remover (usually a disposable item). Staple removal is simple, fast, and usually painless if done carefully.

There are four major skin stapler manufacturers, each with its own line of staplers. United States Surgical Corporation, Norwalk, CT, has the largest line, with the Royal, Signet, and Concord disposables, as well as the Premium and Multifire Premium. The 3M Corporation has three staplers: the Multishot, Vista, and PGX. Ethicon staplers include the Proximate and Proximate II. The Davis+Geck line of Appose skin staplers includes the Unity, ULC, and Ultra.

Each stapler has its own handling characteristics, staple-release mechanism, and wound visibility at the staple insertion site. There are three basic types of staplers. The smallest and least expensive is the pinch type, of which the 3M Multishot may be considered a prototype. This small stapler is placed between the thumb and forefinger and then pinched to insert the staple. The second type of stapler resembles a desk stapler and is usually intermediate in price. The most expensive type of disposable skin stapler is the pistol type. Some pistol-type staplers offer the added convenience of a rotating head for hard-to-reach areas or contours.

In most of the product lines, there is a choice of the number of staples per stapler (usually 5 to 15 or 25 to 35) and also a choice in the staple size. There are usually two staple sizes: regular and wide. The wide staples, after insertion, usually range from 6.5- to 7.1-mm wide and from 3.9 to 4.7 mm in height. The regular size staples are usually between 4.8 and 5.7 mm in width and from 3.4 to 4.2 mm in height.

SUMMARY

Many advances have been made in wound closure materials in recent years. Undoubtedly, progress will continue to be made. Newer suture materials offer decreased tissue reactivity and improved handling qualities. A broad range of absorption rates is now available in absorbable sutures. Needle design continues to improve, and several types are available. A wide array of sutureless closure materials is available, including tissue glues, closure tapes, and stapling devices. An understanding of the mechanical and biomechanical aspects of the various materials available is essential in choosing an appropriate closure material for a particular wound. An appropriate closure material, when combined with proper surgical technique, can then lead to the best possible result for the patient.

REFERENCES

1. Whitaker DC et al: Wound infection rate in dermatologic surgery. *J Dermatol Surg Oncol* **14**:525, 1988

2. Howes EL et al: The healing of wounds as determined by their tensile strength. *JAMA* **92**:42, 1929

3. Crikelar GF: Skin suture marks. *Am J Surg* **96**:631, 1958

4. Brunius U: Wound healing impairment from sutures. *Acta Chir Scand Suppl* **134**:395, 1968

5. Postlethwait RW et al: Human tissue reaction to sutures. *Ann Surg* **181**:144, 1975

6. Van Rijssel EJ et al: Tissue reaction and surgical knots: The effect of suture size, knot configuration, and knot volume. *Obstet Gynecol* **74**:64, 1989

7. Postlethwait RW: Further study of polyglycolic acid suture. *Am J Surg* **127**:617, 1974

8. Bourne RB et al: In vivo comparison of four absorbable sutures: Vicryl, Dexon Plus, Maxon, and PDS. *Can J Surg* **31**:43, 1988

9. Trimbos JB et al: Mechanical knot performance of a new generation of polydioxanon suture (PDS-2). *Acta Obstet Gynecol Scand* **70**:157, 1991

10. Moy RL, Kaufman AJ: Clinical comparisons of polyglycolic acid (Vicryl) and polytrimethylene carbonate (Maxon) suture material. *J Dermatol Surg Oncol* **17**:667, 1991

11. Chu CC et al: Newly made antibacterial preliminary biocompatibility study. *J Biomed Mater Res* **21**:1281, 1987

12. Matras H: Fibrin sealant in maxillofacial surgery: Development and indications: A review of the past 12 years. *J Facial Plast Surg* **2**:297, 1985

13. Staindl O: Indications of the fibrin sealant in facial plastic surgery. *J Facial Plast Surg* **2**:323, 1985

14. Lilius P: Fibrin adhesive: Its use in selected skin grafting: Practical note. *Scand J Plast Reconstr Surg Hand Surg* **21:**245, 1987

15. Stuart JD et al: Application of single-donor fibrin glue to burns. *J Burn Care Rehabil* **9:**619, 1988

16. Wilkinson TS: Tissue adhesives in cutaneous surgery. *Arch Dermatol* **106:**834, 1972

17. Dioguardi D, Musajo-Somma A: Treaded tapes for the suture-less closure of skin wounds. *British J Plast Surg* **30:**202, 1977

18. Moy RL, Quan MB: An evaluation of wound closure tapes. *J Dermatol Surg Oncol* **16:**721, 1990

19. Ersek RA: Prosthetic skin for physiologic wound closure. *Contemp Surg* **35:**64, 1989

20. Eldrup J et al: Randomised trial comparing proximate stapler with conventional skin closure. *Acta Chir Scand* **147:**501, 1981

21. Campbell JP, Swanson NA: The use of staples in dermatologic surgery. *J Dermatol Surg Oncol* **8:**680, 1982

22. Kaplan HY: A quick stapler tie-over fixation for skin grafts. *Ann Plast Surg* **22:**173, 1989

23. Hoffman HT, LaRouere M: A simple bolster technique for skin grafting. *Laryngoscope* **99:**558, 1989

24. Stegman SS et al: *Basics of Dermatologic Surgery.* Chicago, Year Book, 1982

Renuka Diwan

8 Instruments for Dermatologic Surgery

"A surgeon's hand would be of little use to him if he was not supplied with a variety of instruments," wrote Heister in the eighteenth century.[1] Hippocrates wrote that "all instruments ought to be well suited for the purpose in hand as regards their size, weight, and delicacy."[1] Most instruments used for dermatologic surgery are especially suited for handling the skin because of their small size and lighter weight, which allows delicate manipulation of tissue. Cutaneous scars are visible and, therefore, a significant part of the surgeon's effort is directed toward minimizing scarring. Precise and delicate tissue handling is central to the design of surgical instruments for skin surgery.[2]

Each instrument has special features designed for specific purposes. Proper selection of instruments for a particular procedure facilitates the operation and optimizes the outcome. A knowledge of the available instruments, their individual features and design, and their optimal use is therefore essential to good surgical technique.

Any basic surgical excision involves certain steps common to all cutaneous surgery, such as incision and excision, undermining, hemostasis, tissue movement for closure, suturing, and suture removal. The right instruments must be selected for performing each of these steps. Certain basic instruments will be appropriate for most cutaneous surgery. Specific procedures or procedures in certain anatomic locations may call for special instruments other than those used routinely. This chapter describes the instruments available to the dermatologic surgeon from which a selection can be made. Basic instruments will be recommended recognizing that individual preference influences the choice of instruments.

Instruments may be categorized according to the purpose for which they are designed (i.e., for which of the above steps of basic cutaneous surgery they are used). Accordingly, there are instruments for cutting, undermining, holding tissue, hemostasis, suturing, and suture removal. In addition, other instruments which cannot be properly assigned to one of the above classes will be considered separately.

CUTTING INSTRUMENTS

Included in this group are scalpels, scissors, punches, curettes, and dermatomes.

Scalpels

A scalpel is constructed of two parts: a handle and a blade. A variety of scalpel handles are available, with corresponding blades to fit each handle. The most commonly used handle is the Bard-Parker no. 3 scalpel handle (Fig. 8-1). The handle is weighted to provide stability to the instrument. When the anterior end bearing the blade is pressed downward, incising the tissue, the weight of the handle posteriorly provides a counterbalance. The handle is made with and without an engraved centimeter scale. The presence of the scale imparts an additional function to the handle which can be used for measuring the size of a lesion, operative defect, or sutured incision sterilely. The handle can also be used to flatten specimens obtained for Mohs micrographic surgery, with its flat surface. Other types of blade handles (Fig. 8-2) are available that fit Bard-Parker blades, such as the longer Bard-Parker no. 7 or

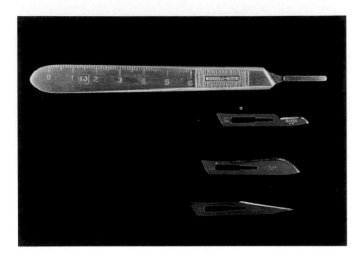

Figure 8-1 Bard-Parker #3 handle with an engraved scale, shown with Bard-Parker #15, #10 and #11 blades, from below upwards.

cylindric handles with a knurled surface (believed to provide a better grip).[3] A variety of handles and blades have been designed over the years by different surgeons in pursuit of the design that is best adapted to the hand.[1] A disposable plastic blade handle is useful when one is operating on patients with transmissible viral infections such as hepatitis B or human immunodeficiency virus (HIV). The plastic blade handle is not weighted and is not as easy to use.

The Bard-Parker no. 3 handle accommodates Bard-Parker nos. 10, 11, and 15 blades (Fig. 8-1). These blades are disposable and made from stainless steel or carbon steel (see discussion below). The no. 15 blade is the most frequently used for making skin incisions which are usually limited in length. The no. 15C blade is a smaller version of the no. 15 that is useful for excising small lesions. The larger no. 10 blade is useful for incising thick skin (e.g., on the back). The tip of the

blade is used to start the incision, which is continued with the belly. The sharpest portion of the no. 15 and no. 10 blades is the belly. The pointed tip provides the precision needed in incising the corners of elliptic excisions or flaps. The blade can also be used for sharp dissection of the skin from subjacent tissue although it is not the ideal instrument for this purpose. The lancet-like no. 11 blade is useful for making small stab incisions for drainage of abscesses and, if necessary, can be used for suture removal although it is not the preferred instrument for this purpose.

Blades are manufactured from stainless steel or carbon steel. Carbon steel is harder than stainless steel. Carbon steel blades are sharper and allow easier incision of loose, poorly supported tissue such as eyelid skin where much pressure cannot be applied. The common razor blade (Fig. 8-3), which is extremely sharp and very thin, is a carbon steel blade.[4] It is very useful for shave excision of skin lesions and incisions of thin skin where a very sharp blade must be used. The blade is inexpensive, disposable, and sharper than other routinely used scalpel blades. The cutting edge of the blade is only a millionth of an inch thick and has a fluorocarbon telomer coating to enhance its incisional ability. The blade can be broken into half and used with one hand for shave biopsies or shave excisions of superficial lesions. The blade can be bent to conform to the contour of the skin surface or to the depth of tissue removal. Precise excision of surface lesions can be achieved without creating a depressed scar. The half-blade is used most commonly in this manner for removal of nevi for cosmetic purposes. However, a corner of the cutting edge of the blade can be broken and engaged by an instrument called the *Castroviejo blade breaker and holder* (Fig. 8-4) for use like a scalpel for eyelid skin incisions.[2] The razor blade can be sterilized when used for sterile procedures.

Besides the workhorse Bard-Parker scalpel, the Beaver scalpel handles and blades (Fig. 8-5) are an option when fine control is necessary for excising very small lesions or work-

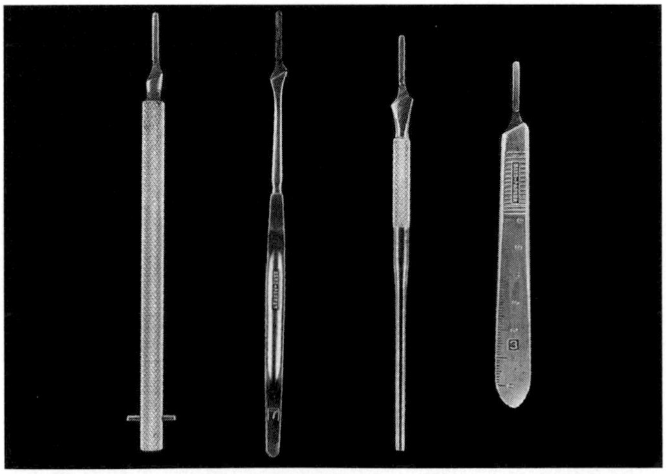

Figure 8-2 Other types of blade handles. From left to right: cylindrical knurled handle; Bard-Parker #7 handle; variation with knurled gripping surface, Bard-Parker #3 handle for comparison.

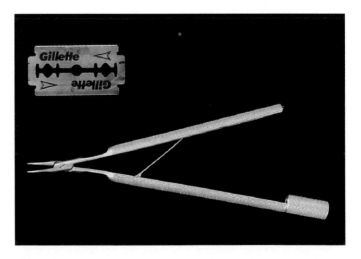

Figure 8-3 Razor blade, top left-hand corner. Castroviejo blade breaker-and-holder, bottom.

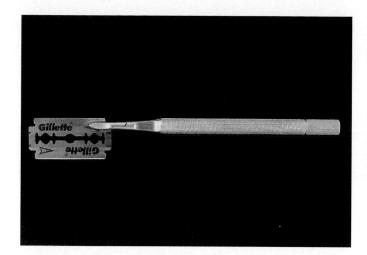

Figure 8-4   Razor blade properly engaged in Castroviejo blade breaker-and-holder for breaking a corner of the blade.

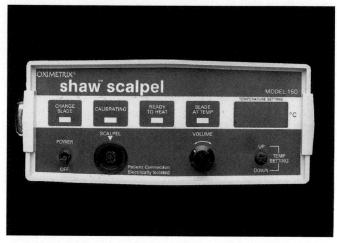

Figure 8-6   Hemostatic Shaw scalpel—the electronic controller box.

ing in areas with confining morphology such as the medial canthus. The Beaver blades, being smaller, can be better suited for small excisions. The Beaver blade no. 67 is a smaller equivalent of a no. 15 Bard-Parker, and the Beaver no. 65 is the smaller version of a no. 11 Bard-Parker blade. Beaver blade handles are hexagonal or cylindric and knurled. The knurled handles are preferred by some who believe that this surface provides a better grip on the instrument.

The Shaw scalpel (Figs. 8-6 and 8-7) is a hemostatic scalpel that has been available since the early 1980s.[5,6] It has the distinct benefit of achieving hemostasis as it cuts tissue and is, therefore, very useful when operating on highly vascular areas such as the scalp or on patients with a coagulopathy. Hemostasis is usually the most tedious and rate-limiting aspect of surgery, and significant time can be saved with the Shaw scalpel. The scalpel blade is sharp, disposable, and Teflon-coated except at the edge. The blade contains copper

electric microcircuits which heat the blade, as well as sensors in its circuit that regulate its temperature at the selected setting. There is no conduction of electricity to the cutting edge of the blade or the tissue. The blade temperature setting can range from 100°C to 270°C. The temperature can be selected by a lever on the electronic controller box itself (Fig. 8-6) or by depressing a button on the distal end of the handle. For cutting, the blade is set at 110° to 150° to seal blood vessels as they are cut. Larger blood vessels must be coagulated at a temperature of 270°C. The blade handle has a thermal coagulation bar (Fig. 8-7) which can be depressed to raise the temperature instantly to 270°C for hemostasis as necessary. The temperature can then be reduced to 110°C for further incisions. The degree of thermal tissue damage resulting from use of the blade is related to the duration of tissue contact with the blade. Expertise in handling the blade is essential to operate quickly and minimize thermal tissue damage. The Teflon

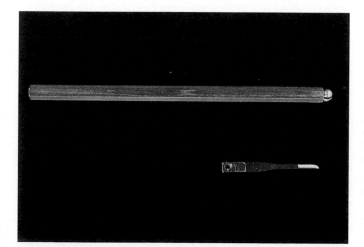

Figure 8-5   Beaver scalpel handle (hexagonal example) and #67 blade.

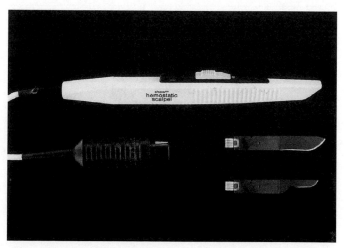

Figure 8-7   Shaw scalpel handle with thermal coagulation bar on its side. Teflon-coated #10 and #15 blades (from above below).

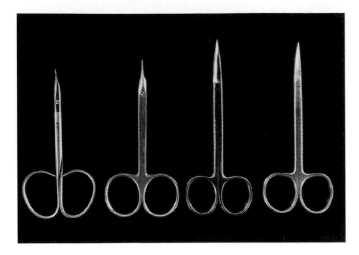

Figure 8-8 From left to right: Gradle; Stevens tenotomy; straight; and curved iris scissors.

coating minimizes adherence of tissue to the blade. The Shaw scalpel should not be used for operating on delicate tissues due to the risk of thermal damage. The blade is available in no. 15, no. 10 (Fig. 8-7) and no. 11 sizes.

Tissue-cutting Scissors

Scissors most commonly used for cutting skin are the Stevens tenotomy, iris, and Gradle (Fig. 8-8). Westcott scissors (Fig. 8-9) are useful for eyelid surgery.

The Stevens tenotomy scissors are available with straight or curved blades and sharp or blunt tips. The straight scissors are useful for cutting straight-line incisions, while the curved scissors are better suited for cutting curved edges (e.g., in an elliptic excision). In addition, the curved blunt-tipped scissors, the blades of which have a 15° to 20° curvature, can be useful for undermining skin. The blades of the scissors, which

dissect bluntly, can be kept parallel to the skin surface, in the plane of undermining, as they are advanced even when the shank of the scissors is held obliquely.

Gradle scissors were designed by Henry Gradle, an ophthalmologist, for suture removal from the eyelids. The Gradle scissors are small, $3^3/4$-in or 4-in long, and have curved blades with small, sharp tips. This makes them less versatile, but the small sharp tips can be easily placed under suture loops which are cut without undue traction on delicate tissue. They may also be used for scissors excision of small lesions such as papillomas.

Iris scissors, curved or straight, have small, sharp tips. The scissors' length ranges from $3^1/2$ in (the very delicate iris scissors) to $4^1/2$ in. The short delicate scissors are especially suited for fine precise work such as suture removal or surgery on delicate structures such as the eyelid. Curved iris scissors are useful for fine dissection for excision of epidermal inclusion cysts. Iris scissors are also available with fine serrations on the edge of one blade (Fig. 8-10). The serrations allow better gripping of the tissue being cut (e.g., fibroepithelial papillomas) between the blades, preventing it from slipping away.[8]

Westcott scissors (Fig. 8-9) have very sharp, small tips and have spring handles. They are used for fine dissection for eyelid surgery where precision is of utmost importance.

All tissue-cutting scissors are also available with tungsten carbide inserts bonded on both blades (Fig. 8-11). Tungsten carbide, being harder than stainless steel, can hold a sharper edge and is more durable.[2] The scissors with tungsten carbide inserts are significantly more costly than regular scissors, but the extra expense is worthwhile in the long run because of less instrument turnover. These extra-sharp scissors are useful for fine work. Scissors with tungsten carbide inserts have gold-plated finger rings for easy identification. Scissors are also available with larger finger rings (ribbon-type scissors) for larger hands.

Tissue-cutting scissors must be sharp and should not be

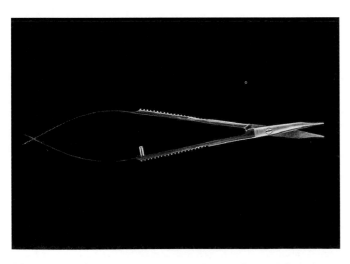

Figure 8-9 Westcott scissors have spring handles and fine, sharp tips.

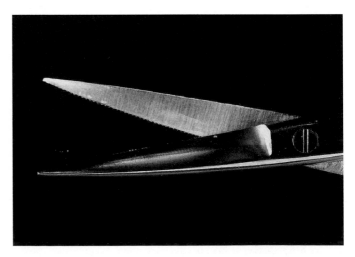

Figure 8-10 Iris scissors with fine serrations on one blade.

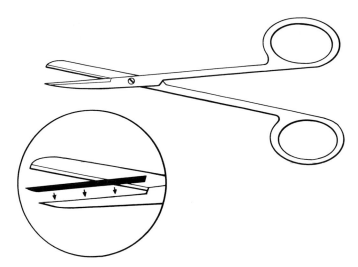

Figure 8-11 Tungsten-carbide inserts on the cutting edges of blades of scissors.

used for cutting suture, which has a dulling effect. A separate pair of scissors (see "Suture-Cutting Scissors" below) should be designated for cutting suture. A pair of curved blunt-tipped Stevens scissors and a pair of straight delicate iris scissors suffice for most surgical procedures on the face. Westcott or delicate curved iris scissors may be added for fine dissection in eyelid surgery.

Punches

A skin punch or trephine is one of the most frequently used dermatologic instruments (Fig. 8-12). A punch is a stainless steel cylinder with a circular cutting edge attached to a handle. Punches are available in incremental diameters (of the cutting edge). One of its earliest descriptions dates to 1887 and is credited to Edward Keyes, a dermatologist, for whom the Keyes punch is named.[9] Its first use was for excision of numerous pinpoint traumatic tattoos from implantation of gunpowder particles in the face. The Keyes punch is still used, being most frequently used now for obtaining biopsy specimens. Modifications of the punch are used for other indications such as excision of small lesions and ice-pick acne scars and hair transplantation.

The Keyes punch is the most familiar of the nondisposable punches, and the size ranges from 1 mm to 10 mm, with 1-mm increments. The walls of the punch are thick and slanted, being wider at the top and narrower at the cutting edge, and the bevel is on the outside of the barrel of the punch. Both of these features are felt to be responsible for the conic specimen obtained.[2] Therefore, the Keyes punch cannot be used for harvesting hair-bearing grafts because the peripheral follicles would be transected.

Different modifications of the punch are available for specific purposes.[10] The Loo trephine (Fig. 8-12) has very thin walls that are more vertical and is attached to a short, knurled handle that is held between the thumb and index finger. It is useful when a vertical incision must be produced in the skin for elevation of the base of depressed scars (e.g., chicken pox scars) or for punch grafts.

Orentreich first described the thin-walled motorized punch for harvesting hair grafts in 1959. The punches used for hair transplantation are attached to a hand engine (Fig. 8-13) for faster harvesting. These punches were beveled on the external surface of the cutting edge. Over the years, attention was focused on the placement of the bevel to improve the quality of the graft harvested.[6,10] Punches with external bevels yield conic grafts. Punches made with an internal bevel yield more cylindric grafts with a greater number of complete hair follicles. The *Australian punch,* (Fig. 8-14) designed for hair transplantation by Australian practitioners, has an internal bevel and also provides more cylindric specimens. Punches

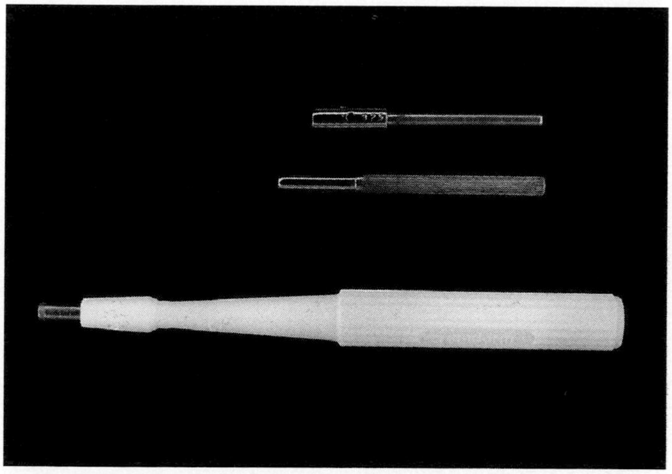

Figure 8-12 Disposable skin punch (bottom); Loo trephine (middle); and the Orentreich punch (top).

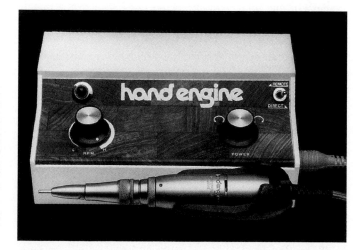

Figure 8-13 Hand engine for motorized harvesting of grafts for hair transplantation, and dermabrasion. Either a punch or dermabrasion fraise is fitted into the tip of the hand engine.

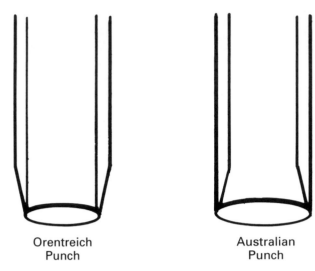

Orentreich
Punch

Australian
Punch

Figure 8-14   The external bevel and the internal bevel of skin punches.

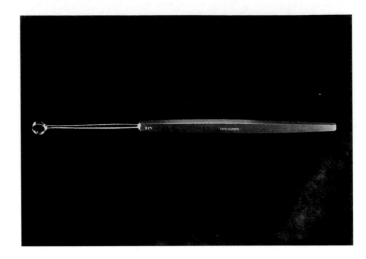

Figure 8-15   Fox curette with circular head and semi-sharp edge.

made for hair transplantation must be very sharp and are made from high-quality carbon steel. Orentreich has also designed a hand-held punch with a short 3-mm-wide knurled handle attached to the punch for creating recipient holes for the hair grafts.[6,10]

Disposable punches are used most commonly for biopsies and small excisions. They are razor sharp, have an external bevel, and are available in sizes ranging from 2 mm to 6 mm, with 0.5- to 1-mm increments in size. Punches are also used for excision of small disks of cartilage to allow placement of a full-thickness skin graft on bare (devoid of perichondrium) cartilage.

When a circular punch is used for excision of small lesions or scars, an elliptic wound that can be sutured without significant dog-ears can be produced by stretching the skin perpendicularly to the relaxed skin tension lines prior to the punch excision. An elliptic wound can thus be created more quickly than with a scalpel.

Besides their use in dermatology, punches are also used in plastic surgery. Large-diameter (40 mm and 50 mm) punches are used for transplanting nipple and areolar tissue for reconstructive surgery of the breast.[10]

Curettes

Dermal curettes are used almost exclusively by dermatologists. The dermal curette was fashioned after a uterine curette. Lesions such as seborrheic and actinic keratoses, molluscum contagiosum, and many basal and squamous cell carcinomas can be readily excised with a curette. The head of a curette is a round [Fox curette (Fig. 8-15)] or an oval (Piffard curette), semisharp blade. The semisharp blade is able to cut through friable or soft tissue of the lesions noted above, but it is not sharp enough to incise normal skin. This allows the curette to

distinguish between normal and abnormal tissue and selectively excise the abnormal tissue. If curettes are resharpened, care must be taken to keep the cutting edge semisharp only.

The Fox curette is available in sizes from 1 mm to 7 mm. Very small curettes, 1 mm to 2 mm in diameter, are important for curetting out small pockets of tumor that cannot be reached by the larger curettes.[11] Heath, Skeele, and Meyhoefer curettes are all small curettes that are not routinely needed.[2] The Heath curette is a smaller version of the Fox curette. The Skeele curette is cuplike with a serrated edge and may be useful for curetting out the cyst walls of small cysts after they are drained.[2]

Dermatomes

Dermatomes are instruments for harvesting split-thickness skin grafts. The two most commonly used for dermatologic surgery are the Brown dermatome and the Davol-Simon dermatome.

The Brown dermatome (Fig. 8-16) is an electric dermatome. The casing of the dermatome is sterilizable but the blade is disposable. The blade must be assembled with the casing prior to use. The blade is $3^3/_8$-in wide, but adjustment screws allow precise alteration of the width of the graft; narrower grafts can be harvested by bringing the screws closer. Calibration screws permit selection of the graft thickness. For medium-thickness grafts, 0.015-in thick, a no. 15 Bard-Parker blade which is approximately 0.015-in thick at its cutting edge can be used to verify the dermatome setting.[12] The space between the blade and the dermatome guard should just allow the insertion of the cutting edge of the no. 3 Bard-Parker blade for harvesting a medium-thickness skin graft.

The Davol-Simon (Fig. 8-17) is also a battery-powered electric dermatome. The unit has a portable, nonsterilizable handle that houses a rechargeable battery. The handle must be covered by a sterile plastic sleeve that is supplied with the dis-

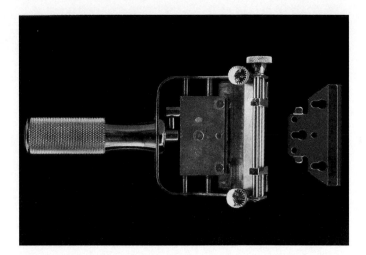

Figure 8-16 Brown dermatome and its disposable blade (right). The end of the handle is connected to an electrical motor. Calibration screws at either end adjust graft thickness.

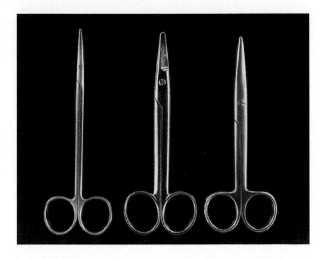

Figure 8-18 Right to left: Straight Metzenbaum (blade-to-handle ratio of 5:1); Castenares; and Mayo (blade-to-handle ratio of 1:1) scissors for undermining.

posable single-use head. The thickness of the graft is fixed at 0.015 in and its width is fixed at 3 cm. It is useful for harvesting small grafts, as it may not have sufficient energy to harvest a long graft.

UNDERMINING INSTRUMENTS

Undermining of the skin is performed with blunt-tipped scissors such as the Stevens tenotomy scissors. Blunt tips are less traumatic than sharp tips, displacing vessels and nerves from their path rather than piercing them. Metzenbaum scissors (Fig. 8-18), having longer handles, are useful in areas where a longer reach is necessary (e.g., for wide undermining on the cheek). The handle-to-blade ratio is 5:1, and the relatively short blades make a small arc when the long handles are

opened, allowing careful undermining. Metzenbaum scissors are available with straight or curved blades.

Mayo scissors (Fig. 8-18) are also blunt-tipped and longer than Stevens tenotomy scissors. The handle-to-blade ratio is 1:1, and the blade tips trace a longer arc. They are therefore not utilized in delicate areas where limited undermining must be performed carefully. They are useful on the trunk where coarser undermining is acceptable and a large area can be undermined quickly. The curved scissors can offer an advantage over straight scissors in maintaining the plane of undermining more easily.

For delicate tissues, fine dissection is best performed with delicate scissors with small sharp tips such as Westcott scissors (see discussion above). Kaye scissors (Fig. 8-19) are blunt-tipped, 4½-in long, and curved. Because these scissors are short, the fingertips can be placed very close to the tips of

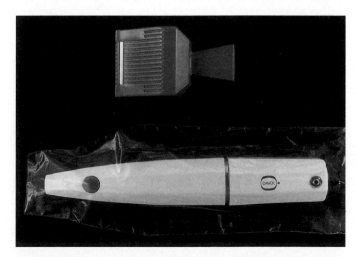

Figure 8-17 Davol-Simon dermatome. The portable handle (bottom) with sterile plastic sheath covering and disposable blade (top).

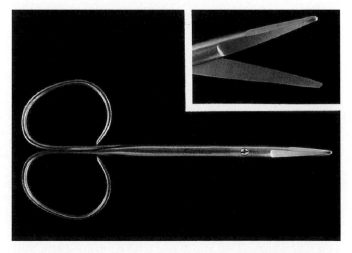

Figure 8-19 Kaye scissors. Inset: One serrated blade, both blades semi-sharp on external edge.

the scissors for close control. The cutting edge of the blades have fine serrations, and the outer edge of the distal half of each blade is semisharp to facilitate undermining. They are felt to be especially useful for blepharoplasty and other situations where fine work is required.[13]

TISSUE-HOLDING INSTRUMENTS

The principle of atraumatic handling of the skin to minimize scarring and optimize the final cosmetic result was established by Halsted. A variety of forceps and skin hooks are available for this purpose. A chalazion clamp is also used to hold tissue in special situations.

Skin Hooks

Skin hooks (Fig. 8-20) are the preferred instruments for tissue holding because they cannot crush the skin edges. Gentle handling prevents devitalization of tissue which invites infection and leads to delayed healing and unnecessary scarring. Since these scars are externally visible, utmost attention must be paid to details of tissue manipulation.

Hooks are available with sharp or blunt prongs. The sharp prongs hold tissue more securely than blunt prongs, which retract but do not actually anchor the tissue. Hooks may be single or double pronged. Skin hooks used commonly for dermatologic surgery are the Tyrell and Guthrie hooks (Fig. 8-20). The Tyrell hook has a small single prong which may be sharp or blunt. The sharp hook is commonly used. The Guthrie hook has two sharp prongs 1.5 mm apart. Larger double- or triple-pronged retractors may be necessary for large flaps on the trunk. Retractors with more than two prongs are also called *rakes*.

Skin hooks are easy to use and are very versatile instruments.[14,15] A hook can be used to lift out a punch biopsy specimen without damaging it or altering histologic details. A skin hook is used to retract the edges of a wound to expose bleeding sites for obtaining hemostasis. A skin hook is also used to place traction on a wound edge or flap as it is being undermined and thus provides countertraction against the forward force of the undermining scissors. For placement of buried subcutaneous sutures, a skin hook everts the skin edge. A skin hook applied to a dog-ear at the pole of a wound demonstrates the degree of cutaneous redundancy that needs to be excised and helps to define the length of the incision needed for its excision.

Forceps

The variety of tissue handled in dermatologic surgery calls for a variety of forceps. The most commonly used forceps are the toothed Adson forceps (Fig. 8-21). They have broad handles that taper to long, narrow tips. There may be one tooth on one tip fitting into two on the opposite or two on one tip fitting into three on the opposite. In addition, the tips may bear a tying platform (Fig. 8-21) proximal to the teeth. The tying platform allows the surgeon to easily grasp the needle when tying knots, these being difficult to hold with the forceps' teeth. Adson forceps with serrated tips (Fig. 8-22) are used for sterile handling of gauze and dressing material. Their use for grasping skin edges is not recommended because the tissue is easily crushed between the tips. Brown-Adson forceps (Fig. 8-21) have a row of seven or eight interdigitating teeth on the tips and are useful for holding thick subcutaneous tissue or cartilaginous tissue on the nose or ears which is difficult to hold with Adson forceps.

The Lalonde forceps, a new forceps with hooks instead of teeth at the tips and a tying platform proximal to the hooks, have been introduced to combine the benefits of a skin hook (atraumatic handling) with the ease of using a forceps for suturing.[16]

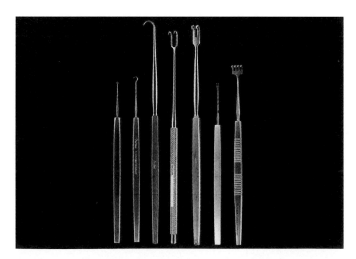

Figure 8-20   Left to right: 1) Frazier hook; 2) Tyrell hook; 3) sharp single-pronged retractor; 4–5) sharp double-pronged retractors; 6) Guthrie hook; and 7) rake.

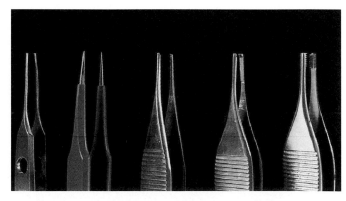

Figure 8-21   Left to right: Bishop-Harmon forceps; Jewelers forceps; Adson toothed forceps; Adson forceps with tying platform; and Brown-Adson forceps.

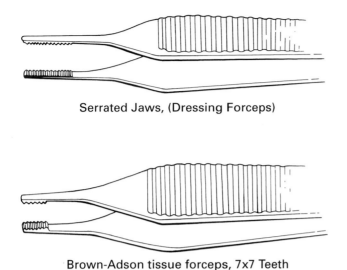

Serrated Jaws, (Dressing Forceps)

Brown-Adson tissue forceps, 7x7 Teeth

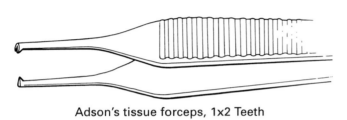

Adson's tissue forceps, 1x2 Teeth

Figure 8-22 Adson forceps with serrated tips. Brown-Adson forceps with seven interdigilating teeth. Toothed Adson forceps with one tooth fitting into two.

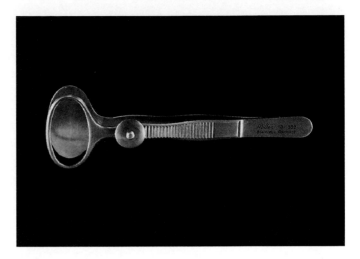

Figure 8-23 Chalazion clamp for holding eyelid or lip.

For delicate handling of thin tissue such as eyelid skin, the Bishop-Harmon forceps (Fig. 8-21) are useful. They are small, have three holes on each handle for a better grip, and have very delicate teeth on fine tips.

Graefe forceps have wide jaws with fine teeth and are useful for holding cartilage.[17]

Jeweler's forceps (Fig. 8-21) have very fine tips that are useful for point cauterization of bleeding vessels but are too fine for grasping tissue. They can also be used for removing suture fragments or splinters.

Chalazion Clamp

A chalazion clamp (Fig. 8-23) is a modification of a forceps. The tips of the forceps are replaced by an oval plate on one side and an apposing oval ring on the opposite. When the plate and the ring are apposed, a curvature in the long axis of the oval is apparent and is meant to conform to the curvature of the eyelid, for which it is specifically designed. In addition, the forceps are tightened by a thumb screw between the two sides.

The chalazion clamp is designed specifically for use in treating a chalazion on the eyelid. The eyelid is held and sta-

bilized with the chalazion clamp, the oval ring being placed around the lesion to be excised with the oval plate behind it. The screw is tightened so that the tissue is firmly held. Overtightening should be avoided to prevent crushing the skin. The tissue enclosed is thus stabilized, making the clamp useful in areas like the eyelid and lip which are difficult to grasp. Due to the circumferential pressure around the lesion, hemostasis is also achieved. This makes it a useful instrument for lip biopsies or excisions when an assistant is unavailable to occlude the labial arteries on either side of the operative site.

SUTURING INSTRUMENTS

Instruments used for suturing are needle-holders, forceps or skin hooks (discussed above), suture-cutting scissors, and staplers.

Needle-holders

Needle-holders selected for dermatologic surgery are meant to hold small needles and fine suture used in most instances. The jaws of the needle-holder must, therefore, be small so that the small needles are not damaged. When larger needles must be used (e.g., for surgery on thick tissue of the trunk), a larger needle-holder is more appropriate so that the needle does not slip. The Webster needle-holder (Fig. 8-24) is most commonly used. The jaws of the needle-holder are narrow and may be smooth or finely toothed. Holding suture ends in toothed jaws for tying knots may result in fraying, and smooth jaws are, therefore, preferred. The jaws are available with tungsten carbide inserts which provide a harder surface (Fig. 8-24). The inserts are thought to give a more secure hold on the needle and decrease instrument wear. Such instruments have gold-plated finger rings and are much more expensive than those without the tungsten carbide inserts.

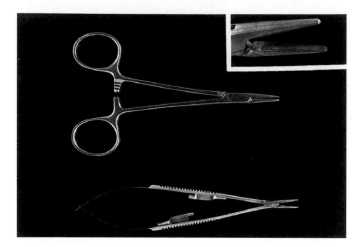

Figure 8-24   Needle-holders: Webster and Castroviejo. Inset: Tungsten-carbide inserts on needle-holder tips.

Suture-cutting Scissors

A variety of scissors may be used for this purpose, some made specifically for this use. The delicate iris scissors (Fig. 8-25) with fine, narrow tips that can be easily inserted under the suture loop, are very well suited for this purpose. The angled iris scissors (Fig. 8-25) are also very useful. Gradle scissors which have sharp narrow tips were originally designed for suture removal. Spencer suture scissors (Fig. 8-25) have a hook on the tip of one blade by which the suture loop can be picked up easily. The loop is then cut by the opposite blade as the scissors are closed. The hook is blunt-tipped to prevent trauma to the skin during suture removal.[17] As mentioned above, a designated pair of scissors should be used for cutting suture so that tissue-cutting scissors are not dulled.

The Castroviejo needle-holder (Fig. 8-24) is an alternative when operating on delicate tissue like eyelid skin. The jaws of this needle-holder are narrower and more delicate than the Webster needle-holder and do not damage the fine needles used on eyelids. The jaws are available with tungsten carbide inserts. It has spring handles with an optional lock. The lock can be set or released with a single press on the spring handle and is easier to operate than the lock on the Webster needle-holder, although it takes some practice to become comfortable with it. The instrument may be used with ease by both right- and left-handed operators. It is significantly more expensive than the Webster needle-holder and is not necessary for routine use.

Staplers

Sutures can be substituted by steel staples for approximation of wound edges in locations where detailed closure and cosmetic outcome are not critical. Such instances include fixation of large split-thickness grafts, where coverage rather than cosmetic result is the goal, and long incisions on the scalp, extremities, or trunk. Staples are placed across the wound edges by a stapler (Fig. 8-26) which dispenses sterile staples. Stainless steel causes very little tissue reaction.

Stapled wound closure is more expeditious than suturing and saves time when closing long incisions. When the wound has healed, staples can be removed with a staple remover (Fig. 8-26). When an occasional improperly placed staple must be removed while the physician is stapling, a hemostat placed and opened under the staple is a handy improvised sta-

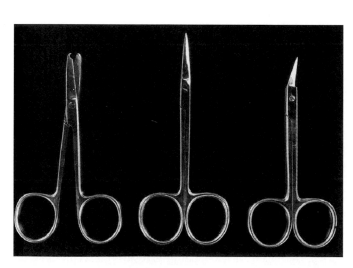

Figure 8-25   Suture-cutting scissors. From left to right: Spencer; straight delicate iris; and angled scissors.

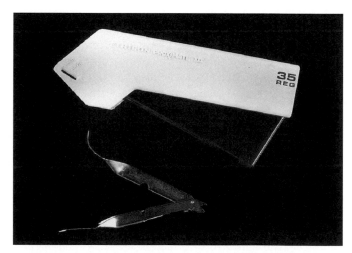

Figure 8-26   Stapler and staple-remover. The hooked jaw of the staple-remover is placed under the staple to be removed.

ple remover and avoids wasting a staple remover just for limited use.

Staplers may be disposable or reusable. Reusable staplers can be autoclaved and are used with sterile cartridges of staples. The Proximate II stapler (Ethicon, Sommerville, New Jersey) is available with staples that are 0.53-mm wide (regular) or 0.58-mm wide (wide).[17]

HEMOSTATIC INSTRUMENTS

These include Hartman and Halsted hemostats (hemostatic forceps), electrocoagulation devices, and heat cautery.

Hemostats

In dermatologic surgery, hemostats are needed for clamping small bleeding vessels that cannot be coagulated by electrodesiccation. Those with fine, narrow tips allow focal isolation of small vessels for ligation without damage to surrounding tissue. The small Halsted and Hartman hemostats (Fig. 8-27), also known as *mosquito hemostats,* are best suited for cutaneous surgery. The Halsted mosquito hemostat is curved or straight, 5-in long, light, and has narrow, serrated blades with fine tips. The serrations provide a better grasp of tissue. It is appropriate for most procedures performed by the dermatologic surgeon. The Hartman mosquito hemostat is similar to the Halsted hemostat except that it is only 3½-in long. It is particularly useful for clamping the orbital fat pads when these are being excised during blepharoplasty. This small, light instrument can be gently supported with less risk of traction on the fat pads and consequent retroorbital bleeding.

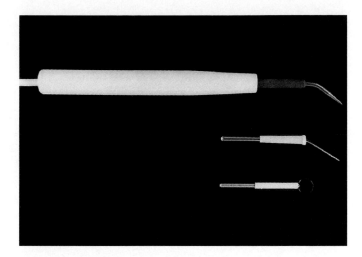

Figure 8-28   Hand unit of Birtcher hyfrecator with resterilizable tip attached (top), and disposable tip (middle) used with hyfrecator. Cutting loop (bottom) used only with Bovie for electrotomy.

Electrocoagulation Devices

The Birtcher hyfrecator is the most popular with dermatologists. It is a portable monopolar, monoterminal device (Fig. 8-28) used for electrodesiccation, electrofulguration, and electrocoagulation. It cannot be used for electrotomy. Bipolar forceps (Fig. 8-29) are available for use with the hyfrecator. A 5-in Adson forceps or 4-in jeweler's forceps can be used to localize the electric current as much as possible. Less current conduction occurs with bipolar forceps than with a monoterminal tip. A dry field is necessary when one is using either the monopolar tip or biterminal forceps to achieve hemostasis.

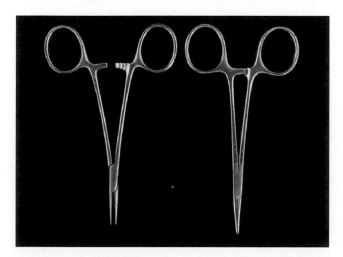

Figure 8-27   Straight (left) and curved (right) Halsted "mosquito" hemostats.

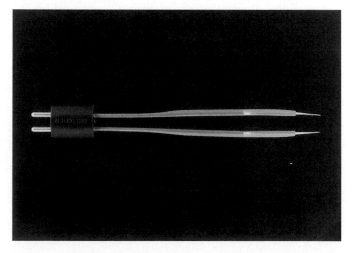

Figure 8-29   Bipolar forceps can be used with hyfrecator to localize electrical current for hemostasis.

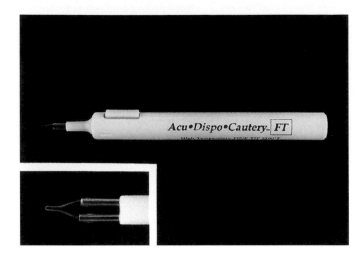

Figure 8-30 Disposable battery-powered heat cautery.

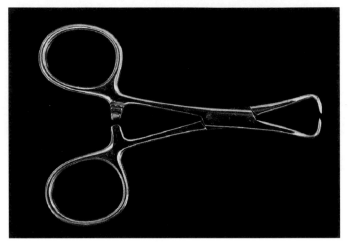

Figure 8-31 Backhaus towel clamp with ratchet clamp.

The electrode can be activated either by a foot control or a switch on the hand unit. The voltage used can be adjusted on a dial on the face of the hyfrecator unit. The hyfrecator tip as well as the cord that attaches it to the hyfercator can be sterilized by autoclaving for use in a sterile field. Alternatively, the hand unit can be placed within a sterile sleeve (e.g., a Penrose drain).

A fresh monoterminal tip, such as a disposable tip (Fig. 8-28), should be used for each patient because the potential for transmission of hepatitis B virus by a tip used on an infected patient has been demonstrated.[18] The smoke generated by use of the electrocautery on viral lesions has been shown to contain infectious papillomavirus particles.[19] A smoke evacuation device is now available for use with the hyfrecator to remove the smoke generated from the surgical field.

The Bovie electrosurgical unit is used for all the functions of a hyfrecator and also for electrotomy (cutting) (Fig. 8-28). The advantage of a Bovie unit is that it can be used for the entire range of electrosurgical functions. It is a monopolar biterminal unit, a grounding pad being used with it.

The heat cautery achieves hemostasis by heat coagulation of the bleeding vessels without transmission of any electric impulses through the tissue. It produces more focal thermal tissue damage than an electric cautery. A disposable battery-powered penlike unit (Fig. 8-30) is available. It is particularly useful in delicate areas like the eyelid where thermal damage needs to be minimized.[19] The cautery has also been recommended for use as a cutting tool for dissection of the orbicularis oculi and orbital fat pads during blepharoplasty.[20]

TOWEL CLAMPS

The Backhaus towel clamp (Fig. 8-31) is commonly used. A towel clamp is used to anchor sterile drapes over the surgical field. It can also be used to anchor a sterile hyfrecator cord in

the operative field. Towel clamps have also been used to approximate wound edges on thick scalp tissue when there is significant tension across the wound. A towel clamp thus applied provides sustained limited traction on the wound edges, helping to recruit additional tissue for wound closure through the phenomenon of creep. However, this results in large holes in the skin edges where the clamp was placed and therefore should be used only on thick tissue for this purpose.

BANDAGE SCISSORS

The Lister bandage scissors (Fig. 8-32) are designed specifically for cutting bandages wrapped around wounds. The scissors are angled, and one tip has a large blunt end that the physician inserts under the bandage, without the fear of cutting the patient's skin. The angled blades allow for easy pas-

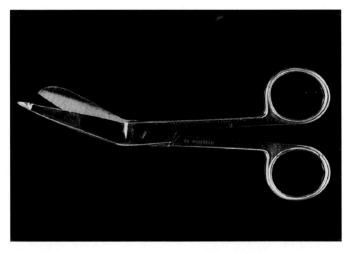

Figure 8-32 Lister bandage scissors with blunt end (in horizontal plane) on lower blade.

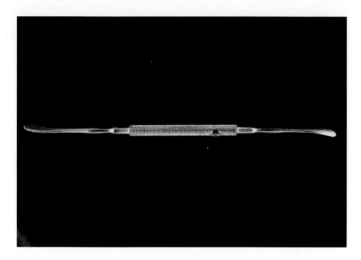

Figure 8-33   Freer periosteal elevator.

sage of the scissors under the bandage. The blades are thick and cut gauze bandages easily. The Universal bandage scissors are a modification and have serrated blade edges with extra cutting power and greater durability.

PERIOSTEAL ELEVATORS:

The Freer periosteal elevator (Fig. 8-33) is used for removing periosteum or perichondrium, usually to ensure tumor-free margins during Mohs surgery. It is a double-ended instrument with a gently curved spatula-like tip at either end. On one end, the edge is sharp and on the other it is blunt. The blunt end is also very useful for separating the nail plate from the nail bed or the proximal nail fold from the nail plate under it during a nail avulsion procedure.

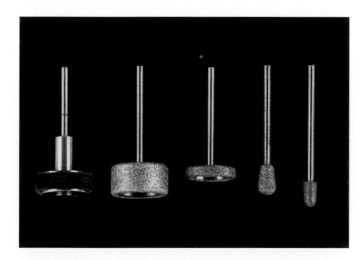

Figure 8-34   Left to right: Wire brush; wide coarse fraise; narrow coarse fraise; pear-shaped fraise; and bullet-shaped fraise.

DERMABRASION FRAISES AND WIRE BRUSH

The basic instrument for dermabrading the skin is the diamond fraise. A diamond fraise (Fig. 8-34) is a stainless steel wheel, the surface of which is studded with minute diamond chips to make it rough.[6] The skin is abraded as the rapidly rotating rough surface touches it. The wheel diameter varies from 1 cm to 1.7 cm. The different wheel thicknesses (widths) available are 2.5 mm, 4 mm, 6 mm, 8 mm, and 10 mm. Wheels with greater thickness provide a larger abrading surface and, therefore, abrade more quickly. The degree of coarseness of the wheel is described as fine, coarse, or extra coarse. Dermabrasion fraises are also available in other shapes (Fig. 8-34) such as the pear-shaped fraise, the cone-shaped fraise, and the bullet-shaped fraise. These modified fraises are preferred for dermabrasion of small areas (e.g., the tragus of the ear), for concave areas such as the root of the nose, or for the finer abrasion of feathering.[6]

Diamond fraises are used mounted on the handpiece of a hand engine and can be safely rotated at speeds up to 60,000 to 85,000 rpm. The direction of rotation of the fraise can be clockwise or anticlockwise. The ability to change the direction of rotation of the fraise allows the surgeon to dermabrade safely over free edges such as the lip or nasal alar rim without changing position with respect to the patient.

The Kurtin wire brush (Fig. 8-34), described originally in 1953, is another device used for dermabrasion.[6] The wire brush is also a stainless steel wheel, but instead of diamond chips the surface of the wheel bears numerous stainless steel wires. The ends of the wires are bent to a 30° angle so that they can cut the skin as the rotating wheel makes contact with it. The wheel diameter is 1.7 cm and is available in two thicknesses: 3 mm and 6 mm. The thickness of the wires themselves varies from fine (0.0025 in) to medium (0.003 in) to coarse (0.004 in). The wire brush produces a much deeper and more uneven dermabrasion than the diamond fraise and should only be used by experienced dermabraders trained in its use. Due to the angulation of the wires, the wire brush can be rotated in one direction only. The brush cannot be balanced to provide safe use at over 25,000 rpm.[6]

INSTRUMENT CARE

The proper care and sterilization of instruments are important not only for their longevity but also for the safety of the patient and staff. Transmission of infection by contaminated instruments to staff or other patients is an important concern.

The steps for sterilizing instruments include an initial physical cleaning of the instruments, followed by wrapping them in sealed packages, and then sterilization. A number of different techniques are available for each of these steps. Each method has its advantages and disadvantages.

Physical cleaning of instruments is necessary to remove debris such as blood and the bulk of contaminating bacteria harbored in this debris. Instruments should be washed as soon as possible to prevent drying of blood or other debris on them. A thorough cleaning with a brush is essential for cleaning irregular surfaces or crevices (e.g., between the teeth of forceps). Physical cleaning can also be accomplished with an ultrasonic instrument cleaner. Sound waves with a frequency of 20,600 to 38,000 are generated by a transducer in a metallic tank in which the instruments are placed. Air bubbles generated by the vibrations dislodge debris from instruments when they collapse (implode). Ultrasonic cleaning decreases the risk of injury to personnel as compared to hand cleaning and also damages bacterial cell walls. Some debris may loosely remain on the instruments and needs to be washed off.

Lubrication of instrument joints is then done, as necessary, prior to sterilization. Oil is not recommended for lubrication as bacterial spores are more resistant to heat sterilization with an oil film. Oil-in-water emulsions are available which can be used for this purpose. Instruments are then packed in paper or cloth before placing them in the sterilizer. Instruments are placed in the open position for complete sterilization.

Sterilization is most frequently achieved in the office setting with a steam-pressure autoclave. Bacteria are more easily destroyed with moist heat rather than dry heat. An autoclave indicator tape is included with the instrument to verify proper sterilization. Instruments contaminated with HIV should be washed and autoclaved for at least 10 min.[2] Inactivation of the hepatitis B virus can be accomplished at 121°C in less than 10 min.[2] Unusual pathogens such as the scrapie disease virus survive autoclaving for 1 h, and standard sterilization techniques are inadequate for such organisms. Time and pressure instructions provided by the manufacturer should be followed.

A disadvantage of moist heat sterilization is that sharp instruments are dulled. Flash sterilization can be performed if a dirty instrument is needed quickly. Steam sterilization for 3 to 5 min can be performed at a higher temperature (as recommended for the particular model).

Besides steam sterilization, other methods are available. Dry heat sterilization offers the advantage of less dulling of sharp instruments but takes longer to kill bacterial spores. Gas sterilization is performed with ethylene oxide and is useful for sterilization of those materials that cannot be heat sterilized (e.g., plastic tubing). Such sterilizers are manufactured for office use as well.

Chemical disinfection (destruction of pathogens but not necessarily all organisms) is frequently used for disinfection of instruments in offices. A 2% glutaraldehyde solution (Cidex) is most commonly used. HIV is inactivated rapidly by soaking instruments in Cidex.[21] A 0.5% sodium hypochlorite solution (a 1:10 dilution of household bleach) inactivates viral agents in 1 min.[22,23] Full-strength bleach corrodes and dissolves instruments and should never be used since it is an effective disinfectant when diluted 1:10 with water.[24]

CONCLUSION

Surgical procedures are greatly facilitated by the use of proper instruments. The choice of instruments is influenced by individual preference. Instruments with tungsten carbide inserts may be worth the additional expense because they are more durable and less time is spent on replacing instruments. Good-quality instruments that are properly cared for provide the best value in the long term.

REFERENCES

1. Thompson CJS: The evolution and development of surgical instruments. *Br J Surg* **25**:1–5, 1937

2. Bennett RG: Instruments and their care, in *Fundamentals of Cutaneous Surgery.* St. Louis, Mosby, 1988 pp 240–273

3. Field LM: Surgical gem: A new, rounded scalpel handle. *J Dermatol Surg Oncol* **8**:918, 1982

4. Shelley WB: The razor blade in dermatologic practice. *Cutis* **16**:843–845, 1975

5. Salyer KE: Use of a new hemostatic scalpel in plastic surgery. *Ann Plast Surg* **13**:532–538, 1984

6. Goldman MP et al: Instrumentation for cosmetic surgery. *Clin Dermatol* **6**:108–121, 1988

7. Gibbs RC: Surgical gem: A love affair with a Gradle scissors. *J Dermatol Surg Oncol* **7**:531, 1981

8. Koranda FC, Luckasen JR: Instruments and tips for dermatologic surgery. *J Dermatol Surg Oncol* **8**:451–454, 1982

9. Keyes EL: The cutaneous punch. *J Cutan Genitourin Dis* **5**:98–101, 1887

10. Stegman SJ: Commentary: The cutaneous punch. *Arch Dermatol* **118**:943–944, 1982

11. Krull EA: Surgical gems: The "little" curette. *J Dermatol Surg Oncol* **4**:656–657, 1978

12. Vecchione TR: A technique for obtaining uniform split-thickness skin grafts. *Arch Surg* **109**:837, 1974

13. Kaye BL: Useful scissors for fine dissecting. *Br J Plast Surg* **24**:319–320, 1971

14. Popkin GL, Brodie SJ: The versatile skin hook. *Arch Dermatol* **86**:343–344, 1962

15. Popkin GL, Gibbs RC: Surgical gems: Another look at the skin hook. *J Dermatol Surg Oncol* **4**:366–368, 1978

16. Lalonde DH: Hook forceps. *Ann Plast Surg* **26**:597–599, 1991

17. Grande DJ, Neuberg M: Instrumentation for the dermatologic surgeon. *J Dermatol Surg Oncol* **15**:288–297, 1989

18. Sherertz EF et al: Transfer of hepatitis B virus by contaminated reusable needle electrodes after electrodessication in simulated use. *J Am Acad Dermatol* **15**:1242–1246, 1986

19. Sawchuk WS et al: Infectious papillomavirus in the vapor of warts treated with carbon dioxide laser or electrocoagulation: Detection and protection. *J Am Acad Dermatol* **21**:41–49, 1989

20. Kaye BL: Two helpful technical aids in blepharoplasty. *Plast Reconstr Surg* **71:**714–715, 1983

21. Spire B et al: Inactivation of lymphadenopathy associated virus by chemical disinfectants. *Lancet* **2:**899–901, 1984

22. Resnick L et al: Stability and inactivation of HTLV-111/LAV under clinical and laboratory environments. *JAMA* **255:**1887–1891, 1986

23. Recommendations for prevention of HIV transmission in health-care settings. *MMWR* **36:**S2–S18, 1987

24. Wesley RE: Destruction of surgical instruments following use of disinfectants to eradicate human immunodeficiency virus. *Ophthalmic Surg* **21:**453–454, 1990

II Evaluation a Management of the Surgical Patient

Timothy H. McCalmont
Barry Leshin

9 Preoperative Evaluation of the Cutaneous Surgery Patient

Careful and comprehensive preoperative planning and evaluation are essential to superlative surgical care. The surgeon must consider three main factors: the nature of the presenting problem or lesion, the anatomic structures that may be affected by the lesion or the surgical procedure, and other medical conditions of the patient that may affect the procedure and its outcome. The time and thought invested in a comprehensive review will yield a better surgical outcome and a decreased complication rate.

Preoperative patient education may also facilitate the actual surgical procedure. An understanding of the nature of a procedure assuages patient fears and thus increases cooperation and rapport. Similarly, if a patient comprehends fully why surgery is necessary and comes to grips with the inherent risks of a particular procedure, there will be no postoperative surprises and fewer postoperative disappointments, even in the face of complications.

THE MEDICAL HISTORY

It is obviously important to obtain an accurate and detailed history of the presenting problem. The value of a careful and complete past medical history and review of systems may be overlooked, however. Patients generally do not volunteer important medical historical information, thus such data must be extracted through direct questioning. It is appropriate to obtain a screening history through a written questionnaire. However, a patient interview by the surgeons and their staff regarding selected important topics will maximize the information yield. The general factors of importance in the medical history are listed in Table 9-1.

Drug Reactions

Inquiry should be made regarding any previous reactions to local anesthetics, sedatives, analgesics, and antibiotics. The true nature of any reported adverse reaction should be ascertained (if possible), as many patients consider themselves "allergic" to important medications, and the "allergy" may consist of nothing more than mild gastric distress. Prior hypersensitivity to topical agents or dressings should also be recorded, as this information may permit avoidance of morbidity in the postoperative period.

Medications That May Affect Surgery

Several classes of medications may predispose the patient to increased operative risk, and thus a careful drug history is imperative. Particular attention must be paid to medications with anticoagulative, anti-inflammatory, beta-blocking, immunosuppressive, or neurologic effects.

TABLE 9-1

Medical Historical Factors of Importance to the Cutaneous Surgeon

Previous drug reactions

Medications

    Anticoagulants

    Aspirin

    Nonsteroidal anti-inflammatory drugs

    Beta-blockers

    Immunosuppressive drugs

    Neuroleptic drugs

Cardiac disease

    Atherosclerosis

    Valvular heart disease

    Congenital heart disease

    Cardiac pacemaker

Vascular disease

Diabetes mellitus

Nutritional disorders

Cigarette smoking

Pregnancy

Chronic infectious diseases

Anticoagulants

Prolonged bleeding is one of the most disturbing surgical complications. Problems in achieving hemostasis may prolong the surgical procedure, and bleeding tends to be unsettling or alarming to the patient. Additionally, hematomas may form due to bleeding or oozing after closure and may contribute to delays in wound healing and create an environment that predisposes the patient to wound infection.[1] Aspirin, nonsteroidal anti-inflammatory drugs (NSAIDs), heparin, and coumarin derivatives may all adversely affect surgery through their anticoagulant effects. Aspirin and NSAIDs will be discussed further in the following section.

Patients with a history of venous thrombosis, thromboembolism, or valvular heart disease may be receiving heparin or coumarin derivatives. Recipients of systemic heparin are in general not candidates for cutaneous surgery. Warfarin, the most common coumarin derivative, interferes with clot formation by inhibiting the synthesis of the vitamin K–dependent coagulation factors, including factors VII, IX, X, and prothrombin. Coumarin derivatives have relatively long half-lives (1 to 6 days, with great variation between patients), and thus their anticoagulant effects may persist for several days after discontinuation.[2]

Ideally, all medications with anticoagulant properties should be interrupted in the perioperative period. Any changes in a patient's medications should be done with the guidance and approval of the primary care physician. Warfarin must be discontinued several days preoperatively to allow the coagulation system to normalize. If more rapid correction of the anticoagulant effect of a coumarin derivative is necessary, vitamin K may be administered intravenously or orally. For emergent bleeding, administration of fresh whole blood or fresh frozen plasma may be necessary to reverse anticoagulant effects. If anticoagulation cannot be interrupted and dermatologic surgery is essential, limited surgery should be performed using meticulous hemostatic technique, and a secure pressure dressing should be affixed postoperatively.

Aspirin and nonsteroidal anti-inflammatory drugs

Aspirin impairs platelet aggregation by irreversibly acetylating platelet prostaglandin G/H synthase 1, yielding loss of cyclooxygenase activity.[3] Aspirin is present in a wide variety of over-the-counter medications, and patients may not be aware that they are consuming the drug if it is one of several components in a product designed for multisymptom relief. Increasing numbers of patients are also taking daily aspirin (on their own or on the advice of a physician) for its putative salutary effects on coronary artery disease. As aspirin's effect on platelet cyclooxygenase activity is irreversible, substantial platelet turnover (requiring 1 to 2 weeks) must occur before the anticoagulant effect abates. Ibuprofen and other NSAIDs also inhibit platelet cyclooxygenase activity, but the effects can be reversible and short lived.[4] For aspirin, discontinuation 2 weeks preoperatively should prevent bleeding difficulties. A shorter drug-free period can be acceptable for some NSAIDs. NSAIDs have also been suggested as a potential cause of increased postoperative morbidity in the cutaneous surgical patient due to delayed wound healing.[5] This report remains unconfirmed, however, and recent experimental evidence suggests that NSAIDs may have no deleterious effects on the duration of healing and the final tensile strength of healing tissues.[6,7]

Beta-Blockers

Malignant hypertension and cardiovascular collapse developed in a small number of patients taking nonselective beta-blockers (such as propranolol) who were given intradermal epinephrine as a component of local anesthesia.[8] Ten patients taking propranolol who received intradermal epinephrine in conjunction with other elements of local anesthesia during Mohs micrographic surgery experienced no adverse effects, however, and thus the risk of this complication during routine procedures is probably very low.[9] The mechanism of this reaction is theorized to be unopposed alpha-receptor stimulation by epinephrine after complete beta-blockade by the nonselective agent. Intravenous chlorpromazine (in 1-mg increments up to a total dose of 5 mg) or intravenous hydralazine may be administered if a hypertensive crisis develops.[8] Emergent general medical consultation should be considered in such an event.

Immunosuppressive agents

Patients taking oral corticosteroids, cytotoxic agents, or other immunomodulatory agents for chronic inflammatory or neoplastic diseases are commonly encountered in modern medical practice. The number of organ transplant recipients has also increased, due to the advent of cyclosporine A and other advances in transplantation methodology. Clearly, these drugs cannot be discontinued perioperatively because of their critical importance to the patient's overall medical well-being.

All of these agents are administered for their immune system-inhibiting effects, and theoretically an increased incidence of surgical wound infections may be expected. Perioperative antibiotic administration can be considered on an individualized basis to compensate for the risk of infection. Drugs from this group may also delay wound healing. Systemic glucocorticosteroids are the most notorious offenders, and agents such as prednisone (especially when administered chronically) interfere by inhibiting necessary inflammatory responses and decreasing protein synthesis.[10,11] Methotrexate may have mild (and possibly clinically insignificant) effects on wound healing, and the inhibitory effects may be reversed or ameliorated with the administration of folic acid.[12] The effect of cyclosporine A on wound healing remains controversial in that either normal or mildly retarded wound healing has been observed in animal and clinical studies.[13]

Neuroleptic agents

Inquiry should be made regarding use of phenothiazines, monoamine oxidase inhibitors, and tricyclic or other antidepressants. Since the mechanism of action of many of these agents is to increase endogenous catecholamine levels, the added burden of the catecholamine epinephrine present in local anesthetic preparations may predispose the patient to the development of a hypertensive crisis.[14]

Cardiac Disease

The dermatologic surgeon must be aware of cardiac symptoms or a history of coronary artery disease. As standard care, sublingual nitroglycerin should be available in the surgical suite for administration intraoperatively should chest pain or other symptoms of myocardial ischemia occur.

Because of the potential toxicity of its cardiostimulatory effects, the epinephrine component of standard local anesthetic formulations deserves extra consideration in the patient with atherosclerotic heart disease. Despite the theoretical risks, no adverse effects from the administration of local anesthesia which incorporated epinephrine (1:50,000 dilution) were observed in 40 patients with coronary atherosclerosis during oral surgery.[15] Since 0.5 mg (approximately 50 mL of a 1:100,000 solution) of epinephrine is required to produce systemic effects, adverse sequelae are unlikely to be encountered in routine procedures.[14] Nonetheless, limitation or omission of epinephrine in local anesthesia may be appropriate in patients with severe or unstable ischemic cardiac disease.

Awareness of a past history of congenital or valvular heart disease is also important, as these lesions increase a patient's risk of developing bacterial endocarditis. Although all authorities agree (and American Heart Association guidelines state) that patients with prosthetic valves merit prophylactic antibiotics during excisional surgery of noninfected lesions, whether or not the dermatologic surgeon should administer prophylactic antibiotics to other patients with structural cardiac lesions for routine cutaneous surgical procedures remains controversial.[16–19] Additional data important to the surgeon's consideration of this controversy includes the facts that significant bacteremia apparently rarely if ever occurs after excisional surgery but that manipulation of infected lesions such as abscesses may yield significant bacteremia.[20,21]

For procedures involving grossly infected or purulent lesions, it is clear that even patients at low risk for endocarditis (valvular disorder, congenital malformation, or history of endocarditis) should receive antibiotic prophylaxis. Patients with prosthetic valves or other prosthetic vascular devices should be prophylaxed for virtually any procedure. In light of the very low incidence of bacteremia after routine excisional surgery, the administration of preventive perioperative antibiotics to patients with other valvular or congenital lesions can be considered optional.

The patient with a cardiac pacemaker should be identified, especially in the setting of electrosurgery. Electrosurgical techniques may be employed safely in paced patients, if proper grounding techniques are followed and short current bursts are used.[22–24] Most of the reported complications of electrosurgery have occurred in patients exposed to prolonged bursts of "cutting" current. Problems can be circumvented by using lower currents and avoiding electrosurgery directly over the pacemaker site.[23,24]

Periodic checks of level of consciousness should be made intraoperatively in all dermatologic surgery patients. In cardiac patients, particularly patients with paced rhythms, intermittent monitoring of pulse rate may also be appropriate.

Vascular Disease

Reduced blood flow yields local hypoxia, and therefore vascular disorders such as atherosclerosis, venous stasis, and diabetic vasculopathy may impair wound healing. Patients with occlusive vascular disease or vasoreactive processes such as Raynaud's phenomenon may also be adversely affected by epinephrine in local anesthesia. Epinephrine is generally to be avoided in surgery involving acral sites, particularly in procedures involving the digits in which nerve blocks are employed, and especially in patients with peripheral vascular disorders.[14,25] As anesthesia duration will decrease due to loss of vasoconstriction if epinephrine is omitted, long-acting local anesthetics such as prilocaine, bupivacaine, or etidocaine should be considered.

Diabetes Mellitus

Wound healing in the diabetic patient is probably slowed both by decreased blood flow due to vasculopathy and metabolic abnormalities, and the risk of postoperative wound infection is high. Defects in opsonization, chemotaxis, and phagocytosis have been documented in diabetic patients and may account for the increased infection rate.[26] Consideration should be given to the administration of prophylactic antibiotics in the perioperative period in this population, particularly if there is any question of contamination of the surgical wound or if it appears wound care may be less than optimal.

Nutritional Factors

Insufficient dietary protein limits the pool of amino acids, and thus many steps in inflammatory, coagulative, and healing reactions may be slowed. Structural protein synthesis may be impaired, but a wide variety of energy- and protein-dependent processes such as cell proliferation, neovascularization, and phagocytosis may also be adversely affected. Vitamins A, C, and K are important cofactors in synthetic pathways vital to hemostasis, protein synthesis, and the local immune response, and thus vitamin deficiencies may potentially compromise wound healing.[26] Zinc and other trace minerals play vital roles in complex processes such as protein synthesis, cell proliferation, and cell motility, and these substances must be present at appropriate levels for normal healing.[26]

From a theoretical point of view, all of these nutritional factors are important in wound healing. However, from a practical standpoint, deficiencies will be rarely seen in patients who consume anything close to an average diet. Some strict vegetarians may be at low risk for protein malnutrition, and patients with severe alcohol dependency are at risk for a variety of nutritional deficiencies. These risk factors can be assessed in the preoperative questionnaire or review.

Cigarette Smoking

In addition to the widely known general health risks of cigarette use, there are also increased risks in dermatologic surgery. One major negative factor is a delay in wound healing, which is probably attributable to nicotine-induced cutaneous vasoconstriction and decreased microvascular oxygen transport due to carboxyhemoglobin formation (because of the presence of carbon monoxide in cigarette smoke).[27] The cigarette smoker is also at an increased risk for flap and graft necrosis.[28,29] In one study, smokers of one or more packs of cigarettes per day showed threefold increases in risk of flap or graft necrosis in comparison to nonsmokers or low-level smokers, and the extent of necrosis was also approximately three times greater in these patients.[28] Former smokers and low-level smokers also showed a slightly increased risk of necrosis in comparison to nonsmokers.

Wound healing in smokers apparently improves within several weeks of cessation of smoking. Therefore, patients should be strongly encouraged to quit smoking for a minimum of several weeks pre- and postoperatively. The risks of delayed healing and the increased risks of graft or flap necrosis should also be explained.

Pregnancy

When dealing with women in the reproductive years, the possibility of pregnancy should be addressed by direct questioning. If there is any possibility of the patient's being pregnant, appropriate testing (if not previously performed) should be obtained before further management. For any patient known or proven to be pregnant, consultation with an obstetrician prior to the time of surgery, if possible, is optimal. In general, the patient should be encouraged to delay elective procedures until after delivery.

For the diagnosis and treatment of cutaneous malignancies or symptomatic neoplasms, surgery during pregnancy may be necessary. Procedures should not be performed during the first trimester if possible, and surgery should be avoided during organogenesis (weeks 3 to 8) unless imperative.[30] If surgery is necessary, informed consent should be obtained, and additional time should be devoted to the answering of questions to alleviate anxiety. The history should include the careful documentation of nonsurgical risk factors (such as illicit drug, alcohol, or tobacco use) that may also affect the fetus.[30] Positioning of the patient is important, particularly in the second and third trimesters, and the patient should rest on the left side to prevent vena caval compression by the gravid uterus. Local anesthesia should be minimized, as is the case with all medication in pregnancy. However, the use of lidocaine in the pregnant patient is generally regarded as safe.[25,30] For brief procedures, tumescent anesthesia using normal saline may be considered as an alternative to conventional medications.[30] Consideration should be given to omitting the epinephrine component of local anesthetic preparations in the pregnant patient, as epinephrine has the potential to cause uterine artery spasm and thus compromise placental perfusion. Although the low doses of epinephrine employed by the dermatologic surgeon are unlikely to create problems, a conservative approach seems warranted.

If perioperative antibiotics are necessary in the care of the pregnant patient, erythromycin (excluding the estolate salt) or penicillin may be safely recommended. For postoperative analgesia, acetaminophen is acceptable. Salicylates and NSAIDs are to be avoided, as they may interfere with fetal growth and development or alter the onset of labor.[30]

Infectious Diseases

Patients with chronic viral diseases such as chronic hepatitis due to hepatitis B virus (HBV) or patients who are seropositive for the human immunodeficiency virus (HIV) pose operative risks to the surgeon and the health care team. This risk is best addressed through the adherence to universal precautions by the surgeons and their staff.[31] Masks, protective eyewear, hats, gowns, and gloves should be used by all personnel during all procedures. Surgeons and staff members should avoid the temptation to use incomplete precautions for small procedures such as diagnostic biopsies or intralesional injections. Double gloving offers extra protection to both the surgeon and the patient against the transfer of bodily fluids, although the surgeon may expect slight decreases in sensation and manual dexterity due to the thickness of the double layer.[32]

Surgeons should also consider preventive safety measures. Viral hepatitis presently poses the largest infectious risk to the surgeon. A substantial proportion of this morbidity is preventable through vaccination for HBV. Surgeons should obtain HBV immunization, and surgical staffs should also be encouraged to pursue vaccination.

THE LESION

Dermatologic surgeons provide an ever-expanding spectrum of services and perform a variety of procedures, including sophisticated cosmetic and laser therapies. The mainstay of dermatologic surgery remains the treatment of cutaneous neoplasms, however. Subtle histologic features separate certain types and patterns of cutaneous neoplasms, and often significantly different surgical approaches are warranted based on these slight differences. The cutaneous surgeon must demand a high level of expertise in histopathologic interpretation, and sections should be interpreted by a dermatopathologist prior to the time of surgery, if possible.

Basal Cell Carcinoma

Basal cell carcinoma (BCC) is by far the most common malignancy in humans, with nearly half a million new cases diagnosed annually. BCCs show little tendency to metastasize; rather, locally aggressive growth is characteristic. The surgeon must evaluate a number of clinical and histologic variables preoperatively that signal lesions requiring special consideration.

Size

Large lesions recur more frequently after surgical extirpation, even when primarily excised by Mohs micrographic surgery.[33] The rate of recurrence appears to be roughly proportional to the diameter of the primary tumor. Lesions greater than 4 cm in diameter must be treated aggressively in light of their relatively high rates of persistence.[33]

Location

Most of the recurrences of BCC occur in periauricular, perinasal, or periorbital skin.[33–36] In particular, central facial car-

cinomas may be highly invasive and destructive and may show substantial subclinical extension (discussed further below). The invasiveness of central facial carcinomas has long been attributed in part to extension of cancer along planes of tissue weakness created by embryologic fusion, although reassessment of this concept has shown it to be fallacious.[37] The cosmetic and functional importance of the midfacial region may result in hesitancy on the part of the surgeon to perform sufficiently aggressive ablative procedures to eliminate the cancer. Primary therapy by Mohs micrographic surgery should be strongly considered.[38]

Duration

As might be expected, tumors of long duration may invade deeply and involve soft tissue and musculoskeletal structures.[38] Nonetheless, the duration of the lesion had no effect on the recurrence rate of primary BCCs after treatment with various conventional therapies.[36,39,40]

Subclinical extension

The size of a BCC may be deceptive, if measurement is based on the visible extent of the lesion, as carcinoma may extend into clinically normal surrounding skin for distances ranging from several millimeters to greater than 1 cm.[34,41] The degree of subclinical extension increases with the size of the primary tumor and in lesions that display aggressive histologic patterns of growth. The greatest degree of subclinical extension may be expected in recurrent carcinomas.[41] It makes sense, therefore, that lesions with ill-defined borders may be more difficult to treat and may have a greater potential to recur. Intraoperative curettage has been forwarded as an effective means to "see" subclinical spread.[42,43] Conceptually, the technique is based on the observation that carcinomas tend to "peel away" from normal structures when curetted. For BCCs, this ease of separation may be related to the fact that the aggregates of carcinoma are often surrounded by abundant mucinous stroma. The act of curettage more precisely defines the extent of the carcinoma than is possible by visual inspection; removal of the curettage site by the planned surgical excision follows. In a recent study of 40 primary BCCs excised by the elliptic technique, negative surgical margins were obtained in all cases in which extent of tumor was defined by curettage in comparison to a 30 percent positive margin rate in a noncuretted control group.[43] Because of the depth of invasion and associated stromal sclerosis, curettage may be less applicable to defining recurrent BCCs and primary BCCs that show aggressive histologic patterns.

Recurrent BCC

Although conventional therapies such as curettage and electrodesiccation, elliptic excision, and radiation therapy yield cure rates of greater than 90 percent for primary BCCs, recurrent lesions treated by these same modalities show significantly higher recurrence rates.[36,39,40] For this reason, most

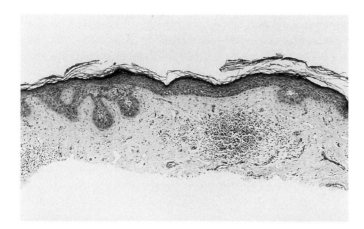

Figure 9-1 Superficial basal cell carcinoma. Small aggregates of basaloid cells exhibiting peripheral palisading are present at the epidermal undersurface. Adjacent mucinous stroma, which is often separated from the tumor by small clefts, is also characteristic.

recurrent lesions warrant Mohs micrographic surgery. Most recurrences of BCC can be expected in the first 4 years following initial therapy.[44]

Histologic growth pattern

Numerous subtypes of BCC have been described. Many of these variants are histologic curiosities which carry no clinical significance. Knowledge of the growth pattern of a carcinoma is a valuable factor in preoperative planning, and certain histologies may have strong impact on the decision regarding therapeutic approach.[34] Active communication between the surgeon and the dermatopathologist is imperative so that the histologic features of clinical importance are relayed. A surgeon who accepts interpretation merely as "basal cell carcinoma," without asking for an analysis of the histologic pattern of the tumor, cheats himself or herself out of some of the most valuable information that can be obtained preoperatively regarding the expected behavior of the lesion. There are five common growth patterns that encompass most BCCs.[45]

Superficial BCC (Fig. 9-1). This relatively indolent form of BCC is characterized histologically by buds of carcinoma extending from the epidermal undersurface. Superficially ablative therapies (including those in which margins are not evaluated) are often appropriate, depending on the site of occurrence. Subclinical lateral extension may lead to recurrence if ablation is incomplete.

Nodular BCC (Fig. 9-2) Large and rounded aggregates of carcinoma are present in the papillary and reticular dermis in this variant, which is often amenable to excisional surgery. For large primary tumors or tumors situated in the high-risk locations discussed above, primary excision by Mohs micrographic surgery should be strongly considered.

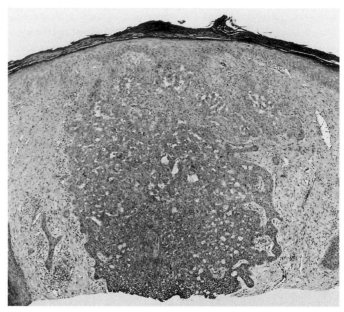

Figure 9-2 Nodular basal cell carcinoma. Atypical basaloid cells are arranged in large aggregates in the dermis, and peripheral palisading and mucinous stroma are generally apparent. Some of the large aggregates may show central necrosis, creating a cystic microscopic appearance.

Infiltrative BCC and Micronodular BCC (Figs. 9-3 and 9-4) Carcinomas showing these histologic patterns are more aggressive than conventional nodular tumors. The infiltrative pattern is characterized by small, angulate and irregular nests

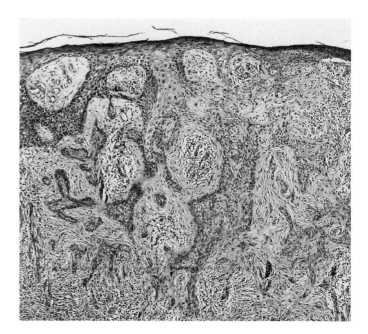

Figure 9-3 Infiltrative basal cell carcinoma. Angulate aggregates of carcinoma are positioned haphazardly in the dermis. The adjacent stroma is mucinous to fibrotic, and peripheral palisading may be only focally apparent.

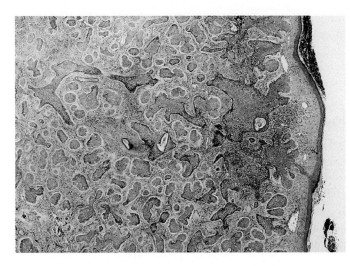

Figure 9-4 Micronodular basal cell carcinoma. Small, rounded aggregates of carcinoma are positioned between collagen bundles in the dermis. Peripheral palisading can be poorly developed and mucinous stroma can be scant, particularly at the advancing edge of the tumor.

of carcinoma that invade between collagen bundles and fibrotic stroma. Micronodular lesions show small, rounded aggregates that percolate between dermal structures. In both of these patterns, peripheral palisading may be poorly developed, and little mucinous stroma may be evident at the advancing edge of the neoplasm.

Morpheic (Morpheaform) BCC (Fig. 9-5)   In the past, many pathologists have loosely used the adjectives *sclerotic* or *sclerosing* to refer to any BCC with a focally irregular pattern of growth. However, a diagnosis of morpheic BCC is far more useful if it is reserved for lesions showing specific histologic

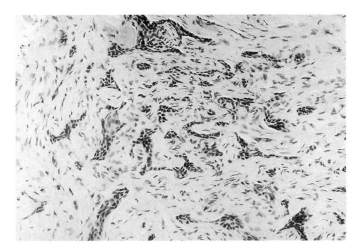

Figure 9-5 Morpheic basal cell carcinoma. Thin strands of hyperchromatic basaloid cells are embedded in a fibrotic stroma. The presence of clefting between the carcinoma and its stroma is a helpful diagnostic clue.

features, which correspond to a lesion with considerable local aggressiveness. Microscopically, morpheic BCCs show thin strands of carcinoma arranged between thickened collagen bundles, with scant amounts of mucinous stroma and with focal clefting of tumor from stroma.

Some authorities refer to the infiltrative, micronodular, and morpheic patterns of BCC collectively as *aggressive-growth BCC*.[46] This approach ignores the behavioral differences among these patterns and is thus less desirable. Because of the aggressive nature of these three patterns of BCC, Mohs micrographic surgery should always be considered in the therapeutic approach, regardless of the site of the lesion. If conventional excision is pursued, careful microscopic evaluation by a reputable pathology laboratory is essential. Surgical techniques in which margins are not evaluated (such as electrodesiccation and curettage) should not be employed in the treatment of carcinomas with high-grade histologic growth patterns.[34]

Other Histologic Considerations in the Management of BCC
BCCs of all histologic patterns not infrequently show foci of squamous differentiation. Some observers have suggested that these *metatypical* BCCs have a malignant potential closer to that of squamous cell carcinoma (SCC). A literature review of all reported cases of metastasizing BCC did not support this view, but the issue remains controversial.[47] In the experience of one of the authors (THM) and other dermatopathologists, keratinization is commonly encountered in BCCs that have ulcerated or have been recently irritated, and the squamous differentiation is thought to represent a reactive change.[48] In contrast, tumors with squamous differentiation have at times exhibited highly aggressive growth in the experience of the other author (BL) and surgical colleagues.[49] Clearly, the issue warrants further study.

Perineural invasion may be noted in approximately 1 percent of BCCs, and lesions with perineural spread are probably best approached therapeutically through Mohs micrographic surgery.[50] In this setting, the Mohs surgeon often obtains additional tissue for paraffin-embedded sections after obtaining negative margins in frozen sections.[50] The examination of the additional tissue may help prevent overlooking the presence of small foci of residual carcinoma situated occultly along the affected nerve. If perineural spread is detected, postoperative radiation therapy may also be considered.

Imitators of BCC

Benign adnexal neoplasms and proliferations are generally readily distinguished from BCC. However, the distinctions at times may be subtle, and the dermatologic surgeon should keep potential pitfalls in mind. This is particularly true for the referral surgeon, who may encounter biopsy results from a number of unfamiliar laboratories during preoperative patient visits. *Trichoepithelioma,* particularly the desmoplastic variant, may show the greatest degree of resemblance to BCC.

Criteria have been assembled to facilitate the distinction of desmoplastic trichoepithelioma from the very similar morpheic variant of BCC, and this distinction is generally made with ease by the experienced dermatopathologist.[51] Obviously, radically different therapeutic approaches are indicated, depending on the correct histopathologic diagnosis.

Age of the patient

Although BCC has historically been a disease of middle and old age, increasing numbers of carcinomas are being identified in younger individuals, perhaps because of increased and excessive sun exposure during adolescence. One recent study has suggested that BCCs with aggressive histologic patterns of growth are more common in younger patients, in comparison with an older control group, but a subsequent study failed to corroborate this view.[46,52] The chief point to the dermatologic surgeon derived from both of these studies is an increased awareness that BCC may be seen through a broad spectrum of patient ages. The tissue-sparing nature and high cure rate of Mohs micrographic surgery may be of particular benefit to younger patients.

Squamous Cell Carcinoma

Cutaneous SCC is a diagnosis that refers to a spectrum of malignant keratinocytic neoplasms.[53] SCCs are of variable malignant potential. The most common type of SCC encountered by the dermatologic surgeon is SCC arising de novo in sun-damaged skin or in association with a solar keratosis. These tumors are generally regarded as low-risk malignancies, although large, poorly differentiated, deeply invasive lesions may exhibit highly invasive behavior.[53]

Selected variants of SCC have greater malignant potential and require aggressive dermatologic surgery. SCCs of the lip and other mucous membranes are relatively common malignancies that may show a greater tendency to metastasize when compared to cutaneous SCC from other sites. The most important microscopic prognostic factors of SCC of the lip are the presence of perineural invasion, depth of penetration greater than 6 mm, a dispersed pattern of growth, and high-grade (poorly differentiated) histologic features.[54] In lesions showing these features, metastatic spread is relatively common; metastatic rates greater than 50 percent have been observed in one study.[54]

A recently characterized and uncommon variant of cutaneous SCC that is important to the surgeon is *adenosquamous carcinoma*.[55,56] Adenosquamous carcinoma is a highly aggressive form of cutaneous SCC showing true glandular differentiation. A dispersed and infiltrative pattern of growth, prominent cytologic atypia, and a tendency to perineural invasion are characteristic.[56] Roughly 80 percent of these tumors occur in the central facial region, based on current data.[55,56] The importance in recognizing adenosquamous carcinoma is its very poor prognosis. A high mortality rate, attributable to uncontrolled and recurrent local disease, is common. Aggressive extirpation via Mohs micrographic surgery is warranted. A multidisciplinary approach should also be considered. Radiation therapy or radical surgical excision may be required to control deeply invasive growth.

Melanocytic Nevi and Malignant Melanoma

If malignant melanoma is a significant consideration in the clinical differential diagnosis of a cutaneous pigmented lesion, primary elliptic excision with a clinical margin of several millimeters should be the diagnostic procedure of choice. If a partial biopsy of a pigmented lesion must be performed, a punch rather than a shave biopsy is preferable. Clinically atypical melanocytic nevi (*dysplastic* or *Clark's nevi*) should be approached in a similar fashion. Excisional biopsy provides adequate material for appropriate histopathologic examination, and thus the patient is ensured every opportunity for an accurate diagnosis and assessment of prognosis. If such an approach is followed, the need for reexcision of lesions with borderline histologic features will be reduced. If the lesion proves to be melanoma in situ or a thin invasive melanoma, current guidelines suggest reexcision with a margin of 5 mm (for in situ disease) or 1 cm (for melanomas up to 1 mm in thickness) of clinically normal skin.[57]

BRIEF ANATOMIC CONSIDERATIONS

In general, dermatologic surgeons confine their interventions to the cutis, subcutis, and superficial soft tissues. For procedures involving the trunk and extremities, the anatomic considerations are relatively less important, as vital structures tend to be deeply situated in these regions. Precise knowledge of pertinent aspects of the anatomy of the head and neck is critical to high-quality surgical care, however, particularly in light of the fact that more than 90 percent of nonmelanoma skin cancers arise in these areas. The density of vital and delicate neurovascular structures is greater on the head and neck in comparison to other regions of the body, and many of the structures are superficially located and are therefore more susceptible to surgical trauma. Only with a clear understanding of the pertinent anatomy can the dermatologic surgeon adequately prepare and plan for such surgeries. Additionally, the patient can be more easily alerted to and adequately informed of the potential complications of the planned procedure.

The structures that will be discussed in this section are illustrated in Fig. 9-6.

Vascular Structures

The blood flow to the skin of the head is largely contributed by the external carotid arterial system. Several branches of this system and the corresponding veins are superficially located. The superficial temporal artery and vein exit the supe-

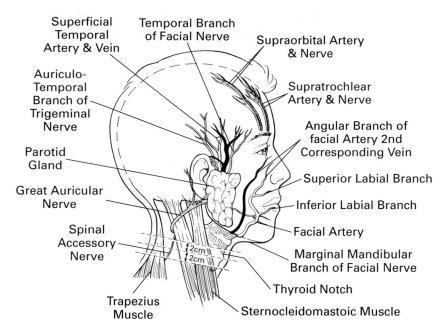

Figure 9-6 Anatomical structures of importance in cutaneous surgery of the head and neck.

rior aspect of the parotid gland at the approximate level of the external auditory meatus and course superficially over the temple toward the scalp.[58] Branches of the facial artery and vein may be superficially located at the point at which these vessels cross the midsection of the mandible. Three other facial arterial tributaries are potentially at risk. The angular artery may be encountered in the lateral paranasal region. The superior and inferior labial branches of the facial artery are superficially located in the lips.

The only portions of the face and scalp supplied by the internal carotid system are the forehead and the frontal scalp. These zones are supplied by supraorbital and supratrochlear branches.[58] Both vessels arise superficially in the region of the medial supraorbital rim and are at risk during deep forehead surgery.

Suction, an electrosurgical unit, hemostats, and sutures for ligature must always be readily available intraoperatively to enable the surgeon to promptly control bleeding.

Neural Structures

Motor nerves

Cranial nerve VII, the facial nerve, supplies motor signals to the muscles of mastication and facial expression. Although the parotid gland and various muscles provide a protective buffer, superficial branches are focally vulnerable. The main trunk of the facial nerve may also be vulnerable as it exits the stylomastoid foramen in children under the age of 5 years.[49] The stylomastoid process protects the nerve at this point in adults, but nerve damage is possible in young children before the process is fully developed.

The temporal branch of the facial nerve, which innervates the muscles of the forehead, ascends across the temple in the deep subcutis. The path of the nerve falls roughly within a narrow triangle in which the earlobe defines the triangular apex, and a line between the lateral aspect of the eyebrow and the lateral aspect of the superior forehead crease defines its base.[58] The nerve shows its greatest vulnerability at the point where it crosses the zygomatic arch. Injury to the nerve may yield loss of ability to wrinkle and move the forehead, as well as eyebrow ptosis. The latter defect is the most disconcerting, as upper visual field defects may result. In instances in which this defect has occurred, a conservative therapeutic approach is warranted. Taping (if necessary) and observation should be pursued for at least 6 to 12 months to permit a maximal degree of nerve healing or axonal regeneration to occur.[59] If a defect persists, browplasty techniques can be considered.[59]

The marginal mandibular branch of the facial nerve also shows segmental vulnerability. This nerve twig exits the inferior border of the parotid gland near the mandibular angle and then lies superficially as it courses medially over the masseter muscle.[58] After a short vulnerable zone, the nerve subsequently dives beneath the platysma muscle. If an injury to the nerve occurs, a limitation in movement of the corner of the mouth and the lower lip may result.

It is also vital to be aware of the spinal accessory nerve (cranial nerve XI). As this nerve is situated away from the face, its vulnerability is easily overlooked. The nerve descends through the posterior triangle of the neck, emerging from the protection of the sternocleidomastoid muscle approximately 2 cm above a horizontal line drawn through the thyroid notch. A 4-cm zone of susceptibility in which the nerve is positioned just inferior to the subcutis ensues.[60] The nerve then dives deep to the trapezius muscle. Nerve injury may initially manifest as shoulder ache (due to fatigue of compensatory muscles) or paresthesias (due to traction on the brachial plexus). Later, the patient may develop shoulder droop and atrophy of the trapezius. If such defects persist, the Henry sling operation has been used as an effective procedure for palliation.[60] In this operation, a fascial sling is created to facilitate shoulder suspension.

Sensory nerves

The skin of the face, anterior scalp, and neck is richly innervated by small branches of the trigeminal nerve (cranial nerve V) and upper cervical nerves. As these nerve branches are ubiquitous on the face, small nerve twigs are unavoidably sacrificed during cutaneous surgery. As an expected consequence, many patients report small areas of numbness or minor paresthesias in the vicinity of their surgical scar. Some of these minor deficits resolve or dissipate with time postoperatively due to axonal regrowth.

In contrast to these minor injuries, keeping the sites of some key larger sensory nerve segments fresh in mind may help avert injuries that have the potential to lead to more substantial sensory alterations or deficits. The supraorbital and supratrochlear nerves are terminal branches of the ophthalmic (first) division of cranial nerve V. These segments exit the supraorbital foramen and ascend superiorly and posteriorly, innervating the forehead and scalp to the vertex. Deep forehead surgeries, especially in the immediate supraorbital region, provide the greatest risk to these structures.[58]

The auriculotemporal branch of the mandibular (third) division of the trigeminal nerve ascends along the course of the superficial temporal artery and vein, just posteriorly to the triangular zone containing the temporal branches of the facial nerve (described above). If the auriculotemporal nerve is injured, altered sensation of the external ear, auditory canal, and adjacent zones of the temporal scalp are possible sequelae.

The great auricular nerve arises from branches of the second and third cervical nerves and supplies sensory input to the skin overlying the mandibular angle, as well as the skin of the retroauricular region.[58] This nerve is most vulnerable as it crosses over the sternocleidomastoid muscle in its midsection, roughly inferior to the angle of the mandible.[58]

Other Structures

The dermatologic surgeon should be ever mindful of the relatively superficial location of the parotid gland. This structure blankets the preauricular region and the angle of the mandible, sandwiched between the subcutis and fascia. A tail of the gland extends posteriorly into the infra- and postauricular region. The parotid tail connects to the body of the gland through a narrow isthmus in the region of the angle of the mandible.[61] The chief risk of surgery in the region of the parotid gland, however, is damage to the body of the gland, which may eventuate in formation of a parotidocutaneous fistula. Fortunately, the delicate parotid (Stensen's) duct is

deeply situated as it crosses the masseter muscle, and the structure is rarely susceptible to injury.

Excessive serous drainage postoperatively may be a clue to underlying parotid gland damage, particularly if the drainage is accentuated postprandially. As with most postoperative complications, a conservative approach is warranted. If only exocrine elements have been damaged, spontaneous healing (after a period of drainage) is the rule.[61] If Stensen's duct or a tributary has been injured, a parotidocutaneous fistula may form and require surgical repair.

THE DAY OF SURGERY

An amicable staff is a tremendous asset in the surgical suite. Warm interactions with the ancillary members of the surgical team help alleviate the patient's anxiety from the time he or she arrives at the office. Friendliness must be supplemented by efficiency and adequate education. If the patient's disease process and the treatment options available have been fully explained, the patient will be able to make truly informed decisions regarding his or her own care or will feel comfortable accepting the surgeon's recommendations regarding care. Some aspects of education regarding different procedures and treatment options can be delivered through pamphlets and other printed materials.

The patient should clearly understand that bleeding, scarring, nerve damage, or infection may occur with any surgical procedure but must also be aware that these complications rarely play an important role in the postoperative course of most surgeries. Although the potential problems and the nature of the procedure are generally discussed with the patient during preoperative visits, a quick review should be performed at the time the consent form is signed.

For the excessively anxious patient or for patients undergoing prolonged and complicated procedures, preoperative sedation may be considered.[14] Unless intravenous access and monitoring equipment is available in the surgical suite, only simple, low-dose regimens should be employed.[14] Diazepam in doses of 5 to 10 mg, either orally or sublingually, is one of the most useful agents in this setting. Meperidine hydrochloride and morphine sulfate are useful alternatives, and one advantage to narcotic preanesthesia is that any effects may be rapidly reversed by administering naloxone hydrochloride (intramuscularly in 0.4-mg increments, every several minutes to a maximum dose of 10 mg).[14] For preanesthesia in children, chloral hydrate (20 to 40 mg/kg, orally or rectally) has long been the medication of choice. If eutectic mixture of local anesthetics (EMLA) is employed as a topical premedication in children, the need for systemic premedication may decrease. For the older child, a 1-h preapplication of EMLA followed by conventional anesthesia may be a productive approach.

Supplemental sedation must be used cautiously in the older patient or the patient on multiple medications because of the possibilities of excessive sedation, a drug interaction, or other adverse effects. Vital signs and the patient's level of consciousness should be frequently monitored. Patients who have been sedated must always be discharged into the care of a friend or relative, and the patient should not be permitted to be responsible for his or her own transportation.

After the procedure, additional education and instructions regarding postoperative care are essential. The patient should view the surgical site, and a relative or friend who will be involved in postoperative care should also see the postoperative changes. If the parties who are caring for the wound have seen it at its baseline, they will be better able to identify any changes in the wound that may signal a need for additional medical attention. The patient should be instructed specifically to watch closely for bleeding, erythema, swelling, excessive tenderness, or purulence, as these factors suggest the impending development of complications. If such features develop, the patient should feel comfortable about contacting the surgeon at any hour, and phone numbers permitting around-the-clock contact with the surgeon should be included in the discharge materials. Written materials describing wound care should be distributed to supplement verbal instructions.

Postoperative analgesia should also be discussed. The patient with untreated postoperative pain will not be able to perform or tolerate wound care and will feel dissatisfied with the surgical experience. Restlessness, vomiting, or hypertension may all potentially be triggered by severe or prolonged pain, and these factors may predispose the patient to excessive postoperative bleeding.

In summary, a comprehensive preoperative review is rewarding for the patient and the surgeon. The patient will be reassured by the surgeon's attention to detail, and patient confidence will rise. A complete assessment of the patient's risks permits the surgeon to take a conservative approach and employ preventive measures, and the risk of operative complications should fall. The end result is an efficient and pleasant surgical experience which is less stressful and taxing for both the patient and the surgeon.

REFERENCES

1. Salasche S: Acute surgical complications: Cause, prevention, and treatment. *J Am Acad Dermatol* **15:**1163, 1986

2. Majerus PW et al: Anticoagulant, antithrombotic, and thrombolytic drugs, in *Goodman and Gilman's The Pharmacologic Basis of Therapeutics,* 8th ed., edited by AG Gilman et al. New York, Pergamon Press, pp 1311–1331, 1990

3. Patrono C: Aspirin as an antiplatelet drug. *N Engl J Med* **330:**1287, 1994

4. Flower RJ: Drugs which inhibit prostaglandin biosynthesis. *Pharmacol Rev* **26:**33, 1974

5. Proper SA et al: Compromised wound repair caused by perioperative use of ibuprofen. *J Am Acad Dermatol* **18:**1173, 1988

6. Dahners LE et al: The effect of a nonsteroidal antiinflammatory drug on the healing of ligaments. *Am J Sports Med* **16:**641, 1988

7. Thomas J et al: The effect of indomethacin on Achilles tendon healing in rabbits. *Clin Orthop* **272:**308, 1991

8. Foster CA, Aston SJ: Propranolol-epinephrine interaction: A potential disaster. *Plast Reconstr Surg* **72:**74, 1983

9. Dzubow LM: The interaction between propranolol and epinephrine as observed in patients undergoing Mohs surgery. *J Am Acad Dermatol* **15:**71, 1986

10. Goslen JB: Wound healing for the dermatologic surgeon. *J Dermatol Surg Oncol* **14:**959, 1988

11. Pessa ME et al: Growth factors and determinants of wound repair. *J Surg Res* **42:**207, 1987

12. Falcone RE, Nappi JF: Chemotherapy and wound healing. *Surg Clin North Am* **64:**779, 1984

13. Ryffel B: Cyclosporine and wound healing. *Urol Res* **17:**27, 1989

14. Winton GB: Anesthesia for dermatologic surgery. *J Dermatol Surg Oncol* **14:**41, 1988

15. Elliott GD, Stein E: Oral surgery in patients with atherosclerotic heart disease: Benign effect of epinephrine in local anesthesia. *JAMA* **227:**1403, 1974

16. Wagner RF et al: Antibiotic prophylaxia against bacterial endocarditis in patients undergoing dermatologic surgery. *Arch Dermatol* **122:**799, 1986

17. Lycka B: Antibiotic prophylaxis and dermatologic surgery. *Arch Dermatol* **123:**424, 1987

18. Wagner RF et al: Antibiotic prophylaxis and dermatologic surgery. *Arch Dermatol* **123:**425, 1987

19. Shulman ST et al: Prevention of bacterial endocarditis: A statement for health professionals by the Committee on Rheumatic Fever and Infective Endocarditis of the Council on Cardiovascular Disease for the Young. *Circulation* **70:**1123A, 1984

20. Sabetta JB, Zitelli JA: The incidence of bacteremia during skin surgery. *Arch Dermatol* **123:**213, 1987

21. Fine BC et al: Incision and drainage of soft tissue abscesses and bacteremia. *Ann Intern Med* **103:**645, 1985

22. Sebben JE: Patient "grounding." *J Dermatol Surg Oncol* **14:**926, 1988

23. Sebben JE: The hazards of electrosurgery. *J Am Acad Dermatol* **16:**869, 1987

24. Sebben JE: Electrosurgery and cardiac pacemakers. *J Am Acad Dermatol* **9:**457, 1983

25. Grekin RC, Auletta MJ: Local anesthesia in dermatologic surgery. *J Am Acad Dermatol* **19:**599, 1988

26. Reed BR, Clark RAF: Cutaneous tissue repair: Practical implications of current knowledge. *J Am Acad Dermatol* **13:**919, 1985

27. Mosely LH, Finseth F: Cigarette smoking: Impairment of digital blood flow and wound healing of the hand. *Hand* **9:**97, 1977

28. Goldminz D, Bennett RG: Cigarette smoking and flap and full-thickness graft necrosis. *Arch Dermatol* **127:**1012, 1991

29. Rees TD et al: The effect of cigarette smoking on skin flap survival in the face lift patient. *Plast Reconstr Surg* **73:**911, 1984

30. Gormley DE: Cutaneous surgery and the pregnant patient. *J Am Acad Dermatol* **23:**269, 1990

31. Vaughn RY et al: HIV and the dermatologic surgeon. *J Dermatol Surg Oncol* **16:**1107, 1990

32. Cohen MS et al: Efficacy of double gloving as a protection against blood exposure in dermatologic surgery. *J Dermatol Surg Oncol* **18:**873, 1992

33. Rigel DS et al: Predicting recurrence of BCCs treated by microscopically controlled excision: A recurrence index score. *J Dermatol Surg Oncol* **7:**807, 1981

34. Lang PG, Maize JC: Histologic evolution of recurrent basal cell carcinoma and treatment implications. *J Am Acad Dermatol* **14:**186, 1986

35. Mora RG, Robins P: BCCs in the center of the face: Special diagnostic, prognostic, and therapeutic considerations. *J Dermatol Surg Oncol* **4:**315, 1978

36. Silverman MK et al: Recurrence rates of treated BCCs, pt 2: Curettage-electrodesiccation. *J Dermatol Surg Oncol* **17:**720, 1991

37. Wentzell JM, Robinson JK: Embryologic fusion planes and the spread of cutaneous carcinoma: A review and reassessment. *J Dermatol Surg Oncol* **16:**1000, 1990

38. Swanson NA: Mohs surgery: Technique, indications, applications and the future. *Arch Dermatol* **119:**761, 1983

39. Silverman MK et al: Recurrence rates of treated BCCs, pt 3: Surgical excision. *J Dermatol Surg Oncol* **18:**471, 1992

40. Silverman MK et al: Recurrence rates of treated BCCs, pt 4: X-ray therapy. *J Dermatol Surg Oncol* **18:**549, 1992

41. Breuninger H, Dietz K: Prediction of subclinical tumor infiltration in BCC. *J Dermatol Surg Oncol* **17:**574, 1991

42. Johnson TM et al: Combined curettage and excision: A treatment method for primary BCC. *J Am Acad Dermatol* **24:**613, 1991

43. Geisse J et al: Curettage prior to excision of basal cell carcinoma maximizes margin control (abstract). Poster presentation, American Society of Dermatologic Surgery, Scottsdale, AZ, March, 1992

44. Silverman MK et al: Recurrence rates of treated BCCs, pt 1: Overview. *J Dermatol Surg Oncol* **17:**713, 1991

45. Sexton M et al: Histologic pattern analysis of BCC: Study of a series of 1039 consecutive neoplasms. *J Am Acad Dermatol* **23:**1118, 1990

46. Leffell DJ et al: Aggressive-growth BCC in young adults. *Arch Dermatol* **127:**1663, 1991

47. Domarus HV, Stevens PJ: Metastatic BCC: Report of five cases and review of 170 cases in the literature. *J Am Acad Dermatol* **10:**1043, 1984

48. Freeman RG: Histopathologic considerations in the management of skin cancer. *J Dermatol Surg* **2:**215, 1976

49. Pena YM et al: Basosquamous cell carcinoma with leptomeningeal carcinomatosis. *Arch Dermatol* **126:**195, 1990

50. Carlson KC, Roenigk RK: Know your anatomy: Perineural involvement of basal and SCC of the face. *J Dermatol Surg Oncol* **16:**827, 1990

51. Takei Y et al: Criteria for histologic differentiation of desmoplastic trichoplastic trichoepithelioma (sclerosing epithelial hamartoma) from morphea-like BCC. *Am J Dermatopathol* **7:**207, 1985

52. Dinehart SM et al: BCC treated with Mohs micrographic surgery: A comparison of 54 younger with 1050 older patients. *J Dermatol Surg Oncol* **18:**560, 1992

53. Barr RJ: Classification of cutaneous SCC. *J Cutan Pathol* **18:**225, 1991

54. Frierson HF, Cooper PH: Prognostic factors in SCC of the lower lip. *Hum Pathol* **17:**346, 1986

55. Weidner N, Foucar E: Adenosquamous carcinoma of the skin: An aggressive mucin- and gland-forming SCC. *Arch Dermatol* **121:**775, 1985

56. Banks ER, Cooper PH: Adenosquamous carcinoma of the skin: A report of 10 cases. *J Cutan Pathol* **18:**227, 1991

57. NIH Consensus Development Panel on Early Melanoma: Diagnosis and treatment of early melanoma. *JAMA* **268:**1314, 1992

58. Phillips JH et al: Key anatomic structures of the face and neck for the dermatologic surgeon: Their relationship in a cadaver dissection. *J Dermatol Surg Oncol* **15:**1101, 1989

59. Grabski WJ, Salasche SJ: Management of temporal nerve injuries. *J Dermatol Surg Oncol* **11:**145, 1985

60. King RJ, Motta G: Iatrogenic spinal accessory nerve palsy. *Ann R Coll Surg Engl* **65:**35, 1983

61. Bernstein G: Surface landmarks for the identification of key anatomic structures of the face and neck. *J Dermatol Surg Oncol* **12:**722, 1986

Rufus M. Thomas
Rex A. Amonette
John L. Buker

10 Perioperative Emergencies

Dermatologists today spend many hours in courses and independent study in order to become more proficient with surgical procedures. Equal attention should be given to the preparation for potential perioperative emergencies. This is particularly true with the increasingly complex procedures being performed coupled with an increasingly older patient population. These patients are frequently on multiple medications and have multiple medical problems.

Preparation for emergencies begins with proper training and planning. Preparation for the most feared emergency, cardiac arrest, involves specific training known as basic life support (BLS) and advanced cardiac life support (ACLS). These courses are available locally through the American Red Cross, American Heart Association, and hospitals. All members of the office staff, including physicians, nurses, and clinical assistants, should have, as a minimum, training in the BLS course and preferably training in the ACLS course.[1] Annual refresher courses are necessary to maintain proficiency. BLS refresher courses are often given in a single afternoon in the familiar office environment by a certified instructor using the "Annie" mannequin.

Preparation for emergencies also involves proper planning. It is advisable to have a written plan stating the role of each staff member in the event of an emergency. One staff member would be assigned the responsibility of notifying 911 or the local emergency medical service. Others would begin cardiopulmonary resuscitation (CPR) in the case of a cardiac arrest, while another would act as a recorder of events. One person should be responsible for securing the emergency medication and equipment cart, starting intravenous (IV) infusions, and administering medications. Regular office drills

simulating emergency situations can sharpen the skills, confidence, and response time of the office staff.

In order to achieve a successful outcome in an emergency, it is essential to stabilize and transport the patient to an emergency care facility as quickly as possible. The telephone numbers for the local emergency systems should be posted by all office telephones. Arrangements can be made in advance with an internist or critical care specialist, possibly in an adjacent office, who would be able to assist in the care of emergency patients.

Prevention of emergencies is equally as important as training and preparation for emergencies. Many emergencies are preventable by taking a good medical history preoperatively. This history should include information concerning past and present illnesses, including a history of cardiovascular, pulmonary, hepatic, or renal disease. In cardiac pacemaker patients, electrocoagulation or electrodesiccation should be used with caution since these forms of electrosurgery potentially cause electric interference with demand pacemakers. To prevent this potential emergency, electrosurgery should be avoided in patients with external or demand-type pacemakers. The cutting current should not be used and bursts of current should be kept under 5 s.[2] Grounding should be at a site distant from the heart and pacemaker, and, similarly, electrosurgery should not be performed near the heart or pacemaker. Use of the carbon dioxide laser for either cutting or coagulation is a consideration.

It is important to record all medications, both prescription and over the counter, as well as any adverse reactions to any medications in the past. It is important to ask whether there is a past history of local anesthetic, paraben, or epinephrine sensitivity, and the offending agents should be avoided. The physician may wish to discontinue aspirin, anti-inflammatory, or anticoagulant medication before surgery to prevent problems with hemorrhage. For patients who are taking beta-blockers, epinephrine should be used only in low concentrations, if at all.

Intraoperatively, emergencies may be prevented by paying close attention to the patient's vital signs and level of consciousness. In some instances, depending on the procedure or the patient's medical condition, monitoring devices such as a pulse oximeter may be necessary. Local anesthetics should be injected slowly with care to avoid IV injection. Keeping an accurate account of the total amount injected is necessary to avoid toxic levels. Meticulous detail must also be given to intraoperative hemostasis.

SPECIFIC EMERGENCIES

Vasovagal Syncope

Vasovagal syncope is one of the more common emergencies encountered in dermatologic surgery. It is frequently seen in young healthy adults and may occur during minor surgical procedures such as a shave biopsy. The patient often exhibits extreme apprehension about the possibility of pain associated with a procedure or may rise too quickly from the sitting or recumbent position. Patients frequently give a history of syncopal episodes associated with vaccinations, venipuncture, or seeing trauma or blood. A family history of similar episodes is not uncommon. Vasovagal syncope, also known as *vasodepressor syncope*, is caused by excessive vagal stimulation resulting in loss of peripheral vasomotor tone with secondary visceral blood pooling and inadequate return to the heart. Without an adequate increase in cardiac output, cerebral hypoperfusion and unconsciousness result.

Certain measures can effectively prevent syncopal episodes. Speaking in a calm, reassuring tone to the patient is important as well as taking the time prior to procedure to explain in detail to the patient what to expect. Procedures generally should be done with the patient in a reclining position rather than sitting or standing, and the patient should not be allowed to view the procedure or to view the specimen that has been removed.[3] Family members or friends that accompany the patient should also be restricted from viewing the procedure as they, too, may experience vasovagal syncope. After the procedure is completed, the patient should be assisted slowly into a sitting position and observed for signs and symptoms of syncope before standing is allowed.

Early signs and symptoms of impending vasovagal syncope include tachycardia, hypertension, and increased cardiac output, which is clinically expressed as apprehension. This is followed by hypotension and a fall in cardiac output which produces pallor, profuse sweating, weakness, nausea, and occasionally vomiting.[4] The loss of consciousness which follows is very transient when appropriate measures are taken.

Treatment includes protecting the patient from a fall, immediately placing the patient in the Trendelenburg position, applying cool compresses to the face and neck, and administering oxygen at 4 to 6 L per min if readily available. Spirits of ammonia may be used to stimulate the patient. Vital signs should be taken and recorded. Full restoration of mental status and cardiopulmonary function should occur quickly— within seconds to minutes. Atropine, 0.5 mg IV should be considered if the syncopal episode is severe or prolonged and associated with bradycardia.[5] If the patient does not promptly return to full mental and cardiopulmonary status, other more serious causes of syncope must be considered.[6] These include stroke, seizure, cardiac arrhythmias, myocardial infarction, and hypoglycemia.

Hemorrhage

Significant hemorrhage occurring intraoperatively or postoperatively can have devastating results if not handled properly. Persistent bleeding can lead to infection, hematoma, and wound dehiscence. Although hemorrhage is most often due to the inadequate intraoperative hemostasis or drug-induced coagulopathy, a preexisting bleeding disorder should be ruled out before surgery.

A family or personal history of bleeding problems such as prolonged bleeding after trauma, unprovoked nosebleeds, or bleeding from the gums would raise suspicions for a hereditary or acquired coagulopathy. A thorough review of all the medications that the patient takes, including both prescription and over-the-counter products, should be carried out, as many patients unknowingly take over-the-counter products which contain aspirin. On physical examination, petechiae and ecchymoses may indicate a significant bleeding diathesis.

Screening laboratory tests used to evaluate a hereditary or acquired coagulopathy include a complete blood count, platelet count, peripheral smear for platelet morphology, a prothrombin time, partial thromboplastin time, and bleeding time. A simple bleeding time is an effective office screening tool that will detect most major potential bleeding problems.

Drug-induced coagulopathy is the most common cause of perioperative problems from hemorrhage. Aspirin, nonsteroidal anti-inflammatory drugs such as ibuprofen, and anticoagulants are frequent causes of drug-induced coagulopathy. Elective dermatologic surgery is generally not done on patients who are undergoing parenteral anticoagulation with heparin.[7] When possible, surgery should be deferred until a more stable condition exists. Many patients require chronic anticoagulation with a coumarin-type drug because of transient ischemic attacks, chronic atrial fibrillation, cardiac valve prostheses, or recurrent thrombophlebitis. These patients may be able to undergo dermatologic surgical procedures with certain precautions. In consultation with the patient's internist, the surgeon frequently stops coumarin several days prior to a surgical procedure and then reinstitutes it within a few days after surgery. When the patient's medical condition does not allow discontinuation of the anticoagulant, often the procedure may still be performed but with meticulous attention given to the intraoperative hemostasis and application of a postoperative pressure dressing.

The use of specialized cutting instruments, such as the carbon dioxide laser and certain electrosurgical units, offers the advantage of rapid hemostasis since small capillary vessels are sealed immediately, resulting in a relatively bloodless incision. Oral or parenteral vitamin K can be administered to help control persistent bleeding.

Aspirin and aspirin-containing products account for most of the perioperative bleeding problems. A single aspirin severely affects platelet aggregation. This decrease in platelet aggregation can be seen over the lifetime of the platelet which is 6 to 10 days. Whenever possible, and particularly with complex surgical procedures, aspirin should be discontinued 7 to 14 days prior to surgery and should not be reinstituted for 5 to 7 days after surgery.[7] Nonsteroidal anti-inflammatory drugs and dipyridamole also have an effect on platelet aggregation but not as severely as that of aspirin. Alcohol is another drug that should be avoided during the perioperative period as it is a potent vasodilator.

Hemorrhage secondary to inadequate intraoperative hemostasis is a preventable problem. Before closure of a wound, meticulous attention should be given to thorough cautery or ligation of all bleeding points. An excellent review by Larson[1] describes where and when to use topical hemostatic agents such as absorbable gelatin sponges, oxidized cellulose, microfibrillar collagen, and thrombin.[8] These agents may be very helpful for the control of capillary and small-vessel bleeding associated with drug-induced coagulopathy. Adequate closure of all dead space should be performed using subcutaneous, dermal, and skin sutures as necessary. An effective layered pressure dressing should be applied and kept in place for the first 24 h postoperatively. Postoperative hemorrhage necessitating a return visit to the physician requires a complete examination of the surgical wound.[1] Expansile hematomas may develop within hours of surgery and constitute an emergency situation. The immediate treatment includes removal of sutures and evacuation of the hematoma as well as ligation of all bleeding points. The wound is then resutured and a drain may be left in for 24 h. Antibiotic therapy would be indicated at this time if not already instituted.

Seizures

The incidence of seizures in the general population is 1 or 2 percent.[9] A variety of disorders can be associated with seizures, including metabolic disorders such as hyponatremia, hypocalcemia, or hypoglycemia, drug or alcohol withdrawal or overdose, infections such as meningitis or encephalitis, cerebral vascular accidents, drug reactions and anesthetic toxicity, and primary convulsive disorders. Signs and symptoms include auras, excessive salivation, convulsive movements of the extremities, incontinence, unresponsiveness, and loss of consciousness.

The vast majority of seizure episodes are benign in nature and short in duration, and therapy is primarily aimed at protecting the patient from personal injury. Patients should be placed in a position in which they cannot be hurt. If possible, they should be kept in a side-lying position so that mucus and saliva do not block the airway. The most common serious threat to life during grand mal seizures is vomiting followed by aspiration of gastric contents.[10] Turning the patient on one side will help prevent this complication. Some recommend that a plastic airway be inserted between the teeth to prevent trauma to the tongue and cheeks. Hard or wooden objects should not be used nor should the closed tonic jaw be forced open because these measures can produce dental or soft-tissue injuries and possible tooth aspiration.[11]

Most convulsions are self-limiting, and no further intervention may be necessary. However, status epilepticus of the grand mal type constitutes a potentially life-threatening medical emergency. Grand mal status epilepticus refers to repeated generalized seizures without intercurrent recovery. The tonic and clonic limb movements are continuous or are closely coupled episodes. Normal respirations are compromised during the seizure activity and hypoxic insult can result.

No prior seizure disorder is known in 50 percent of patients with status epilepticus.[12] It is essential to search for and correct metabolic disturbances as well as other causes such as drug overdose.

In the outpatient setting, when status epilepticus is encountered, the physician should have office staff activate the 911 emergency response system. Immediate actions to be taken include establishing an IV access and the administration of 50 mL of 50% dextrose in water for possible hypoglycemia. Diazepam should be given IV, 5 to 10 mg, at a maximum rate of 1 to 2 mg per min in adults.[13] Diazepam should not be mixed with IV fluids because it adheres to the tubing. Because of the significant incidence of cardiac and respiratory depression, vital signs should be monitored closely.

Diazepam is useful in the acute treatment of status epilepticus because of its potency and rapid onset of action; however, its duration is short, lasting only 15 or 20 min. If the seizures have not stopped within 10 min, another 5 to 10 mg should be administered at 2 mg per min. If the status is not terminated, administration of phenobarbital and/or phenytoin should be considered. Blood samples for glucose, blood chemistries, anticonvulsant drug levels, and a toxicology screen can be obtained if time permits prior to the patient's transport to an emergency room.

Cerebrovascular Accident

Cerebrovascular accident (CVA) is a common life-threatening disease which accounts for 10 percent of all deaths.[14] Also commonly referred to as a stroke, CVA is a syndrome consisting of a number of neurologic findings which are usually sudden in onset and which persist for more than 24 h. Strokes are caused by (1) the thrombotic or embolic occlusion of a cerebral artery resulting in infarction or (2) the spontaneous rupture of a vessel resulting in intracerebral or subarachnoid hemorrhage. Ischemic strokes, which include those caused by thrombi and emboli, account for 75 to 85 percent of all strokes.[14] Thrombotic strokes are frequently preceded by one or more transient ischemic attacks (TIAs). TIAs are focal neurological deficits that last minutes to an hour and fully resolve in less than 24 h. Thrombotic stroke patients frequently have a history of hypertension, diabetes, or show evidence of atherosclerotic vascular disease elsewhere such as a past history of myocardial infarction, intermittent claudication, or angina. Thrombotic strokes commonly occur during sleep or shortly after arising. The neurologic picture for thrombotic strokes as well as other types of strokes depends upon the artery involved and the site of the obstruction.

Carotid circulation involvement commonly causes contralateral hemiparesis, hemisensory loss, and permanent or temporary ipsilateral monocular visual loss (amaurosis fugax). Involvement of the vertebral-basilar circulation causes neurologic deficits referable to the brainstem or occipital cortex which can result in ataxia, nystagmus, vertigo, dysarthria, dysphagia, or homonymous visual field loss.

Embolic strokes may occur at any time of day or night and are distinct in that they evolve most rapidly, being complete in seconds to minutes. Cardiac sources of emboli include rheumatic heart disease, especially with atrial fibrillation; recent myocardial infarction; valve prostheses; bacterial endocarditis; and mitral valve prolapse. Noncardiac sources of emboli include foreign bodies, air, nitrogen, fat or tumor cells, and atheromatous material from the aorta or carotid artery.

Strokes secondary to intracranial hemorrhage are often associated with abrupt change in mental status, severe headache, and vomiting. However, in many instances, hemorrhagic strokes cannot be differentiated from ischemic stroke without the aid of a computed tomography (CT) scan. Intracerebral hemorrhage is most frequently associated with chronic systemic hypertension, while subarachnoid hemorrhage can result from saccular or berry aneurysms.

Treatment of CVA in the office is mainly supportive until emergency medical service (EMS) personnel arrive. The surgical procedure would be suspended and bandages applied as necessary. Vital signs should be obtained promptly and frequently. Greatly elevated blood pressure can be seen in all types of stroke, but no attempt to lower the blood pressure should be made.[15] The airway must be kept open by using the head-tilt/chin-lift maneuver if necessary. If available, a cardiac monitor should be placed to monitor for arrhythmias. Oxygen may be given by mask or nasal cannula. All staff members should speak to the patient in a calm and reassuring tone regardless of whether the patient is able to communicate.

Drug Toxicity

In office surgery, toxic reactions to drugs are most commonly related to local anesthetics or vasoconstrictive agents used with local anesthetics. Toxic reactions may be either localized at the site of the injection or generalized. Local toxicity may be manifested by cellulitis, ulceration, abscess formation, and tissue slough. Local toxicity is uncommon and is usually due to traumatic or improper injection technique; however, it may be due to contamination of the anesthetic agent or a reaction to the anesthetic itself, preservatives, or vasoconstrictors.

General toxicity is due to excessive dosage, rapid absorption of the drug, inadequate metabolism and redistribution of the drug, or unintentional intravascular injection. Systemic or generalized toxic reactions to local anesthetics are almost always due to overdose and are entirely preventable. The physician should always be aware of the toxic dose of the anesthetic being used, and the dosage used should be compatible with the body weight of the patient. For example, the toxic dose of the most commonly used anesthetic, 1% lidocaine, is 300 mg (30 cc) when used without epinephrine and 500 mg (50 cc) when used with epinephrine in a healthy adult patient of average weight (70 kg). Aspiration should be performed prior to injecting, especially in mucous membranes.

Systemic toxicity to local anesthetics at lower blood levels often produces symptoms which should alert the physician to a possible toxic reaction. These include yawning, drowsiness, numbness of the tongue or perioral tissues, ringing in the ears, nausea, vomiting, and a metallic taste in the mouth. As blood levels increase, signs such as nervousness, diplopia, and fine tremors of the face and hands may appear. These tremors can eventuate into grand mal seizures. As the blood levels of the anesthetics continue to climb, the next manifestation of toxicity may be depression of the central nervous system (CNS) characterized by extreme drowsiness merging into unconsciousness, respiratory depression, and arrest. Respiratory arrest is the most common cause of death directly attributable to reactions to local anesthetics. The cardiovascular effects of anesthetic toxicity are usually manifested by myocardial depression with peripheral vasodilation, hypotension, bradycardia, and cardiovascular collapse leading to cardiac arrest.

Prevention of local anesthetic emergencies begins first with careful visual monitoring of the patient after each local anesthetic injection. Early CNS abnormalities can be reversed by the simple administration of oxygen.[16] If the patient is symptomatic, attention should also be given to the maintenance of a patent airway and beginning an IV infusion. Diazepam (2.5 to 5 mg) may be given very slowly IV for persistent seizures. This should be done cautiously as diazepam may inhibit respirations. Treatment of circulatory depression may require administration of IV fluids and a vasopressor as directed by the clinical situation. In severe toxic reactions leading to respiratory or cardiac arrest, standard cardiopulmonary resuscitative measures should be instituted.

Vasoconstrictive agents, most commonly epinephrine, are frequently administered with local anesthetics and may also cause toxic reactions. Vasoconstrictors are used primarily to lessen bleeding at the surgical site; however, the vasoconstriction also inhibits absorption of both the vasoconstrictor and the local anesthetic, thereby minimizing the possibility of systemic toxicity of both agents. However, toxic reactions can occur with epinephrine when a high dosage is used, with accidental intravascular injection, or in patients who are very sensitive to the effects of epinephrine. Some of the manifestations of vasoconstrictor toxicity include palpitations, throbbing headache, tremor, tachycardia, tachypnea, and cardiac arrhythmias. Fortunately, these effects are usually short lived as the serum half-life of epinephrine is short, and usually only supportive therapy is needed.[17]

Epinephrine should be used with caution or avoided in those patients who give a history consistent with an epinephrine sensitivity. Absolute contraindications to the use of epinephrine are hyperthyroidism and pheochromocytoma. Epinephrine should also be used with caution in patients with a history of cardiac disease. In addition, a possible life-threatening interaction between epinephrine and propranolol has been described.[18,19] Propranolol is a broad beta-antagonist affecting both $beta_1$ and $beta_2$ receptors. The proposed mechanism of the interaction is thought to be propranolol-induced blockade of the $beta_2$ vascular bed receptors, with resultant unopposed alpha-pressor effect. This effect may lead to marked hypertension followed by a reflex bradycardia which ultimately can lead to cardiac arrest or stroke. The serious reactions that have been reported have occurred primarily with higher doses of epinephrine. In patients taking propranolol, epinephrine concentrations of 1:200,000 or less should be used, especially if a large volume of anesthesia is needed. For large procedures it may be prudent to discuss with the patient's internist the possibility of discontinuing propranolol prior to the procedure.

Allergic Reactions and Anaphylaxis

Type I allergic reactions are mediated by IgE and involve the release of chemical mediators from mast cells and basophils. Substances such as pollen, drugs, insect stings, vaccines, local anesthetics, and food products may induce allergic reactions in susceptible individuals. In the perioperative setting, the most common cause of allergic reactions is the injection of medications or local anesthetics. A broad spectrum of clinical manifestations can occur ranging from pruritus and urticaria to laryngeal bronchospasm, hypotension, and cardiovascular collapse. Anaphylaxis, the most severe form of allergic reaction, can result in death within minutes.

Local anesthetic agents fall into two groups: those with an ester-linkage group and those with an amide linkage. Those from the ester-linkage group are rarely used for local anesthesia of the skin today but previously were associated with allergic reactions at a rate of 1 percent. This group includes procaine, chloroprocaine, and tetracaine. They have been replaced by the amide group of local anesthetics that include lidocaine, bupivacaine, carbocaine, etidocaine, and prilocaine. True allergic reactions to this group of anesthetics appear to be exceedingly rare.[20] Of the few allergic reactions that have been reported in recent years, most may be attributable to the preservatives methylparaben or metabisulfite which are used in multidose vials.[16,21] Single-dose vials do not contain these preservatives. Also, ready-to-inject cardiac lidocaine (1% or 2%), which is used in cardiac resuscitation, contains neither epinephrine nor preservatives. It may be used cautiously as the local anesthetic in patients who give a history of reactions to local anesthetics.[22] Normal saline or diphenhydramine may also be used, and both are very effective for brief procedures such as a shave or punch biopsy. An allergist should evaluate patients who have a history of severe reactions occurring after local anesthetics. These patients can be approached by using a standardized drug selection and drug-challenge protocol to determine which local anesthetic can be safely used.[23]

In the treatment of allergic reactions, epinephrine is the initial drug of choice.[24] In the adult, 0.3 to 0.5 mL of a 1:1000 solution should be administered subcutaneously every 10 to 20 min as needed for up to three doses. The dosage in a child is 0.01 mL/kg of a 1:1000 solution. For life-threatening anaphylactic reactions, 5 mL of a 1:10,000 solution should be given IV and repeated every 5 to 10 min as needed. The sublingual or endotracheal routes of administration may be used if an IV line cannot immediately be established. A continuous infusion of epinephrine may be preferable to bolus administration as it may allow for more careful titration of dosage. Given in this way, 1 mL of a 1:1000 dilution of epinephrine is placed in 500 mL of 5% dextrose in water. This is then given IV at a rate of 0.5 to 5 µg per min. A venous tourniquet proximal to the injection site may be used to delay the absorption of an injected antigen, and epinephrine, 0.3 mL of a 1:1000 solution, may be injected subcutaneously into the site.

Maintenance of a patent airway along with the administration of oxygen is critical. With signs of upper airway compromise, endotracheal intubation should be performed, and, in cases of severe laryngeal edema, cricothyrotomy or tracheostomy may be necessary. Initially, bronchospasm may be treated with inhaled bronchodilators such as metaproterenol or albuterol. Secondary treatment of bronchospasm would include aminophylline 6 mg/kg infused IV over 20 to 30 min. Volume expansion with normal saline or Ringer's lactate solution may be needed as large losses of fluid from the intravascular compartment commonly occur. Hypotension unresponsive to volume expansion may require the use of a vasopressor such as dopamine hydrochloride.

Antihistamines and corticosteroids, although of little value in treating the acute episode, should both be considered for use in secondary therapy as they may shorten the duration of the reaction and prevent life-endangering recurrences.[25]

Diphenhydramine hydrochloride, 25 to 50 mg, can be administered IV over several minutes, although intramuscular or oral routes may be used.

Hydrocortisone sodium succinate or its equivalent should be administered IV for serious or prolonged reactions. As life-endangering manifestations of anaphylaxis can appear up to 8 h after apparent remission, it is recommended that all patients experiencing anaphylaxis be admitted to the hospital for careful monitoring and observation.[24]

Myocardial Infarction

Myocardial infarction occurs in approximately 1.5 million Americans each year and is responsible for about 25 percent of all deaths in the United States.[26] More than 50 percent of deaths associated with acute myocardial infarction occur within the first 2 h after the onset of symptoms and are related to ventricular arrhythmias, particularly ventricular fibrillation. Therefore, early recognition and careful management during the acute phase of this emergency is essential.

Signs and symptoms of acute myocardial infarction include crushing substernal chest pain, diaphoresis, cyanosis or pallor, and nausea or vomiting. The chest pain associated with myocardial infarction may resemble angina pectoris but is usually greater in severity and duration and not relieved by nitroglycerin. The pain has been described as crushing, pressing, constricting, oppressive, or heavy, and there may be radiation to one or both shoulders or arms or to the neck, mandible, or back.

If myocardial infarction is suspected, surgery should be terminated and the emergency medical system should be activated. Because of the high incidence of ventricular fibrillation and other life-threatening arrhythmias, electrocardiographic monitoring should be initiated immediately if available. Oxygen should be administered to all patients with myocardial infarction as there is some evidence that an elevation of PaO_2 may reduce the size of the infarction.[27] The oxygen should be administered by mask or nasal cannula at a flow rate of 1 to 4 L per min. IV lines should be established promptly. Vital signs should be measured frequently and recorded by one member of the office staff.

Relief of pain should be given a high priority. Nitroglycerin 0.4 mg can be administered sublingually in an attempt to relieve the pain if the patient is normotensive or hypertensive. This may be repeated at 5-min intervals, or, if the pain is severe or unremitting, morphine sulfate can be administered IV at titrated doses of 2 to 5 mg as often as every 5 to 10 min. Many experts feel that prophylactic therapy with lidocaine should be started at the earliest possible time as ventricular fibrillation may occur suddenly and without preceding arrhythmias.[28] A bolus of 1 mg/kg of 1% lidocaine IV is administered initially, followed by a continuous infusion of 2 mg per min. In the presence of decreased cardiac output, or patients older than 75 years old, or with hepatic dysfunction, the dosage of lidocaine should be reduced by half.

Surgery should not be carried out in patients who have suffered a myocardial infarction within the past 6 months. This is due to a significantly increased risk of reinfarction.[29] Precautions should be taken with patients with serious ischemic heart disease such as unstable angina.

Fortunately, reversal of coronary artery thrombosis and successful reperfusion of myocardium can often be accomplished when patients are stabilized and transported in a rapid fashion to a cardiac care center. These methods include enzymatic thrombolysis and transluminal coronary angioplasty.[26] Thrombolysis agents include streptokinase, urokinase, and tissue-plasminogen activator which are given IV and can lyse clots in 70 to 90 percent of patients. Coronary angioplasty can be used emergently or when thrombolytic therapy has failed, and it has a success rate of 75 percent.

Cardiac Arrest

More Americans die of cardiovascular disease than from any other cause. Nearly 1 million deaths in the United States each year result from cardiovascular disease, primarily due to underlying coronary and ischemic heart disease. It has been estimated that up to 1000 cardiac arrests occur every day in the United States alone, and 60 to 70 percent of these occur outside the hospital setting.[30] Cardiac arrest survival is dramatically increased when early CPR is coupled with an efficient emergency medical system and ACLS capability. This is often referred to as the *chain of survival* and involves four links: early access to the EMS system, early CPR, early defibrillation, and early advanced cardiac care.[31] The BLS and ACLS courses strengthen each link of this chain. The National Conference of Cardiopulmonary Resuscitation and Emergency Cardiac Care develops and publishes standards and guidelines for the proper training in and performance of CPR and emergency cardiac care (ECC).[30] The most recent standards and guidelines were published in 1985, with previous guidelines having been published in 1974 and 1980.

The first priority in cardiac arrest is initiating CPR. The sequence of BLS is often simplified as the ABC's of CPR and includes *airway, breathing,* and *circulation.* Each of the ABC's begins with an assessment phase: evaluate for unresponsiveness, evaluate for breathlessness, and evaluate for pulselessness, in that order. Determining unresponsiveness is important to prevent injury from attempted resuscitation of a patient who is not truly unconscious. This can be done by tapping or shaking the patient. If the patient is unresponsive, a member of the office team should be sent to activate the EMS. If the patient is determined to be unconscious, the airway should be opened immediately using the head-tilt/chin-lift maneuver (Fig. 10-1). The previously recommended head-tilt/neck-lift maneuver is no longer recommended.[30]

The assessment for breathlessness includes (1) looking for the rise and fall of the patient's chest, (2) listening for air escaping during exhalation, and (3) feeling for the flow of air from the patient's nose or mouth. This should be done while

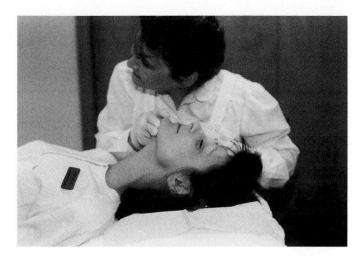

Figure 10-1   The head-tilt/chin-lift maneuver.

the airway is opened and maintained and should take no more than 5 s. If there are no signs of spontaneous respiration, two initial breaths of 1 to $1\frac{1}{2}$ s each should be given. This is a change from the former recommendations of four quick initial ventilations.

An excellent alternative to mouth-to-mouth is mouth-to-mask ventilation.[32] Advantages of mouth-to-mask ventilation are: (1) It eliminates direct contact with the patient's mouth and nose, (2) administration of supplemental oxygen is easy, (3) it diverts the patient's exhaled gas away from the rescuer when a one-way valve is used, (4) it is easy to teach and learn, and (5) it provides effective ventilation and oxygenation. The mask is placed on the face of the patient while the head-tilt maneuver is applied (Fig. 10-2). Oxygen tubing is connected to the port on the mask, with an oxygen flow rate of 10 L per min. The one-way valve is connected to the mask and the rescuer may then administer ventilations through it, observing the rise and fall of the chest. A bag-valve-mask device with supplemental oxygen may also be used for ventilation. However, proper training and practice in the use of the bag-valve-mask system is required as it may be difficult to provide a seal to the face while maintaining an open airway in a patient who is not intubated.[30]

Assessment of circulation should be performed carefully, checking the carotid pulse for 5 to 10 s. If a pulse is present but there is not spontaneous breathing, rescue breathing should be done at a rate of 12 times per minute (once every 5 s) after the initial two ventilations. If no pulse is detected, the diagnosis of cardiac arrest is confirmed, and external chest compressions should be instituted. If not previously done, the EMS system should be activated.

Proper hand-positioning and chest compression techniques are both critical in performing effective CPR.[30] The heel of the hand nearest the patient's head is placed over the lower half of the sternum, and the other hand is placed on top of the hand on the sternum. The fingers may be either extended or interlaced but must be kept off the chest. Elbows are locked

and the shoulders positioned directly over the hands so that each chest compression is directed down on the sternum. In the normal-sized adult, the sternum must be depressed $1\frac{1}{2}$ to 2 in. External chest compressions must be released completely, allowing the chest to return to its normal position after each compression. The time allowed for release should equal the time required for compression. The hands should not be lifted from the chest or the position changed in any way. The current recommendation for compression rate is 80 to 100 per min for both single- and double-rescuer CPR. The proper compression/ventilation ratio for one rescuer is 15:2 and 5:1 for two rescuers. The mnemonic "one and, two and, three and, four and . . ." helps establish the proper compression rate of 80 to 100 per min. Following a series of compressions, the airway should be opened again and rescue breaths delivered, two for the single rescuer and one for double rescuers. One to $1\frac{1}{2}$ s should be taken to deliver each breath. CPR should not be interrupted for more than 5 to 10 s to check for spontaneous breathing or for return of the carotid pulse.

Endotracheal intubation combined with oxygen will provide the best delivery of oxygen to the lungs. However, endotracheal intubation should only be attempted by personnel who are highly trained in that technique and who either use endotracheal intubation frequently or are retrained frequently.[30] A suction apparatus should be available to remove oral and gastric secretions prior to placement of an endotracheal tube. Once an endotracheal tube is in place, ventilation need not be synchronized to chest compressions but should be performed at a rate of 12 to 15 per min. Other adjuncts for ventilations include oropharyngeal, nasopharyngeal, and esophageal obturator airways. These airways also require proper training in their use and may be necessary whenever a bag-valve-mask device is utilized. Ventilations should never be interrupted for more than 30 s when placing an airway or during endotracheal intubation.[30,32]

After early access and early CPR, early defibrillation is the

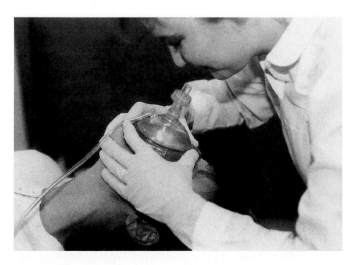

Figure 10-2   Mouth-to-mask ventilation.

TABLE 10-1

Management of Ventricular Fibrillation (VF) and Pulseless Ventricular Tachycardia (VT) in Adults

1. In a witnessed arrest, if no pulse is present, a single precordial thump should be delivered.

2. If there is still no pulse, begin CPR until a defibrillator arrives.

3. If a monitor confirms VF (pulseless VT treated identically), defibrillate with 200 J. Repeat a second time with 200–300 J and a third time with up to 360 J if VF persists.

4. Establish IV, if possible, while continuing CPR. Give epinephrine, 1:10,000, 5–10 mL IV and repeat every 5 min during resuscitation attempt.

5. Endotracheal intubation should be done, if possible. Do not interrupt CPR for more than 30 s.

6. Defibrillate again with up to 360 J.

7. Lidocaine should be given 1 mg/kg IV push. Defibrillate again with 360 J.

8. If VF persists, give bretylium 5 mg/kg IV push or first repeat doses of lidocaine 0.5 mg/kg every 8 min to a total dose of 3 mg/kg.

9. After 1–2 min, defibrillate again with up to 360 J.

10. If VF persists, give bretylium 10 mg/kg IV push. After 1–2 min, defibrillate with up to 360 J. Bretylium may be repeated at 15–30 min intervals to a maximum dose of 30 mg/kg.

11. Boluses of lidocaine or bretylium may be repeated at the recommended intervals to the maximum limit. Each bolus should be followed by defibrillations.

---

next link in the chain of survival for cardiac arrest patients. The electrocardiographic patterns of cardiac arrest most frequently encountered include ventricular fibrillation, pulseless ventricular tachycardia, asystole, and electromechanical dissociation. The success of resuscitation of patients with ventricular fibrillation and pulseless ventricular tachycardia is directly related to the rapidity of defibrillation.[33] A monitor defibrillator unit is generally necessary to determine which cardiac arrest pattern is present. However, many emergency personnel today are using automated external defibrillators. These are highly sophisticated devices which, when attached to the patient, record the rhythm, analyze the rhythm, and if ventricular fibrillation is present will deliver the appropriate shock.[31,33]

After appropriate rhythm diagnosis using a cardiac monitor and prompt defibrillation as indicated, the next priority should be the establishment of a reliable IV line to administer medications. Antecubital veins should be the first choice to establish venous access since cannulation of either the jugular or subclavian veins not only interrupts CPR but is also associated with significant complications if improperly performed. Five percent dextrose in water is generally used to keep the IV line open.

The three drugs of most value in the acute management of cardiac arrest are epinephrine 1:10,000, lidocaine 1% or 2%, and atropine. These three medications have a distinct advantage in that they can be administered via an endotracheal tube

if difficulty has been encountered in establishing an IV line. All cardiac medications should be purchased in premixed, ready-to-inject syringes. Calcium chloride and sodium bicarbonate, which had previously been used routinely in the treatment of cardiac arrest, are now used infrequently or in very specific settings.[34] Calcium chloride is indicated only in specific situations such as cardiac arrest related to hyperkalemia, profound hypocalcemia, or calcium channel-blocker toxicity. Sodium bicarbonate should only be used after defibrillation, chest compressions, and ventilatory support (including intubation, epinephrine, and antiarrhythmics) have been used; and then it is used only when blood gases are available and indicate a profound acidosis.

The great majority of outpatient cardiac arrests are due to ventricular fibrillation.[34] Treatment of this rhythm disturbance begins with CPR and activation of the emergency medical system (Table 10-1). A precordial thump has been shown to convert ventricular fibrillation and is recommended in patients with monitored ventricular fibrillation or in witnessed cardiac arrest when a defibrillator is unavailable. A precordial thump is delivered to the center of the sternum with the hypothenar aspect of the fist from a height of no more than 12 in. If a defibrillator is available, immediate defibrillation is critical and is carried out initially with 200 J. If fibrillation is persistent, a second shock should be administered at a strength of 200 to 300 J. If the first two shocks are ineffective in establishing a life-sustaining rhythm, a third shock not exceeding 360 J should be delivered immediately.

Proper paddle electrode positioning is important. One electrode should be placed to the right of the upper sternum and below the clavicle; the other should be placed to the left of the nipple, with the electrode in the center of the midaxillary line (Fig. 10-3). Approximately 25 lb of pressure should be applied to each paddle. In patients with permanent pacemakers, the electrodes should not be closer than 5 in from the pacemaker generator.[30]

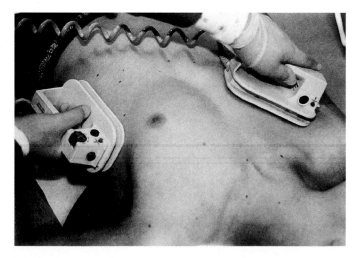

Figure 10-3 Proper position of defibrillator electrodes.

If initial defibrillation is unsuccessful, epinephrine should be administered immediately after establishing an IV line. Epinephrine is administered in a dose of 5 to 10 mL of a 1:10,000 solution every 5 min during resuscitation. Intracardiac administration of epinephrine should be avoided unless both IV and endotracheal routes are not readily available. This is because of the risk of coronary artery laceration, cardiac tamponade, or pneumothorax. When epinephrine is administered in an intracardiac fashion, there is also an interruption of external compression and ventilation. Epinephrine, with its potent alpha-adrenergic receptor-stimulating properties, increases myocardial and CNS blood flow during ventilation and chest compression.

Lidocaine is the second drug which would be administered during ventricular fibrillation or pulseless ventricular tachycardia when these arrhythmias are resistant to defibrillation. In controlled studies, lidocaine is as effective as other agents in improving the response of these arrhythmias to electric therapy. An initial dose of 1 mg/kg of lidocaine is administered by IV push. After this dose, additional boluses of 0.5 mg/kg can be administered every 8 to 10 min, if necessary, up to 3 mg/kg. Only bolus therapy should be used in the cardiac arrest setting. After successful resuscitation, continuous infusion of 2 to 4 mg per min should be started. The dose should be reduced to half the normal bolus dose in the presence of decreased cardiac output, in patients older than 70 years, or in patients with hepatic dysfunction. Also, the dosage should be reduced immediately if signs of lidocaine toxicity (slurred speech, altered consciousness, muscle twitching, seizures) are observed.[30]

Bretylium is the drug of choice in ventricular fibrillation that is refractory to both defibrillation and lidocaine. Bretylium is administered in an IV bolus of 5 mg/kg and is followed in 1 to 2 min by a single electric defibrillation of up to 360 J. The dose can be increased to 10 mg/kg and repeated at 15- to 30-min intervals until the maximum dose of 30 mg/kg is administered.

In cardiac arrest due to ventricular asystole, the prognosis is poor.[34] Frequently, patients with asystole have end-stage cardiac disease or have had a prolonged arrest and are not resuscitatable. The diagnosis of asystole should be confirmed in at least two different lead configurations, and, if there is any uncertainty as to the rhythm, the rhythm should be treated as though it were ventricular fibrillation. If asystole is present, CPR should be continued, and, when an IV line has been established, epinephrine should be given in the same dosage and frequency as for ventricular fibrillation. Intubation should be carried out if possible, and then atropine is administered (1-mg IV push). Atropine, as a parasympatholytic agent, enhances sinus nodes' automaticity and atrioventricular conduction via its direct vagolytic effect. If asystole persists, a second dose of atropine (1 mg IV) is repeated in 5 min. Full vagal blockade occurs after a total dose of 2 mg. Epinephrine should be administered prior to atropine and should be repeated every 5 min if ventricular asystole persists.

Cardiac arrest associated with electromechanical dissociation carries an exceedingly poor prognosis.[34] In this setting, the electrocardiogram shows organized electric activity but without effective myocardial contraction. This rhythm disturbance is frequently fatal and can be due to many causes, including severe acidosis, hypovolemia, hypoxemia, cardiac tamponade, tension pneumothorax, or massive myocardial damage from infarction, prolonged ischemia during resuscitation, or pulmonary embolism.[30,34] This is a very difficult rhythm disturbance to treat. Meticulous CPR should be maintained, IVs should be established, and epinephrine should be administered 5- to 10-mL IV push every 5 min during which an aggressive search to identify a correctable cause is undertaken.

BASIC EQUIPMENT AND MEDICATIONS

Successful outcome in emergencies requires both knowledge in the recognition and treatment of various emergencies and the availability of basic equipment and medications (Table 10-2). Oxygen is probably the most essential part of the basic emergency equipment.[35] A small portable oxygen tank with regulator, tubing, and a mask or nasal cannula would be sufficient. Also, pocket masks with ports for oxygen administration and one-way valves are necessary. Surgical tables which can be manually or automatically placed into a Trendelenburg position are recommended. A cardiac board may be needed if the surgical table is not firm. Many would consider the combination cardiac monitor and defibrillation unit a nonoptional, essential piece of equipment for the office. An alternative to

TABLE 10-2

Basic and Optional Equipment and Supplies

Basic

Oxygen tank with adapter, tubing, and mask or nasal cannula

Pocket masks and/or bag-valve mask (Ambu bag)

Suction device, tubing, Yankauer catheter

IV pole, tubing, catheters, and fluids (D5W, normal saline, Ringer's lactate)

Cardiac arrest board

Cardiac defibrillator-monitor

ECG paste

Tourniquet

Stethoscope

Sphygmomanometer

Optional

Airways (oropharyngeal, nasopharyngeal, or esophageal obturator)

Endotracheal tubes

Laryngoscope

this would be the automatic defibrillator units that were previously discussed. Various airways, laryngoscope, and different sizes of endotracheal tubes are important optional pieces of equipment that should be restricted to medical personnel who are trained in their use. An optional piece of equipment that is very helpful in the prevention of emergencies is the pulse oximeter. Newer pulse oximeters are noninvasive, highly accurate, and provide early detection of even small levels of hypoxia.[36] A pulse oximeter is particularly useful when surgery is being performed on a patient with a complicated medical history and certainly those undergoing procedures with IV sedation.

Essential medications as well as optional medications are listed in Table 10-3. These medications along with other equipment can be kept in an emergency tray or rolling cart.[1] IV fluids such as dextrose 5% in water, normal saline, and Ringer's lactate, along with IV tubing and IV catheters, are necessary for delivery of medications. A chart outlining the appropriate adult and pediatric dosages for emergency medications can be very useful and can be attached to a clipboard on the emergency cart along with a flow sheet for recording the events in a cardiac arrest. It is necessary on a regular basis to review the contents, expiration dates, and potency of all medications and fluids on the emergency cart. Likewise,

equipment checks, such as testing the charging and the discharging of the defibrillator and checking the pressure and the volume of the oxygen tank and oxygen delivery system, should be done at regular intervals. A logbook should be kept, documenting that the medications are current and that all emergency equipment is functioning well and in working order.

SUMMARY

Although perioperative emergencies in dermatologic surgery are relatively rare, the physician must be knowledgeable in the early recognition and treatment of various emergencies. Many simple steps can be taken to prevent emergency situations from arising. However, when an emergency does arise, nothing can replace the time that has been spent planning, training, and practicing to handle these situations. Training and retraining in BLS and ACLS are especially important in the management of cardiac emergencies. The physician should stay abreast of changes in the standards and guidelines that might effect techniques or medication dosages.

There are two examples of recent studies which could potentially change future standards and guidelines. One involves the medication epinephrine as used in the resuscitation of cardiac arrest. Some studies and anecdotal reports have suggested that high-dose epinephrine might be better for resuscitation rather than the standard dose currently recommended.[37,38] In the second example, a recent study indicated that the addition of interposed abdominal counterpulsation during CPR improved survival in cardiac arrest patients.[39] In this study, abdominal compressions centered over the umbilicus were interposed between chest compressions at the same rate of 80 to 100 per min.

Lastly, the physician should have basic emergency equipment and supplies on hand and should be knowledgeable in the proper use of this equipment.

TABLE   10-3

Basic and Optional Emergency Medications

Basic*

Epinephrine	1:1000
	1:10,000
	1% or 2%

Lidocaine

Atropine

Diazepam

Diphenhydramine

Hydrocortisone sodium succinate

Dextrose 50%

Optional*

Sodium bicarbonate

Calcium chloride

Bretylium

Dopamine

Aminophylline

Morphine sulfate

Other

Nitroglycerin tablets

Metaproterenol or albuterol inhaler

* Many of these are injectable medications that can be purchased in preloaded, ready-to-inject syringes.

REFERENCES

1. Larson PO: Review: Topical hemostatic agents for dermatologic surgery. *J Dermatol Surg Oncol* **14:**623, 1988

2. Amonette RA, Thomas RM: Emergencies in skin surgery, in *Dermatologic Surgery: Principles and Practice,* edited by RR Roenigk, HH Roenigk. New York, Marcel Dekker, 1989, pp 71–84

3. Sebben JE: Electrosurgery and cardiac pacemakers. *J Am Acad Dermatol* **9:**456, 1983

4. Castrow FF: Office Emergencies. *Dialogues in Dermatology* **12**(4):1983

5. Schultz KE: Vertigo and syncope, in *Emergency Medicine: Concepts and Clinical Practice,* edited by P Rosen et al. St. Louis, Mosby, 1987, pp 1359–1388

6. Bennett RG: Appendix F, in *Fundamentals of Cutaneous Surgery.* St. Louis, Mosby, 1988, pp 780–783

7. Donahue JH, Schrock TR: Emergencies in outpatient skin surgery, in *Skin Surgery,* 6th ed, edited by EE Epstein, EE Epstein Jr. Philadelphia, Saunders, 1987, pp 71–77

8. Salasche SJ: Acute surgical complications: Cause, prevention and treatment. *J Am Acad Dermatol* **15:**1163, 1986

9. Menzer L: Convulsions, in *Principles and Practice of Emergency Medicine,* 2d ed, edited by GR Schwartz et al. Philadelphia, Saunders, 1986, pp 773–777

10. Wolpow ER: Neurologic emergencies, in *MGH Textbook of Emergency Medicine,* 2d ed, edited by E.W. Wilkins. Baltimore, Williams & Wilkins, 1983, pp 338–368

11. Tomlanovich MC, Yee AS: Seizure, in *Emergency Medicine: Concepts and Clinical Practice,* edited by P Rosen et al. St. Louis, Mosby, 1987, pp 1339–1358

12. Pruitt AA: Neurologic emergencies, in *Emergency Medicine,* 3d ed, edited by EW Wilkins. Baltimore, Williams & Wilkins, 1989, pp 336–384

13. Applegate CN, Fox PT: Neurologic emergencies in internal medicine, in *Manual of Medical Therapeutics,* 26th ed, edited by WC Dunagan, ML Ridner. Boston, Little, Brown, 1989, pp 463–481

14. Jacobs FL: Stroke, in *Emergency Medicine: Concepts and Clinical Practice,* edited by P Rosen et al. St. Louis, Mosby, 1987, pp 1325–1338

15. Bergey GK, Tuhrim S: Neurologic assessment and management, in *Medical Perioperative Management,* edited by SD Wolfsthal. Norwalk, Conn, Appleton & Lange, 1991, pp 243–263

16. Grekin RC, Auletta MJ: Local anesthesia in dermatologic surgery. *J Am Acad Dermatol* **19:**599, 1988

17. Winton GB: Anesthesia for dermatologic surgery. *J Dermatol Surg Oncol* **14:**41, 1988

18. Foster CA, Aston SI: Propranolol-epinephrine interaction, a potential disaster. *Plast Reconstr Surg* **72:**74, 1983

19. Dzubow LM: The interaction between propranolol and epinephrine as observed in patients undergoing Mohs surgery. *J Am Acad Dermatol* **15:**71, 1986

20. Giovenniti JA, Bennett CR: Assessment of allergy to local anesthetics. *J Am Dent Assoc* **98:**701, 1979

21. Schwartz HJ et al: Metabisulfite sensitivity and local dental anesthesia. *Ann Allergy* **62:**83, 1989

22. Thomas RM: Local anesthetic agents and regional anesthesia of the face. *J Assoc Military Dermatol* **8:**28, 1982

23. Anderson JA, Adkinson NF: Allergic reactions to drugs and biologic agents. *JAMA* **258:**2891, 1987

24. Bochner BS, Lichtenstein LM: Anaphylaxis. *N Engl J Med* **324:**1785, 1991

25. Wasserman SI, Marquardt DL: Anaphylaxis, in *Allergy: Principles and Practice,* 3d ed, edited by E Middleton et al. St. Louis, Mosby, 1988, pp 1365–1476

26. Hupp JR: Myocardial infarction: Current management strategies. *J Oral Maxillofac Surg* **47:**1070, 1989

27. *Textbook of Advanced Cardiac Life Support: American Heart Association,* 2d ed. Dallas, American Heart Association, 1981, pp 11–26

28. Klopf F, Ridner ML: Ischemic heart disease, in *Manual of Medical Therapeutics,* 26th ed, edited by WC Dunagan, ML Ridner. Boston, Little, Brown, 1989, pp 90–113

29. Perioperative myocardial ischaemia and noncardiac surgery (editorial). *Lancet* **337:**1516, 1991

30. Standards and guidelines for cardiopulmonary resuscitation (CPR) and emergency cardiac care (ECC). *JAMA* **255:**2905, 1986

31. *Textbook of Advanced Cardiac Life Support: American Heart Association,* 2d ed. Dallas, American Heart Association, 1981, pp 287–299

32. *Textbook of Advanced Cardiac Life Support: American Heart Association,* 2d ed. Dallas, American Heart Association, 1981, pp 27–39

33. Cummins RO, Thies W: Encouraging early defibrillation: The American Heart Association and automatic defibrillators. *Ann Emerg Med* **19:**1245, 1990

34. Serota H: Basic and advanced cardiac life support, in *Manual of Medical Therapeutics,* 26th ed, edited by WC Dunagan, ML Ridner. Boston, Little, Brown, 1989, pp 175–184

35. Nagi C, Greenway HT: Emergency airway assessment and management: Guide for office practice. *J Assoc Military Dermatol* **9:**66, 1985

36. Lopert H: The pulse oximeter in dental surgery. *Anesth Prog* **36:**140, 1989

37. Burnette DD, Jamesson SJ: Comparison of standard versus high-dose epinephrine in the resuscitation of cardiac arrest in dogs. *Ann Emerg Med* **19:**8, 1990

38. Kosgrove EM, Paradis NA: Successful resuscitation from cardiac arrest using high-dose epinephrine therapy: Report of two cases. *JAMA* **259:**3031, 1988

39. Sack JB et al: Survival from in-hospital cardiac arrest with interposed counterpulsation during cardiopulmonary resuscitation. *JAMA* **267:**379, 1992

Thomas H. King
Donald J. Grande

11 Postoperative and Ongoing Care Following Surgery

The postoperative period is experienced differently by the surgeon and the patient, and this difference in perspective strongly influences the surgical outcome. To the surgeon, who has conscientiously applied his or her clinical judgment and technical skills to the surgical challenge, the deftly sutured wound seems almost an end in itself. Events following the procedure, while not ignored, seem anticlimactic by comparison. Because the actual process of wound healing is slow, incremental, and, frankly, unglamorous, the surgeon may be tempted to devote less attention to this aspect of the patient's care. The reason is obvious: The surgeon creates the wound, but it is the patient who does the healing. Wound healing takes place not in the relatively short time that it took to create and repair the surgical wound but in the days, weeks, and years following the day of surgery. Thus it is important that the surgeon consider the fact that the patient views events through a different lens. To the patient, postoperative events assume enormous importance because he or she deals with the consequences in an extremely personal way. Especially in an ambulatory setting, where the patient leaves the medical facility soon after the operation is completed, the immediate postoperative period is often fraught with anxiety and uncertainty.[1] Minor problems, such as postoperative swelling or ecchymosis, seem gravely serious. The wise surgeon, recognizing that the patient views events differently, establishes a trusting relationship with the patient beforehand, explaining the procedure, its risks and complications, and the natural history of postoperative wound healing.

In the context of western medicine, the surgeon involved in postoperative care practices applied human biology to the known scientific principles of wound healing.[2-11] However, while recent advances in our understanding of the biology of wound healing may have changed certain aspects of postoperative care, nothing has changed the ancient ethic of duty to the patient. An ideal outcome of the surgical encounter would dictate that both the surgeon and the patient are satisfied with the result. This chapter attempts to focus attention on rational management of expected issues which commonly occur in the postoperative setting and of the unexpected complications, recognizing that sometimes an expected result to the surgeon may be viewed as a complication by the patient.[12]

ROUTINE POSTOPERATIVE CARE

Wound Care Principles

Rational postoperative wound care aims at ensuring the unimpeded progression of the healing process as we understand it and at intervening when obstacles to proper healing occur. The major objectives of postoperative wound care are to reestablish surface continuity and development of sufficient tensile strength to withstand normal stress. Ideally, any surgical decision in the postoperative period with successful wound healing as its goal should have a rationale founded in the known physiology of wound healing.[11]

Care of the postoperative wound really begins in the preoperative period. Careful patient selection and identification of factors which may inhibit normal healing (Table 11-1) are

TABLE 11-1

Factors Hindering Normal Wound Healing

Systemic disease
 Diabetes mellitus
 Uremia
 Cachexia
 Cushing's syndrome
Hematoma
Infection
Necrosis
Foreign body
Pharmacologic agents
 Corticosteroids
 Colchicine
 D-penicillamine
 Isoniazid
 Chemotherapeutic agents
Genetic defects
 Ehlers-Danlos
 Marfan's syndrome
Factitia
Malignancy
 Squamous cell carcinoma (Marjolin's ulcer)
 Basal cell carcinoma
 Malignant melanoma
Radiation injury

essential. Proper surgical technique is the single most important contribution a surgeon makes in ensuring a successful outcome.

Another important consideration is the type of wound resulting from surgical intervention.[10] Partial-thickness wounds, such as those created by dermabrasion, curettage and electrodesiccation, laser vaporization, or split-thickness skin graft donor sites, heal by the relatively rapid process of epithelialization from adnexal structures. Full-thickness wounds which are closed immediately or in a delayed manner by sutures heal mainly by the process of collagen deposition. Wounds which are left to heal by secondary intention require that relatively prolonged process of complex interrelated events which comprise normal wound healing: inflammation, epithelialization, wound contraction, and collagen synthesis.

Fortunately, wound aftercare is remarkably uncomplicated. Winton[13] has described three simple rules governing the aftercare of wounds: Keep the wound clean, moist, and covered. A daily dressing change is usually adequate. Choice of topical antibiotics is often a matter of the individual surgeon's preference.[14] Studies suggest that occlusive dressings afford quicker healing.[15,16] Many surgeons employ other topical therapies, including plant-derived drugs, which they and the patient believe may enhance wound healing.[17] An example is the commonplace use of aloe vera, in which the evidence of efficacy is conflicting.[18] In truth, there seem to be many postoperative wound care regimens used, based on the individual surgeon's preference, which eventuate in satisfactory outcomes.

Instructions to Patients

Postoperative instructions must be given in a lucid, understandable manner, and all of the patient's questions must be answered. Common postoperative issues, such as pain, bleeding, bruising, swelling, etc., should be explicitly discussed with the patient. Moreover, the surgeon should emphasize that the postoperative wound heals in stages and often over many months. A helpful device to reinforce wound care instructions is a written wound care instruction sheet (Fig. 11-1). Such a handout should include phone numbers the patient may use to contact the surgeon in the event of a problem or question. In an ambulatory surgery setting, it is imperative that the surgeon be available to the patient for emergencies, as well as to address the myriad unexpected situations which may develop postoperatively. It is often best for the patient to arrive and de-

Department of Dermatology
Dermatologic Surgery

POST-OPERATIVE WOUND CARE INSTRUCTIONS

1. Keep initial dressing dry and do not remove for 24 hours. You may shower after the initial 24 hours.

2. If bleeding starts, keep continuous pressure on area for 15 minutes without removing the bandage. You should contact us if this occurs.

3. Depending upon the location and nature of your surgery, there may be activity restrictions which will be specified to your case.

4. Sleep with 2-3 pillows and on unaffected side for the first few nights as this helps to minimize swelling.

5. **No aspirin** or **aspirin containing products** until stitches or staples are removed. Take **Tylenol** or **Extra Strength Tylenol** for pain.

6. Change the dressing daily using the following steps:

 a. Wash hands before and after each dressing change.

 b. Remove old bandage for first dressing change. You may want to shower with the old dressing on so it is easier to remove.

 c. Wash area gently with sterile gauze using **Hydrogen Peroxide** to remove any crusting along suture line/wound. (If you had a skin graft, gently wash along the perimeter of the bolster. Do not try to wash underneath or to remove the bolster).

 d. Dab dry with sterile gauze.

 e. Apply **Bacitracin** or **Polysporin** ointment to keep wound moist for better healing.

 f. Cover with dry sterile gauze and Bandaid.

 g. It is not necessary to cover the wound if you will be staying indoors as long as Bacitracin has been applied. A dressing must be applied when you are outdoors.

7. If your wound becomes red, warm, painful or begins to drain, or if you develop a fever of 101° or greater, please contact us.

8. **No alcohol** for 48 hours after surgery.

 ❏ Apply ice once every 2 hours for 10 minutes at a time for the rest of the day.

 ❏ No bending, lifting or strenuous exercise until sutures are removed.

If you have any further questions or problems, call the dermatologic surgery division at (617) 273-8457, Monday through Friday 9:00 a.m. to 5:00 p.m. If problems occur at night or during weekend hours, page the dermatologic surgeon on-call at (617) 273-8300.

Sutures/staples to be removed in _____ days at _____ office.

LAHEY CLINIC

12540 12/94

Figure 11-1 Wound care instruction sheet given to patients at the Lahey Clinic.

part the ambulatory surgical facility accompanied by a supportive relative or friend who can provide comfort, transportation, and other needed assistance.

Basic wound aftercare is very simple, and most patients have no difficulty performing the tasks expected of them at home. Sometimes it is helpful to demonstrate a dressing change to the patient or the relative who will care for the wound at home. The complexity of wound care required varies, and the surgeon should gauge the ability of the patient to perform wound aftercare. Often, elderly patients living alone are unable to satisfactorily care for even simple wounds. Arranging for the assistance of visiting nurse services is invaluable for these situations.

Pain Management

Postoperative pain following cutaneous surgery is relatively minor, although the perception of pain intensity varies among patients. Pain is commonly manageable with over-the-counter analgesics, usually acetaminophen. Aspirin and aspirin-containing products should be avoided because of their antiplatelet activity and the possibility that they might enhance postoperative bleeding. Other nonsteroidal anti-inflammatory drugs may also lead to bleeding sequelae.[19] Certain procedures, by virtue of their location (e.g., frontotemporal scalp) or their nature, may result in more severe pain. In the case that minor analgesics are ineffective, use of narcotic analgesics, such as pentazocine or propoxyphene, or narcotic combinations, such as codeine or hydrocodone combined with acetaminophen, are almost always adequate for postoperative pain relief. The surgeon should be alert to the possibility that severe pain following skin surgery may often signal a complication, such as hematoma or wound infection, and necessitate further evaluation of the wound.

Antibiotic Prophylaxis

Bacteremia does occur in clean skin surgery but with very low frequency.[20,21] For this reason, the use of prophylactic antibiotics is usually not necessary. Prophylaxis should be confined to those instances in which there is a high risk of postoperative infection or in which the consequences of an infection might be catastrophic (e.g., bacterial endocarditis).[22] In addition, some advocate use of antibiotic prophylaxis in contamination-prone areas such as the nose, groin, axilla, and perineum.[23] When choosing an antibiotic, the surgeon must consider the type of organisms usually responsible for infections, the route of administration, adequate dosage, and timing of administration.[24–27]

Drains

Drains are rarely used in dermatologic surgery and justifiably so.[12] These can be a route of entry of pathogenic bacteria into the wound. Occasionally, a drain is employed and the basic

principle governing its postoperative management is to remove it as soon as is practical, usually within 24 to 48 h.

Suture Removal

There is no strict rule as to the appropriate time to remove sutures.[6] The judgment of the individual surgeon often decides this issue. As a general rule, sutures should be removed when they have served their purpose and before they themselves become a cause of potential complications (i.e., suture sinus tract formation occurring between the third and the eighth postoperative day).[4] In most cases in dermatologic surgery, skin sutures are employed to carefully approximate wound edges during the relatively rapid process of wound healing, the task of wound apposition being subserved by buried absorbable sutures. In the case where the skin sutures are themselves responsible for tensile strength in the healing wound, sutures should obviously be retained longer. After sutures are removed, the wound edges are best supported with wound-closure tapes to minimize the potential for wound dehiscence. Commonly accepted time intervals for cutaneous suture removal include 3 to 7 days for the head and neck, 7 to 14 days for the trunk, and 14 days or greater for the extremities.

Follow-Up Visits

Follow-up visits are normally required for the surgeon to ensure that the postoperative wound is healing properly (and to monitor the dermatologic condition which required surgical intervention). Very little follow-up is necessary in the case of a primarily closed wound resulting from the removal of a benign lesion. Usually, in this instance, a single visit at the appropriate time for suture removal is all that is required. Complicated wounds require more frequent follow-up. For example, a wound resulting from Mohs micrographic surgery for an aggressive basal cell carcinoma allowed to heal by secondary intention will obviously require much more aftercare by the patient and more frequent follow-up by the surgeon in order to ensure that proper wound healing is occurring and also to monitor for possible recurrence of the tumor.

Adequate follow-up requires a well-organized record-keeping system. Operative notes, pre- and postoperative drawings, and photographs are invaluable aids in documenting the postoperative course.[28] Collection and careful analysis of data are integral to the surgical process.[29] Use of clinical data with a pragmatic, problem-solving attitude and a humane concern for the patient's comfort often leads to improvements in postoperative care.[30]

Ongoing Care

The surgeon must continue to address underlying conditions which may or may not have contributed to the need for surgical intervention. In the patient with chronic sun-damaged skin (a complex of findings termed *dermatoheliosis* by Fitzpatrick[31]) who has had a basal cell carcinoma removed surgically still requires follow-up for his or her underlying condition. Repeated cutaneous examinations are necessary for early detection of new cancers. Preventive measures, such as avoidance of sunbathing and use of topical suncreens, should also be encouraged since there is evidence that educational measures are effective in changing patient behavior.[32]

COMPLICATIONS

The best method of avoiding postoperative complications is prevention through judicious preoperative patient selection, adherence to meticulous intraoperative surgical technique, and insistence upon appropriate follow-up. However, every surgeon must be prepared for the unexpected result or complication (to the patient these are often synonymous) of the operation. Despite the best of intentions and surgical technique, the unexpected may occur. The surgeon should inform the patient of potential complications which occur relatively frequently, such as bleeding, infection, undesirable scar, nerve damage, etc. The patient who is mentally prepared for the possibility of complications and who trusts the surgeon's judgment will be more likely to accept such circumstances with equanimity than one who is not. Moreover, because frequent reassessment of results and complications is a necessary part of the surgical process, the surgeon who forthrightly confronts postoperative complications with a positive, problem-solving approach will benefit himself or herself and the patients the most.

Surgical complications, discussed below, do not occur in a vacuum. In the complex series of interrelated events which comprise wound healing, one complication will almost inevitably contribute to the development of another.[33] For example, a wound closed under excessive tension without subcutaneous sutures is at risk for development of distal wound edge necrosis, which predisposes the wound to infection and dehiscence, which can lead later to unsightly scarring (Fig. 11-2). For this reason, when a complication occurs, decisive early intervention is essential to interdict this cascade effect.

Bleeding

Postoperative bleeding of any extent is alarming to the patient, but it is not uncommon for postoperative wounds to bleed a little. In the great majority of cases, this will be minor postoperative oozing from the wound edges. This often occurs after trauma to the area following surgery. In other cases, bleeding may occur in patients occultly using aspirin, aspirin-containing medications, or nonsteroidal anti-inflammatory drugs. Operative procedures performed in skin with relatively thin dermis, such as the periorbital region, may result in considerable ecchymosis. Patients should be forewarned of this possibility.

Before the patient leaves the site of ambulatory surgery,

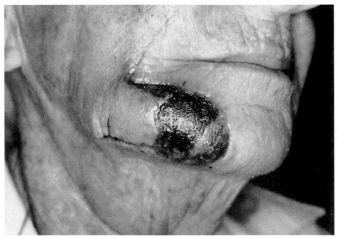
a

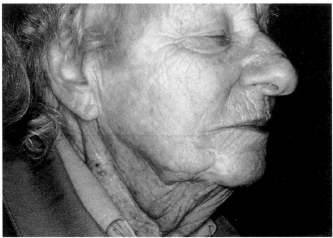
b

Figure 11-2   (*a*) Partial necrosis occurring in the distal tip of a reverse nasolabial flap; (*b*) surgical result 13 months later. Note the atrophic scar corresponding to the original region of necrosis.

specific instructions should be given in the event that postoperative bleeding occurs. In most cases, application of firm constant pressure to the bleeding point for at least 15 min will result in hemostasis.

Significant bleeding almost always results from ineffective intraoperative hemostasis or preexisting clotting disturbances, chiefly, aspirin ingestion.[34] In other cases, hematologic disorders may exist which may potentiate postoperative bleeding. Ideally, the surgeon should identify patients who are at risk for bleeding and defer elective procedures. In the vast majority of cases, significant bleeding may be prevented by careful intraoperative hemostasis and preoperative instructions to discontinue aspirin and aspirin-containing compounds. In patients who continue to ooze from skin edges despite all efforts to stop bleeding, placement of a drain should be considered (Fig. 11-3).

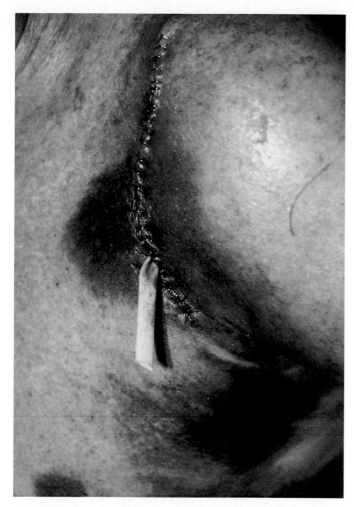

Figure 11-3   Extensive ecchymosis adjacent to anterior axillary wound. Note that a drain has been placed.

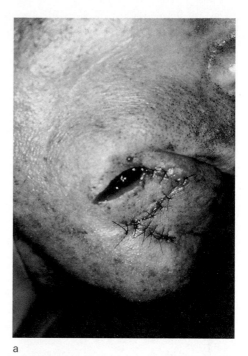

a

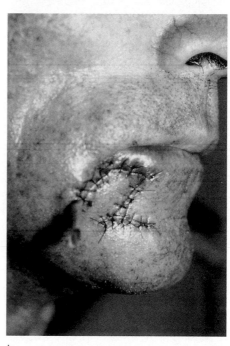

b

Figure 11-4   (*a*) Acute hematoma formation following transposition flap repair. The repair has been taken down partially preparatory to hematoma evacuation; (*b*) following evacuation of the hematoma and establishment of adequate hemostasis, the wound has been resutured. Note that a surgical drain has been placed.

Hematoma

Acute expanding hematomas (Fig. 11-4) in the postoperative setting can be dramatic and anxiety provoking for patient and surgeon alike but are rarely life threatening.[33] More importantly, wound security may be threatened significantly by hematomas, which are space-occupying and exert pressure on the wound edges, rendering the wound more susceptible to dehiscence, infection, and flap or graft necrosis.[35] Hematoma is best prevented by careful attention to hemostasis during the operative procedure.

Treatment of hematoma is straightforward: evacuation of the clot, identification of bleeding vessels, and meticulous hemostasis. Often, small hematomas may be expressed through the incision line without completely taking down the entire surgical repair. Krugman has described use of a suction-assisted lipectomy apparatus in managing auricular hematomas.[36] If further bleeding is feared, placement of a drain may be warranted.

Infection

Wound infection (Fig. 11-5), which occurs in approximately 1 percent of clean dermatologic surgical cases, often results from intraoperative lapses in sterile technique.[37] Wound in-

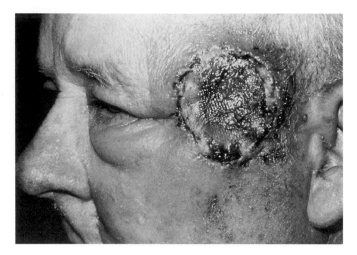

Figure 11-5   Wound infection.

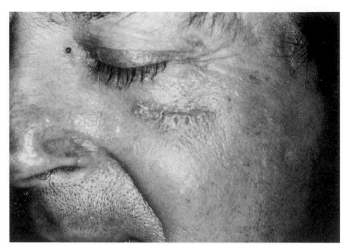

Figure 11-6   Suture reaction.

fection is frequently the ultimate result when other complications occur. Hematoma, dehiscence, and necrosis often contribute to development of a wound infection. Important factors implicated in subsequent development of surgical wound infection include elderly patients, long procedures (especially longer than 3 h), types of procedures (clean versus contaminated wound) and, most importantly, the presence of bacteria in the wound.[38,39] Signs and symptoms usually become manifest during the fourth to the eight postoperative days.[33] Typical symptoms include increasing redness, tenderness, and swelling of the wound, infrequently accompanied by chills and fever. Purulent drainage is often noted. In advanced cases, lymphangitis or cellulitis may be present.

When wound infection is suspected, appropriate cultures should be taken. Antimicrobial therapy should be prescribed, based on the anticipated pathogen.[24,25,27] Therapy is best instituted promptly, not only to prevent more severe infection but also to prevent other complications, such as wound dehiscence and necrosis, which may later ensue.

Suture Reactions

Even the least reactive of suture materials are foreign material, and one must anticipate potential adverse reactions (Fig. 11-6).[40,41] The surgeon must balance the need for sutures for wound strength against the need to remove skin sutures in order to prevent suture reactions. No simple rules apply here, only sound surgical judgment.

When the suture is placed, epidermal keratinocytes migrate along the puncture wound created by the needle.[4] If the suture is left in too long, stitch abscesses with subsequent scarring may result. If the sutures are tied too tightly, a railroad-track appearance may result. Infection may also result from suture material.[42] Subcutaneous sutures which are placed too high in the dermis may "spit," or physically extrude from the wound. These are best treated by extraction.

Contact Dermatitis

Dermatologic surgeons are particularly aware of the potential for development of contact irritation or hypersensitivity to materials used in preoperative skin preparation, such as povidone-iodine or chlorhexidine, and those used in wound dressings, such as topical antibiotics.[43–46] The distinctive appearance of a pruritic eczematous eruption in pattern on or near the wound which suggests an extrinsic source is diagnostic (Fig. 11-7). If applicable, the presumed offending agent should be discontinued immediately and replaced with an alternative. Use of compresses and topical corticosteroid preparations is usually effective in resolving contact dermatitis. Patch testing should be considered to identify the offending substance if allergic contact hypersensitivity is suspected.

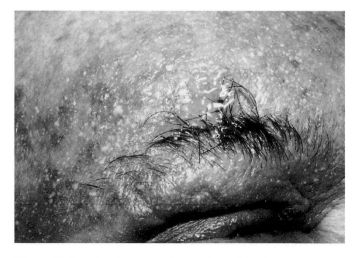

Figure 11-7   Allergic contact dermatitis resulting in severe edema, erythema, and vesiculation surrounding a sutured wound in the right eyebrow. Patch testing confirmed delayed hypersensitivity to compound tincture of benzoin.

Dehiscence

Failure of the wound to heal, manifested by wound dehiscence (Fig. 11-8), is disconcerting. Predisposing factors include advanced age, chronic illness, medications, and poor nutritional status. In some cases, dehiscence may result from events occurring subsequently to surgery, such as trauma, hematoma, or infection. Infection in particular is frequently present in dehisced wounds. In most cases, however, dehiscence results from surgical errors, such as allowing excessive tension on the wound, using inadequate suture material, and premature suture removal.[47] Dehiscence most frequently occurs soon after suture removal, particularly in cases where no buried absorbable sutures have been used. At this stage in wound healing, intrinsic wound strength is minimal because collagen deposition and cross-linking, which supplies wounded tissue with strength and integrity, requires weeks to

reach clinically meaningful levels.[48] An often-cited surgical dictum states that without inflammation there is no healing. Since many dehisced wounds fail to exhibit the healing ridge (representing inflammation) characteristic of primarily closed wounds at 5 to 8 days postoperatively, consideration should be given in these cases to delaying suture removal in order to prevent dehiscence. As with most postoperative complications, dehiscence is best treated by prevention through good surgical technique.

When wound dehiscence occurs, the dermatologic surgeon has two options. The wound may be left open and left to heal by secondary intention. This option is obviously more desirable in the presence of wound infection. The other option, particularly in clean wounds, is to anesthetize the dehisced wound and resuture it after "freshening" the edges. Resutured wounds are known to rapidly acquire increased tensile strength.[49–51]

Necrosis

When tissue is deprived of oxygen, necrosis may occur. As with dehiscence, necrosis may result from factors occurring subsequent to surgery. Many believe that heavy smokers are especially at risk to develop wound necrosis, particularly in flaps.[52,53] However, the main cause of wound necrosis is failure of circulation at distal wound margins (Fig. 11-9), usually resulting from technical errors by the surgeon. Excessive tension on the wound edges, excessive undermining, and superficial undermining may compromise circulation, leading to tissue necrosis.[33] Random flaps and grafts, by their very nature, are especially at risk to necrotic sloughs.[54–56] The best way to prevent tissue necrosis is good intraoperative technique: Avoid excessive tension on the wound, and handle tissues gently.

The degree of necrosis will vary, but the treatment of all tissue sloughs is similar. Basic wound care should be prescribed and careful debridement performed when the tissue forms an eschar and separates easily. Wound healing will then proceed by the more prolonged process of granulation and epithelialization. Since such wounds are prone to infection, early use of appropriate antibiotics seems a wise choice. Scar revision should be considered later, if necessary.

Abnormal Surface Scar

If the final surface scar resulting from dermatologic surgery is inconspicuous, patient and surgeon are usually extremely pleased with the result. All scars resulting from an operative procedure undergo somewhat of a metamorphosis from a raised purple-red in the first few weeks to flat, pale, and thin months to years later. Because the surface scar is often viewed by the patient as the "bottom line," this gradual transformation process should be explained in advance. An important corollary is that scar revision should be delayed until maturation occurs. Often, an unsightly scar will mature and

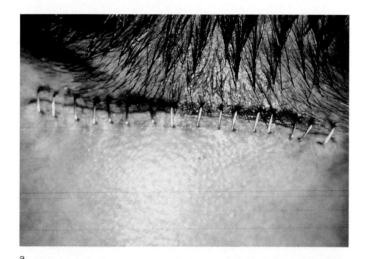

a

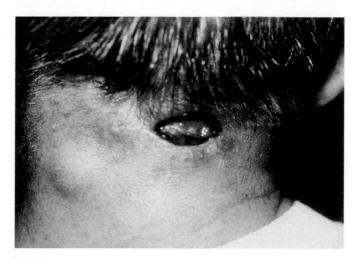

b

Figure 11-8   (*a*) Linear closure of a surgical wound on the posterior neck; (*b*) wound dehiscence following removal of staples used for skin closure.

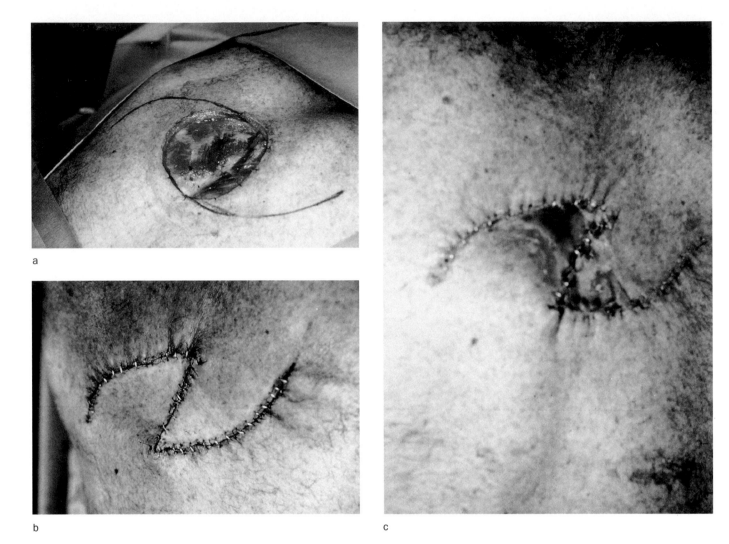

a

b

c

Figure 11-9 (*a*) Large surgical defect on the back prior to repair; (*b*) bilateral rotation flap used to close the defect; (*c*) after 10 days, obvious necrosis of the distal tips of both flaps has occurred. The resulting wound required prolonged secondary intention healing.

gradually become much less obvious. Many surgeons advocate spot dermabrasion of cutaneous scars at approximately 8 weeks following surgery to improve the scar's cosmetic appearance.[54]

Spread scars are not uncommon. Certain anatomic regions seem to be more prone to develop spread scars, especially the chest, back, and shoulders. In addition, when other complications such as necrosis, dehiscence, or infection occur, spread scars may often result. Spread scars also commonly develop in wounds which are closed under a great deal of tension. Buried absorbable sutures have been recommended as a way to prevent this result. Moreover, a recent study suggests that when the dermis is supported by a subcuticular nonabsorbable suture for a prolonged period, there is a considerable reduction of scar spread when compared with conventional interrupted skin suture.[57] Early spread scars are best left alone unless the patient is insistent upon treatment. Surgical scar

revision may be helpful in more mature lesions. Spot dermabrasion may also be helpful.

Depressed scars may often accompany spread scars but occur with much less frequency. A common site for depressed scars is tissue replete with sebaceous glands, such as the nose. Depressed scars may be revised surgically or dermabraded to improve the cosmetic appearance. Alternative treatments involve use of filler substances, such as bovine collagen or injection of gelatin matrix implants.[58]

Dog-ears, or standing cones of tissue, occur occasionally. Proper surgical technique will prevent these but, occasionally, small dog-ears are inevitable. Often, in these cases, smaller dog-ears will flatten with the passage of time. Otherwise, spot dermabrasion or surgical revision is indicated.

Other commonly occurring events which render scars more obvious are pigmentary abnormalities. In persons with darker constitutive pigmentation, scars often develop significant hyperpigmentation.[60] In other cases, hypopigmentation of scars may result. In either case, treatment should be expectant; often over time the dyspigmentation will spontaneously improve.

Pruritus of surgical scars is common. Some have speculated on the etiologic significance of elevated histamine levels in scars.[61,62] Treatment with bland emollients or low-potency topical corticosteroids is effective.

Milia, small superficial 1 to 4 mm cysts, often develop in scars following dermatologic surgery, particularly after dermabrasion.[63] Experimental evidence has established that cysts may result from dermal implantation of epidermis.[64] Treatment is straightforward: incision and expression of the cyst contents. Topical tretinoin and use of mild abrasive pads are often useful in treating milia.

Keloids and hypertrophic scars differ clinically, histologically, and biochemically from normal scarring.[65–67] Not only are such lesions unsightly, but they are often pruritic, painful, and may even interfere with function. These lesions, like spread scars, appear more frequently in certain regions, such as the chest, shoulders, and upper back. Hypertrophic scarring and keloid formation seem to occur despite proper surgical technique. Some patients are predisposed to forming hypertrophic scars and keloids. Recently, atypical keloids have been reported in patients who underwent dermabrasion after treatment with isotretinoin.[68] The surgeon must carefully consider the potential risks when contemplating surgery on a patient who may be predisposed to hypertrophic scars or keloids.

Because the treatment for keloids and hypertrophic scars is similar, they are often considered identical for purposes of discussion. However, keloids differ clinically from hypertrophic scars because they are often familial, occur more commonly in blacks than whites, spread beyond the site of injury (often with characteristic clawlike projections), and, most importantly, are persistent. Hypertrophic scars, on the other hand, may regress significantly over time. Scar revision of hypertrophic scars should thus be delayed as long as possible to await further maturation of the scar.

Numerous therapies have been advocated for treatment of hypertrophic scars and keloids.[69] Although use of pressure or massage on the scar and intralesional repository steroids are most commonly employed, other proposed therapies include kilovoltage radiation, cryotherapy, interferon alfa-2b, recombinant interferon gamma, exogenous electric current, and silicon gel.[70–76] Some authors have reported successful surgical excision with flap or graft repairs.[77] Often, repository steroids and pressure are employed as adjunctive measures. Some have advocated use of the carbon dioxide laser to vaporize and excise keloids.

Miscellaneous Complications

It is beyond the scope of this discussion to catalog all of the myriad possible complications which may result from a dermatologic surgical procedure. Obviously, some are rare, such as lint granulomas, or talc granulomas.[78,79]

Many complications are more particularly associated with the procedure performed. For example, unique problems are often encountered after dermabrasion, chemical peels, and laser surgery.[63,68,80–83] Flaps, by virtue of their often tenuous blood supply and novel shapes, may lead to specific complications.[55,84] A good example would be the *trapdoor effect* seen commonly following nasolabial flap repairs.[85] Similarly, cutaneous grafts may be prone to certain complications.[56,86]

Certain anatomic sites, such as the eye or the ear, have complications peculiar to the region.[87–89] Adequate knowledge of regional anatomy and wound healing is essential in preventing such complications. Management of such complications (e.g., ectropion) may entail appropriate referral to a surgeon with specific expertise.

Inadvertent damage to underlying structures may result in postoperative complications. A common example is injury to cutaneous sensory nerves during dermatologic surgery. Persistent numbness at the surgical site, while usually harmless, may be upsetting to some patients. These patients should be reassured that, often, numbness or hypesthesia related to surgery will improve over months to years. Injury to motor nerves, especially the facial nerve, is more serious but, fortunately, occurs with much less frequency. Similarly, injury to the lacrimal drainage system and the parotid duct is uncommon but potentially serious. Referral should be made to a surgeon experienced in dealing with these complications.

CONCLUSION

A good patient history, careful preoperative planning, painstaking surgical technique, and careful follow-up are the best ways to ensure normal wound healing. Wound care in the postoperative period should be based on the known biology of wound healing. Developing a rapport with the patient and discussing expected and unexpected issues regarding the postoperative course are helpful should surgical complications ensue. Since one complication often leads to another, prompt intervention is essential.

Finally, the postoperative course is viewed from the differing perspectives of the patient and the surgeon, each often using subjective criteria. The ideal outcome of a procedure is not easily defined, other than that circumstance in which everyone is satisfied with the result. For the surgeon pleased with the well-healed, barely perceptible, surgical scar, nothing is more disconcerting than a patient's apparently trivial complaint. A defensive response is inadvisable because the patient must then assume that the minor side effect is of greater importance than previously realized. Such assumptions often form the basis for litigation. An open, honest, and problem-solving approach is much more likely to result in successful resolution of the problem.[89]

REFERENCES

1. Peacock EE: Major ambulatory surgery of the plastic surgical patient. *Surg Clin North Am* **67**(4):865–879, 1989

2. Moore FD: Teaching the two faces of medical history. *Surg Clin North Am* **67**(6):1121–1126, 1987

3. Ordman LJ, Gillman T: Studies in the healing of cutaneous wounds, pt 1: The healing of incisions through the skin of pigs. *Arch Surg* **93**:857, 1966

4. Ordman LJ, Gillman T: Studies in the healing of cutaneous wounds, pt 2: The healing of epidermal, appendageal, and dermal injuries inflicted by suture needles and by the suture material in the skin of pigs. *Arch Surg* **93**:883, 1966

5. Ordman LJ, Gillman T: Studies in the healing of cutaneous wounds, pt 3: A critical comparison in the pig of the healing of surgical incisions closed with sutures or adhesive tape based on tensile strength and clinical and histological criteria. *Arch Surg* **93**:911–927, 1966

6. Peacock EE Jr: Wound healing and wound care, in *Principles of Surgery,* 4th ed, edited by SI Schwartz. New York, McGraw-Hill, pp 301–312, 1984

7. Peacock EE Jr: Wound healing and care of the wound, in *Manual of Preoperative and Postoperative Care,* 2d ed, edited by JM Kimney et al. Philadelphia, Saunders, pp 3–18, 1971

8. Harris DR: Healing of the surgical wound, pt 1: Basic considerations. *J Am Acad Dermatol* **1**:197–207, 1979

9. Harris DR: Healing of the surgical wound, pt 2: Factors influencing repair and regeneration. *J Am Acad Dermatol* **1**:208–215, 1979

10. Cohen IK: Complications of wound healing, in *Complications in Surgery and Trauma,* 2d ed, edited by LJ Greenfield. Philadelphia, Lippincott, pp 3–9, 1990

11. Goslen JB: Wound healing for the dermatologic surgeon. *J Dermatol Surg Oncol* **14**:959–972, 1988

12. Bennett RG: *Fundamentals of Cutaneous Surgery.* St. Louis, Mosby, 1988

13. Winton GB, Salasche SJ: Wound dressings for dermatologic surgery. *J Am Acad Dermatol* **13**:1026–1044, 1985

14. Feingold DS: Antibacterial agents, in *Dermatology in General Medicine,* 3d ed, edited by TB Fitzpatrick et al. New York, McGraw-Hill, pp 2550–2552, 1987

15. Nemeth AJ et al: Faster healing and less pain in skin biopsy sites treated with an occlusive dressing. *Arch Dermatol* **127**:1679–1683, 1991

16. Hien NT et al: Facilitated wound healing using transparent film dressing following Mohs micrographic surgery. *Arch Dermatol* **124**:903–906, 1988

17. King TH, Perez-Figaredo RA: Plant-derived dermatologic drugs. *J Assn Milit Dermatol* **14**(1):26–31, 1988

18. Shelton RM: Aloe vera: Its chemical and therapeutic properties. *Int J Dermatol* **30**:679–683, 1991

19. Connelly CS, Panush RS: Should non-steroidal anti-inflammatory drugs be stopped before elective surgery? *Arch Intern Med* **151**:1963–1966, 1991

20. Sabetta JB, Zitelli JA: The incidence of bacteremia during skin surgery. *Arch Dermatol* **123**:213–215, 1987

21. Halpern AC et al: The incidence of bacteremia in skin surgery of the head and neck. *J Am Acad Dermatol* **19**:112–116, 1988

22. Wagner RF Jr et al: Antibiotic prophylaxis against bacterial endocarditis in patients undergoing dermatologic surgery. *Arch Dermatol* **122**:789–901, 1986

23. Bencini PL et al: Antibiotic prophylaxis of wound infections in skin surgery. *Arch Dermatol* **127**:1357–1360, 1991

24. Roth RR, James WD: Microbiology of the skin: Resident flora, ecology, infection. *J Am Acad Dermatol* **20**:367–390, 1989

25. Feingold DS, Wagner RF: Antibacterial therapy. *J Am Acad Dermatol* **14**:535–548, 1986

26. Nichols RL: Use of prophylactic antibiotics in surgical practice. *Am J Med* **70**:686–692, 1981

27. Abramowitz M: The choice of antimicrobial drugs. *The Medical Letter* **32**(817):41–48, 1990

28. Sebben JE: Office photography from the surgical viewpoint. *J Dermatol Surg Oncol* **9**:763–768, 1983

29. Collison DW et al: Data collection and analysis, in *Mohs Micrographic Surgery,* edited by GR Mikhail. Philadelphia, 1991, Saunders pp 309–328

30. Freitag DS, Bennett RG: Postoperative elevation of eyeglasses from the nasal bridge. *J Dermatol Surg Oncol* **17**:906–908, 1991

31. Pathak MA et al: Preventive treatment of sunburn, dermatoheliosis, and skin cancer with sun-protective agents, in *Dermatology in General Medicine,* 3d ed, edited by TB Fitzpatrick et al. New York, McGraw-Hill, pp 1507–1522, 1987

32. Robinson JK: Behavior modification obtained by sun protection education coupled with removal of a skin cancer. *Arch Dermatol* **126**:477–481, 1990

33. Salasche SJ: Acute surgical complications: Cause, prevention, and treatment. *J Am Acad Dermatol* **15**:1163–1185, 1986

34. Moake JL, Funicella T: Common bleeding problems. *Clin Symp* **35**:1–32, 1983

35. Straith RE et al: The study of hematomas in 500 consecutive face lifts. *Plast Reconstr Surg* **59**:694, 1977

36. Krugman M: Management of auricular hematomas with suction assisted lipectomy apparatus. *Otolaryngol Head Neck Surg* **101**:504–505, 1989

37. Whitaker DC et al: Wound infection rate in dermatologic surgery. *J Dermatol Surg Oncol* **14**:5, 1988

38. Davidson AIG et al: A bacteriological study of the immediate environment of the surgical wound. *Br J Surg* **58**:326–333, 1971

39. Cruse PJE, Foord R: A five-year prospective study of 23,649 surgical wounds. *Arch Surg* **107**:206, 1973

40. Postlewait RW et al: Human tissue reaction to sutures. *Ann Surg* **181**:144, 1975

41. Madsen ET: An experimental and clinical evaluation of surgical suture materials. *Surg Gynecol Obstet* **97**:73, 1953

42. Edlich RF et al: Physical and chemical configuration of sutures in the development of surgical infection. *Ann Surg* **177:**679–687, 1973

43. Marks JG Jr: Allergic contact dermatitis to povidone-iodine. *J Am Acad Dermatol* **6:**473, 1982

44. Osmundsen PE: Contact dermatitis to chlorhexidine. *Contact Dermatitis* **8:**81, 1982

45. Fisher AA: *Contact Dermatitis,* 3d ed. Philadelphia, Lea & Febiger, 1986

46. Grandinetti PJ, Fowler JF Jr: Simultaneous contact allergy to neomycin, bacitracin, and polymyxin. *J Am Acad Dermatol* **23:**646 647, 1990

47. Hunt TK: Wound complications, in *Management of Surgical Complications,* 3d ed, edited by CP Artz, JD Hardy. Philadelphia, Saunders, pp 21–32, 1975

48. Clark RAF: Cutaneous tissue repair: Basic biologic considerations, pt 1. *J Am Acad Dermatol* **13:**701–725, 1985

49. Botsford TW: The tensile strength of sutured skin wounds during healing. *Surg Gynecol Obstet* **72:**690–697, 1941

50. Madden JW, Smith HC: The rate of collagen synthesis and deposition in dehisced and resutured wounds. *Surg Gynecol Obstet* **130:**487–493, 1970

51. Peacock EE Jr: Some aspects of fibrinogenesis during the healing of primary and secondary wounds. *Surg Gynecol Obstet* **115:**408–414, 1962

52. Goldminz D, Bennett RG: Cigarette smoking and flap and full-thickness graft necrosis. *Arch Dermatol* **127:**1012–1015, 1991

53. Nolan J et al: The acute effects of cigarette smoke exposure on experimental skin flaps. *Plast Reconstr Surg* **75:**544–549, 1985

54. Katz BE, Oca GS: A controlled study of the effectiveness of spot dermabrasion ("scarabrasion") on the appearance of surgical scars. *J Am Acad Dermatol* **24:**462–466, 1991

55. Kerrigan CL: Skin flap failure: Pathophysiology. *Plast Reconstr Surg* **72:**766–774, 1985

56. Smith F: A rational management of skin grafts. *Surg Gynecol Obstet* **42:**556–562, 1926

57. Elliot D, Mahaffey PJ: The stretched scar: The benefit of prolonged dermal support. *Br J Plast Surg* **42:**74–78, 1989

58. Millikan L et al: Treatment of depressed cutaneous scars with gelatin matrix implant: A multicenter study. *J Am Acad Dermatol* **16:**1155–1162, 1987

59. Dzubow LM: The dynamics of dog-ear formation and correction. *J Dermatol Surg Oncol* **11:**722, 1985

60. Mosher DB et al: Disorders of pigmentation, in *Dermatology in General Medicine,* 3d ed, edited by TB Fitzpatrick et al. New York, McGraw-Hill, pp 794–876, 1987

61. Fitzpatrick DW, Fisher H: Histamine synthesis, imidazole dipeptides, and wound healing. *Surgery* **91:**430, 1982

62. Kahlson G et al: Wound healing as dependent on rate of histamine formation. *Lancet* **2:**230, 1960

63. Monash S, Rivera RM: Formation of milia following abrasive treatment for postacne scarring. *Arch Dermatol Syph* **68:**589, 1953

64. Epstein WL, Kligman AM: Epithelial cysts in buried human skin. *Arch Dermatol* **76:**437, 1957

65. Arnold HL et al: *Andrew's Diseases of the Skin: Clinical Dermatology,* 8th ed. Philadelphia, Saunders, 1990

66. Lever WF, Schaumburg-Lever G: *Histopathology of the Skin,* 7th ed. Philadelphia, Lippincott, 1990

67. Bailey AJ et al: Characterization of the collagen of human hypertrophic and normal scars. *Biochim Biophys Acta* **405:**412–421, 1975

68. Rubenstein R et al: Atypical keloids after dermabrasion of patients taking isotretinoin. *J Am Acad Dermatol* **15:**280–285, 1986

69. Ceilley RI: The treatment of hypertrophic scars and keloids, in *Skin Surgery,* 6th ed, edited by EE Epstein, EE Epstein Jr. Philadelphia, Saunders, pp 580–586, 1987

70. Golladay ES: Treatment of keloids by single intraoperative perilesional injection of repository steroid. *South Med J* **81:**736–738, 1988

71. Doornbos JF et al: The role of kilovoltage irradiation in the treatment of keloids. *Int J Radiat Oncol Biol Phys* **18:**833–839, 1990

72. Mende B et al: Treatment of keloids by cryotherapy. *Z Hautkr* **62:**1348–1355, 1987

73. Berman B, Duncan MR: Short-term keloid treatment in vivo with human interferon alfa-2b results in selective and persistent normalization of keloidal fibroblast collagen, glycosaminoglycan, and collagenase production in vitro. *J Am Acad Dermatol* **21:**694–702, 1989

74. Granstein RD et al: A controlled trial of intralesional recombinant interferon-gamma in the treatment of keloidal scarring. *Arch Dermatol* **126:**1295–1302, 1990

75. Weiss DS et al: Exogenous electric current can reduce the formation of hypertrophic scars. *J Dermatol Surg Oncol* **15:**1272–1275, 1989

76. Mercer NSG: Silicone gel in the treatment of keloid scars. *Br J Plast Surg* **42:**83–87, 1989

77. Pollock SV, Goslen BJ: The surgical treatment of keloids. *J Dermatol Surg Oncol* **8**(12):1045–1048, 1982

78. Amromin G et al: Lint granuloma. *Arch Pathol* **60:**467, 1958

79. Eiseman B et al: Talcum powder granuloma: A frequent and serious postoperative complication. *Ann Surg* **126:**820, 1947

80. Fulton JE: The prevention and management of postdermabrasion complications. *J Dermatol Surg Oncol* **17:**431–437, 1991

81. Ship AG, Weiss PR: Pigmentation after dermabrasion: An avoidable complication. *Plast Reconstr Surg* **75:**528–532, 1985

82. Brody HJ: Complications of chemical peeling. *J Dermatol Surg Oncol* **15:**1010–1019, 1989

83. Olbricht SM et al: Complications of cutaneous laser surgery: A survey. *Arch Dermatol* **123:**345–349, 1987

84. Salasche SJ, Grabski WJ: Complications of flaps. *J Dermatol Surg Oncol* **17:**132–140, 1991

85. Koranda FC, Webster RC: Trapdoor effect in nasolabial flaps. *Arch Otolaryngol* **111:**421–424, 1985

86. Gilman T et al: Reactions of healing wounds and granulation tissue in man to anti-Thiersch, autodermal, and homodermal grafts. *Br J Plast Surg* **6:**153, 1953

87. Baylis HI, Cies WA: Complications of Mohs' chemosurgical excision of eyelid and canthal tumors. *Am J Ophthalmol* **80:**116–122, 1975

88. Leshin B et al: Unusual auricular complications in cutaneous oncology. *J Dermatol Surg Oncol* **17:**891–896, 1991

89. Larson PO: Surgical complications, in *Mohs Micrographic Surgery,* edited by GR Mikhail. Philadelphia, Saunders, pp 193–206, 1991

Abel Torres

12 Medicolegal Issues for the Dermatologic Surgeon

It is important to understand that the legal responsibilities of physicians will be determined by a combination of federal and state laws. The term *laws* is used in a generic sense to encompass legislative statutes, administrative rules and regulations, and common law (law promulgated by the courts). Any discussion regarding the legal rights and responsibilities of physicians and patients must be interpreted with the realization that those rights and responsibilities may vary from state to state. Although this chapter can serve as an educational tool for the physician, it is no substitute for the advice of an attorney when potential and/or actual medicolegal issues arise.

Although medical malpractice is at the forefront of medicolegal issues, the dermatologic surgeon has many other legal responsibilities of equal importance. Among those that will be discussed are establishing a physician-patient relationship, consent to treatment, contracts with patients, disclosures about patients, proper management of medical records, management of patients with HIV, and alternative dispute resolution (arbitration).

ESTABLISHING OR TERMINATING A PHYSICIAN-PATIENT RELATIONSHIP

A physician-patient relationship usually creates a contractual relationship where both the physician and patient have du-ties.[1] The physician is implied to promise to use the degree of skill, care, and knowledge of practitioners in good standing in the community, and the patient promises to behave as a reasonable person would in undergoing treatment.[2] The creation of a physician-patient relationship usually requires some form of contact with the patient, but this contact can also consist of gratuitous advice or service.[3] The contact can also consist of a telephone conversation or even no physical contact.[4] The courts will determine whether a physician-patient relationship exists, and usually imply it, if there is a physician-patient contact where the physician undertakes to treat the patient or his or her action creates a reasonable expectation of treatment by the patient.[5] Thus, in telephone or other contacts, if the physician doesn't want to establish a relationship, he or she or the staff must be careful not to give advice or directions upon which the person may rely for treatment.

Physicians are not obligated to give gratuitous advice and are free to choose their patients unless qualified by a specific statute.[6] They can also limit the relationship to treat the patient to one particular treatment, procedure, time, or place.[7] An appointment is usually considered to be an agreement to see a patient and not sufficient to establish a relationship.[8] However, if the appointment is for treatment of a specific problem, some courts have decided that this constitutes an agreement to treat a specific illness and thus implies a relationship.[3] It would be wise, therefore, for the dermatologic surgeon to follow up on appointments missed by patients referred for specific problems. Once a relationship is established with a patient, he or she may use a substitute physician, but the substitute physician must be qualified and competent, and the patient must be aware of a possible substitution.[9]

Once the physician-patient relationship is established, it can't be terminated unless one of the following occurs: (1) There is a mutual consent of the parties, (2) the services are no longer needed, (3) it is limited or conditioned by agreement, (4) the physician is dismissed by the patient, or (5) the physician unilaterally but properly withdraws.[10] A caveat is that if the patient refuses further treatment or dismisses the physician, the patient must be advised of the risks, prognosis, possible complications, and alternatives to that decision.[11] If the physician chooses to unilaterally withdraw from the relationship, he or she must afford the patient a reasonable opportunity to obtain the services of another physician and must continue to care for the patient for the time it will reasonably take the patient to secure replacement care.[12] Failure to properly withdraw from a patient's care can lead to a physician's being found liable for malpractice, abandonment, and/or breach of contract.[13] When a physician wants to withdraw from the care of a patient, he or she would be prudent to document the notice to the patient (in writing and preferably by certified mail), assist the patient in finding other care (refer to the local medical society, etc.), and provide the patient with ongoing care for a reasonable amount of time.[13]

Contracts

The physician-patient relationship is a contractual relationship. Thus, when a physician acts negligently, he or she may be liable for both professional negligence (malpractice) and for breach of his or her contractual duty to render care according to accepted practices.[14] However, the courts do not consider that a physician guarantees the success of treatment unless that physician promises a cure, a certain result, or to perform in a certain manner.[15–17] Thus, although physicians do not normally guarantee results, it is important that they and their staff be careful about making statements that might be interpreted as guaranteeing an outcome. The use of words such as *routine, rare, common, infrequent, likely,* etc., should be used with care to avoid creating a false reassurance that might be interpreted as a guarantee.[18]

Consent to Treatment

Any intentional touching of, or use of force upon, another person without that person's consent, no matter how slight, may constitute a battery even if the person suffers no physical injuries.[19] A battery action can result in punitive or compensatory damages from a defendant. If the dermatologic surgeon performs a procedure without the patient's consent, unless it's an emergency, this may constitute a battery.[20] There need not be any actual body contact since even the administration of a medication without consent can constitute a battery. However,

absent some misrepresentation by the physician, if the patient consents to the touching (treatment), this will be a complete defense to an action for battery.[21] This is true even if the patient is not happy with the results.[21]

Most physicians realize that it is prudent to obtain a consent from a patient before proceeding with any treatment. However, if the surgeon extends the surgery beyond the limits previously discussed with the patient, this may exceed the scope of consent and constitute a battery.[21,22] Yet, if the surgeon gets consent to remedy a medical condition rather than just for a procedure, this will be less likely to be considered exceeding the scope of the consent.[23] The latter gives the physician more leeway in how he or she approaches the treatment although he or she will still have a duty to give the patient informed consent. Also, although consent may be implied by the courts from the patient's conduct, it is prudent for the physician to get written consent when feasible or at least carefully document the circumstances of treatment in the patient's record.[24]

Obtaining consent to treatment may avoid an action for battery, but it still doesn't eliminate the duty by the physician to obtain informed consent to treatment. Failure to obtain informed consent can bring about an action in negligence.[25] Informed consent carries the obligations of (1) obtaining the patient's consent prior to the treatment and (2) disclosure of sufficient information so that the patient can decide whether the treatment is in his or her best interest.[26] Informed consent requires the disclosure of (1) uncommon but material (serious) risks and (2) common risks even if not material (serious). Informed consent doesn't require the diclosure of (1) uncommon and not material (serious) risks and (2) risks that are common knowledge to laypersons.[27] Thus, it is not necessary for the physician to read the Physicians' Desk Reference (PDR) to the patient. Four exceptions to informed consent are (1) when the patient waives the right to informed consent or disclosure (i.e., doesn't want to know), (2) when disclosure of the risks to the patient could harm the patient or impair his or her ability to make a rational decision, (3) if the patient is incompetent, and (4) in an emergency situation.[20]

The problem with informed consent is that since each circumstance is different, the courts can't disclose exactly how much disclosure is "adequate" for informed consent to exist. To judge whether disclosure is adequate, the physician can look at the two standards that the courts use. One standard is the *legal standard* or, that is, that the physician reveal all the information that a reasonable person would consider material in deciding whether or not to undergo treatment.[28] The other standard is the *professional standard* or, that is, that the physician reveal the same information that other physicians would disclose to the patient in the same or similar circumstances.[29] The standard used by the courts will vary according to the laws of that jurisdiction. Under both standards, the courts will require that the accusing party (plaintiff) show that he or she would have refused treatment if disclosure had been adequate. However, once again, the states will vary as to whether the test will be what would a reasonable person have done versus what would that particular patient have done.[30] Dermatologic surgeons should be familiar with the standard used in their jurisdiction so that they can be assured that their disclosure has been adequate.

MEDICAL MALPRACTICE

One in five dermatologists has faced a medical liability claim.[31] However, 35 percent of the claims are either dropped or dismissed in favor of the physician, and, as a whole, the risk of a suit is considerably higher for other medical specialists such as plastic surgeons.[32] A significant number of those claims against dermatologists are related to conditions and procedures dealing with skin cancer management and surgical procedures.[33] Thus, it would behoove the dermatologic surgeon to be familiar with the elements of medical malpractice since it is more likely to impact on him or her.

Medical malpractice law is based on a number of causes of action (theories) which the plaintiff (accuser) can use to bring an action against the defendant (doctor, hospital, etc.). The author has already discussed some of these causes of action such as failure to obtain consent or informed consent, the duty not to abandon the patient, and breach of contract. This section concentrates on medical malpractice as it relates to the *tort law of negligence* which compensates individuals for the losses they suffer due to the negligent acts of another person.

Negligence is a conduct which involves the breach of a duty to conform to a certain standard which in turn results in a foreseeable harm to another.[34] The requirements for medical negligence are (1) the establishment of a duty by the physician, (2) the breach of a duty by the physician, (3) a reasonably close casual connection between the conduct and the resulting injury, and (4) an actual injury (damages).[34]

The duty that a physician owes to his or her patients is to act with the knowledge, care, and skill exercised by reasonable and prudent practitioners under similar circumstances.[34] At one time, the standard was to conform to the knowledge, care, and skill exercised by local practitioners. Increasingly, because of modern communication and modern technology, that standard is now held to be to conform to the knowledge, care, and skill practiced by physicians nationally.[35] It is important for the dermatologic surgeon to note that if a physician performs a procedure that is traditionally performed by a specialist in another medical field, the physician will be held to the standard of that other field.[36] The fact that the physician owes a duty to a patient will be established when, as discussed above, the physician-patient relationship is established. Also, as discussed previously, that duty will not cease to exist until the physician-patient relationship is properly terminated.

That a duty was breached by a physician requires a showing that the physician deviated from the standard of care.[37] Expert testimony by another physician is required to show that a breach of duty occurred, unless the act is one that is within the common knowledge of a nonmedical person.[38] Thus, if the dermatologic surgeon gives the patient a medication which he or she knows the patient has an allergy to or fails to make sure that his or her autoclave is working properly, there may not be a requirement for expert testimony. It is also important for the dermatologic surgeon to realize that "doing what the majority of surgeons do" is not determinative of whether he or she will prevail. What is determinative is which expert the jury believes. In other words, the breach of the standard of care has essentially become that established by the winner of the battle of the experts. The dermatologic surgeon would be best served by familiarizing himself or herself with the literature and choose what is in the patient's best interests rather than what the majority of the surgeons would do.

Even if there is a breach of duty by the physician, there is no medical negligence unless the patient-plaintiff can establish that he or she was actually damaged (injured).[39] This damage can be physical such as a scar or damage to a nerve. It can also be due to a psychological damage such as anxiety or depression, and most recently there have been suits based on "fear of" contracting a disease such as AIDS. It would be prudent for the physician to communicate with the patient and address these anxieties and fears.

The last element of negligence that the patient-plaintiff must prove is causation; that is, that there was a foreseeable and actual causal link between the breach of the standard of care and the injury to the patient.[38,39] Every time that a duty is breached, liability may not exist if a damage did not actually occur. With the increasing emergence of such intangible damages such as "anxiety" and/or "fear of," it is less likely that no damages will be found by the jury.

The elements that have been discussed above are those that the patient-plaintiff must prove to establish that there was medical malpractice by a physician. However, the physician has defenses that he or she can raise even if those elements are found to be present.[40]

One defense to damages is that if the damage suffered is covered by a disability plan or a settlement with another physician, the physician-plaintiff may not be able to recover any further damages. One defense to causation is called *abreaction* or, that is, an abnormal reaction to treatment resulting in damages unexpected from the actual breach of duty that occurred.[41] Yet, physicians will still need to take reasonable precautions such as properly assessing the patient and obtaining informed consent. Furthermore, in some jurisdictions, the abnormal sensitivity of the patient will not reduce the damages (the eggshell doctrine).[41] Even if the physician is found to be negligent, the damages may be reduced or negated if the patient-plaintiff is found to have also been negligent either in helping to cause the injury or not taking steps to mitigate it. The result will depend on whether the jurisdiction follows the doctrine of *contributory* (a complete bar to recovery) versus *comparative* negligence (diminish the damages).[41] Thus, if a patient fails to follow instructions or doesn't advise the physician that there is a problem, the patient may be held accountable for his or her own negligence. It is prudent for the physician to closely follow up on his or her patients or be readily available so that the patients are likely to be held accountable for their actions.

One important defense for the physician is the statute of limitations to a cause of action.[36] The reasoning for statute of limitations is that punishment must be within a reasonable time and that after a period of time defending a suit may be an unreasonable burden.[41] The length of statute of limitations varies between jurisdictions. In the past, the statute of limitations started to run when the injury actually occurred. However, many jurisdictions have adopted the *discovery rule* which states that the statute of limitations runs from the time that the patient-plaintiff discovers the injury.[36] As is evident, this could be a burden for defendants, since discovery may not take place for years. As a result, many other jurisdictions have adopted *statutes of repose,* which place an outer limit on the time needed to discover and injury or the time to file a negligence claim.[36] Statutes of limitations may be tolled (suspended) by actions such as a continued relationship between the physician and patient, fraudulent concealment by the physician, and, in some jurisdictions, the physician's silence as to an act of possible negligence.[36,41] In other words, if the physician continues to see the patient or tries to hide the negligent act, the statute of limitations will be found not to have expired. A physician should not try to conceal a possible negligent act, but it is controversial whether there is a duty to inform the patient of the act if it doesn't appear that the patient was harmed. Similarly, if an unhappy patient stops coming for care and later reappears, this should alert the physician as to the possible attempt by the patient to restart the statute of limitations. Whether to see the latter patient or discuss possible negligent actions with a patient is ultimately a decision that must be made by the physician and his or her attorney and/or malpractice carrier.

Regardless of what defense the physician asserts, his or her defense will rely largely on the completeness and accuracy of his or her medical records. It may well be that a physician's best defense is his or her medical records.

Medical Records

A physician's medical records serve as a chronologic record of the patient's medical care as well as a tool for evaluating and planning a patient's care. The contents of a medical record are usually admitted as evidence for or against a hospital and/or physician.[42] In fact, many times the medical record will be the only credible evidence available. Thus, the completeness and accuracy of the medical records are very important not only for the well-being of the patient but also for the protection of the physician.

General correspondence and billing records should be kept separate from the medical records.[18,43] A record should document all positive and negative findings which are essential to or customarily recorded for a patient's care.[18,43] All sources of information should be documented in order to establish the source of any inaccuracies. Consistency of the record will increase its credibility. The record should be complete but concise since a voluminous record impairs its usefulness as a treatment tool and may provide a plaintiff's lawyer with abundant material that may help build a case against the physician.[43] Any discussions with the patient or related third parties should be recorded in the medical record whether they occur in the office, on the telephone, or outside of the office.[43] All diagnostic considerations and treatment plans should be well documented as well as any instructions or warnings given to the patients and related third parties.[43] Any lists written in the records should either be complete or include a general inclusive statement.[43] Always document informed consent and patient noncompliance.[43]

A medical record will have a high degree of credibility if it includes mainly information for the patient's care and avoids self-serving entries.[18,43] Expressions which imply a frustration with or disapproval of the patient or another health care provider should be avoided.[18,43] If a patient is being manipulative, describe your assumptions as possibilities rather than statements of fact.[18,43] Document medical complications, mishaps, or unusual occurrences in the records using terms that describe the event but avoid premature conclusions as to the cause.[18,43] Risk-prevention activity by the physician, economic issues (failure of the patient to pay you), and legal matters (e.g., who was at fault in an accident) should be omitted from the records unless they have a bearing on the course of treatment.[18,43] Threats and complaints by the patient should be recorded in a manner that reflects patient care such as documenting that it may create a problem with future patient care.[18] Avoid statements that imply carelessness or that something has gone wrong, but do not make statements that are inaccurate or deliberately misleading.[18,43] Respond to record entries by others, such as a nurse; if you disagree with an entry, give an explanation.[18,43]

Altering the medical record can have severe consequences in addition to affecting its credibility and the credibility of the physician.[18] If an error is recognized while you are making an entry in a new page that has no other entries, then it may be appropriate to rewrite the page.[18] Otherwise, a prior record shouldn't be altered unless for the protection of the patient (e.g., to note that the patient *does* have an allergy).[18,43] Any correction should be initialed and dated with the previous entry lined out. Preferably, any corrections should be made in a new note, since this avoids giving the impression of altering the record, but avoid defensive entries since these will be looked upon with suspicion.[18,43] Prior records must be presumed to have been photocopied by a patient-plaintiff's lawyer, and any alteration attributable to the physician may undermine his or her defense even if the facts support a lack of findings of malpractice.

A physician's medical records are his or her private property. Most states statutorily allow the patient access to the records either directly or through an authorized representative such as another physician or a lawyer or the patient's insurance company.[43] In addition, there may be other statutory exceptions for the release of records, and, if the physician has any doubts, he or she should consult his or her lawyer. Any release of information should be authorized in writing by the patient and carefully documented. A copy and not the original record should be released since the record could get lost and result in inadequate care for the patient or lack of evidence for the support of the physician. The patient's record is subject to an ethical and legal duty of confidentiality, and unauthorized release of that information can have serious civil and/or criminal consequences for a physician.

Litigation Versus Arbitration

It is hoped that a physician educated about his or her legal responsibilities will be better able to avoid the litigation process. Nevertheless, in a less-than-perfect world, and with one in five dermatologists facing medical liability claims, the physician should be familiar with the litigation process.

Warning signs that a suit may ensue are communications from an attorney, threats by the patient, and unanticipated untoward results.[30,44] When the lawsuit is filed, the physician will be formally served with what in legal terminology is called a *complaint*.[30,44] The physician should contact the malpractice insurance carrier immediately, since there is a limited time in which to answer the complaint or face forfeiting the right to litigate.[30,44] The insurance company will then usually appoint an attorney who will assist the physician in answering the complaint. The discovery process begins after the complaint is answered and consists of both sides' investigating the facts of the case. This process consists of attorneys,' for either side, using interrogatories or requests for admissions, requests for production of documents, and depositions.[30,44] Interrogatories or requests for admission are written questions addressed to the opposing side, which the physician is obligated to answer under penalty of perjury.[30,44] Requests for documents may be for medical records and have to be promptly complied with, although the originals do not have to be supplied, and the opposing side can be charged the reasonable expenses of copying the records.[30,44] Depositions are conducted under oath in the presence of a court reporter.[30,44] They consist of question-and-answer sessions conducted in person by an attorney and anyone (physician) who knows about the facts of the case.[30] Depositions are often fishing expeditions where the opposing attorney is looking for possible new legal theories, further clarification of the facts, and assessing the credibility of the deposed. Thus, the physician should always be represented by counsel and though he or she must tell the truth, he or she should be as concise as possible, volunteering little information and not making any hasty conclusionary statements. If the physician is unsure of or unable to recall some facts, he or she should consult with his or her attorney before answering. A hasty answer can undermine the physician's credibility at a later trial. During the entire litigation process, the physician should always check with his or her lawyer before attempting to communicate with the opposing side.

An insurance carrier's defense attorney may recommend that a physician settle a case rather than go through the expense of a trial.[30,44] However, depending on the terms of the policy, it is the physician and not the carrier who has the ultimate say as to whether a settlement or a trial will take place. Yet, the physician, if he or she proceeds to trial despite the advice to settle, risks liability for any damages in excess of what the policy covers. Similarly, if the physician is unhappy with the appointed counsel and the carrier refuses to provide a different attorney, the carrier may be liable for damages in excess of the policy's limits.

An increasingly popular alternative to conventional litigation is *voluntary binding arbitration*.[45] Arbitration is a contractual agreement between the physician and patient that serves as a complete substitute for trial. Usually, the opposing sides will either agree on a neutral arbitrator, or each will choose an arbitrator who in turn selects a neutral arbitrator.[45] There are multiple arbitration formats which are subject to the statutes and state laws of the individual states but usually consist of (1) no pretrial proceedings, (2) hearings by arbitrators chosen from a AAA panel or designees of the parties, (3) no rules of evidence, (4) informal private hearings with the results not published, and (5) review of the decision usually limited to errors of process.[45] The courts generally accept binding arbitration agreements where patient protection exists such as (1) treatment is not used in an emergency situation, (2) the physician's language is understandable, (3) there is a clear waiver of jury trial, and (4) the patient has an escape clause within 30 to 90 days of signing the agreement.[45]

In comparing binding arbitration to conventional litigation, there are compelling differences. Voluntary binding arbitration is efficient, rapid, less costly emotionally and economically (awards are usually one-third the size of jury awards), and the arbitrator's decision may not be published, thus affording privacy for the physician.[45] However, voluntary binding arbitration also lacks awards that can be appealed, and usually favors defendants, and there is the belief that arbitrators always award something.[45] In fact, some feel that binding arbitration may be more conducive to malpractice claims because it is less expensive and faster.[45] However, the experience with health maintenance organizations (HMOs) and other health care providers seems at present to be that arbitration is less expensive and more efficient with little loss of the substance of conventional litigation.[45] The dermatologic surgeon faces a greater risk of medical malpractice claims and might benefit from looking into the feasibility of voluntary binding arbitration for his or her practice.

HUMAN IMMUNODEFICIENCY VIRUS (HIV) INFECTION

It is not uncommon for some dermatologic surgeons to require information of a patient's HIV status before performing any type of surgery or other surgical treatment. However, the legality of this practice is unclear. In California, the California Unruh Civil Rights Act, Civil Code S51, forbids a physician from arbitrarily discriminating against a patient.[46] A physician can probably order the test in order to take steps to prevent HIV transmission but, if he or she uses the test as a basis of denying therapy, this may raise serious legal questions about liability.[46] Furthermore, in ordering the test in California, the physician must take very specific steps to obtain informed consent, meet mandatory reporting requirements, and protect confidentiality.[46] Confidentiality is an especially important issue since it encompasses limited disclosure of the results to third parties, segregating the results so as to prevent inadvertent disclosure and even limiting access of the test results to selected office staff.[46] Thus, before a dermatologic surgeon in California or any other state decides to order an HIV test, he or she should become knowledgeable as to what the law is in his or her state or face the prospect of significant civil or criminal penalties.[46]

REFERENCES

1. Annotation, *What Constitutes Physician-Patient Relationship for Malpractice Purposes,* 17 ALR 4th, 132 (1982).
2. *Thomas v Corso,* 265 Md. 84, 288 A 2d 379 (1972)
3. *Hiser v Randolph,* 617 P.2d 774 (Ariz 1980)
4. *Hamil v Bashline,* 305 A2d 57 (1973)
5. *Betesh v United States,* 400 F Supp. 238 (D.C. 1974)
6. *Oliver v Brock,* 342 So. 2d (Ala. 1976)
7. *Osborne v Frazor,* 425 S.W. 2d 768 (1968)
8. *Lyons v Grether,* 239 S.E. 2d 103 (1977)
9. *Perna v Pirozzi,* 457 A.2d 431 (N.J. 1983)
10. *Millbaugh v Gilmore,* 285 Del. 19 (1972)
11. *Truman v Thomas,* 27 Cal 3d 285 (1980)
12. *Miller v Dore,* 154 Me. 363, 148 A.2d 692 (1959)
13. 61 Am. Jur. 2d *Duty Not To Abandon Case* sec. 236 (1981)
14. *Alexandridis v Jewett,* 388 F.2d 829 (1968)
15. *Guilmet v Campbell,* 188 N.W, 2d 601 (1971)
16. *Stewart v Rudner,* 84 N.W. 2d 816 (1957)
17. *Greenstein v Fornell,* 257 N.Y.S. 673 (1932)
18. Tennenhouse J, Kasher MP: *Risk Prevention Skills,* San Rafael, Tennenhouse Professional Publications, p 69, 1988
19. *Black's Law Dictionary,* St. Paul, West Publishing Co. (Rev. 5th Edition) p 139, 1979
20. Meisel A, Kabnick L: The Exceptions to the Informed Consent Doctrine: Striking A Balance Between Competing Values in Medical Decision Making. *Wisconsin Law Rev* **2:**413, 1979
21. Keeton, PW et al.: *Prosser and Keeton on the Law on Torts,* St Paul, West Publishing Co. (5th Edition) p 113, 1984
22. *King v Carney,* 204 P. 270 (1922)
23. *McGuire v Rix,* 118 Neb. 434, 22 N.W. 120 (1929)
24. Bianco, EA: *Consent to Treatment,* in Legal Medicine: Legal Dynamics of Medical Encounters, Chapter 21 (pp 216–226), edited by American College of Legal Medicine, developmental ed Kathryn H. Falk, St Louis, C.V. Mosby, 2nd Edition, 1991
25. Waltz & Sheuneman, Informed Consent to Therapy, *Nw. UL Rev* Vol. 64, **5:**628, 1970
26. Meisel A, Kabnick L: Informed Consent to Medical Treatment; An Analysis of Recent Legislation. *U Pitt Law Review* **407:**410, 1980
27. *Cobbs v Grant,* 8 Cal 3d. 229, 502 P.2d 1, (1972)
28. *Canterbury v Spence,* 150 U.S. App. D.C. 263, 464 F2d 772 (1972)
29. *Natanson v Kline,* 350 P2d 1093 (1960)
30. Redden EM, Baker BC: *Medicolegal Problems in the Management of Patients with Skin Cancer,* in Cancer of the Skin, Chapter 41 (pp 603–610), Edited by Friedman RJ, et al., Philadelphia, W.B. Saunders, 1991
31. Altman J: One in Five Hit with Malpractice Claims in past Ten Years. *Dermatology Marketing and Practice Management* **2:**2 1988
32. Altman J: The National Association of Insurance Commissioner's (NIAC) Medical Malpractice Closed Claim Study, 1975–1978. *J Am Acad Dermatol* **5:**721, 1981
33. Physicians Insurers Association of America: PIAA Data Sharing Reports: January 1, 1985–December 31, 1987, Lawrenceville, N.J., Copyright Physicians Insurers Association of America, 1988
34. Keeton PW et al.: *Prosser and Keeton on the Law on Torts,* St Paul, West Publishing Co. (5th Edition) p 164, 1984
35. Keeton PW et al.: *Prosser and Keeton on the Law on Torts,* St Paul, West Publishing Co. (5th Edition) p 188, 1984
36. Keeton PW et al.: *Prosser and Keeton on the Law on Torts,* St Paul, West Publishing Co. (5th Edition) p 187, 1984
37. Fiscina FS: *Medical Law for the Attending Physician,* Carbondale, Southern Illinois Press, 1982
38. Sills H: What is the Law? *Dental Clin North Am* **26:**256, 1982
39. Rapp JA, Rapp RT: *Medical Malpractice: A Guide for the Health Sciences,* St Louis, C.V. Mosby Co., 1988
40. Keeton PW et al: *Prosser and Keeton on the Law on Torts,* St Paul, West Publishing Co. (5th Edition) pp 166, 451, 1984
41. Flamm MB: *Medical Malpractice: Physician as Defendant,* in Legal Medicine: Legal Dynamics of Medical Encounters, Chapter 41 (pp 525–534), edited by American College of Legal Medicine, developmental ed Kathryn H. Falk, St Louis, C.V. Mosby, 2nd Edition, 1991

42. Holder AR: The Importance of Medical Records *JAMA* **228:**118–119, 1974

43. Moorman CT et al.: *Medical Records,* in Legal Medicine: Legal Dynamics of Medical Encounters, Chapter 23 (pp 237–253), edited by American College of Legal Medicine, developmental ed Kathryn H. Falk, St Louis, C.V. Mosby, (2nd Edition, 1991)

44. *The Anatomy of a Lawsuit,* New York, Medical Liability Mutual Insurance Company, 1984

45. Ladimer I: *Alternative Dispute Resolution,* in Legal Medicine: Legal Dynamics of Medical Encounters, Chapter 12 (pp 111–128), edited by American College of Legal Medicine, developmental ed Kathryn H. Falk, St Louis, C.V. Mosby, (2nd Edition, 1991)

46. Crooks PL, Tocker MW: *AIDS/HIV,* California Physicians Legal Handbook, San Francisco, California Medical Association, 1991

III Procedures and Technical Aspects

David A. Kriegel
Daniel M. Siegel

13 Electrosurgery

Electrosurgery is an integral tool in the treatment of skin disease. It involves the transmission of electric energy to destroy benign and malignant growths, to control bleeding, and to cut tissue. The majority of electrosurgery is high-frequency electrosurgery which employs the use of generators which can convert alternating current into high-frequency oscillating fields.[1] In this chapter, the authors will also discuss the clinical significance of galvanic surgery which uses devices that convert alternating current to direct current in order to produce heat for tissue destruction.

GALVANIC SURGERY

The electric current used in galvanic surgery is a low-voltage, low-amperage, direct electric current in which electrons flow unidirectionally from the negative electrode to the positive electrode. The circuitry consists of a loop which includes a current source, a positive electrode (dispersive electrode), a negative electrode (treatment electrode), and the patient. The source of the current may be a low-voltage battery or any instrument that can convert alternating current to a low-voltage direct current. The negative electrode is in contact with the area to be treated and the positive electrode is held by the patient away from the treatment site.

Mechanism of Action of Galvanic Surgery

Galvanic surgery involves a series of chemical interactions, including ionization, acid formation, metallic ion release, and liquefaction of the target tissue at the tissue site.[2] More specifically, the negative electrode is applied to the target tissue where electrons are released. The electrons interact with the tissue to produce sodium hydroxide and hydrogen gas which cause liquefaction of the tissue.[3] At the same time, acids are produced at the positive electrode which causes protein coagulation and deposition on the electrode. This electrode is usually held by or attached to the patient to complete the circuit loop.

Clinical Applications of Galvanic Surgery

The primary clinical applications of galvanic surgery include electrolysis and iontophoresis. The most common application is that of electrolysis. This process involves inserting the negative electrode (treatment electrode) into the hair follicle while the patient holds the larger positive electrode. With a gradual increase in current through the circuit, electrons are slowly released and cause hydroxides to be released which liquefy the hair follicle protein.[4]

Iontophoresis, which is used to treat hyperhidrosis, also involves a galvanic current. This process involves twice-a-day application of water-soaked pads to the areas of hyperhidrosis. The current flows through these pads and causes protein liquefaction within the eccrine glands.

ELECTROCAUTERY

Electrocautery utilizes a heating filament tip which transfers heat to the target tissue to produce thermal destruction. There is no electric current transfer to the target tissue. When the current is passed through the needle, heat is produced by the resistance to the current flow, analogous to the heating of a filament in a light bulb. The electric current is direct or alternating and has a low voltage and high amperage.[5] Unlike galvanic surgery, the patient is not part of the circuit loop in electrocautery. The electrocautery circuit consists of a treatment filament tip connected to a current source consisting of a step-down 110 V alternating current transformer or a battery.[2]

TABLE 13-1

Characteristics of High-Frequency Electrosurgery

	Electrodesiccation/ electrofulguration	Electrocoagulation	Electrosection
Wave:	Highly damped	Moderately damped	Undamped
Type of current:	Current is alternating consisting of high frequency, high voltage, and low amplitude.	Current is alternating consisting of high frequency, low voltage, and high amplitude.	Current is alternating consisting of high frequency, low voltage, and high amplitude.
Clinical result:	Pure coagulation	Combination of cutting and coagulation	Pure cutting
Tissue effect:	Superficial destruction	Deep extensive destruction	Localized destruction

Mechanism of Action of Electrocautery

The mechanism of action involves heat transfer from the filament to the target tissue causing protein denaturation and tissue coagulation. The thermal tissue damage which is induced in this reaction will often cause significant heat damage to the adjacent tissue. The intensity of tissue coagulation may tend to retard wound healing.

Clinical Applications of Electrocautery

Despite the negative consequences of electrocautery, it has a very definite role in electrosurgery. It is an extremely safe modality since the patient is not included in the electric current circuit. Therefore, when a patient is a high-risk candidate for receiving electrosurgery (i.e., cardiac pacemaker patients), or the region of the body being operated on is an area of high electrosurgical risk (i.e., surgery in the region of the eye), electrocautery is the option of choice. In addition, electrocautery works well in areas of nonconductive material such as bone, cartilage, and nails.[3] Since the technique is purely one of heat transfer and thermal destruction, and does not require tissue conduction of the current, these materials are not a hindrance to this form of electrosurgery. Finally, when most electrosurgical techniques are used in bloody fields, there is a dissipation of the energy over a large surface area which limits the efficacy of the desired hemostasis. However, electrocautery does not include the field in its circuit and therefore can be used in such conditions with reasonable efficacy.

The technique used for electrocautery is relatively simple. The heated treatment electrode is applied to the target tissue. The setting used is dependent on the cautery unit as well as on the desired result. If the electrode is not heated sufficiently, the charred tissue will adhere to the metal surface making further treatment ineffective. However, an electrode which is too hot will create increased tissue damage and slower healing.

The Shaw scalpel consists of a scalpel blade with a copper wire which acts as a heating element on the side of the blade. The mechanism of action is as follows: The scalpel edge cuts the tissue and the heated sides cauterize the blood vessels, al-

lowing for immediate hemostasis. This instrument is useful when the surgeon is operating in very vascular areas such as the scalp and the nose. The main advantage of this unit is the immediate hemostasis obtained which allows for a drier surgical field and better visibility for precise cutting. Also, as in all electrocautery, the patient is not part of any electric current, which allows one to use this device in higher-risk electrosurgery patients. The disadvantages of this instrument are those of increased heat-induced tissue coagulation and damage from the cautery as well as increased wound healing time, along with the added cost of the specialized blade electrodes.

PHYSICS OF HIGH-FREQUENCY ELECTROSURGERY

High-frequency electrosurgery uses an alternating current from a standard outlet and boosts the voltage and frequency levels while decreasing the amperage. This type of electrosurgery acts by generating an oscillating radio wave which may be either damped or undamped sine waves.[3,5,6] This oscillating current produces molecular movement which causes friction and subsequent heat production. Heat is also generated through electric fields in the tissue itself. It is this heat production which causes the desired effect of coagulation and dehydration.

A damped sine wave can be generated by means of a high-frequency generator, a charged capacitor, and the use of a spark gap. When the capacitor is charged, the charge jumps the spark gap. The current is caused to oscillate through the circuit causing the sine wave. (Table 13-2) The damped com-

TABLE 13-2

Waveforms

Highly damped	
Moderately damped	
Undamped	

ponent of the sine wave is caused by the diminishing oscillations over time, providing hemostasis without providing a good cutting current.[3,5,6]

An undamped sine wave consists of a continuous oscillation of current without peaks and troughs. This continuous oscillation is produced by a vacuum tube or, more commonly, by a transistor. This type of undamped sine wave, in its strictest sense, is more commonly associated with a cutting current that provides no hemostasis. An effective electrosurgical cutting current requires some hemostasis, and thus it is a combination of a damped and undamped current that will provide the best cutting current.[2]

The spark gap width has a direct effect on the current. With a widened spark gap, a greater current is required in order to jump the increased air space. A higher voltage will therefore be necessary to produce this increased current. The frequency of sparks will decrease as a result of this higher voltage. The initial wave of the current will have a greater amplitude which will cause more of a dampening effect and thus will increase hemostasis. If the spark gap is narrowed, the current necessary to jump this decreased air space will be less and will require a decreased voltage. This decrease in voltage will allow for an increase in frequency of the sparks with a decreased amplitude producing less dampening of the wave.[6]

High-frequency electrosurgery involves current transfer by the use of either a monoterminal or a biterminal modality. A *monoterminal* modality implies the use of a single treatment electrode, while a *biterminal* modality implies the use of two treatment electrodes. Monoterminal high-frequency electrosurgery can be used with or without the use of a dispersive electrode. Although this dispersive electrode is a second electrode in the circuit, it is still considered to be a monoterminal circuit since there is only one treatment electrode. The terms *bipolar* and *monopolar* electrosurgery are often used interchangeably with monoterminal and biterminal electrosurgery. However, purists will argue that monopolarity and bipolarity are not appropriate terms when discussing alternating current since there are no poles with this type of current.[7]

TECHNIQUES OF HIGH-FREQUENCY ELECTROSURGERY

The various high-frequency electrosurgical techniques include: electrofulguration, electrodesiccation, electrocoagulation, and electrosection. Each technique is defined by a specific waveform and a specific mechanism of action.

Electrofulguration involves a damped sine wave whereby a spark is generated through the air from the electrode to the tissue. There is no contact between the electrode and the tissue. This method uses high voltage, low amperage, and high-frequency energy. The advantages of this method include rapid tissue healing secondary to minimal deep tissue damage as there is less heat penetrance with this modality.

Electrodesiccation is similar to electrofulguration with the only difference being that the electrode comes in contact with the tissue. Desiccation occurs by transfer of heat to the tissue. Since there is contact between the electrode and the tissue, the tissue damage is greater than that seen in electrofulguration. The extent of tissue damage has a direct relationship with the time that the electrode is in contact with the tissue.

Electrocoagulation involves a moderately damped waveform. Its function is to provide tissue coagulation through the generation of heat in the tissue. The mechanism of action of this technique involves incorporating the patient into the circuit, which allows one to use a lower voltage and higher amperage and thereby generate a greater degree of coagulation. A dispersive electrode is used for this modality. Although electrofulguration and electrodesiccation will also coagulate blood vessels, the hemostatic effect is greater with electrocoagulation since the patient is incorporated into the circuit. This method is most commonly used for coagulating bleeding in a surgical site.

Electrosection is the cutting current discussed previously. This current is either a pure sine wave or a modulated sine wave, which is a blend of a cutting current and a coagulating current. The pure sine wave allows for ease in tissue cutting without the benefit of hemostasis, and the modulated sine wave induces an increase in tissue resistance when cutting but allows for some hemostasis.

DANGERS WITH HIGH-FREQUENCY ELECTROSURGERY

Although high-frequency electrosurgery is very safe, there are some dangers which should be elucidated. The risks of electrosurgery are uncommon; they include burns and ignition, electrocution, and cardiac pacemaker interference.

Burns and Ignition

Burns can occur from the treatment electrode, from the dispersive electrode, or from an "accidental" electrode. The treatment electrode burn can occur mostly through carelessness. If the treatment electrode is inadvertently activated by a pedal or handpiece while it is in contact with the patient, it will cause a burn. The dispersive electrode burn occurs as a result of inappropriate attachment of the electrode. When this electrode is only partially attached to the skin, the current is not dispersed over a wide area but rather concentrated only in the area of the electrode that is in contact with the skin. This can cause a large amount of current to be concentrated over a small area, causing a burn in this area. The accidental electrode is a conducting surface which is accidentally in contact with the patient while the designated dispersive electrode is either not connected or connected incorrectly. This conducting surface acts as a ground, localizing the flow of electric energy, thereby causing a burn.[8]

Ignition is a significant hazard of electrosurgery. The use

of flammable chemicals such as alcohol and skin disinfectant tinctures which contain alcohol, can ignite with the spark of an electrosurgical instrument. Also, the use of electrosurgery around some anesthetic agents and oxygen, or in the perianal area during expulsion of colonic gas, may cause combustion and significant burns.[9]

Finally, burns can be caused by a process called *channeling,* whereby current is concentrated in a very small area away from the intended treatment zone. When channeling occurs, the current travels through tissue that is more conductive than the intended treatment area and the heat produced may cause burns.[10]

Electrocution

Electrocution can occur in situations where there are faulty electric connections and a high voltage is being used to produce a high-amperage current. When this current is directed through the patient rather than through the typical grounded pathway, electrocution can result. Although this is a very uncommon consequence of electrosurgery, the operator must be sure that the patient is not connected to an unearthed ground. If the patient is accidentally connected to an unearthed ground, the patient could serve as an electric pathway for current in the event of machinery malfunction.[10]

Pacemakers

In rare circumstances, pacemakers have been reported to be affected by electrosurgery. This interaction is less common today as pacemakers are being produced with insulated protective material. The reported adverse effects involve electrosurgical current affecting the pacemaker's sensing device, causing premature firing or inhibition of firing.[11,12]

The electric interference is greater with the use of demand pacemakers compared with fixed-rate pacemakers. This is because a demand pacemaker has a sensing device which has potential to pick up erroneous impulses for electrosurgical devices. A demand pacemaker can be converted to a fixed-rate pacemaker by the use of a magnet. This may be a reasonable option for very unstable cardiac patients who require the use of electrosurgical devices.[11,12]

Other precautionary measures can be employed to improve the safety profile in patients with pacemakers. The use of electrocautery in place of high-frequency electrosurgery is recommended. Electrocautery does not transmit current to the patient and is therefore safe in pacemaker patients. Biterminal electrosurgery allows for the flow of electricity to occur between terminals without involving the pacemaker. The use of a dispersive electrode will decrease the chances of adverse effects of electrosurgical current on a pacemaker. The dispersive electrode should be placed close to the treatment electrode but in a different direction from the heart and pacemaker. Short bursts of electricity will diminish the chances of adverse effects on the sensing device of the pacemaker.

Avoidance of high-frequency electrosurgery on skin which overlies the pacemaker will decrease the chance of current flow to the pacemaker. Cardiac monitoring will increase the safety profile. When the surgeon is operating in the office, following the pulse rate and rhythm is adequate monitoring for detection of pacemaker malfunction.[11,12] Finally, pacemaker patients are equipped with a magnet in order to set the rate of the unit. If one places the magnet over the pacemaker, this will allow the unit to function at an automatic rate of 70 and will prevent electrosurgical interaction with the pacemaker.

CLINICAL APPLICATIONS

Electrosurgery has many clinical applications. It can be used on its own as an electric scalpel to excise benign and malignant lesions, as well as for cosmetic reconstruction, or as a destructive tool to eradicate benign and malignant lesions. This method has the advantages of immediate hemostasis, efficiency, and low cost.

Electrosurgery is more commonly used in conjunction with another surgical modality such as a scalpel or curette. It provides hemostasis for elliptic and shave excisions and tissue destruction for treatment of malignancies.

Electrosurgery for Removal of Benign Lesions

Electrosurgery can be used to remove benign lesions. The surgeon can do this with the electrode alone or in conjunction with another instrument such as a curette or scalpel.

Electrosurgery is best used on its own when the surgeon is removing pedunculated lesions such as skin tags or pedunculated verrucae as well as for treatment of facial telangiectasias. To remove pedunculated lesions, one should grasp the lesion at the distal end and gently stretch the stalk. The current is set on low and is then applied to the base of the lesion in a circumferential fashion. The lesion is left alone until it falls off a few days later. Sometimes a second treatment is required at a higher setting if the lesion does not fall off. This is not acceptable treatment if malignancy is suspected (Fig. 13-1).[2]

To treat telangiectasias, spider nevi, and senile angiomas requires minimal intervention and often results in good clearance of these benign vessels. One should use the smallest treatment electrode available to start and increase the size for larger vessels. A monoterminal electrode set at the lowest current setting is usually sufficient for treatment of these vessels. The technique involves flattening the area to be treated with two fingers and inserting the treatment needle into the vessel. Current should be applied at this time which should obliterate the vessel. Angiomas should be treated with a more superficial approach without actually entering the vessel. Rarely, one may need to increase the current settings or even add a dis-

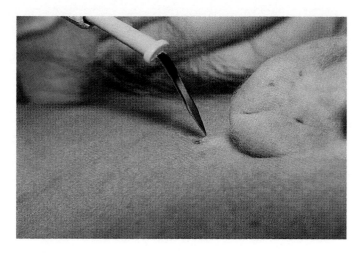

Figure 13-1 Electrosurgical removal of a pedunculated lesion below left ear.

persive electrode for more effective electrocoagulation. In these situations, one must be very cautious and be aware of the increased risk of scarring with increased current application.[13]

Once the electrode and current settings are chosen, the obliteration procedure may begin. The treatment electrode is lightly applied to the vessel and the current is activated. The electrode is then carefully moved along the pathway of the vessel. A gray charring is sometimes produced which can be curetted away to see the effect of the chosen current. For very apprehensive patients, it is prudent to treat a test site, preferably not in a noticeable part of the face.[13]

Electrosurgery and curettage are an excellent combination therapy for many benign lesions such as seborrheic keratoses, verrucae vulgaris, flat warts, condyloma acuminata, dermatosis papulosis nigra, molluscum contagiosum, and lentigines. These lesions can be successfully eradicated with light electrodesiccation of the surface of the lesion followed by curettage with a curette or even a firm wiping with a cotton gauze. An alternative way of treating seborrheic keratoses is to first curette this very easily detachable lesion and then lightly electrodesiccate the base for hemostasis and further destruction of any remaining lesion.

Electrodesiccation is an excellent modality to be used in conjunction with a scalpel or razor blade. When removing raised melanocytic nevi, one can obtain an excellent cosmetic result using the following technique: After anesthetizing the region, the nevus is shaved flush with the skin by using a scalpel or razor blade. There is often a lip of residual tissue after this shaving technique is implemented as there is a natural tendency to lift up with the blade as the shave is being completed. This residual tissue can be gently destroyed with the use of light electrodesiccation. Alternatively, a blade can then be used obliquely as a dermabrader to smooth out the surface of the wound (Fig. 13-2, *a-d*).

Vascular lesions such as hemangiomas, pyogenic granulomas, and venous lakes can also be treated with a shave/electrodesiccation technique. As with nevi, the hemangioma is shaved flush with the skin. Residual destruction of blood vessels and hemostasis may then be accomplished with electrosurgery. Unfortunately, there may be a tendency for atrophic scarring with this technique as aggressive electrosurgery is recommended to achieve destruction of the residual vascular bed and prevent recurrence.

Another benign hyperplasia which responds very well to electrosurgery is rhinophyma. This condition is due to sebaceous gland hyperplasia. Given the significant vascularity of this area, a cutting-current electrosurgical technique is far superior to cold steel excision of this tissue.[14]

To perform a rhinophymectomy on the entire nose, one needs to anesthetize the region through a field block. The electrosurgical unit is set on cutting current and a wire loop electrode or a Shaw scalpel is often used as the treatment electrode. As previously mentioned, the Shaw scalpel consists of a heated scalpel blade that cuts and cauterizes at the same time. More specifically, the blade acts as the cutting instrument, while the heat of the blade allows for thermal cautery. The scalpel can be adjusted to various temperatures as needed for the specific clinical scenario (i.e., the vascularity of the tissue).[14,15,16]

The sebaceous tissue is excised in layers with a gentle fluid motion by using the chosen cutting electrode. The nose is sculpted to the desired shape using this technique. When a final desirable shape is obtained, the resultant wound should be allowed to heal for 4 to 6 weeks. After this period of time, an evaluation for final contour touch-ups can be made. If further refinements are deemed necessary, they can often best be obtained with the use of dermabrasion.[14–16]

Electrosurgery for Hemostasis

Electrosurgery can provide hemostasis in an operative field through two methods. The simplest approach is direct contact of the treatment electrode with the bleeding points providing direct heat to the bleeding area. This can be performed with either a single treatment electrode or the combination of a treatment and dispersive electrode (Fig. 13-3).

A more effective approach involves the use of a metal instrument such as a hemostat or forceps. The instrument grasps the bleeding vessels by its two prongs. The active electrode is applied to the metal instrument, and heat is conducted through the metal to the bleeding site providing electrocoagulation (Fig. 13-4). This technique can only be implemented with the use of both a treatment and dispersive electrode since a single treatment electrode does not provide sufficient current. In addition, "bipolar" forceps are an effective tool to achieve hemostasis. These consist of forceps connected to a power source which provides current to the tips. The current flows from one tip of the forceps to the other, and, at variable times, each tip acts as both the active and dispersive electrode. The

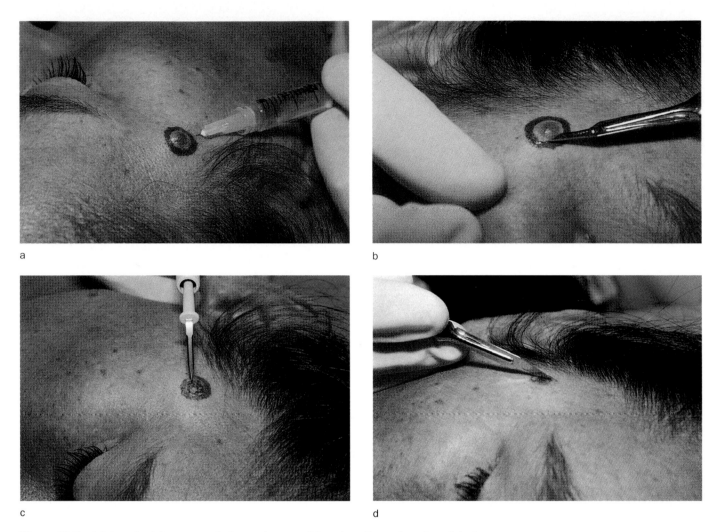

a

b

c

d

Figure 13-2   (*a*) Anesthetizing a nevus before a shave excision also allows plumping of the lesion and facilitates removal; (*b*) shaving nevus flush with the skin; (*c*) gentle electrodesiccation to destroy residual tissue; (*d*) a no. 11 blade is used to smooth out surface of skin.

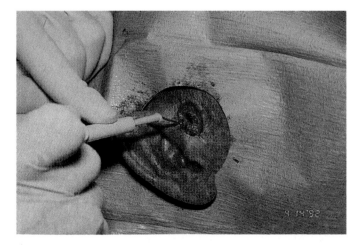

Figure 13-3   Treatment electrode is applied to individual bleeding points.

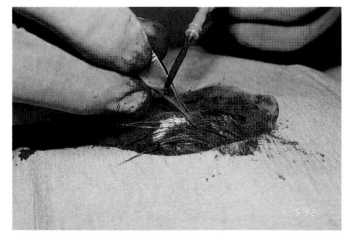

Figure 13-4   The use of forceps to facilitate current conduction and provide hemostasis.

tissue damage is restricted to the small area of tissue between the two tips.[17]

Electrosurgery for Removal of Malignant Lesions

The three most common dermatologic malignancies are basal cell carcinomas, squamous cell carcinomas, and malignant melanomas. Electrosurgery with curettage is appropriate treatment for some basal cell carcinomas and squamous cell carcinomas but should not be used for malignant melanomas. Those basal cell carcinomas appropriate for treatment by curettage and electrosurgery will usually have a cure rate in the 90 percent range. The cosmetic results after curettage and electrosurgery are most often quite acceptable.[18]

Tumors which are acceptable for treatment by curettage and electrodesiccation are determined based on size, location, and histologic subtype. In order to obtain a high cure rate, the tumor should be a primary lesion less than 2 cm in diameter. The location of the tumor is a significant factor for recurrence rates. Tumors on the trunk and extremities have high treatment success rates when treated with curettage and electrosurgery. Some areas on the face are appropriate for this method of treatment as well. Areas on the face which are embryonic fusion planes are not appropriate for curettage and electrodesiccation. These areas include the midnose, ala nasi, medial canthi, periauricular area, and nasal labial folds. In addition, squamous cell carcinomas of the lip and helix of the ear have a higher rate of metastases and should not be treated with curettage and electrodesiccation. Excision with histologic control is the treatment of choice for squamous cell carcinomas in these locations. Squamous cell carcinomas arising in scars or ulcers are also a more aggressive subtype and should not be treated with curettage and electrosurgery.[18,19]

Finally, some histologic subtypes of basal cell carcinomas and squamous cell carcinomas should not be treated with curettage and electrosurgery. Specifically, basal cell carcinomas of the morpheaform variety or those with an aggressive pattern, as well as poorly differentiated aggressive-appearing squamous cell carcinomas, are best treated with excision with histologic guidance.

The technique for curettage and electrodesiccation is easily learned but is most successfully performed by an experienced clinician. The malignancy to be treated should be anesthetized with local anesthesia. The lesion should then be firmly curetted in multiple directions with a firm scraping movement until all of the soft tissue is removed. The remaining base is then treated with electrocautery at a power just above that which would be used for hemostasis. The peripheral rim of normal tissue should also be treated with electrocautery. This curettage and electrodesiccation procedure should be repeated twice more in order to achieve a high cure rate. There are many acceptable individual variations to the approach that also have merit.

Electrosurgery is an important treatment modality in cutaneous surgery. The process of transforming electrical energy into heat thereby inducing cell injury, allows for hemostasis, tissue destruction and tissue cutting.[20,21,22] In order to obtain the desired effect from electrosurgery, an understanding of the physics as well as the technical principles of treatment are recommended. As the physician becomes more experienced and comfortable with electrosurgical techniques, he will be able to apply his expertise to a countless number of clinical situations.

REFERENCES

1. Bodian EL: Electrosurgery by bipolar modalities. *J Dermatol Surg Oncol* **4**(3):235, 1978

2. Blankenship ML: Physical modalities, electrosurgery, electrocautery and electrolysis. *Int J Dermatol* **18**:443, 1979

3. Sebben JE: *Cutaneous Electrosurgery*. Chicago, Year Book, 1989

4. Wagner RF et al: Electrolysis and thermolysis for permanent hair removal. *J Am Acad Dermatol* **12**:441, 1985

5. Boughton RS, Spencer SK: Electrosurgical fundamentals. *J Am Acad Dermatol* **16**:862, 1987

6. Sebben JE: Electrosurgery: High frequency modalities. *J Dermatol Surg Oncol* **14**:367, 1988

7. Sebben JE: Electrodes for high frequency electrosurgery. *J Dermatol Surg Oncol* **15**(8):805, 1989

8. Battig CG: Electrosurgical burn injuries and their prevention. *JAMA* **204**:91, 1968

9. Rugins H et al: The explosive potential of colonic gas during colonoscopic electrosurgical polypectomy. *Surg Gynecol Obstet* **138**:554, 1974

10. Sebben JE: The hazards of electrosurgery. *J Am Acad Dermatol* **16**:869, 1987

11. Sebben JE: Electrosurgery and cardiac pacemakers. *J Am Acad Dermatol* **9**:457–463, 1983

12. Krull EA et al: Effects of electrosurgery on cardiac pacemakers. *J Dermatol Surg Oncol* **1**(43):45, 1975

13. Robinson JK: Electrodesiccation of nevi aranei ("spiders") and senile angiomas. *J Dermatol Surg Oncol* **6**(10):794, 1980

14. Clark DP, Hanke CW: Electrosurgical treatment of rhinophyma. *J Am Acad Dermatol* **22**:831, 1990

15. Verde SF et al: How we treat rhinophyma. *J Dermatol Surg Oncol* **6**(7):560, 1980

16. Greenbaum SS et al: Comparison of CO_2 laser and electrosurgery in the treatment of rhinophyma. *J Am Acad Dermatol* **18**:363, 1988

17. Bennet RE: *Fundamentals of Cutaneous Surgery*. St. Louis, Mosby, 1988

18. Kopf AW et al: Curettage/electrodesiccation treatment of basal cell carcinomas. *Arch Dermatol* **113**:439, 1977

19. Whelan CS: Electrocoagulation and curettage for carcinoma involving the skin of the face, nose, eyelids and ears. *Cancer* **31**:159, 1973

20. Sebben JE: Electrosurgery principles: Cutting current and cutaneous surgery, pt 1. *J Dermatol Surg Oncol* **14**(1):29, 1988

21. Popkin GI: Electrosurgery, in *Skin Surgery,* edited by E Epstein. Springfield, Ill, Charles C Thomas, 1987 p 164–183

22. Wheeland, RG: *Cutaneous Surgery.* WB Saunders and Company, 1994.

Rodney P. R. Dawber

14 Cryosurgery

There is undoubtedly more information and experience regarding the effects of cold on the skin than any other organ—both from observation in cold climates and environments and from its many uses in cryosurgical practice in humans and in other animals.[1-3] Since the skin has long been known to heal well after cold injury, a vast array of conditions have been treated by cryosurgery—often amounting to overuse and misuse.[4] The comprehensive lists in Tables 14-1 and 14-2 reflect those conditions for which good results have been recorded, though this is not to imply that cryosurgery is the treatment of choice for all these entities. Cutaneous cryosurgery has come more into the fore during the last 15 years, partly because of improved cryobiological background knowledge but more because in the pragmatic arena of everyday dermatology, with the ready availability of liquid nitrogen, it has become cheap, quick, easy to perform, and can usually be carried out without surgical theater facilities and even in the patient's home under certain circumstances.[5]

MECHANISM OF DAMAGE DUE TO COLD INJURY[6]

Cryosurgery can be loosely defined as the deliberate destruction of diseased tissue by freezing in a controlled manner—the controversy regarding whether *cryotherapy* would be a more representative term can safely be left to the "semantologists." Many well-recognized events follow the rapid lowering of temperature in biologic systems.

Factors Causing Cellular Injury

Extracellular Ice

When cryosurgery was first introduced, it was thought that the main cause of cell death was the formation of ice in the tissues and the mechanical damage produced as the ice crystals formed. Observation has demonstrated that if cells are frozen in vitro, extracellular ice forms first, which gradually squeezes the cells together. It has been difficult to demonstrate actual disruption of membranes by this means; however, volume changes in the extra- and intracellular compartments have been measured during freezing and thawing and the conclusion drawn that disruption of cell membranes must occur. It appears that extracellular ice formation alone is not sufficient to kill cells. The temperature changes during cryosurgery are so rapid that intracellular ice formation is inevitable as well, this being physically very destructive.

Hypertonic Damage

When extracellular ice is formed in association with cell suspension in vitro, the amount of extracellular water decreases, causing an increase in concentration of solutes in the remaining fluid. Changing osmotic gradients between cells and extracellular fluids are therefore produced, which lead to passage of electrolytes out of the cells, causing a decrease in cell volume and a disruption of cell membranes. It has been shown that when a certain concentration is reached, normally intracellular components, for example, hemoglobin in red blood cells, pass out of the cell, causing irreversible damage. Rapid electrolyte transfer has also been incriminated as the cause of damage to cell proteins and enzyme systems, and it is generally accepted that the temperature gradients produced during cryosurgery cause damage by this means, especially during the reverse process of thawing.

Sensitization

In experiments using red blood cells, it has been shown that gross cell damage is produced even if hypertonic conditions necessary for disruption are not achieved. It has therefore been postulated that this sensitization damage is the result of disruption of phospholipids in cell membranes, but this has

TABLE 14-1

Some Skin Conditions Treatable by Cryosurgery[3,22,34]

Acne vulgaris[35,36]

Acrochordon[2]

Adenoma sebaceum[34]

Angiofibroma[38,39]

Angiokeratoma

Angiomas[37]

Basal cell carcinoma[10,16,20,27,60] (see Figs. 14-2a–b—14-4a–b)

Bowen's disease (skin and mucosal surfaces)[3,18,21] (see Figs. 14-1a–b and 14-5a–b)

Carbuncle

Chloasma (melasma)

Chondrodermatitis nodularis helicis[2]

Clear cell acanthoma

Cryoanesthesia[26,42,43]

Cutaneous horn (see Fig. 14-2a–b)

Cylindroma

Dermatofibroma[44]

Digital myxoid cyst[45]

Eccrine poroma

Elastosis perforans serpiginosa

Eosinophilic granuloma

Granuloma annulare

Granuloma (mycobacterial)

Hidradenitis suppurativa

Hidradenoma

Histiocytoma[44]

Hyperhidrosis

Ingrowing toenail[32]

Keloid[1,3]

Keratoacanthoma[3,21]

Keratoses[46]

    Actinic

    Arsenical

    Seborrheic (see Figs. 14-6a–b)

Leiomyoma

Leishmaniasis[7,47]

Lentigo maligna[20]

Lentigo maligna melanoma[3,23] (see Figs. 14-7a–b)

Lentigo simplex

Lichen simplex

Lupus erythematosus

Lupus vulgaris

Mastocytoma

Molluscum contagiosum

Mucocele

Neurofibroma

Nevoid basal cell epithelioma (Gorlin's syndrome)

Nevus

    Epidermal

    Sebaceous

Palliation[27]

Porokeratosis

Prurigo nodularis granuloma[48]

Pruritus ani[49]

Pseudopyogenic granuloma[50]

Pyogenic granuloma (see Figs. 14-8a–b)

Rhinophyma[51]

Sarcoid

Sebaceous hyperplasia[52]

Squamous cell carcinoma[3,13] (see Figs. 14-9a–b)

Steatocystoma multiplex

Syringoma

Tattoos[53]

Trichoepithelioma

Warts (viral)[54–59]

Xanthelasma

---

not been confirmed by other workers. It may be that events taking place during thawing, for example reversed osmotic gradients, may give rise to this form of damage.

Intracellular Ice

Extracellular ice formation and sensitization damage can only occur when freezing is slow (i.e., when differential freezing in different parts of a system is allowed to occur). When very rapid freezing takes place, intracellular ice formation occurs, and it is widely believed that this gives rise to cellular death even though cells assume a remarkably normal appearance immediately after thawing. Damage to cell organelles such as

mitochondria and endoplasmic reticulum has been postulated to be the cause of injury by intracellular ice. The size of the ice crystals is probably important; the larger the crystals, the greater the damage. Most of the evidence supports the general principle that intracellular ice is lethal. It is probably that recrystallization of ice during the slow thaw time after cryosurgery is responsible for tissue destruction, this process being as important as the initial freeze in causing cell death.

Circulatory Changes

Many authorities feel that as important as the initial freeze-thaw events in causing cell and tissue death are: (1) the circu-

TABLE 14-2

Statistics for Treatment of Some Benign Lesions

Viral warts (hand)	Bunney et al[54]	75% cure if treated at either 2- or 3-week intervals
Tattoos	Colver, Dawber[53]	54% clear after one treatment (see Figure 14-4a–b)
Myxoid cysts	Dawber et al[45]	86% cure rate
Rhinophyma	Sonnex, Dawber[51]	Five patients, all with good improvement
Dermatofibroma	Lanigan, Robinson[44]	90% good or excellent results (of 35)
Actinic keratosis	Lubritz, Smolewski[46]	99% cure rate (of 1018)
Ingrowing toenail	Sonnex, Dawber[32]	54% cure; increased to 64% after treatment
Seborrheic warts		Despite widespread use of cryotherapy, little data available; except for grossly hyperkeratotic or thick lesions, cryotherapy nearly always successful

latory (capillary and lymphatic) malfunction associated with the early endothelial damage and edema and (2) the capillary and venous occlusion seen several days after treatment, leading to anoxia, further cell death, and tissue necrosis.

Immunologic Events

Cryosurgery has been shown to excite immunologic reaction against tumor cells. Lymphocytes and serum from tumor-bearing animals receiving a single cryosurgical dose have demonstrated greater cytotoxicity to an identical tumor in a syngeneic animal than lymphocytes and serum from an untreated animal. This response has been shown to be tissue specific and stimulated by the release of tumor-specific antigen either during or after freezing. Other workers have observed the effects of an immune reaction after cryosurgery of tissues such as the prostate. Whether such events are important in human cutaneous cryosurgery remains to be proven.

EQUIPMENT AND METHODS

The most common equipment in use for routine clinical practice is designed to utilize liquid nitrogen as a refrigerant since it is almost universally available. It is essential for the treatment of premalignant and malignant skin lesions, giving the most consistent "cell killing."

The simplest technique is the dipstick method. This long-used method employs either a cotton-wool swab or copper disk with insulated handles.

The swab or disk is dipped into a robust metal Dewar flask containing liquid nitrogen and then applied to the area to be treated. The time of application depends on the size and nature of the lesions to be treated; to maintain relatively long tissue freezing, repeat dipping and reapplication may be necessary. It is very difficult to standardize this technique in view of the many variables—ambient temperature, the pressure applied, distance the dip instrument travels from the Dewar flask to the lesion, and "dripping" of liquid nitrogen. This

technique is considered to be only suitable for small benign superficial conditions, which include very many conditions listed in Table 14-1. "Artistry" and experience are essential if consistently good cure rates are to be achieved with this method that has been used successfully by dermatologists for many decades. If premalignant and malignant integumentary lesions are to be treated, then modern standardized equipment is required.[3,8]

For routine outpatient cryosurgery, most dermatologists prefer a small hand-held spray unit or a compact tabletop unit, capable of either spray or cryoprobe application; the former are by far the most commonly used in clinical practice. For details of the various commercially produced units available, the reader is referred to more detailed text.[3] Most units allow for variation in the width of the spray and have probe attachments of different sizes to equate with the size of the area to be treated. The probes are generally cylindric, preferably with flat contact surfaces; they are particularly useful when pressure is needed, for example, with vascular lesions and for areas where open spray is a problem (around the eye, the mouth, and the vagina). Also, very small lesions can be treated with pointed probes since spray techniques give too wide of an icefield and therefore greater morbidity. Instruments utilizing carbon dioxide snow or nitrous oxide cooling (Joule-Thomson effect) for dermatologic lesions will not be considered in this chapter. These techniques are described in detail elsewhere.[3]

Various items of auxiliary equipment are important if the full range of cryosurgical techniques is to be employed:

1. Truncated nonconducting cones are frequently employed (Fig. 14-1) to limit surface application of the spray.[2,9] For small lesions, if carefully localized spray is required, auriscope cones can be used. This method gives a very rapid rate of temperature decrease which is probably more destructive than the open spray technique.[10] Some recently introduced machines have an attachable closed cone that sprays liquid nitrogen (N_2) into the cone, which is pressed onto the skin.

2. To protect the orbit of the eye when eyelid tumors are to be treated, a plastic eyelid retractor is essential; if one is not available, a plastic spoon without coarse edges may suffice.
3. Monitoring devices are necessary.[3] If only benign and relatively flat and small premalignant and malignant lesions are to be treated, and liquid N_2 is the refrigerant, then monitoring equipment is unnecessary since no physical instrument can measure adequate cell death. The treatment of deep or large tumors requires careful depth-dose monitoring equipment. This equipment most commonly is a pyrometer-thermocouple combination; some methods employ electric impedance or tissue resistance-measuring devices which in principle have the advantage of measuring actual freezing; only thin, inexpensive electrodes are needed, and many areas of the tumor can be monitored with a single probe.

In an attempt to standardize the treatment used for different lesions at varying sites, and so that surgeons can further their knowledge of the relative sensitivity or resistance of different lesions to cryosurgery, the author has adopted a spot-freeze technique; this enables medical personnel of varying degrees of experience to obtain the same results.[11]

The spot freeze technique involves first defining the size of the field to be treated (as with radiotherapy) and then inducing ice formation within that field by liquid N_2 spray. Large lesions are divided into overlapping circles of 2-cm diameter by using a skin marker. The liquid N_2 spray (e.g., S spray of CryAC Units, Brymill Corp., USA) is held approximately 1 cm from the skin surface in the center of a 2-cm circle and spraying commences; the white "iceline" is allowed to extend outward until it fills the circle. This ice field is then "held" for a measured time by continuing the spray with a sufficient jet pressure to maintain the iceline. The measured time will depend entirely on the nature of the lesion; once the time is completed, spraying is stopped and thawing commences. Each 2-cm circle is treated similarly.

A single freeze and thaw is termed a *freeze-thaw cycle* (FTC). Malignant lesions usually receive two, sometimes three, FTCs, the intervening thaw time being at least three times the duration of the initial freeze. Evidently, treatment fields of less than 2-cm diameter do not require to be divided up.

The time added after ice field formation must be learned by experience but will vary with the size, site, and type of pathology. The record in the hospital notes is usually made, for example, as follows:

LN$_2$:   Single ice field: 1   × 15 s

(Liquid nitrogen):   Single < 2 cm :1 FTC × (Time after
                                                           ice formed)

This schedule is typical of that used for a small flat plaque of Bowen's disease of the skin. Viral warts may require as little as 4 to 5 s, while malignant lesions need up to 30 s. Times of less than 30 s do not usually cause connective tissue distortion and scarring.[12]

The author has tested the adequacy of the spot freeze method in experiments on the flank skin of pigs and has shown consistent cell killing and satisfactory temperature levels within the field of treatment. The method is exactly repeatable from patient to patient and site to site; if, following a particular schedule, the treated lesion is not cured, the time of treatment can be lengthened. Also, whichever physician sees the case at follow-up, the exact treatment procedure is known and can be specifically modified.

Many other techniques are available involving varying spray methods for treating large lesions and liquid N_2 probe methods. The important factor is to gain experience with whatever techniques are to be learned by (1) experimenting on skin of cheap meats or other animal tissue (e.g., pigs' feet or hock available from most meat retailers), (2) working with an animal "model" where possible, and (3) observing experienced operators in practice. This is particularly important if malignant lesions are to be treated since much of the therapeutic failure with small basal and squamous epitheliomas can be ascribed to poor technique.

As with all surgical treatments, accurate diagnosis is essential before cryosurgery is used. This evidently does not mean biopsy of all lesions prior to freezing, since clinical diagnosis will often be adequate, particularly with benign lesions (Table 14-1) and many basal cell carcinomas (BCCs). As with radiotherapy, wrong diagnosis may lead to blurring of physical signs, for example, with melanotic lesions, and may facilitate tumor spread before the diagnosis becomes obvious.

Treatment of Malignant Skin Lesions (Table 14-3)

Theoretically, as with x-irradiation, all skin malignancies could be treatable by appropriate cryosurgical techniques, but, like radiotherapy, in clinical practice, certain tumor types have been found to be amenable to *cold killing* with high cure rates and relatively low morbidity indices.[7,13] The malignancies which are often treated by cryosurgery are BCC (Figs. 14-1–14-3), squamous cell carcinoma [SCC (Fig. 14-9)], carcinoma in situ [Bowen's disease (Fig. 14-5)] of the skin and adjacent epithelial surfaces, lentigo maligna [LM (Hutchinson's freckle)], and some cases of lentigo maligna melanoma [LMM (Fig. 14-7 and Table 14-3)]. In general, malignancy requires two FTCs to ensure consistent cell killing and good success rates. Apart from the examples to be mentioned, it is mandatory to perform a biopsy to obtain tissue diagnosis prior to treatment.

Those who are only used to using cryosurgery for benign lesions should start by treating tumors which might otherwise be treated by curettage and cautery or simple excision and primary closure. Also, until the physician acquires greater cryosurgical skill, sites which have the highest recurrence

TABLE 14-3

Statistics for Treatment of Malignant Tumors

BCC eyelid	Biro, Price[42]	3.4% recurrence (of 87): 5 years
BCC nose	Biro, Price[42]	2.6% recurrence (of 155): 5 years
BCC		39% recurrence: 1 year
BCC	Graham[13]	2.5% recurrence (of 623): 5 years
BCC and SCC	Graham[36] (quoting Zacarian's figures)	2.7% recurrence (of 4379): 5 years
Lentigo maligna and lentigo maligna melanoma	Dawber, Wilkinson[23]	100% clearance (of 22): up to 21 1/2 years
BCC and SCC of ears	Kuflik,[40] Webb[31]	5% recurrence (of 180)
BCC head and neck	McIntosh et al[41]	5% recurrence (of 34)
BCC	Holt[38]	2.7% recurrence (of 225): 5 years
SCC	Holt[38]	2.9% recurrence (of 34): 5 years
Bowen's diseases	Holt[38]	0.8% recurrence (of 128): 5 years

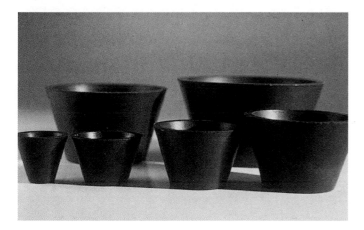

Figure 14-1 Cryosurgery cones of various sizes used in the Torre cone spray technique.

rates whatever the method of treatment, bar Mohs surgery, are best avoided (i.e., inner canthus, nasolabial folds, and periauricular lesions). In general, one can state that the ear, eyelid, and cartilaginous parts of the nose are relatively good sites for cryosurgery because cartilage necrosis is not likely with routine methods.[14] Also, connective tissue damage and distorting scars are rare.[12]

Basal Cell Carcinoma (Figs. 14-2–14-4)

Superficial spreading BCC of the type often seen on the trunk in the elderly (sun exposure not a factor), lesions of the basal cell nevus (Gorlin's syndrome), and small lesions on x-ray-damaged skin are treatable with a single FTC (i.e., there is less inflammatory morbidity from this than with the two FTCs used most frequently in the rodent ulcer or cystic types

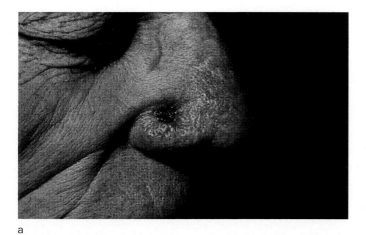

a

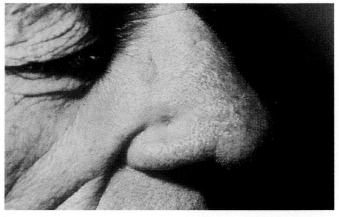

b

Figure 14-2 (a) Basal cell carcinoma of the nose; (b) 3 weeks after two freeze-thaw cycles of liquid nitrogen spray.

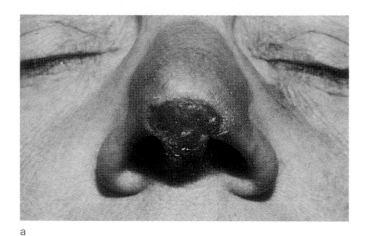
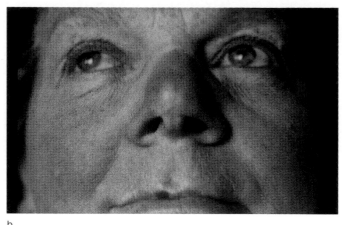

a   b

Figure 14-3   *(a)* Basal cell carcinoma of the tip of the nose with crust removed; *(b)* 4 weeks after two freeze-thaw cycles of liquid nitrogen spray.

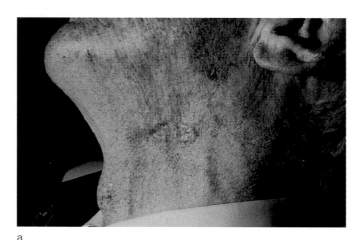
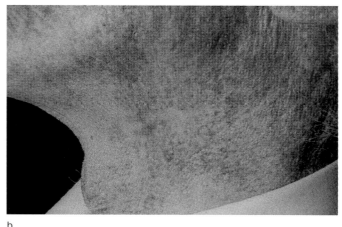

a   b

Figure 14-4   *(a)* Basal cell carcinoma of neck occurring on x-ray-damaged (acne therapy) skin; *(b)* 6 weeks after a single freeze-thaw cycle of liquid nitrogen spray.

mostly seen on the face). With careful case selection, cure rates of greater than 97 percent can be obtained.[10,13,15] Particularly gratifying are the cure rates and excellent cosmetic results obtained for lesions on the nose and the ear.[10,16] The latter is important because only rarely BCCs invade the underlying cartilage. This type of tumor tends to spread horizontally, superficially to the cartilage; SCC, however, may invade and therefore, if cryosurgery is used after healing and cure, a structural defect may remain forever.[14]

Squamous Cell Carcinoma (Fig. 14-9)

It is the author's opinion that cryosurgery is the treatment of choice for carcinoma in situ (Bowen's disease) of the skin, ex-

ternal genitalia in the female, and penis [erythroplasia of Queyrat (Fig. 14-5)].[17–19] Of considerable advantage regarding genital skin Bowen's disease is that the freezing methods used do not cause connective tissue scarring, and contracture is a major advantage.[1]

Well-differentiated SCCs related to sun damage require two FTCs to avoid treatment failure or frequent recurrences.[20–22]

Unlike BCC, SCC more often invades underlying tissues such as cartilage; lesions on the ear are thus better not treated by freezing. Even though good cure rates can be obtained, loss of ear cartilage and poor cosmetic results are common. The clinical signs of SCC in the early stages are less clear-cut than BCC. Therefore, prior to treatment of SCC, a diagnosis is crucial. Evidently, this leads to the conclusion that very

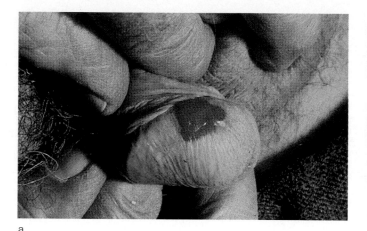

a

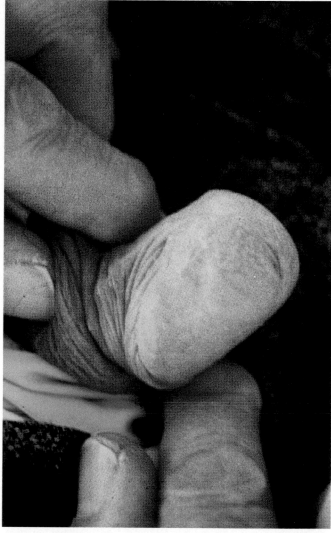

b

Figure 14-5 *(a)* Bowen's disease of the penis (erythroplasia of Queyrat); *(b)* 4 weeks after cryosurgery (one freeze-thaw cycle).

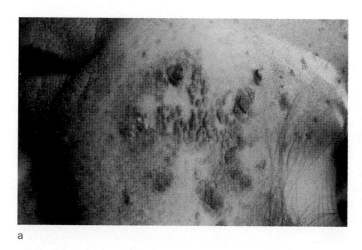

a

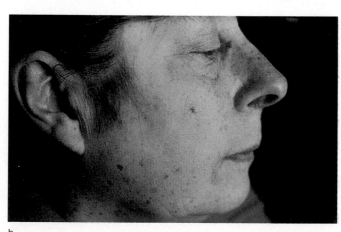

b

Figure 14-6 *(a)* Multiple coalescing benign seborrheic keratoses of the face; *(b)* 8 weeks after treatment.

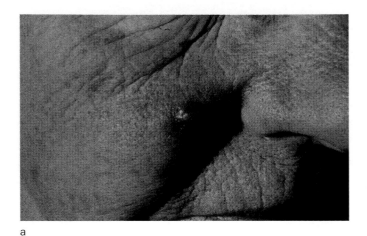
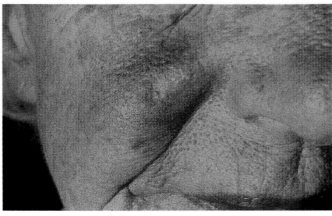

a   b

Figure 14-7   *(a)* Lentigo maligna melanoma; *(b)* 11 weeks after two freeze-thaw cycles of liquid nitrogen spray.

small lesions are better treated by excision biopsy if primary closure is possible.

Lentigo Maligna and Lentigo Maligna Melanoma (Fig. 14-7)

Dermatologists have in practice been using various freezing techniques for LM and LMM for many decades; anecdotal reports have always appeared good. Dawber and Wilkinson[23] published a series with long follow-up observations confirming the long held view that aggressive cryosurgery gives satisfactory cure rates (Table 14-3). It is important to note that cryobiological research has confirmed the ease with which normal melanocytes are killed by short freezes as used in clinical practice, fully justifying pilot studies in malignant

melanoma of the good prognostic group such as biopsy-proven early malignant melanoma.[24] Studies are continuing in other types of melanoma.[3]

Palliation

Arnott[26] showed the value of freezing temperatures applied to surface malignant lesions—decreasing the size of primary and secondary (often fungating) malignancies in the skin. Also, pain in such tumors was often decreased and any chronic bacterial infection usually improved or was cured. In parts of the world where surgical facilities and radiotherapy are not available, such palliative methods are still useful, since liquid N_2 is a better killing refrigerant than Arnott's salt-ice mixtures. Kuflik[27] has shown that it is still a useful prin-

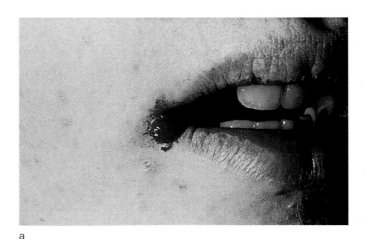
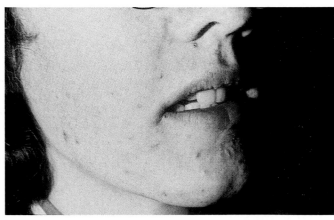

a   b

Figure 14-8   *(a)* Pyogenic granuloma (eruptive hemangioma); *(b)* 3 weeks after freezing.

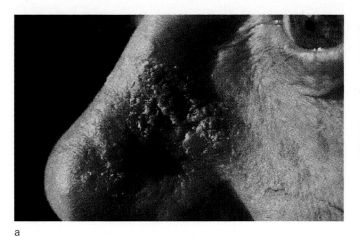

a

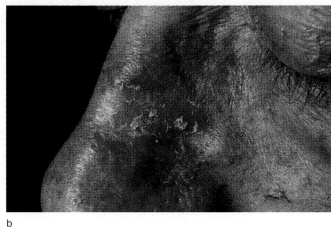

b

Figure 14-9 *(a)* Well-differentiated squamous carcinoma of the nose; *(b)* 13 weeks of cryosurgery (two freeze-thaw cycles).

ciple to use for many incurable malignant skin lesions. Liquid N_2 is so widely available around the world in hospitals, veterinary and other biologic units (mostly for tissue preservation), and other industries that even in third world countries, liquid N_2 can usually be obtained.

SOME ADVANTAGES, SIDE-EFFECTS, AND DISADVANTAGES

The patient usually feels a burning sensation during freezing and thawing. Any pain experienced is usually transient due to the anesthetizing effect of freezing.[28,29] Local anesthesia is not required for short freeze times but may be indicated when one is treating malignant lesions or for patients thought to have a low pain threshold. Deep treatments on the forehead may occasionally produce migraine-like headaches, and periungual treatment produces relatively greater discomfort than other digital sites.

Some degree of erythema and edema is to be expected with cryosurgery treatments, and, in areas where the skin is lax (periorbital skin, lips, labia majora, and penis), edema may be pronounced. Prolonged freezing schedules may produce blister formation (Fig. 14-10); even short freeze times may cause such changes in atrophic skin.

Because this acute inflammation was thought to be unnecessary to obtain good cure rates, for many years the author advocated pre- and posttreatment (3 to 5 days) anti-inflammatory therapy with oral aspirin 300 to 600 mg up to four times daily and Dermovate (clobetasol propionate) cream daily to the treated area. The value of this, and sometimes oral steroids, has been confirmed by objective assessment.[30,31]

Obviously many of the conditions listed in Tables 14-1–14-3 as being curable by cryosurgery are also amenable to other surgical methods; the modality chosen will often de-

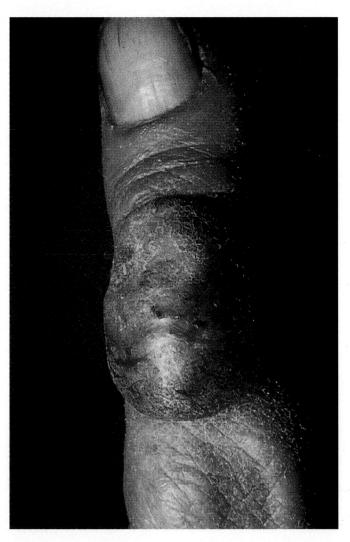

Figure 14-10 Hemorrhagic blister 2 days after cryosurgery of common (viral) wart.

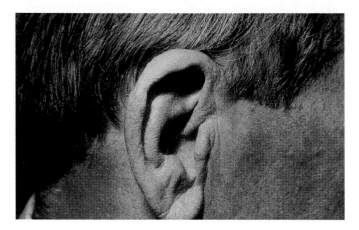

Figure 14-11 Slight epithelial atrophy at the ear margin 8 weeks after cryosurgery to a basal cell carcinoma.

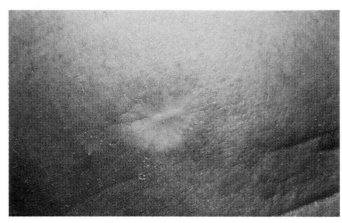

Figure 14-12 Hypopigmentation following two freeze-thaw cycles of liquid nitrogen spray to a basal cell carcinoma.

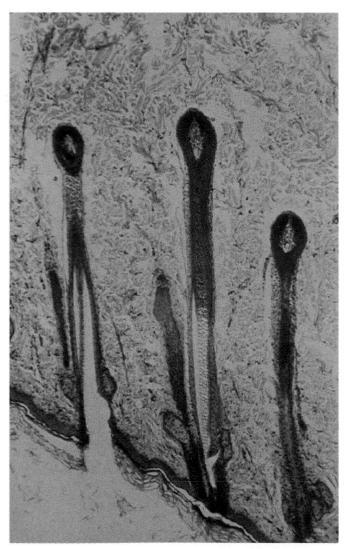

a

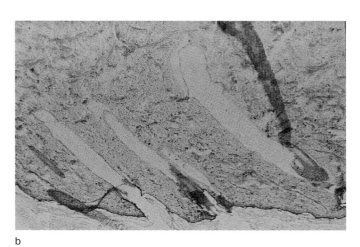

b

Figure 14-13 *(a)* Mature anagen hair follicles; *(b)* 2 weeks after a single 10-s spray of liquid nitrogen.

pend on the skills available in the department to which the patient has been referred. Cryosurgery has the advantage over all other modes of being quick, cheap, and easy to learn and to carry out; usually sterile surgical facilities are not required and treatment can be initiated even in the presence of bacterial infection (e.g., ingrowing toenail).[32] The fact that post-treatment connective tissue distortion does not generally occur makes cryosurgery advantageous where scarring would be progressively troublesome (e.g., perianal, penile, vulval, and periorbital skin) and also over joints where a full range of movement can be expected to be retained even after treatment of malignancy with two or three FTCs.

Cartilage necrosis is extremely rare after freezing; therefore, ear (Fig. 14-11), eyelid, and many nasal lesions give good cosmetic results after cryosurgery. It should be remembered that the only consistent exception to this dogma is cartilage already invaded by tumor—even if good cure is obtained, a cartilage defect may occur.

Anything but the shortest freeze schedules will give pigment changes in the treatment area—hyperpigmentation with very short freezes and at the edge of more aggressively treated areas.[24,25] Hypopigmentation (Fig. 14-12) occurs after prolonged freezing (e.g., > 5 s after ice field formation) and may be permanent; therefore, cryosurgery is less valuable in patients with racially dark skin (e.g., Asian or Negroid and exposed-part lesions in Caucasians who tan darkly on sun exposure).

In general, cryosurgery is not recommended for the treatment of lesions on sites with coarse terminal hair. Hair follicles are easily damaged by cryosurgery (Fig. 14-13) and permanent alopecia is not uncommon.[33]

Temporary impairment of sensation in the treatment area is common after freezing; only rarely will the patient be aware of this.[28,29] Such nerve ending damage can be expected to disappear within a few months, apart from malignancy regimes using two or three FTCs. At sites such as the finger pulp and lip margin, permanent sensory loss may give important functional impairment, but in other sites it is generally of no significance. Though nerve trunk damage and "distant" sensory and motor loss have been recorded, they are very rare and reversible, usually within a few months.

A rare side effect of cryosurgery is delayed bleeding; this may be due to granulation tissue formation, as in pyogenic granuloma, or from erosion of a small artery. The former may require no more than pressure to abort it or chemical treatment (e.g., silver nitrate), or an electrocautery-patent bleeding artery requires tying off with an appropriate suture.

It is now evident that cryosurgical equipment and skill are essential in all dermatology and surgical departments which regularly treat lesions, benign and malignant, of the type noted in Tables 14-1–14-3. There are many skin conditions in which excision, radiotherapy, and cryosurgery may be alternative modes of treatment under consideration. Clearly, for many of these lesions, cryosurgery is now the treatment of choice.

REFERENCES

1. Shepherd JPL, Dawber RPR: Cryosurgery: History and scientific basis. *Clin Exp Dermatol* **7**:321, 1982

2. Torre D: Cutaneous cryosurgery: Current state of the art. *J Dermatol Surg Oncol* **11**:292, 1985

3. Zacarian SA: *Cryosurgery for Skin Cancer and Cutaneous Disorders.* St. Louis, Mosby, 1985

4. Dawber RPR, Walker NPJ: Physical and surgical procedures, in *Textbook of Dermatology,* 5th ed, edited by RH Champion et al. Oxford, Blackwell Scientific, 1992, pp 3113–3114.

5. Shepherd JP, Dawber RPR: The response of hypertrophic and keloid scars to cryosurgery. *Plast Reconstr Surg* **70**:677, 1982

6. Torre D et al: *Practical Cutaneous Cryosurgery,* 1st ed. New York, Appleton & Lange, 1985

7. Dawber RPR: Cold kills! *Clin Exp Dermatol* **13**:137, 1988

8. Breitbart EW: Cryosurgery: Method and results. *Hautarzt* **34**:612, 1983

9. Torre D: Cryosurgical treatment of epitheliomas using the cone-spray technique. *J Dermatol Surg Oncol* **4**:561, 1978

10. Kuflik EG: Treatment of basal cell carcinoma with open spray technique. *J Dermatol Surg Oncol* **12**:125, 1986

11. Colver GB, Dawber RPR: Cryosurgery: The principles and simple clinical practice. *Clin Exp Dermatol* **14**:1–6, 1989

12. Shepherd JP, Dawber RPR: Wound healing and scarring after cryosurgery. *Cryobiology* **21**:157, 1984

13. Graham GF: Statistical data on malignant tumours in cryosurgery. *J Dermatol Surg Oncol* **9**:238, 1982

14. Burge SM et al: Effect of freezing the helix and the rim or edge of the human and pig ear. *J Dermatol Surg Oncol* **10**:816, 1984

15. Torre D: Cryosurgery of basal cell carcinoma. *J Am Acad Dermatol* **15**:917, 1986

16. Kuflik EG: Cryosurgery for multiple basal cell carcinomas on the nose. *J Dermatol Surg Oncol* **10**:16, 1984

17. Dawber RPR: Cryosurgery for Bowen's disease of skin. *Br J Dermatol* **103**:14, 1980

18. Mortimer PS et al: Cryotherapy for multicentric pigmented Bowen's disease. *Clin Exp Dermatol* **8**:319, 1982

19. Sonnex T et al: Erythroplasia of Queyrat: Treatment by liquid nitrogen cryosurgery. *Br J Dermatol* **106**:581, 1982

20. Kuflik EG: Treatment of basal and squamous cell carcinoma of the nose by cryosurgery. *J Dermatol Surg Oncol* **6**:811, 1980

21. Zacarian SA: Cryosurgery of cutaneous carcinoma. *J Am Acad Dermatol* **9**:947, 1983

22. Torre D, Lubritz RR: Special issue: Cryosurgery. *J Dermatol Surg Oncol* **9**:183, 1983

23. Dawber RPR, Wilkinson JD: Melanotic freckle of Hutchinson: Treatment of macular and nodular phases. *Br J Dermatol* **101**:47, 1979

24. Burge SM et al: Pigment change and melanocyte distribution after cutaneous freeze injury. *Br J Dermatol* **113**:770, 1985

25. Burge SM et al: Pigment changes in human skin after cryotherapy. *Cryobiology* **23:**111, 1986

26. Arnott J: *On the Treatment of Cancer by the Regular Application of an Anaesthetic Temperature.* London, Churchill, 1851

27. Kuflik EG: Cryosurgery for palliation. *J Dermatol Surg Oncol* **11:**867, 1985

28. Sonnex TS et al: Long term effects of cryosurgery on cutaneous sensation. *Br Med J* **290:**188, 1985

29. Faber WR et al: Sensory loss following cryosurgery of skin lesions. *Br J Dermatol* **117:**343, 1987

30. Hindson TC et al: Clobetasol propionate ointment reduces inflammation after cryotherapy. *Br J Dermatol* **112:**599, 1985

31. Kuflik EG, Webb W: Effect of corticosteroids on post-cryosurgical oedema and other manifestations of the inflammatory response. *J Dermatol Surg Oncol* **11:**464, 1985

32. Sonnex TS, Dawber RPR: Treatment of ingrowing toenails with liquid nitrogen spray cryotherapy. *Br Med J* **291:**173, 1985

33. Burge SM, Dawber RPR: Hair follicle destruction and regeneration in guinea-pig skin after cutaneous freeze injury. *Cryobiology* **27:**153–163, 1990

34. Dawber RPR: Cryosurgery, in *Dermatological Surgery,* edited by JL Verbov. Lancaster, UK, MPT Press, 1986, p 79

35. Graham G: Cryosurgical treatment of acne. *Cutis* **16:**509, 1975

36. Graham GF: Cryosurgery for acne, in *Cryosurgery for Skin Cancer and Cutaneous Disorders,* edited by AN Other. St. Louis, Mosby, 1985, p 59

37. Castro-Ron G: Cryosurgery for angiomas and birth defects, in *Cryosurgery for Skin Cancer and Birth Defects,* edited by SA Zacarian. St. Louis, Mosby, 1985, p 77

38. Holt PJA: Cryotherapy for skin cancer: Results over a 5-year period using liquid nitrogen spray cryosurgery. *Br J Dermatol* **119:**231–240, 1988

39. Jackson AD: Treatment of skin cancers in general practice. *Br J Gen Pract* **41:**213, 1991

40. Kuflik EG: Cryosurgery for tumors of the ear. *J Dermatol Surg Oncol* **11:**1165, 1985

41. McIntosh GS et al: Basal cell carcinoma: A review of treatment results with special reference to cryotherapy. *Postgrad Med J* **59:**698, 1983

42. Biro L, Price E: Cryogenic anaesthesia and haemestasis. *J Dermatol Surg Oncol* **61:**608, 1980

43. Spiller WF, Spiller RF: Cryoanaesthesia and electrosurgical treatment of benign skin tumours. *Cutis* **35:**551, 1985

44. Lanigan SW, Robinson TWE: Cryotherapy for dermatofibromas. *Clin Exp Dermatol* **12:**121, 1987

45. Dawber RPR et al: Myxoid cysts of the finger: Treatment by liquid nitrogen cryosurgery. *Clin Exp Dermatol* **8:**153, 1982

46. Lubritz RR, Smolewski SA: Cryosurgery cure rate of actinic keratoses. *J Am Acad Dermatol* **7:**631, 1982

47. Al-Gingan Y et al: Cryosurgery in old world cutaneous leishmaniasis. *Br J Dermatol* **118:**851, 1988

48. Waldinger TP et al: Cryotherapy improves prurigo nodularis. *Arch Dermatol* **120:**1598, 1984

49. Detrano SJ: Cryotherapy for chronic non-specific pruritus. *J Dermatol Surg Oncol* **10:**483, 1984

50. Leonard JN et al: Pseudogenic granuloma. *Clin Exp Dermatol* **6:**215, 1981

51. Sonnex TS, Dawber RPR: Rhinophyma. *Dermatology Digest* **1:**31, 1984

52. Wheeland RG, Wiley MD: Q-tip cryosurgery for the treatment of senile sebaceous hyperplasia. *J Dermatol Surg Oncol* **13:**729, 1987

53. Colver GB, Dawber RPR: Tattoo removal using liquid nitrogen cryospray. *Clin Exp Dermatol* **9:**364, 1984

54. Bunney MH et al: An assessment of various methods of treating virus warts. *Br J Dermatol* **94:**667, 1976

55. Ghosh AK: Cryosurgery of genital warts in cases in which podophyllin treatment failed or was contraindicated. *Br J Vener Dis* **53:**49, 1977

56. Bashi A: Cryotherapy versus podophyllin in the treatment of genital warts. *Int J Dermatol* **24:**535, 1985

57. Masters NJ: An audit of wart cryotherapy. *Modern Medicine* **8:**581, 1987

58. Masters NJ: Dermatologists and warts. *Br Med J* **296:**570, 1988

59. Steele K: Dermatologists and warts. *Br Med J* **296:**569, 1988

60. Graham G: Unusual difficult to treat skin tumours seen as possible cryosurgery candidates. *Dermatology News* **12:**2, 1979

Leonard H. Goldberg

15 Cold Steel Surgery: The Ellipse

THE ELLIPSE

The ellipse is the workhorse of dermatologic excisional and reconstructive surgery of the skin. Nearly all simple excisions of the skin are done through the performance of the ellipse. Understanding and execution of the ellipse is a fundamental building block for performing more complicated dermatologic surgery procedures.

The basic principle of the ellipse is to close a round-to-oval defect in the skin by sewing the edges together (side to side); however, this will cause folds (dog-ears, darts) to form at either end (Fig. 15-1).

These folds do not resolve spontaneously and require excision and lengthening of the scar line in order to obtain a smooth skin surface, thereby achieving good cosmesis. The excision of these folds turns the round-to-oval defect into an ellipse, which, on closure, will allow the skin to lie flat. The resulting closure line varies from a straight line to a curve, depending on the angle of the excision of the dog-ears from the closure line (Fig. 15-2).

Cosmesis is best (a hidden, fine-line scar) when the final suture line is placed in a major skin fold, wrinkle line, or in the imaginary minimum skin tension line (MSTL). This makes the planning of the placement of the ellipse a most important stage in the procedure and probably the most important determinant to the achievement of excellent long-term cosmesis.

The determination of the MSTL for each procedure is based on a number of factors (Table 15-1). These include Langer's lines, gravity, direction of hair, wrinkle lines, and MSTL. The MSTLs usually agree with Langer's lines (Fig.

15-3a–b) but may vary from patient to patient, depending on age, obesity, laxity of the skin, gravity, and the muscles of expression (in the face).[1]

MSTLs are determined by pinching the skin lightly between the fingers in different directions and noting where the resulting skin folds are finest [thin] (Fig. 15-3c).

The length of the ellipse is approximately three times the diameter of the primary excision defect. This differs from place to place on the surface of the skin, being less with thin skin (eyelid) and more with thick skin (back). Initially, a short ellipse can be planned and then, after the excision is completed, the flatness of the skin surface can be observed. Further lengthening of the ellipse may be necessary if dog-ears are apparent, indicating the presence of excess skin.

The shape of the ellipse may vary from tangent-to-circle to fusiform. Figure 15-4a gives a narrower tip angle versus the wide tip angle of Fig. 15-4b. Less excess skin needs to be removed to achieve a flat surface when dog-ears are removed with the tangent-to-circle technique.

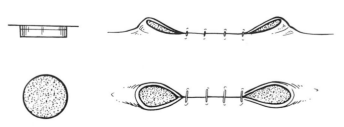

Figure 15-1 Horizontal and vertical views of the dog-ears formed by an elliptical closure.

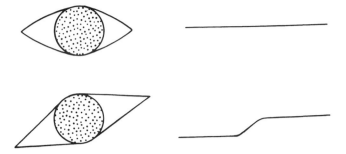

Figure 15-2 Example of closure lines resulting from the angle of excision of the dog-ears.

TABLE 15-1

Factors Influencing the Optimal Placement of an Ellipse

Major skin folds

Langer's lines

Wrinkle lines

Influence of underlying muscle groups on the skin

Patient positioning (gravity)

Direction of hair growth

SURGICAL METHOD

First, determine the direction and placement of the ellipse. The proposed elliptic incision lines are then marked with a marking pen. Local anesthesia is injected to encompass the area of the ellipse as well as an area up to 1 cm around the ellipse. Xylocaine 1% with 1:100,000 epinephrine is the standard solution used for anesthesia. It is preferable to buffer the solution with NaHCO$_3$ to reduce the pain during injection. It is important not to hurt the patient during the injection, and time should be taken injecting the anesthetic slowly, explaining the procedure to the patient, and engaging the patient in conversation to take his or her mind off what is going on, as well as to determine if the patient feels pain. When pain is felt, stop injecting and wait for several seconds for the pain to subside before resuming the injection process.

The injection is made into the dermis and less into the subdermal fat. Injecting into the subdermal fat is less resistant than the dermal injection, and there is no blanching of the skin, but the anesthetic effect is less.

The skin is then *cleansed* with Betadine, alcohol, or any antibacterial solution or soap of preference. The area may be draped and sufficiently bright lighting of the area arranged.

The skin to be excised is stabilized by the assistant's or surgeon's hands; the patient is asked to keep still and is advised that cutting is about to begin. The skin is then carefully incised through the full thickness of the dermis down to the

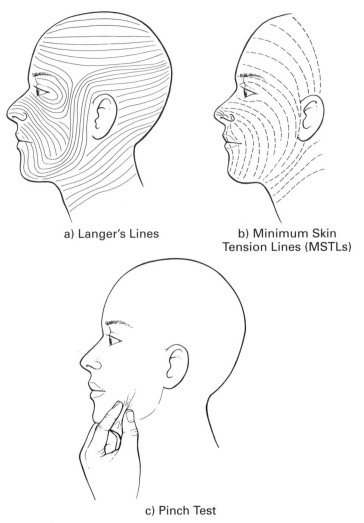

a) Langer's Lines

b) Minimum Skin Tension Lines (MSTLs)

c) Pinch Test

Figure 15-3 *(a, b)* Langer's lines and Minimum Skin Tension Lines (MSTLs) are used to determine the excision lines. *(c)* The "pinch test" is used to determine MSTLs.

subcutaneous fat. The incision is made at a 90° angle to the skin surface, providing right-angle skin edges. This is important so that closure of the edges will be perfect. If 90°-angled skin is approximated to 100°-angled skin, perfect closure will not be obtained (Fig. 15-5). Ask any carpenter to verify this!

In order to cut the ellipse, the sharp end of the blade is pushed into the skin and pulled over the line of the ellipse. It is important to aim the blade over the line of the ellipse, mov-

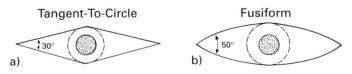

Tangent-To-Circle   Fusiform

a) 30°   b) 50°

Figure 15-4 *(a)* Tangent-to-circle excision of dog-ears with 30° tip angle. *(b)* Fusiform excision of dog-ears has a wider angle at the tip and more skin is removed.

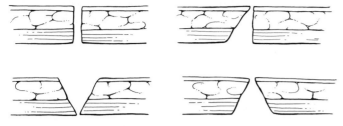

Figure 15-5 Illustration of the possible angles of excision to demonstrate the necessity of a 90° angle for perfect closure.

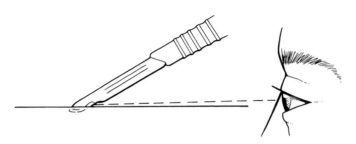

Figure 15-6 The scalpel blade handle is pulled over the line of the ellipse.

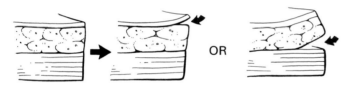

OR

Figure 15-7 Undermining may be done at the dermal/fat junction or the fat/muscle junction.

ing the blade handle as the blade moves over the skin (Fig. 15-6).

The scalpel handle must be kept parallel to the line that is being cut. If this is not done, a perfectly sharp 90° cut will not be made. When the entire ellipse is incised through the dermis into the fat, the elliptic skin is lifted up with toothed forceps and, by using either scissors or the blade, is dissected at the level of the dermal-fat junction.

Bleeding points are cauterized using the available method of electrocautery.* It is preferable to pick up each bleeding vessel in the dermis with fine-toothed forceps, gently pull the vessel away from the base of the defect, and then cauterize the vessel by applying current to the forceps. The author's surgical unit uses a Valley Lab electrocautery machine. It is not necessary to cauterize all the small vessels of the dermis. These will stop bleeding when pressure is applied to them by approximation and sewing of the wound edges.

---

* Be sure to confirm that the patient does not have a cardiac pacemaker which would make electrocautery hazardous.

UNDERMINING

Undermining is a method of detaching the dermis and epidermis from the subcutaneous fat and fascia (Fig. 15-7). This is done to achieve greater movement of the dermal-epidermal unit (skin) over the underlying and less movable fat, fascia, and muscle, thus facilitating advancement, approximation, and closure of the wound edges.

Undermining is usually done at the dermal-fat junction or the fat-muscle junction with a blade or a scissors. When hair-bearing skin is to be moved (e.g., scalp, eyebrows, or beard), it is necessary to undermine below the level of the hair follicles which can be seen in the upper or midfat. The skin is lifted with a skin hook and the incision is made right under the dermis. The width of undermining is determined by the smoothing/flattening of the skin surface needed, the necessity to move the skin to obtain closure based on the size and location of the defect, and the surgeon's preference and experience. Undermining may need to be continued beyond the tip of the ellipse and up to 1 cm beyond the edges of the ellipse (Fig. 15-8). Undermining of the skin is not always necessary for exact placement of sutures.

After the skin is undermined, the blood vessels that have been severed in the process should be cauterized before closure is begun. A hook is used to lift up the skin edge. The light is shone under the skin surface, and bleeding points are sought and cauterized or, rarely, tied. When the wound is ready for closure, it is washed with saline which removes any debris that may have accumulated.

CLOSURE

Almost all closures are done in two layers, beginning with subcutaneous absorbable sutures which hold the dermis to-

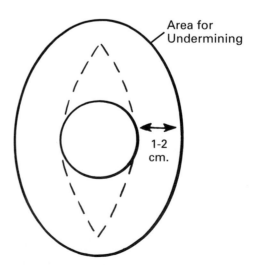

Area for Undermining

1-2 cm.

Figure 15-8 Hypothetical area for undermining, determined by amount of flattening needed, size and location of the defect, and surgeon preference.

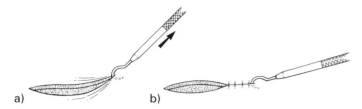

Figure 15-9   *(a, b)* The action of pulling the tip of the ellipse upwards and away from the center tends to approximate the edges, making closure easier.

gether and followed by epidermal sutures which evert and close the skin edges.

Appropriate absorbable suture materials for subcutaneous placement include: PDS (polydioxanone), Vicryl, or Dexon. Five-0 or 4–0 strength should be adequate for dermatologic surgery. Generally, the suture is swaged onto a reverse-cutting, three-eighths circle, P1- or P3-size needle. When there is tension on the wound edges, 4–0 or 3–0 suture may be used. If too much tension is applied to the skin, it will blanch and may necrose over the subsequent day or two due to lack of blood supply.

Commencing the Closure

A skin hook is placed at the end of the ellipse, and the edge is pulled upward and away from the center of the ellipse in the line of the closure (Fig. 15-9). This action will approximate the edges closer together and allow exact placement of the sutures. Subcutaneous sutures may be either individual or running, horizontal or vertical (Fig. 15-10). The methodology of each of these types is explained in Suturing Techniques, Chap. 16. Superficial "cutaneous" sutures are then placed on the surface to get exact leveling of the skin edges.

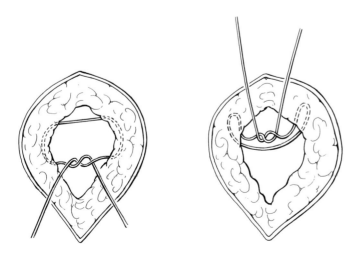

Figure 15-10   Horizontal and vertical subcutaneous sutures.

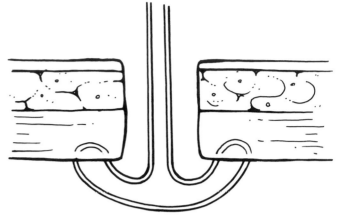

Figure 15-11   Proper placement of subcutaneous suture for perfect eversion of the skin edges.

Careful placement of these sutures is very important, as they achieve the leveling of the skin edges and the smoothness of the skin, which determines the final cosmetic result.

When the subcutaneous suture is placed correctly at the *undersurface* of the dermis (Fig. 15-11), the skin edges will evert and approximate perfectly. This makes placement of the cutaneous or surface sutures very easy and exact. The subcutaneous suture is buried, does not show on the skin surface, and is absorbed over time. This suture pulls the skin edges together and holds the tension. It is easier to do interrupted subcutaneous stitches, as each suture may exert a different amount of tension. These sutures stay in place for weeks, giving the skin edges ample time to knit together and reducing to almost nil the risk of dehiscence (separation) of wound edges. The mastery of placement and tying of this stitch is an essential part of technique in dermatologic surgery.

Based upon the surgeon's personal preference, the skin surface of an ellipse may be closed from one tip to the other, or the method of halving may be used (Fig. 15-12).

Closure of the Skin Surface

The surface suture is used to level the epidermal surfaces so that the two edges are the same and healing will occur with a

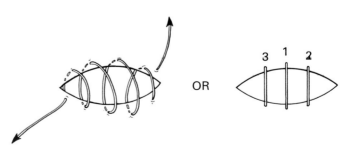

Figure 15-12   Closure of an ellipse may be accomplished by suturing from one tip to the other or by the method of halving.

resulting smooth surface. This suture is placed very loosely in the skin, as it is not used as a tension suture to close the wound edge. Start the suture *beyond* the wound edge and end it beyond the wound edge on the other side. The progression of the suture may be made by any one of the three patterns in Fig. 15-13. A 6–0 nylon suture on a P1 or P3 needle is effective for closing the skin surface, using running sutures, which save time, or interrupted sutures.

A tip suture has recently been described which may assist in leveling dog-ears and thus may allow the surgeon to keep the length of the wound as short as possible. The author has not used this suture personally, but it may possibly be used fairly routinely in the future.

When the final sutures have been placed, gently squeeze the wound between gauze swabs for a few seconds to extrude any collected blood between the wound edges.

Drains: Drains are not routinely required; however, they are required when it is suspected that there may be oozing of blood or tissue fluid postoperatively because:

1. Not all of the dead space of an excision has been closed.
2. The excision is very large.
3. The patient has a tendency to bleed.
4. The patient has a possibility of having an infected wound. In this case, the drain may be placed and left in for 48 h and then removed. The drain can be constructed from the finger of a sterile glove or a Penrose drain can be used. It is also effective to leave a piece of sterile Vaseline or Xeroform gauze sticking into the wound to act as a wick and soak up any fluid which may collect within the wound.

It is helpful to photograph all excisions preoperatively and postoperatively for personal, teaching, and medicolegal reasons.

A pressure dressing is then placed over the ellipse consisting of a layer of antibiotic ointment covered with a Telfa (optional) gauze and silk tape, paper tape, or some form of elastic tape.

Instruct the patient to leave the operated area undisturbed for 48 h and then do postoperative wound cleaning and dressing once or twice daily for a week.

Remove cutaneous sutures at 5 to 7 days for convenience. Sutures may be removed from 3 to 14 days or even longer. Using this technique prevents both dehiscence of the wound and permanent suture marks in the skin from occurring.

Routine oral postoperative antibiotics are not necessary except under the following circumstances:

1. Patient's request
2. Cardiac valve disease
3. Permanent foreign body (e.g., pacemaker, artificial joint, etc.)
4. Immunosuppressed patient
5. Infected wound at time excision is performed
6. Long, arduous surgery under less than ideal conditions

Under these special circumstances, a broad-spectrum antibiotic is recommended, and very often the patient's cardiologist or internist will play a role in the choice of antibiotic. The antibiotic is taken 1 day prior to surgery and for 3 to 7 days postoperatively. Patients with frequently recurring herpes simplex outbreaks may be given acyclovir (Zovirax) orally starting on the day of surgery. A dose of 400 mg twice daily is recommended.

Given this course of care, at the time of suture removal, the wound will have healed with little or no redness at all. Although complications are rare, marked tenderness, swelling, oozing, pus formation, abscess, or symptoms of systemic infection can occur and must be promptly and appropriately handled.

PATIENT COMMUNICATION

It is appropriate to prescribe oral pain medication for the night of the surgery. Patients may be advised to apply an ice pack over the dressing for 15 min every hour and to apply pressure for any bleeding problems. Should bleeding occur and continue so that the bandage becomes soaked or drips with blood, the patient should be seen that night or as soon as possible. Calling patients after surgery at home the night of surgery to inquire about bleeding, pain, or other problems can be comforting for the patient and informative to the physician. If the patient describes acute swelling of the wound (possible hematoma), it is advisable to see the patient immediately. If a patient complains of swelling, redness, or pain prior to suture removal, it is wise to see the patient to rule out the possibility of wound infection.

Patients should be provided with a telephone number which will give them contact with the physician concerning any problem in the immediate postoperative period. It is preferable to examine a patient with a complaint of postoper-

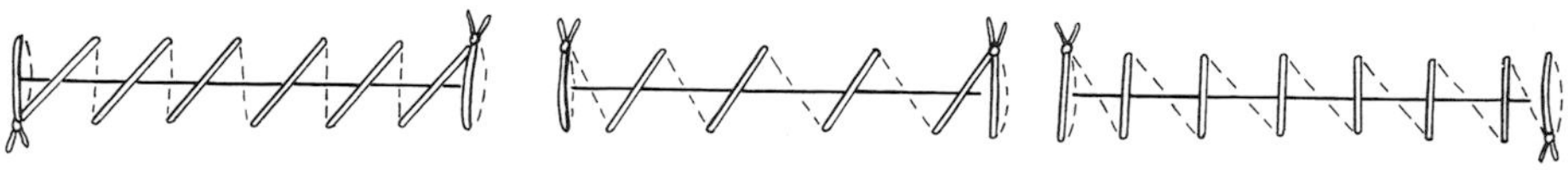

Figure 15-13 Suture progression patterns for the ellipse.

ative conditions which might signal complications as quickly as possible so that treatment can be undertaken before a serious condition develops (e.g., hematoma, infection, or dehiscence). Patients are greatly relieved to know that they have access to the physician if the need should arise.

The long-term (3 months and above) cosmesis and patient's acceptance of the ellipse depends on two major factors:

1. The smoothness of the surface
2. The fineness of the closure line

The smoothness of the surface depends on:

1. Complete removal of all excess skin (dog-ears)
2. Perfect approximation of skin edges from the horizontal viewpoint

The fineness of the scar line depends on:

1. Subcutaneous sutures that provide sufficient approximation of the dermis for adequate closure strength and approximation of the epidermis while assuring a lack of tension on the epidermal closure.
2. Placement of the ellipse exactly in the MSTL, causing the scar to be under no tension to open. If the resulting scar is under continuous, long-term tension, a thicker or even hypertrophic scar will form. It is clear that the thicker scar will be much less acceptable to the patient.

The scar resulting from an ellipse or a simple side-to-side closure, which is basically an ellipse, is usually superior to that of any other closure because:

1. The suture lines can be placed completely within the MSTL and thus be almost completely invisible.

2. Less excess skin (dog-ears) needs to be removed with the closure.
3. Skin is not rotated, resulting in no additional skin folds which may need to be excised.
4. The direction of hair growth in the surrounding skin is not altered.

If the tip of the ellipse needs to be carried to an undesirable area such as the eyelid or other major cosmetic point, the direction of the point of the ellipse may be changed, or the ellipse may be shortened by an M-plasty or a O-T closure. These are described in detail elsewhere in the text.

Suture and scalpel techniques are learned skills which need to be honed and practiced on a regular basis if excellence of performance is to be obtained and maintained. Students, residents, and fellows are advised to practice these techniques at home, regularly, as would a musician or an athlete who practices to achieve and maintain peak performance. Fruit, especially oranges, bananas, and other thick-skinned and pliable fruits can be very effectively used to practice scalpel and suture technique. Keeping an instrument kit at home for practice is useful. Surgery, like other arts, must be practiced; it is not sufficient to do surgery only occasionally when the occasion presents itself.

REFERENCE

1. Meirson D, Goldberg LH: The influence of age and patient positioning on skin tension lines. *J Dermatol Surg Oncol* **19**:39–43, 1993

George J. Hruza

16 Suturing Techniques

Correct suture technique is crucial for functionally and cosmetically outstanding results in skin surgery. In addition to approximation of wound edges, properly placed sutures are important for skin edge eversion, minimization and redistribution of tension, elimination of dead space, and maintenance or restoration of natural anatomic contours while avoiding the formation of permanent suture marks on the skin surface. The suture technique chosen for a specific wound closure will depend on which of the above functions are most important as well as the anatomic location and wound edge thickness. Considering the importance of correct suture technique for successful wound closure, very little scientific study has been done on this subject. Most of the medical literature on suture techniques is based only on uncontrolled clinical studies.

INSTRUMENT TIE

Proper knot tying is of paramount importance for correct suturing. Except for suture ligatures, sutures are tied with a needle-holder. The knot should be tied so as to lie flat against the surface with perfect apposition of the wound edges and without any significant tension or tightness. This will minimize the risk of wound edge strangulation and possible necrosis.

The instrument tie (Fig. 16-1) is started by pulling the long end of the suture taut. The needle-holder is looped once for a regular knot and twice for a surgeon's knot (Fig. 16-2a) around the suture pointing toward the suture's end. Next, the short end of the suture is grasped with the needle-holder and pulled through the loop(s) and pulled across the wound so that the loops lie flat against the wound without any bunching.

The tightness of the tie should take account of anticipated postoperative wound edge swelling (Fig. 16-2b–c). A square knot is created by looping the needle-holder around the long end of the suture in the opposite direction, grabbing the short end of the suture, pulling it through the loop, and tying it flat on the previous knot (Fig. 16-2b). Depending on the memory and thickness of the suture material being used, three to six knots may be needed to properly secure the suture in place. Thicker sutures and sutures with greater memory require more knots to be reliably secured in place. Tying the knot too tightly and failing to take account of expected wound edge edema may result in ischemia and permanent suture mark formation.[1] To minimize this problem, the second knot may be tied loosely, leaving a small loop with the remaining knots squared off in the usual fashion (Fig. 16-2b). This loose loop allows the suture to adjust to any wound edema that may develop.[2]

When suturing flaps or grafts in position, place the knot away from the flap or graft so as to minimize compression of the wound edge with compromised circulation. The knots are squared off to minimize the risk of suture loosening as well as strangulating. Granny knots should not be used because they are less secure and are easily tied too tight.

Some surgeons advocate the use of the surgeon's knot (Fig. 16-2a), in which the first knot consists of two loops, because of increased knot security before the knot is "locked" in place with the next squaring-off knot. This is especially helpful with monofilament sutures that have a lot of memory. Others feel that single-loop knots afford better control of knot placement and tightness. For buried sutures, the additional loop results in more foreign body material being buried in the wound. In most situations, the knot used is a matter of personal preference.[3,4]

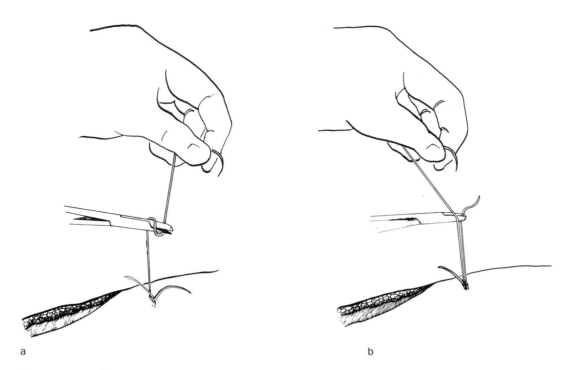

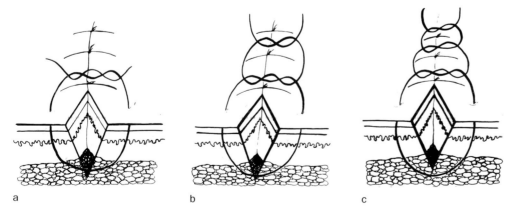

Figure 16-1   The instrument tie. *(a)* The needle-holder is ready to grasp the short end of the suture; *(b)* the suture has been tied down and is being held taut to make cutting it easier.

Figure 16-2   Loop throw. *(a)* Surgeon's knot; *(b)* second loop tied looser; *(c)* additional knots tied tighter. This allows the second loop to accommodate postoperative wound edge edema.

INTERRUPTED SUTURE

Simple Interrupted Suture

The simple interrupted suture is the most basic and versatile suture used by dermatologic surgeons. If the suture is placed close to the wound edges, very precise coaptation of the wound edges can be achieved even in wounds with edges of unequal thickness. If it is placed farther from the wound edges, deeper tissues can be pulled in with redistribution of tension across the wound. When the suture is properly placed in a flask-shaped configuration, wound edge eversion can be achieved.[5]

The suture is placed by passing the needle through the epidermis into the deep dermis or subcutaneous fat, across the wound bed, and back up through the dermis and epidermis (Fig. 16-3). In order to maximize wound edge eversion, the suture starts close to the wound edge and moves farther away as it travels deeper. On the opposite side, the suture starts farther away from the wound edge and moves closer in as it travels toward the epidermis. This flask-shaped configuration brings in more deep tissue than superficial tissue to the wound

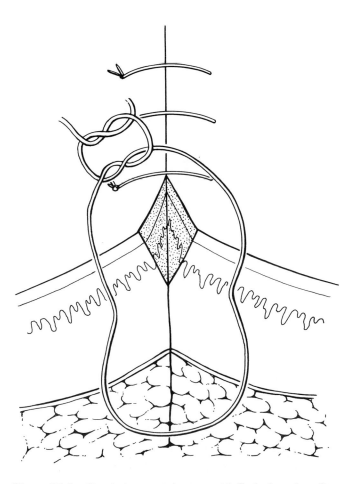

Figure 16-3   Simple interrupted suture with flask-shaped configuration to maximize wound eversion.

edge with resulting wound edge eversion. One way to achieve this is to start the suture with the needle pointing away from the wound edge as it enters the skin and, on the opposite side, to consciously pull in deep tissue with the needle before piercing the epidermis on the way out. Wounds in which the edges are of unequal thickness can be aligned by taking a larger bite from the thinner edge and a smaller bite from the thicker edge. Wounds in which one edge appears higher than the other can be similarly aligned. The simple interrupted suture can also be used as a temporary tacking suture to align complex wound edges or to properly position a flap.[4]

The main disadvantage of the simple interrupted suture is the risk of crosshatch marks across the suture line. This problem can be minimized by removing the sutures within 5 to 7 days before the formation of epithelial suture tracks is complete. Using minimally reactive monofilament suture such as polypropylene reduces suture marks. Elimination of tension across the wound with appropriate wound closure planning, adequate undermining, and the use of buried sutures will also reduce crosshatch marks.

This suture has a tendency to cause wound edge inversion with resultant slowing or re-epithelialization and a noticeably depressed or grooved scar. This is most frequently seen when the skin is very thin or after the removal of a large amount of subcutaneous tissue as occurs in the removal of a large lipoma or epidermal cyst. This problem can be minimized by careful flask-shaped placement of the suture (Fig. 16-3). However, in extreme cases, an everting mattress suture may have to be substituted at strategic locations along the suture line.[6]

A minor problem when compared to a running suture is that the simple interrupted suture is more time consuming to place and remove especially for long suture lines. In settings where wound healing may be impaired due to advanced age or underlying disease, interrupted suture techniques may be preferred as interrupted sutures may have, with all other factors being equal, greater tensile strength, less edema, less induration, and less impaired microcirculation than running sutures.[7]

Vertical Mattress Suture

The vertical mattress suture is one of the best sutures for wound edge eversion and that is the main indication for its use by dermatologic surgeons. It also reduces dead space and minimizes tension across the wound, doing the job of both a buried dermal suture and a skin suture. Because this suture requires four entry points in the skin, significant crosshatching can be expected if the suture is not removed within 5 to 7 days. Even though the vertical mattress suture can be used anywhere on the body, its use on the trunk and extremities results in significant suture marks because it has to be left in place longer than 7 days. On the face, some surgeons use vertical mattress sutures instead of two-layer closure, while others prefer two-layer closure of surgical defects. Even when deep dermal sutures are used, a few vertical mattress sutures can be placed along the wound for maximal wound edge eversion, while the intervening areas can be precisely approximated with simple interrupted sutures.[5]

The vertical mattress suture (Fig. 16-4) is started by passing the needle into the skin 5 to 10 mm from the wound edge into the depth of the wound. Next, it is passed across the wound, entering the deep surface of the wound edge and passing up through the skin equidistant from the entry point. The needle is reversed on the needle-holder and the skin is entered 1 to 3 mm from the wound edge, passing superficially into the opposite side and exiting at a point equidistant from the entry point. The suture is then tied slowly so as to gather the tissue in without undue puckering. In the event when the suture is used for tension reduction rather than just wound edge eversion, a bolster should be placed between the suture and the skin so as to prevent the suture from digging into the skin which could lead to suture marks and wound edge necrosis. Whether to start the suture with the far or the near part first is a matter of personal preference.[4,8] In either case, this is a relatively time-consuming suture to place.

Another variation of the vertical mattress suture is the near-far suture. The needle enters the skin 1 to 3 mm from the wound edge and passes out through the opposite side, wide of the wound edge. The needle is reversed entering near the wound edge and leaving the skin across the wound, wide of the wound edge. This modification may be helpful in elevating deep tissue.[9,10]

Half-buried Vertical Mattress Suture

The half-buried vertical mattress suture is a modification of the standard vertical mattress suture designed to eliminate one-half of the four suture marks in areas such as the face where minimal scarring is important. This suture is intermediate between a simple interrupted and standard vertical mattress suture in terms of relieving tension across the wound and achieving eversion of the wound edges. It is sometimes used along the hairline where the buried component is placed on

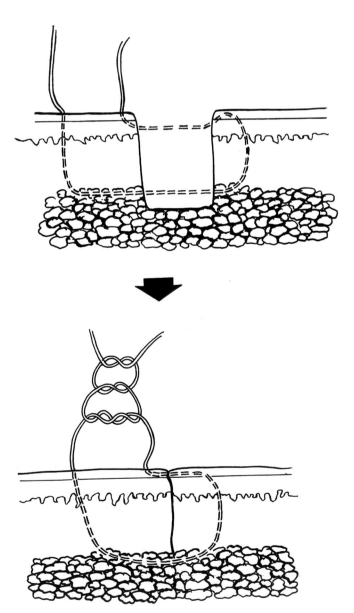

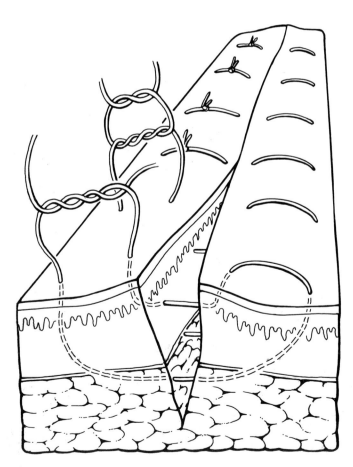

Figure 16-4   Vertical mattress suture.

Figure 16-5   Half-buried vertical mattress suture.

the face and the exposed part of the suture is placed in the hairline.[4]

The half-buried vertical mattress suture (Fig. 16-5) is placed with the needle entering on one side of the wound edge, passing through the deep tissue on the opposite side, and back out through the side of entry. It is relatively difficult to properly align wound edges with this suture and as a result it is rarely used in dermatologic surgery.

Horizontal Mattress Suture

Classically, the horizontal mattress suture has been used for reducing tension across wound closures under significant tension. This suture can be placed as an initial tension-reducing or holding suture and to bring the wound edges closer together so that subcutaneous sutures can be placed to distribute tension and close the wound. At this point, if the tension has been adequately distributed, the horizontal mattress suture may be removed. If tension across the wound persists, the horizontal mattress suture may be left in place for a few days while early wound healing proceeds and removed before suture tracks have had a chance to form. In areas at high risk for wound dehiscence, such as the lower extremities, the horizontal mattress suture may even be left in place for a few days after the skin sutures have been removed. However, when the horizontal mattress suture is left in place for more than 7 days and sometimes even less time, significant suture tracks are almost certain to form.[5,6]

Alternatively, the horizontal mattress suture may be used to presuture 12 to 24 h before a proposed excision that may be under considerable tension. This short-term tissue expansion may allow as much as 30 percent more tissue to be removed at the time of definitive excision.[11] Presuturing has been used successfully in alopecia reduction, rhytidectomy, and congenital nevus excision.[11–13]

The suture is started a fair distance from the wound edge, with the needle passing deeply across the wound edge and exiting across the wound equidistant from the wound edge (Fig. 16-6). Next, the needle enters the skin some distance parallel with the wound edge and equidistant from the wound edge, crossing deeply under the wound to the opposite side where it is tied. If this retention suture is to be left in place, bolsters should be placed under the visible suture line on each side of the wound (Fig. 16-6b) so as to prevent the suture from cutting into the skin.[4] Buttons can be very effective bolsters.[14]

The main disadvantage of this suture is the possibility of wound edge necrosis as this suture can easily strangulate the dermal plexus between its limbs. This problem is minimized by taking large bites with the needle to encompass large amounts of tissue, by using bolsters, by tying the suture only as tight as necessary to accomplish the task of bringing the wound edges together, and by removing the suture as soon as possible, ideally within 2 days of wound closure. Prior to contemplating the use of a horizontal mattress suture for tension reduction, the surgeon should consider other means of reduc-

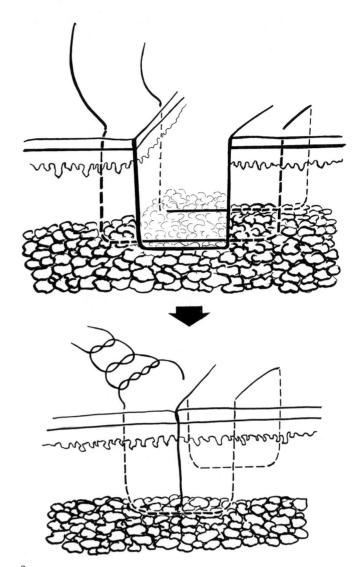

a

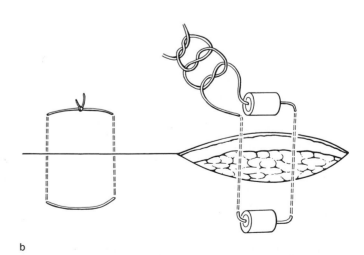

b

Figure 16-6 (a) Horizontal mattress suture; (b) horizontal mattress suture with a bolster in place.

ing tension across the wound, including appropriate undermining and closure orientation, the use of flaps from areas of tissue excess, the use of preoperative or intraoperative tissue expanders, the use of serial excisions, and the use of subcutaneous sutures.

Another effect of the horizontal mattress suture is prominent wound edge eversion. This property can be utilized by using a relatively fine suture material and taking relatively small bites when the suture is placed across a tension-free wound that has been closed with buried sutures. This achieves wound edge eversion, and, if the suture is not tied too tightly, wound edge necrosis is unlikely to develop.[15]

A cross-stitch variant of the horizontal mattress suture has been described to secure individual hair transplant punch grafts in their recipient holes. The suture is placed similarly to a regular horizontal mattress suture except that whenever the suture crosses the wound it is placed diagonally across instead of directly across. The suture enters the skin only in the donor site dermis and only crosses across the punch graft. Thus, trauma to the graft is minimized. This time-consuming suture technique minimizes *cobblestoning* or elevation of the punch grafts and there is no need for postoperative dressings.[16]

Half-buried Horizontal Mattress Suture

The half-buried horizontal mattress suture is primarily indicated for the positioning of various corners and tips, including flap tips, M-plasty tips, and V-Y closure tips. It can also align the edges of tangential flaps and flaps with ischemic wound edges. The buried limb of this suture is placed in the potentially ischemic area in order to minimize interference with the dermal vascular plexus.[15] This reasoning has been challenged because a superficial simple interrupted suture through a flap tip does not appear to result in increased risk of flap tip necrosis.[17]

The half-buried horizontal mattress suture should only be placed after all tension at the wound edge has been eliminated with other sutures. The needle enters the skin on the wound edge away from the tip and passes into the wound relatively superficially adjacent to the tip (Fig. 16-7). Next, the needle is passed horizontally through the tip at the same level. The suture is completed by passing through the opposite wound edge at the same level. The suture is tied very gently under minimal tension to minimize any trauma to the flap tip. Very fine 5–0 or 6–0 suture should be used for most tip stitches. The portion of the suture lying on the surface should not cross the tip itself as this may increase the risk of tip necrosis.[6]

Interrupted Subcutaneous Suture

A wound gains only 7 percent of its final strength after 2 weeks.[18] As most skin sutures are removed within 1 week of placement, absorbable buried sutures are used as part of layered wound closure. This provides support for the wound until tensile strength has increased sufficiently to prevent wound dehiscence.

Deep, buried sutures are placed into wounds to reduce or eliminate tension on the wound edges. On the trunk and extremities, where tension across wounds is greatest, the use of buried sutures may reduce the amount of scar spread. Buried sutures can align the wound edges so that the skin edges are closely approximated even before the placement of skin sutures. Deep sutures can eliminate dead space and align deep structures such as skeletal muscle or fascia. Deep sutures can also be used to anchor overlying tissue to underlying fixed structures such as periosteum to maintain proper facial contour and function. This is exemplified by the anchoring to the maxillary periosteum of a meilolabial flap used to close a nasal defect.

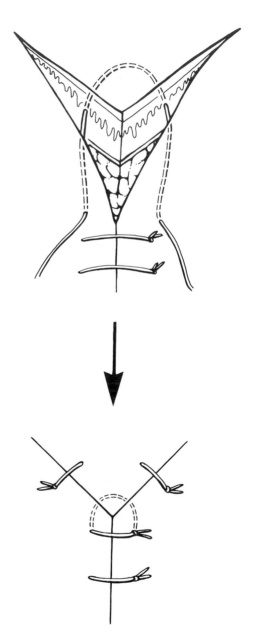

Figure 16-7 Half-buried horizontal mattress suture used to secure a corner in place.

Buried Dermal Suture

The buried dermal suture is used routinely as part of layered closures in dermatologic surgery to eliminate tension across the superficial wound edges and to properly align the wound edges. A properly placed buried dermal suture will allow the easy placement of skin sutures without tension. As this suture is placed at the dermis-fat junction, the knot has to be buried so as to minimize tissue reaction to the suture and extrusion through the wound.

The suture is started with the needle entering the undermined deep surface of the wound up into the deep reticular dermis, across the wound, entering the opposite reticular dermis at the same level, and passing down into the subcutaneous fat (Fig. 16-8). Therefore, when the knot is tied, it will be buried away from the surface of the wound.

If several buried sutures are placed in a wound with stiff and thick edges, the last few buried sutures may be difficult to place as the wound edges become closely approximated. In such cases, it may be easier to place all of the deep sutures before tying any of them. This allows better access to the wound as the wound edges remain separated.[19]

Deep Subcutaneous Suture

The deep subcutaneous suture is entirely subcutaneous. It is used to decrease the amount of dead space, to anchor flaps, and to align deep structures. Because it is deep, tissue reaction to the suture or suture extrusion through the wound is very unlikely even if nonabsorbable suture material is used. Therefore, the knot need not be buried.

The suture is placed by passing the needle through the subcutaneous tissue from superficial to deep, across the wound, and up through the subcutaneous tissue on the other side (Fig. 16-9). In order to minimize fat necrosis and maximize the amount of tissue moved, the bite should be relatively large and ideally some fibrous tissue such as fascia should be in-

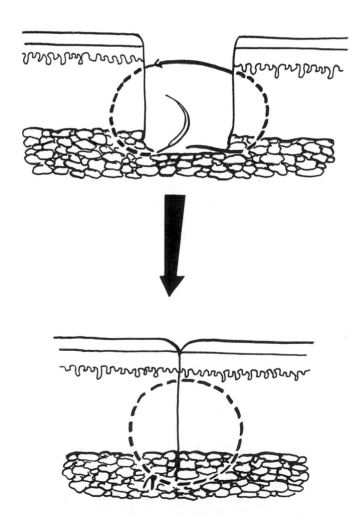

Figure 16-8   Standard buried dermal suture.

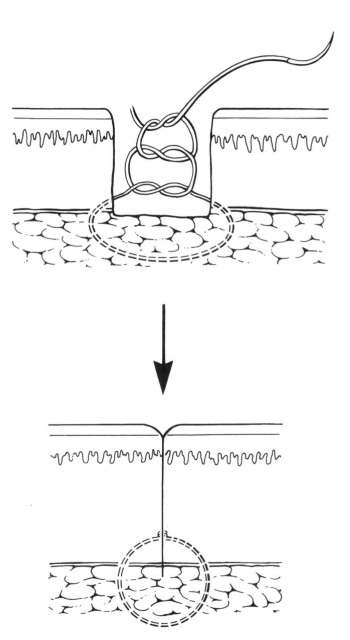

Figure 16-9   Deep subcutaneous suture.

cluded. To maximize the amount of dead space eliminated as the needle is passed across the floor of the wound, additional tissue may be picked up from the wound base before proceeding to the other side, resulting in a three-pointed vertical suture.

Buried Horizontal Mattress Suture

The buried horizontal mattress suture is a purse-string suture that is occasionally used to eliminate dead space or reduce tension across wounds in areas where there is not enough room to place vertical sutures such as defects on the nose with its stiff dermis and minimal subcutaneous tissue. Also, it can be used as a purse-string suture to close off dead space such as is seen after the removal of an epidermal cyst. This suture has to be placed deeply and tied not too tightly as the enclosed tissue can become easily strangulated.[20]

The needle enters the deep dermis or subcutaneous fat and is passed horizontally to pass back into the wound at the same level (Fig. 16-10). Next, it crosses the wound and passes horizontally through the opposite wound edge. Care is taken not to tie the suture too tightly.[5]

Buried Vertical Mattress Suture

One disadvantage of the standard buried dermal suture is that the wound edges are pulled flat without significant wound edge eversion.[21] The buried vertical mattress suture incorporates a modification of the buried dermal suture that maximizes prolonged wound edge eversion with resulting improved wound healing.[22]

The buried vertical mattress suture (Fig. 16-11) can be visualized as a standard vertical mattress suture that is completely moved below the skin surface while maintaining its shape. The suture is more superficial farther from the wound edge than at the wound edge. The needle enters the wound edge from the deep undermined surface and is passed superficially and then turned to move toward the deep dermis where it reenters the wound. Next, it passes across the wound,

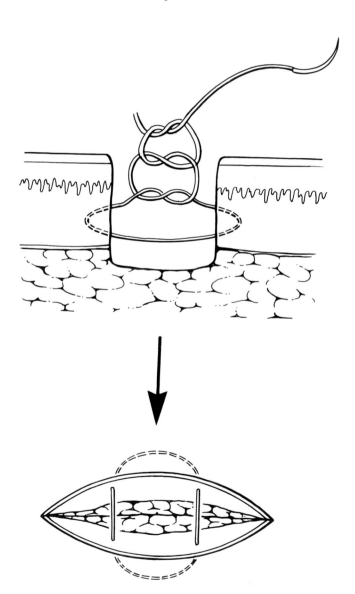

Figure 16-10 Buried horizontal mattress or purse-string suture.

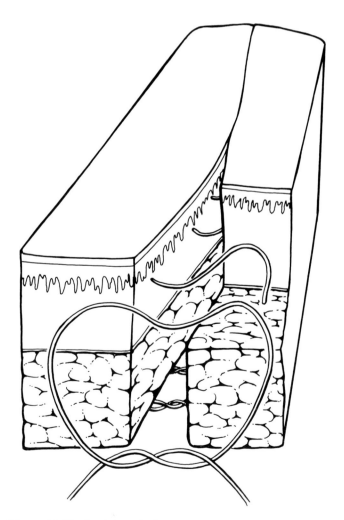

Figure 16-11 Buried vertical mattress suture.

entering the deep dermis, and passing first superficially and then deeply into the subcutaneous fat at the base of the undermined wound edge. As the suture is tied with a buried knot, the enclosed tissue from the superficial lateral sides is pulled in, resulting in significant wound edge eversion. It is important to avoid coming too closely to the underside of the epidermal surface with the suture as this may result in puckering, suture extrusion, and necrosis in the area. In order to successfully place this suture, a half-circle needle is necessary.[21,23]

RUNNING SUTURE

Simple Running Suture

The simple running suture can be used in situations where the wound edges are of equal thickness without tension, closely approximated, and with an absence of subcutaneous dead space. This usually implies that the wound has been substantially closed with buried sutures.

The simple running suture is started as a simple interrupted suture that is tied, but the end with the needle is not cut (Fig. 16-12a). The suture is continued by passing the needle through the dermis or into the subcutaneous fat from side to side, over and over, until the end of the wound has been reached (Fig. 16-12b). The suture is tied to the final loop of suture (Fig. 16-12c). It is important to constantly keep adjusting tension on the suture so that it is even without puckering or gaping of the wound edges. An assistant may be helpful in maintaining an appropriate amount of tension on the suture line and keeping the suture out of the surgeon's way by gently pulling on the loose suture material. The placement of the bites should be evenly spaced from the wound edges and along the suture line. Whether the perpendicular limb of the suture crosses the wound within the wound or along the surface is a matter of the surgeon's personal preference.

This suture is most useful for wounds that have already been closed by buried sutures, for the attachment of full-thickness or split-thickness skin grafts, and in areas of thin skin such as the eyelids, ears, neck, and scrotum. This suture is relatively quick and easy to place, making it an ideal suture to close long suture lines.[24] By eliminating all but two knots, there is less suture material resting against the skin, resulting in the development of less suture mark scars. However, fine adjustments along the suture line are difficult to make, and the suture has a tendency to pucker when one is suturing very lax and thin skin such as eyelid skin. In thin skin, the knots at each end may be tied over small bolsters to prevent the knots from cutting into the tissue.[4–6]

Running Locked Suture

The running locked suture (Fig. 16-13) is a variant of the simple running suture in which, after the placement of each loop,

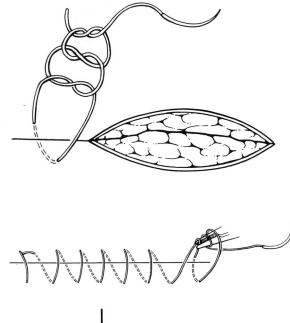

a

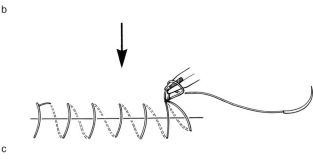

b

c

Figure 16-12   Simple running suture. *(a)* Start with simple interrupted suture; *(b)* continue with over-and-over running suture; *(c)* finish by tying the suture to the last preceding loop.

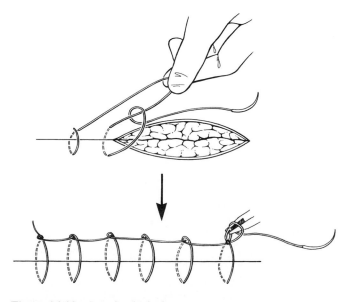

Figure 16-13   Running locked suture.

the needle is passed through the previous loop prior to starting the next loop. It is also known as a *baseball stitch*. It is intended for the closure of well-vascularized wounds under a moderate amount of tension. The wound edges should be stiff and of equal thickness without a tendency for inversion. It is stronger than a simple running suture, but, if placed too tightly or if significant postoperative swelling develops, tissue strangulation with wound edge necrosis may ensue. Once a loop is locked in place, it is extremely difficult to adjust tension. It is used primarily on the scalp for the closure of scalp reduction defects and hair transplant donor sites. Occasionally, it has been used for defects of the forehead, back, and proximal thighs. This suture is strong and rather quick and easy to place but should be used sparingly and only when clearly indicated because of the potential for tissue strangulation if not placed properly.[5,6]

Running Horizontal Mattress Suture

The running horizontal mattress suture is primarily a skin edge everting suture. It is the ideal suture for closure of wounds with a significant tendency for wound edge inversion such as the thin skin of the eyelids, neck, scrotum, or dorsa of hands. In addition, by pulling in additional tissue to the wound edge, spreading of facial scars as seen in young patients can be minimized. At the other end of the age spectrum, surgical defects in elderly patients with very lax thin skin have naturally inverting wound edges. They may benefit from the maximal wound edge eversion achieved with a running horizontal mattress suture.

The running horizontal mattress suture (Fig. 16-14) is

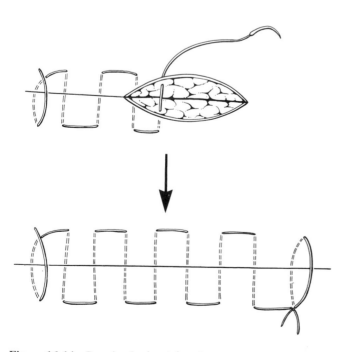

Figure 16-14   Running horizontal mattress.

started as a simple running suture, but, instead of crossing the wound with each loop, the needle reenters the skin farther along the wound on the same side where it exited the skin. Next, the needle passes in the dermis to the opposite side, exits the skin, and reenters on the same side. This is repeated along the entire suture line with the suture tied to the last loop that was placed.

This suture should be used only for wounds where the wound edges are relatively well approximated with buried sutures when maximal wound edge eversion is desired. If the suture is tied too tightly, wound edge strangulation and necrosis may develop. Therefore, meticulous placement is required, and the suture should be used sparingly in wounds that may be ischemic such as skin flaps and wounds on the trunk and extremities.

Running Subcuticular Suture

The running subcuticular suture is basically a buried running horizontal mattress suture. It is one of the more difficult sutures to place, but properly placed it results in a most elegant closure. It is ideal for the closure of wounds in areas where the suture has to remain in place for more than 7 days. As the suture is buried, there are no suture marks to worry about, and the suture may be left in place for several weeks without difficulty, or when absorbable suture material is used the suture may be left in place until it is absorbed. It is most useful for the closure of wounds on the trunk and extremities where prolonged wound support is essential to avoid wound dehiscence and to minimize scar spreading.[25] As this suture is capable of only modest wound edge alignment, it should be reserved for wounds in which the tension has been eliminated with deep sutures and the wound edges are closely approximated and of approximately equal thickness. Even though it can be used on the face, other suture techniques provide better wound edge alignment and eversion. Also, as sutures are usually removed within 7 days on the face, suture marks are rarely a problem when nonreactive monofilament sutures are used.

The running subcuticular suture should be placed with a nonreactive monofilament suture such as polypropylene to facilitate suture removal and to prevent suture breakage within the wound.[26] The needle enters the skin 5 to 10 mm from one end of the wound and is passed into the wound at the tip (Fig. 16-15). Next, the needle is passed from one side of the wound to the other in the mid-dermis, taking a horizontal bite on each side and continuing down the length of the wound, backtracking slightly with each pass across the wound. As the distal end of the wound is reached, the needle is passed out from the wound, exiting approximately 5 to 10 mm from the edge. The smaller the bites that are taken with each pass, the better the wound edge approximation. If no wound gaping is evident, the two suture ends can be tied loosely together or affixed to the skin with surgical tapes. If any gaping is evident, each suture end is tied to itself, taking out any laxity as needed with multiple slipknots. Some surgeons prefer to tie

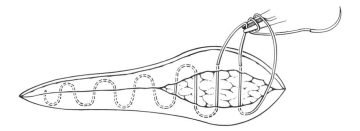

Figure 16-16 Running subcutaneous suture.

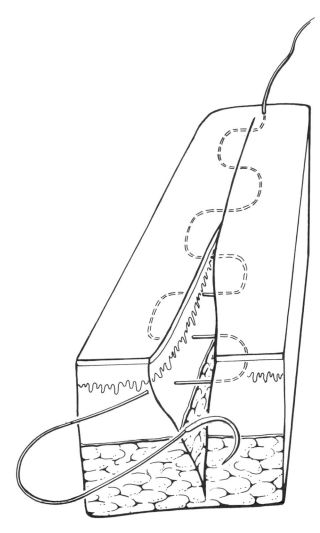

Figure 16-15 Running subcuticular suture.

the suture ends over a small bolster to minimize suture slippage and the possibility of the knots' sinking under the skin surface which would make suture removal difficult. Another alternative is to tie the suture ends to a metallic suture tensor device that pulls the suture ends in opposite directions, maintaining the closure properly aligned.[27] If some gaping still persists, it can be closed with a small simple interrupted suture that is removed within 7 days. For long wounds, one loop of suture should be brought out every 2 cm to the skin surface to facilitate suture removal.

An alternate method for running subcuticular suture placement is the use of absorbable sutures. In this case, the suture is started within the wound at one end as a buried dermal suture, but only one end is cut. The suture is continued as a regular running subcuticular suture. At the other end of the wound, the suture is ended by tying it to the last loop that has been placed. Thus, this suture is entirely buried, not requiring suture removal.[28,29] However, if the patient develops a suture reaction, pruritus, suture abscesses, and suture spitting may

develop. Some surgeons advocate the use of permanent sutures left in place indefinitely as this can reduce scar stretching.[30] If nonabsorbable sutures are to be used for totally buried sutures, clear nonreactive suture material such as polypropylene should be used.[5,6]

Running Subcutaneous Suture

The running subcutaneous suture is designed for the closure of the deep component of relatively long surgical defects that are only under moderate tension. It replaces the buried dermal interrupted suture in selected situations.

The suture is started with a buried dermal suture that is tied, but only one end is cut (Fig. 16-16). The other end with the needle is used for a vertical running suture starting in the subcutaneous fat and moving up into the reticular dermis. Next, the needle crosses across to the other wound edge and enters the reticular dermis, moving down into the subcutaneous fat. This is repeated over and over until the wound is closed. At each step, the suture is tightened to eliminate tension and gaping of the wound. The suture is completed by tying the loose end to the last loop placed.

The main advantage of this suture is the speed of placement over that of interrupted sutures. However, if the suture material were to rupture anywhere along the suture line, the entire wound might dehisce or a subcutaneous dead space could form under the skin edge without being apparent at the surface. Therefore, this suture should be reserved for wounds under a relatively small amount of tension.[5,31]

BASTING SUTURE

Interrupted Basting Suture

The interrupted basting suture is designed to help a skin graft adhere to its wound bed, especially when the surgeon is grafting a concave wound bed.

After the periphery of the graft has been sutured in place, the suture is placed vertically through the graft into the wound bed, taking a bite of tissue from the wound bed and exiting back out through the graft. The suture is tied snugly. To maximize graft adherence to the wound bed, the suture is often

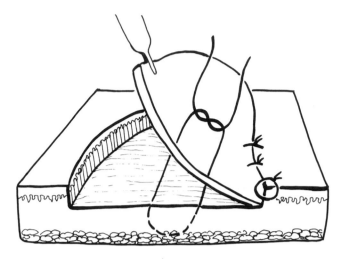

Figure 16-17 Visualized basting suture.

tied over a bolster such as a piece of cotton or a dental roll covered with antibacterial ointment.[32]

When a basting suture is placed blindly, a blood vessel may be lacerated in the wound bed with resulting bleeding and possible hematoma formation. To eliminate this possibility, the suture should be placed under direct visualization (Fig. 16-17). The graft edge is only partially sutured in place, and the basting suture is placed through the graft and, with the graft elevated, the bite through the wound bed is made under direct visualization. After all of the basting sutures have been placed, the remainder of the graft margin is sutured in place. The basting suture can be placed by using either an absorbable or nonabsorbable suture material such as polypropylene or mild chromic gut, respectively.[33]

Buried Basting Suture

The buried basting suture is used as a flap- or skin graft-anchoring suture. The needle is passed under direct visualiza-

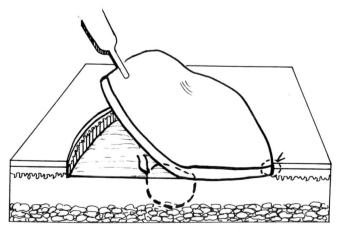

Figure 16-18 Buried visualized basting suture.

tion horizontally through the undersurface of the flap or graft, staying relatively deep (Fig. 16-18). Next, the needle is passed horizontally, taking a bite through the wound bed, and is tied in place.[33] If anchoring is necessary to maintain a concavity, the deep bite has to encompass some immobile structure such as the periosteum. In anchoring a flap, the suture has to be placed along the long axis of the flap so as not to compromise the vascular pedicle.[34]

Running Basting Suture

The running basting suture is designed to quickly secure large skin grafts to the wound bed so as to minimize the risk of grafts shearing from the wound bed. The suture is started as an interrupted basting suture, but the needle end of the suture is not cut and the suture is continued. The needle enters through the graft, into the wound bed, and back out farther along. This is repeated until the graft is secured in numerous locations, and the suture is finally tied to the last preceding external loop or to the starting point of the suture. The most common suturing design is a spiral basting suture from the center of the graft to its periphery. To eliminate the need for suture removal with the risk of graft displacement, this suture is usually placed by using absorbable suture material.[32]

A variant of this technique, called the *upper dermal running stitch,* has been described to secure rows of standard hair transplant grafts in their recipient sites, prevent cobblestoning of the grafts, and eliminate the need for postoperative dressings. The suture is run through the dermis of the recipient area between each recipient hole, and each graft is placed under the suture into each recipient hole with the overlying suture securing it in place without passing through the graft itself.[35,36]

SUTURE REMOVAL

Suture marks are due to epidermal downgrowth along the suture track seen within 5 to 7 days of suture placement and aggravated by sutures being tied too tightly.[6,15] Sutures should be removed at the earliest possible time to prevent or minimize suture reaction and suture marks. However, they should remain in place long enough to prevent wound dehiscence and scar spread. In general, the less blood supply to an area and the greater tension across a wound, the longer the sutures should be left in place. On the face and ears, most skin sutures should be removed within 5 to 7 days, with eyelid sutures being removed in 3 to 5 days. Neck sutures should be removed in 7 days and scalp sutures in 7 to 10 days. On the trunk and extremities, risk of wound dehiscence takes precedence over suture marks. Sutures on the trunk and upper extremities should be left in place for 10 to 14 days. Lower extremities may require 14 to 21 days of suture support.[37]

For proper suture removal, the suture line should be cleansed with an antiseptic. The interrupted suture is grasped

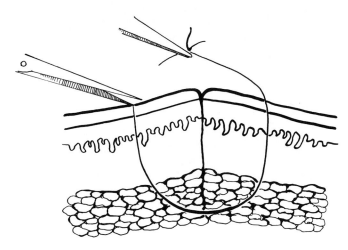

Figure 16-19   Correct suture removal.

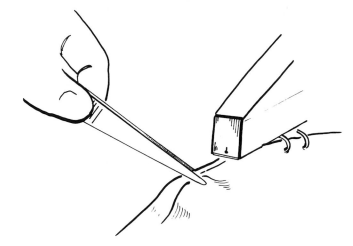

Figure 16-20   Staple wound closure. Skin edges are everted with forceps, and the staples are placed by squeezing the staple gun while straddling the incision line.

with fine forceps at the knot, and it is cut on the side opposite the knot at the suture entry point into the skin. Next, the suture is gently pulled out by pulling toward the wound edge (Fig. 16-19). This will minimize tension away from the wound edge that could possibly cause the wound to dehisce, and no exposed and possibly contaminated suture will pass through the wound. A running suture is removed by cutting it at every other loop and grasping the intervening loop with forceps and pulling it out. This will minimize shearing forces across the wound and contamination of the wound. A running subcuticular suture is removed by cutting the knot at one end and pulling the suture out slowly from the other end to minimize the risk of suture breakage in the wound.[38]

Absorbable sutures are left in place. However, some patients develop suture reactions consisting of suture abscesses and suture extrusion through the wound. If this happens, the suture should be carefully picked up with small forceps and cut out of the wound. Any purulent material should also be drained.

STAINLESS STEEL STAPLE CLOSURE

Staple closure of wounds is an alternative to suture closure. The staples have the advantage of very quick placement, minimal tissue reaction to the staples, and a very strong wound closure.[39,40] It is most often used for closure of long wounds, especially on the scalp where the suture line is hidden by scalp hair. Potentially contaminated wounds that are closed with staples appear to be more resistant to infection than wounds closed with sutures.[41]

Proper placement of staples requires careful alignment and eversion of wound edges before the staple gun is placed firmly against the skin and discharged (Fig. 16-20). As the staple closes, it pulls tissue toward the wound edge, closing the wound and everting the wound edges. Staples are removed with a staple remover. If a staple remover is not available, they can be removed with a hemostat. The hemostat is inserted closed under the visible staple and forcefully opened, releasing the staple from the skin. Staples provide efficient wound closure, but when exact wound edge alignment is required sutures should be used instead. Also, surgical staples are far more expensive than suture material.[40]

WOUND CLOSURE TAPES

Wound closure tapes are used to provide additional support to a suture line, especially when a running subcuticular suture has been used.[6] In addition, they are helpful in supporting the wound edges after the skin sutures have been removed. Wounds closed with wound closure tapes have a lower risk of wound infection than sutured wounds.[42,43] However, as they fail to achieve adequate wound edge eversion and tension reduction, wound closure tapes are rarely used as primary wound closure materials.

Wound closure tapes are applied after the surface has been prepared by painting with Mastisol or tincture of benzoin to improve adhesion. Many surgeons prefer Mastisol as it provides stronger adhesion, and tincture of benzoin has been associated with allergic contact dermatitis.[44] The tape is applied perpendicularly to the suture line on one side of a wound and pulled toward the opposite side where it is attached to the surface (Fig. 16-21a). Whether the tapes are placed purely perpendicularly across the wound or in a crisscross pattern is a matter of personal preference, but it is important to use numerous tapes so as to maximize wound support. As the wound closure tapes become dislodged, the patient may be instructed in applying new ones for several weeks after the sutures have been removed. Wound closure tapes are removed by picking up one edge and lifting it off toward the suture line and then picking up the opposite edge and lifting it also toward the su-

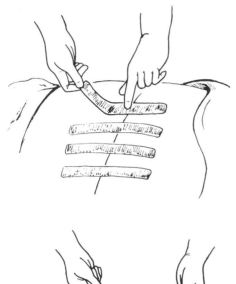

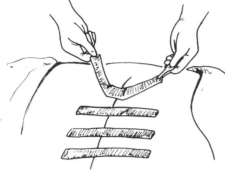

a

b

Figure 16-21 Wound closure tapes. *(a)* Placement; *(b)* removal.

ture line until the two loose tape edges meet and the tape is lifted off the skin (Fig. 16-21*b*). Removing the wound closure tape all from one side generates undesirable shearing forces on the immature and relatively weak suture line as the tape is pulled off the opposing wound edge away from the suture line.

Wound closure tapes will rarely provide sufficient support, wound edge alignment, and eversion to replace skin sutures but can be used as an adjunct.[45] Keeping them in place for several weeks may reduce the amount of scar spreading.[46]

COMBINATION CLOSURES

Combination closures utilizing more than one suture technique are used very often. Most dermatologic surgeons combine buried sutures for tension reduction and gross wound edge approximation, and skin sutures for wound edge alignment and eversion. A few vertical mattress sutures may provide wound edge eversion, while numerous intervening simple interrupted sutures may provide exact wound edge alignment. The only limit to combination closures are the demands of the individual situation and the imagination of the dermatologic surgeon.[47]

REFERENCES

1. Crikelair GF: Suture marks. *Am J Surg* **96:**631, 1958
2. Bernstein G: The loop stitch. *J Dermatol Surg Oncol* **10:**587, 1984
3. Edgerton MT: *The Art of Surgical Technique.* Baltimore, Williams & Wilkins, 1988
4. Lober CW: Suturing techniques, in *Dermatologic Surgery: Principles and Practice,* edited by RK Roenigk, HH Roenigk Jr. New York, Marcel Dekker, Inc, 1989, p 205
5. Stegman SJ et al: *Basics of Dermatologic Surgery.* Chicago, Year Book, 1982
6. Stegman SJ: Suturing techniques for dermatologic surgery. *J Dermatol Surg Oncol* **4:**63, 1978
7. Speer DP: The influence of suture technique on early wound healing. *J Surg Res* **27:**385, 1979
8. Snow SN et al: The shorthand vertical mattress stitch: A rapid skin everting suture technique. *J Dermatol Surg Oncol* **15:**379, 1989
9. Bernstein G: The far-near/near-far suture. *J Dermatol Surg Oncol* **11:**470, 1985
10. Knowles WR: Wedge resection of the lower lip. *J Dermatol Surg* **2:**141, 1976
11. Meirson D et al: Presuturing in alopecia reductions. *J Dermatol Surg Oncol* **16:**818, 1990
12. Hedén P: Presuturing in rhytidectomy: A case report. *Aesthetic Plast Surg* **15:**161, 1991
13. Liang MD et al: Presuturing: A new technique for closing large skin defects: Clinical and experimental studies. *Plast Reconstr Surg* **81:**694, 1988
14. Adnot J et al: Button bolsters in dermatologic surgery. *J Dermatol Surg Oncol* **15:**59, 1989
15. Perry AW, McShane RH: Fine tuning of the skin edges in the closure of surgical wounds: Controlling inversion and eversion with the path of the needle: The right stitch at the right time. *J Dermatol Surg Oncol* **7:**471, 1981
16. Orentreich N, Orentreich DS: Cross-stitch: Suture technique for hair transplantation. *J Dermatol Surg Oncol* **10:**970, 1984
17. McQuown SA et al: Gillies' corner stitch revisited. *Arch Otolaryngol* **110:**450, 1984
18. Harris DR: Healing of the surgical wound, pt 1: Basic considerations. *J Am Acad Dermatol* **1:**197, 1979
19. Albom MJ: Dermo-subdermal sutures for long, deep surgical wounds. *J Dermatol Surg Oncol* **3:**504, 1977
20. Presser SE: The subcutaneous stitch revisited. *J Dermatol Surg Oncol* **15:**342, 1989
21. Davidson TM: Subcutaneous suture placement. *Laryngoscope* **97:**501, 1987
22. Zitelli JA: TIPS for a better ellipse. *J Am Acad Dermatol* **22:**101, 1990
23. Zitelli JA, Moy RL: Buried vertical mattress suture. *J Dermatol Surg Oncol* **15:**17, 1989

24. McLean NR et al: Comparison of skin closure using continuous and interrupted nylon sutures. *Br J Surg* **67:**633, 1980

25. Clayer M, Southwood RT: Comparative study of skin closure in hip surgery. *Aust N Z J Surg* **61:**363, 1991

26. Pham S et al: Ease of continuous dermal suture removal. *J Emerg Med* **8:**539, 1990

27. Weber PJ et al: Suture tensor. *J Dermatol Surg Oncol* **16:**535, 1990

28. Sanders RJ: Subcuticular skin closure: Description of technique. *J Dermatol Surg* **1:**61, 1975

29. Herron J: Skin closure with subcuticular polyglycolic acid sutures. *Med J Aust* **2:**535, 1974

30. Elliot D, Mahaffey PJ: The stretched scar: The benefit of prolonged dermal support. *Br J Plast Surg* **42:**74, 1989

31. Ftaiha Z, Snow SN: The buried running dermal subcutaneous suture technique. *J Dermatol Surg Oncol* **15:**264, 1989

32. Glogau RG et al: Refinements in split-thickness skin grafting technique. *J Dermatol Surg Oncol* **13:**853, 1987

33. Adnot J, Salasche SJ: Visualized basting sutures in the application of full-thickness skin grafts. *J Dermatol Surg Oncol* **13:**1236, 1987

34. Salasche SJ et al: The suspension suture. *J Dermatol Surg Oncol* **13:**973, 1987

35. Borges AF: Prevention of cobblestoning in hair transplantation. *J Dermatol Surg Oncol* **4:**168, 1978

36. Weber PJ: Hair transplantation (a new method for recipient site suturing): The upper dermal running stitch. *J Dermatol Surg Oncol* **17:**80, 1991

37. Chernosky ME: Scalpel and scissors surgery as seen by the dermatologist, in *Skin Surgery,* 6th ed, edited by E Epstein, E Epstein Jr. Philadelphia, Saunders, 1987, p 88

38. Koruth NM, Jones PF: Removal of drains and sutures. *Br Med J* **281:**45, 1980

39. Roth JH, Windle BH: Staple versus suture closure of skin incisions in a pig model. *Can J Surg* **31:**19, 1988

40. Gatt D et al: Staples for wound closure: A controlled trial. *Ann R Coll Surg Engl* **67:**318, 1985

41. Stillman RM et al: Skin wound closure: The effect of various wound closure methods on susceptibility to infection. *Arch Surg* **115:**674, 1980

42. Moy RL et al: Commonly used suturing techniques in skin surgery. *Am. Fam. Physician* **4:**1625, 1991

43. Edlich RF et al: Wound healing and wound infection, in *Wound Healing and Wound Infection: Theory and Surgical Practice,* edited by TK Hunt. New York, Appleton-Century-Crofts, 1980

44. Mikhail GR et al: Reinforcement of surgical adhesive strips. *J Dermatol Surg Oncol* **12:**904, 1986

45. Bunker TD: Problems with the use of Op-Site sutureless skin closures in orthopaedic procedures. *Ann R Coll Surg Engl* **65:**260, 1983

46. Hodges JM: Management of facial lacerations. *South Med J* **69:**1413, 1976

47. Talamas I: A fast and good way of suturing the skin. *Aesthetic Plast Surg* **6:**59, 1982

Daniel E. Gormley

17 Management of Excess Tissue: Dog-ears, Cones, and Protrusions

The cutaneous surgeon strives for the most unobtrusive wound closure possible. In order to achieve this, wound edges must be carefully apposed in order to facilitate healing and to preserve normal contours. Occasionally, the surgeon is frustrated by the appearance of folds or protrusions of skin (*dog-ears*) which usually appear at the ends of the wound. A number of strategies have been developed in order to prevent or eliminate these unsightly appendages. It is essential, however, that the principles underlying these methods be understood if they are to be successfully used.

The etiology of dog-ears is derived from a variety of factors: (1) the geometry of the wound, (2) the dynamics of wound closure, (3) the contours of the operative field, and (4) surgical technique.

THE GEOMETRY OF THE WOUND IN THE HORIZONTAL PLANE

In the horizontal plane there are three important geometric factors which determine whether or not a crimp or protrusion (dog-ear) will form along the sides of an excisional wound:[1]

1. The ratio of the length of the sides of the wound to the length of the central axis along which closure is accomplished*

   * Also occasionally expressed as the width/length ratio.

2. The ratio of the lengths of the sides of the wound with respect to one another
3. The size of the apical angle

Side/Length Ratio

Except for the special case of the simple linear incision in which no tissue is excised, there is always a disparity between the length of the skin at the edges of the wound and the length of the line of closure which lies along the central axis of the wound (Fig. 17-1). The ratio of these two lengths determines the amount of excess tissue that will be available for crimp or dog-ear formation. The ratio can vary within wide limits from 1.0 for a linear excision, to 1.57 for a circular defect,[1] or 2.0 for a square wound, assuming that the edges are moved perpendicularly to the longest midline axis of the wound during closure.

Side/Side Ratio

If a wound is asymmetric, the excess length on the longer side will express itself as crimps or folds at the time of closure somewhere along the length of the longer side (Figs. 17-2 and 17-3).

The Apical Angle

The geometry of an excisional defect between the end of the wound and the suture nearest to it is important regardless of

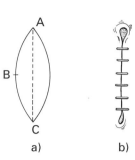
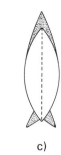
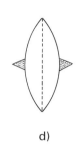

a)   b)   c)   d)

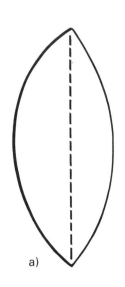

a)

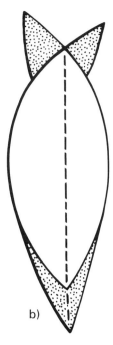

b)

Figure 17-1   Excess tissue ("dog-ears") and symmetric wounds. *(a)* The curved length of the sides of a fusiform wound is greater than the length of its straight central axis (arc ABC > line AC); *(b)* when the sides are brought together along the central axis at the time of closure, excess length will manifest itself in the form of folds, crimps, or cones which usually appear at the wound apices; *(c)* dog-ears are avoided by creating wounds in which the ratio of the length of the side and wound axis approach unity. When protrusions occur at the ends or edges of a symmetric wound, symmetric corrective steps are required. These are designed to bring the side axis length ratio closer to unity either by lengthening the wound (top of *c*) or by removing excess length from the edge of the wounds (bottom of *c* or *d*). Apical maneuvers are often favored since they maintain the axis of closure in the most desirable direction.

Figure 17-3   Dog-ears and the asymmetric overly short wound. A differential maneuver may be required in order to eliminate excess tissue and create symmetry. Dog-ears are managed by reducing the differences in length of the sides with respect to one another and the length of the midline.

overall side and axis length considerations (Fig. 17-4). In Fig. 17-4*a* the difference between lengths (AB + BC + CD) and AD is slight, and the ratio of the two values is close to one. Nevertheless, a suture placed along FE would obviously generate a dog-ear at the end of the wound. The dog-ear in this case would be due to the difference in the length of 2AB + BF as compared to AE. Conversely, however, an ideal apical angle cannot be expected to cancel the geometric effects of an excessive side/axis length ratio as demonstrated in Fig. 17-4*b*.

Wound Design

It can be appreciated that all of the geometric factors discussed above are important determinants of dog-ear formation. They must be dealt with in advance in the form of adequate planning, or corrective measures may be required afterward.

The optimal wound from the standpoint of dog-ear pre-

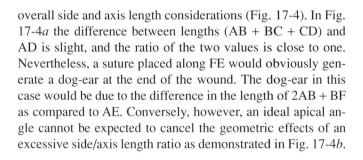
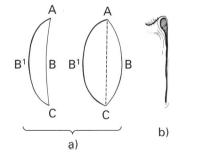
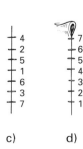
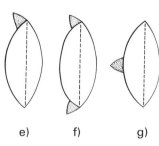
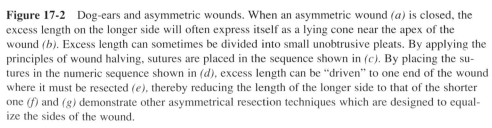

a)   b)   c)   d)   e)   f)   g)

Figure 17-2   Dog-ears and asymmetric wounds. When an asymmetric wound *(a)* is closed, the excess length on the longer side will often express itself as a lying cone near the apex of the wound *(b)*. Excess length can sometimes be divided into small unobtrusive pleats. By applying the principles of wound halving, sutures are placed in the sequence shown in *(c)*. By placing the sutures in the numeric sequence shown in *(d)*, excess length can be "driven" to one end of the wound where it must be resected *(e)*, thereby reducing the length of the longer side to that of the shorter one *(f)* and *(g)* demonstrate other asymmetrical resection techniques which are designed to equalize the sides of the wound.

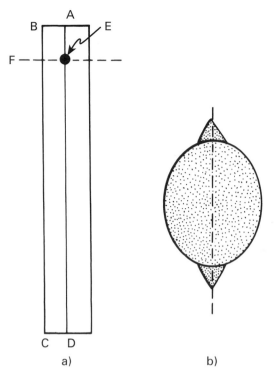

Figure 17-4   Importance of local geometric factors in the genesis of excess tissue folds. *(a)* In spite of the fact that the side to axis length ratio of this figure approaches unity, the difference in length between lines 2AB + BF as opposed to AE will find expression in dog-ear formation; *(b)* conversely, a marked disparity between the length of the sides and the axis length cannot be canceled out by an "ideal" apical angle.

vention will be symmetric, will be fusiform in shape, and will have gently tapering sides with apical angles of approximately 30°. Dog-ears that appear in symmetric wounds that are too short (high side/axis ratio) or which have excessively wide apical angles will usually appear at the wound apices. They are eliminated by a symmetric maneuver which reduces the side/axis ratio either by making the wound longer (Fig. 17-1) or by reducing the length of the edges that must be moved to the central axis at the time of closure.

When asymmetric wounds are created either accidentally or intentionally, there is a disparity between the lengths of the sides of the wound with respect to one another. Asymmetry may make it possible for the surgeon to meet an important goal. In the case of a crescentic-shaped wound, for example, a wound closure might be caused to lie in a curvilinear wrinkle and thereby be camouflaged. The penalty for such a maneuver or error appears in the form of an excess fold of skin which will appear along the longer side usually, but not invariably, near the wound apex. Sometimes the extra length can be subdivided into unobtrusive pleats by applying the principles of wound halving (Fig. 17-2). Often, tissue must be

excised from the longer side in order to bring side/length ratios closer to unity (Fig. 17-2).

The wound that is simultaneously plagued by asymmetry and excessive length/axis ratios (Fig. 17-3) will require asymmetric corrective steps, with the greatest amount of tissue being removed from the longer side.

Crimp formation that results from a wide apical angle in the absence of coexistent length ratio problems is often readily correctable by creating a tapering 30° apical angle at the end of the wound. Other techniques may have to be used if lengthening of the wound for the creation of an optimal apical angle is not feasible.

GEOMETRIC CLASSIFICATION OF DOG-EARS

Other authors have classified dog-ears by their geometric properties (Fig. 17-5).[2] Such an exercise is of more than academic interest. A cone of tissue which has been dubbed a *standing cone* tends to develop at the ends of symmetric wounds and/or at the ends of wounds on convex surfaces. (This is not however an absolute rule.) Correction would require a symmetric maneuver (i.e., wound lengthening or symmetric excision from each side of the wound). *Lying cones* often develop at the ends of asymmetric wounds on the longer side, mandating asymmetric excision of tissue from that edge. First mention will be made here of the *inverted cone* or *negative dog-ear* (Figs. 17-5c and 17-6). In this instance, the excess tissue manifests itself as a depression at one end of the wound with the apex of the cone lying deeper than the skin

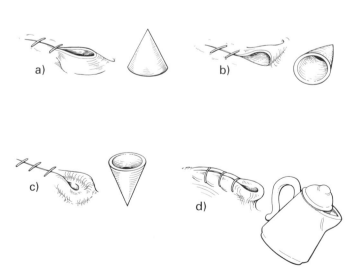

Figure 17-5   Geometric classification of dog-ears. *(a)* standing cone; *(b)* lying cone; *(c)* inverted cone, umbilicated; *(d)* inverted cone, pitcher lip.

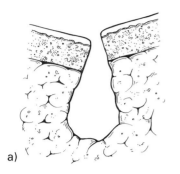 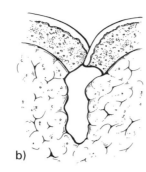

Figure 17-6 Genesis of umbilicated variant of inverted-cone dog-ear. If skin is rigid or edges are bound down by collagen or fibrosis, edges will roll inward. Apposition of epithelialized surfaces will impair wound healing.

surface. An inverted cone is more likely to occur in skin that is thick, comparatively rigid, or inadequately undermined. Under these circumstances, attachments deep in the wound may prevent the free incised edges from everting. The forces of closure may then cause the apposing edges to roll inward. The existence of dead space deep in the wound may also facilitate the formation of such umbilications. These deformi-

ties result in the apposition of epithelialized surfaces which impair healing. The edges of the dog-ear should be everted with a skin hook after undermining and mobilization. The appendage is converted into a standing or lying cone whereupon it can be managed more readily using standard methods.

A second type of inverted cone or *pitcher lip* deformity (Figs. 17-5*d* and 17-6) is discussed in a subsequent section.

TISSUE DYNAMICS

Forces Generated by Closure

It is instructive to place a loop of suture in material (cloth or elastic bandage) on which a grid has been inscribed in order to obtain a graphic representation of the forces and counterforces generated by the dynamics of closure (Fig. 17-7). From a graphic representation of the material compressed and displaced by the loop as it closes, the following dynamic factors can be identified:

1. Displacement Forces: Material is pulled or displaced by the traction forces of the suture as it is tightened. With the exception of the force vector that coincides with the mo-

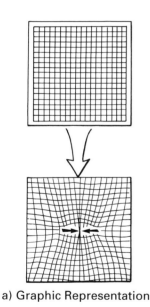 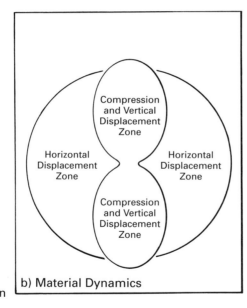 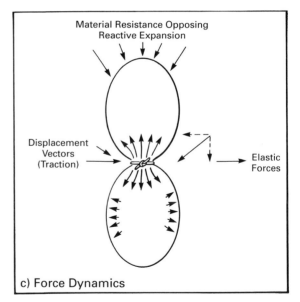

a) Graphic Representation b) Material Dynamics c) Force Dynamics

Figure 17-7 Dynamics of wound closure. *(a)* Graphic representation of configuration of material on which a grid has been inscribed and in which a loop of suture has been placed and tightened. Note material has been pulled toward the suture loop generating zones of tension and compression; *(b)* a representation of material dynamic zones: displacement, compression and vertical displacement. *(c)* Force dynamics: traction in displacement area and reactive expansion above and below the suture loop. These forces operate in three dimensions. Displacement (traction) vectors pull material from areas both lateral to and below the suture loop. Reactive expansion forces will push material above and below the suture loop as well as along a primary axis of force perpendicular to the plane of the suture loop. Material resistance forces operate in opposition to the dynamic vectors both within (in opposition to traction vectors) and beyond (opposing reactive expansion forces) the zone of compression. Protrusions that form will be proportional to (1) the displacement and compression forces of the suture and (2) the volume of material in the compression zone.

tion of the suture as it is drawn in, these forces are diagonal to the axis of closure and operate through an arc. (For purposes of discussion, the axis of closure is defined as that axis which lies 90° to the long axis of the suture and is the axis toward which material is drawn as the suture loop is closed.) These diagonal forces can be reduced to their component vectors which lie perpendicular and parallel to the axis of closure. Those vectors which lie 90° to the axis of closure, which could be called the *displacement forces,* will compress any tissue that lies between them and the axis of closure (vector X in Fig. 17-9). Those vectors which lie parallel to the axis of closure are usually of less significance but can contribute to tissue compression to some extent.

2. Tissue Compression and Reactive Expansion: When the suture loop is tightened, tissue will be compressed within its confining loop. As a result of the pressure that is generated by this event, reactive expansion will occur along vectors that are mostly perpendicular to the plane of the suture loop.

3. Reactive Forces: For every action there is an equal and opposite reaction. All matter resists compression and displacement. This resistance will be proportional to the volume of tissue affected. These resistance forces will oppose the displacement and reactive expansion vectors described above. These opposing force vectors will cause the tissue to buckle in a direction perpendicular to the plane of the surface.

4. Elastic Forces: Elastic forces generated by the closure will operate maximally along the axis of displacement and minimally perpendicular to them and will serve to partially efface tissue mounds.

5. Force Vectors: Force vectors operate along *straight* lines, a factor that is important when wounds are closed along curved surfaces.

These basic forces, while always present, will express themselves in different degrees and ratios depending upon the properties and volume of the material or tissue upon which the surgeon is working. Variables such as elasticity, tissue thickness and rigidity, and the relationship of the axis of closure to the maximal and minimal skin tension lines are obviously important. The basic conclusion of this analysis is, however, clear: Dog-ears and tissue mounds will form to the extent that wound design allows for the inclusion and compression of tissue within the displacement and reactive expansion zones described above.

The Relationship Between Geometry and Dynamics

Surgeons are accustomed to speaking of dog-ears as a function of length/width ratios. While such plane geometric constructs are important, all surgeons recognize that dog-ears are basically a volumetric or three-dimensional problem. As has already been discussed, dog-ears have been described as conic structures. Closure dynamics and geometric factors interact in important ways.

Displacement Vectors and Wound Edges

If displacement vectors intersect with a free edge at 90°, there will be rippling and wrinkling of the material as it is compressed but there will be little effect on the edge per se (Figs. 17-8 and 17-9).

Contrariwise, if the displacement vectors intersect with a free edge in a direction parallel with it, the edge will be buckled in a vertical direction as a result of opposing internal anticompression forces. Thus, the problem for the surgeon who wishes to close the wound is compounded. Not only has an unsightly volume of tissue been created, but the displaced or buckled edge will complicate wound closure and impair wound healing. Such buckled free edges will form to the extent that the opposing displacement and reactive forces are parallel to the free wound edge (Figs. 17-8 and 17-9). It is for this reason that local factors (i.e., those that exist between the wound apex and the suture loop that lies nearest to it) are important determinants of dog-ear formation. As has already been discussed, these operate independently of other geometric factors such as the overall axis/side length ratio.

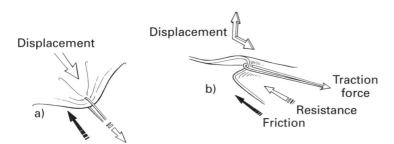

Figure 17-8   *(a)* Forces operating on a free wound edge. Forces applied at right angles to a free edge will encounter little material resistance. The edge will be altered only slightly, and displacement forces will express themselves primarily in the form of motion. *(b)* Forces applied parallel to the edge will be opposed by material resistance, and displacement is more likely to express itself in a vertical direction in the form of buckling.

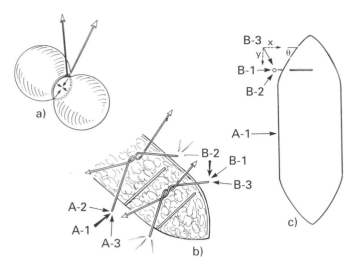

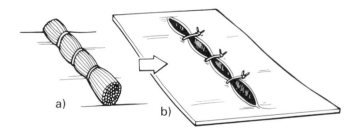

Figure 17-9 Effects of compression and displacement. *(a)* "Suture" placed around a cylindric balloon demonstrates compression forces of confining loop as it is tightened and reactive expansion displacement forces beyond the loop. Forces operate in three dimensions, resulting in projection and elevation of reactively expanding material. *(b)* Displacement or traction vectors caused by sutures at various points along a wound margin. Those perpendicular to the margin (vector A-1) cause no buckling. *(c)* Vectors that are more parallel to the wound edge near the apex of a wound with a wide apical angle are more likely to cause elevation of an edge. (Note B2 or the x component of B-3). To the extent that these vectors and the wound margins between the suture and the apex are parallel (i.e., the more acute angle theta is), the greater will be the tendency for the sides to be elevated. These dynamics are analogous to those shown in Figure 17-8.

In the asymmetric wound, the disparity of length factors described above will be augmented by the fact that displacement vectors and the edge of the longer side are more nearly parallel, contributing to free edge displacement in a vertical dimension.

As will be seen subsequently, analogous force vectors operating in the vertical plane are particularly important when wounds on convex surfaces are closed.

Tissue Elasticity

The skin is a forgiving material with which to work. Those who doubt this need only perform a number of surgical excisions on nonelastic cloth. It will be noted that any fusiform closure will generate excess folds at the wound apices or along the sides. The elastic forces which counter the vectors of closure will efface many of the crimps or folds generated by the geometric properties of the skin. The clinical implications of this are obvious: Skin with little elasticity will be more likely to generate dog-ears than skin with great elasticity.

It is for this reason that apical cones and/or crimps are more likely to form in the presence of tissue that is loose, flaccid, or rigid. Flaccidity is more commonly encountered by the cutaneous surgeon. However as is discussed below, when wounds are closed under tension, apical protrusions can also

form (see "The Role of Surgical Technique" below). Problems can also arise in the presence of thick rigid tissue as in the skin of the back. Bulky rigid wound apices are less likely to be influenced by elastic forces. They also contribute to tissue volume. Thick rigid tissue, particularly when it is poorly undermined or mobilized, may form inverted cones as described above. Trimming and tissue volume reduction usually are remedial.

Rigidity is also an important consideration in the management of wounds and cartilaginous tissue (see "Three-Dimensional Considerations and the Role of Contour" below).

THREE-DIMENSIONAL CONSIDERATIONS AND THE ROLE OF CONTOUR

Wounds on convex surfaces are more likely to develop apical crimps if the long axis of the wound lies parallel to the arc of the convexity. When sutures are placed along the length of a wound, they form a series of constricting bands.[1] The fibrillar material of the skin can be molded into a sheath or fascicle of fibers if there is a significant degree of tissue compression. This compressed sheath of tissue, because of its greater density and rigidity, will be less likely to conform to the curved convex surface and will appear to elevate itself away from the contours curving away below the wound apices (Fig. 17-10).

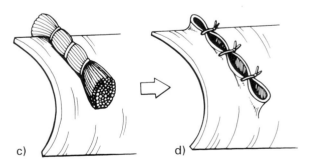

Figure 17-10 *(a)* Tissue compressed into a fascicle of fibers by confining loops of suture; *(b)* edges gaping above diverging fibers in zones of reactive expansion; *(c)* dense fascicle of fibers failing to conform to a convex contour; *(d)* forces combined to produce an inverted cone dog-ear deformity, a pitcher lip. *(From Gormley DE: The dog-ear: Causes, prevention and correction. J Dermatol Surg Oncol 3:194–198, 1977. Used with permission.)*

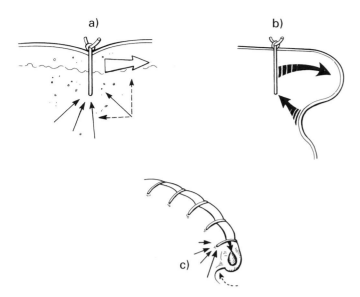

Figure 17-11 Vertical dynamics of wound closure. *(a)* Traction vectors from below (thin solid lines) are developed as suture loop is closed. Dotted lines represent components of vectors showing how tissue is displaced toward the loop and away from the apex. Reactive expansion forces tend to project wound apex (heavy arrow). *(b)* Summation of forces tend to create a curling-wave configuration which tends to amplify dog-ears on convex surfaces. *(c)* Genesis of the pitcher-lip variant of the inverted-cone dog-ear on the markedly convex surface (e.g., lip). Epidermal surface at point of dotted line is pulled toward the suture loop nearest the apex by vertical traction vectors. Dense fascicle of fibers within confining loop of suture is projected outward by reactive expansion forces.

If a sufficient volume of tissue has been displaced in the apical region, a cone or crimp of tissue will form. This phenomenon will be augmented by the gaping of the fibers and skin edges that occurs beyond the suture loop nearest the apex and by an absence of countervailing elastic forces. Thus, a variety of forces summate to amplify a trend toward apical dog-ear formation which might be overlooked in a wound on a less curved surface.

All of the above will be amplified in the absence of countervailing elastic forces (i.e., if the skin is flaccid and if the absence of subcutaneous tissue mandates the creation of a shallow wound).

It must be remembered that when a suture loop is closed, force vectors are generated in the *vertical* dimension and along the longitudinal axis of the wound (Fig. 17-11). These vectors are the vertical counterpart of the horizontal displacement vectors shown in Fig. 17-9*b*. When a wound is closed, tissue is pulled from beyond the wound apex by vectors which lie *below* the suture loop. On a flat surface, these vectors are relatively unimportant. On the curved surface, however, the tissue that is influenced by these forces is the skin that lies beyond and below the wound apex on the convex anatomic surface. Combined vectors operate to displace the apical and subapical tissues upward (Fig. 17-11). At the same time, suture loop compression reaction forces push tissue to-

ward the wound apex as it is being elevated by forces from below. These dynamic factors combine with the increased density and rigidity of the tissue that has been compressed by the suture loops to contribute to apical protrusion and dog-ear formation.

In the markedly convex surface (e.g., the lip or the radial and ulnar aspects of the forearm), the arc described by the long axis of the wound may equal or exceed 180°. Under these circumstances, the force vectors of reactive expansion will tend to project the wound apex while vertical displacement vectors pull tissue from directly below the wound. The result can be an inverted cone or a pitcher lip deformity (Fig. 17-5*d* and 17-11*b*).

Conversion of the wound into a wedge excision will usually be preventive. This deepens the wound and eliminates much of the tissue compression that can impede closure and contribute to dog-ear formation. Such an option is most easily exercised on the lip. In the case of the lip, attempts to prevent extension of the wound below the vermilion border are often best avoided (1) if the vermilion line that remains is distorted, (2) if tissue that remains impedes closure, and/or (3) an inverted cone remains at the apex. If a distorted vermilion (with or without an inverted cone) and a high degree of compression are the prices that must be paid for the conservation of tissue, a wedge excision with an incision through the vermilion with careful reapposition of this important margin will be preferable in most cases.

The conversion to a wedge may not be an option that can be exercised on the forearm where deep tissue reserves are usually limited. Here, wound lengthening or symmetric side length resections must be used for correction.

THE ROLE OF SURGICAL TECHNIQUE

Technique in addition to that of creating a properly configured wound can often prevent problems from arising, particularly in borderline situations. Many difficulties arise because of a failure to appreciate the importance of technique with respect to both the horizontal and vertical dimensions.

Tension and Tension Avoidance

If a wound is closed under tension, the midportions of the length of the wound will sometimes be depressed with respect to the wound apices. Pointing of tissue at the wound apices may create the appearance of dog-ears (pseudo dog-ears) when, in fact, none exist. Existing protrusions may be amplified. The role of tension in the depression of the midportion of the wound and the relative elevation of the apices is understood if the following is remembered:

1. Tissue volume is lost when an excision is done.
2. Very few contours on the body are perfectly flat, with most being convex.
3. When tension is applied from one side of a wound to the other, the force vectors that develop will follow a *straight*

line as the edges are pulled into the wound to fill the void left by the tissue that has been excised. The tissue that is pulled into the wound will be molded by these forces into a less convex, flat, or even concave configuration. The tissue beyond the apices will retain its normal convexity and appear to be raised with respect to the midportion of the wound. The tendency for dog-ears to form under these circumstances will be further amplified by the dynamics that operate on convex surfaces.

Steps that can be taken to reduce wound tension include preoperative planning and undermining.

Preoperative Planning

If the wound can be closed without tension, it should be possible to slide skin from both edges of the area to be excised to a line beyond the planned midline of the wound before excision is undertaken. If this cannot be accomplished, a more complex repair method may have to be selected. While such preoperative estimates of tissue mobility and elasticity are helpful, beginners are nonetheless sometimes dismayed by the loss of elasticity from its preoperative to its intraoperative state. It must be remembered that the elasticity of the skin is in part a function of its compressibility. This property can be temporarily diminished if the skin is engorged with large volumes of local anesthetic or edema fluid because water is not, for practical purposes, compressible. A small reduction in tissue mobility and a corollary increase in rigidity and tension can be expected unless steps are taken to keep skin edema to a minimum. This is particularly true on the back where the dermis is thick. While the fluid content of the skin will rarely make the difference between a failed and successful closure, allowances for the avoidance of fluid-related phenomena will help. The use of minimal amounts of local anesthetic agent in the skin per se and the placement of solution in the subcutaneous fatty layer instead will often help facilitate closure and avoid the creation of deceptively large protrusions at the wound apices.

Undermining

Adequate undermining of wound edges will prevent tissue deep in the wound from being pulled into the closure. Vertical traction vectors and tension are eliminated. The bulkiness of the tissue that is confined within the suture loops is diminished. Such tissue bulk at the wound apices contributes to protrusion formation, particularly, as was previously mentioned, in wounds on convex surfaces.

Wound Depth

Many of the events that occur on the horizontal plane are duplicated in the vertical dimension (Fig. 17-12). A shallow

* Or long side-length/axis-length ratio.

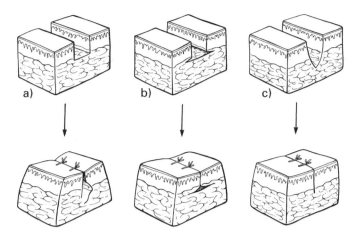

Figure 17-12 (a) Schematic representation of closure of a shallow flat bottom wound which has not been undermined. Excess tissue bulk causes distortion; (b) closure of an undermined wound results in little distortion; (c) closure of wedge-shaped wound results in almost no distortion.

wound with a high width/depth ratio is the vertical analog of the wound with a high width/length ratio.* As the wound edges are drawn toward the center of the wound, excess tissue volume is compressed by the suture loop. Tissue compression distorts the wound edges and enhances dog-ear formation, especially on convex surfaces. When possible (in the lip or in the presence of an ample subcutaneous fatty layer), the wound should be configured so that it is wedge or triangular in shape and symmetric in the vertical as well as the horizontal direction.

Obviously, other factors will often influence the configuration of the wound in the vertical dimension (i.e., the proximity of underlying structures, etc.). Nevertheless, the principles outlined above should be followed to the greatest extent possible.

Whether or not the wedge or transected elliptic configuration can be used, undermining will alleviate the factors that lead to tissue compression and apical gaping that can lead to a "bulk" *dog-ear.*

Suturing Technique

It was already noted that sutures placed in accordance with principles of wound halving will often prevent the collection of excess tissue at the wound apices. Conversely, certain techniques such as the use of running sutures may "drive" the excess length to one end of the wound, making a corrective excision mandatory.

Angled sutures, particularly if they are placed so that the long side of an asymmetric wound is drawn toward the wound apex, can create or enhance a dog-ear (Fig. 17-13).

Suture placement in the *vertical* plane can also contribute to dog-ear formation. Sutures must be placed perpendicularly to the skin surface, a point sometimes overlooked by begin-

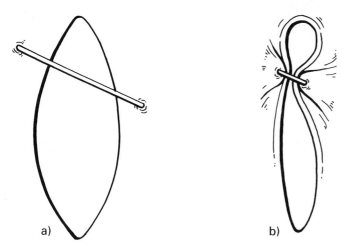

Figure 17-13   Suture placed at an angle other than 90° to the long axis of the wound will contribute to dog-ear formation. *(From Gormley DE: The dog-ear: Causes, prevention and correction. J Dermatol Surg Oncol 3:194–198, 1977. Used with permission.)*

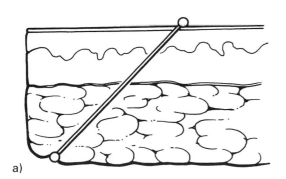

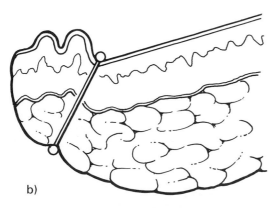

Figure 17-14   Sutures must be placed 90° to the epidermal surface. Errors in this regard, particularly near the wound apex, can contribute to buckling and dog-ear formation. *(From Gormley DE: The dog-ear: Causes, prevention and correction. J Dermatol Surg Oncol 3:194–198, 1977. Used with permission.)*

ners (Fig. 17-14). This is an error which is particularly common on curved surfaces (Fig. 17-15). Such erroneous suture placement results in the compression of tissue at the wound apices which can contribute to dog-ear formation.

OTHER TECHNIQUES FOR THE AVOIDANCE AND CORRECTION OF DOG-EARS

Benign neglect is an option that occasionally works (i.e., sometimes even the worst crimp or protrusion will disappear over time). The risk, of course, is that this gambit may not work and a repeat procedure may be required. Such an alternative should be used only in those instances in which there are compelling reasons for keeping the wound as small as possible and/or in which there is a need to finish the procedure quickly.

The M-Plasty

The M-plasty is a surgical maneuver which is designed to make it possible to shorten the wound. Properly used, it is a helpful tool. Unfortunately, it is often misused and the resulting disappointments have caused misunderstanding to the point of controversy.[3] A basic problem derives from the preoccupation with the maxim that the angles at the ends of the modified wound must be 30°. While this is true, there are other geometric requirements that must be met (Fig. 17-16). In the final analysis, the geometric configuration of the M-plasty is helpful because it reduces the apical compression zone. Reference to Fig. 17-16 will show that half of the tissue

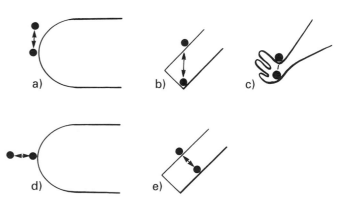

Figure 17-15   Errors in suture placement with respect to the vertical angle are particularly common on convex surfaces. *(a, b, c)* Such mistakes, particularly near the wound apex, can cause buckling and can contribute to protrusion formation *(d, e)* correct placement of sutures with respect to the skin surface. *(From Gormley DE: The dog-ear: Causes, prevention and correction. J Dermatol Surg Oncol 3:194–198, 1977. Used with permission.)*

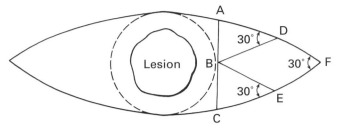

Figure 17-16 The M-plasty. A circular margin of appropriate width is drawn around the lesion to be excised and incorporated into a standard fusiform excisional figure which is approximately three times as long as it is wide with apical angles of 30°; a tangent is drawn to the circular margin which is perpendicular to the long axis of the wound; points D and E, which are halfway between the tangent AC and the apex at F, are connected to the midpoint of AC at B by lines DB and BE; the incision is made along lines AD, DB, BE, and EC, defining the angles at D and E which are 30°. *(From Bennett RG: The Fundamentals of Cutaneous Surgery, St. Louis, Mosby, 1988, pp 486–487. Used with permission.)*

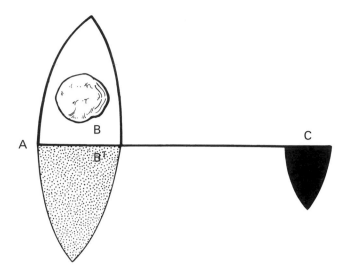

Figure 17-17 Burow's closure (see text).

in this zone (triangles ADB and BEC) is eliminated. The distance that sides AD and EC must move toward the central wound axis is also reduced. The geometric requirements described in Fig. 17-16 also prescribe that the wound must be closed so that points A, B, and C are brought together along line AC without compressing triangle BDE. These are important points that are occasionally overlooked. As Bennett[4] points out, point B will tend to be pulled away from line AC by contractile forces. If point B is sutured in place closer to the wound apex than line AC, problems arise. The angles at D, B, and E will be widened and this will generate excess tissue length along the sides of the now distorted apical triangles. More importantly, a greater volume of tissue will be compressed within the suture loop nearest the wound apex. Such compressions, for reasons already outlined, will generate a protrusion. If point B is sutured at a point farther from point F than line AC, this will cause a bowing of apices, increased apical angles, and increase the side-length/axis-length ratio. It will also cause a reduction in the angle of the displacement vectors (running perpendicularly to the long axis of the wound) with respect to sides AD and EC. For reasons already reviewed, this will result in buckling of the free edges at the sides of the wound. Proper suturing is also important. The apex at B must be secured with a corner suture. An excessive amount of tension along line ABC will cause tissue compression and the vertical displacement of the tissue in angle DBE. This point will also tend to protrude if it is placed upon a convex surface. Poor results are often the result of simple technical errors (poor suturing or poor angle formation).

In the properly designed M-plasty angles ADB, BEC, and DBE are 30°. If the angles are made too large, the triangle of tissue DBE will be much wider and shorter. This will cause length ratio and tissue compression problems which will lead to at least partial dog-ear formation.

Burow's Flap: The Dog-ear Transplant

Flaps are generally regarded as devices for procuring tissue so that it can be moved from an area of tissue abundance to an area of scarcity. Certain flap options, however, can be regarded as methods of transplanting portions of excisional wounds or *their equivalent tissue excesses* to more convenient locations.[5] This is particularly true of the sliding, stretching (Burow's) flaps which are modifications of the simple fusiform closure (Fig. 17-17). It may, for one reason or another, be advantageous to avoid extending the wound below line AB. The ellipse is, therefore, reconfigured into a triangle. If corners A and B are apposed, the tissue between these two points will be converted into an unsightly crimp or fold (dog-ear). If line AB is extended to point C, however, when A is apposed to B, an interesting thing happens. From a purely geometric standpoint, AB'C is greater than BC and the excess length along the lower line (equal to the difference between AB'C and BC) might be expected to show up as a dog-ear equal in magnitude to that which would have occurred if A had been sutured to B. If the defect is created in cloth, this is what happens. Since the skin is elastic, much of the excess skin that would have found expression as a dog-ear is effaced. Much of the remaining excess can be disposed of by dividing it into small pleats by applying the principles of wound halving. The dog-ear can sometimes be eliminated effectively if line AC is long enough. At a minimum, the triangle below line B'C which represents the much atrophied transplanted lower half of the ellipse (represented by the stippled area below line AB) can often be made much smaller than the portion of the wound above line AC.

Burow's Triangle and Multiple Excisions

The "rubber duck" technique described by Cronin[6] allows for the simultaneous excision of two lesions. It might be regarded

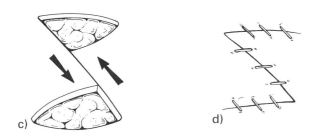

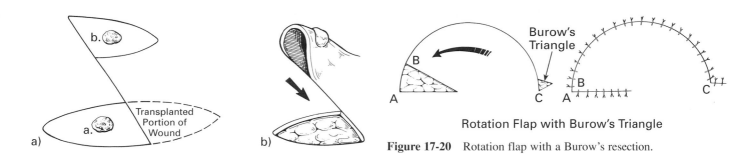

Rotation Flap with Burow's Triangle

Figure 17-20   Rotation flap with a Burow's resection.

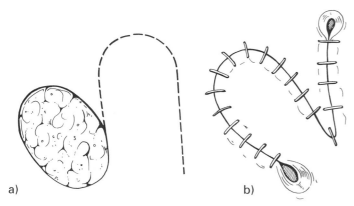

Figure 17-18   Cronin's "rubber duck" technique for concomitant excision of two lesions.

either as a mechanism for transplanting a dog-ear to the site of the second lesion or the removal of a transected half of an elliptic excision to the same location. This approach allows for closure along minimal skin tension lines (Fig. 17-18). Often, the dual resection can be accomplished with a greater conservation of normal tissue as compared to other options.

OTHER COMPLEX WOUNDS

The same principles that operate to create dog-ears in simple closures are apparent with other closures in which flaps and grafts are employed. While a detailed discussion of such repairs is beyond the scope of this chapter, a few relevant points can be made.

Transposition Flap

In this context, excess crimps of tissue can occur at two locations: (1) at the proximal leading edge of the transposed flap and (2) at the apex of the donor area (Fig. 17-19).

The crimp at the base of the flap is best left undisturbed for at least 3 to 4 weeks. Attempts to remove it may compromise the vascularity and viability of the flap. Dog-ears at the apex of the donor area are avoided by designing the wound with the desired fusiform configuration.

Rotation Flap

It can be anticipated that arc ABC will be longer than arc BC (Fig. 17-20). Often, this excess length can be distributed by applying the principles of wound halving. If the length differential is excessive, however, this can cause an unsightly pleated appearance along the longer side of the wound. A length-equalizing resection of tissue from the longer side may be required.

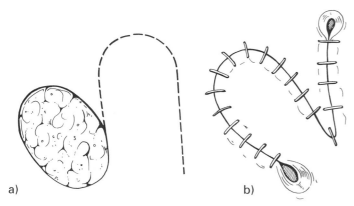

Figure 17-19   When transposition flaps are mobilized, dog-ears will tend to form at two locations: (1) at the proximal leading edge of the flap and (2) at the apex of the donor area. Resection of excess tissue at the base of the flap should be delayed for a period of at least 3 to 4 weeks lest the viability of the flap be compromised.

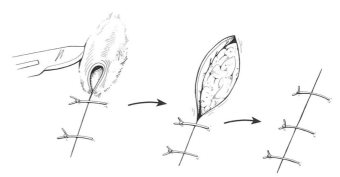

Figure 17-21   Removal of standing cone (straight dog-ear excision). After the wound is closed, the margins of the standing cone can be defined with a gentian violet dye marker. It is then excised with a scalpel or scissors. The limits of the area to be excised often can be estimated before wound closure.

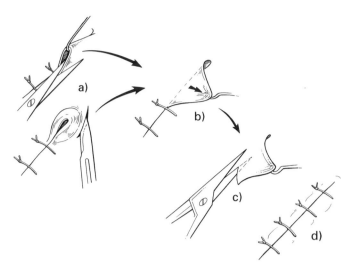

Figure 17-22   Alternate method for removal of standing cone. *(a)* The amount of tissue can be more accurately estimated if an incision is made on one side of the standing cone. *(b)* The attached edge is mobilized over the incised edge. *(c)* The pedicle is amputated along the previous incision line. *(d)* The wound is then closed. Occasionally, slight angling at the end of the wound may result if the estimated amount of tissue is less than perfect.

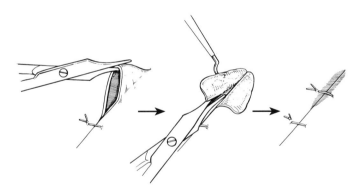

Figure 17-23   Standing cone (symmetric straight dog-ear excision). Split and amputate method.

S-Shaped Wounds

S-shaped wounds can shorten the axis of a wound and redirect the forces of closure in an advantageous way. They may be visualized as two crescentic wounds laid end to end, and the principles outlined above for such excisions can be applied.

Cartilage

Cartilage is relatively rigid and displays few of the forgiving qualities of skin. The surgeon who resects cartilage from the auricle will encounter problems akin to those of the sheet metal worker who must rely to a greater extent upon geometric precision for a good result. While a detailed description of techniques for auricular excisions is beyond the scope of this chapter, it must be anticipated that the forgiving compress-

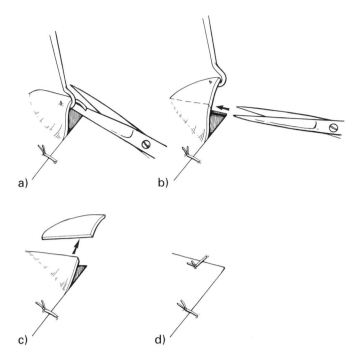

Figure 17-24   *(a–d)* Lying cones which usually develop along the sides of asymmetric wounds are excised in a manner analogous to standing cones. The amount of tissue to be excised can be defined by premarked boundaries or estimated with the mobilization and amputation method. Angling of the end of the wound is inevitable. Often the angle of the incision can be made to conform to wrinkle lines in the area, thereby camouflaging the incision line. Regardless of technique used, incisions should be made 90° to the surface of the skin. Trimming of excess subcutaneous fat may also be required.

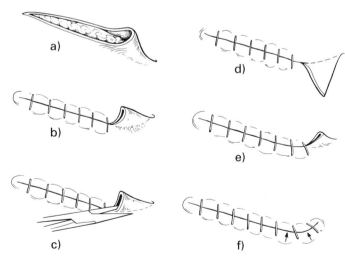

Figure 17-25   Curved dog-ear repair. *(a)* Dog-ear at end of symmetric wound; *(b)* planned excision designed to curve incision along wrinkle line. Note, however, some excess tissue remains beyond outside of angle of incision; *(c)* first incision made along desired line of angulation or curvature; *(d)* flap mobilized over incision line and amputated; *(e, f)* residual excess tissue may be insignificant or require additional resection at angle deviating from desired incision line. This problem would be amplified in an asymmetric curved crescentic wound in which there would be additional length along the longer inferior margin.

ibility and elasticity that characterize skin will be found wanting in cartilage. Apical angles and side/axis length ratios must be planned carefully if dog-ear equivalents in the form of unsightly buckling are to be avoided.

CONCLUSION

The appearance of dog-ears is such a common event it should not be regarded as a product of failure on the part of the surgeon. While their avoidance, when possible, is desirable in the interest of saving time, their removal should be regarded as an integral part of the surgical process. Remedial action will be faster and easier if the factors leading to their creation are understood. In some cases, they are inevitable and can be anticipated. Suggestions for corrective action are reviewed in Figs. 17-21–17-25.

REFERENCES

1. Gormley DE: The dog-ear: Causes, prevention and correction. *J Dermatol Surg Oncol* **3:**194–198, 1977

2. Borges AF: Dogear repair. *Plast Reconstr Surg* **69:**707–713, 1982

3. Borges AF: Pitfalls in flap design. *Ann Plast Surg* **9:**201–210, 1982

4. Bennett RG: *The Fundamentals of Cutaneous Surgery.* St. Louis, Mosby, 1988, pp 486–487

5. Gormley DE: A brief analysis of the Burow's wedge/triangle principle. *J Dermatol Surg Oncol* **11:**121–123, 1985

6. Cronin TA: *Surgical Approach to Multiple Cutaneous Malignancies.* Presented at Third Annual Meeting, Florida Society of Dermatologic Surgeons, Vero Beach, Fla, Apr 14, 1984

Peter B. Odland
Brian H. Kumasaka

18 Fusiform (Elliptic) Excision and Variations

The ellipse, or fusiform, excision is a time-honored surgical technique utilized for the removal of lesions of the skin. Conceptually, the ellipse is quite simple. However, unless the cutaneous surgeon develops a clear understanding of the basic elements required for correct design and execution, the simple ellipse can become a very complicated, anxiety-provoking procedure to perform. Any discussion of the design and execution of the standard ellipse and its variations (including the crescentic modification, S-plasty, M-plasty, and circumferential excision) would be incomplete without reviewing the subjects of relaxed skin tension lines (RSTLs), undermining, and suturing.

Furthermore, the surgeon and the patient are more reliably rewarded when standard perioperative patient management is practiced. This includes thorough preoperative patient evaluation (history and physical, planning and discussing the proposed surgery), application of appropriate intraoperative techniques (analgesia, anesthesia, sterility, design and execution of the excision, suturing, and bandaging), and postoperative patient care. These aspects are fundamental to the practice of cutaneous surgery and are discussed in detail elsewhere in the text.

RELAXED SKIN TENSION LINES

A clear understanding of RSTLs is crucial to effect the proper design of an excision. The importance of RSTLs to the subject of this chapter warrants a brief description. Complete discussion is found in Chap. 19.

It has been determined that forces (or tensions) affecting any one point on the skin pull in virtually every direction.[2] However, these forces are usually greatest along just one axis. For example, the defect that results from a perfectly circular full-thickness excision of skin from the abdomen will immediately assume the shape of an ellipse. A fusiform excision designed properly should have its long axis oriented parallel to the forces that tend to pull a circular excision into an ellipse. The effect this will have is to reduce the tension on the wound edge when closure is completed, which serves to reduce the risk for wound dehiscence and scar spread.

RSTLs as a concept, then, describe the most favorable direction along which one should orient the long axis of a proposed ellipse. They tend to run parallel to the direction of greatest force, or tension, acting upon any point on the skin at rest. RSTLs usually follow a predictable distribution, but variations exist.[3] Passive tissue manipulation, palpation, and pinching the skin allow proper identification of RSTLs (Fig. 18-1). For example, "wrinkle" lines generally follow RSTLs, but because wrinkles are in large part determined by muscle pull, they may be perpendicular to RSTLs. This is especially apparent with the muscles of facial expression.[4]

PREOPERATIVE EVALUATION

The goal of the preoperative history and physical examination is to identify surgical risks and contraindications. Evaluation should include assessment of the cardiopulmonary, hematologic, endocrine, renal, and neurologic systems. Pertinent history regarding current drug therapy, drug allergies, immune

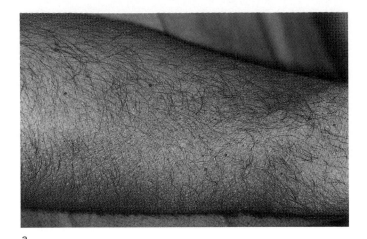

a

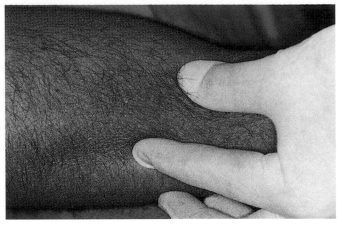

c

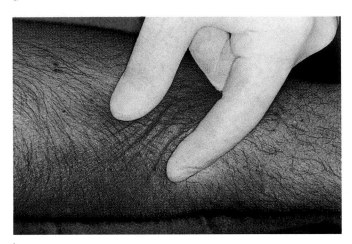

b

Figure 18-1 *(a)* Identification of the RSTLs is not readily recognized visually in the resting state; *(b)* a pinch test oriented parallel to RSTL creates linear folds; *(c)* oriented perpendicularly to RSTL, the pinch creates irregular bulging.

status, and prior surgeries and wound healing should be elicited.[5]

Physical examination, as well as appropriate laboratory tests, will identify high-risk patients. The preoperative visit should also include patient education. Preoperative, intraoperative, and postoperative expectations should be discussed with the patient in full detail. Well-informed patients will tend to develop less anxiety about the procedure. Written information will enhance patient retention and understanding and further alleviate the fear of the unknown. Patient consent should be obtained following explanation of treatment options, including no treatment or alternatives to the elliptic excision. The planned procedure should be diagramed in full scale and side effects, potential negative outcomes, anticipated limitations in activity, including duration, explained to the patient. Preoperative evaluation is an important aspect of any surgical procedure and should not be overlooked.

ELLIPSE EXCISION

The ellipse, or fusiform, excision is a fundamental technique with which all cutaneous surgeons should be familiar. By fol-

lowing a few basic principles, this straightforward procedure can be executed efficiently with reliably successful results. Establishing a routine for all surgeries will enhance physician confidence, will help eliminate overlooking important details, and will result in a satisfying surgical experience for patient and physician.

The initial step in designing a standard elliptic excision is to analyze the lesion. Close inspection with good lighting, and magnification if necessary, will assist the surgeon in determining the appropriate clinical, and therefore surgical, margins. Evaluation of surrounding skin and consideration of how the surgery will affect surrounding anatomic structures must be accomplished. The RSTLs should be identified. Following standard sterile preparation of the operative site and appropriate draping, the planned excision is marked out on the skin. The goal of the procedure is to excise the lesion and allow closure of the resulting defect with minimal or no noticeable functional or cosmetic defect. The long axis of the defect should be oriented parallel to the RSTLs (see "Relaxed Skin Tension Lines" above). The outer border of the proposed surgical margin is drawn; this shape is usually circular. The classic elliptic excision requires that the length be three to four times the measured width. This ratio forms angles at the

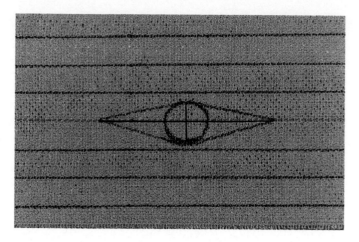

Figure 18-2 The standard ellipse. Tangents drawn to the circular lesion form the elliptic or fusiform shape. The length measures three to four times the width of the lesion.

end (or apex) of the ellipse of 30° or less, an angle which nearly always allows primary closure without dog-ear formation.[6] The length should be drawn perpendicularly to and bisecting the width of the lesion. Finally, drawing a tangent-to-circle or standard fusiform shape completes the outline (Fig. 18-2). Once the outline is completed, the field should be anesthetized. If epinephrine is used with the anesthetic, several minutes should be allowed before incision to allow maximal vasoconstriction.

The incision should be made with countertraction (Fig. 18-3) in three directions, following the outline. The scalpel is usually held as a pencil or in some other secure fashion. Use of a no. 15 blade is customary. The scalpel tip is used to make the initial penetrating incision at the apex of one of the angles on the outline. With the blade perpendicular to the surface of the skin (no bevel) and the scalpel handle straight up, gently

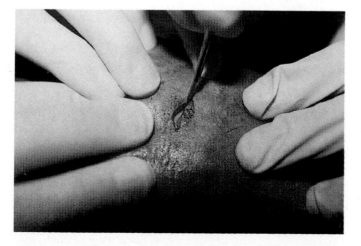

Figure 18-3 Three-way countertraction during incisions facilitates clean penetration to the desired plane.

penetrate the surface. Effective stretching through countertraction applied in concert by the surgeon and the surgical assistant aids tremendously in this and all subsequent steps of the excision. After insertion, the scalpel is rotated from the tip to the belly of the blade to extend the incision along the full length of the outline. It must be emphasized that to avoid a beveled cut, the orientation of the blade should be perpendicular to the skin surface throughout the incision. With proper countertraction, the blade will penetrate the depth of the dermis and the subcutaneous fat will "herniate" through the wound. This is the desired plane for simple excisions. Repetitive strokes may be required to reach the adipose tissue. Crosshatching of the ellipse can be avoided by rotating the blade back to the perpendicular position as the end of the arc is approached. Once the incision is completed, an apex of the specimen is reflected using a skin hook or forceps and is dissected towards the other apex at the dermal-subcutaneous plane with scissors or a scalpel. A conscious effort must be made to avoid dissecting deeply toward the center and shallow toward the ends by intermittently checking the thickness of the specimen and adjusting as necessary. Failure to maintain a uniformly thick specimen can result in the development of *standing cones* (dog-ears) upon attempted closure.[7]

In some instances there is enough tissue laxity so that the edges of the excisional defect can be reapposed and everted without undermining. In most cases, however, a better scar results from undermining 5 to 15 mm in every direction. The tissues slide more easily and the platelike scar that is produced redrapes over the contours more evenly. The resulting increase in dead space requires adequate attention to hemostasis and subcutaneous closure.

Undermining is accomplished by using a skin hook(s) to gently elevate and reflect the wound edges. Blunt and sharp dissection may be done with undermining scissors, or sharp dissection may be done with the scalpel. The optimal plane for undermining varies with the anatomic site.[8] The best plane for undermining the scalp is deep to the galea; for the forehead, it is below the deep fat; and for extremities, it is between the deep fat and fascia. Review of important anatomic structures is important to minimize risk of neurovascular compromise.

The most desirable immediate postoperative closure of the ellipse produces apposition with epidermal eversion but without constriction. This may be accomplished with a variety of suture materials and specific techniques that will be discussed in greater detail in Chap. 16. There are very few situations in which one can justify not using a layered closure for ellipse excisions. In areas where the skin is thin (e.g., eyelid), where there is extra tissue so the closed wound is under vanishingly small amounts of tension (e.g., aged patients; the scrotal skin), and in areas where wounds closed under very little tension will not be subjected to exogenous forces acting to separate the edges (e.g., scalp), a nonlayered simple closure can be considered the most advantageous.

Variations of the Ellipse

The simple, standard fusiform shape is adequate for the vast majority of excisions and is flexible enough to allow adaptation to needs in various anatomic areas. These are the variations of the ellipse that will be discussed in the following sections. The fundamentals of ellipse design and execution apply for these variations. Following removal of the lesion, standard closure techniques should be employed.

Crescentic Ellipse

Many regions on the body have RSTLs that follow curves rather than straight lines. To accommodate these natural bends in the RSTLs, slight curves may be incorporated into the long axis of the excision. When done properly, this crescentic variation can produce an outcome that is more aesthet-ically pleasing than a standard ellipse. (A crescent is described as a blunted or incomplete *C* shape). This procedure can be achieved in a variety of ways.

One effective way to design this excision is to draw the arc (or line) that the suture line will follow (Fig. 18-4a). Ideally, this will fall into or run parallel to the RSTLs or the junction lines of the regional (aesthetic) subunits of the face.[9] The arc may course through or next to the lesion to be excised and may extend beyond the anticipated length of the proposed excision (Fig. 18-4b). As with any excision, appropriate margins are marked around the lesion. At this point, lines are drawn to outline the proposed excision (Fig. 18-4c). They will trace circles of different radii in order to best result in a scar that falls into the desired arc of closure. The curves may be in the same or opposite orientation depending on the lesion and its relative position to the desired arc. These designs will neces-

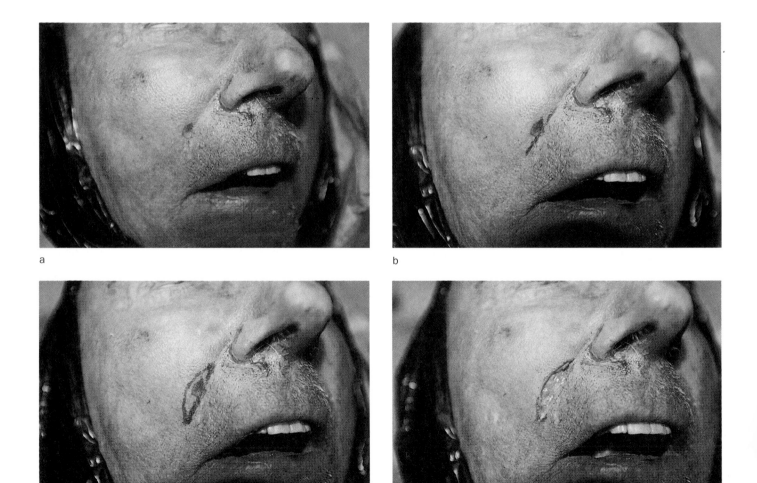

a

b

c

d

Figure 18-4   The crescentic ellipse. *(a)* Cutaneous lesion of right cheek; *(b)* proposed suture line; *(c)* crescentic ellipse; *(d)* crescentic ellipse excised. (*Continued*)

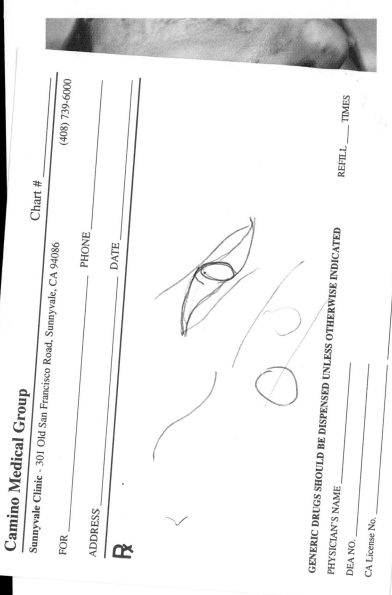

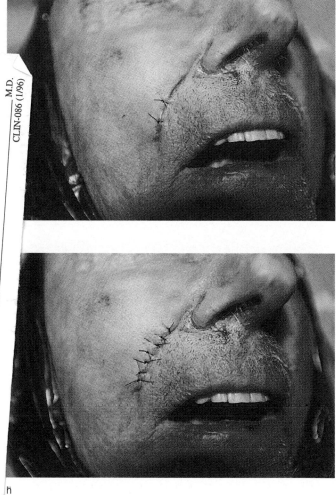

by using rule of halves.

sarily result in sides of unequal length and will require closure of the resulting defect using the *rule of halves* (Fig. 18-4*e–h*).[10] The degree of undermining will be dictated by the orientation of the excision to the desired line of closure. In most cases, one side of the defect will require slightly to substantially more undermining than the other to minimize displacement of the scar from the desired orientation. After adequate hemostasis is achieved, the deep tissues can be closed by using the above-mentioned rule of halves in the following fashion: The first buried suture is placed in the center of the wound. Each subsequent suture bisects the remaining defect until the wound is completely apposed. This acts to distribute the excess tissue on the longer side of the defect equally along the shorter side which effectively eliminates the need for a dog-ear repair. The resulting scar should ultimately redrape (in several weeks to months) to conform with the natural RSTLs and creases in that part of the body.

S-Plasty

Convex or concave surfaces pose unique challenges in designing an ellipse excision. Because wounds contract during healing in all directions, a straight wound on a convex or concave surface, theoretically, may result in a depressed or elevated scar, respectively.[11] The S-plasty can be used to minimize such undesirable contour irregularities. Its double convex shape (Fig. 18-5) outlines an excision the length of which is greater than the distance between its two ends. As contraction of the wound occurs in the horizontal plane, the increased length in the curves of the S-plasty serves as a reservoir of tissue that can be absorbed. As a result, the maturing scar effectively straightens rather than becoming depressed or elevated (webbing). Vertical displacement (contraction) is theoretically opposed by everting the wound edges at the time of closure. It is important to note that the S-plasty

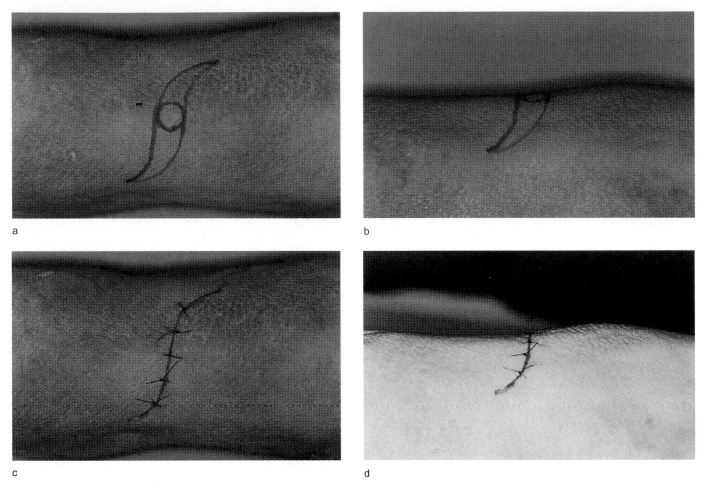

a   b

c   d

Figure 18-5   *(a–d)* The S-plasty. Double convex shape serves as a reservoir for scar contraction on convex or concave surfaces to avoid depressed or elevated scars, respectively.

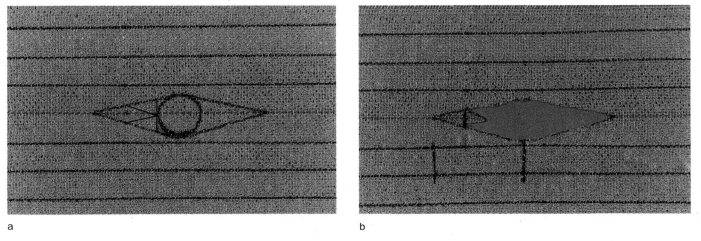

a   b

Figure 18-6   The M-plasty. *(a)* An isosceles triangle is outlined by drawing its base tangentially to the circle outlining the surgical margin and perpendicularly to the long axis of the ellipse. Lines drawn connecting the midpoints of the sides and the base of this isosceles triangle complete the *M* to be excised. *(b)* So marked, this unilateral M-plasty excision is performed.

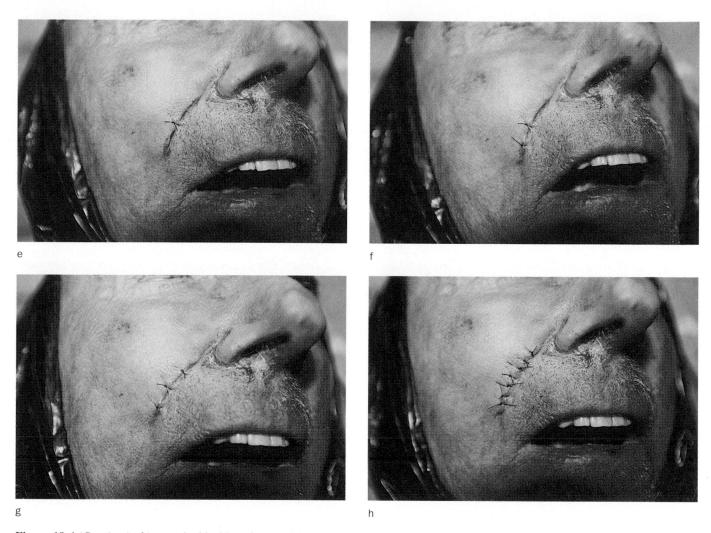

e

f

g

h

Figure 18-4 (*Cont.*)   (*e–h*) wound with sides of unequal length closed by using rule of halves.

sarily result in sides of unequal length and will require closure of the resulting defect using the *rule of halves* (Fig. 18-4*e–h*).[10] The degree of undermining will be dictated by the orientation of the excision to the desired line of closure. In most cases, one side of the defect will require slightly to substantially more undermining than the other to minimize displacement of the scar from the desired orientation. After adequate hemostasis is achieved, the deep tissues can be closed by using the above-mentioned rule of halves in the following fashion: The first buried suture is placed in the center of the wound. Each subsequent suture bisects the remaining defect until the wound is completely apposed. This acts to distribute the excess tissue on the longer side of the defect equally along the shorter side which effectively eliminates the need for a dog-ear repair. The resulting scar should ultimately redrape (in several weeks to months) to conform with the natural RSTLs and creases in that part of the body.

S-Plasty

Convex or concave surfaces pose unique challenges in designing an ellipse excision. Because wounds contract during healing in all directions, a straight wound on a convex or concave surface, theoretically, may result in a depressed or elevated scar, respectively.[11] The S-plasty can be used to minimize such undesirable contour irregularities. Its double convex shape (Fig. 18-5) outlines an excision the length of which is greater than the distance between its two ends. As contraction of the wound occurs in the horizontal plane, the increased length in the curves of the S-plasty serves as a reservoir of tissue that can be absorbed. As a result, the maturing scar effectively straightens rather than becoming depressed or elevated (webbing). Vertical displacement (contraction) is theoretically opposed by everting the wound edges at the time of closure. It is important to note that the S-plasty

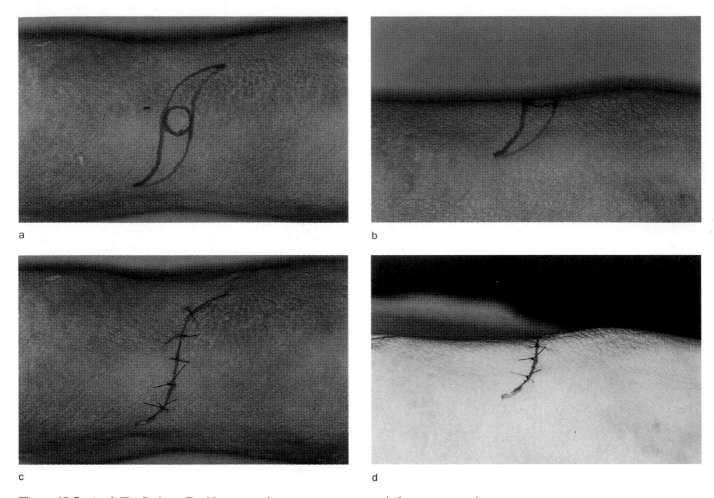

Figure 18-5 *(a–d)* The S-plasty. Double convex shape serves as a reservoir for scar contraction on convex or concave surfaces to avoid depressed or elevated scars, respectively.

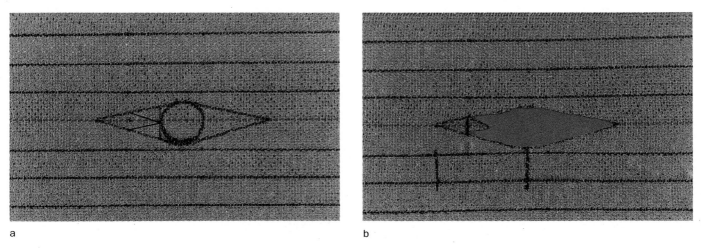

Figure 18-6 The M-plasty. *(a)* An isosceles triangle is outlined by drawing its base tangentially to the circle outlining the surgical margin and perpendicularly to the long axis of the ellipse. Lines drawn connecting the midpoints of the sides and the base of this isosceles triangle complete the *M* to be excised. *(b)* So marked, this unilateral M-plasty excision is performed.

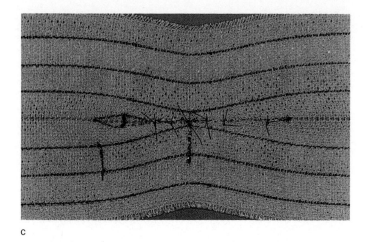

c

Figure 18-6 (Cont.) *(c)* The resulting defect is closed with a layered linear closure utilizing a tip-stitch for the *M* portion of the repair.

cannot be formed by obliquely joining the sides of a straight incision—it must be planned in advance.[12] The convexities and concavities of the face and extremities are sites where this technique may be useful.

M-Plasty

To avoid the formation of dog-ears, the design of a standard elliptic excision calls for a length/width ratio of 4:1. Although this requires sacrifice of normal tissue at the apices of the ellipse, it produces an acceptable surgical outcome. If the lesion closely approximates sensitive anatomic structures, a variation of the 4:1 ratio of the standard ellipse called an *M-plasty* can be employed.[10] This variation acts to effectively shorten the overall length while maintaining the width of the ellipse. In planning the M-plasty, the ellipse is divided into two isosceles triangles, with each base drawn as a vertical tangent to the circle that identifies the lesion. The length of the sides of the triangles are divided into halves and a line is drawn

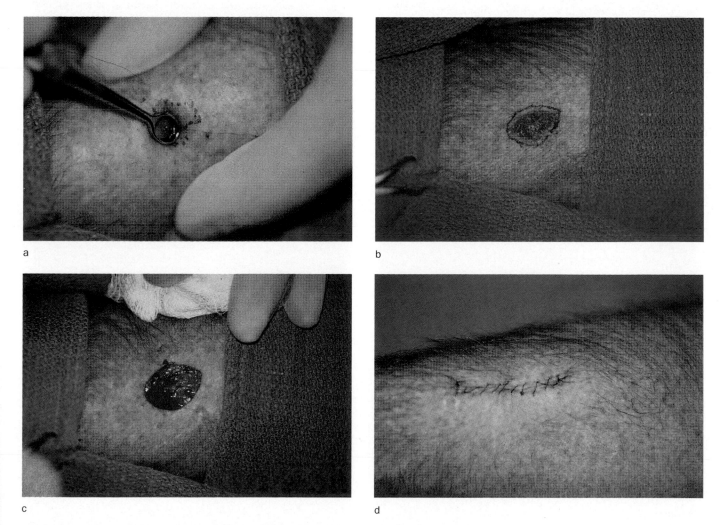

a

b

c

d

Figure 18-7 The circumferential excision. *(a)* The tumor is debulked with curettage. *(b)* Then a 1–3 mm margin is marked and *(c)* excised. *(d)* After undermining, the defect will assume an elliptic shape, which directs the orientation of closure.

from the midpoint of these lines to the midpoint of the base of each triangle (Fig. 18-6). The resulting *M* shape forms angles of 30° or less that should allow primary closure.[13] If one is removing a malignant lesion, care must be taken to allow for adequate surgical margins when planning the middle point of the *M*.

Circumferential Excision

In some cases, the ideal orientation of the long axis of the proposed excision cannot be determined in a reliable way preoperatively. In such cases, one can proceed with a circumferential excision of the lesion. Then, if one undermines several millimeters in every direction, the defect will respond to the forces acting upon the wound and will create an ellipse, the long axis of which will be oriented naturally along RSTLs. To complete this excision, redundant tissue is excised in the standard dog-ear repair fashion, adequate hemostasis is achieved, and then a layered linear closure is completed.[14] Another application for this technique is for certain skin cancers that can be effectively treated with standard excisional techniques. In such cases, debulking the tumor, usually with curettage, precedes the above described circumferential excision (Fig. 18-7). Although this technique requires an additional surgical step, it produces higher cure rates than other non-margin-controlled techniques.[15]

REFERENCES

1. Borges AF, Alexander JE: Relaxed skin tension lines, z-plasties on scars, and fusiform excision of lesions. *Br J Plast Surg* **15**:242, 1962

2. Stegman SJ: Excisions on the face. *Dermatology* **3**(4):43, 1980

3. Borges AF: *Elective Incisions and Scar Revision,* 1st ed. Boston, Little, Brown, 1973

4. Gross DA: On history-taking before surgery. *J Dermatol Surg Oncol* **7**:71, 1981

5. Webster RC et al: M-plasty techniques. *J Dermatol Surg* **2**:393, 1976

6. Robbins TH: Elliptical excision and closure. *J R Coll Surg Edinb* **25**:59, 1980

7. Stegman SJ et al: *Basics of Dermatologic Surgery,* 1st ed. Chicago, Year Book, 1982

8. Salasche SJ et al: *Surgical Anatomy of the Skin,* 1st ed. Norwalk, Conn, Appleton & Lange, 1988

9. Bennett RG: Complex closures, in *Fundamentals of Cutaneous Surgery,* 1st ed, edited by RG Bennett. St. Louis, Mosby, pp 473–491

10. Zitelli JA: Wound healing for the clinician. *Adv Dermatol* **2**:243, 1987

11. Zitelli JA: TIPS for a better ellipse. *J Am Acad Dermatol* **22**:101, 1990

12. Hanke CW: Repair of surgical defects. *Dermatol Clin* **5**:287, 1987

13. Davis TS et al: The circular excision. *Ann Plast Surg* **4**:21, 1980

14. Johnson TM et al: Combined curettage and excision: A treatment method for primary basal cell carcinoma. *J Am Acad Dermatol* **24**:613, 1991

Gerald Bernstein

19 Lines of Elective Incision on the Skin

It has been generally accepted that finer, more cosmetically acceptable scars will be achieved if incisions are placed along or within certain lines that have been shown to exist in the skin.[1–3,7,9–22] The two main categories of lines are the contour lines and the skin tension lines (STLs).[2]

CONTOUR LINES

The contour lines mainly consist of those lines which divide the facial skin into anatomic or cosmetic units, such as the cheeks, nose, lips, etc.[7] On most individuals they are well defined and clearly identifiable. On the face, they include the vermilion line, the alar fold, the nasolabial fold, and the junction of the eyebrow of the forehead and the eyelid margin (Fig. 19-1). Contour lines also include the junction of hair-bearing skin with glabrous skin, the contour of the nose, and shape of the ears. The contour line which marks the junction of the nose and cheek is less obvious. The subtle angles and proportional relationships which have been measured on the face and neck by cosmetic surgeons can also be included in the concept of contour lines.[4,6] Contour lines are also present on the skin of the trunk and extremities. Examples are the antecubital fold, the creases of the wrist and hands, as well as creases and furrows over other articular surfaces.

As the contour lines contribute to a person's appearance, they must be regarded as the predominant lines of the skin. They generally take preeminence over the STLs which will be described in "Skin Tension Lines" below. Alterations in these aesthetic proportions and angles can have a profound impact on an individual's appearance. Individuals tend to be very intolerant of even small changes in their contour lines. These lines should be changed or altered in ablative or reconstructive surgery only when there is an overriding medical condition, such as a malignancy. By contrast, cosmetic surgery is largely concerned with enhancing or restoring contour lines to achieve a more aesthetically pleasing appearance. Moreover, there are functional complications which may result from violating some contour lines, such as those over joints. Incisions placed across the creases of the fingers or wrists, for example, can produce contractures and impairment of function. Thus, recognition and identification of the contour lines on the head and neck, as well as the extremities, is an essential part of preoperative planning.

The contour lines also serve as important aids to scar enhancement and camouflage. Placing a surgical incision within or along a contour line tends to produce a less obvious or often invisible scar.[1,3,5] The nasolabial fold is an example of an ideal location for placement of an elective incision. Incisions situated in the nasolabial fold will tend to disappear with healing. Similarly pleasing results can be anticipated by placing incisions along other contour lines such as the junction of the ear and cheek or at the junction of glabrous skin with the hair-bearing skin of the eyebrow or sideburn, etc. The adept surgeon will utilize every effort to place incisions within the contour lines whenever feasible.

The anatomic units are frequently further divided into cosmetic subunits.[3,6] The defining lines are usually less well developed and more variable than the contour lines. The cosmetic subunits share similarities in texture, color, pore size, degree of "sebaceousness," etc., often to a greater degree than

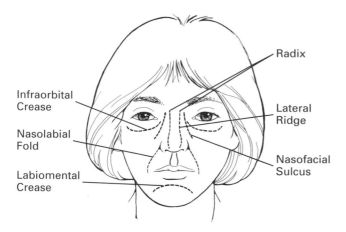

Figure 19-1 Examples of contour lines of the face.

do the cosmetic units. The nose, for example, can be divided into cosmetic subunits which include the root, the dorsum, the lateral sidewalls, the ala nasi, the soft triangle, the tip, and the columella (Fig. 19-2*a*).[3,6] The cosmetic subunits of the lip include the vermilion, the upper lip (infranasal area), the philtrum, and the lower lip [separated from the chin by the labiomental line (Fig. 19-2*b*)]. The glabella is a subunit of the forehead.

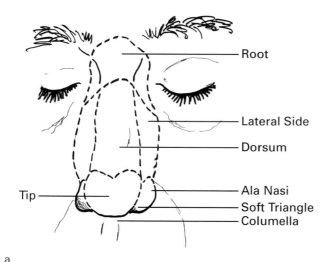

a

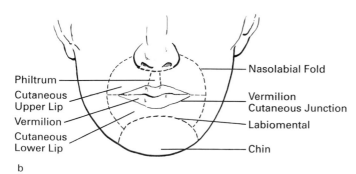

b

Figure 19-2 (*a*) Cosmetic subunits of the nose; (*b*) cosmetic subunits of the lips.

The cosmetic subunits of the eyelids are the canthi, brow, upper lid, lower lid, and medial canthus. The lids can be further divided into the orbital and palpebral portion. Ophthalmologists have defined the pretarsal and preseptal areas of the palpebral portions of both the upper and lower lids.[8]

Examination of many faces will demonstrate differences in definition and prominence of the various cosmetic subunits. There is substantial variation in the prominence of the nasal tip. Some individuals have a flat nasal dorsum with clear lines demarcating the dorsal from the lateral aspects of the nose. In others, the nasal dorsum is rounded and the lines defining the dorsal and the lateral aspects of the nose are less clear.[6] The chin may be sharply divided into two clearly separated mounds by a vertical furrow (cleft chin) or have a solitary bulbous mound with no furrow. The placement of elective incisions will vary in either case.

Incisions placed along the junctions of cosmetic subunits also tend to heal with more cosmetically pleasing results than when situated within the subunits.[3,6] For example, one should try to place an incision along the junction of the dorsum and side of the nose rather than within these subunits. Also, because of the similar physical characteristics of the skin, flaps and grafts taken from the same subunit tend to produce superior aesthetic results. If skin is not available from the subunit, one would next try to find available skin from the same anatomic unit before utilizing skin from a different anatomic unit. Many reconstructive surgeons have demonstrated superior cosmetic results when they replace an entire cosmetic subunit rather than simply closing a wound within a subunit. To achieve this, they must excise the normal tissue surrounding the defect to the margins of the subunit.[6]

SKIN TENSION LINES

The STLs are frequently called *Langer's lines* because of his major work on this subject in 1861.[9] However, many other names have been utilized to identify the STLs, such as crease lines (Cox), dynamic facial lines (Stark), lines of elasticity (Conway), elective lines (Kocher), increased skin tension lines (Cox), maximum tension lines (Gibson and Kennedi), minimal skin tension lines (Converse), relaxed skin tension lines [RSTLs (Borges)], and tension lines and wrinkle lines (Webster).[5,7,18] They have also been referred to as lines for elective surgical incision (Kraissl).[5,9–11,13–18] The STLs are considered to be identical to *wrinkle lines,* a term also used in this chapter.[8]

The STLs are usually less well defined than the contour lines, especially in young individuals. Similar to contour lines, incisions placed in or parallel to these lines will tend to heal with a finer, more cosmetically pleasing scar than incisions placed across or at angles to the STLs. The forces which result in the STLs remain a source of debate and their exact direction is similarly contested.[7] Although many investigators have created contour maps which purport to indicate the correct pattern or direction of the skin lines, it appears that there

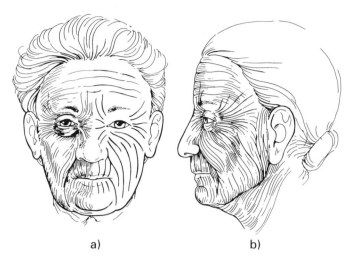

Figure 19-3   *(a, b)* Diagram of skin tension lines of the face.

is marked individual variation in the direction of the STLs (Fig. 19–3). Thus, most skin line contour maps are unlikely to accurately depict the actual STLs in the individual patient.[3,7,18]

HISTORICAL ASPECTS

The first description of the STLs was made by Dupuytren in 1834.[19] He noted linear wounds which resulted from stabs made with a thin, round leather awl in a suicide attempt. Subsequent research on cadavers by Dupuytren demonstrated that circular incisions produced linear wounds. The direction of the wounds varied with the location on the body. However, Langer is credited with the major definitive work on this subject. In 1861, he performed extensive experiments on cadavers, working on the skin of the face, as well as on the trunk and extremities. He demonstrated the presence of the adult pattern of STLs in the first year of life.[9,10] Of interest was his observation that while STLs are very prominent over the joints of the extremities, they tend to become progressively less so between joints. Despite the thoroughness and scope of his work, Langer's lines are not now generally believed to accurately describe the direction of the lines of tension in the skin. Most surgeons would rarely elect to place incisions along the lines depicted by Langer.

Many other investigators have contributed to the work on STLs. In 1941, Cox noted the persistence of STLs in excised skin. He postulated the existence of intrinsic forces within the skin which contribute to the creation and maintenance of the STLs.[17] At that time, however, Gibson noted that ultrastructural examination did not confirm the existence of spatially oriented fibers.[18]

In 1954, Ragnall demonstrated that the skin was three times more extensible at right angles to the STLs.[20] Thus, incisions placed parallel to the STLs would have an equivalent reduction in tension on the wound edges. Reuben in 1948 and

Kraissl in 1951 related the STLs to the contraction of the underlying musculature and equated these lines with the wrinkle lines.[16,21] They demonstrated that the STLs were therefore perpendicular to the direction of contraction of the muscle fibers. Kraissl further demonstrated fibers attaching the skin to the muscles. The pull of the muscles was thus postulated to throw the skin into folds (i.e., the STLs) which ultimately became visible as the wrinkle lines. Kraissl, however, took the position that the STLs were uniform and followed a universal pattern.

In 1973, Borges published drawings of, what he termed, RSTLs. Borges felt that the RSTLs originated from universal forces which resulted from the skin's being stretched tentlike over the bony and cartilaginous structures.[11] He differentiated the RSTLs from the wrinkle lines which he felt were related to muscle pull. However, he felt the RSTLs were of greater importance than the wrinkle lines and indicated that they were identical for all individuals. He constructed detailed line maps which have been referred to as the *correct* direction for the placement of incisions.[11,22]

More recently, Bulacio Nunez attempted to identify the direction of the STLs by cutting circular incisions and observing the circles pull into ovals along what he took to be the correct tension lines.[23] He also related the formation of these lines to the contracture of the superficial musculature of the skin of the face. Stegman,[24] also using circular incisions, confirmed Bulacio Nunez's work. In addition, he demonstrated areas of neutral tension in some individuals. The neutral tension often appeared in areas that usually have directional lines in most individuals. He further demonstrated individual variations in the direction of the STLs.[24] Similarly, Gibson and Kennedi,[18] in their extensive work on the biomechanical properties of the skin, indicated their inability to produce a "tension contour map" of the body because of the marked variation in the STLs from person to person as well as in the same individual.

In 1976, Mitz and Peyronie[25] described the superficial musculoaponeurotic system (SMAS) in the skin of the face. The SMAS has been further described by many investigators.[3,26,28] While there is disagreement as to the exact details of the character of the SMAS, it is generally understood to be a broad fibrofascial band surrounding and interconnecting the muscles of facial expression. Understanding the anatomic and biophysical aspects of the SMAS is pivotal to the understanding of facial dynamics, as well as the performance of facial surgery, especially cosmetic surgery. The interested reader is referred to current reviews of this subject.[3,26,28,29] The SMAS lies within the superficial fatty layer and has been shown to integrate and harmonize the action of the facial muscles and to create the incredible array of human facial expressions and movements. Of importance to the concept of the STLs is the demonstration of fibrous septa extending from the surface of the SMAS to the dermis.[26] The existence of fibrous attachments to the dermis has also been demonstrated by Pierard and LaPierre.[30,31] Similar ultrastructural changes have been demonstrated in wrinkles as well.[32,44] These findings support the earlier work of Kraissl and provide support for the concept of the development of wrinkles from the tethering effect of fibrous bands on the dermis.

FACTORS IN THE DEVELOPMENT OF SKIN TENSION LINES

The STLs are a result of a complex interaction of intrinsic and extrinsic factors acting on the skin. The intrinsic factors include the extensibility, elasticity, and tension of the major biostructural elements of the skin (i.e., the dermal collagen and elastic tissues). The extrinsic factors are the action of the underlying muscles of facial expression on the skin of the face and neck, as well as solar damage, gravity, and aging of the facial skin.

Intrinsic Factors

Collagen is the major structural component of the dermis, comprising approximately 70 to 80 percent of its volume. Collagen consists of a "family of related proteins which are genetically distinct."[45] It consists of long, thin fibers made up of smaller fibrils. The basic microfibrillar unit is a helical structure consisting of three identical cross-linked strands of polypeptide chains.[34,35,45] In the skin, types I and III collagen predominate and provide the tensile properties of the skin. *Tension* is defined as a force tending to elongate, deform, or stretch the skin. *Extensibility* is the property of the skin which allows it to be stretched. *Elasticity* is the ability of the skin to return to its original stage after being deformed.

Collagen is very flexible but resists either extensibility or stretch under sudden tension. However, with prolonged tension, such as occurs with pregnancy, obesity, serial excision, and tissue expansion, the collagen fibers will slowly accommodate to these forces by elongating. When the skin is at rest, the collagen fibers are convoluted and intertwined in a random fashion. With tension and elongation of the skin, increasing numbers of fibers become straightened and aligned. Under maximum tension, all the collagen fibers become aligned and the skin will not stretch farther. With aging, the collagen becomes increasingly cross-linked, elongated, and reduced in volume, and there is diminished collagen synthesis.[18,33–35,45]

The second major fibrous component of the dermis is the elastic tissue. These fibers are normally thinner than the collagen and consist of elastin molecules which have both fibrillar and amorphous elements. They are easily extensible under minimal tension but are highly elastic; that is, they have the capacity to resume their original shape when the tension is released.[34,36,45]

Elastic fibers are responsible for maintaining static tension on the skin and for restoring the deformed or stretched collagen to its original state. Even at rest, the elastic fibers maintain static tension on the skin of the face. Although the elastic fibers are arranged in a random pattern, they have a functional

direction as demonstrated by the increased tension vectors parallel to the STLs and by the diminished tension perpendicular to the STLs.[1,33,34] This tends to be confirmed by the observation that round wounds tend to pull into ovals parallel to the STLs after undermining. Age-related changes in the mechanical properties of the skin are mostly a result of degenerative changes in the elastic network of the skin.[36] With progressive aging and prolonged sunlight exposure, the elastic fibers undergo progressive structural and functional deterioration. Aging and ultraviolet light have different effects on the collagen. Aging in sunlight-protected skin results in fragmentation and loss of elastic fibers. In contrast, in sun-damaged skin there are increased amounts of elastotic material which consists, at least in part, of cross-linked elastic fibers.[45] The elastic fibers lose their ability to return to their original length and the skin begins to deform under its own weight.[37] This results in wrinkled and sagging skin.[45]

Extrinsic Factors

The muscles of facial expression appear to be the dominant factor in the creation of the STLs. The muscles of facial expression are unique in that they originate and/or insert directly onto the skin, fascia, and superficial muscles of the facial skin.[38,39] This is in contrast to most other voluntary muscles which originate and insert into bones. Moreover, along the entire course of the muscles, fibrous septa connect the dermis to the SMAS. Thus, contracture of the muscles has a continuous integrated effect on the overlying skin. Over a period of years, repeated muscular contraction can be seen to produce a gradual stretching of the collagen in the direction in the action or pull of the muscle.[44]

In younger individuals, the elastic tissue is able to maintain the shape of the skin and to reform the skin to its original smooth appearance. With aging and deterioration of the elastic fibers, the skin is thrown into folds and wrinkles with the deep part of the wrinkles corresponding to the fibrous attachments of the dermis to the fascia [SMAS (Fig. 19-4)].[31,43] These wrinkles are, in fact, the STLs.[1,2,15] Although these lines are clearly apparent as wrinkles in aged people, this adult pattern has been shown to be present in childhood.[10,18] The STLs are therefore at right angles to the direction of the line of action of the muscles. Also, as a consequence of the lengthening of the skin, the skin tension is reduced in the direction of the action of the facial muscles and perpendicular to the STLs. [the so-called line of maximum extensibility (LME)].[17,22,24]

Other factors which can influence the STLs include sun damage, aging, and smoking.[40] It is interesting to speculate on possible effects of occupation or personality traits on the STLs. For example, a person who is chronically depressed may have STLs which are in a totally different direction than one who does not suffer that trait. Advanced age, dermal and fat atrophy, plus the effect of gravity may produce dependency lines creating a crosshatch of wrinkle lines.

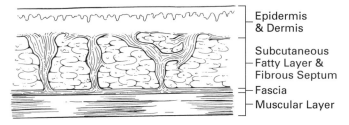

Figure 19-4 Diagram demonstrates fibrous septa connecting SMAS to dermis. Elongation of collagen and deterioration of elastic fibers lead to formation of wrinkles at site of dermal insertion of fibrous septa.

CAUSES OF VARIABILITY IN THE DIRECTION OF THE STLs

There is marked variation in the muscles of facial expression among individuals.[3,7,16,18,21] The platysma muscle provides a striking example of the variation in facial musculature. This muscle is situated in the most superficial muscular layer of the face; its insertion can vary from the level of the mandible to that of the zygomatic arch.[3,7] In some individuals, the platysma muscle is virtually absent. Other muscles of facial expression can show similar anatomic variations and can thus effect the direction of the STLs (Figs. 19-5a–b). While the

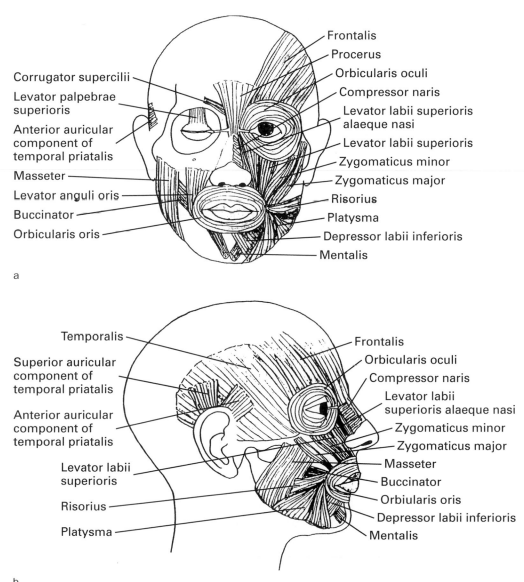

a

b

Figure 19-5 *(a)* Facial musculature, frontal view. Superficial muscles are demonstrated on the left; deep muscles are on the right *(used with permission of Mosby-Year Book. Current Issues in Dermatology, vol 2, 1984. Jeffery P. Callen, Sam Stegman, eds. Forces in Skin Tension Lines by Gerald Bernstein, M.D.); (b)* facial musculature, lateral view. The platysma and risorius muscles are highly variable. The risorius may be entirely absent.

amount of solar elastosis, which is a function of sunlight exposure and intrinsic melanin protection, may effect the degree of wrinkling, it should have little effect on the direction of the STLs.

Sleep Lines

Stegman[41] postulated the existence of what he called "sleep-induced (facial) lines." He considered sleep lines to be a result of constant pressure of the facial skin against the pillow and bedding repeated over years of sleeping in the same position. However, investigators into the physiology of sleep have demonstrated that there is frequent body movement during periods of sleep.[42] This suggests that individuals do not sleep in one position throughout the night. Therefore the amount of unrelieved tension on one area would appear to be inadequate to create permanent sleep lines. However, at present, there is insufficient evidence to either support or refute the existence of sleep lines.

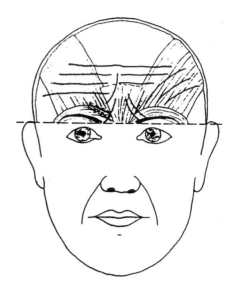

Figure 19-6 The relationship of STLs of the forehead to the overlying muscles.

Direction of the STLs

The author has attempted to show that variation exists in the direction of the STLs from one individual to another. Nonetheless, there appear to be some areas of the face where the STLs tend to be in general conformity between individuals, while in other areas there is likely to be greater diversity in the direction of the STLs. Familiarity with the anatomy of the underlying muscles of facial expression will allow one to more accurately predict areas of uniformity and diversity.[3,7] Where a single muscle or muscle group exerts its action in one direction, there will tend to be uniformity in the direction of the STLs. However, in those areas where there are multiple muscles or muscle groups acting in different directions, there will tend to be greater individual variation in the direction of the STLs. Examples of the former are found on the forehead and medial cheek. On the forehead there is a solitary muscle, the occiptofrontalis, acting in a vertical direction. Thus, horizontal lines on the forehead can usually be predicted with confidence. Similarly, on the medial cheek, where the elevators of the lips and mouth all act in a vertical and diagonal direction, the curved diagonal lines of the medial cheek are usually seen. The contracture of the solitary procerus muscle at the nasal root produces the transverse lines of the nasal muscle, while the corrugator supercilii acts at the upper medial orbit forming the oblique lines which commonly extend from the orbit to the glabella (Fig. 19-6). Greater variation in the direction of the STLs is expected around the mouth and chin where there are different muscles and muscle groups acting in different directions on the same area (elevators of the mouth, depressors of the mouth, risorius, platysma, buccinator, orbicularis oris). The STLs in this area are expected to result from the action of the muscles or muscle groups which are dominant in that individual. Thus, substantial individual variation is expected in these lines (Fig. 19-7a). The skin of the

lips themselves tends to show radial lines because of the sphincter-like effect of the orbicularis oris. Here, the purselike action on the orbicularis oris muscle is dominant.

As the muscles of facial expression predominate in the central face, there is little significant muscular action on the skin of the lateral face and temples. Here, STLs can also show marked variation. The muscles acting on the ear (auricularis anterior, superior, and posterior) are undeveloped in most individuals and have little effect on the overlying skin. Other factors such as aging and mechanical factors will have a greater influence on the STLs in these locations. In many individuals a crosshatch effect is seen where both horizontal and diagonal lines intersect on the lateral forehead and temple. Uncommonly, individual predominance of the temporoparietalis muscle (superior and anterior parietal muscles in conjunction with the temporal fascia) may be sufficiently well developed to influence the forehead lines.[7,35] It is the author's opinion that in this instance diagonal lines will develop extending from the eyebrow to the scalp (Fig. 19-6a). Virtually all diagrams of the STLs show a concave line or furrow extending from the alar fold around the oral commissure to the chin.[6,16] However, examination of elderly individuals will demonstrate that the lower portion of this line often extends laterally from the oral commissure toward the midmandible rather than medially to the mental area (Fig. 19-7c,e). Following a contour map in this area may result in the incision crossing the STLs.

On the skin of the lateral neck, the STLs tend to parallel the crease lines which run in a diagonal direction from the posterior triangle to the anterior midline. This would appear to result from the contraction of the platysma muscle. On the nuchal area, the lines may be horizontal but often the skin tends to form intersecting diagonal lines creating rhomboids

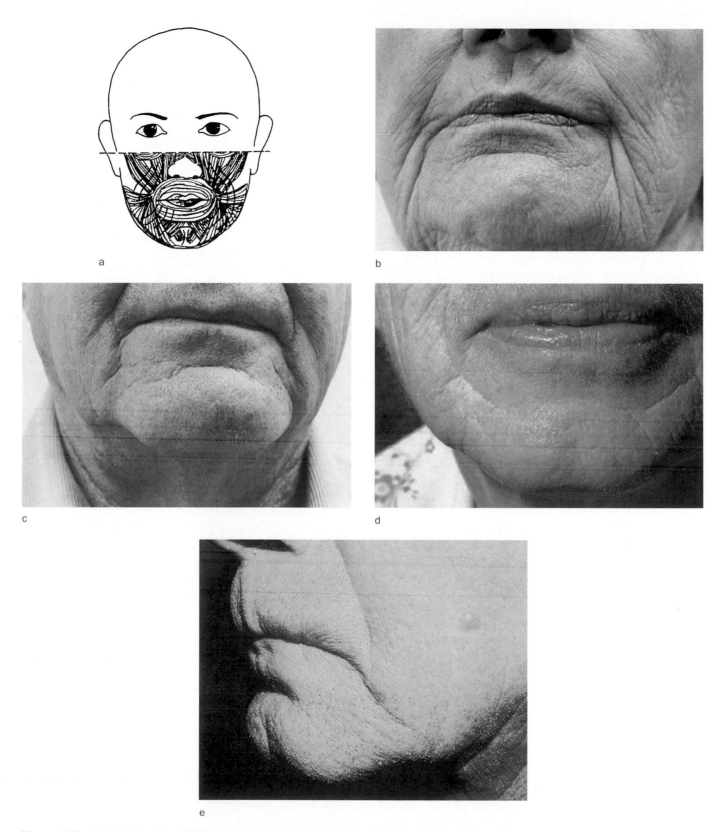

Figure 19-7 *(a)* Relationship of STLs of the cheeks, perioral area, and chin to the underlying muscles. Note variation of STLs about mouth and chin. STLs on upper cheeks tend to be constant *(used with permission of Mosby-Year Book. Current Issues in Dermatology, vol 2, 1984. Jeffery P. Callen, Sam Stegman, eds. Forces in Skin Tension Lines by Gerald Bernstein, M.D.); (b–e)* variations in direction of STLs around the mouth. *(Used with permission of Mosby-Year Book. Current Issues in Dermatology, vol 2, 1984. Jeffery P. Callen, Sam Stegman, eds. Forces in Skin Tension Lines by Gerald Bernstein, M.D.)*

or a diamond-shaped pattern. In this area, a diagonal incision may be more appropriate depending on the individual pattern.

The STLs on the trunk and extremities tend to be highly variable. While the STLs over the joints are more well defined, in other areas of the trunk and extremities they are highly variable and change with shifts of position. Also, as noted in "Contour Lines" above, incisions over joints should be aligned parallel to the flexion (contour) lines to avoid contractures and impairment of function.

Determining the Direction of the STLs

Identifying the STLs is easy in adults or elderly individuals in whom a highly developed wrinkle pattern exists (Fig. 19-8). The surgeon merely places the incision in, or parallel to, the prominent wrinkle lines in the adjacent skin. If a tumor deforms the skin and obliterates the lines at the operative site, the skin of the contralateral side or the adjacent skin may be used as an aid to finding the direction of the STLs. When operating on younger individuals or those who do not have well-developed wrinkle lines, there are several techniques which can help to identify the direction of the STLs for those individuals. These include:

1. Having the patient exercise the skin (by grimacing, smiling, frowning, etc.)
2. Pinching the skin
3. Performing a circular incision

Exercising the facial muscles will throw the skin into easily discernible folds. However, the folds that are created are forced and will not necessarily depict the RSTLs. Moreover, in areas such as the mouth, where multiple muscles act in different directions, the skin lines caused by one action, such as frowning, will produce lines which vary 180° from those produced by another action, such as smiling. Thus, the lines created by forced muscle contraction may not be accurate (Figs. 19-9a–b).

Another way to determine the direction of the skin lines is to gently pinch the skin between the thumb and forefinger.[24] This will create parallel lines when the direction of the pinch is perpendicular to the existing STLs. If one pinches across or at angles to the STLs, a twisting or S-shaped series of lines will appear (Figs. 19-10a–b). By carefully repeating this procedure both on the operative site and the contralateral skin, one can often accurately determine the correct direction of the STLs. The author believes this can be a highly effective technique when properly executed.

Perhaps the most accurate technique to identify the direction of the STLs is to excise the tumor in the shape of circle.[3,7,23,24] The skin is then undermined and hemostasis achieved. After a variable waiting period of up to 10 mins, the skin will often be spontaneously pulled into an oval with its long axis parallel to the STLs. This is likely to be the direc-

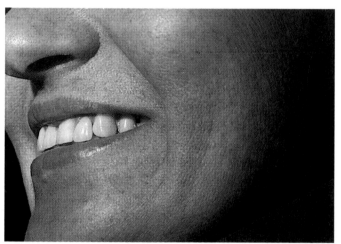

a

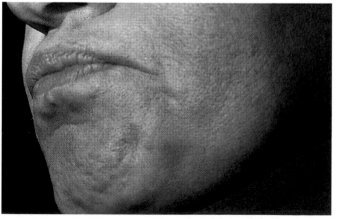

b

Figure 19-9 Effect of exercising facial muscles to determine direction of STLs. Note variation in direction of lines during smiling (*a*) as compared with frowning (*b*).

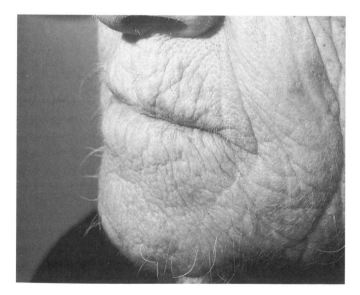

Figure 19-8 The prominent wrinkle pattern in an elderly individual.

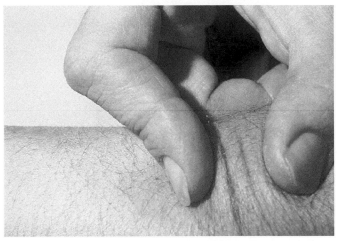

a

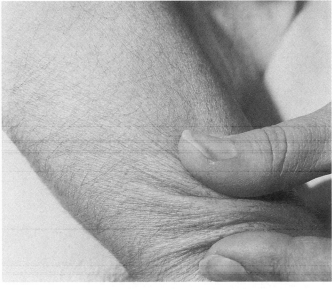

b

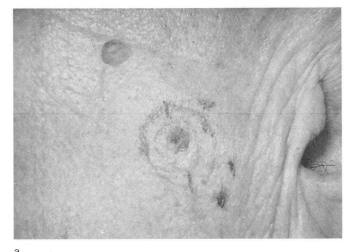

a

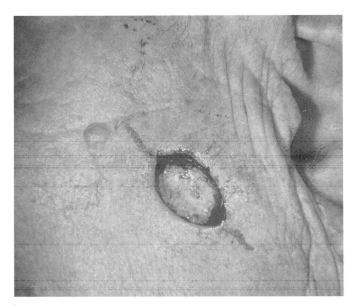

b

Figure 19-10 *(a)* Pinching the skin gently between the thumb and forefinger causes fine parallel wrinkles that indicate the direction of the STLs; *(b)* when the fingers are not pinching the skin at right angles to the STLs, twisted or crinkled lines appear. *(Used with permission of Mosby-Year Book. Current Issues in Dermatology, vol 2, 1984. Jeffery P. Callen, Sam Stegman, eds. Forces in Skin Tension Lines by Gerald Bernstein, M.D.)*

Figure 19-11 Determining direction of STLs by excising a circle. *(a)* wound is excised in a circular fashion as outlined on the skin; *(b)* after one undermines the wound and waits up to 10 min, the wound pulls up into an oval along direction of STLs.

tion of the actual STLs for that patient (Figs. 19-11*a–b*). One then simply closes the wound along the long axis of the oval and removes the resultant dog-ear deformity at each pole. However, in order for this maneuver to be effective, the facial musculature must be relaxed and in an anatomically neutral position. Twisting to obtain an optimally exposed operative site can distort the skin and produce inaccurate STLs (Figs. 19-12*a–b*). Exercise or contracture of the facial muscles can have the same effect. The surgeon may need to take off the surgical drapes and have the patient relax and assume an anatomically neutral position; it may be even necessary to have the patient sit up. The excellence of the resultant scar

more than justifies the expenditure in time. If the procedure is performed on skin with neutral tension, excising a circle will not result in an oval. In this instance, one should try to gently close the wound with fingers or skin hooks, in all directions, to determine the direction with the least tension. Although these techniques can help to accurately identify the STLs, they are not infallible, and, in some individuals, it will be difficult or impossible to find the STLs with certainty.

Not infrequently, the long axis of a lesion may be situated perpendicularly to the STLs. In this instance, it is often more appropriate to excise the tumor parallel to its long axis rather than to the STLs in order to keep the incision from being too long. The incision can be redirected during surgery by the use of one or more Z-plasties or, if necessary, later with running W-plasties (Fig. 19-13*a–b*).

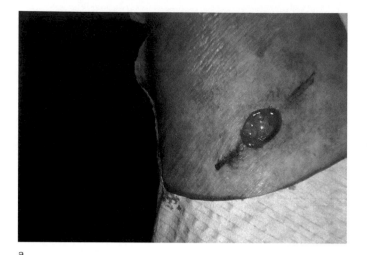

a

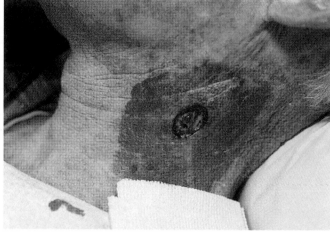

a

b

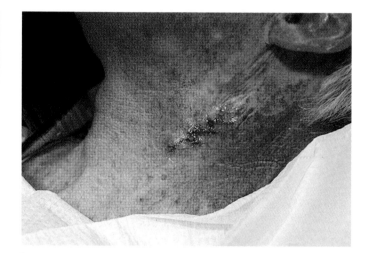

b

Figure 19-12   Effect of movement on STLs. *(a)* A circular incision was made on the forearm. After it was undermined, wound pulled into an oval. This figure demonstrates direction of the oval in a relaxed normal anatomic position; *(b)* same wound when the extremity is moved to obtain optimal exposure. *(Used with permission of Mosby-Year Book. Current Issues in Dermatology, vol 2, 1984. Jeffery P. Callen, Sam Stegman, eds. Forces in Skin Tension Lines by Gerald Bernstein, M.D.)*

Figure 19-13   *(a)* Wound directed across rather than parallel to STLs. *(b)* Z-plasty is used to redirect incision along STLs.

Special attention must be given to the direction of the line of elective incisions at free edges, such as the lips, the alar rim, and the eyelid margins. Incisions made parallel to the free margin are likely to result in retraction of the free margin. In these areas the incisions should be made perpendicularly to the free margin. This is true even when, as in the eyelid, the STLs run parallel to the lid margin (Fig. 19-14).[3]

Incisions made over concavities must be placed perpendicularly to the direction of the concavity. As wounds contract along their long axis, incisions placed in the long axis of a concavity will tend to shorten and form a web (Fig. 19-15). Placing the incision across the concavity can help prevent this complication.[3]

On the trunk and extremities, determining the optimal direction of elective incision may be very difficult. Pinching the skin gently between the thumb and forefinger will often demonstrate favorable lines. Also, excising the lesion in a circular fashion, as described above, can help. Again, for these maneuvers to reproduce the STLs accurately, it is important that the patient be relaxed and in an anatomically neutral position. Even with these precautions, the skin lines may be difficult to find on the trunk and extremities because of the changes in tension with movement and changes in position.

Also, while surgeons generally agree that placing incisions parallel to the STLs will produce a finer surgical result, it is not inevitably so. Adherence to the principles of hemostasis, dead space closure, careful suturing, and other technical aspects of wound closure are also critical elements to the creation of a fine scar. Thus, cutting across an STL will not inevitably produce a cosmetically unacceptable scar.[7,16]

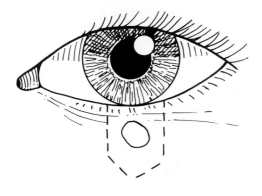

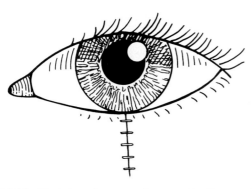

Figure 19-14   Excision of tumor at free margin. Correct direction of excision of tumor at eyelid margin is perpendicular to the free edges, even though this crosses the STLs.

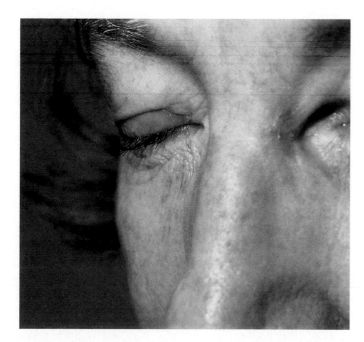

Figure 19-15   Web forming at medial canthus. This wound healed by secondary intention. Directing incision parallel to rather than across concavity of medial orbit would produce a similar unsatisfactory result.

SUMMARY

The optimal placement of an elective incision depends on several factors. The most important of these are the contour lines and the STLs. The contour lines are boundaries which define major facial anatomic structures and cosmetic units, such as the eyes, lips, nose, cheeks, etc., as well as flexural creases. Contour lines also include the shapes of these structures and the depressions, concavities, and proportional relationships of the structures of the head and neck. Contour lines are generally uniform for most people and are ordinarily easy to identify. These lines are of cosmetic and often functional importance. The surgeon should attempt to maintain the contour lines by appropriate placement of elective incisions. Also, these lines can be utilized to hide or camouflage surgical scars.

Most facial anatomic structures are further divided into cosmetic subunits by usually less well-defined boundaries or lines. Utilization of these lines can similarly enhance a surgical result. Grafts and flaps taken from the same cosmetic subunit as the wound tend to heal with cosmetically superior results.

In contrast to the contour lines, the STLs tend to be variable and are often difficult to define, especially in younger people or those with smooth skin. The STLs appear to be a result of long-term contraction of the underlying musculature on the overlying skin, especially on the face. Other factors include loss of elasticity, solar damage, aging, gravity, smoking, and mechanical factors. The STLs are felt to be equivalent to the wrinkles. The STLs can be variable and their direction cannot be confidently determined by examining a standard contour map; they must be identified for each individual. Techniques to help identify the STLs on an individual include exercising the muscles of facial expression, pinching the skin, and excising a circle.

Placement of the incision along rather than across or at angles to the STLs will tend to result in a more cosmetically acceptable scar. By placing an elective incision in or parallel to a contour line or an STL, one can enhance the cosmetic appearance of the surgical scar. However, careful placement of an incision does not guarantee a perfect scar nor does violation of these lines invariably produce a bad scar.

REFERENCES

1. McGregor IA: *Fundamental Technics of Plastic Surgery and Their Surgical Applications,* 6th ed. Baltimore, Williams & Wilkins, 1975, pp 1–5

2. Grabb WC, Smith JE: *Plastic Surgery: A Concise Guide to Clinical Practice,* 2d ed. Boston, Little, Brown, 1968, pp 3–6

3. Salasche J et al: *Surgical Anatomy of the Skin.* Norwalk, Conn, Appleton & Lange, 1988, pp 13–35

4. Powell N, Humphreys B: *Proportions of the Aesthetic Face.* New York, Thieme-Stratton, 1984

5. Converse JM: Introduction to plastic surgery, in *Reconstructive Plastic Surgery,* 2d ed, edited by JM Converse. Philadelphia, Saunders, 1977, pp 38–44

6. Burget GC, Menick FJ: The subunit principal in nasal reconstruction. *Plast Reconstr Surg* **76:**239, 1985

7. Bernstein G: Forces in skin tension lines of the face, in *Current Issues in Dermatology,* edited by JP Callen. Boston, CK Hall, 1984, pp 213–235

8. Reeh MJ et al: *Ophthalmic Anatomy.* Rochester, American Academy of Ophthalmology, 1981

9. Langer K: On the anatomy and physiology of the skin, pt 1: The cleavability of the cutis. *Br J Plast Surg* **31:**3–8, 1978

10. Langer K: On the anatomy and physiology of the skin, pt 2: Skin tension. *Br J Plast Surg* **31:**93–106, 1978

11. Borges AF: *Elective Incisions and Scar Revisions.* Boston, Little, Brown, 1973, pp 1–14

12. Malgaigne JF: *Manuel d'Medicine Operatoire.* Paris, JB Bailliere, 1849

13. Conway JH: Note on cutaneous healing in wounds. *Surg Gynecol Obstet* **66:**140–144, 1938

14. Stark RB: *Surgery.* New York, Harper & Row, 1962, pp 38–40

15. Kocher T: *Textbook of Operative Surgery,* vol 1, 3d English ed. New York, Macmillan, 1911, pp 30–32

16. Kraissl CJ: The selection of appropriate lines for elective surgical incisions. *Plast Reconstr Surg* **8:**1–28, 1951

17. Cox HP: The cleavage lines of skin. *Br J Surg* **29:**234–240, 1941

18. Gibson T, Kennedi RM: Biomechanical properties of skin. *Surg Clin North Am* **47:**279, 1969

19. Dupuytren JF: *Traite Théorique et Practique des Blessures par Arnes de Guerre* volume 1, p 66. Paris, JB Bailliere, 1834

20. Ragnell A: The tensibility of the skin: An experimental investigation. *Plast Reconstr Surg* **14:**317–323, 1954

21. Ruben LR: Langer's lines and facial scars. *Plast Reconstr Surg* **3:**147–155, 1948

22. Becker FF: *Facial Reconstruction with Local and Regional Flaps.* New York, Thieme-Stratton, 1985, pp 45

23. Bulacio Nunez AW: A new theory regarding the lines of skin tension. *Plast Reconstr Surg* **53:**663–669, 1974

24. Stegman SJ: Guidelines for the placement of elective incisions. *Dermatol Allerg* **3:**43–52, 1980

25. Mitz V, Peyronie M: The superficial musculoaponeurotic system (SMAS) in the parotid and cheek area. *Plast Reconstr Surg* **58:**80, 1976

26. Rees TD: Aesthetic plastic surgery, in *The SMAS and the Platsyma,* vol 2. Philadelphia, Saunders, 1980, pp 634–683

27. Dzubow LM: A histologic pattern approach to the anatomy of the face. *J Dermatol Surg Oncol* **12:**712, 1986

28. Jost G, Levet Y: Parotid fascia and facelifting: A critical evaluation of the SMAS concept. *Plast Reconstr Surg* **74:**72, 1984

29. Jost G, Lamouche G: SMAS in rhytidectomy. *Aesthetic Plast Surg* **6**(2):69, 1982

30. Pierard GE, Lapierre CM: Microanatomy of the dermis in relation to relaxed skin tension lines and Langer's lines. *Am J Dermatopathol* **9:**219–224, 1987

31. Pierard GE, Lapierre CM: Micro and anatomical basis of facial frown lines. *Arch Dermatol* **125:**1090–1092, 1989

32. Tsuji T: Ultrastructure of deep wrinkles in the elderly. *J Cutan Pathol* **14:**158–164, 1987

33. Gibson T: The physical properties of skin, in *Reconstructive Plastic Surgery,* 2d ed, edited by JM Converse. Philadelphia, Saunders, 1977, pp 69–77

34. Gibson T, Kennedi RM: The structural components of the dermis, in *The Dermis,* edited by W Montagna, JP Bentley & RL Dobson. New York: Appleton-Century-Crofts, 1970 p 19

35. Montagna W, Parakkal PF: *The Structure and Function of the Skin,* 3d ed. New York, Academic Press, 1974, pp 96–137

36. Braverman IM, Fonkerko E: Studies in cutaneous aging, pt 1: The elastic fiber network. *J Invest Dermatol* **78:**434–443, 1982

37. Daly CH, Odland GF: Age-related changes in the mechanical properties of human skin. *J Invest Dermatol* **73:**84–87, 1979

38. *Gray's Anatomy,* 27th ed, edited by CM Goss. Philadelphia, Lea & Febiger, 1965

39. Hollinshead WH: *Anatomy for Surgeons,* vol 1, 2d ed. New York, Harper & Row, 1968

40. Kadunce DP et al: Facial skin wrinkling in "crow's foot." *Ann Intern Med* **114:**840–844, 1991

41. Stegman S: Personal communication, July 1987

42. *The Anatomy of Sleep.* Nutley, NJ, Roche Labs, Division of Hoffman-LaRoche, 1966

43. Lapierre CM: The aging dermis: The main cause for the appearance of "old" skin. *Br J Dermatol* **122**(suppl):35–11, 1990

44. Tsuji T et al: Light and scanning electronmicroscopic studies on wrinkles in aged person's skin. *Br J Dermatol* **114:**329–335, 1986

45. Uitto J: Connective tissue biochemistry of the aging dermis: Age-related alterations in collagen and elastin. *Dermatol Clin* **4**(3):433–446, 1986

IV Chemical Destructive Techniques

Harry M. Humeniuk
Gary P. Lask

20 Surgical and Medical Treatment of Benign Cutaneous Lesions

This chapter addresses the management of benign cutaneous lesions. Such tumors are brought to the dermatologic surgeon's attention for one of several reasons: The patient may notice a new lesion or a change in a previously static one. There may be an associated functional or mechanical problem or removal may be requested for purely cosmetic reasons. Regardless, the method chosen to remove the growth must take into consideration the banality of the lesion. Whether cosmesis was of the patient's initial concern or not, the resultant scar from a procedure should not be less desirable than the preexisting lesion.

A sound understanding of surgical anatomy and basic surgical technique is prerequisite for many of the procedures described hereafter. Some lesions described in this chapter may require more complicated closures than are discussed. Expertise in the use of various flaps may be necessary to achieve results that are cosmetically acceptable. Proper selection and execution of complicated cutaneous flaps are best left in the hands of the advanced dermatologic surgeon.

Although each benign cutaneous lesion amenable to surgery is not addressed in this chapter, the techniques described are adaptable to most benign lesions presenting to the dermatologist. Brief clinical descriptions precede outlined therapeutic modalities. Generally, simple procedures are discussed first followed by techniques of increasing complexity.

VERRUCAE

Warts are probably the most common virally induced cutaneous tumors in humans. Greater than 60 in number, subtypes of human papilloma virus (HPV) can be identified by DNA hybridization. Subtypes of HPV causing condyloma acuminatum have been identified in cervical carcinoma. Keratoacanthomas have also been associated with HPV. Subtype identification of condyloma acuminatum in females may be warranted as it will help identify a population at risk for development of squamous cell carcinoma (SCC).[1,2]

Immunocompromised individuals have an increased susceptibility to HPV. Organ transplant patients on immunosuppressives are often plagued by recalcitrant verrucae. Multiple keratoacanthomas have also been seen to arise in these individuals.

As grouped subtypes of HPV induce different types of verrucae, their number, location, and type may dictate the form of therapy chosen.

Verrucae Vulgaris

Although this form of wart may arise at any age, it is generally found in children and younger teens. These well-circumscribed, brown-to-black, rough-surfaced papules may arise on any cutaneous surface. However, sites of predilection include the dorsum of the hands and fingers. Lesions tend to be relatively asymptomatic unless they are located on pressure points or are periungual.

Management

A conservative initial approach to the treatment of verrucae vulgaris is usually recommended.

Liquid Nitrogen Cryotherapy causes a split at the dermal-epidermal junction resulting in a blister. Blister formation usually begins in 8 to 24 h. Since the HPV is limited to the epidermis, the wart should theoretically be shed with the blister roof. As an adjunct to cryotherapy, paring down thick warts may be done with a no. 10 blade. This is done to a level where the dilated capillaries are just visible. Care should be taken not to cause bleeding. Paring down lesions in this fashion will allow for shorter freeze times. A few small lesions may be treated by repeated alternating cotton tip-swab applications of liquid nitrogen. A 1 to 2 mm rim of freeze should be achieved. Thaw times vary depending on lesion size and range from 3 to 30 s. Larger lesions may be treated in a similar fashion by utilizing a gynecologic cotton swab (lollipop) applicator. This large swab holds more liquid nitrogen as will loosening the cotton tip on conventional 6-in applicators. Liquid nitrogen spray provides slightly less fine control than cotton tip application. However, it may be more applicable if there are numerous or very large lesions. Cryotherapy of periungual warts can be exquisitely painful and frequently provides inadequate results. Often this is due to a wart's subungual extension or too short a freeze time by the sympathetic operator. Cryotherapy may require several treatment sessions.[3,4]

Electrodesiccation and Curettage Local anesthetic with or without ephinephrine is injected beneath the wart, raising the lesion with a small bleb. The verrucous mass is curetted or shaved off providing a specimen for biopsy. The base of the lesion is then destroyed by electrodesiccation or electrofulguration and repeated curettage. Both steps may need to be repeated several times to eradicate the lesion and a final electrodesiccation is performed for hemostasis. Topical antibiotics should be applied daily to the treated area until they are completely healed. A no. 4 or larger curette is generally used in removing verrucae in this fashion. However, small

periungual extensions may be removed by utilizing a small no. 1 or 2 curette while leaving the nail intact.[5]

Extensive subungual extension of the wart requires nail avulsion before adequate therapy can be provided. Anesthesia is provided with a ring block. The nail may be bluntly dissected from the nail bed with a hemostat, grasped, and removed.

Topical Agents Many topical agents previously available by prescription only are now available as over-the-counter preparations. Of these, the salicylic acid-impregnated films allow for easy and accurate application by the patient. As described in "Liquid Nitrogen" above, thick lesions may be pared down on the initial office visit and the patient given visual instruction as to the medication's application. The film is cut to a size 1 to 2 mm larger than the lesion and applied directly to its surface. Occasionally, waterproof tape is necessary to keep the film in place. The film is removed every 2 to 5 days, and the soft white tissue is gently removed with clean gauze or a pumice stone. The process is then repeated.

Laser CO_2 laser can be effective. The power setting is from 3 to 20 W utilizing a continuous wave and defocused mode. Multiple passes are made over the wart to produce a char. The char is then removed with hydrogen peroxide-soaked gauze by gentle rubbing. Any remaining portion of the lesion may then be retreated.[6]

Bleomycin Recently, this chemotherapeutic agent has become popular in the treatment of verrucae. Bleomycin, although very effective, is expensive and once reconstituted has a short shelf life. Initially, reconstituted bleomycin was injected directly into warts. Treatment sessions were restricted to 2 mL total volumes, a maximum of 1 mL single largest dose per lesion, and often were painful.[7]

Another technique developed by the Shelleys[8] causes less pain and utilizes smaller dosages. A warm-water soak of the wart for 10 min hydrates the overlying keratin. Lidocaine 2% with or without epinephrine is used for anesthesia. Bleomycin (1 U/mL) is dropped from a tuberculin syringe onto the wart's surface (0.02 mL/5 mm^2). A bifurcated vaccination needle is then rapidly punctured through the wart's base. About 40 such punctures are performed in a 5 mm^2 area. A dry dressing is applied over the treated area. Minimal discomfort may be noted for the following 24 h. This technique was met with a 92 percent cure rate in the study quoted.[8]

Verrucae Planae

Also known as *flat warts,* these 0.1 to 0.3 cm flat papules are usually flesh to tan in color. They commonly arise on the dorsum of the hands and are extremely problematic when found in the beard area or on the legs where shaving can lead to extensive autoinoculation.

Management

A conservative approach is generally warranted as aggressive therapy may produce cosmetic results less satisfactory than the lesion itself.

Topical Tretinoin   Tretinoin cream in a concentration of 0.025% is applied daily. The patient should be instructed to apply the cream to *areas* of flat warts rather than treating lesions individually since new lesions may arise. Response to this form of therapy is variable and may require an extended treatment period.

Electrodesiccation   A disposable pointed tip or metal-hubbed 30-gauge 1/2-in needle with adapter is used. The hyfrecator is turned to the "just on" position. The flat wart's surface is then painted to a gray-white color. Lesions crust over and are shed in a few days.

Liquid Nitrogen   See "Liquid Nitrogen" above in "Verrucae Vulgaris." Freeze times are 5 to 10 s.

Trichloroacetic Acid (TCA)   Precise application of TCA in concentrations of 10 to 35% may be efficacious. This form of treatment, as the previous two, may be repeated every 2 to 3 weeks.

Plantar Warts

This form of wart, affecting the soles, can achieve an impressive size. Thickened keratotic plaques often produce pain over pressure points of the heel and metatarsals. Plantar warts often persist for years and may be recalcitrant to many forms of therapy.

Management

Initially a nonsurgical approach may be warranted. Scarring is not an uncommon side effect from aggressive surgery of the soles resulting in life long pain.

Topical Agents   See "Management" above in "Verrucae Vulgaris." An alternative is to apply 70 to 90% TCA to the lesion followed by covering the lesion with a salicylic-impregnated plaster and waterproof tape. This is left in place for a 5- to 7-day period. This process results in a soft white lesion which often blisters. The mass can then be removed by blunt dissection.[9] This form of therapy would be best avoided if there is a concomitant fungal infection.

Bleomycin   Planter warts may be the best candidates for this form of therapy. See "Management" above in "Verrucae Vulgaris."[8]

CO_2 LASER/LIQUID NITROGEN   See "Management" above in "Verrucae Vulgaris."

Condylomata Acuminata

This form of wart is generally considered a sexually transmitted disease. Condylomata tend to arise on moist surfaces of the genitalia. They appear as soft, fleshy, skin-colored papules that may be pedunculated with a broad base. Multiple flat lesions can become confluent. Several considerations must be addressed prior to treating these lesions which include:

1. Large lesions may represent giant condylomata of Buschke-Löwenstein. This tumor has a distinct clinical appearance, described as a cauliflower-like exophytic mass generally localized to the glans penis. This tumor should be classified as a verrucous carcinoma of the anogenital mucosa and therefore treated as a malignancy.[10,11]
2. Female patients with condylomata may be at additional risk for the development of cervical carcinoma. A gynecologic consultation can assist in the search for internal lesions and provide the follow-up necessary for screening for SCC. Subtypes that have been implicated include HPV 16, 18, 31, 32, 33, 35, 39, 42, and 51 to 54.[1]
3. Perianal condylomata may recur after apparently adequate therapy. These recurrences may not necessarily represent reinfection but seeding from deeper internal lesions. Consultation with gastrointestinal (GI) or colorectal surgery are necessary for the search for these hidden lesions.

Management

Excision   A few lesions may be treated by simple excision. Local anesthetic is injected beneath the lesion. The wart is held with fine forceps and removed by either shave excision or with sharp curved iris scissors. The base is then lightly electrodesiccated to destroy any remaining viral particles. Scarring is usually minimal.

Liquid Nitrogen   See "Management" above in "Verrucae vulgaris." Pedunculated lesions may be somewhat difficult to treat with cryotherapy and care should be taken to achieve an adequate freeze at the base of the lesion. Pain and mild scarring can be infrequent side effects.

Topical Preparations   Podophyllin is a derivative of the mayapple, available in various concentrations. Application is performed in the office and allowed to remain for a period of 6 to 8 h and then washed off. Pain and burning are common side effects but rarely necessitates premature removal. Removal is accomplished by soaking in a tub of warm water while gently cleansing the area. The concentration of Podophyllin can vary from lot to lot as well as with shelf life.

Condylox   Condylox is an at-home application of podofilox by the patient. An in-office initial application will give the patient a better understanding of its use. As with podophyllin, once an applicator has been used, it should not be reintroduced into the solution. Removing most of the cotton from the applicator tip allows for less waste and more precise application. Condylox is applied daily for 3 consecutive days. After a 4-day holiday, the sequence is repeated. Several days later the patient is reevaluated and, if necessary, a second course is prescribed.[12]

Laser See "Management" above in "Verrucae Vulgaris." As is the case with cryotherapy, attention to the base of pedunculated lesions is a must.

Interferon Alpha and beta forms of interferon can be injected intralesionally or intramuscularly. Flulike symptoms and prolonged treatment sessions are limitations.[1,13]

ACROCHORDONS

These filiform flesh-colored lesions are also known as *fibroepithelial polyps* or *skin tags*. Acrochordons generally measure between 0.1 to 0.4 cm in length. However, large pedunculated cerebriform lesions may arise with narrow stalks. Most commonly these lesions are localized to areas where skin rubs against skin, including the neck, axilla, below the breasts, and on the inner upper thigh. This latter location is a site of predilection for the larger pedunculated forms. These giant acrochordons often produce mechanical problems and are routinely traumatized by underclothing or by merely walking. A common presentation is an acrochordon that twisted on its stalk and infarcted.

There may be a loose association between acrochordons and the development of colon polyps.

Management

Excision Multiple small acrochordons can be removed by simple scissor excision. The lesion is grasped with fine-tipped forceps and snipped flush with the skin with sharp curved iris scissors. This is a relatively painless procedure and local anesthetic is rarely necessary. If required, cautery is achieved by application of 20% aluminum chloride or light electrodesiccation.

Large pedunculated acrochordons may not be amenable to scissor excision. Under local anesthetic, with or without epinephrine, a small, tight elliptic excision at the base of the stalk is followed by simple closure.

Electrodesiccation A hyfrecator set at a low current is used along with a fine tip. The hyfrecator tip is placed on the upper outer edge of the acrochordon and power is applied for 0.5 to 2 s. The skin tag and its associated vessel is thermally destroyed resulting in a minute char. The coagulated remnant will drop off in a few days.

SEBORRHEIC KERATOSES

These lesions are sharply demarcated and vary in color from gray-white to brown to black. Seborrheic keratoses are generally less than 1 cm in diameter but occasionally measure up to several centimeters. Sites of predilection are the back and face; however, they may be commonly found elsewhere. Lesions generally appear in the fourth and fifth decades of life and gradually increase in number with age.

The sign of Leser-Trélat is the abrupt onset of multiple seborrheic keratoses heralding an internal malignancy. Seborrheic keratoses may be dominantly inherited or spontaneous.

Clinically, seborrheic keratoses can be confused with verrucae or acrochordons.

Management

Curettage Curettement can be a simple, rapid treatment for seborrheic keratosis. A local anesthetic is injected underneath the lesion. A no. 4 or larger curette is used and the curettement is begun at the edge of the lesion closest to the operator. A

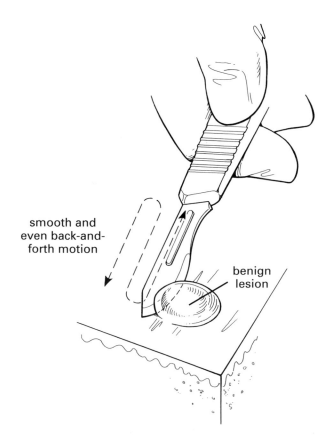

Figure 20-1 Technique for shave excision.

quick rotational flick of the currette away from the operator completes the lesion's removal. Soft lesions may be pre-treated with liquid nitrogen rendering the lesion more firm and easier to remove. Freezing may also obviate the need for a local anesthetic.

Cautery is achieved with aluminum chloride, TCA, or light electrodesiccation.

Liquid Nitrogen   Cryotherapy alone may be used in the re-moval of seborrheic keratosis. However, incomplete removal of the lesion is common as is postinflammatory hyperpig-mentation. Curettement therefore should accompany this form of treatment.

Excision   Shave excision is done under a local anesthetic. The shave is begun at the edge of the lesion farthest from the operator. With the blade's surface horizontal to the patient's skin, the shave is performed by a smooth back-and-forth saw-ing motion of the blade as it is advanced toward the operator. The procedure is completed by applying gentle pressure with a finger from the free hand on the lesion's surface while com-pleting the blade's advancement (Fig. 20-1).

Scissor excision may be performed for the pedunculated variety of seborrheic keratosis. See "Management" above in "Acrochordons."

Electrodesiccation   Local anesthesia is recommended for this form of treatment. Electrodesiccation may be used alone or in combination with curettage.

DERMATOSIS PAPULOSA NIGRA

These smooth, brown-black papules resemble seborrheic ker-atosis histologically. They are found most commonly in dark-skinned individuals about the face, neck, and upper trunk. Le-sions tend to be multiple and measure 0.1 to 0.4 cm.

Management

Curettage   Light curettement of multiple lesions may pro-vide excellent results. Lesions need not be completely re-moved, only "roughed up" to provide adequate treatment. A few test areas may be treated initially. If results are satisfac-tory, large areas may be treated in this fashion. Local anes-thetic is only rarely required.[14]

With electrosurgery, multiple lesions may be ablated with low-current electrodesiccation.

MELANOCYTIC NEVI

Nevocytic nevi are common benign lesions of the skin. His-tologically, these lesions consist of grouped nevus cells.

Melanocytes and nevus cells are both dopa-positive; they dif-fer in that nevus cells lack dendrites and also tend to form "nests."

Clinically, benign nevi are symmetric, evenly pigmented, and maintain a regular order. Nevi may be flat, dome shaped, cerebriform, or pedunculated. Pigmentation may be flesh-colored in dome-shaped or pedunculated forms of nevi. When pigmentation is present, it is generally uniform and lesions may appear tan, brown, or black.[15]

Dysplastic nevi (Clark's nevus) and nevi with features of a lentigo may be difficult to distinquish clinically. Whether or not dysplastic nevi represent markers or precursors of melanoma is beyond the scope of this discussion and is ad-dressed elsewhere in this text. The episcope, once reliable standardized criteria are established, should be a valuable tool in the evaluation of these pigmented lesions.[16]

Nevi are brought to the attention of the dermatologist for various reasons. Often times the patient wishes the lesion to be removed for cosmetic reasons alone. Elevated lesions may be subject to trauma and therefore be mechanically problem-atic. Biopsy of the nevus is a must if there has been irregular growth, change in color, ulceration, and/or bleeding. If the le-sion can be easily removed in toto, it should be done. An in-cisional biopsy is a plausible alternative for lesions that are very large or on cosmetically significant locations.

Management

Local anesthetic is required for all of the methods of removal described below.

Excision   Scissor excision may be performed as described for pedunculated nevi above in "Acrochordons." One or two simple interrupted sutures may be necessary to close the de-fect.

Shave excision may be performed as described above in "Seborrheic Keratoses." Flesh-colored lesions should be out-lined or painted with a surgical marking pen before the infil-tration of local anesthetic. Care should be taken not to shave too deeply as this will likely result in a depressed scar. The patient should be made aware that a portion of the lesion can remain and be slightly elevated (Fig. 20-2). Repeat shave ex-cision may then produce a satisfactory result. The patient should also be informed that shave excision of dome-shaped, pigmented nevi may result in a flat pigmented macule. Pa-tients must be made aware that future biopsies at sites where nevus cells are left behind can be histologically misinter-preted as a melanoma. Therefore, this erroneous diagnosis can be avoided with adequate information.

Excisional surgery followed by closure often provides an excellent result. This method also provides the dermato-pathologist with an adequate specimen for diagnosis. Exci-sional surgery is strongly recommended for a suspected ma-lignancy. Shave excision and biopsy may provide an adequate specimen for the diagnosis of melanoma; however, it may

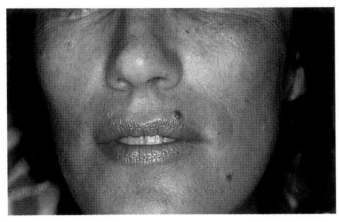

a

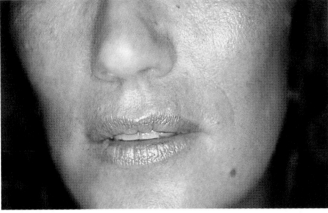

b

Figure 20-2 *(a)* Compound nevus left upper lip. *(b)* After removal by shave excision.

eliminate the ability to make an accurate measurement of depth of invasion and hence prognosis.

LENTIGINES

Simple lentigines (lentigo simplex) are tan, evenly pigmented to black-colored macules that may arise on any mucocutaneous surface. Typically, these lesions are first noted in childhood and measure 0.1 to 0.2 cm in diameter. As the individual ages, the lesions may enlarge, become confluent, or regress. There are multiple syndromes which have lentigo simplex as a component.

Solar lentigines, as their name suggests, are induced by ultraviolet irradiation. They are typically tan to brown in color and may reach several centimeters in diameter. These lesions are commonly found on the dorsum of the hands and on the face. These are the lesions which the layperson commonly refers to as *age* or *liver spots*.[17]

Lentigo maligna is the transformation of a solar lentigo into a melanoma in situ. Since solar lentigines often have ir-

regular borders, this criteria is often not useful in the detection of lentigo maligna. However, alterations as well as irregularities in pigmentation can be diagnostic aids. Biopsy should be performed in all suspected lesions and, if positive, they should be managed as a de novo malignant melanoma. The episcope may become a valuable tool in the evaluation of lentigenes.[16]

Management

Topical Therapy Daily application of hydroquinone, a tyrosinase inhibitor, may slowly fade the lesion. Prescription forms of hydroquinone are available in greater concentrations than the over-the-counter formulations and are available combined with a sunscreen. This form of therapy may be extremely arduous if multiple lesions necessitate treatment. Application of the hydroquinone should be strictly limited to the lesion as it may cause hypopigmentation of surrounding normal skin, creating a bull's-eye effect.

Topical tretinoin 0.1% applied daily may lead to a significant decrease in pigmentation of lentigenes. Results are often seen after only one month of therapy and lightening continues with further treatment.[18]

Liquid Nitrogen Cryotherapy can produce excellent results in the treatment of lentigines. An initial conservative light freeze is suggested. Although this technique usually requires several treatment sessions, it permits the adjustment of freeze times to more resistant areas within a single lesion. This stepwise approach can leave the lesion nearly indistinguishable from adjacent normal skin. If freeze and thaw times are too excessive, irregular hypopigmentation is likely to occur. The alternating cotton tip application method, as described above in "Liquid Nitrogen" for the treatment of verrucae vulgaris, allows precise application of liquid nitrogen. Thaw times should be brief (less than 20 s) as not to induce blister formation. Treatment evaluation and retreatment should be in 2- to 3-week intervals.

Pretreatment of lentigines with topical tretinoin cream 0.025% daily for a 6-week period can decrease the necessary freeze times by 50 percent.

Trichloroacetic Acid A cotton-tip swab is utilized in applying a 10 to 50% concentration of TCA. The solution should be applied evenly to the lesion until an *acid frost* is achieved. Scarring is almost never observed.

CYSTS

Cystic lesions that occur as midline nasal masses may represent dermoids, hemangiomas, nasal gliomas, or encephaloceles. Subcutaneous masses that arise at the base of the nose, along suture lines of the skull, or along the spinal column should be evaluated by appropriate radiographic studies. The

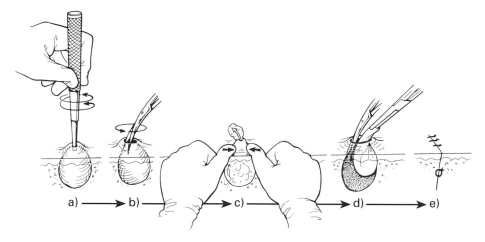

Figure 20-3 Removal of cyst through a small incision.

aforementioned tumors warrant evaluation by the neurosurgeon.[19]

Epidermoid Cysts

Epidermoid cysts are most commonly found on the face, neck, and trunk. Clinically, these cysts are freely movable in the subcutaneous tissue and measure from 0.5 cm to 5 cm in diameter. The overlying epidermis may appear smooth and shiny secondary to the outward pressure caused by the subcutaneous mass. A comedo or dilated core may commonly be found on the distended epidermis.

Cysts can rupture secondarily to incidental trauma or when the patient attempts to manually express the cyst's contents. An intense foreign body reaction may ensue once the macerated keratin and sebaceous products are introduced into the dermis. Ruptured cysts are more difficult to remove as their once pristine, definable wall becomes obliterated by fiberous scar tissue.

Management

Mildly inflamed cysts may be made quiescent with the use of intralesional steroids and oral antibiotics. Triamcinolone in a concentration of 2.5 to 3.3 mg/mL can be injected directly into the cyst. An alcohol swab is used to cleanse the skin overlying the cyst. If a dilated pore can be identified, this should be used as the entry point for the hypodermic needle and 0.05 to 0.25 mL of steroid is slowly infiltrated into the cyst.[20] Upon removal of the needle, a small amount of the cyst's contents may exude through this opening and a culture may be done to help direct antibiotic therapy. However, one of the cephalosporins or erythromycin is a good initial choice.

The patient is instructed to return in 2 weeks' time for evaluation, and retreatment or excision of the cyst may be performed. Occasionally, cysts treated in this fashion may completely resolve or they may become asymptomatic so that the patient requests no further treatment.

Excision Piezosurgery is a technique for the removal of small cysts that can produce excellent cosmetic results. As it was initially described, anesthesia is achieved by infiltrating 2% lidocaine without epinephrine just below the epidermis and above the cyst. A small, linear incision is made to a depth of the most superficial aspect of the cyst. Bilateral pressure is then applied perpendicularly to the incision which generally provides adequate exposure of the small cyst. The exposed lesion is grasped with toothed forceps and excised from below with curved iris scissors. The resultant defect may be closed with Steri-Strips or by a simple interrupted sutures.[21] A vertical mattress stitch may be preferred as it will help compensate for the space defect and evert the wound edge.

Enucleation is another popular approach to the removal of small-to-medium-sized cysts, particularly in cosmetically significant locations. Local anesthetic with or without epinephrine is infiltrated around the periphery of the lesion, creating a field block. Care should be taken not to infiltrate anesthetic directly into the lesion as this may expand and rupture the cyst wall. A 2 to 4 mm punch biopsy is used to create the defect to encounter the cyst. Larger cysts may require incision and expression of their contents prior to removal through the small defect. The glistening capsule is grasped with either toothed forceps or a hemostat and the sac is carefully dissected out with curved iris scissors. Gentle rotation of the sac in a clockwise and counterclockwise fashion often interrupts the weak adhesions and the sac is removed in toto. Complete removal of the lesion is necessary to prevent recurrence. The defect is sutured as described above (Fig. 20-3).

Larger lesions may be approached in a similar fashion when exposure is provided by the removal of a small ellipse of tissue overlying the cyst. Anesthesia is accomplished as described immediately above in "Excision." Removal of the small ellipse provides greater exposure to the larger cyst while removing expanded tissue caused by the large subcutaneous mass. Once the cyst wall is encountered, it is gently dissected out with curved iris scissors and the defect is closed with simple interrupted sutures. If a large space defect is created by the cyst removal, buried absorbable sutures are recommended.

Larger inflamed and possibly infected cysts may require an alternative approach. Incision and drainage of the lesion can often produce dramatic resolution of pain. The purulent material encountered should be cultured to ensure appropriate antibiotic coverage. Erythromycin or one of the cephalosporins should be started directly. A local anesthetic with or without epinephrine should be utilized as this procedure can be accompanied with extreme discomfort. Iodoform tape may be utilized as a packing for the created defect. A 1- to 2-in wick of tape is left exposed and either steri-stripped or paper-taped to the skin. This wick is withdrawn 1 to 2 inches daily until it is completely removed. Excision may then be followed as described above in 3 to 4 weeks. Delineation of the cyst may be difficult secondary to extensive fibrosis and inflammation that is common with these lesions.

Dana's Procedure This is a method of ablation of cysts by utilizing electrocautery. The electrocautery probe is introduced into the cyst through intact skin. Theoretically, the cyst wall is destroyed by maneuvering the electrocautery probe while it is inside the cyst. This procedure is included for historic reasons as previously described techniques are likely to cause less damage to adjacent adnexa.

Pilar Cysts

Other names for pilar cysts include *trichilemmal cysts, isthmus catagen cysts,* and *wens.* Clinically these cysts may resemble epidermal cysts; however, they arise primarily on the scalp. Pilar cysts are often very firm nodules that may be multiple. Occasionally, alopecia may appear to be overlying the lesion.

Proliferating pilar cysts can mimic SCC both clinically as well as histologically. This clinical entity has been associated with *satellite cysts* as well as lymph node metastases. If the diagnosis is unclear, these lesions should be managed as a malignancy.[22–24] These lesions tend to occur more commonly in women.

Management

As with epidermal cysts, the size of a pilar cyst can be extremely variable. As a pilar cyst matures, the cyst wall tends to become somewhat thickened and less pliable than in epidermoid cysts. The decrease in pliability of the cyst wall may obviate certain surgical approaches.

Excellent cosmetic results are not necessarily limited by the incisional approach to pilar cysts. Adequate exposure can be hindered by approaches such as piezosurgery and the use of the punch biopsy technique.

Hair overlying the cyst need not be widely shaved or cut short. An adequate field of exposure can be achieved by carefully separating the hair away while paper tape keeps it in place.[25] As described above, anesthesia is then infiltrated around the lesion to create a field block. A small amount of anesthesia may then be injected into the dermis overlying the cyst. A 5- to 10-min wait between injection of anesthesia and the initiation of removal provides an interval for the epinephrine to induce a hemostatic effect. A linear incision may be made over the dome of the cyst or a small ellipse of tissue is excised. The latter technique is preferred as it helps compensate for the expansile effect of the underlying cyst. The length of incision should approximate the diameter of the cyst. Curved iris scissors are utilized to dissect any adhesions to the cyst wall and the subcutaneous mass may be delivered in toto.

Steatocystoma Multiplex

This form of cyst can arise spontaneously or may be inherited as in an autosomal dominant trait. Histologically, steatocystomas have a flattened sebaceous gland in the cyst wall periphery. The commonly misused term *sebaceous cyst* would seem applicable to steatocystoma multiplex. Clinically, these cysts may reach several centimeters in size and are most commonly located on the chest. The proximal extremities, neck, and external genitalia are also sites common to this form of cyst.[26]

Management

These lesions may be approached by any of the methods described above in "Epidermoid Cysts." The enormous number of cysts that can be present may preclude the removal of each individual lesion. If only a few lesions are present and the patient opts for their removal, he or she should be informed that new lesions are likely to arise. Since the majority of these lesions arise on the chest, the patient should also be informed that surgery in this area often provides a poor cosmetic result.

Digital Mucoid Cysts

These cysts may arise from a herniation of the joint lining or secondarily to a metabolic disarrangement of fibroblasts. They are typically located between the distal interphalangeal joint and the proximal nail fold. A thinned epidermis covers these cystic lesions which tend to be solitary, shiny, smooth, and translucent to flesh-colored. Pain may be a presenting symptom.

Management

Intralesional Steroids Anesthesia may not be necessary in the performance of this procedure. A large-bore needle equipped with a Luer-Lok syringe is utilized to aspirate the mucinous fluid from the cyst. Triamcinolone, in a concentration of 5 to 10 mg/mL, is then infiltrated into the cyst. This form of therapy is often fraught with recurrence of the cyst; however, retreatment may lead to its resolution.

Cryotherapy The cyst is first punctured with a hypodermic needle and its contents are either aspirated or expressed by manual pressure. Liquid nitrogen may be applied by either spray or by alternating cotton-tip swabs while a 2-mm rim of freeze is achieved. Freeze times should range between 15 and 30 s. Best results are achieved when a second freeze is performed of similar duration once the initial thaw is complete.[27]

Surgical Excision A digital block should be performed to achieve adequate anesthesia for this procedure. The epidermis overlying the lesion is incised and the cyst and any synovial connections must be carefully dissected out. A method to help define the extension of the cyst is to first evacuate the cyst contents with a large-bore needle and syringe and inject methylene blue. Adjacent advancement flaps may be necessary to close the defect. Surgical excision of digital mucous cysts is not recommended for the novice surgeon. Complications can include joint stiffness and diminished mobility.

Hidrocystoma

This form of cyst may arise from either the apocrine or eccrine gland. The apocrine form of hidrocystoma tends to arise on the medial lower eyelid but can be found on other areas of the face, ears, scalp, chest, or shoulders (Fig. 20-3). Clinically, these firm blue papules may be confused with blue nevi. Eccrine hidrocystomas are clinically similar in appearance and generally arise over the cheeks. Interestingly, the number of eccrine hidrocystomas in a given individual may increase during exposure to excessive humidity and heat.

Management

Excision Simple excision with primary closure as described above in "Epidermoid Cysts" generally provides good cosmetic results.

Electrosurgery Multiple eccrine hidrocystomas may be ablated with low-current electrodesiccation.

Milia

Milia are small globoid papules that typically arise about the eyelids and cheeks. This form of cyst generally measures only a few millimeters in diameter, is white to yellow in color, and lacks a central umbilication which helps differentiate milium from molluscum contagiosum.

Management

Extraction Anesthesia is not necessary. The epidermis over the small cyst is nicked with either a no. 11 blade or a hypo-

dermic needle. The minute cyst is then plucked out with the hypodermic needle or expressed with a comedo extractor. Closure is not necessary and cosmetic results are generally excellent.

Destruction of multiple lesions may be accomplished with the use of a topical keratolytic, light electrodesiccation, or cryotherapy.

Lipomas

Lipomas are common lesions that are usually solitary and confined to the subcutis. These lesions can vary in size from less than 1 cm in diameter to greater than 5 cm in diameter. They rarely alter the overlying epidermis and may require tangential lightening to appreciate their space effect on the overlying epidermis. Lipomas are soft to palpation and can be surprisingly mobile, particularly in the mobile encapsulated form.[28] Lipomas have infrequently been found to be infiltrative. Dumbbell-shaped lipomas of the thorax apparently infiltrate through an intercostal space. Lipomas have also been found to infiltrate between large groups of muscle fascicles such as those found on the forearm.

Angiolipomas, as their name suggests, have a prominent vascular component. Clinically, angiolipomas differ from common lipomas in that they tend to be multiple and frequently are associated with pain.[29]

A lipoma that is located midline in the sacrococcygeal region should not be attempted to be removed or even biopsied. This lesion may represent a lipomeningocele that communicates with the dura.[30]

Excessively large lipomas (i.e., greater than 10 cm in diameter) may represent a malignancy. A biopsy of these lesions should be performed to identify their nature, particularly if they are located on the upper thigh.[31] If atypical fat is encountered during the removal of any lipoma, of any size, a biopsy should be performed rather than complete removal of the lesion.

Management

Many of the same surgical techniques described above in "Epidermoid Cysts" can be applied to the removal of lipomas.

Excision Since lipomas rarely alter the overlying epidermis, palpation of the lesion and outlining with a surgical marking pen prior to the infiltration of anesthetic is recommended. The blanching and induration caused by field anesthesia can obliterate the soft clinical signs of the lipoma's location.

Small lipomas may be approached by making a 2- to 3-mm incision directly over the lesion. A no. 2 cutting currette is introduced into the defect and is utilized to free and deliver the lipoma through the incision.[32] Although sutures are not required for closure, they are preferred by the authors.

Larger lesions may be approached by removing a small ellipse of tissue directly over the lipoma. This ellipse of tissue generally does not have to exceed 2 cm in length. Although very large lipomas may be enucleated through very small incisions, the subcutaneous space defect created may be difficult to close adequately. Once the lipoma is encountered, it is grasped with toothed forceps and curved iris scissors are used to dissect any adhesions. Layered closure with absorbable deep sutures is generally recommended. A pressure dressing reduces the chance of hematoma formation.

Excision from a Distance   This is a technique for the removal of subcutaneous masses in cosmetically significant locations. Areas of consideration for the use of this technique include the scalp, eyelids, preauricular region, nasolabial folds, oral mucosa, and the inframammary folds. The incision made for this approach should approximate its distance from the lesion.[33] A lighted retractor and bipolar bayonet forceps are suggested by this technique.

Liposuction   Suction-assisted lipectomy can provide excellent cosmetic results in nearly any location with a small incision.

Dermatofibromas

These firm, smooth nodules are the result of a reactive proliferation of fibroblasts or histiocytes. Although dermatofibromas may reach several centimeters in size, they usually are less than 1 cm in diameter (Fig. 20-4). These lesions may arise on any cutaneous surface, with the anterior lower extremities as a common site. The exact etiology of dermatofibromas is unclear. They may arise spontaneously or secondarily to trivial trauma, such as an insect bite. The overlying epidermis may vary in color from red to dark purple or dark brown and be flat or slightly elevated. A characteristic clinical feature of these lesions is central dimpling with the application of lateral pressure.[34]

Dermatofibrosarcoma protuberans (DFSP) is a malignant, invasive tumor of the dermis. DFSP rarely metastasizes but is locally invasive. This lesion can achieve an enormous size and occurs most commonly on the trunk.

All lesions suspected of being a DFSP should be completely excised to the level of the deep fat. Conservative excision is often met with recurrence as these lesions are usually wider than they appear clinically. The depth of invasion can also be extensive involving fascia and underlying muscle. Mohs micrographic surgery is a viable alternative to wide excision.

Management

The following discussion addresses only the treatment of dermatofibroma.

Excision   Local anesthetic is infiltrated around the lesion to produce field anesthesia. An elliptic excision of tissue is made to the superficial fat and the lesion is removed completely. Smaller lesions may be closed with simple interrupted sutures. Larger lesions are best closed in a layered fashion with deep absorbable sutures.

Cryotherapy   Satisfactory cosmetic results can sometimes be achieved with liquid nitrogen therapy. See "Management" above in "Verrucae Vulgaris." An adjunctive approach is to perform a punch biopsy at the center of the lesion prior to cryotherapy. This technique accomplishes several things. It provides the dermatopathologist with a specimen to adequately evaluate the lesion and increases the surface area of this dermal lesion for cryotherapy.[3,35]

Angiofibromas

These lesions tend to be less than 0.5 cm in diameter and are red-brown to flesh in color. Angiofibromas appear as small dome-shaped papules that have a smooth surface and occasionally have associated telangiectasias. A solitary angiofibroma may occur anywhere on the face and be clinically confused with a basal cell carcinoma. The nose is a common location for solitary angiofibroma and the lesion is then referred to as a *fibrous papule* of the nose. As a part of the triad of tuberous sclerosis, multiple angiofibromas are localized to the nasolabial folds, cheeks, and chin.

Management

Excision   See "Excision" above in "Seborrheic Keratoses." As previously described, these lesions should be marked with a surgical marking pen prior to the injection of local anesthetic. The anesthetic can cause blanching which renders the lesion nearly indistinguishable from the surrounding normal epidermis.

The Gillette Super Blue blade may provide greater flexibility for shave excision. This blade is very sharp and provides the ability to contour its shape to anatomic structures.[36]

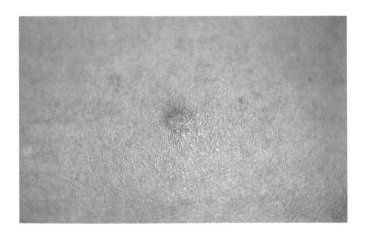

Figure 20-4   Dermatofibroma.

Its advantages become obvious when attempting removal of lesions on the dorsum of the nose, the ala, or the alar grove.

Dermabrasion   The inherited form of multiple angiofibromas may be best approached by dermabrasion. The patient should be informed that new or recurrent lesions are apt to form necessitating repeat dermabrasion.[37,38] For technique, see the methods for dermabrasion described in Chap. 36.

Laser   Multiple lesions may also be approached by the use of CO_2 or argon laser. The CO_2 laser is used with a power setting between 5 and 10 W with a spot size of 1 to 2 mm in a continuous wave defocused mode. The argon laser power setting is used at 0.8 to 1.2 W with a spot size of 0.2 to 2 mm. Pulse duration should be 0.2 to continuous wave.

Sebaceous Hyperplasia

Although these lesions are generally seen in individuals beyond their fifth decade, they may be noted as early as the second and third decade. Sebaceous hyperplasia clinically appear as grouped, confluent, yellowish papules on the forehead and cheek but may be found elsewhere. Lesions generally measure less than 0.5 cm in diameter and frequently have associated telangiectasias. Scrutiny of the lesion will usually reveal a central punctum. The main differential diagnosis for these lesions is basal cell carcinoma.

Fordyce's granules or spots are the oral equivalent of cutaneous sebaceous hyperplasia.

Management

As is the case with most of the lesions discussed in this section, the removal of sebaceous hyperplasia is purely cosmetic. However, if the diagnosis is suspect, biopsy must be performed to rule out malignancy.

Excision   Shave excision, as described above in "Seborrheic Keratoses," can provide excellent cosmetic results. This technique also provides an adequate specimen for the dermatopathologist to evaluate.

Curettage   Under a local anesthetic, light electrodesiccation followed by curettage often provides adequate results.

Cryotherapy   As described above in "Liquid Nitrogen" used for the treatment of verrucae vulgaris, a 1-mm rim of freeze is generally sufficient for these lesions. Freeze times should be 5 to 10 s.[39]

Dermabrasion   See Chap. 36 for techniques of dermabrasion.

CO_2 Laser   A 1- to 2-mm spot size with a power setting of 5 to 10 W is used in a continuous wave defocused mode for the ablation of multiple lesions.

Syringomas

These lesions commonly arise in a bilaterally symmetric fashion on the lower eyelids. Syringomas are of eccrine gland origin, are red-yellow to flesh in color, and measure only a few millimeters in diameter. Singular lesions are infrequently seen. The eruptive form of syringoma, also known as *eruptive hidradenoma of Darier en Jaquet,* appears as crops of small papules on the chest and abdomen (Fig. 20-5). This form is more common in young women and is seen in a greater than expected frequency in patients with Down's syndrome.[40,41]

Management

See "Management" above in "Angiofibromas." Since eruptive syringomas may spontaneously resolve, observation rather than treatment is suggested.

Trichoepithelioma

Solitary, multiple, and desmoplastic forms of this lesion occur. The solitary trichoepithelioma occurs spontaneously and is usually found on the face. It may achieve a size of 2 cm or greater in diameter.[42] The multiple form of trichoepithelioma arises as an autosomal dominant trait. This was first described by Brooke and called *epithelioma adenoides cysticum.* They appear as multiple cystic or smooth nodules measuring 0.2 to 0.8 cm about the nasolabial folds, cheeks, and eyelids. This form of trichoepithelioma may also be associated with cylindroma. The desmoplastic type of trichoepithelioma occurs on the cheek and is most common in young women. Clinically this form of trichoepithelioma can be difficult to distinguish from a morpheaform basal cell carcinoma.[43]

Management

The distinction between desmoplastic trichoepithelioma and morpheaform basal cell carcinoma can be difficult. A diagnostic biopsy is suggested when these lesions are encountered.

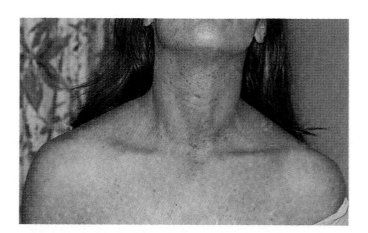

Figure 20-5   Eruptive Syringomas.

Excision Shave excision as described above in "Seborrheic Keratoses" may provide an excellent cosmetic result. Larger lesions such as the solitary or desmoplastic form of trichoepithelioma may be more amenable to the use of the Gillette Super Blue blade subsection or simple excision followed by primary closure.

CO₂ Laser See the parameters for laser treatment above in "Angiofibromas."

Curettage Light electrodesiccation followed by curettage may provide adequate results.

Xanthelasma

These lesions are also known as *xanthelasma palpebrarum.* They are common lesions mostly affecting the elderly patient. Xanthelasmas appear as smooth papules and plaques about the medial canthi and eyelids. Normal serum lipid levels are found in the majority of patients with xanthelasma. However, familial hypercholesterolemia, hepatobiliary disease, myxedema, and diabetes may manifest xanthelasma.

Management

Excision As these lesions tend to occur in elderly individuals, the associated lid laxity with advanced age permits simple excision with primary closure to produce excellent results.

Trichloroacetic Acid Ten to 35% TCA may be applied and repeated in 1 to 2 weeks. Occasionally, large xanthelasmas may be recalcitrant to this form of therapy and TCA in a concentration of 50 to 100% may then be effective.[44] An infrequent side effect is hypopigmentation.

CO₂ Laser Spot size of 1 to 2 mm with a power level of 5 W in a continuous wave mode may produce acceptable results.

REFERENCES

1. Cobb MW: Human papillomavirus infection. *J Am Acad Dermatol* **22:**547–566, 1990

2. Jablonska S, Orth G: Warts/human papillomaviruses. *Clin Dermatol* **3:**1–220, 1985

3. Torre D et al: *Practical Cutaneous Cryosurgery.* Norwalk, Conn, Appleton & Lange, 1988

4. Bolton RA: Nongenital warts: Classification and treatment options. *Am Fam Physician* **43:**2049–2056, 1991

5. Krull EA: Surgical gems: The "little" curet. *J Dermatol Surg Oncol* **4:**656–657, 1978

6. Street ML, Roenigk RK: Recalcitrant periungual verrucae: The role of carbon dioxide laser vaporization. *J Am Acad Dermatol* **23:**115–120, 1990

7. Shumer SM, O'Keefe EJ: Bleomycin in the treatment of recalcitrant warts. *J Am Acad Dermatol* **9:**91–96, 1983

8. Shelley WB, Shelley ED: Intralesional bleomycin sulfate therapy for warts. *Arch Dermatol* **127:**234–236, 1991

9. Varuch K: Blunt dissection of treatment of plantar verrucae. *Cutis* **46:**145–152, 1990

10. Schwartz RA: Buschke-Löewenstein tumor: Verrucous carcinoma of the penis. *J Am Acad Dermatol* **23:**723–727, 1990

11. Wick MR et al: Histopathologic considerations in the management of skin cancer, in *Skin Cancer: Recognition and Management,* edited by RA Schwartz. New York, Springer-Verlag, 1988, pp 246–275

12. Greenberg MD et al: A double-blind, randomized trial of 0.5% Podofilox and placebo for the treatment of genital warts in women. *Obstet Gynecol* **77:**735–739, 1991

13. Niimura M: Application of beta-interferon in virus-induced papillomas. *J Invest Dermatol* **95:**149S–151S, 1990

14. Kauh YC et al: A surgical approach for dermatosis papulosa nigra. *Int J Dermatol* **22:**590–591, 1983

15. Beare JM, Koblenzer PJ: Nevi, melanocytic, in *Practical Management of the Dermatologic Patient,* edited by AJ Rook et al. Philadelphia, Lippincott, 1986, pp 138–142

16. Pehamberger H et al: In vivo epiluminescence microscopy of pigmented skin lesions, pt 1: Pattern analysis of pigmented skin lesions. *J Am Acad Dermatol* **17:**571–591, 1987

17. Hodgson C: Lentigo senilis. *Arch Dermatol* **87:**197–207, 1963

18. Rafal ES et al: Topical tretinoin (retinoic acid) treatment for liver spots associated with photodamage. *N Engl J Med* **326:**368–374, 1992

19. Kennard CD, Rasmussen JE: Congenital midline nasal masses: Diagnosis and management. *J Dermatol Surg Oncol* **16:**1025–1036, 1990

20. Strauss JS: Sebaceous glands, in *Dermatology in General Medicine,* 2d ed, edited by TB Fitzpatrick et al. New York, McGraw-Hill, 1979, pp 437–458

21. Shelley ED, Shelley WB: Piezosurgery: A conservative approach to encapsulated skin lesions. *Cutis* **38:**123–126, 1986

22. Holmes EJ: Tumors of the lower hair sheath: The common histogenesis of certain so-called "sebaceous cysts," adenomas, and "sebaceous carcinomas." *Cancer* **21:**234–248, 1968

23. Barr RJ et al: Pseudomalignant and pseudobenignant lesions of the skin and subcutaneous tissues. *Dermatology Update—Reviews for Physicians,* 275–279, 1979

24. Gordon CJ: Proliferating trichilemmal cyst in an organoid nevus. *Cutis* **48:**49–52, 1991

25. Witkowski JA, Parish LC: Taping of a cyst: A method to facilitate removal of a scalp cyst. *Int J Dermatol* **13:**226, 1974

26. Jaworsky C, Murphy GF: Capsule dermatology: Cystic tumors of the neck. *J Dermatol Surg Oncol* **15:**21–26, 1989

27. Bohler-Sommeregger K, Kutschera-Hienert G: Cryosurgical

management of myxoid cysts. *J Dermatol Surg Oncol* **14:**1405–1412, 1988

28. Trapp CF, Baker EJ: Mobile encapsulated lipomas. *Cutis* **49:**63–64, 1992

29. Howard WR, Helwig EB: Angiolipoma. *Arch Dermatol* **82:**924–930, 1960

30. Harrist TJ: Unusual sacrococcygea embryologic malformations with cutaneous manisfestations. *Arch Dermatol* **188:**643, 1982

31. Goldschmidt H, Grekin RC: *Lipomas in Andrews' Diseases of the Skin.* Philadelphia, Saunders, 1990, pp 734–735

32. Hardin FF: Surgical gem: A simple technique for removal of lipomas. *J Dermatol Surg Oncol* **8:**316–317, 1982

33. Peinert RA, Courtiss EH: Excision from a distance: Removal of benign subcutaneous lesions. *Plast Reconstr Surg* **72:**94–96, 1983

34. Niemi KM: The benign fibrohistiocytic tumours of the skin (review). *Acta Derm Venereol* (Stockh) **50**(suppl 63):1–66, 1970

35. Lubritz RR: Cyrosurgery. *Clin Dermatol* **5:**120–127, 1987

36. Shelley WB: The razor blade in dermatologic practice. *Cutis* **16:**843–845, 1975

37. Roenigk HH Jr: Dermabrasion: State of the art. *J Dermatol Surg Oncol* **11:**306–314, 1985

38. Epstein E, Epstein E Jr: *Techniques in Skin Surgery.* Philadelphia, Lea & Febiger, 1979, pp 171–176

39. Zacarian SA: *Cryosurgery.* St. Louis, Mosby, 1985, pp 51–52

40. Hashimoto K et al: Eruptive hidradenoma and syringoma. *Arch Dermatol* **96:**500–519, 1967

41. Urban CD et al: Eruptive syringomas in Down's syndrome. *Arch Dermatol* **117:**374–375, 1981

42. Lever WF, Schaumburg-Lever G: *Histopathology of Skin,* 7th ed. Philadelphia, Lippincott, 1990, pp 582–586

43. Brownstein MH, Shapiro L. Desmoplastic trichoepithelioma. *Cancer,* **40:**2979–2986, 1977

44. Stegman SJ, Tromovitch TA: *Cosmetic Dermatologic Surgery.* Chicago, Year Book, 1984, pp 20–21

Christine M. Hayes
Duane C. Whitaker

21 Surgical Treatment of Malignant Lesions

The skin manifests a wide range of malignant lesions and signs of neoplastic processes. These range from primary skin tumors on one hand to cutaneous metastases from distant organs on the other. With few exceptions, surgery plays a therapeutic role only in tumors which arise from skin and its adnexa and supporting structures. The vast majority of cutaneous malignancies are accounted for by basal cell carcinoma (BCC), squamous cell carcinoma (SCC), and malignant melanoma (MM). Over the past two decades, there has been a marked increase in the incidence of BCC, SCC, and MM. Surgical management of other malignancies will be considered as well, but most of the authors' discussion will be devoted to these malignancies which account for over 99 percent of cutaneous oncology.

Dermatologic surgery encompasses electrosurgery, curettage, cryosurgery, laser surgery, and scalpel surgery which includes excisional surgery (ES) and Mohs micrographic surgery (MMS).[1,2] The techniques of these procedures are described in detail elsewhere in this text. The purpose of this chapter will be to outline and explain where these procedures are best applied in the management of cutaneous malignancies. For completeness, the authors will refer to other modalities such as radiation therapy (RT), chemotherapy, and molecular techniques where they play a role but will not discuss them in detail.

BASAL CELL CARCINOMA

Readers will be familiar with much of the general data regarding incidence, risks, and morphology of BCC, the most common of all malignancies in humans. However, some review is in order. BCC has an approximate incidence of 600,000 new cases yearly in the United States. The true incidence is difficult to determine since many which are diagnosed and treated in private offices are never reported. Risk factors for BCC include skin types I and II, genetic factors (e.g., basal cell nevus syndrome), and cumulative sun exposure.[3]

The clinical presentation of BCC is a pearly pink or red papule with rolled borders, telangiectasias, and a rodent ulcer at the center. Morpheaform BCC clinically appears as a sclerotic, white-to-yellow, indurated plaque with ill-defined borders.

The characteristic histology of nodular BCC shows basophilic islands of cells in the dermis which may be solid or cystic, with peripheral palisading. The stroma embedding the tumor nests may be desmoplastic. The histology of morpheaform BCC shows individual strands of cells, spicular in configuration, extending into the dermis, surrounded by a dense fibrous stroma. Micronodular BCC may show architectural similarities to morpheaform tumors but lacks a stromal response. Superficial BCC displays basaloids budding off the epidermis with minimal dermal invasion.

The most common location of BCC is the head and neck, with 85 percent of the tumors being found there. The other 15 percent can be found anywhere on the body, with the trunk and arms being frequent locations. BCC is a locally aggressive tumor which generally has a slow growth rate and rarely metastasizes. Therefore, the major risk is local invasion which may extend into deeper tissue, including fascia, muscle, perichondrium, periosteum, cartilage, bone, and nerve.[4] BCC rarely invades cartilage unless previous irradiation has occurred but rather migrates over the perichondrium.[5] In a series of 183 patients, the cartilage was invaded in 1.7 percent of the cases.[5] BCC of the eyelid may spread along the tarsal plate with an affinity for the cilia margin. BCCs may spread via nerve sheaths, lymphatic vessels, and blood vessels.[2,4]

The literature suggests that all surgical modalities, electrodesiccation and curettage (ED&C), cryosurgery, ES, and MMS, provide a 90 percent or better cure rate.[6–9] Therefore the physician must possess the knowledge and judgment to choose appropriate therapy for a given tumor and patient. Four factors which are critical in that choice are: location, size/duration, histologic type, and previous treatment. Patient characteristics of age, health, longevity, and predisposing factors of irradiation or history of multiple tumors will also be important.

High-risk locations include the nasal ala, columella, septum, and tip; nasofacial groove; melolabial fold; upper lip; anterior ear and pre- and postauricular sulci; medial canthus and eyelid margin; scalp and forehead.[6,10,11] Figure 21-1 outlines these areas which represent high risk of recurrence in the central and lateral face. Some authors have included the temple as a high-risk area.[12] BCC is the most common tumor of the

eyelid and treatment failure increases the risk of lid dysfunction and orbital invasion.[12,13] One series found that large, aggressive tumors of the scalp were more common in women and may present prior to age 40.[14] Because of the tendency of tumors in this location to spread widely at the base, periosteal, bone, and even dura invasion have been documented.

Tumors greater than 2 cm diameter may have more extensive subclinical infiltration. Size of the tumor is important as it has been shown that tumors that are greater than 2 cm have a 46 percent recurrence rate when treated by non-Mohs modalities.[10] Tumors greater than 2 cm in diameter in any location should be considered for excisional rather than destructive techniques. A cancer that has recurred despite previous treatment portends a worse prognosis. The causes of recurrent tumors may include incomplete excision and inapparent perineural spread of the tumor.[4]

Morpheaform BCC extends an average of 7.2 mm beyond the apparent clinical margins.[15] Based on this evidence, morpheaform tumors of the head and neck require wider margin excision or MMS because of the higher risk of recurrence.[15] Figures 21-2 and 21-3 display a morpheaform tumor and the defect necessary to obtain clear margins by MMS.

Primary, nodular tumors in noncritical locations offer the widest range of options regarding therapy. Tumors that are less than 2 cm in diameter and not in high-risk sites may be treated with any of the surgical options available as long as good follow-up examination is performed. Figure 21-4 demonstrates an example of a BCC in a noncritical location amenable to various types of treatment. On the other hand, morpheaform BCC in high-risk locations requires frozen section margin control techniques as afforded by MMS.[4,16,17]

Tumors that are most amenable to ED&C are small, primary nodular tumors not in critical anatomic locations. Ideal

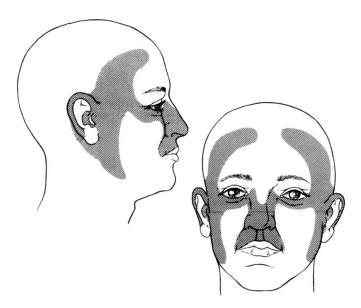

Figure 21-1 High-risk locations for facial tumors are illustrated. *(Figure courtesy of NA Swanson and Archives of Dermatology.)*

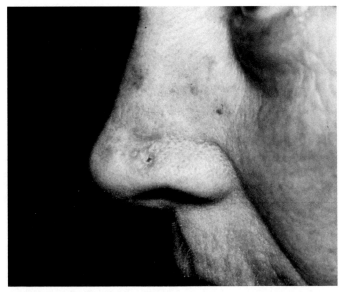

Figure 21-2 A morpheaform basal cell carcinoma on the left nasal ala and tip.

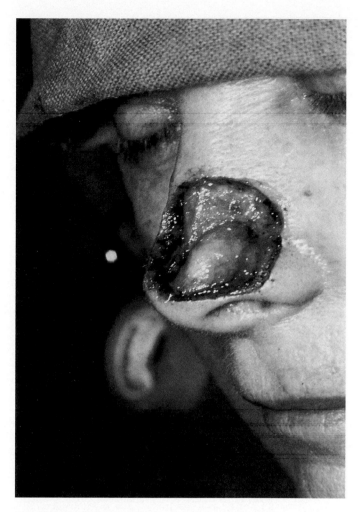

Figure 21-3 The defect seen after Mohs micrographic surgery for the lesion in Figure 21-2, extended to cartilage.

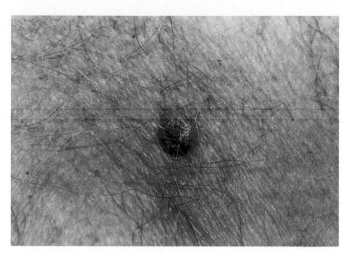

Figure 21-4 A nodular basal cell carcinoma is shown on the presternal area amenable to many surgical modalities.

locations are the trunk and proximal extremities. The reported cure rate is greater than 90 percent with carefully chosen tumors.[7,18] With the cautious selection of tumors and execution of ED&C by a skilled practitioner, high cure rates are reported for selected facial lesions. Tumors of the head and neck may be more resistant to ED&C than those on the trunk and extremities.[19] The 5-year recurrence rate has been found to be 26 percent for ED&C when these criteria were not used.[20] The cosmetic result is usually satisfactory and improves with time although a depressed or hypertrophic scar can occur. Therefore, age and cosmetic concerns of the patient as well as cure rate should be evaluated in treatment selection.

Cryosurgery, while not widely practiced for malignancy, has advocates who report similar cure rates to ED&C for properly selected lesions.[21,22] Criteria outlined by experienced cryosurgeons include a well-defined, primary lesion less than 2 cm in diameter. Some practitioners feel that cryosurgery can be used in certain high-risk locations in elderly patients, with cure rates approaching 90 percent. Since

destructive techniques do not allow a microscopic examination of the surgical margin, outcome is correlated with clinical skill and experience.

Excision is an excellent option for tumors which are primary, well defined, less than 2 cm in diameter, and not morpheaform.[7,8,23] One study has shown that nonmorpheaform BCCs less than 2 cm require at least a 4-mm circumferential margin to achieve a greater than 90 percent cure.[24] Recurrent tumors treated by standard excision without margin control have a reported cure of 80 percent.[16]

MMS offers the highest documented cure rate for all types of BCC. There are no absolute contraindications to MMS in the treatment of BCC based on tumor or patient characteristics. Limitations are related to factors of medical resources available (time, expense, and availability of a trained surgeon) and presumed longevity of the patient. It is clear that not all BCCs require MMS but rather the technique should be employed for those tumors or patients who have decreased chances of cure by other methods. These include all recurrent tumors, primary tumors greater than 2 cm, all morpheaform tumors, and primary BCCs which are in high-risk locations with a high recurrence rate as outlined above.[10,15–17]

The 5-year recurrence rate for recurrent tumors treated with MMS is 5.6 percent as compared to 19.9 percent when treated with non-Mohs modalities.[16] As noted above, morpheaform BCC may extend well beyond clinically estimated borders.[15] Thus microscopic control plays a special role in the treatment of recurrent and morpheaform BCC. Large or aggressive BCCs are best treated with a multidisciplinary surgical approach.[25] A cutaneous oncologic surgeon, reconstructive surgeon, neurosurgeon, and oculoplastic surgeon may work together to extirpate these tumors.[25,26] Most tumors treated with MMS can have optimal reconstruction immediately. However, tumors which are a product of multiple treatment failures may be managed by functional reconstruction on a temporary basis.[27] Recurrent tumor is less easily detected under a flap or full-thickness skin graft. Closure by second intention healing or split-thickness skin graft may be recommended since flaps alter tissue planes.[28] After the patient is tumor free for 12 to 24 months, more elegant and aesthetic reconstruction can be considered if the patient desires.

Carbon dioxide laser can be used to excise (with or without MMS) or vaporize a tumor.[29–32] Laser vaporization has the drawback of other destructive techniques: There is no histologic specimen to verify adequacy of treatment. Successful treatment of multiple superficial BCCs with vaporization followed by ED&C has been reported with relatively short follow-up period.[20] ES performed with the laser in the cutting mode may decrease perioperative bleeding but any other advantage remains to be proven.[29]

RT is not suitable primary treatment for BCC in patients 50 years of age or younger because of the significant risk of secondary malignancy.[33] If patients are unable or refuse to undergo surgery, RT may be the only approved option available to them. Although some literature suggests a 90 percent or greater cure rate, it appears that fewer patients are now referred for RT than in the past.[8] This may be in part due to the public's fears over the dangers of radiation but also due to increased life expectancy. Older patients now survive long enough so they experience complications and malignancy in radiated fields. Cosmetic results of RT diminish significantly over time. A study of tumor recurrences in failed RT patients has documented that these are frequently devastating tumors to treat.[34] Tumors appear to be more aggressive and some patients are not resectable. At the present time, RT appears to play a role of adjunctive therapy or offers an avenue for those patients who refuse surgery for BCC.[35]

Nonsurgical methods of BCC treatment include systemic retinoids, topical 5-fluorouracil, intralesional 5-fluorouracil, intralesional interferon, and hematoporphyrin-derivative photoradiation therapy.[36–43] The latter two techniques are presently investigational in BCC therapy but may offer additional nonsurgical alternatives in the future.

Metastatic BCC is exceedingly rare but tends to occur in males with tumors of long-standing duration. There are over 200 cases in the literature. The reported rate of metastases ranges from less than 0.01 percent to 0.1 percent.[44,45] The primary tumor is usually located on the head and neck.[46] The distant sites of metastases include the lymph node, lung, bone, liver, and spleen.[44,46] Once metastases occur, the prognosis is poor with approximately a 10 percent 5-year survival.[46] Treatment consists of surgery, RT, chemotherapy, or a combination.[47–49]

The risk of skin cancer, either new or recurrent, in patients with a previous skin cancer is estimated to be at least 22 percent and may be as high as 50 percent.[50,51] This underscores the importance of regular skin examinations for these patients, with some authors recommending examinations every 6 months for 2 years and then yearly.[52]

SQUAMOUS CELL CARCINOMA

SCC is the second most common type of cutaneous neoplasm with a yearly estimated rate of 100,000 to 150,000 cases. Known etiologic factors include skin type; radiation, both ultraviolet and ionizing; carcinogens, such as coal tar and arsenic; human papilloma virus (HPV); immunosuppression; and certain chronic inflammatory/ulcerative processes of the skin.[53–57]

SCC clinically appears as a red- to flesh-colored, indurated papule, plaque, nodule, or ulceration. More commonly located on sun-exposed surfaces, SCCs have been described anywhere on the body, at both cutaneous sites and mucous membranes. Figure 21-5 shows a primary SCC of the temple. Growth rate is highly variable and may simulate BCC behavior or may grow rapidly and become locally invasive with early spread to adjacent tissues or regional nodes. SCC histologically demonstrates full-thickness atypia of the keratinizing squamous cells with invasion into the dermis. Large, abnormal cells with bizarre mitoses and dyskeratotic cells may be present. SCC are graded by their differentiation and sometimes by depth of invasion as well.

SCC may develop from actinic keratoses (AK) or de novo.[58] Because of the malignant potential, AK may be treated by numerous modalities, including topical 5-fluorouracil, topical tretinoin, cryosurgery, laser surgery, or ED&C.[36,37] Actinic damage on the lip, actinic cheilitis, is also premalignant and must be closely monitored as labial SCCs behave in an aggressive manner. Surgical treatment options for actinic cheilitis, after a biopsy is performed to exclude SCC, consist of ablation of the lip with cryosurgery, electrosurgery, carbon dioxide laser, or scalpel vermilionectomy.[59] Nonsurgical therapy includes topical 5-fluorouracil.[37]

In the treatment of SCC, the physician must evaluate and consider the potential for metastatic disease. Metastases are

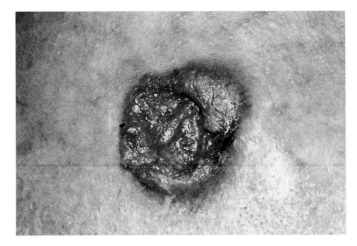

Figure 21-5 A nodular squamous cell carcinoma with central ulceration.

more common in men.[60] Tumors at greatest risk are those on the lip or adjacent to mucous membranes, ear SCCs, and large (greater than 2 cm) or recurrent lesions.[60] The metastatic rate reported in the literature for all SCCs varies widely based on the population studied but may range from 0.5 to 16 percent for all populations combined.[60] Local recurrence and metastatic disease may in part be due to the tendency for neurotropism. The incidence of perineural invasion has been reported to be approximately 2.4 to 4.9 percent.[4] SCC metastasizes to regional lymph nodes most commonly and to the lung, liver, bone, brain, and mediastinum less commonly.[60,61] Location on the ear and the lip may increase the metastatic rate to 11 and 13 percent and greater, respectively.[61,62]

Identification of high-risk SCC (i.e., those tumors more likely to recur or metastasize) has been studied in detail.[61] Variables which have been identified as prognostic risk factors include size, depth of invasion, histologic differentiation, rapid growth, etiology, anatomic site, immunosuppression, histologic evidence of neurotropism, and recurrence after treatment.[61] Lesions greater than 2 cm in diameter and 4 mm in depth which are poorly differentiated and grow rapidly are at higher risk. Also, tumors which arise in a scar or primary tumors of the ear or lip have a higher risk profile.

Evaluation of SCC arising in actinically damaged skin has shown that both the level of dermal invasion and the vertical tumor thickness correlates with disease-free survival, rate of recurrence, metastatic disease, and poorer prognosis.[63] In fact, destructive techniques such as ED&C and cryosurgery should be reserved for those tumors which are confined to the dermis. Large tumors, male patients, and lower extremity location were noted to be risk factors for recurrence.[64] Recurrent SCC is a difficult tumor to treat because of the risk for metastatic disease; it has a 3.4 percent recurrence rate after treatment with MMS as compared to a 23.3 percent recurrence rate after all non-Mohs modalities.[61,64] Therefore, the treatment of choice for recurrent SCC may be MMS with evaluation and treatment for regional or distant metastatic disease.

MMS for SCC has a reported cure rate of 93.3 percent.[65] Many authors recommend excising a larger margin around SCC or taking an additional layer after a "clear margin" has been obtained by frozen sections.[61,65] The rationale is excision of a margin of apparently normal tissue which may harbor discontiguous tumor cells more distant from the clinical mass. The advantage of MMS is that it serves as a continual histological monitor during the surgery. The surgeon does not determine a set margin preoperatively but has the option of extending an additional margin based on microscopic findings at the time of surgery. In many instances, inflammatory cells at the margin which cannot be explained on other grounds should be included in the excision. Tumors which are poorly differentiated, recurrent, and 2 cm or greater in diameter should have MMS or margin determination at the time of surgery. Primary tumors which are 1 to 2 cm with invasion

into the reticular dermis should have excision with a 1-cm or more margin or margin control surgery.

Labial SCC represents a good model of SCC with a higher metastatic rate. The higher-risk tumors which arise from keratinized epithelium both in sun- and nonexposed areas can metastasize as well. The primary risk of recurrent SCC is spread to regional lymph nodes, distant tracking along neurovascular bundles, and widespread metastatic disease. In large or recurrent tumors, histologic study of the mental nerve at or before its entrance to the mental foramen is recommended because of the neurotrophic potential.[66] When any of these treatment complications occur, the patient must be reevaluated and a combined treatment plan involving head and neck oncologists, radiation oncologists, and chemotherapists is necessary. In most instances, therapy will be directed toward reexcision of the primary tumor and either surgery or radiation for lymph node disease. Patients who are treated with high-risk tumors should be considered for prophylactic radiation to the nodal basin draining the involved area. Once regional nodal disease has developed, surgery and/or RT will be necessary for nodal treatment. In general, chemotherapy has a small role except in disease which has spread beyond the regional nodes.[48] The 5-year survival for metastatic SCC is 25 percent, which stresses the importance of optimal first-line treatment.[59]

RT, because of the risk of metastatic disease, plays a greater role in the treatment of SCC than BCC.[34] It is unclear which patients will benefit from adjunctive RT to the surgical site or regional nodes. Systemic retinoids may play a chemoprevention role in SCC and also an adjunctive chemotherapy role in widespread disease.[67] However, retinoids or chemotherapeutic agents are not a first-line treatment for SCC. Other nonsurgical methods have not proven useful for SCC at the present time.

MARJOLIN'S ULCER, VERRUCOUS CARCINOMA, AND BOWEN'S DISEASE

Marjolin's ulcer tumor is an SCC arising in a site of previous injury, chronic ulceration, or certain inflammatory skin conditions. Characteristic settings are ulcers, draining sinuses, and burn scars. While the specific etiology is unclear, these tumors are aggressive in behavior. The metastatic rate has been reported to range from 10 to 34.8 percent.[62,68] They have a poor prognosis, with overall mortality of 32.5 percent in one series.[68] They must be considered high risk for metastatic disease on presentation and the workup directed appropriately. Even when no evidence of widespread cancer is found, occult disease may be present and therapy planned with this in mind. Usually treatment is wide excision (3 to 5 cm) with histologic control of deep and peripheral margins. Preservation of questionable tissue may sacrifice the opportunity to cure. Delayed reconstruction and functional graft coverage rather than flap

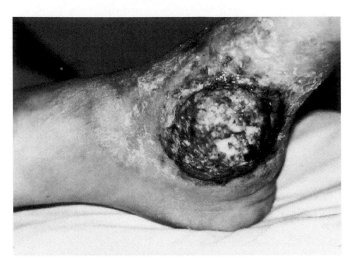

Figure 21-6 Large verrucous carcinoma of medial malleolus is shown.

repair may be preferable when recurrence is a concern. RT is not recommended and benefit is not apparent from chemotherapy in localized disease.[68]

The term *verrucous carcinoma* encompasses oral florid papillomatosis, giant condyloma acuminatum of Buschke and Löewenstein, and epithelioma cuniculatum.[69] Figure 21-6 shows a verrucous carcinoma of the ankle. Verrucous carcinoma refers to a histopathologic picture of a well-differentiated SCC which requires clinical correlation in order to establish diagnosis. These tumors tend to invade locally and have little tendency to metastasize. Primary treatment is usually surgical, either with cold steel or a cutting laser.[70] Since it is difficult to estimate tumor extent, MMS is a good method for total tumor ablation with margin control and maximal preservation of normal tissue structure and function.[69,71–73] Although ES is usually required, cryosurgery has been used in conjunction with 5-fluorouracil in one report with good results.[74] RT is contraindicated as these tumors may become more atypical, aggressive, and metastasize after radiation. Chemotherapy is indicated only for palliation of nonresectable disease.

Bowen's disease (BD) is SCC in situ and review of both the clinical and histopathologic picture are necessary in order to determine treatment. BD can be treated by ED&C, cryosurgery, scalpel excision, MMS, laser surgery, and possibly topical chemotherapy.[37,38,75] Patients should be questioned regarding arsenic ingestion and thoroughly examined for other lesions. BD which is large (3 cm or greater in diameter), thick or indurated on physical examination, and shows invasion into follicular and eccrine structures has potential to behave more aggressively. These lesions should be excised with margin control. Smaller lesions without these features can be treated by the surgical or destructive method of the clinician's choosing. Topical 5-fluorouracil, when employed,

should be followed with a posttreatment biopsy to assess cure. Recurrent tumors can be treated with excision or MMS.

KERATOACANTHOMA

Keratoacanthoma (KA) clinically and histologically resembles SCC. It is differentiated from SCC by a characteristic history, appearance, and histopathologic architecture. KA often develops rapidly, on sun-exposed skin, and the typical appearance is a dome-shaped nodule with a keratin-filled central crater. Figure 21-7 shows a KA of the lower lip. Though certain histopathologic features may distinguish KA from SCC, it appears that this diagnosis is rendered less frequently than in the past. In general, primary treatment for KA is excision with adequate margin control. However, the behavior of KA is variable, and some may resolve with no treatment while others are in fact invasive SCC. Management is challenging when the tumor cannot be excised with a primary closure. Tumors which occur on the nose, eyelid, or critical locations present special difficulties. Size, location, pathology, and patient characteristics must all be considered. If nonsurgical management is chosen, the patient should be followed closely for evidence of malignant changes. 5-Fluorouracil has the longest history of intralesional use in KA; however, this may not be effective for lesions which are not in a proliferating phase.[76] More recently, intralesional methotrexate has been reported as efficacious and may require fewer treatments.[77] Treatment parameters for 5-fluorouracil include a concentration of 50 mg/mL, 1 to 3 mL injected every 1 to 4 weeks for two to six treatments.[76] Guidelines for methotrexate are 12.5 to 25 mg/cc with 0.4 to 1.5 mL injected every 2 weeks for two treatment sessions.[77] For multiple eruptive KA, both systemic 13-cisretinoic acid and etretinate have been used for 12 weeks with fair results.[78] Intralesional and systemic therapy may also be combined.

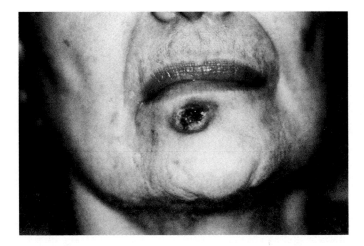

Figure 21-7 Characteristic appearance of keratoacanthoma on the lower lip.

MALIGNANT MELANOMA

There are approximately 32,000 new cases of MM yearly which cause approximately 6,500 deaths.[79] The incidence rate has been steadily increasing, faster than any other cancer, and has tripled in the last four decades.[80] An even greater rate of increase has been observed in young women.[80] The survival rate has improved, however, and this may be due to earlier diagnosis.[81] Risk factors associated with the development of MM include ultraviolet radiation (UVR) exposure, type I and II skin, family history of melanoma, and the presence of dysplastic or congenital nevi.[80] The four types of MM (lentigo maligna melanoma, superficial spreading melanoma, acral lentiginous melanoma, and nodular melanoma) have a characteristic clinical and histopathologic picture.

The best indicator of survival is the clinical stage of disease and the Breslow depth measurement. Other features such as evidence of regression, Clark's level, anatomic location, and presence of ulceration may also be useful in identifying higher-risk populations.[82] Males have a worse prognosis even when other factors are controlled.[79] The issue of pregnancy affecting the prognosis has been recently examined and no correlation with long-term survival was found.[83] The prognosis of MM worsens with increasing tumor thickness. In patients with tumors less than 0.75 mm thick, the 5-year survival rate is 96 percent. This decreases to 47 percent in patients with MM greater than 4 mm thick. The 5-year survival rate declines to 36 percent in patients with nodal metastases and to less than 5 percent in those with distant metastases.[84] High-risk locations for MM on the head and neck include the scalp, ears, and posterior and lateral neck.[85] Other areas of high risk include the upper back, posterolateral arms, and acral areas (e.g., the subungual area, palms, and soles).[82,86]

Because of the importance of establishing a prompt diagnosis in MM, a few comments regarding biopsy are relevant. When a lesion is suspicious for MM, it is preferable to perform an excisional biopsy if possible. A minimal margin can be taken at this time until the diagnosis is established. Figure 21-8 is an example of an MM marked for an excisional biopsy. If it is not possible to excise the suspicious lesion or the effect would be detrimental if the lesion proves benign, then incisional or punch biopsies may be done to sample the tumor. There is no evidence that incising into an MM increases the risk of spreading the tumor. In all cases, the specimen submitted must be full-thickness dermis with subcutaneous tissue.

The authors' discussion will concentrate on the treatment of clinical stage I MM; that is, disease confined to the primary site. Surgery with excisional margin determined by tumor depth is the primary treatment for stage I MM. Lesions that are under 0.76-mm depth can be excised with a 1-cm margin, including the subcutaneous tissue.[87–89] There are no clear recommendations for tumors that are of intermediate depth (0.76 to 1.5 mm) though they are generally excised with a 1.5- to

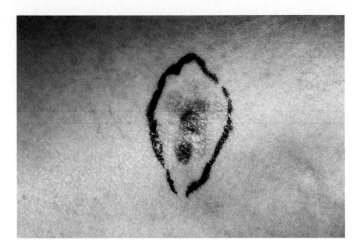

Figure 21-8 Malignant melanoma outlined for an excisional biopsy.

2-cm margin.[84] Many authors recommend that MMs which are greater than 1.5 cm in depth should undergo an excision with 3-cm margins, including subcutaneous tissue.[84,88,90] There is no evidence that wider margins or excision of underlying fascia increases survival of these patients.[84,88–91]

All patients should be evaluated for adenopathy although patients with lesions less than 1.5 mm in depth are unlikely to present with clinical stage II disease. Patients with stage I disease and lesions 1.5 mm or less in depth do not benefit from elective lymph node dissection.[89,92–94] Selective cases of intermediate depth lesions (1.5 to 3 mm) may benefit from node dissection, though this is a controversial issue beyond the scope of the authors' discussion.[89,94–97] The thickness of the primary MM correlates with risk of lymph node metastases. Fifty percent of presenting lesions which are greater than 4 mm in depth will have metastases.[98] Intermediate and deeper lesions should be reviewed in a consultative setting so that surgical, medical, and radiation oncologists can be involved in the planning.

MM metastasizes to local skin, regional lymph nodes, distant skin, liver, lung, and the central nervous system. Metastatic MM may be palliated by excision of cutaneous, nodal, or pulmonary metastasis.[99] Nonsurgical modalities utilized for the treatment of metastatic MM include adjunctive chemotherapy, hormonal therapy, isolated regional perfusion, and adjunctive immunotherapy.[100–103] While RT is rarely a primary treatment for MM, this modality often has a role in metastatic disease and can be adjunctive in regional treatment of stage II disease.[104,105]

The follow-up period for MM should be life, and frequency tailored to the lesion depth. Even patients with thin MM are at increased risk of developing a secondary MM. Patients should be seen at a minimum of 3-month intervals in the first postoperative year. The second and third year, the follow-up should be at 4- to 6-month intervals and subsequent follow-up at 6- to 12-month intervals.

Lentigo Maligna

Lentigo maligna occurs usually in elderly persons, on any sun-exposed area, though more commonly on the malar and temporal areas of the face. This premalignant lesion may be present for many years and can attain a large size prior to malignant progression. Estimations of lifetime progression to invasive MM vary widely in the literature from 2.2 to 50 percent.[106,107] With this potential, removal is often desirable but the location and size may be an obstacle. Also, it may be difficult to discern the accurate borders, even with Wood's lamp examination. Atypical melanocytes may extend well beyond the apparent clinical margins, though rush permanent sections appear to be a reliable method for directing excisional margins.[108,109] Destructive modes of therapy which have been used for lentigo maligna include argon laser, cryotherapy, ED&C, and RT.[107] Patients treated with nonexcisional methods should be followed and rebiopsied if recurrent disease is suspected.

DERMATOFIBROSARCOMA PROTUBERANS

Dermatofibrosarcoma protuberans (DFSP) is a relatively rare, malignant tumor of the skin which may arise from fibroblasts in the dermis and is locally invasive but rarely metastasizes.[110,111] One series of 86 patients showed a 6 percent metastatic rate which usually occurs only after local recurrence or severe neglect of the tumor.[112] Clinically, DFSP presents as an ill-defined, firm plaque or nodule. The most common location is the trunk, followed by the proximal extremities, and head and neck. Figure 21-9 demonstrates a nodular DFSP of the abdomen. DFSP is more common in males, presenting in early to mid-adult life.[112,113] Histologically, a cartwheeling pattern is seen extending laterally in the dermis and into the subcutis and skeletal muscle.[113]

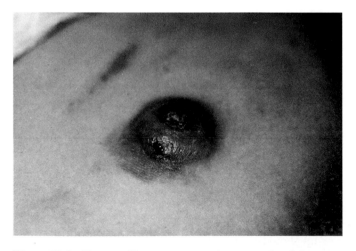

Figure 21-9 Dermatofibrosarcoma protuberans on the abdomen.

Treatment of choice is complete wide excision, extending to and, if necessary, including fascia and muscle. A 3-cm margin or more may be necessary to achieve a tumor-free plane.[114] Still these tumors have a high recurrence rate of close to 50 percent.[111,113] Recent series have shown MMS to be of value due to the microscopic margin control as the tumor may extend up to four times the surface area of the clinically evident lesion.[110] MMS may be especially valuable on the head and neck where 3-cm margins would cause severe disfigurement. When these tumors are excised with margin control, it is imperative that all reactive fibrous or inflammatory tissue be resected otherwise the risk of recurrence is increased.

MALIGNANT ADNEXAL TUMORS

Microcystic adnexal carcinoma

Microcystic adnexal carcinoma (MAC) is a rare, locally aggressive tumor which shows both pilar and eccrine differentiation. Clinically, MAC presents as a flesh- to yellow-colored nodule or plaque on the upper lip, periorbital skin, or other head and neck locations. MAC is seen in middle-aged adults. Histopathology shows both squamoid and basal cells, horn cysts, ducts, and a desmoplastic stroma. MAC may also have a tendency for perineural invasion. Complete surgical excision is recommended; however, approximately 40 percent of patients suffer a local recurrence from simple excision.[115] Due to the highly infiltrative nature of MAC, MMS appears to be ideally suited for this tumor. Neurophilic behavior of the tumor should be anticipated and traced out surgically where possible since this tumor may not be radiosensitive.[115]

Sebaceous carcinoma

Sebaceous carcinoma (SC) may arise from sebaceous glands at any cutaneous location; however, SC of the eyelid and periocular skin presents special management difficulties. SC in this region can originate from the meibomian glands of the tarsal plate; the glands of Zeis, which are eyelash associated; the caruncle; or the skin of the brow and canthi. This tumor, which is deceptive in its clinical presentation, may exhibit diffuse spread along the lid or conjunctival margin or directly invade the orbit. Figure 21-10 shows an SC of the upper lid.

Complete surgical excision is the treatment of choice; however, this is complicated by the possible multifocal origin of SC. The pagetoid spread of atypical sebaceous cells may necessitate extensive surgery so that preservation of the eye is in doubt. While the tumor mass of SC can be seen on frozen sections, intraepithelial pagetoid spread may be barely discernible even on paraffin sections.[116] Oil red O stains of fresh frozen tissue have been recommended to aid in establishing diagnosis. ES with frozen sections can be followed with permanent sections to ensure the highest-quality margin assess-

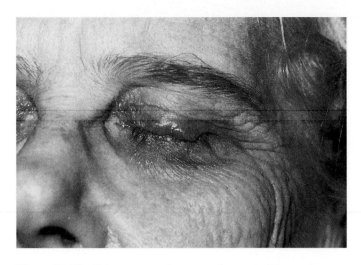

Figure 21-10   Sebaceous carcinoma on the upper lid.

ment. Patients should be evaluated and followed for nodal disease. RT is not a primary treatment modality for SC but may be employed if the patient refuses surgery or has recurrent disease. Orbital invasion and nodal metastases may occur in 10 to 35 percent of patients.[117,118] Follow-up examinations must be directed toward these complications as well as early local recurrence.

ATYPICAL FIBROXANTHOMA AND MALIGNANT FIBROUS HISTIOCYTOMA

It may not be possible to distinguish these two tumors on standard microscopic examination. Atypical fibroxanthoma (AFX) or malignant fibrous histiocytoma (MFH), which occurs superficially in the dermis, probably is a tumor of the same or similar origin. AFX was first described as a malignant-appearing mesenchymal tumor most commonly seen in elderly males with a history of radiation, either ultraviolet or ionizing.[119] Sun-exposed skin is often involved, the most common sites being the face, ears, hands, and arms. Clinically, the tumor appears as a flesh- to red-colored papule or nodule which may ulcerate or bleed. Histologically, pleomorphic anaplastic cells with multiple mitoses are seen in the dermis.

While some authors have suggested that AFX tends toward benign behavior, this is not always the case. The reported recurrence rate for AFX is approximately 6 percent following all modalities and is 50 percent for deep MFH.[119,120] The correct figure is probably somewhere in between. Some AFXs simulate an aggressive SCC, and patients should be evaluated for potential of regional or metastatic spread as there are reports in the literature of metastases from AFX to lymph nodes and lung.[121] Surgery should involve complete excision with margin control and close follow-up. Some physicians may have treated AFX by destructive modes with acceptable re-

sults. However, this tumor is unpredictable enough that the authors recommend excision with submission of a pathologic specimen.

MFH which arises from muscle fascia or deep subcutaneous tissue carries a poor prognosis. These deeper tumors often involve skeletal muscle and may be entirely within the muscle. Even with seemingly adequate margins, the recurrence rate is almost 50 percent, presumably because of poor demarcation.[120] MFH not infrequently metastasizes to the regional lymph nodes or lungs. The leading cause of death in these patients is pulmonary metastases.

EXTRAMAMMARY PAGET'S DISEASE

Extramammary Paget's disease (EMPD) occurs in elderly persons; women are more commonly affected than men. Clinically, it presents as a slowly enlarging, pruritic, erythematous, eczematous plaque, most commonly in the anogenital area. Figure 21-11 demonstrates the clinical appearance of EMPD. Histopathologically, it appears similar to Paget's disease of the breast, with large rounded cells seen in the epidermis. The etiology of EMPD is controversial. EMPD is frequently associated with a subjacent or regionally proximate visceral carcinoma.[122–124] Other studies have shown an underlying carcinoma in situ of sweat gland origin.[125] Therefore an evaluation to rule out underlying malignancy is required.

Treatment of EMPD is primarily surgical; however, the extent of surgery is controversial. In general, the more radical the surgery, the higher the cure rate. Treatment varies from laser ablation and local excision to radical surgical resection for very extensive disease. However, in more limited disease, ES may result in similar survival. MMS may be a reliable method of treating EMPD by removing all the diseased tissue and preserving as much normal tissue as possible.[126,127] EMPD is felt to be multifocal in origin; therefore, marginal

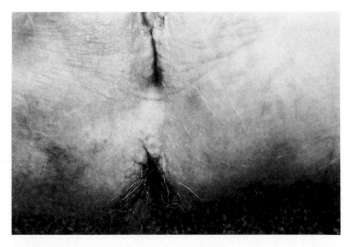

Figure 21-11   Extramammary Paget's disease of the anogenital area.

recurrence or residual disease is a complication of all localized therapy. Nonsurgical methods have included topical bleomycin; however, long-term benefit was not documented.[128] Local recurrences range from 31 to 61 percent for conventional surgery; therefore, long-term follow-up is necessary. Mortality is correlated with the presence of a proximate invasive carcinoma.[123]

MERKEL'S CELL CARCINOMA

Merkel's cell carcinoma (MCC) is a rare malignancy which may present as a red-to-pink, firm nodule of the face or extremities, though there is no reliable clinical picture. Histopathologically, anastomosing bands of deeply basophilic cells are seen in the dermis. On electron microscopy, neurosecretory granules are seen in the cells.

Treatment of MCC consists of complete wide excision as it has a high local recurrence rate ranging from 30 to 60 percent.[129,130] The average time to local recurrence was 4.3 months.[131] MCC metastasizes to regional lymph nodes, central nervous system, and viscera. Some authors recommend elective lymph node dissection as the metastatic rate is over 40 percent.[130,131] The death rate was shown to be 40 percent with a short follow-up period.[129] RT and chemotherapy appear to have minimal effect on this tumor.[129] These patients need close monitoring after surgical excision.

ANGIOSARCOMA

Angiosarcoma (AS) is a vascular malignancy seen in the elderly, often on the scalp and face. AS can also occur in the setting of chronic lymphedema (Stewart-Treves syndrome) or postradiation. Clinically, red-to-purple macules, plaques, and nodules develop on the face and scalp. Figure 21-12 demonstrates the clinical appearance of angiosarcoma on the scalp.

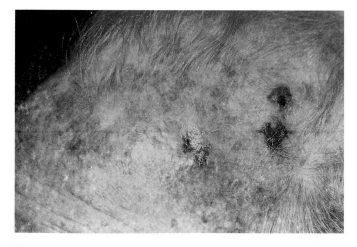

Figure 21-12 Angiosarcoma of the scalp in an elderly male.

Histopathologically, irregular anastomosing vascular channels and atypical cuboidal endothelial cells are seen.

Surgical excision, if possible, is the ideal treatment. Unfortunately, at time of diagnosis, the tumor frequently has spread widely beyond the apparent clinical margin. The tumors are locally invasive, extending into underlying bone or muscle, and may metastasize to regional lymph nodes, lungs, and liver. While no treatment is uniformly successful, surgery and RT are the most commonly used, though these modalities as well as chemotherapy are often palliative. The role of dermatologic surgery is to establish tissue diagnosis and arrange consultants to determine therapy as appropriate. At present there is no convincing evidence that tissue-sparing techniques or well-executed margin control surgery increases survival.

REFERENCES

1. Cottel WI et al: Essentials of Mohs micrographic surgery. *J Dermatol Surg Oncol* **14**:11–13, 1988

2. Swanson NA: Mohs surgery: Technique, indications, applications, and the future. *Arch Dermatol* **119**:761–773, 1983

3. Vitaliano PP, Urbach F: The relative importance of risk factors in nonmelanoma carcinoma. *Arch Dermatol* **116**:454–456, 1980

4. Hanke CW et al: Chemosurgical reports: Perineural spread of basal cell carcinoma. *J Dermatol Surg Oncol* **9**:742–747, 1983

5. Robinson JK et al: Invasion of cartilage by basal cell carcinoma. *J Am Acad Dermatol* **2**:499–505, 1980

6. Mora RG, Robins P: Basal cell carcinomas in the center of the face: Special diagnostic, prognostic and therapeutic considerations. *J Dermatol Surg Oncol* **4**:315–321, 1978

7. Reymann F: Basal cell carcinoma of the skin: Recurrence rate after different types of treatment. *Dermatologica* **161**:217–226, 1980

8. Freeman RG et al: The treatment of skin cancer: A statistical study of 1,341 skin tumors comparing results obtained with irradiation, surgery, and curettage followed by electrodesiccation. *Cancer* **17**:535–538, 1964

9. Chernosky ME: Squamous cell and basal cell carcinomas: Preliminary study of 3,817 primary skin cancers. *South Med J* **71**:802–803, 1978

10. Roenigk RK et al: Trends in the presentation and treatment of basal cell carcinomas. *J Dermatol Surg Oncol* **12**:860–865, 1986

11. Salasche SJ: Curettage and electrodesiccation on the treatment of midfacial basal cell epithelioma. *J Am Acad Dermatol* **8**:496–503, 1983

12. Carruthers JA et al: Basal-cell carcinomas of the temple. *J Dermatol Surg Oncol* **9**:759–762, 1983

13. Cielley RI, Anderson RL: Microscopically controlled excision of malignant neoplasms on and around eyelids followed by immediate surgical reconstruction. *J Dermatol Surg Oncol* **4**:55–62, 1978

14. Binstock JH et al: Large, aggressive basal cell carcinoma of the scalp. *J Dermatol Surg Oncol* **7:**565–569, 1981

15. Salasche SJ, Amonette RA: Morpheaform basal-cell epitheliomas: A study of subclinical extensions in a series of 51 cases. *J Dermatol Surg Oncol* **7:**387–394, 1981

16. Rowe DE et al: Mohs surgery is the treatment of choice for recurrent (previously treated) basal cell carcinoma. *J Dermatol Surg Oncol* **15:**424–431, 1989

17. Lang PG, Maize JC: Histologic evolution of recurrent basal cell carcinoma and treatment implications. *J Am Acad Dermatol* **14:**186–196, 1986

18. Kopf AW et al: Curettage-electrodesiccation treatment of basal cell carcinomas. *Arch Dermatol* **113:**439–443, 1977

19. Suhge d'Aubermont PC, Bennett RG: Failure of curettage and electrodesiccation for removal of basal cell carcinoma. *Arch Dermatol* **120:**1456–1460, 1984

20. Salasche SJ: Status of curettage and desiccation in the treatment of primary basal cell carcinoma. *J Am Acad Dermatol* **10:**285–287, 1984

21. Kuflik EG: Cryosurgery for carcinoma of the eyelids: A 12-year experience. *J Dermatol Surg Oncol* **11:**243–246, 1985

22. Kuflik EG: The five year cure rate achieved by cryosurgery for skin cancer. *J Am Acad Dermatol* **24:**1002–1004, 1989

23. Popkin GL, Bart RS: Excision versus curettage and electrodesiccation as dermatologic office procedures for the treatment of basal cell carcinomas. *J Dermatol Surg Oncol* **1:**33–35, 1975

24. Wolf DJ, Zitelli JA: Surgical margins for basal cell carcinoma. *Arch Dermatol* **123:**340–344, 1987

25. Baker SR et al: An interdisciplinary approach to the management of basal cell carcinoma of the head and neck. *J Dermatol Surg Oncol* **13:**1095–1106, 1987

26. Baker SR, Swanson NA: Complete microscopic controlled surgery for head and neck cancer. *Head Neck Surg* **6:**914–920, 1984

27. Barton FE et al: The principle of chemosurgery and delayed primary reconstruction on the management of difficult basal cell carcinomas. *Plast Reconstr Surg* **68:**746–752, 1981

28. Albom MJ: The management of recurrent basal cell carcinomas: Please, no flaps or grafts at once. *J Dermatol Surg Oncol* **3:**382–384, 1977

29. Bailin PL et al: CO_2 laser modification of Mohs' surgery. *J Dermatol Surg Oncol* **7:**621–623, 1981

30. Wheeland RG et al: Carbon dioxide laser vaporization and curettage in the treatment of large or multiple superficial basal cell carcinomas. *J Dermatol Surg Oncol* **13:**119–125, 1987

31. Goldman L: Laser surgery for skin cancer. *N Y State J Med* **10:**1897–1900, 1977

32. Adams EL, Price NM: Treatment of basal cell carcinomas with a carbon dioxide laser. *J Dermatol Surg Oncol* **5:**803–806, 1979

33. van Vloten WA et al: Radiation-induced skin cancer and radiodermatitis of the head and neck. *Cancer* **59:**411–414, 1987

34. Smith SP, Grande DJ: Basal cell carcinomas recurring after radiotherapy: A unique, difficult treatment subclass of recurrent basal cell carcinoma. *J Dermatol Surg Oncol* **17:**26–30, 1991

35. Chahbazian CM, Brown GS: Radiation therapy for carcinoma of the skin of the face and neck: Special considerations. *JAMA* **244:**1135–1137, 1980

36. Hodak E et al: Etretinate treatment of the nevoid basal cell carcinoma syndrome: Therapeutic and chemopreventive effect. *Int J Dermatol* **26:**606–609, 1987

37. Peck GL: Topical tretinoin in actinic keratosis and basal cell carcinoma. *J Am Acad Dermatol* **15:**829–835, 1986

38. Goette DK: Topical chemotherapy with 5-fluorouracil: A review. *J Am Acad Dermatol* **4:**633–649, 1981

39. Ebner H: Treatment of skin epitheliomas with 5-fluorouracil ointment: Influence of therapeutic design on recurrence of lesions. *Dermatologica* **140:**42–46, 1970

40. Avant WH, Huff RC: Intradermal 5-fluorouracil in the treatment of basal cell carcinoma of the face. *South Med J* **69:**561–563, 1976

41. Greenway HT et al: Treatment of basal cell carcinoma with intralesional interferon. *J Am Acad Dermatol* **15:**437–443, 1986

42. Cornell RC et al: Intralesional interferon therapy for basal cell carcinoma. *J Am Acad Dermatol* **23:**694–700, 1990

43. Robinson JK: Advances in the treatment of non-melanoma skin cancer. *Dermatol Clin* **9**(4):757–764, 1991

44. Domarus HV, Stevens PJ: Metastatic basal cell carcinoma: Report of 5 cases and review of 170 cases in the literature. *J Am Acad Dermatol* **10:**1043–1060, 1984

45. Bennett RG: *Fundamentals of Cutaneous Surgery,* 1st ed. St. Louis, Mosby, 1988

46. Farmer ER, Helwig EB: Metastatic basal cell carcinoma: A clinicopathologic study of seventeen cases. *Cancer* **46:**748–757, 1980

47. Robinson JK: Use of a combination of chemotherapy and radiation therapy in the management of advanced basal cell carcinoma of the head and neck. *J Am Acad Dermatol* **17:**770–774, 1987

48. Coker DD et al: Chemotherapy for metastatic basal cell carcinoma. *Arch Dermatol* **119:**44–50, 1983

49. Guthrie TH et al: Cisplatin and doxorubicin: An effective chemotherapy combination in the treatment of advanced basal cell and squamous carcinoma of the skin. *Cancer* **55:**1629–1632, 1985

50. Robinson JK: Risk of developing another basal cell carcinoma. *Cancer* **60:**118–120, 1987

51. Bergstresser PR, Halprin KM: Multiple sequential skin cancers: The risk of skin cancer in patients with previous skin cancer. *Arch Dermatol* **111:**995–996, 1975

52. Robinson JK: What are adequate treatment and follow-up care for nonmelanoma cutaneous cancer? *Arch Dermatol* **123:**331–333, 1987

53. Stern RS et al: Cutaneous squamous cell carcinoma in pa-

tients treated with PUVA. *N Engl J Med* **310:**1156–1161, 1984

54. Martin H et al: Radiation induced skin cancer of the head and neck. *Cancer* **1:**61–71, 1970

55. Aubry F, MacGibbon B: Risk factors of squamous cell carcinoma of the skin: A case-control study in the Montreal region. *Cancer* **55:**907–911, 1985

56. Lutzner MA: Skin cancer in immunosuppressed organ transplant recipients. *J Am Acad Dermatol* **11:**891–893, 1984

57. Eliezri YD et al: Occurrence of human papilloma virus type 16 DNA in cutaneous squamous and basal cell neoplasms. *J Am Acad Dermatol* **23:**836–842, 1990

58. Fukamizu H et al: Metastatic squamous cell carcinomas derived from solar keratosis. *J Dermatol Surg Oncol* **11:**518–522, 1985

59. Stanley RJ, Roenigk RK: Actinic cheilitis: Treatment with the carbon dioxide laser. *Mayo Clin Proc* **63:**230–235, 1988

60. Dinehart SM, Pollack SV: Metastases from squamous cell carcinoma of the skin and lip. *J Am Acad Dermatol* **21:**241–248, 1989

61. Johnson TM et al: Squamous cell carcinoma of the skin (excluding lip and oral mucosa). *J Am Acad Dermatol* **26:**467–484, 1992

62. Moller R et al: Metastases in dermatological patients with squamous cell carcinoma. *Arch Dermatol* **115:**703–705, 1979

63. Friedman HI et al: Prognostic and therapeutic use of microstaging of cutaneous squamous cell carcinoma of the trunk and extremities. *Cancer* **56:**1099–1105, 1985

64. Robins P et al: Squamous cell carcinoma treated by Mohs surgery: An experience with 414 cases in a period of 15 years. *J Dermatol Surg Oncol* **7:**800–802, 1981

65. Dzubow LM et al: Risk factors for local recurrence of primary cutaneous squamous cell carcinomas: Treatment by microscopically controlled excision. *Arch Dermatol* **118:**900–902, 1982

66. Brown RG et al: Advanced and recurrent squamous carcinoma of the lower lip. *Am J Surg* **132:**492–497, 1976

67. Meyskens FL et al: Activity of isotretinoin against squamous cell cancers and preneoplastic lesions. *Cancer Treat Rep* **66:**1315–1319, 1982

68. Novick M et al: Burn scar carcinoma: A review and analysis of 46 cases. *J Trauma* **17:**809–817, 1977

69. Mohs FE, Sahl WJ: Chemosurgery for verrucous carcinoma. *J Dermatol Surg Oncol* **5:**302–306, 1979

70. Japaze H et al: Verrucous carcinoma of the vulva: Study of 24 cases. *Obstet Gynecol* **60:**462–466, 1982

71. Swanson NA, Taylor WB: Plantar verrucous carcinoma: Literature review and treatment by the Mohs' chemosurgery technique. *Arch Dermatol* **116:**794–797, 1980

72. Padilla RS et al: Verrucous carcinoma of the skin and its management by Mohs' surgery. *Plast Reconstr Surg* **73:**442–447, 1984

73. Mora RG: Microscopically controlled surgery (Mohs' chemosurgery) for treatment of verrucous squamous cell carcinoma of the foot (epithelioma cuniculatum). *J Am Acad Dermatol* **8:**354–362, 1983

74. Carson TE: Verrucous carcinoma of the penis: Successful treatment with cryosurgery and topical fluorouracil therapy. *Arch Dermatol* **114:**1546–1547, 1978

75. Landthaler M et al: Laser therapy of bowenoid papulosis and Bowen's disease. *J Dermatol Surg Oncol* **12:**1253–1257, 1986

76. Parker CM, Hanke CW: Large keratoacanthomas in difficult locations treated with intralesional 5-fluorouracil. *J Am Acad Dermatol* **14:**770–777, 1986

77. Melton JL et al: Treatment of keratoacanthomas with intralesional methotrexate. *J Am Acad Dermatol* **25:**1017–1023, 1991

78. Street ML et al: Multiple keratoacanthomas treated with oral retinoids. *J Am Acad Dermatol* **23:**862–866, 1990

79. Rigel DS et al: Factors influencing survival in melanoma. *Dermatol Clin* **9**(4):631–642, 1991

80. Sober AJ et al: Epidemiology of cutaneous melanoma: An update. *Dermatol Clin* **9**(4):617–629, 1991

81. Day CL et al: Narrower margins for clinical stage I malignant melanoma. *N Engl J Med* **306:**479–482, 1982

82. Slingluff CL et al: Lethal "thin" malignant melanoma. *Ann Surg* **208:**150–161, 1988

83. Slingluff CL et al: Malignant melanoma arising during pregnancy: A study of 100 patients. *Ann Surg* **211:**552–559, 1990

84. Koh HK: Cutaneous melanoma. *N Engl J Med* **325:**171–182, 1991

85. Wanebo HJ et al: Prognostic factors in head and neck melanoma: Effect of lesion location. *Cancer* **62:**831–837, 1988

86. Hudson DA et al: Subungual melanoma of the hand. *J Hand Surg* **15-B:**288–290, 1990

87. Veronesi U et al: Thin stage I primary cutaneous malignant melanoma: Comparison of excision with margins of 1 or 3 cm. *N Engl J Med* **318:**1159–1162, 1988

88. Kelly JW et al: The frequency of local recurrence and microsatellites as a guide to reexcision margins for cutaneous malignant melanoma. *Ann Surg* **200:**759–763, 1984

89. Rogers GS: Surgical management of stage I malignant melanoma. *Dermatol Clin* **9**(4):649–655, 1991

90. Aitken DR et al: The extent of primary melanoma excision: A re-evaluation—how wide is wide? *Ann Surg* **198:**634–641, 1983

91. Kenady DE et al: Excision of underlying fascia with a primary malignant melanoma: Effect on recurrence and survival rates. *Surgery* **92:**615–618, 1982

92. Crowley NJ, Seigler HF: The role of elective lymph node dissection in the management of patients with thick cutaneous melanoma. *Cancer* **66:**2522–2527, 1990

93. Binder M et al: Elective regional lymph node dissection in malignant melanoma. *Eur J Cancer* **26:**871–873, 1990

94. Coit DG, Brennan MF: Extent of lymph node dissection in

melanoma of the trunk or lower extremity. *Arch Surg* **124:**162–166, 1989

95. Roses DF et al: Selective surgical management of cutaneous melanoma of the head and neck. *Ann Surg* **192:**629–632, 1980

96. Olson RM et al: Regional lymph node management and outcome in 100 patients with head and neck melanoma. *Am J Surg* **142:**470–473, 1981

97. Balch CM: The role of elective lymph node dissection in melanoma: Rationale, results, and controversies. *J Clin Oncol* **6:**163–172, 1988

98. Roses DF et al: Primary melanoma thickness correlated with regional lymph node metastases. *Arch Surg* **117:**921–923, 1982

99. Karp NS et al: Thoracotomy for metastatic malignant melanoma of the lung. *Surgery* **107:**256–261, 1990

100. Wiernik PH et al: Phase I trial of Taxol given as a 24-hour infusion every 21 days: Responses observed in metastatic melanoma. *J Clin Oncol* **5:**1232–1239, 1987

101. McClay EF, Mastrangelo MJ: Systemic chemotherapy for metastatic melanoma. *Semin Oncol* **15:**569–577, 1988

102. Baas PC et al: Hyperthermic isolated regional perfusion in the treatment of extremity melanoma in children and adolescents. *Cancer* **63:**199–203, 1989

103. Franklin HR et al: To perfuse or not to perfuse? A retrospective comparative study to evaluate the effect of adjuvant isolated regional perfusion in patients with stage I extremity melanoma with a thickness of 1.5 mm or greater. *J Clin Oncol* **6:**701–708, 1988

104. Cooper JS et al: Present role and future prospects for radiotherapy in the management of malignant melanomas. *J Dermatol Surg Oncol* **5:**134–139, 1979

105. Cooper JS: Radiation therapy for cancers of the skin. *Dermatol Clin* **9**(4):683–687, 1991

106. Weinstock MA, Sober AJ: The risk of progression of lentigo maligna to lentigo maligna melanoma. *Br J Dermatol* **116:**303–310, 1987

107. Arndt KA: Argon laser treatment of lentigo maligna. *J Am Acad Dermatol* **10:**953–957, 1984

108. Dhawan SS et al: Lentigo maligna: The use of rush permanent sections in therapy. *Arch Dermatol* **126:**928–930, 1990

109. Grande DJ et al: Surgery of extensive, subclinical lentigo maligna. *J Dermatol Surg Oncol* **8:**493–496, 1982

110. Robinson JK: Dermatofibrosarcoma protuberans resected by Mohs' surgery (chemosurgery): A 5-year prospective study. *J Am Acad Dermatol* **12:**1093–1098, 1985

111. Burkhardt BR et al: Dermatofibrosarcoma protuberans: Study of 56 cases. *Am J Surg* **111:**638–644, 1966

112. McPeak CJ et al: Dermatofibrosarcoma protuberans: An analysis of 86 cases—five with metastasis. *Ann Surg* **166:**803–816, 1967

113. Taylor HB, Helwig EB: Dermatofibrosarcoma protuberans: A study of 115 cases. *Cancer* **15:**717–725, 1962

114. Roses DF et al: Surgical treatment of dermatofibrosarcoma protuberans. *Surg Gynecol Obstet* **162:**449–452, 1986

115. Mayer MH et al: Microcystic adnexal carcinoma (sclerosing sweat duct tumor). *Plast Reconstr Surg* **84:**970–975, 1989

116. Folberg R et al: Recurrent and residual sebaceous carcinoma after Mohs' excision of the primary lesion. *Am J Ophthalmol* **103:**817–823, 1987

117. Kass LG, Hornblass A: Sebaceous carcinoma of the ocular adnexa. *Surv Ophthalmol* **33:**477–490, 1989

118. Yeatts RP, Waller RR: Sebaceous carcinoma of the eyelid: Pitfalls in diagnosis. *Ophthal Plast Reconstr Surg* **1:**35–42, 1985

119. Detlefs RL: Atypical fibroxanthoma. *Arch Dermatol* **120:**782–785, 1984

120. Enjoji M et al: Malignant fibrous histiocytoma: A clinicopathologic study of 150 cases. *Acta Pathol Jpn* **30:**727–741, 1980

121. Glavin FL, Cornwell ML: Atypical fibroxanthoma of the skin metastatic to a lung: Report of a case, features by conventional and electron microscopy, and a review of the relevant literature. *Am J Dermatopathol* **7:**57–63, 1985

122. Rosen L et al: Bowen's disease, Paget's disease and malignant melanoma in situ. *South Med J* **79:**410–413, 1986

123. Pitman GH et al: Extramammary Paget's disease. *Plast Reconstr Surg* **69:**238–244, 1982

124. Chanda JJ: Extramammary Paget's disease: Prognosis and relationship to internal malignancy. *J Am Acad Dermatol* **13:**1009–1014, 1985

125. Lee SC et al: Extramammary Paget's disease of the vulva: A clinicopathologic study of 13 cases. *Cancer* **39:**2540–2549, 1977

126. Mohs FE, Blanchard L: Microscopically controlled surgery for extramammary Paget's disease. *Arch Dermatol* **115:**706–708, 1979

127. Coldiron BM et al: Surgical treatment of extramammary Paget's disease: A report of six cases and a reexamination of Mohs micrographic surgery compared with conventional surgical excision. *Cancer* **67:**933–938, 1991

128. Watring WG et al: Treatment of recurrent Paget's disease of the vulva with topical bleomycin. *Cancer* **41:**10–11, 1978

129. Domarus H et al: Merkel cell carcinoma of the face, case report and review of the literature. *J Maxillofac Surg* **13:**39–43, 1985

130. Ecker HA et al: Trabecular or Merkel cell carcinoma of the skin. *Plast Reconstr Surg* **70:**485–489, 1982

131. Meland NB, Jackson IT: Merkel cell tumor: Diagnosis, prognosis and management. *Plast Reconstr Surg* **77:**632–638, 1986

David J. Leffell

22 Scar Revision

The art of successful scar revision requires knowledge of the biology of wound healing, the aesthetics of the affected region, and the dynamics of scar contracture as they affect functional regions.[1,2] Perhaps most importantly, it requires patience and judgment. For example, a scar that is so subtle that the patient must identify it to you should not be revised.

Scar revision is often considered in dermatologic surgery when the physician or patient believes that an unsatisfactory result has been obtained, either in a repair of trauma or as the result of an elective intervention, whether for the treatment of cancer or for cosmetic improvement. In some ways, the process of scar revision really begins at the time of the initial procedure. It is at this point that the patient must be advised of realistic expectations. The patient's satisfaction with the final result will largely be influenced by the expectations that are established at the consultation. A similar consultative appointment should take place prior to any scar revision so that the patient can again be advised of what the surgery can reasonably be expected to accomplish. It is to the surgeon's benefit to ensure that the patient embarking on surgery, especially if elective, has a realistic understanding of the possible results. It is helpful to use a mirror to demonstrate to the patient the likely extent of the scar and to outline any other surface or free-margin changes that might take place. Explicit discussion of the potential need for additional scar revision at a later date, if an unsatisfactory result occurs, is beneficial to the patient and confirms for the patient that certain aspects of the healing process are beyond the surgeon's control. The unpredictable elements in any surgical procedure must be conveyed with confidence to the patient so that, having listened to extensive disclaimers, he or she does not begin to lose faith in the ultimate skill of the surgeon.

Scar revision is necessarily a broad topic. This chapter will review functional and cosmetic issues, principles of scar revision, scar analysis (in preparation for revision), surgical methods of revision, and nonsurgical revision.

SCAR REVISION: FUNCTIONAL AND COSMETIC CONCERNS

In general, scar revision is requested by the patient or recommended by the surgeon for functional or cosmetic reasons. Functional problems include distortion of free margins of important organs such as the eyelids. This particular complication can result from poor selection of scar orientation prior to repair of a defect, improperly performed blepharoplasty, unanticipated hypertrophic scarring, or exaggeration of natural senile laxity of the lower lid. As a result of ectropion, keratitis may develop which can lead to significant corneal injury.

Adverse effects on the eye needn't occur only at the free margin. Scarring in the region of the lacrimal duct, perhaps secondary to a cheek advancement flap under tension in which hypertrophic scarring has occurred, can lead to epiphora. The patient may have blurred vision from the pooling of tears rather than intrinsic ophthalmic pathology.

Perioral distortion usually leads to cosmetic rather than functional impairment. Because of the constant tension on wounds in this cosmetic unit secondary to the underlying activity of the orbicularis oris muscles, hypertrophic scarring on the upper lip and even on the chin can be marked. Functional deficits from distortion of the lip include perlèche secondary to drooling and an inability to drink from certain cups which can lead to spilling of liquids.[3,4]

Scarring in the region of the ear can affect hearing, and perioperative injury to nerves around the eye may lead to lid droop. Similarly, unsatisfactory healing of reconstructive procedures around the ala may lead to distortion or collapse of the nostril along with difficulty in breathing.

Keloids and hypertrophic scars, which can cause chronic itching or pain, may occasionally be amenable to revision, but the biology of the process, still incompletely understood, makes attempts at improvement less successful than desired.[5]

PRINCIPLES OF SCAR REVISION

The cardinal principle of scar revision is best summarized by the dictum "examine, think, wait." The most critical consideration in the evaluation of a scar for revision is the amount of time that has elapsed since the original unsatisfactory surgery.[6] Examination of the scar will help determine if it has matured completely or whether any additional improvement can be expected. It is also important to think about the problem scar itself and to know whether it can be improved with revision. Scars with malaligned edges usually benefit from re-

vision. However, those on presternal and shoulder regions can rarely be improved unless the history suggests that the poor result may have been due to infection, bleeding, or some other perioperative complication. This method of assessment applies to any widened scar or spread scar.

An excellent bedside manner, disposed to hand-holding, is very helpful in the management of the patient when there is cause for dissatisfaction. "Time heals all scars" is an axiom with practical underpinnings. The need for patience is supported by knowledge of the biology of wound healing. Collagen remodeling and maturation continue actively for many months after the original surgery, so natural resolution of many problem scars can be expected.[7,8] A photographic review of the sequential healing of a dehisced flap demonstrates the remarkable ability of the skin to heal and of scar tissue to remodel (Fig. 22-1).

Scars appear worst from 2 weeks to 4 months postopera-

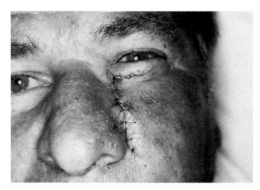

a

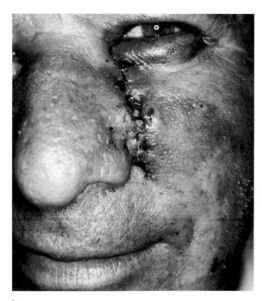

b

c

Figure 22-1   (*a*) Cheek advancement flap performed on sebaceous facial skin with moderate tension; (*b*) early wound dehiscence at 1 day, with purulent drainage; (*c*) wound was opened and packed with iodoform gauze. (*Continued*)

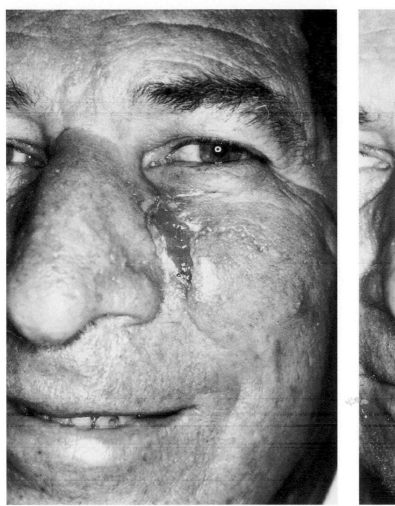

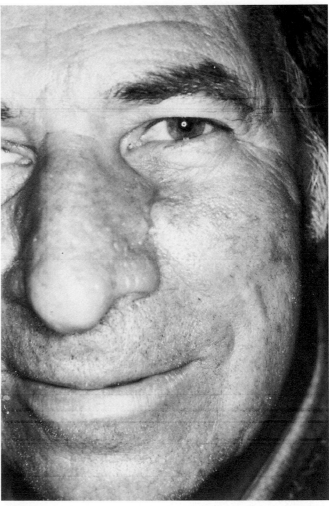

d

e

Figure 22-1 (*Cont.*)   (*d*) second intention healing at 2 weeks; (*e*) second intention healing at 6 weeks demonstrating remarkable ability of facial skin to heal secondarily, even in the setting of preceding infection.

tively, so a revision performed during this interval will appear to the patient to be improved compared with the original scar. Similarly, a revision done after the original scar has already started to mature may look worse than if it had been left alone, and the patient may wonder if revision was truly required.[9]

It is best to advise the patient prior to surgery that the final functional and cosmetic result cannot be guaranteed or predicted but that the techniques used have been developed over many years to optimize the chance of an ideal outcome. It should be emphasized to the patient that individuals heal differently over time, and a final judgment about the appearance of the scar cannot be made until 6 to 12 months after the repair. The importance of waiting before proceeding with revision is highlighted by the bulky appearance of the melolabial flap in Fig. 22-2. For the first 3 months after surgery, it was puffy and unsightly but at 4 months began to soften quickly and intervention was not required.

Scar Analysis

Prior to revision surgery it is helpful to evaluate the patient for hints of potential adverse outcomes: Signs of hypertrophic scarring, persistent redness of remote surgery sites, and a history of past healing experiences are especially important.[6]

Determination of final maturation of the scar may be based on hallmarks which include the absence of redness, pliable tissue around the scar, and low scar tissue volume as estimated by palpation. This last feature is best judged by comparison with previous examinations of the same scar over time.

When a scar revision is being considered because of cosmetic concerns, texture, color, size, and contour of the scar under study must be evaluated. When functional issues are involved, the added considerations of orientation and hypertrophy are important to note.[10]

Skin type often has predictive value about scar outcome.

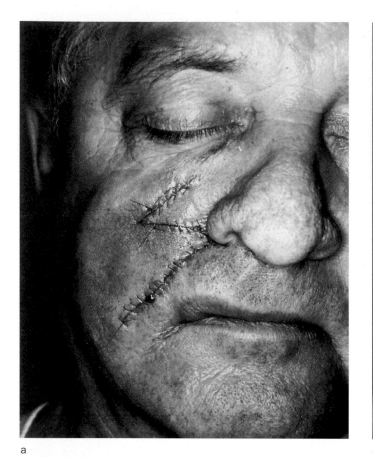

a

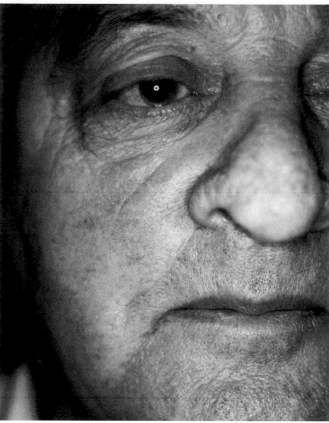

c

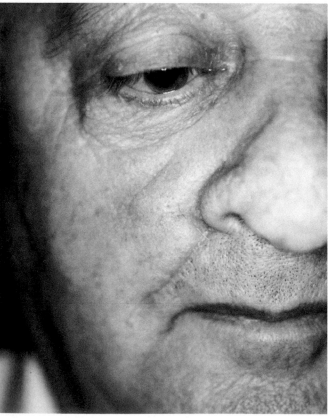

b

Figure 22-2   (*a*) Transposition flap of cheek-lip margin to repair large defect that traversed two cosmetic units; (*b*) at 4 weeks, flap is well healed but bulkiness (early trapdoor effect) is unsightly. Revision at this point would be premature; (*c*) spontaneous resolution of trapdoor effect at 4 months postoperatively.

Fair-skinned individuals are at less risk of developing keloids and hypertrophic scarring, but their scars will tend to stay red for many months. Scar erythema is a function of the neovascularization that occurs in the healing process and can be affected by the degree of tension under which the wound is closed. Scars in more darkly pigmented individuals are less likely to demonstrate postoperative erythema but are at greater risk for pigmentary change, including hyper- and hypopigmentation.

The degree of scar elevation and its shape are important to note as a distinction between hypertrophic scar and keloid will be helpful in planning the revision. A keloid is a tumor of fibrous tissue which overgrows its incisional scar and invades surrounding normal tissue. A hypertrophic scar represents proliferative scar tissue limited to the repair site itself which usually resolves over time.[5]

Because unsatisfactory scars may be due to poor initial design with respect to relaxed skin tension lines (RSTLs), the orientation of the scar to be revised should be noted and reoriented if necessary.[11] For example, ectropion may have resulted from poor placement of the scar, and repositioning the scar by making intelligent use of RSTLs will correct the problem. In this particular situation though, endogenous factors, such as the laxity of the senile lid, may not permit complete repair of the ectropion. Analogously, a wide scar which is of concern for cosmetic reasons may be so configured because of failure to take into account RSTLs, and reorientation may be beneficial in this case (Fig. 22-3).

Regional factors, however, may make successful revision difficult. For example, revision in the lower medial segment of the cheek often heals well, but revisions in other facial regions such as the lateral submandibular region are disposed to hypertrophic scarring. Skin tension on the upper back is so great, especially in young, active patients, that spreading of the scar is unavoidable.

The sebaceous skin of the face, especially the nose, often heals with obvious depressed scar lines. This can be compounded, in the case of a transposition flap, by the development of the trapdoor effect. The resulting bulkiness of the flap can be unsightly and is thought to be due to insufficient undermining of adjacent tissue and the loss of contact inhibition between the flap and the base of the wound.[12] Fortunately, scar revision in this case is relatively simple. It involves incision along the original scar line, broad undermining at the level of the scar tissue plane, and removal of fat and excess scar tissue with a blunt scissors.

A transposition flap in the region of the nose can be complicated by bulkiness and by loss of the meloalar angle. This too can be repaired by combining defatting of the flap with excision and repositioning of the inferior margin of the healed flap superior to the natural angle (Fig. 22-4).

Reconstruction after skin cancer surgery can sometimes best be done in stages. The patient should understand this from the outset. In Fig. 22-5, a large nasal defect is presented for repair. The reconstructive options included a forehead flap

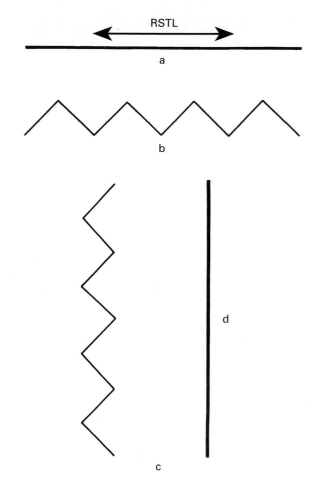

Figure 22-3 Reorientation of a scar can be accomplished by the use of Z-plasty. The Z-plasty is an array of rhombic transposition flaps. *(a)* Horizontal linear scar. *(b)* Multiple 60° rhombic flaps have elongated the scar and reoriented the lines of tension. This revision would only be beneficial if *a* was not in the RSTL or one was revising a free margin distortion. *(c)* A similar Z-plasty has been used to elongate a linear vertical scar *(d)* such as one might note on an extremity. The buckling from contracture of the original scar can be corrected to some degree by elongating as shown in *(c)* and the spreading of the scar may also be minimized.

or a full-thickness skin graft. In either case, the patient was advised that reconstruction of the soft triangle of the nose would be difficult. The patient opted for the skin graft, which did well except for the anticipated notch for which the patient was well prepared. The notch was repaired by using a composite graft from the helix of the right ear. A triangular defect at the recipient site was excised to match the donor graft which was sutured in place with 6-0 Prolene sutures and mild chromic sutures. The final result was very satisfactory and obviated the need for hospitalization and extensive forehead scarring. The second procedure was a scar revision but one for which the patient had been prepared from the beginning.

Occasionally a patient will present who has undergone surgery elsewhere and was reconstructed suboptimally. In Fig. 22–6, a circular defect of the glabella was repaired with

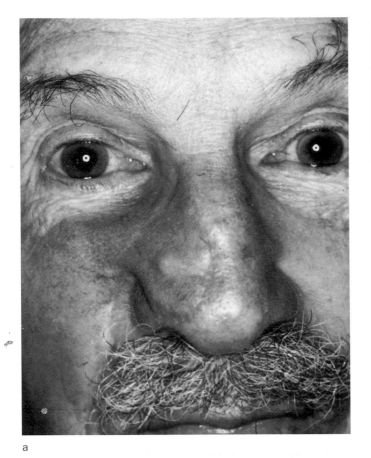

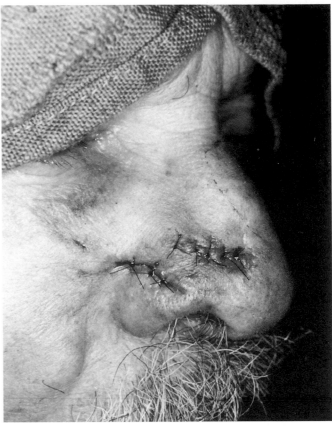

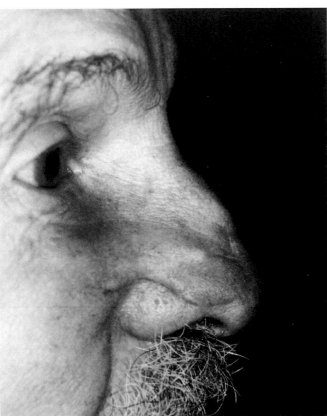

a

c

b

Figure 22-4   (*a*) Nasolabial transposition flap to repair nasal defect has healed, as predicted, with blunting and webbing in region of superior alar margin and loss of distinction between cheek and nose cosmetic units. Trapdoor effect is also noted; (*b*) 45° view; (*c*) at 6 weeks postoperatively the flap was incised along inferior margin, undermined broadly at the level of the scar. Excess fatty tissue and scar was removed. The flap in the region of the lateral ala-cheek interface was incised and trimmed and the scar repositioned more medially and superiorly. (*Continued*)

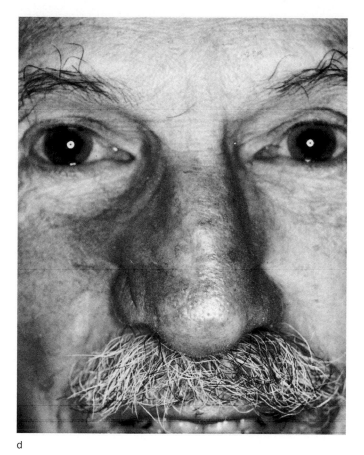
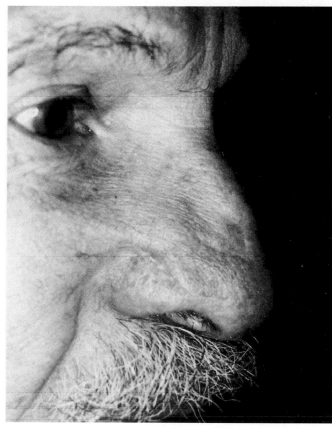

d

e

Figure 22-4 (*Cont.*)   (*d*) 2 months post-revision, frontal view; (*e*) post-revision, 45° view.

a skin graft when an adjacent tissue transfer would have been less noticeable. The mismatch of texture, tissue depth, and lines of expression necessitated a revision. The graft was removed and a classic O to T advancement flap was performed so that the vertical component would blend into the glabellar lines and the horizontal component would be camouflaged in the root of the nose. No spread of scar was noted because the majority of closure forces were perpendicular to the contraction lines of the procerus muscle.

Other cosmetically important problems that may present for revision include track marks. These result from epithelial channels which form because sutures have been allowed to stay in too long or have been tied too tightly. This complication, which resembles a row of snake fang marks, is unsightly and is completely avoidable if the surgeon has an understanding of wound-healing biology. In general, sutures on the face should be removed within 3 to 5 days.

Methods of Scar Revision

The key technical objectives of scar revision include improvement in the orientation of the scar; division into smaller, less noticeable components; and refinement of surface irregularities.

There are several principles that direct the methods which have evolved for scar revision. For example, when a linear scar cannot be hidden in a natural fold or at the border of a cosmetic unit, such as a vertical repair in the brow line of the forehead, a broken line is likely to be less noticeable. Similarly, a 5-inch vertical linear scar on the cheek is likely to be more prominent than an even longer scar which has been broken up into many jagged components. The Z-plasty and the W-plasty have evolved as a means of breaking up such lengthy linear scars so that they will be less noticeable. The application of the Z-plasty double transposition flap technique to the revision of linear scars for cosmetic improvement was first described in 1954.[13] A few years later, the W-plasty was described for facial scars. It minimized the protrusions and trapdoor effect that had been a disadvantage of multiple Z-plasties. In general, scars that do not follow the RSTLs on the eyelids, nose, nasolabial folds, and lips can be repaired by Z-plasty (Fig. 22-7).

The Z-Plasty

Although the Z-plasty was originally used to correct malaligned anatomic areas, it is probably most helpful in lengthening a scar, where wound contracture over time has caused buckling. Such buckling, in part the result of natural

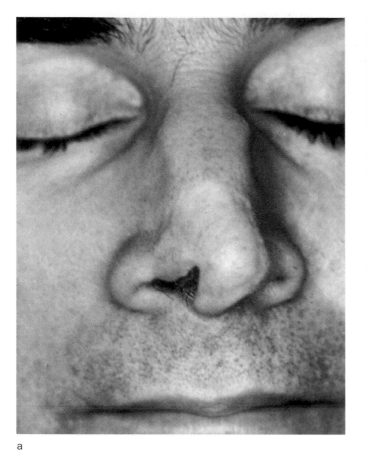

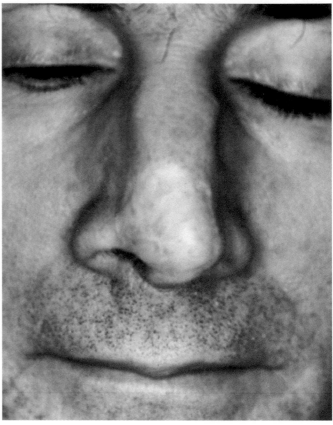

Figure 22-5   (*a*) Soft-triangle defect after nasal reconstruction with full-thickness graft; (*b*) composite graft from the right helix was used to recreate soft triangle; (*c*) revision 6 weeks post-composite grafting.

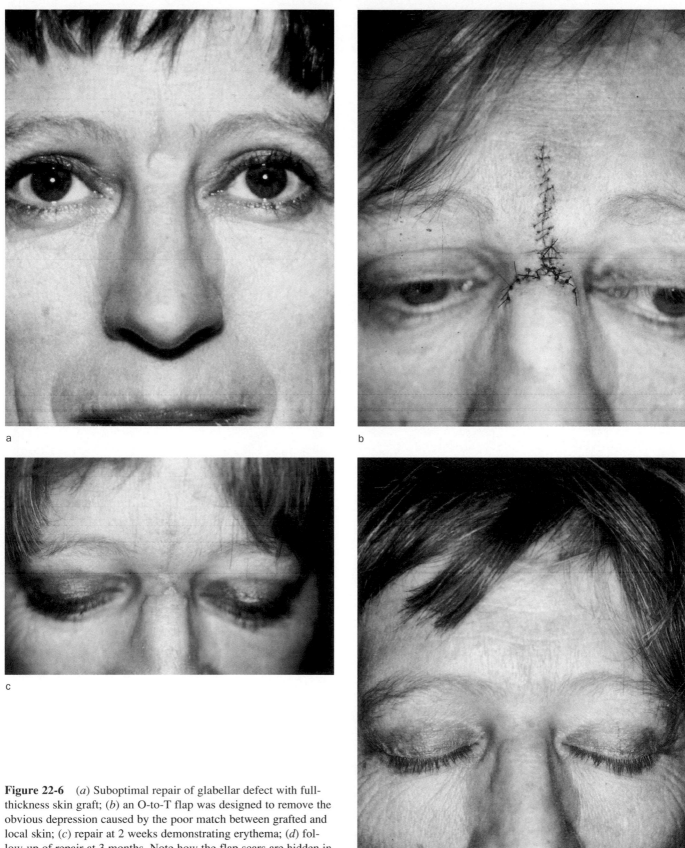

Figure 22-6   (*a*) Suboptimal repair of glabellar defect with full-thickness skin graft; (*b*) an O-to-T flap was designed to remove the obvious depression caused by the poor match between grafted and local skin; (*c*) repair at 2 weeks demonstrating erythema; (*d*) follow-up of repair at 3 months. Note how the flap scars are hidden in natural creases in this region. Transverse scar across the root of the nose is also well concealed.

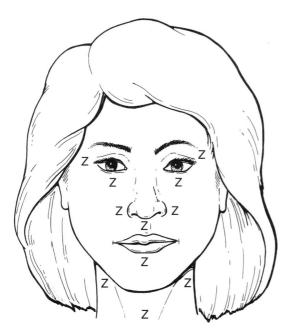

Figure 22-7 Diagram denotes locations in which Z-plasty may be most beneficial to reorient scar or correct functional problem.

linear scar contraction, which can be as high as 30 percent, occurs most frequently when a linear repair is performed over a convex surface.[14] This complication can sometimes be obviated by performing the original repair with a lazy-S fusiform incision which, through its intrinsic length, will accommodate tightening of the scar over convex surfaces.

Although the Z-plasty is routinely used and often discussed, its applications are not always agreed upon. One concern is that the Z-plasty may excessively elongate a scar, and, if done for cosmetic improvement, the opposite effect may occur. That is, multiple small irregular scars may well be more noticeable than a single thin linear scar. For example, a Z-plasty constructed of 60° flaps may lengthen a scar by 40 percent. Pincushion effect, dehiscence, and infection are just a few of the complications that can be associated with Z-plasty. Because the repair consists of multiple small flaps, tip necrosis may also occur.[6] Although there is debate about the utility of the Z-plasty for cosmetic revision, there is less disagreement about its use to correct webbing over a concavity, such as in the medial canthus, or where binding down and contraction has occurred over a convexity, such as the forearm. One of the concerns about the Z-plasty and the W-plasty is that the very small flaps which comprise them may result in multiple small trapdoor effects.[10]

In effect, the Z-plasty is an array of rhomboid flaps designed to reorient the scar so that it takes advantage of the RSTLs in the region (Fig. 22-8). By spreading the forces of contracture over many directions, a Z-plasty can redirect tensions and minimize scar diameter.[15]

Figure 22-9 demonstrates the use of multiple Z-plasties to elongate a nasal repair which had resulted in an alar notch.

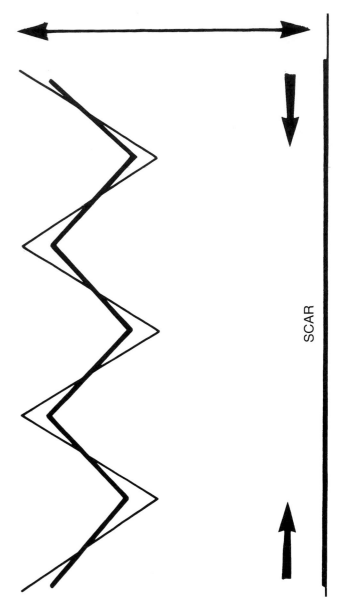

Figure 22-8 The Z-plasty spreads the forces of scar contracture over a larger area, minimizing spreading of the scar. In addition, by altering the angle of each flap, the length of the scar can be increased proportionately (thin-line z-plasty versus thick-line z-plasty). This diagram demonstrates how the orginal scar (Scar) with vertical forces of contracture is changed to a scar in which the forces of contracture are along RSTL. From Borges, AF: *Elective Incisions and Scar Revision,* Boston, 1973, Little, Brown & Co.

This vertical repair was just one component of a complex advancement flap from the lip to reline the nose and a transposition flap from the cheek, but revision of just the latter component improved the final result.

In the classic Z-plasty, the flap has 60° angles and two sides of equal length. Undermining the two flaps that are created and transposing them increase flap length by 75 percent. Two 30° angles will yield a 25 percent increase in length and two 45° flaps will increase the length of the scar by 50 per-

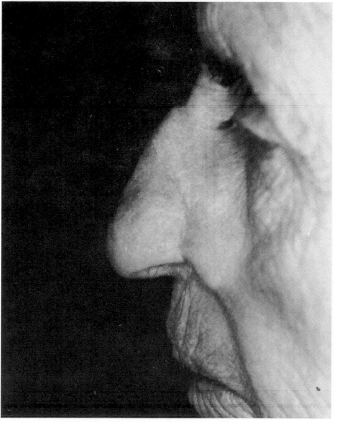

a

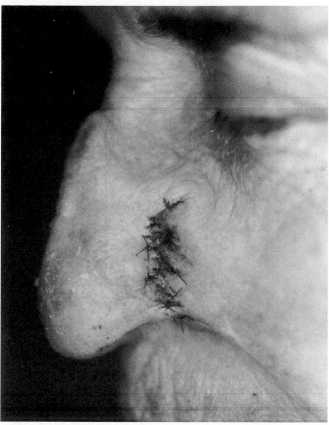

b

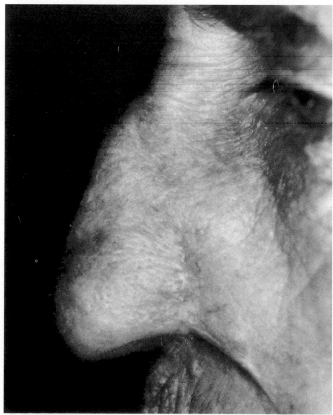

c

Figure 22-9 (*a*) Notched ala after complex repair of complete nostril loss. The nasal lining had been re-created with a V-to-Y flap from the upper lip, which was advanced superiorly. A nasolabial flap was then used to resurface the newly created ala. The notching was predicted, and, despite the minimally evident new ala, is cosmetically disturbing; (*b*) multiple Z-plasties were designed along vertical scar to lengthen scar and allow notch to drop. Z-plasties were created through and through; (*c*) relaxation of notch as a result of Z-plasty at 2 months. The patient was pleased with the elimination of the notch.

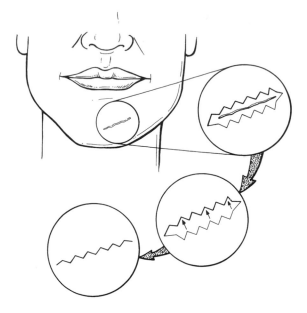

Figure 22-10 This diagram demonstrates the W-plasty method. The original scar is excised in the fashion described so that the flaps may interdigitate, creating repeating "W"s. Although tensions are not significantly changed, the smaller scar lines may minimize puckering and be less obvious, especially if combined with dermabrasion.

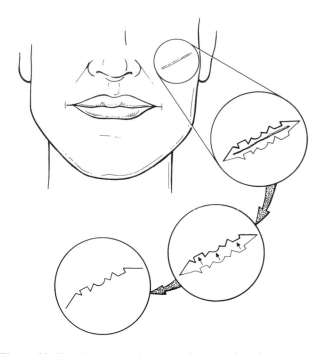

Figure 22-11 The geometric broken line technique is an extension of the W-plasty technique and is based on the principle that multiple small, uneven lines are better camouflaged than a single straight line. Although there is some debate about this, and the trapdoor effect can make this revision worse, there are times when scars excised in the fashion shown here—and resutured—may be improved.

cent. When the angle is less than 30 percent, tip necrosis may result. Dog-ear deformities are a complication when angles greater than 75 percent are used. The Z-plasty may be used to increase the base of a rhomboid flap to provide more mobility although the base of the flap may then be compromised. Z-plasty followed by light dermabrasion may be especially helpful.

The W-Plasty

A variation of the Z-plasty is the W-plasty. Although the W-plasty lies in the same general direction as the linear repair, the vectors of the closure contraction forces are different and minimize the risk of scar contracture.[16] The W-plasty is preferred on the face and when the wound is over 1.5 cm in length. Because the W-plasty often requires excision of more skin than is required when performing a Z-plasty, it is not the preferred procedure near free margins where distortion may occur (Fig. 22-10).

The Geometric Broken Line

Another variation of the Z-plasty is the geometric broken line technique which results in an irregular scar pattern.[17,18] It is intended to conceal a lengthy linear repair. Again, the rationale is that a long scar is less perceptible if it consists of multiple small scars. The geometric broken line technique consists of designing a random array of geometric shapes on each side of the scar to be revised (Fig. 22-11). In the case of all scar revisions, the final result of this approach may be op-

timized by light dermabrasion of the repair 4 to 6 weeks after excision.

Specialized Techniques

A variety of other scar revision approaches can be used for specialized situations. Acne scars and pox scars can be treated by punch excision with suturing.[19,20] In this case, a punch trephine is used that is large enough to include the whole scar. Tension is applied to the scar perpendicularly to the final desired axis. The punch excision is made through to the subcutis. The wound is then closed with 6-0 Prolene by using simple interrupted sutures. If vertical mattress sutures are used to aid in eversion, they should be removed in 3 days. There is a risk in this technique that the final scar may resume a circular appearance if healing is inadequate. To avoid this problem, punch grafting can be done.[21] The small defect is removed by using a punch trephine, and a punch graft, usually from the postauricular area, is obtained and sutured into the revision site by using 6-0 Prolene sutures. Following healing, the punch graft can be smoothed by gentle dermabrasion of the area. Although the technique has been widely published and is reportedly successful in experienced hands, a highly satisfactory result is a challenging goal.

Certain skin types present unavoidable problems during wound healing. Revision of acne scars after cystic acne has become quiescent must be approached cautiously.[22] First, the multiple areas of scar tissue along the depressed scar make it difficult to appose the tissue well. Second, the epidermis is usually irregular, so obtaining a fine scar can be difficult. Third, the presence of large follicles may also inhibit healing and can lead to dehiscence. Moreover, revision of serious acne scars must take into account the effect of skin aging. Laxity of the skin, even in a 20 year old, can accentuate scars, which will not be improved by excision. In selected cases, rhytidectomy may provide some improvement in the appearance of the scars exacerbated by the effects of photoaging.

With the exception of major revisions of bulky or irregular scars, a great deal of cosmetic improvement can be obtained by using dermabrasion or shave abrasion.[23] Full-thickness skin grafts, which can be raised at their edges, benefit by shave abrasion at 6 weeks postoperatively. In this case, a sterile razor blade is gently bent to match the contour of the skin, and, by using the blade in a sawing motion, the excess tissue, including the graft and some adjacent skin, is removed as though planing wood (Fig. 22-12). A coarse diamond fraise on a hand engine can be used to accomplish the same effect but is more involved and has the added risk of generating airborne blood particles. The dermabrasion technique is very helpful in smoothing the edges of flaps as well.

NONSURGICAL SCAR REVISION

Often an unsatisfactory scar develops that is not amenable to surgical intervention. It is important to be very judicious about which scars may actually be improved by scalpel surgery.

Hypertrophic scarring is probably the most common problem that skin surgeons encounter. Individual disposition aside, it occurs most often when wounds are closed under tension, especially in highly mobile areas. Such scarring is common on the upper and lower lip, the angle of the jaw, postauricular area, and upper torso. Constant tension due to mouth movement, neck mobility, and truncal motion probably accounts for a large number of cases of hypertrophic scarring. Weight lifters, for example, seem especially prone to presternal hypertrophic scars following surgery in that area. Interestingly, other regions at risk for developing keloid or hypertrophic scars are the earlobes, which are not normally under tension stresses, and the nostrils. Such scarring will resolve over time, but patients should be warned that the natural biology of scarring is such that it is likely to worsen during the first 6 months and then improve over time.

For the patient's comfort and for that of the surgeon, it is necessary to intervene. Intralesional triamcinolone is well documented as a successful approach to the problem of hypertrophic scarring. Low doses of intralesional steroid are thought to be successful (2.5 to 5 mg/cc) in inhibiting fibroblast production of collagen.[24,25] Forty milligrams of triamcinolone (TAC) per cc has, in the author's experience, provided the most dramatic results in refractory cases of hypertrophic scarring and keloids. Regular retreatment every 4 to 6 weeks with up to 0.3 cc of the suspension is unlikely to have systemic effects.[26] Technique is very important to keep the steroid confined to the dense scar tissue and avoid the side effects of soft tissue and epidermal atrophy.

Control of the injection is provided by using a tuberculin syringe and a 30-gauge, 1/2-in needle. The proper method for intralesional injection includes grasping the scar with both fingers so that the borders of the tumor may be identified by palpation and injection directly into the scar tissue by using a fanning motion. Sometimes, manipulation of the scar permits easier introduction of the material which otherwise might meet with stiff resistance. While the danger of atrophy is less with large scars, and one must use this technique carefully on the face where atrophy and telangiectasia would be especially unwelcome, the results can be dramatic. In the author's experience, the worst cases of atrophy with intralesional steroids have occurred on the shoulders and back where atrophy has been noted after just a single injection.

Hypertrophic scarring which results from regional effects, suture reaction, or endogenous disposition can be improved by simple massage. Proper use of this technique may minimize the need for steroid injection. Massage should be done at least once a day, by applying firm circular compressive motion, for at least 10 min. When there is a hard surface against which to press the scar, such as the maxilla, this should be encouraged. Patients should be advised to use a lubricating agent such as Vaseline, and many will ask if they can use vitamin E cream, whose reparative powers have been more highly touted than the objective data support. Nonetheless, the patient's belief that vitamin E cream may well improve the scar appears in many cases to enhance compliance and should not be discouraged unless a contact dermatitis develops.

Recently, silicone gel sheeting has been used to aid in the treatment of keloids and hypertrophic scarring.[27] This material, first used in Great Britain to prevent hypertrophic scarring in burn patients, is now generally available.[28] The sheeting is manufactured as a rectangle of silicone polymer which is thought to be biologically inert; no significant absorption has been documented. Application of the sheeting over a hypertrophic scar, or developing hypertrophic scar, appears to decrease scar volume (Fig. 22-13). In a recent study, patients noted that itching, scar swelling, and redness all decreased as a result of regular use. Side effects were few. The main problem was in making the sheeting adhere in concave areas. When silicone gel sheeting is combined with TAC injections, many hypertrophic scars seem to respond well to the sheeting therapy. Use for longer than 2 months does not seem to be necessary and, if the scar responded to therapy, further retreatment with the sheeting is not necessary.

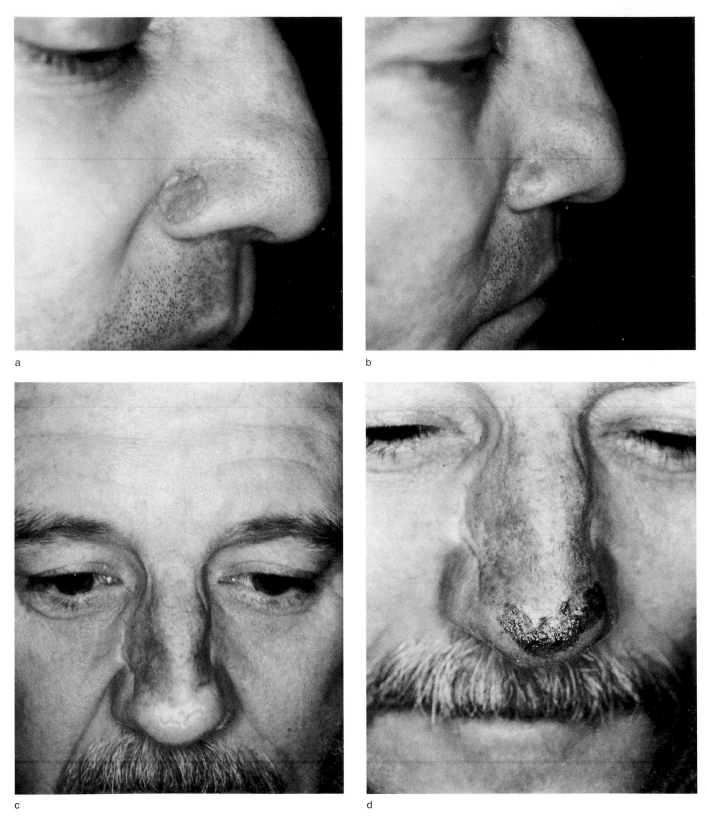

Figure 22-12 *(a)* Full-thickness graft of nostril demonstrating elevation at margin of graft; *(b)* after shave abrasion performed at 6 weeks, contour is natural and appearance of graft is excellent; *(c)* uneven graft margin at inferior pole of graft on nose. Dermabrasion was used in this case rather than shave abrasion; *(d)* hemostasis was obtained with ferric chloride. Aluminum chloride provides less risk of tattoo.

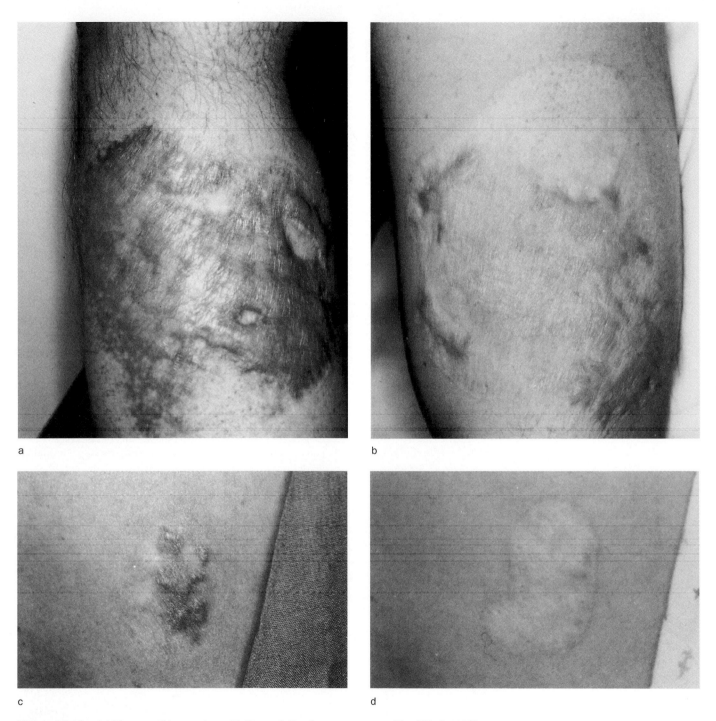

a

b

c

d

Figure 22-13   *(a)* Hypertrophic scarring of left arm following tattoo removal by CO_2 laser. Patient refused other laser modalities; *(b)* after 6 weeks of silicone gel sheeting and Kenalog injections, dramatic reduction in scar tissue is noted; *(c)* hypertrophic scar on breast; *(d)* after 2 months of silicone gel sheeting and Kenalog injections.

SUMMARY

Scar revision is performed for functional or cosmetic reasons. When function is impaired due to a poorly healed scar, careful analysis of the repair is required to ensure that the revision will improve the functional deficit. When scar revision is being considered to address cosmetic concerns, complete communication between the surgeon and patient is required to be certain that patient expectations are realistic and that the patient is aware that the revision result may be less acceptable than the original scar. Patience is critical in both situations as scar maturation over 6 to 12 months often resolves healing problems before the surgeon must intervene.

REFERENCES

1. Edlich RF et al: Biology of wound repair: Its influence on surgical decision. *Facial Plastic Surgery* **1:**169–180, 1984

2. Reed BR, Clark RAF: Cutaneous tissue repair: Practical implications of current knowledge, pt 2. *J Am Acad Dermatol* **13:**919, 1985

3. Wilkie TP: Surgical treatment of drooling: Follow-up report of five years' experience. *Plast Reconstr Surg* **45:**459, 1970

4. Fairbanks GR, Dingman RD: Restoration of the oral commissure. *Plast Reconstr Surg* **49:**411, 1972

5. Brown LA, Pierce HE: Keloids: Scar revision. *J Dermatol Surg Oncol* **12**(1):51–56, 1986

6. Lacy GM, Hemphill JE: Facial scar revision. *Surg Clin North Am* **49**(6):1343–1350, 1969

7. Howes EL, Harvey SC: The age factor in the velocity of the growth of fibroblasts in the healing wound. *J Exp Med* **55:**577–590, 1986

8. Wolfe D, Davidson TM: Scar revision. *Arch Otolaryngol Head Neck Surg* **117**(2):200–204, 1991

9. Borges AF: Timing of scar revision techniques. *Clin Plast Surg* **17**(1):71–76, 1990

10. Borges AF: Scar analysis and objectives of revision procedures. *Clin Plast Surg* **4**(2):223–237, 1977

11. Onizuka T: Scar revision. *Aesthetic Plast Surg* **6**(2):85–89, 1982

12. Koranda FC, Webster RC: Trapdoor effect in nasolabial flaps: Causes and corrections. *Arch Otolaryngol* **111:**421–424, 1985

13. Borges AF: The W-plastic versus the Z-plastic scar revision. *Plast Reconstr Surg* **44**(1):58–62, 1969

14. McGrath MH, Simon RH: Wound geometry and the kinetics of contraction. *Plast Reconstr Surg* **72:**66–72, 1983

15. Yanai A et al: Direction of suture lines in Z-plasty scar revision. *Aesthetic Plast Surg* **10**(2):97–99, 1986

16. Webster RC, Smith RC: Scar revision and camouflaging. *Otolaryngol Clin North Am* **15**(1):55–68, 1982

17. Harnick DB: Broken geometrical pattern used for facial scar revision. *Laryngoscope* **94**(6):841–842, 1984

18. Webster CC et al: Broken line scar revision. *Clin Plast Surg* **4**(2):247–254, 1977

19. Orentreich D, Orentreich N: Acne scar revision update. *Dermatol Clin* **5**(2):359–368, 1987

20. Eiseman G: Reconstruction of the acne-scarred face. *J Dermatol Surg Oncol* **3:**332–338, 1977

21. Dzubow LM: Scar revision by punch-graft transplants. *J Dermatol Surg Oncol* **11**(12):1200–1202, 1985

22. Ellis DA, Michell MJ: Surgical treatment of acne scarring: Non-linear scar revision. *J Otolaryngol* **16**(2):116–119, 1987

23. Roenigk HH Jr: Scar camouflage using dermabrasion. *Facial Plastic Surgery* **1:**3-10, 1984

24. Booth BA et al: Steroid-induced dermal atrophy: Effects of glucocorticosteroids on collagen metabolism in human skin fibroblast cultures. *Int J Dermatol* **21:**333, 1982

25. Bauer EA et al: Glucocorticoid modulation of collagenase expression in human skin fibroblast cultures: Evidence of inhibition of transcription. *Biochim Biophys Acta* **825:**227, 1985

26. Callen JP: Intralesional corticosteroids. *J Am Acad Dermatol* **4:**149, 1981

27. Ahn ST et al: Topical silicone gel: A new treatment for hypertrophic scars. *Surgery* **106:**781-6, 1989

28. Perkins K et al: Silicone gel: A new treatment for burn scars and contractures. *Burns Incl Therm Inj* **9:**201-204, 1983

Bernard I. Raskin

23 Nails

W hile the nail is little emphasized and certainly less glamorous than other regions in dermatologic surgery, even complex nail reconstructions are within the purview and training of surgical dermatologists.

Nail and paronychia surgery is delicate but rarely difficult. But, and the author places great emphasis on this point, *even the simplest nail surgery becomes a challenge when poor or dull instrumentation is used.* Dull punches, lack of fine-point sharp scissors, and poor-quality nail nippers contribute to suboptimal results. The surgical nail tray should have its own instruments, including a blunt nail elevator and a good-quality nail nipper.

Next, attention to developing a bloodless field beforehand facilitates an effortless surgery. Additionally, aseptic sterile technique is a must since surgery may result in osteomyelitis or a septic joint. Attention to postoperative pain relief is mandatory since nail surgeries often result in considerable pain. Finally, patients must understand the limitations of nail surgery and the results that may be expected.

CLINICAL TERMINOLOGY

Onychoschizia	distal horizontal splitting
Onychauxis	surface irregularity and thickening, hypertrophy
Onychogryposis	curvature and hornlike hypertrophy of the plate
Onychocryptosis	ingrown nail
Onychomadesis	separation of the nail plate proximally
Onychomycosis	fungal nail
Onychorrhexis	superfacial longitudinal striation
Macronychia	widened nail
Trachyonychia	roughened nails

PRE-OPERATIVE STATUS

Medical and laboratory evaluation pre-operatively is based on the physician's judgment. However, because of tissue oozing, aspirin should be discontinued 7 to 10 days prior. Nonsteroidals are generally not considered problematic in this author's experience. Pre-operative or intraoperative antibiotics for surgically created clean wounds are not considered necessary, and use depends on physican's judgment. Traumatic or contaminated wounds warrant a tetanus toxoid injection if none within the last 5 to 10 years, along with antibiotic consideration. X-ray is recommended prior to excising distal digit tumors.

ANESTHESIA

Digital blocks represent the most effective approach, sparing discomfort. For fingers, injections along the sides of the digit, proximally, are adequate. For the great toe, a ring block is helpful. Generally non-epinephrine agents are utilized, although some authors maintain that epinephrine is safe in most patients.[1] While distal nerve block is easily obtained by injecting adjacent to the proximal nail fold, this approach is painful. A more proximal injection is recommended along the proximal phalanx. Generally 10–20 min are required for proximal blocks to be effective.

Like all procedures, skill in anesthesia improves with repetition.

Supplies Needed

1 or 2% lidocaine (Xylocaine)®

30-gauge needle, Luer-Lok syringe

0.25% bupivacaine (Marcaine)®

Procedure

With the patient supine, since vasovagal reactions are common, a 30-gauge needle is used to inject approximately 1.5 cc on each side of the proximal phalanx. This may be injected adjacent to the bone or within the dermis. The needle is inserted into the dorsum of the digit. Either small amounts are injected ahead of the needle as it advances to the plantar aspect, or the needle is inserted from the dorsal digit and immediately advanced to the skin under the plantar aspect and injected as the needle is withdrawn. Some authors recommend aspiration before injection, but a 30-gauge needle makes aspiration difficult. If the needle is continuously moving during the injection, then the chance of injecting any significant amount intra-arterially is low.

Adequate volume is necessary to achieve digital block anesthesia. For the great toe, a ring block is often needed. It is sometimes helpful to dorsiflex the patient's great toe when one is injecting horizontally on the superior (dorsal) aspect and direct the needle under the tendon. Ten to 20 min is required after a digital block until adequate anesthesia has supravened. Even if full anesthesia has not occurred by this time, enough partial anesthesia has resulted so that local injection adjacent to the surgical site will be minimally felt.

The bipuvicaine may be injected at the completion of the procedure directly into the surgical site. Be aware that a prolonged anesthetic finger needs a bulky dressing to prevent subsequent trauma during the 6 to 8 h of anesthesia. The accompanying illustrations (Figs. 23-1 and Fig. 23-2) demonstrate digital block technique.

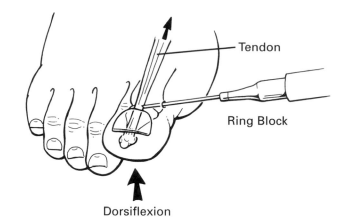

Figure 23-2   Anesthesia; ring block, great toe.

ANATOMY

Surgical Anatomy

The main anatomic aspects are delineated in the illustrations (Figs. 23-3, 23-4, and 23-5).[2,3,9] Proximally, there is the proximal nail fold which overlies the proximal part of the nail plate and the matrix. The proximal nail fold extends to the eponychium and the adjacent cuticle. The matrix is identified as the whitish area beneath the proximal nail plate and nail fold, and it extends distally to the lunula. The nail plate is bordered laterally and medially by the nail fold. Distally, there is the sole horn, distal groove, and hyponychium. Many texts group this distal area as simply the hyponychium.

In sagittal view are two ligaments (Fig. 23-5). The anterior ligament attaches the hyponychium area to the distal phalanx, and the posterior ligament is at the proximal nail fold bone in-

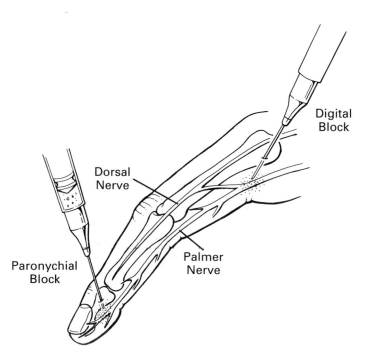

Figure 23-1   Anesthesia; paronychial and proximal digital blocks.

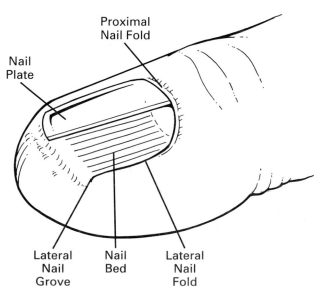

Figure 23-3   Nail unit anatomy.

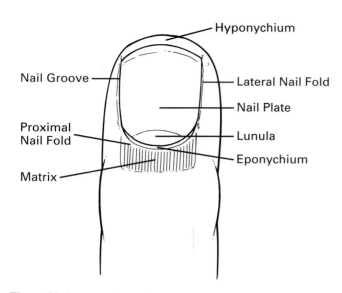

Figure 23-4 Nail unit anatomy.

terface. Note in sagittal view that deep to the nail bed is periosteum; there is no fat under the nail bed or under the matrix. Also be aware that the extensor tendon insertion is at the base of the nail matrix near the midline of the proximal portion of the distal phalanx. For reference, the insertion is usually about 2 or 3 mm distal to the distal interphalangeal (DIP) joint or 12 mm proximal to the cuticle and is generally not a problem unless a large excision is planned.[9]

Blood and Nerve Supply

A dual blood supply occurs from superficial arcades that derive from the lateral digital arteries which form anastomosis with other branches from the main digital arteries directly (Figs. 23-6 and Fig. 23-7). The lateral digital arteries enter the distal phalanx adjacent to the bony volar surface, then form extensive branches within the distal pulp. There is both a proximal and a distal arcade that supplies the matrix and nail

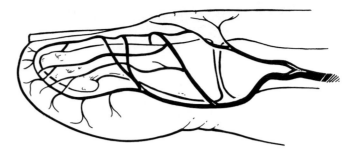

Figure 23-6 Arterial, supply.

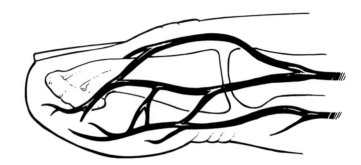

Figure 23-7 Venous architecture.

bed. The blood supply directly from the digital artery arises from the midpoint of the middle phalanx and anastomoses with the lateral digital artery arcades, thus supplying a dual blood supply.

Clinically important is the presence of a visually apparent branch of the digital artery immediately under the matrix.[3] Therefore, there is potential for significant bleeding in fingertip surgery. However, because of the dual supply and interfacing arcades, there is minimal risk of local surgery impairing circulation.

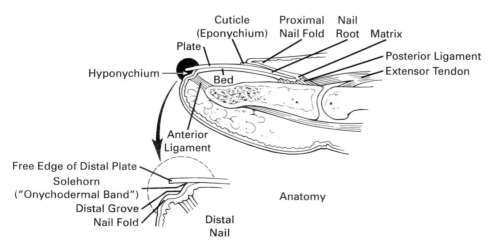

Figure 23-5 Detailed distal digit anatomy.

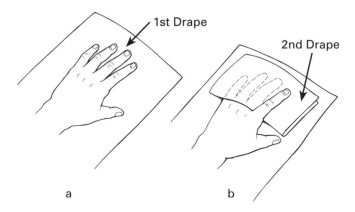

Figure 23-8   *(a, b)* Preparing the field.

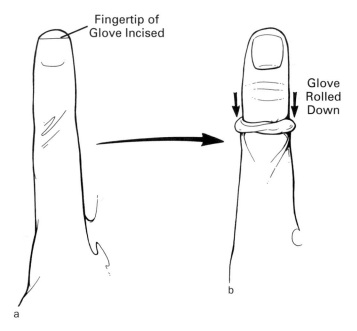

Figure 23-9   *(a, b)* Glove tourniquet.

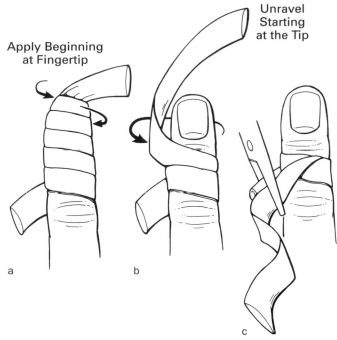

Figure 23-10   *(a–c)* Exsanguination technique.

There are arterial venus anastomoses throughout the circulation within the nail unit and distal digit. Veins are present on both sides adjacent to the nail plate within the nail fold. Extensive lymphatic drainage is also present. Nerves parallel the arterial supply and are both rich and overlapping.

PREPARING THE FIELD

Successful efficient surgery mandates careful pre-operative attention. Suggestions include use of a sterile drape over the extremity and an additional drape underneath to develop a sterile field (Fig. 23-8). Similarly, a fenestrated drape can isolate the affected digit. One common approach is to snip the tip off the "finger" of a sterile glove.

Developing a bloodless field usually involves a tourniquet. Tourniquets may be safely utilized for 15 min, released, then reapplied. Rubber bands, long a favorite, are discouraged since use may result in vascular spasm, or they may be inadvertently left in place postoperatively. Generally, wider tourniquets such as a 3/8-inch Penrose drain held in place with a hemostat are recommended.

Two alternative methods of tourniquet are presented; however, many variations have been offered: Bennett[4] (Fig. 23-9) has espoused incising the tip of a glove, placing the tip over the affected digit, and rolling it back to the base of the finger. A combination tourniquet and exsanguination technique is illustrated (Fig. 23-10) in which a Penrose is wrapped distally to proximally, then unwrapped distally to proximally and secured with a hemostat.

Finally, during surgery, bleeding may be controlled by lateral compression of the distal digit with the thumb and index finger of the free hand.

INSTRUMENTATION

Except for nail cutting or avulsion, distal digit procedures usually require standard, readily available instruments. Importance of a high-quality stainless steel nail nipper is emphasized. For removing partially onycholytic nails without anesthesia, a dual action nail nipper is particularly beneficial as the hinge allows for molding to the nail bed's shape to facilitate correct position for trimming painlessly (Fig. 23-11).

English nail splitters are quite useful due to the anvil-like jaw on the bottom and cutting blade on top so that the instrument is easily inserted under the nail (Fig. 23-12). Some type of blunt elevator is also mandatory. A 2 to 3 mm nail elevator

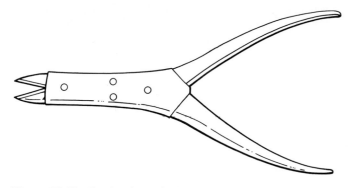

Figure 23-11 Dual-action nail nipper.

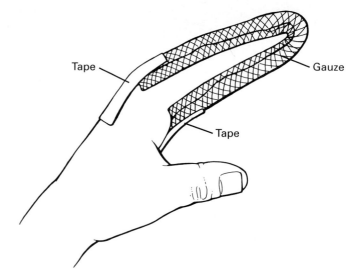

Figure 23-14 Postoperative longitudinal dressing.

is available or similar-sized dental spatula may be used. Freer septum elevators are also popular (Fig. 23-13). For grasping the nail plate, a large-sized hemostat is needed.

POSTOPERATIVE STATUS

Many surgeons recommend that oxidized cellulose (Gelfoam)® or collagen matrix sponges be placed over open digital tip wounds for hemostasis. Alternatively, strips of iodoform gauze may be packed under the nail fold to control postoperative oozing.

While special digital tubing dressings can be purchased, use of everyday immediately available dressings works well. Circumferential wrapping of the digit is to be avoided to prevent pain and vascular congestion. To produce a bulky dressing, standard 2- by 2-in or 3- by 3-in gauze can be unfolded and placed longitudinally over the digit (Fig. 23-14). Tape

should be placed longitudinally also, and care must be taken to avoid tight dressings as noted above.

Postoperative pain may be significant. Locally injecting the site with Marcaine® postoperatively helps, as does postoperative elevation, codeine, and nonsteroidal analgesics. The bulky dressing prevents painful trauma immediately postoperatively. Usually within a day, more routine dressings may be used.

In the author's experience, postoperative infections are infrequent on fingers or toes, and antibiotics are used only when infection is present or suspected at the time of surgery or based on the patient's immune system status. There is no consensus on pre- or postoperative antibiotics and decision for same is best determined by individual judgment. If the patient has a traumatic puncture wound, assessment for tetanus injection is mandatory.

In general, sutures of the digit and nail area are removed after 7 days.

NAIL AVULSION

Simple avulsion routinely takes but a few minutes.[5] After anesthesia, the nail plate is bluntly dissected on both dorsal and ventral aspects. For fingernails, the dental spatula suffices, but for thick horny toenails, a more heavy-duty periosteal elevator may be required. First, dissection is performed by elevating the nail fold overlying the plate. The elevator is pushed firmly, and at first resistance is encountered. Once the area of resistance has been passed, the elevator is advanced a few more millimeters, then withdrawn. This is performed in the nail fold around the entire nail plate; the subungual region is addressed similarly. The elevator is passed with firm pressure under the nail and moderate resistance is encountered, although less resistance is noted when the matrix is reached.

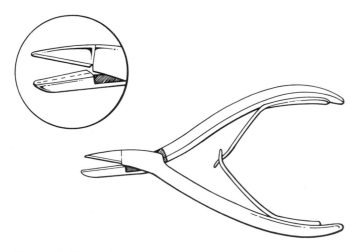

Figure 23-12 Anvil-type nail splitter.

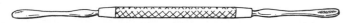

Figure 23-13 Freer septum elevator.

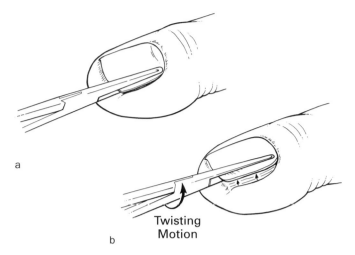

a

b

Twisting
Motion

Figure 23-15 *(a)* Nail avulsion technique. *(b)* Nail avulsion; rotating hemostat to remove nail.

Generally, the dissection is carried out a few millimeters past the proximal nail fold. The nail plate is then grasped firmly on one lateral end with a large hemostat (Fig. 23-15). The least traumatic removal is accomplished by *rolling* the hemostat toward the other lateral aspect. The nail is not pulled out longitudinally or lifted vertically but removed by a rotating wrist movement from one lateral edge to the other. The nail folds are then investigated for any residual nail spicules.

In partial nail avulsion, a nail splitter is used to split the nail first, with care that the split is extended under the nail fold so that the entire nail plate is split. Elevation and under-

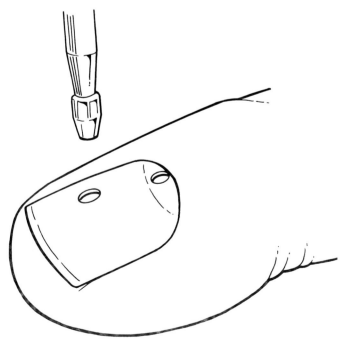

Figure 23-16   Nail and matrix biopsy techniques.

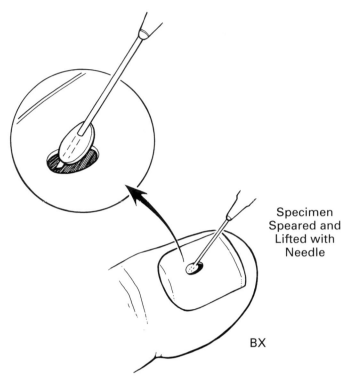

Specimen
Speared and
Lifted with
Needle

BX

Figure 23-17   Specimen removal technique.

mining are carried out as described above only on the portion to be avulsed and then segued with the same rolling motion for removal.

Proximal nail avulsion is accomplished by first retracting the nail fold as outlined below in "Biopsy and Small Excisions" and then sliding the elevator under the nail from the proximal aspect as far as necessary. In cases where the distal nail bed is particularly fibrotic, this may be the preferred method for nail extirpation.

BIOPSY AND SMALL EXCISIONS

Nail Plate and Nail Bed

For diagnosis of onychomycosis or psoriasis, a nail plate-hyponychium biopsy can be performed with shave, punch, or scalpel technique depending on the thickness of the overlying plate. Nail plate and nail bed biopsies should be taken distally of the lunula to avoid matrix damage.

When a punch is used, a 3-mm punch may be taken down to the periosteum (Fig. 23-16). The bound-down tissue is best lifted gently with a 25- to 30-gauge needle (Fig. 23-17), and the base is cut with a fine scissors, with Gelfoam hemostasis. This technique can be utilized on any part of the nail plate and subjacent bed. In some cases, the overlying plate is punched with a 4-mm punch, and then the 3-mm punch is used for the nail bed.

Sometimes a partial or full avulsion is completed before

accessing the nail bed. For larger lesions, a fusiform excision may be necessary (Fig. 23-18). This can be accomplished without avulsion if the plate is thinned, or an avulsion may be necessary to approach the underlying nail bed. This fusiform excision should be directed longitudinally and extends deeply to the bone. Generally for 3 mm of width, primary closure is possible without additional maneuvers. For slightly wider excisions, undermining at the periosteal level a few millimeters in each direction is helpful. Longitudinal, relaxing incisions at the lateral edges of the nail bed helps reduce tension (both the *physician's* and the *wound's*). Closure is with fine absorbable sutures, usually best accomplished with a P or PC needle. When the nail plate is present, sutures may be passed directly through it. As long as the nail matrix is not violated, no permanent nail plate defect will result.

Nail Matrix

When the nail matrix is biopsied, there is a significant chance of a residual nail defect or abnormality such as ridging or thinning or splitting. A 3-mm punch may be used. If the punch is positioned distally without violating the lunular edge, the potential defect will occur on the undersurface of the nail plate. Distal onycholysis will generally not occur if the integrity of the distal lunular curve is maintained.

The nail matrix biopsy is best performed by retracting the overlying nail fold (Fig. 23-18). This is accomplished by bilateral longitudinal incisions approximately 5 mm long at the lateral nail fold aspects. It is best to first place a septal elevator under the nail fold to guide the incision and to avoid inadvertently nicking the matrix. The tissue is then retracted with a suture or hook. Dissection of the proximal nail plate can be performed, leaving the distal plate intact for cosmesis and protection, or the entire nail plate can be avulsed. In the proximal matrix, a punch or small transverse ellipse can be used, and the removal carried deeply to the bone, with actual tissue

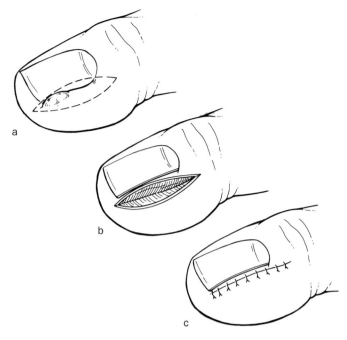

Figure 23-19 *(a–c)* Partial nail excision technique.

removal as described above in "Nail Plate and Nail Bed." Suturing is with 5–0 or 6–0 absorbable suture. Some authors recommend replacing the nail plate or inserting a 0.020-in silicone to prevent adhesion.[6] A small piece of Xeroform gauze may be similarly utilized or oxidized cellulose (Gelfoam®) inserted. The nail fold is steri-stripped or sutured back in place.

Points to remember about matrix biopsies and incisions:

1. Avoid transection of the matrix when possible.
2. Suture the defects when possible.
3. The length of the matrix is responsible for the thickness of the nail so a small sutured defect within the matrix results only in local thinning of the nail plate.
4. A distal rather than proximal biopsy is recommended because the proximal part generates the nail surface. A scar on the distal matrix will affect the underside of the nail.
5. Try to avoid the distal curvature of the nail matrix (lunula).

Orientation of biopsies and small incisions is shown in Figs. 23-16 and 23-18.

PARTIAL NAIL UNIT EXCISION

A longitudinal fusiform excision may be accomplished and is particularly useful in the lateral aspect of the nail unit where any residual nail defect is less noticeable. In this technique (Fig. 23-19), either with or without prior avulsion, a fusiform excision is performed longitudinally beginning at the nail fold or more proximally if combined with matricectomy. The excision is carried deeply to the periosteum. The wound may granulate or be sutured. In cases of lateral nail fold hypertro-

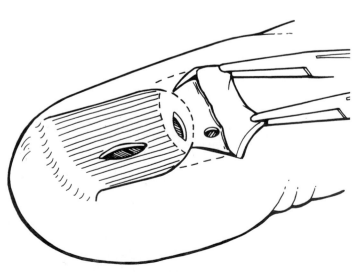

Figure 23-18 Fusiform excision orientation.

phy, or chronic ingrown nail, the lateral fold may be included, again with healing secondarily. If matricectomy is intended, then careful attention must be directed to the proximal aspect of the excision and the lateral horn region of the matrix to make sure all affected tissue is removed. This is further detailed below in "Matricectomy."

MATRICECTOMY

Total matricectomy is useful for pincer nail deformities or disorders of severely thickened nails. Partial matricectomy is particularly beneficial in ingrown nails.

Scalpel Technique

Surgical excision is effective if attention is paid to the lateral nail horn region, which has a tendency to regrow since the area is often overlooked because it is recessed. In partial excision, usually the nail fold is retracted for good visualization. The matricectomy incision is directed longitudinally to encompass the most proximal portion to the most distal portion (lunula) of the matrix. The incision is extended to the lateral nail fold and then proximally along the nail groove to the lateral horn region and deeply to the periosteum. Total matricectomy is completed by a complete removal of the matrix from the proximal nail groove to the distal portion of lunula with second intention healing.

CO$_2$ Laser Technique

The laser is quite effective in this region because the beam can be directed, in contrast to electrocautery, which disperses energy from the tip in all directions. Again, the matrix is exposed, usually by retracting the nail fold, and vaporization is performed generally in a defocused mode at approximately 5 W. Attempts to minimize deeper thermal damage are recommended such as short pulse intervals or lower energies.

Electrosurgery Technique

Curetting and electrodesiccation may be utilized in which the matrix is first vigorously curetted followed by cauterization. As with all techniques, attention must be directed toward the recessed lateral horn region to prevent spicular regrowth. Since the matrix is particularly resistant to destruction, up to 5 s of cauterization is done and then repeated as necessary.[1] The use of Teflon-coated probes allows a more directed flow of energy, thus avoiding the need for proximal nail fold reflection.

Chemical Technique

Podiatrists have long advocated a phenol matricectomy for the great toe.[7] Most commonly utilized is 88% phenol, al-though 10% sodium hydroxide solution has also been suggested.[1,7] The main contraindication is moderate-to-severe vascular disease.[7]

In this technique, a completely bloodless field is necessary (see "Preparing the Field" above). Thick petrolatum is recommended to cover the exposed nail bed and proximal and lateral folds. Eye protection should be worn. After avulsion of the plate, the lateral horn region must be inspected for residual nail plate. A small curette is used to physically debride exposed matrix. Phenol is then directly applied to the exposed matrix by using a cotton applicator. It is extremely important that the applicator not be excessively wet. The applicator is directed into the lateral recesses, usually by twisting motions. Again, by twisting motion the applicator is moved over the other areas of matrix. Three to five 30-second applications are needed.[7] After completion, lavage with alcohol, boric acid, or 3 to 5% acetic acid is needed. Remember, with phenol, because of the chemonecrosis, healing may be a 3- to 6-week process until sloughing and oozing cease. In partial matricectomy with phenol, excess liquid may seep under the adjacent nail plate centrally, resulting in onycholysis, which can be prevented by careful application of the phenol in a rotating fashion directed toward the lateral horn region.

Postoperatively, considerable drainage will occur as outlined above although, generally, postoperative pain is easily controlled.

SUBUNGUAL HEMATOMA

This type of hematoma occurs from trauma. Patients present with severe pain. Unless the trauma is localized and physical findings are minimal, an x-ray for fracture is suggested. Recommendations for instrumentation include a drill, needle, paper clip heated until red hot, small battery-powered microcautery, number 11 blade, electrocautery, or small punch. Most physicians create only a small hole which temporarily decompresses but may allow recurrence when a clot seals the hole; therefore, a hole larger than a paper clip is recommended. Avulsion is recommended if greater than 25 percent of the nail unit is involved, with repair or cauterization of the underlying injury.[6] For a large or distally located subungual hematoma, incising the hyponychium may be preferable for decompression.

CHRONIC PARONYCHIA

This red chronic process results in disappearance of the cuticle and separation of the paronychia from the nail plate, leading to progressive retraction. Medical therapy includes local steroid application, antifungal and antibiotic agents, avoidance of wet exposures, and protective gloves.

Surgically, this condition may be addressed with a crescent-shaped, full-thickness excision of the proximal nail fold (Fig. 23-20).[8,15] This excision begins at the lateral nail fold,

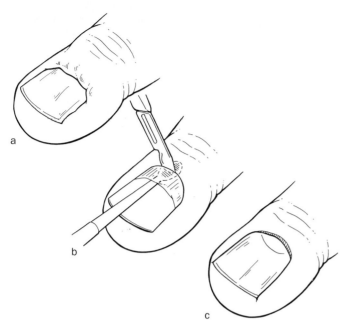

Figure 23-20 *(a–c)* Chronic paronychia excision.

PROXIMAL NAIL FOLD RE-CREATION

If the patient presents with a torn nail fold from minor injury or laceration, the wound may be sutured closed. Depending on the patient's status and mode of injury, a tetanus injection may be required if more than 5 or 10 years have elapsed since previous injection.

Often a deformed proximal nail fold results from cicatrix due to prior injury. The remaining portion can then be excised in a crescent-shaped excision, with second intention healing, as described in "Chronic Paronychia" and illustrated in Fig. 23-20.

PROXIMAL NAIL FOLD LESIONS

When only a small lesion exists at the most distal portion of the fold, a small longitudinally shaped fusiform or wedge excision can be performed as illustrated (Fig. 23-21). It is recommended to have an elevator immediately under the fold to prevent a scalpel incision into the matrix. Frequently, this type of wedge excision may only be closed by freeing up the entire nail fold with the elevator or dental spatula and then making two lateral relaxing incisions of the proximal nail fold. These lateral incisions need only be about 5-mm long and heal quite well by secondary intention.

Small fusiform incisional biopsies or excisions may be performed on the lateral aspect of the proximal nail fold and closed primarily or left to granulate. Incisional biopsies are useful for histologic evaluation of chronic paronychia for fungal infections, atypical mycobacteria, foreign body granuloma, or connective tissue disease.

A crescentic excision of the entire proximal nail fold, with healing by second intention as described earlier in this chapter, is effective for chronic paronychia or larger lesions.

MYXOID CYSTS

Myxoid cysts are well recognized by clinical dermatologists, are known to communicate with the DIP joint, and may result

extends across the midline, and culminates at the opposite lateral fold. Second intention healing requires about 2 months, and the visible difference is a more noticeable lunula.

It is strongly recommended that crescentic excisions be marked first. Extreme caution is advised regarding the extensor tendon which inserts into the phalanx approximately 2 to 3 mm distally of the distal interphalangeal (DIP) joint. Complete release of the tendon may occur with the sweep of a crescentic excision which extends within 2 or 3 mm of the DIP.

Generally, problems with matrix trauma or tendon incision can be avoided if the proximal nail fold is sandwiched between a septum elevator and the scalpel as the blade traverses the planned excision line. Hemostasis is accomplished with cauterization of bleeders and application of oxidized cellulose (Gelfoam® or equivalent).

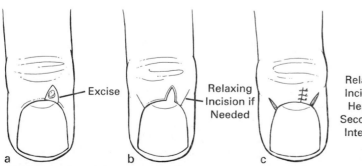

Figure 23-21 *(a–c)* Proximal nail fold lesion excision.

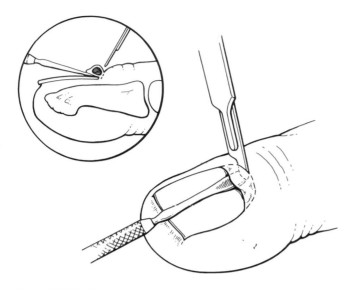

Figure 23-22 Myxoid cyst excision.

in nail plate abnormalities. Many approaches are documented in the literature. Sometimes repeated simple drainage or intralesional injection with triamcinolone, 3 to 5 mg/cc, may effect resolution.[18] Cryosurgery after decompression performed as a single freeze of the cyst is frequently efficacious and bereft of matrix injury.[10,18] Similarly electrosurgery may be used.[15] The cyst may be excised as a crescentic excision of the

entire nail fold and allowed to heal as performed for chronic paronychia (Fig. 23-22).[15]

Larger cysts are best treated by excision. This is performed by first injecting sterile methylene blue intra-articularly, which visualizes the extent of the pseudocyst. Frequently the cyst is demonstrated to be larger than clinically apparent. To be effective, all blue-stained tissue is to be excised, and any stalk which appears to communicate with the DIP joint should be cauterized. The surgery is effected by excising the skin over the cyst and then meticulously dissecting the blue-stained tissue from the surrounding connective tissue. Closure usually requires a rotation flap as illustrated (Fig. 23-23), with the donor area of the flap healing secondarily. A flap can sometimes be avoided by using an arcuate excision over the cyst and dissecting the cyst from the overlying skin. By retracting or folding back the flap, adequate exposure is provided and the deeper part of the cyst may be dissected. Skin is closed by simply folding the flap back over the defect, as illustrated in Fig. 23-24.

For larger cysts located more in relation to the DIP joint than the proximal nail fold, an H-shaped incision is typically used with the transverse portion lying at the level of the extension crease of the DIP joint.[16] Skin flaps are raised proximally and distally for good exposure, and dissection is best accomplished by using surgical loupes magnification. The cyst and stalk connecting to the joint are excised and the stalk base is cauterized. In this type of surgery, the tourniquet is best removed prior to closing to ensure that all bleeders are cauterized. Sutures are removed at 1 week.

Caution: The extensor tendon extends about 3 mm past the DIP joint and may be subject to surgical trauma when procedures are carried out on the most proximal portion of the proximal nail fold. In general, the tendon unit functions well if not completely truncated.

LATERAL NAIL FOLD EXCISIONS

Typically, lateral nail fold excisions are performed for hypertrophic folds, often in relation to chronic ingrown nails. Chronic inflammation is often accompanied by excessive granulation tissue and eventual fibrosis.

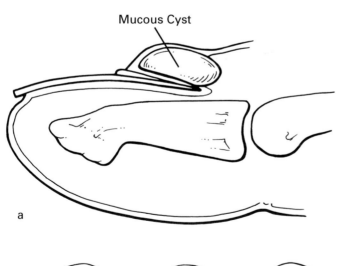

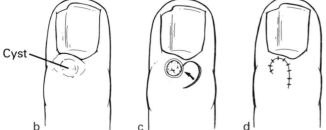

Figure 23-23 *(a–d)* Excision of larger myxoid cyst.

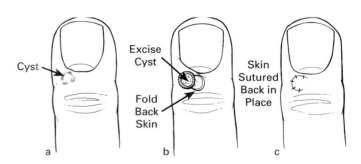

Figure 23-24 *(a–c)* Cyst excision; skin retraction technique.

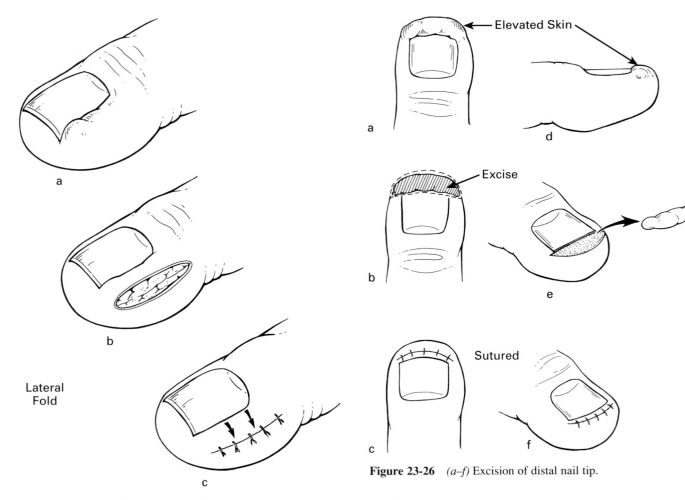

Figure 23-25 *(a–c)* Lateral nail fold reconstruction.

Figure 23-26 *(a–f)* Excision of distal nail tip.

Several options are available for treatment. One approach involves a simple fusiform excision on the lateral aspect of the toe which optimally pulls the lateral nail sulcus away from the plate, as illustrated in Fig. 23-25a. More commonly, direct excision of the fold is performed (Fig. 23-19). In some cases, a simple shave excision of the exophytic tissue may be accomplished without partial nail avulsion, with secondary healing.

In more involved cases, after avulsion, a lateral nail fold excision may be performed down to periosteum and primarily closed. Lateral nail fold excisions may also be combined with partial matricectomy.

For excisional surgery of the fold with matricectomy of the adjacent nail, a partial avulsion of the nail adjacent to the fold is performed first. A longitudinal fusiform excision is initiated beginning approximately 3 mm distally of the nail bed and ending on the proximal nail fold, encompassing the hypertrophic lateral nail fold tissue. The incisions are extended deeply to the periosteum, and the tissue is removed under direct visual control. The excision encompasses the lateral nail fold, adjacent lateral nail bed, and proximal nail fold. By making sure that the incision extends 8 to 10 mm proximally of the cuticle, and extends to the periosteum, the underlying

matrix is excised. The skin on the lateral aspect of the excision is sutured directly to the nail plate (best performed with a 4–0 nylon on a PC3- or PC5-type needle or equivalent). The result is a slightly narrowed nail.

Alternatively, for fold excision and matricectomy, after partial avulsion a debulking excision may be performed of the lateral nail fold, basically excising the skin but not extending to the periosteum. A matricectomy is accomplished by any of the methods available, and the surgical defect is closed with 4–0 sutures (in this case the closure is skin to skin and does not involve the nail plate).

DISTAL NAIL TIP EXCISION

Distortion of the distal tip of the toe may result from repeated avulsions. Without counterpressure from the nail plate, the pulp is gradually distorted dorsally from walking, yielding a distal nail wall. Conservatively, repeated massage of the wall may allow the nail to overgrow, resulting in a return to its normal condition. Alternatively, a crescent-shaped excision can be accomplished parallel to the former hyponychium, starting about 3 or 4 mm proximally to the end of the lateral fold. The width of the excision is empirically determined at surgery and may be as narrow as a few millimeters with primary closure (Fig. 23-26).

THE INGROWN NAIL

The dermatologic, podiatric, and surgical literature is replete with a surfeit of recommendations. The simplest treatment applicable for the occasional ingrown nail where no significant infection has supravened is wedging a small cotton pledget under the corner at the hyponychium and leaving it in place for a few days. In these individuals whose only complaint is usually mild pain, the nail may also be cut back slightly at the corner to remove the ingrown spicule prior to placing the cotton. However, these individuals should be counseled in general not to trim the nail shorter than the hyponychium to avoid recurrences. Any sign of infection in ingrown nails mandates oral antibiotics along with culture, especially in the immunocompromised, diabetic, or vascular insufficiency patients.

For ease of application and of use for nonsurgical candidates, cryosurgery (Fig. 23-27) may be efficacious in circumstances where there are granulomatous infected areas with adjacent tissue hypertrophy.[17] Utilizing a spray-type unit, held 1 cm from the target area, the physician can perform a freeze in a well-defined area without encroaching onto the matrix. A freeze time of 30 s after establishment of an ice field is used and includes all granulomatous and infected areas as well as adjacent nail fold. Aspirin is recommended every 6 h for the subsequent 48 h. Considerable exudation occurs postoperatively which may require frequent dressing changes or soaks. Clinical pain improvement from the underlying condition is reported to occur within 1 to 2 days. Since no nail spicule removal is performed, and because minimal gross morphologic nail fold changes are identified subsequently, it is assumed that clinical benefit results from effects of cryotherapy on the nerve endings locally or from a degree of nail fold retraction during healing.

For deeply ingrown or significantly infected cases, a partial nail avulsion, with or without matricectomy is indicated. Recurrent cases benefit from lateral matrix excision/matricectomy. The technique is described above in "Nail Avulsion," and "Matricectomy." Briefly, a partial or complete avulsion is performed. The proximal nail fold is incised on both lateral

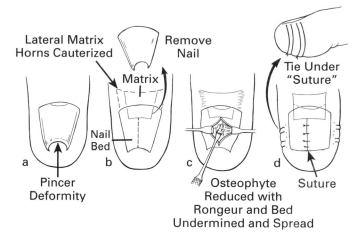

Figure 23-28 (a–d) Pincer nail deformity reconstruction.

aspects and reflected back on itself. The exposed matrix horn is meticulously dissected and excised from the base of the bone, with the physician's taking care to excise the lateral horn aspect. The defect is filled with an antibiotic and oxidized cellulose (Gelfoam® or equivalent), and the proximal nail fold incision is closed or steri-stripped. Phenol or curettage and desiccation of the matrix may also be utilized (see "Nail Avulsion").

PINCER NAIL DEFORMITIES

A *pincer nail* is defined as a transverse curvature. Typically, this is wider at the proximal nail fold, and curvature increases distally to the point where the nail bed is virtually pinched at the hyponychium. This condition appears to result from a matrix widened proximally, but of normal width distally, causing conic growth of the nail plate. An underlying osteophytic elevation occurs and this is thought to result from traction of the plate since the plate is tightly bound to the nail bed, which is adherent to the periosteum. This osteophyte is not always visible on x-ray.

Correction is technically challenging and involves restructuring the anatomy of the underlying osteophyte and reforming the nail bed.[8] The nail is removed, the proximal fold is retracted onto itself, and the lateral matrix horns are cauterized. A longitudinal skin incision is made in the nail bed to expose the osteophyte and the osteophyte is reduced with a bone rongeur; then, the bed is undermined, spread, and sutured. The lateral folds are sutured with a tie-under suture that runs under the toe (Fig. 23-28), and the threads are placed in plastic gutters or other protection to prevent the suture material from cutting through the skin. The tie-under suture is performed to keep the nail bed spread, and the sutures are left in place 2 weeks or longer.

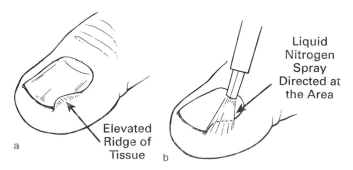

Figure 23-27 (a, b) Cryosurgery of ingrown nail.

SPLIT NAIL DEFORMITIES

Treatment of longitudinally split nails involves narrowing the matrix cicatrix to effect more normal anatomy. Surgical approach depends on the extent of deformity, etiology, and location.

Splits within the lateral third are most effectively excised as a lateral nail excision with matricectomy and primary closure as described previously in this chapter. The boundary of the excision is from the split to the lateral margin of the nail plate. Remember that the excision needs to extend to the periosteum and sufficiently proximally to remove the matrix.

For splits in the middle third (Fig. 23-29), the proximal nail fold is incised at both lateral edges and reflected on itself to expose the base of the nail and entire matrix area. The nail plate in the proximal nail fold region needs to be dissected away with a nipper or strong scissors or blade. Cut the nail plate cautiously in a rectangular shape 1 mm wider than the scar that is to be excised. Then meticulously dissect out the nail bed and adjoining matrix of the defective region. The defect is then sutured with 6–0 resorbable sutures. However, these sutures are prone to pull through, so it is important to oversuture the adjoining nail plate with 3–0 nylon (use a sharp needle) and knot it firmly.[8] This further joins the tissue and relieves stress and pull on the nail bed/matrix region.

For scars too wide for primary closure, relaxing longitudinal incisions on the lateral nail sulcus, extended to the bone, facilitate closure. Alternatively, a small rotation flap of nail bed and matrix can be developed. This is accomplished through an L-shaped incision of the lateral aspect of the finger at the lateral nail wall with secondary healing of the donor site.

For distal fissures, removal of the distal nail plate is needed. Often, these fissures result from a subungual lesion. If no subungual abnormality is present, then the fissure may be from stress on a locally thinned nail plate, resulting from a matrix defect.

LONGITUDINAL MELANONYCHIA

Important in pigment disorders is determining where to biopsy. The anatomic site of involved matrix is determined from Fontana's silver stain of nail clippings. The surface of the nail plate (dorsum) is produced by the most proximal part of the matrix, and the part in contact with the nail bed (ventral) is produced by that portion adjacent to the lunula (see "Anatomy" and "Biopsy and Small Excisions"). Once determination of the anatomic region within the matrix is made, then the proper choice of approach is chosen. For specific techniques, see "Biopsy and small Excisions." The method may be punch biopsy of the proximal matrix, punch of the distal matrix, or longitudinal excision, including proximal and distal matrix and distal nail bed.

EXOSTOSIS

Usually occurring on the great toe, and typically the result of repeated trauma, the underlying bony process causes a heaped-up deformity and pain. Since the exostosis has a fibrocartilaginous cap, the mandatory pre-operative x-ray may not demonstrate the full extent of the enlargement. The procedure used to correct this condition is very similar to the surgery described above in "Pincer Nail Deformities." In general, the nail plate is avulsed, the skin incised and dissected from the bony lesion, and the exostosis debulked with a bone rongeur or bone chisel. Excess skin may then be trimmed if needed, but the matrix and nail bed are to be preserved, and then the wound is primarily sutured.

ONYCHOGRYPOSIS

In this heaped-up nail problem, there is vertical in place of horizontal nail growth with disruption of the plate's cohesion to the bed. The resulting shrinkage and metaplasia of the bed

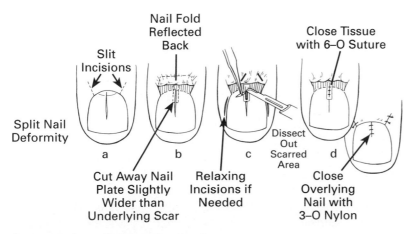

Figure 23-29 *(a–e)* Split nail deformity.

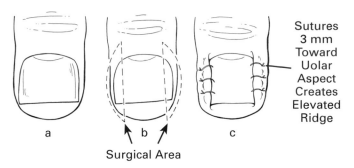

Figure 23-30 *(a–c)* Racquet thumbnail revision.

obviates further nail plate adherence. Treatments are repeated trimmings as needed which are facilitated by 40% urea ointment under occlusion for 48 h prior, or complete avulsion with matricectomy.

RACQUET THUMBNAIL

This short wide nail lacks lateral nail folds. Treatment is cosmetic and consists of narrowing the nail and creating lateral folds (Fig. 23-30). The nail is narrowed on each side by a lateral-longitudinal nail excision, including the matrix. Undermining laterally at the level of the bone is completed, and then backstitches are utilized to create a lateral nail fold. This is accomplished by taking a bite of tissue 2 to 3 mm toward the volar aspect of the thumb with the suture needle and suturing directly through the nail plate. Essentially, this extra bite of tissue forms an elevated ridge along the lateral aspect of the nail, with the sulcus epithelializing secondarily.

NAIL PLATE DEBRIDEMENT

For hypertrophic dystrophies, mycotic infections, nonsurgical candidates, psoriasis, or those with significant vascular impairment, chemical debridement is effective.

The most popular chemical method is a 40% urea, compounded in various mixtures available by direct purchase from companies dealing frequently with dermatologists. It may be compounded as 40% urea, 5% beeswax, 20% lanolin, 25% petrolatum, and 10% silica gel type H, and it has a 4-month shelf life.[1,5] Generally, urea removes dystrophic portions, only leaving the normal nail intact. Other combinations include salicylic acid and urea together to remove nondystrophic nails.

The urea must be occluded, and yet the adjacent skin must be protected. This can be accomplished by applying adhesive felt around the nail plate, usually in several layers to build up a wall which holds the debriding agent in place. The thicker the nail, the more debriding compound is needed. Once applied, the compound is held in place by waterproof tape to provide an occlusive environment. The area must be kept dry. The dressing is left in place usually for 3 to 7 days. Once the

nail has been softened, it is debrided by using a nail elevator and nail nipper. Or the nail may be painlessly avulsed or trimmed to just under the proximal nail fold. Once the nail is avulsed, medical treatments of the underlying condition may segue.

Failure of chemical debridement may occur not uncommonly. Nail plates that are simply thickened but nondystrophic respond minimally to chemical debridement. Water under the dressing dilutes the effect, and inadequate occlusion prevents hydration of the plate. Some individuals require more prolonged occlusion or repeated treatments. Complications include irritant reactions, reactions to adhesives utilized, and bleeding at the time of nail plate removal.

Mechanical debridement is a conservative palliative approach at debulking a nail. This can be completed with a nail nipper, and usually a double-action forceps type is recommended because it conforms to the nail bed and is therefore less painful. Rotary sanding, probably best performed with an inexpensive hobby-type drill (Dremel), is effectively utilized (one should not use delicate high-speed hand engine instruments for this procedure). Low speeds are essential to prevent adjacent tissue injury by heat or trauma. Various burs are available, but significant dust is produced and use of protective eye- and breathing wear is recommended.

ONYCHOSCHIZIA

Brittle and horizontally split nails are common problems, seen frequently in women. One form is caused by breakdown of the intercellular cement substance between the horny lamellae of the nail, leading to layered splitting or a shalelike exfoliation of the nails at the free edge. The term *onychoschizia* refers to this common type of nail brittleness. While systemic diseases or vascular insufficiency may contribute, some believe there is a relation to trace element deficiency.[13] Recently however, repeated water exposure followed by dehydration and caustic exposures have been documented to elicit onychoschizia.[14]

While, generally, onychoschizia is a nonsurgical situation, the evaluation of this condition falls within the purview of the surgical dermatologist since the etiology may not be apparent clinically. Recently, biotin given orally in a daily dose of 2.5 mg for 6 to 9 months has demonstrated clinical efficacy with thickening of the nails and reduction in splitting.[13]

CARCINOMA AND NAIL UNIT EXCISION

Squamous cell carcinoma (SCC) is far more frequent than basal cell carcinoma (BCC) of the nail unit.[18] Diagnoses of carcinoma are frequently delayed as patients are treated empirically under a variety of other diagnoses. The delay in diagnosis may become more frequent as patients are shuttled

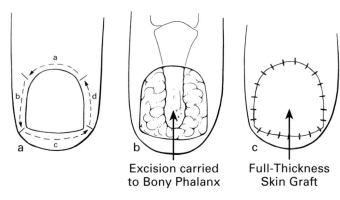

Excision carried
to Bony Phalanx

Full-Thickness
Skin Graft

Figure 23-31 *(a–c)* Nail unit excision.

into gatekeeper systems. However, SCC of the nail unit is generally a slowly progressive lesion with low metastatic rates.[18] Any patient with a diagnosis of carcinoma should have an x-ray of the digit, and, if bone invasion is noted, then the patient should be referred for amputation.

SCC in situ treatments include electrodesiccation and curettage, cryosurgery, excision, and Mohs surgery.[1] For carcinoma involving skin only, Mohs surgery or excisional surgery can be performed. The benefit of Mohs surgery would be in larger lesions or in nail unit preservation for smaller lesions. Other treatments considered appropriate for carcinoma of the nail unit include electrosurgery or radiation.[1] Alternatively, a complete nail unit excision may be performed. Nail unit excision is indicated for SCC, BCC, Bowen's carcinoma in situ, and melanoma in situ.[11,12]

Melanoma treatment is beyond the scope of this chapter; however, current care recommendations usually involve at least disarticulation.[18]

Nail unit excision (Fig. 23-31) and reconstruction can be performed as follows:[1] After anesthesia and tourniquet, an excision is performed extending across the proximal nail fold transversely to the opposite lateral nail fold, then distally along the lateral nail fold to a point 2 or 3 mm distally of the hyponychium, then carried across the tip of the digit, and then proximally back to the starting point. The excision is carried to the bony phalanx and sharply dissected from the underlying bone. Electrocoagulation is utilized for coagulation. Reconstruction is accomplished by full-thickness skin graft which may be harvested from the volar forearm, antecubital fossa, or inner upper arm. Because of location, a tie-over dressing is recommended. While rare, persistent pain or inflammation over the subsequent weeks should alert the surgeon to the possibility of underlying osteomyelitis.

BENIGN NAIL UNIT TUMORS

Acquired digital fibrokeratoma

This may occur on the nail unit as a fibrous smooth exostosis. The process, however, may stay totally hidden within the

proximal nail fold, presenting only as a thinned nail plate or grooved plate. Treatment is surgical removal (Fig. 23-32), and the key is to expose the base of the process, then identify the plane between it and the dermis, and virtually bluntly dissect it out.

Glomus Tumors

This benign painful process may present as a blue, red, or purplish suffusion under the nail and is tender to compression. There may or may not be associated nail plate changes. Pain may be minimal or severe, spasmodic or chronic, and occasionally exacerbated by temperature changes. The tumor is an overgrowth of the arteriolar portion of the arterial-venous shunt thermal regulation unit, known as the Sucquet-Hoyer canal, and the cell or origin is a smooth muscle cell.[18]

Surgery is effective, but there are local recurrences with incomplete excisions. The procedure involves removal of the nail plate, either locally with a punch or as an avulsion. In many cases, a punch excision of the tumor is possible since the tumor is encapsulated, so the integrity of the tumor is maintained as it is taken up by the punch or dissected out. In cases where an enlarged tumor is identified, excision followed by a split-thickness nail bed graft from the great toe may be used.

Giant Cell Tumors of the Tendon Sheath

Typically, this process derives from deeper tissue arising from synovial lining cells. Generally, the overlying skin is movable

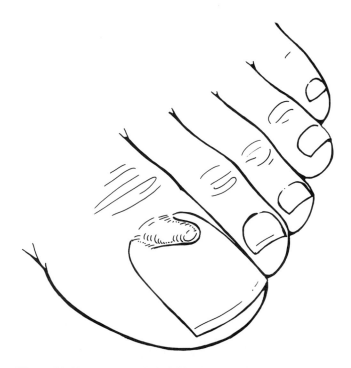

Figure 23-32 Acquired digital fibrokeratoma.

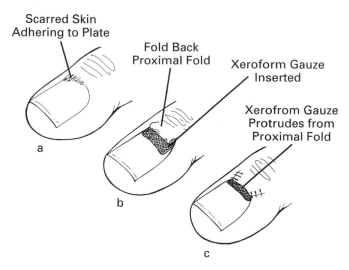

Figure 23-33 *(a–c)* Pterygium reconstruction.

but may become fixed as the tumor enlarges. Often, there is a multilobular quality to the growth. A soft-tissue mass may be present on x-ray.[18] Usually this process is best referred to a hand surgeon for extirpation.

Pterygium

Pterygium may occur secondary to trauma. Pterygium of the hyponychium may be painful and is treated by removing the distal 5 mm of nail from the bed and hyponychial area. A strip of nail bed and hyponychium 3 mm wide is resected and replaced by a split-thickness skin graft, causing nonadherence of the hyponychial area and pain relief.[6] A pterygium of the proximal fold (Fig. 23-33) is treated by freeing the fold from the plate and inserting a small piece of silicone sheet or, alternatively, Xeroform gauze. The undersurface of the fold epithelializes thus releasing the adherence.

SPLIT-THICKNESS GRAFT NAIL BED RECONSTRUCTION

In cases where excision of a lesion, for instance a glomus tumor, results in a significant nail bed defect, a reconstruction can be accomplished by a split-thickness graft from the great toe.[6] In this approach, the toenail is avulsed. A thin split-thickness graft is removed with a surgical blade by using a back-and-forth sawing movement to remove a small area of nail bed. Remember to only harvest nail bed distal of the lunula. Only a small graft is possible because the curve of the nail bed precludes obtaining a large fragment. The graft is sutured into the defect with fine absorbable sutures. The nail can be replaced over the great toe and sutured into position.

MINOR LACERATIONS

Optimally, wounds are treated within hours, but satisfactory repair may still be possible after 1 to 2 weeks.[19] One must evaluate the patient for tetanus injection and for phalanx fracture. Most lacerations are closed primarily or allowed to heal, and many small lacerations of the nail bed do not need repair. For those needing repair (usually lacerations greater than 3 mm in size), the nail plate can be avulsed (Fig. 23-34) and lifted in "car hood" fashion, the laceration sutured, then the nail replaced and lightly sutured into position on both lateral aspects. Typically, the replaced nail is pushed out by regenerating nail in 1 to 3 months. Stellate or complex lacerations are more frequently associated with underlying fracture.

WARTS

Clearly a frustrating problem, periungual verrucae are by far the most common nail problem contended with by dermatologists. Certainly, the tincture-of-time approach may be warranted, as are conservative approaches with keratolytics or cantharidin preparations. Since the keratolytics have been reduced in strength to over-the-counter preparation concentration, and canthariden no longer FDA approved, the more conservative approach has become less efficacious in the experience of the author.

Cryosurgery is often difficult as the lesions are often resistant to freezing and pain on treatment is significant.[1] Digital anesthesia may be necessary, and treatment facilitated by applying salicylic acid preparations to the wart under occlusion for 3 days before. Nail avulsion may be needed to access subungual lesions. Application is by spray or applicator with a freeze-thaw time of 30 to 45 s repeated 2 or 3 times.[1] There may be significant postoperative pain and 2 to 5 weeks until healing.

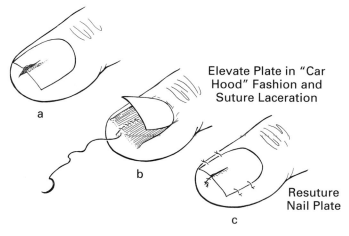

Figure 23-34 *(a–c)* Laceration repair.

Surgical treatment involves isolating the verruca, often requiring avulsion first. In many cases, a plane of dissection can be established by cutting along the entire visible junction of the wart and then bluntly dissecting the tissue.[20] The base is then cauterized as required.

Electrosurgery and curettage is accomplished by first applying saline-soaked dressing to the affected area to hydrate the lesion for 10 min so that tissue vaporization is facilitated.[1] The tissue is vaporized by applying the cautery tip to the hyperkeratotic tissue until a bubble is noted, with resultant char removed by curette or scissor, and repeated as needed until clinically no wart tissue remains. Treatment of subungual warts may result in thermal damage to adjacent tissue which may result in scarring or nail deformity.

CO_2 laser surgery may be particularly effective in treating recalcitrant or recurrent lesions.[1] The modality offers precise control of the destruction depth in practiced hands and offers reduced postoperative pain. The technique involves vaporizing the verruca at a defocused mode with the power at 5 to 10 W. For subungual lesions, the procedure can be performed by directly vaporizing the overlying nail plate and so avoids an avulsion. Char is removed by H_2O_2 gauze, curette, or scissors. Adjacent thermal damage may occur, so care must be exercised. Because of possible viral particles in the air, careful use of a smoke evacuator is required.

REFERENCES

1. Clark, RG: Nail surgery, Wheeland R, *Cutaneous Surgery* WB Saunders, Philadephia, 1994, pp 375–402

2. Scher RK, Daniel CR eds: *Nails: Therapy, Diagnosis, Surgery.* Philadelphia, Saunders, 1990, pp 13, 27, 28

3. Ditre DM, Howe NR: Surgical anatomy of the nail unit. *J Dermatol Surg Oncol* **18:**665–671, 1992

4. Bennett RG: Glove tourniquet for digital surgery. *SurgiGuide Lines* **1:**3, 1987

5. Daniel RC: Basic nail plate avulsion. *J Dermatol Surg Oncol* **18:**685–688, 1992

6. Zook EG: The Perionychium, *Operative Hand Surgery,* edited by DP Green. New York, Churchill-Livingston, 1988, pp 1331–1371

7. Siegle RJ et al: Phenol alcohol technique for permanent matricectomy. *Arch Dermatol* **120:**348–350, 1984

8. Eckart H, Baran R: Nails: Surgical aspects, Parish L, Lask G, *Aesthetic Dermatology* McGraw Hill New York 1991

9. Rich P: Nail biopsy. *J Dermatol Surg Oncol* **18:**673–682, 1992

10. Dawber RPR et al: Myxoid cyst of the finger: Treatment by liquid nitrogen spray cryosurgery. *Clin Exp Dermatol* **8:**153–155, 1983

11. Herndon JH et al: Advanced surgery, in *Nails: Therapy, Diagnosis, Surgery,* edited by RK Scher, CR Daniel. Philadelphia, Saunders, 1990, pp 281–293

12. McLeod GR: Management of melanoma in situ, *Pigment Cell: Surgical Approaches to Cutaneous Melanoma,* edited by CM Balch. Basel, Switz, Karger, 1985, pp 1–7

13. Colombo VE et al: Treatment of brittle fingernails and onychoschizia with biotin: Scanning electron microscopy. *J Am Acad Dermatol* **23:**1127–1132, 1990

14. Wallis MS et al: Pathogenesis of onychoschizia (lamellar dystrophy). *J Am Acad Dermatol* **24:**44–48, 1991

15. Salache SJ: Myxoid cysts of the proximal nail fold: A surgical approach. *J Dermatol Surg Oncol* **10**(1):25–39, 1984

16. Miller PK et al: Focal mucinosis (myxoid cyst) surgical therapy. *J Dermatol Surg Oncol* **18:**716–719, 1991

17. Sonnex TS, Dawber RPR: Treatment of ingrowing toenails with liquid nitrogen spray cryotherapy. *Br Med J [Clin Res]* **291:**173–175, 1985

18. Salashe SJ, Orengo IF: Tumors of the nail unit. *J Dermatol Surg Oncol* **18:**701–700, 1992

19. Melone CP, Grad JB: Primary care of fingernail injuries. *Emerg Med Clin North Am* **3:**255–261, 1985

20. Habif TP, Graf FA: Extirpation of subungual and periungual warts by blunt dissection. *J Dermatol Surg Oncol* **7:**553–555, 1981

David S. Orentreich

24 Punch Graft

Although the precise origin of the surgical punch may never be known, a Dr. B. A. Watson described the use of a punch in two articles published, one in 1878, entitled *Discotome,* and the other in the *St. Louis Medical and Surgical Journal* (volume 35, page 145), entitled *Gunpowder Disfigurements.*[1,2] Apparently, without knowledge of Dr. Watson's reports, a New York dermatologist, Edward Keyes (1843–1925), described the use of small cutaneous trephines or punches to treat a youth (in 1879) whose face was tattooed by an exploding firecracker.[3] He devised these instruments to have a sharp cutting edge and diameters from 1 mm upward in $^1/_2$-mm increments. He punch excised the black pigment by sharply rotating the punch.[4]

Kromayer worked in Germany and published numerous papers on the use of punches for excisional skin surgery from 1905 to 1935.[5] He also described the use of motor-powered punches and reported that the use of 2- or 3-mm punch excisions (without grafting) seldom resulted in scars.[6] Among the conditions he treated were boils, acne cysts, superfluous hair, lentigines, nevi, other tumors, and tattoos. Also treated were deep-seated, crateriform acne and pox scars.

In 1953, Lowenthal, then in South Africa reported on the use of a punch autograft to repair the sites of punch-excised lesions of greater than 2-mm diameter.[7] He used this technique in the treatment of small growths as well as cosmetic blemishes such as isolated scars of varicella. He preferred the submammary fold and behind the ear for donor sites. He also reported the necessity of cutting the donor grafts with a punch of larger diameter than the one used to excise the recipient site and the use of a diathermy needle to flatten slightly protruding grafts several weeks after healing.

In 1953, Norman Orentreich communicated the use of dermabrasion to level punch autografts on the face.[8] Burks confirmed the success of punch autografting for ice pick-type acne scars and small tumors of the face (8 mm or less in diameter).[9] He also observed that "Grafted sites may be superficially planed to yield an almost perfect cosmetic result."[9]

In 1959, Orentreich reported on the use of hair-bearing punch autografts to cosmetically correct androgenic alopecia.[10] Many years later, it was discovered that a Japanese dermatologist, Okuda, in a 1939 report virtually unrecognized in the English-speaking world, described the use of small full-thickness autografts of hair-bearing skin for the correction of alopecia of the scalp, eyebrow, and moustache areas.[11] A total of 200 patients, most of whom had cicatricial alopecia, were successfully treated in this fashion. Okuda did not, however, specifically note the use of his technique in patients with androgenic alopecia.

Skin autografts have been employed in animals to study hair growth, pigment formation, wound healing, and immunity. Exchange autografts were performed in humans to study vitiligo, amyloidosis, morphea, scleroderma, acrodermatitis chronica atrophicans, allergic eczematous dermatitis, fixed-drug eruptions, and hyperhidrosis. The effects of autografts have been observed following plastic repairs for lupus erythematosus.[12]

The success of punch skin autografts in treating a broad spectrum of dermatologic disorders is explained by the principle of "donor dominance."[10] This principle states that when a graft of normal skin is transplanted to an affected site, the transposed, grafted skin maintains its integrity and characteristics independently of the recipient site. When the transposed, grafted skin takes on the characteristics of the recipient site, it is described as being "recipient dominant."[10] Recipient dominant conditions are not ordinarily correctable by autografts.

To achieve a successful transplant, sufficient nourishment (vascular recipient bed), primary tissue contact, asepsis, and control of excess bleeding are necessary. The first nourishment of the graft is plasma. There is an early anastomosis of small capillaries, and then new capillaries proliferate into the older vessels. Vascularization of a graft usually occurs in 3 days, connective tissue attachment in 2 weeks, and fat layer appearance in 3 weeks.[13] Sensation (pain, temperature, tactile) develops in a variable period of months to a year, usually starting at the periphery and proceeding toward the center of the graft.

PUNCH EXCISION WITHOUT AUTOGRAFTING

The punch excision method is very useful as a diagnostic tool. The cylindric piece of skin is simply excised and submitted for histopathologic examination. Depending on the nature of the lesion excised, its location, and size, the surgeon may elect to allow the site to heal by secondary intention or to suture it. A variety of lesions are amenable to punch excision without autografting (Table 24-1).

Punch excisions that are allowed to heal by secondary intention may yield satisfactory results if the diameter of excision is less than or equal to about 2 mm. This includes facial lesions such as ice-pick scars. Hemostasis is usually achieved with manual pressure. Occasionally, a piece of collagen matrix (Gelfoam) may be used; however, hemostatic agents such as ferric subsulfate (Monsel's solution) or aluminum chloride solution are avoided. A comparison of healing of punch biopsy wounds treated with either Monsel's solution or a collagen matrix plug showed that the collagen matrix produced less inflammation, had a lower incidence of wound infection, was associated with a faster re-epithelialization rate, and healed with a modestly better appearance at 4 weeks than did Monsel's solution.[14]

Postoperatively, patients are instructed to treat the excision site with antibiotic ointment or to keep it covered with a dressing such as Micropore skin-toned surgical tape to avoid desiccation necrosis that would accompany dry crust formation.

TABLE 24-1

Indications for Punch Excision Without Autografting

Traumatic tattoos

Boils

Acne nodules

Hypertrichosis

Lentigines

Nevi

Small ice-pick and other scars

Routine biopsy

Biopsy of the nail bed

When a decision has been made to close the punch excision site with a suture, the skin may be stretched prior to punch excision in order to obtain an oval-shaped wound, preferably with the long axis parallel to resting skin tension lines. This maneuver will facilitate closure with a minimum of "dog-ear" formation. The length of time that the suture remains in place will depend on the location of the excision and the age of the patient.

Punch excision without autografting may be a desirable alternative if the recipient site is in an area where punch grafting may yield a suboptimal result. Such areas include thick, sebaceous skin; skin where multiple cysts and epithelialized tunnels exist; surfaces that are highly curved, such as the nasal sulcus; densely bearded skin; and the labial commissures where there is considerable movement. If the final outcome is suboptimal because the healed site is depressed or leukodermic, a punch autograft repair may be performed.

PUNCH ELEVATION

The punch elevation procedure is designed to bring the base of a depressed scar up to the level of the surrounding skin.[15] For this procedure to be successful, the skin comprising the visible base of the scar must be relatively smooth, normal in color, and approximately the same diameter as the ostium. This procedure is better suited to treat relatively circular scars larger than 3 mm in diameter.

A punch with the same diameter as the scar is used to perform a circular incision perpendicular to the skin surface (Fig. 24-1). The punch excision should penetrate the subcutaneous tissue sufficiently to allow the plug to move freely on its pedicle. A fine-toothed forceps or gentle squeezing is employed to manipulate the cylinder upward, without tearing it out completely, until it is aligned with the surface. The skin may be secured with tape or sutures.[16] Several weeks after healing, electrodesiccation may be used to blend the edges. Alternatively, if a dermabrasion is planned as part of a rehabilitative program, that, too, will facilitate blending.

The punch elevation is not used as often as the other methods of punch excision since few scars meet all the criteria. Apart from acne, several other scarring conditions can be treated in a similar fashion: small pox, chicken pox, herpes zoster, and rarer conditions such as necrotic tuberculids.[15] Scars resulting from the excision or destruction of small cutaneous tumors may also be corrected in this manner.[17]

PUNCH EXCISION WITH FULL-THICKNESS AUTOLOGOUS PUNCH GRAFT REPLACEMENT

Punch excision surgery with punch graft replacement is suitable for patients with either a few discrete scars or with numerous scars not amenable to improvement by dermabrasion or soft-tissue augmentation injections.[18] Punch excision is

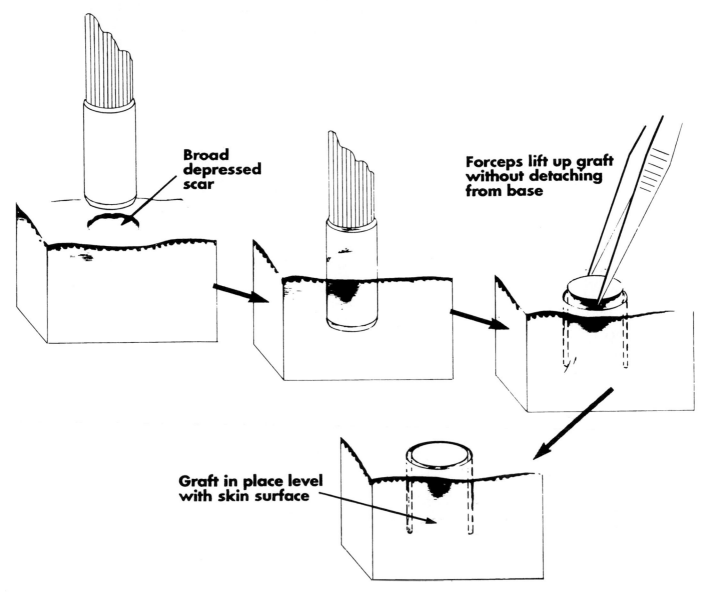

Broad depressed scar

Forceps lift up graft without detaching from base

Graft in place level with skin surface

Figure 24-1 Punch elevation.

ideally suited to treatment of the ice-pick acne scar which is essentially an epithelial tract in which bands of collagen fix the epithelial invagination to the subcutaneous layer. When keratin, sebaceous, and bacterial debris collect in these epithelialized invaginations, episodic inflammatory responses and epithelialized infundibular cysts may result. Usually, the typical acne patient has a variety of scar types, and several different techniques may be required to achieve optimal over-all rehabilitation.[19]

Additional skin lesions amenable to the autologous punch grafting method of rehabilitation include trichostasis spinulosa, isolated large pores, giant comedones, small epidermoid cysts, small steatocystomas, nevi, small skin cancers, stable leukodermas, tattoos, traumatic scars,[20] chicken pox scars, and those scarring conditions treatable by punch elevation (Table 24-2).

T A B L E   2 4 - 2

Indications for Punch Grafting

Skin cancer	Reference 17
Ice-Pick acne scar	Reference 19
Epithelialized sinuses (tunnels)	Reference 27
Leukoderma	Reference 21
Leukoderma and cicatricial alopecia	Reference 12
Piebaldism	Reference 28
Vitiligo	Reference 22–24
Hair transplantation for androgenic alopecia	Reference 10
Hair transplantation for cicatricial alopecia	Reference 29
Facial scar revision	Reference 20
Re-epithelialization of leg ulcers	

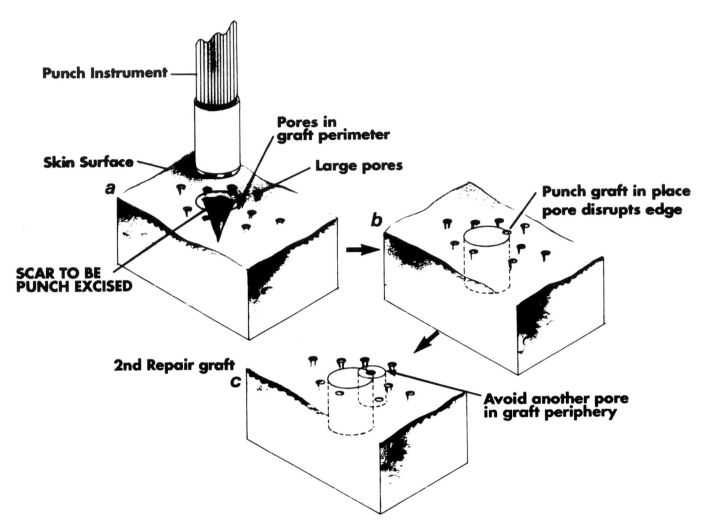

Figure 24-2   Punch graft in sebaceous skin. *(a)* Skin lesion situated within thick sebaceous skin and large pores; *(b)* large pore located in the perimeter of healed punch graft; *(c)* attempt at repair may repeat the problem.

Lesions situated on the face are suitable for punch grafting under appropriate conditions; however, certain locations pose a greater challenge. The thick sebaceous skin of the nose is frequently covered with a multitude of large pilosebaceous orifices, and it may be difficult to excise a lesion without transecting one of these (Fig. 24-2*a*). The problem that may then arise after healing is the occurrence of a large pore in the graft's perimeter (Fig. 24-2*b*). Further correction may be attempted by punch excising this large pore; however, there is a possibility of repeating this sequela in the second graft (Fig. 24-2*c*).

Areas of the face normally subject to a great deal of movement, such as the perioral area, and deeply concave areas, such as the nasal sulcus, are problematic. It may be necessary to secure grafts in these locations if initial attempts prove unsatisfactory.

In the case of ice-pick scar removal, the skin immediately adjacent to the scar is also closely examined for the presence of a connecting epithelialized tunnel (Fig. 24-3*a*). If a tunnel is present, and the entire tunnel is small enough (less than 3 mm), a punch may be used to remove the entire lesion (Fig. 24-3*b*). If the tunnel is greater than 3 mm, then the technique for excision of epithelialized sinuses described below may be used or an alternative method chosen.

Considerable normal skin can be conserved when correcting a linear ice-pick scar by excising it in two stages. Two small-diameter punch excisions are performed adjacently to one another, as opposed to one excision with a large-diameter punch (Fig. 24-4). Usually, 1 month or more is allowed between the first and second stages. A slight overlap of the two grafts assists in obtaining an optimal cosmetic result.

Autologous punch grafting for stable leukoderma

Repigmentation of stable leukodermas can be satisfactorily achieved by implanting autologous punch grafts from nor-

EXCISION OF EPITHELIALIZED TUNNEL

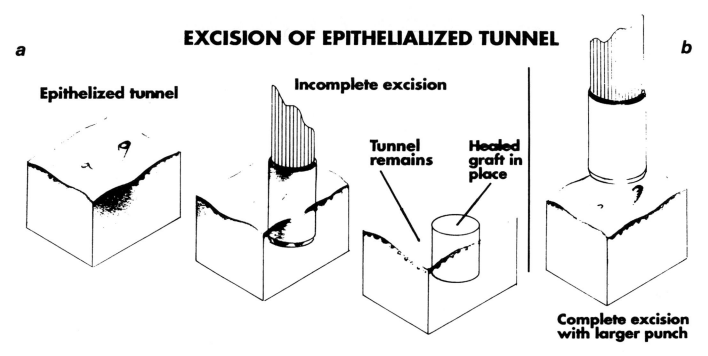

Figure 24-3 Excision of epithelialized tunnel. *(a)* Punch excision and grafting of ice-pick scar that in actuality is part of an epithelialized tunnel; *(b)* punch excision of entire tunnel.

EXCISION OF LINEAR ICE-PICK SCAR IN TWO STAGES

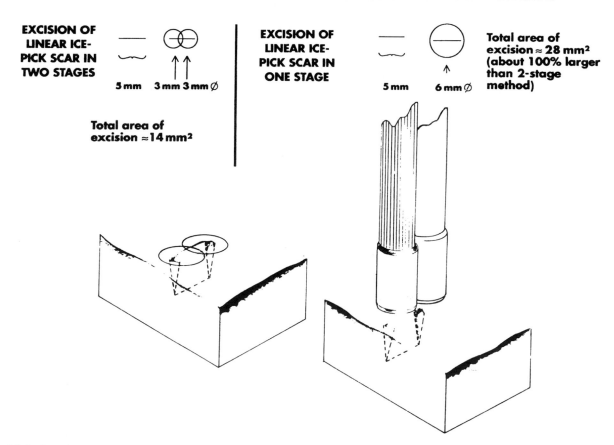

Figure 24-4 Punch excision of ice-pick scar in two stages reduces the area of surrounding normal skin excised.

mally pigmented areas of the body.[21] Donor sites of choice include the posterior earlobe and the medial aspect of the upper arm. Before attempting complete repigmentation of stable leukoderma, it is advisable to treat a small test area.

The radial extension of melanocytes and melanin from the autografts progresses gradually and takes approximately 6 months to attain full pigment spread. Whether 1- or 2-mm diameter grafts are employed, the pigment spread is consistently about 1 mm.[21] In terms of area of pigmentation, the 1-mm diameter normal skin grafts function more efficiently than the 2-mm ones. For 1 mm, the resultant pigmentation is 3 mm in diameter (7 mm^2). From a graft double the diameter (2 mm), the resultant pigmentation is 4 mm in diameter (12.6 mm^2). On the other hand, utilization of grafts larger than 1 mm in diameter would decrease the number of autotransplants to be performed, allow less alteration in skin texture, and may enable a better fit in the repigmentation of a given leukodermatous portion. Grafts are usually placed 5 to 10 mm apart during a single visit. Areas of residual leukoderma remaining between healed autografts are treated on subsequent visits.

The success of this method has been confirmed.[22] Attempts have also been made to repigment areas of segmental vitiligo and localized vitiligo.[23,24] Although autologous minigrafts proved successful in many of the patients reported, the postoperative observation period was not longer than 2 years.

Early investigations into the pathogenesis of vitiligo demonstrated recipient dominance.[10] Normally pigmented skin transplanted to vitiligo skin became vitiliginous. Vitiligo skin transplanted to normally pigmented skin became pigmented. The different clinical, physiologic, and therapeutic characteristics between segmented and generalized vitiligo may account for the different results obtained.

TECHNIQUE

Preoperative Instructions

Prior to punch grafting, it is desirable, but not absolutely essential, that the patient avoid aspirin for 7 to 10 days and alcohol for at least 1 day. Aspirin substitutes such as acetaminophen are permitted. The face and postauricular areas are cleansed thoroughly. It is not necessary for the patient to fast the day of the procedure; a regular breakfast or lunch is recommended. Sedation is rarely necessary in adults.

It is advisable to have preoperative and postoperative photographic documentation when punch surgery is performed in cosmetically significant areas.

Suggested list of instruments and supplies

Orentreich punches, 1 to 6 mm in 0.25-mm increments
Orentreich punches, 6 to 12 mm in 0.5-mm increments
Fine-curved scissors or iris scissors
Fine-toothed forceps (Adson's)

Needle-holder and suture
Liquid adhesive (Mastisol)
Adhesive remover (Detachol)
Steri-Strips, $^1/_8$ in or Micropore® tape
Gauze sponges
Cotton-tipped applicators
Gentian violet
Local anesthetic for injection, usually lidocaine 1 to 2%, with and without epinephrine
Syringe
30-gauge needles ($^1/_2$-in)
Chlorhexidine wash
Petri dishes
Hydrogen peroxide
Antibiotic ointment

Procedure for Punch Grafting

With the patient seated on the examining table, a movable light is positioned overhead to optimally delineate the scars. With the patient looking on in a hand-held mirror, the scars to be treated are selected and circled with gentian violet. The patient is then placed in a recumbent position, and the selected sites are examined with the aid of magnification.

A punch is selected that will encompass an area slightly larger than the lesion, especially when punch excising scars such as ice-pick or chicken pox scars (Fig. 24-5). A punch that is inadequate in size to completely remove the epithelial wall of the scar may result in sinus tract or cyst formation after the graft has healed in place (Fig. 24-6).

Prior to infiltration of the recipient site with a local anesthetic, the appropriately sized punch is used to score the skin. This indelibly marks the site and facilitates accurate excision after the area has been infiltrated with a local anesthetic. The author prefers to use the Orentreich punch (Robbins Instruments, Chatham, NJ), a cylindric stainless steel punch with a knurled handle and a hole in the cylinder for easy cleaning.

The donor and recipient sites are locally anesthetized with lidocaine (1 to 2%), usually containing epinephrine (1:100,000 to 1:200,000), injected through a 30-gauge needle. Five to 10 min is allowed in order to attain maximum vasoconstriction and for dissipation of the anesthetic solution so as to minimize tissue distortion. The punch is held at a right angle to the skin surface, and the defect is excised with a firm, manual rotation of the instrument. The punch should be sharp enough to complete the excision with a single rotation. The depth of excision may be varied; however, for most purposes it is extended into the superficial subcutaneous fat.

When penetrating subcutaneous tissue, the surgeon must take care to avoid damage to underlying blood vessels and nerves whenever possible. This may be unavoidable, however, when excising skin cancers. Infiltration of the subcutaneous tissues with additional local anesthetic solution or sterile physiologic saline just prior to punch excision will lift the skin away from underlying structures and reduce the likeli-

EXCISION OF ICE-PICK SCAR

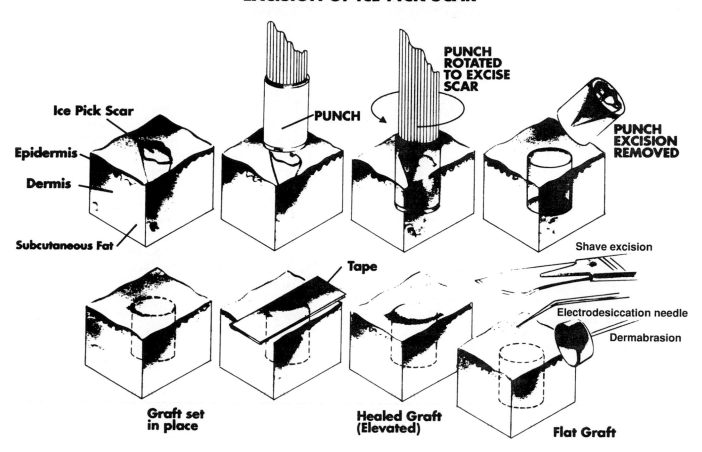

Figure 24-5   Diagram of a punch graft repair of an ice-pick scar. Three commonly used methods to flatten healed grafts are illustrated.

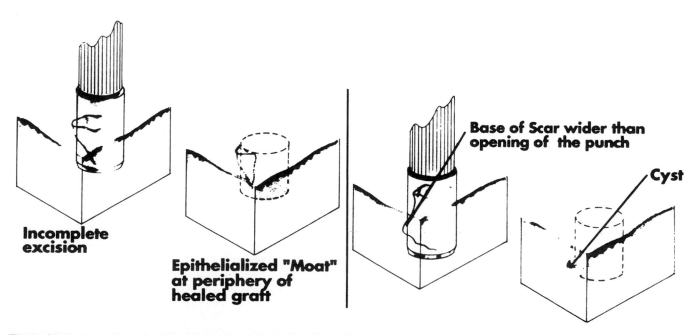

Figure 24-6   Incomplete ice-pick scar excision. The entire epithelial wall of an ice-pick scar must be removed to avoid a sinus tract or epithelial cyst formation after grafting.

hood of damaging them. However, one must account for the consequent distortion of the surface topography. Examples of anatomic areas that require caution include the posterior triangle of the neck where the spinal accessory nerve lies beneath the subcutaneous fat in the fascia and alongside the nose where the angular artery is located.

Care is taken to avoid undue lateral traction on both the recipient and donor sites during punch excision. Undue distortion increases the possibility of producing elliptic rather than circular excisions and grafts. Although saline infiltration of hair transplant donor sites may be used to increase skin turgor, minimize distortion, and maximize yield, it is not usually used for facial punch grafting since hair follicles are not routinely present in the donor skin. It is important to use sharp punches in order to minimize distortion of both donor and recipient sites from the pressure and friction applied to the skin by the instrument.

A graft of normal skin is punch excised from the donor site, usually the posterior earlobe. The entire posterior surface of the ear, the postauricular sulcus, and the immediately adjacent postauricular mastoid-area skin may also be used. Preauricular skin and the skin of the medial upper arm are suitable if the above areas have been exhausted. The donor area is also chosen according to how well it matches the recipient site and its ease of concealment. Even when scars from both sides of the face are being punch excised during a single session, donor grafts may be harvested from a single donor site in order to facilitate postoperative care and the patient's sleeping comfortably on one side.

Removal of the recipient tissue as well as the donor graft is accomplished with a fine, single-toothed forceps. The donor graft is gently grasped on dermal tissue to avoid damaging the epidermis, and the cylinder of skin is gently lifted out. Occasionally, the subcutaneous attachment gives way without cutting; alternately, a fine scissors is used when resistance is met. The recipient site specimen is either submitted for histopathologic examination or discarded as the individual circumstance dictates.

As a result of the skin's elastic recoil property, the recipient site tends to spread open farther after excision, and the donor skin graft contracts. Therefore, the donor skin graft is usually excised with a larger punch than the one used to excise the defect, thereby ensuring a snug fit. A graft taken with a donor punch that has an *area* about 40 to 80 percent larger than that of the punch used to excise the recipient site generally produces an optimal fit (Table 24-3). Adjustments are made on an individual basis. Generally, it is preferable to use a graft that is slightly too large than too small, since it is easier to flatten an elevated graft that has healed well around its perimeter than to correct a depressed graft.

After their removal, the grafts may be placed in a petri dish on top of sterile gauze covered with cool physiologic saline until the surgeon is prepared to place them into the recipient sites. When only one or a few grafts are being performed, they are often placed directly into the recipient site(s).

If the recipient site is within the beard area of a male patient, the punch excision is performed parallel to the hair follicles to avoid ingrown hairs. The posterior hair-bearing scalp may be used for the donor site, and some trimming of the graft's subcutaneous tissue may be required. However, care is taken to avoid inadvertent trimming of the dermal papillae.

If the lesion is elliptic, it can be excised with a circular punch by stretching the lesion across its short axis, thereby creating a "circular" lesion, which assumes an oval configuration upon release. The donor tissue is also excised in a similar manner [i.e., the skin is stretched prior to punch excision in order to produce an oval graft upon release (Fig. 24-7)].

On a patient's first treatment visit, it may be advisable to perform a small number of punch grafts. This affords the surgeon the opportunity to observe the results prior to embarking on further repairs. It also allows the patient to develop familiarity and confidence in the technique, as well as facility in caring for the grafts during the immediate postoperative period.

Multiple autologous punch grafts may be performed conveniently in a single office visit, and these may all be har-

TABLE 24-3

Typical Donor-Recipient Punch Choices*

Diameter of Punch used at Recipient Site (mm)	Area of Recipient Punch (mm²)	Diameter of Punches used at Donor Site (mm)	Area of Donor Punch (mm²)	Ratio of Donor Area to Recipient Area
1.75	2.4	2.25	4.0	1.7
2.00	3.1	2.50/2.75	4.9/5.9	1.6/1.9
2.25	4.0	2.75/3.00	5.9/7.1	1.5/1.8
2.50	4.9	3.00/3.25	7.1/8.3	1.4/1.7
2.75	5.9	3.50/3.75	9.6/11.0	1.6/1.9
3.00	7.1	3.75/4.00	11.0/12.6	1.6/1.8

*As the table shows, an optimal fit will be obtained when the punch used to excise the donor graft has an area approximately 50 to 80 percent larger than the punch used to excise the recipient site.

PUNCH EXCISION & PUNCH GRAFT REPLACEMENT

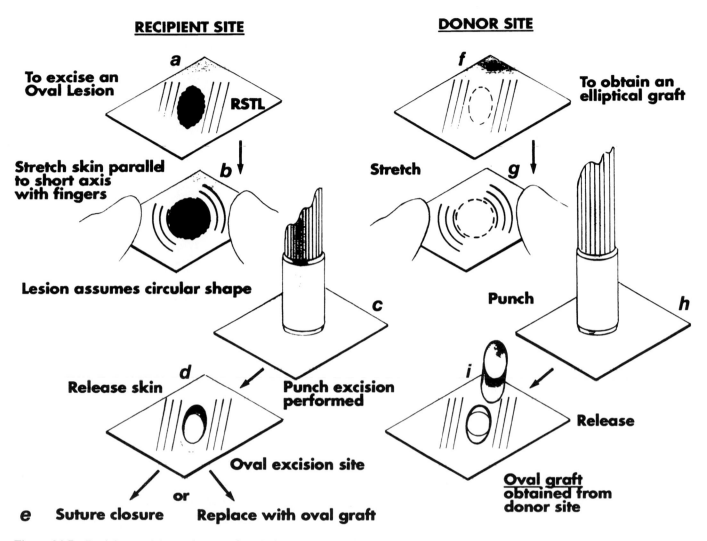

RECIPIENT SITE

a — To excise an Oval Lesion — RSTL

b — Stretch skin parallel to short axis with fingers — Lesion assumes circular shape

c — Punch excision performed

d — Release skin — Oval excision site

e — Suture closure — or — Replace with oval graft

DONOR SITE

f — To obtain an elliptical graft

g — Stretch

h — Punch

i — Release — Oval graft obtained from donor site

Figure 24-7 Recipient and donor sites. *(a)* Oval lesion (e.g., ice-pick scar); *(b)* outward traction applied in order to stretch skin at right angles to relaxed skin tension lines; *(c)* punch excision of lesion; *(d)* skin tension released, punch excision site assumes oval shape; *(e)* excision site sutured closed or replaced with oval graft; *(f)* donor site at rest; *(g)* outward traction applied to donor skin; *(h)* donor punch excision performed; *(i)* skin tension released, oval graft obtained.

vested from one healthy earlobe. On occasion, many dozens of grafts may be performed. It is helpful to have an assistant record the number, size, and location of punch excisions and the number of donor grafts needed in each size. Certain patients with a history of severe acne may have earlobes that are so cystic and scarred as to make them unsatisfactory donor sites. In these patients, the alternative donor sites mentioned above may be used.

When an appropriately sized donor punch has been selected, the donor graft will fit snugly into the recipient site. By slowly rotating the donor graft in the recipient site, a position which provides the best fit will be located. If excessive

subcutaneous fat causes undue elevation of the donor graft, it is trimmed; otherwise, trimming of fat is usually unnecessary. In most cases, the donor graft sits level in the recipient site or is slightly elevated above the surrounding normal skin. A graft is usually not allowed to remain if it sits well below the surface of the surrounding skin.

After the donor graft is placed and hemostasis has been achieved by manual pressure, each graft that is 4 mm or less in diameter is usually secured with a 3M Micropore skin-toned surgical tape dressing. Whenever possible, overlapping the tape strips is avoided to facilitate the later removal of individual strips. An adhesive such as Mastisol (Ferndale Laboratories, Inc., Ferndale, Michigan) may be applied to the skin around the graft prior to taping to prevent it from loosening prematurely. Sutures may be used to hold large grafts in place, but good results have been obtained by taping in place donor autografts, even up to 6 mm. A cross-stitch or steel pin may be used to secure medium-sized grafts (4.5 to 6 mm), while simple sutures into the graft edge are often used for large grafts (greater than 6 mm).[16,25]

Hemostasis at the recipient and donor sites is achieved without hemostatic agents, such as Monsel's solution or aluminum chloride, that may interfere with healing and graft survival by delaying vascularization.[14] A plug of collagen matrix or Gelfoam may be placed in the donor site and a pressure dressing applied to the donor area with either a Telfa pad or other bandage. Healing of the postauricular donor site by secondary intention is usually excellent. A suture may be used to close the donor site if hemostasis is difficult to achieve with manual pressure alone. All sutures are usually removed in 5 to 7 days. Oral antibiotics are prescribed on an individual basis, usually erythromycin 250 mg, 1 po b.i.d. for up to 7 days.

The tape dressing over the recipient site is left in place to protect the graft for about 5 days. The patient is advised to apply direct firm pressure if bleeding occurs from either donor or recipient sites after leaving the doctor's office. Hydrogen peroxide can be used to dissolve clotted blood from under the Micropore tape without disturbing the tape or the graft. Avoidance of excessive facial movement for a few days is helpful, but compliance is problematic. The patient is also advised to avoid activities that may dislodge the grafts. Makeup may be applied over the tape or after the tape has been removed, but the makeup should be removed gently. Removal of tape and dressing is made easier by wetting. After the tape

TABLE 24-4

Sequelae

Sequelae	Possible Causes	Prevention and Treatment in Order of Invasiveness
1. Failure to take	—Excessive facial movement —Excessive bleeding —Infection —Unrecognized associated epithelialized tunnel —Trauma (accidentally dislodged)	—Allow to heal by secondary intention —Regraft +/− suture graft in place
2. Infection	—Possible with any surgical disruption of normal integumentary barrier —Unrecognized epithelialized tunnel	—Antibiotics —Incision and drainage —Regraft later if indicated
3. Persistent erythema	—Sun exposure —Individual variation in wound healing	—Sun protection —Time —Topical/intralesional anti-inflammatory corticosteroids
4. Color discrepancy (hypopigmentation)	—Donor site dissimilar to recipient site —Donor site in sun-protected area	—Sun protection —Time —Mild chemical peeling (20% trichloroacetic acid) of area around graft —Dermabrasion
5. Hyperpigmentation	—Postinflammatory —Seen more often in dark-skinned individuals	—Sun protection —Time —Topical/intralesional anti-inflammatory corticosteroids —Hydroquinone bleaching —20% trichloroacetic acid peels
6. Elevated graft	—Contracture of healing tissues —Graft larger than optimal	—Electrodesiccation —Shave excision —Dermabrasion
7. Depressed graft	—Graft smaller than optimal —Graft thickness inadequate in relation to recipient site depth	—Punch elevation —Injection of soft-tissue augmenting material —Regraft (slightly larger)
8. Depressed groove at junction of graft and surrounding skin	—Graft contracture —Graft size insufficient —Individual wound healing characteristics	—Time (may fade in 6 to 12 months) —Electrodesiccation —Dermabrasion —Regraft
9. Hypertrophic scar	—Rare —Individual wound healing characteristics —Facial movement (location)	—Time —Intralesional corticosteroids (1 to 5 mg/cc triamcinolone acetonide)

EXCISION OF LARGE EPITHELIALIZED TUNNEL

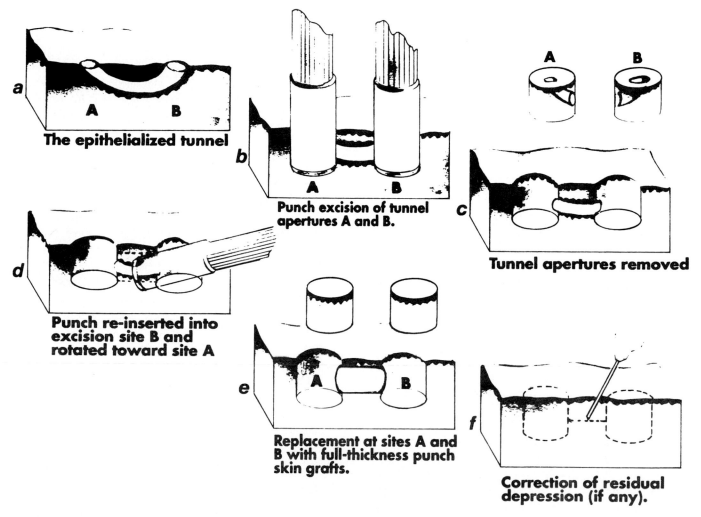

The epithelialized tunnel

Punch excision of tunnel apertures A and B.

Tunnel apertures removed

Punch re-inserted into excision site B and rotated toward site A

Replacement at sites A and B with full-thickness punch skin grafts.

Correction of residual depression (if any).

Figure 24-8 *(a)* The epithelialized tunnel; *(b)* punch excision of sinus apertures A and B; *(c)* excised tissue removed; *(d)* punch inserted into excision site B and rotated toward site A to excise residual epithelial tunnel; *(e)* replacement of punch excision sites A and B with full-thickness punch skin grafts obtained from the posterior earlobe; *(f)* correction of residual depression, if any.

dressings are removed, an antibiotic ointment may be sparingly applied to residual crusts at the donor and recipient sites several times a day to prevent desiccation necrosis. The surgical sites may be gently washed as long as contact with irritating soaps or chemicals is avoided.

Postoperative discomfort is usually minimal, and acetaminophen usually provides adequate analgesia. For those patients who experience greater discomfort, stronger analgesics may be necessary.

Before leaving the office, the patient is given instructions to follow if a graft inadvertently comes out:

1. Handle the graft gently, and cleanse it in an 8-oz glass of tepid water to which ¼ tsp of salt has been added.

2. Wrap the graft in a clean handkerchief saturated with some of the mildly salted water, and place it in a clean plastic bag.

3. Store the wet-wrapped graft in the refrigerator (not the freezer) for no more than 4 days.

4. Call the office for an appointment the same or next day to have the graft replaced. If the graft is lost or cannot be saved, the site can be regrafted either prior to or after healing by secondary intention.

For optimal cosmetic results, a fully healed graft usually requires leveling by either electrodesiccation or tangential shave excision 4 weeks or more after grafting. If the patient has extensive and varied scarring (as from acne) that is suitable for dermabrasion, then a dermabrasion will further blend the grafts.

At least 6 to 8 weeks are allowed after grafting and before dermabrasion in order to prevent the grafts from being avulsed. Alternatively, dermabrasion may be performed first and punch grafting of the remaining ice-pick scars done afterward.

Postoperative sequelae that may be encountered with punch autografting are listed in Table 24-4, along with their possible causes and recommended treatments.

EXCISION OF EPITHELIALIZED SINUSES

Moderate-to-severe acne may result in epithelialized tunnels or sinuses [Fig. 24-8a (see previous page)]. These lesions may be up to 1 cm in length and 1 to 4 mm in width. They are usually large enough to "thread" with a fine scissors or small suture needle. Keratin, sebum, and bacteria often become trapped beneath the surface of the skin in these epithelialized tunnels, leading to recurrent infection and inflammatory necrotic reactions.

Dermabrasion removes superficial sinuses with an excellent cosmetic result; it may also unroof deeper ones that may then require further cosmetic reconstruction, such as soft-tissue augmentation.[26] Small, superficial epithelialized tunnels can also be individually unroofed with a scissors or scalpel.

The correction of large, deep epithelialized tunnels is problematic since their unroofing would leave an unacceptable scar, elliptic excision may leave a linear scar, and they are often too deep for dermabrasion. An Orentreich punch can be used to excise large, deep tunnels in the following manner:[27] Apertures A and B of the sinus are punch excised as though each were a separate ice-pick scar (Fig. 24-8b–c). A punch is then partially reinserted into site B down to the level of the residual sinus and redirected to be parallel with the surface of the skin (Fig. 24-8d). The instrument is then rotated toward site A, thereby excising the remaining sinus tract and a small amount of normal tissue surrounding it, but leaving the skin above intact. Sites A and B are replaced with appropriately sized full-thickness punch skin grafts from the posterior earlobe (Fig. 24-8e). If the skin above the cored-out sinus settles, it may be corrected with injectable soft-tissue augmentation materials (Fig. 24-8f).

REFERENCES

1. Watson BA: Discotome. *The New York Medical Record,* July 27, 1878, p 78

2. Goodman H: Cutaneous punch. *Archives of Dermatology and Syphilology* 56:268–269, 1947

3. Parish LC: Edward Lawrence Keyes. *Cutis* 3:394–401, 1967

4. Keyes EL: The cutaneous punch. *Journal of Cutaneous Genito-Urinary Disease* 5:98–101, 1887

5. Kromayer E: Cosmetic Treatment of Skin Complaints, 2d ed, English translation. New York, Oxford University Press, 1930, p 9

6. Kromayer E: Die Heilung der Akne durch ein neues Narbenloses Operationsverfahren. *Das Stanzen, Illustrierte Monatlische Schreibung, Ärtzlische, Polytech* 27:101, 1905

7. Loewenthal LJA: Punch biopsy with autograft. *AMA Archives of Dermatology and Syphilology* 67:629, 1953

8. Blau S, Rein CR: Dermabrasion of the acne pit. *AMA Archives of Dermatology and Syphilology* 70:754–766, 1954

9. Burks JR: *Wire Brush Surgery.* Springfield, Ill, Charles C Thomas, 1956

10. Orentreich N: Autografts in alopecias and other selected dermatological conditions. *Ann N Y Acad Sci* 83:463–479, 1959

11. Okuda S: Clinical and experimental studies of transplantation of living hairs. *Japanese Journal of Dermatology* 46:135–138, 1939

12. Lobuono P, Shatin H: Transplantation of hair bulbs and melanocytes into leukodermic scars. *J Dermatol Surg* 2:53–55, 1976

13. Converse JM, Rapaport FT: The vascularization of skin autografts and homografts; an experimental study in man. *Ann Surg* 143:306–315, 1956

14. Armstrong RB et al: Punch biopsy wounds treated with Monsel's solution or a collagen matrix: A Comparison of healing. *Arch Dermatol* 122:546–549, 1986

15. Arouete J: Correction of depressed scars on the face by a method of elevation. *J Dermatol Surg Oncol* 2:337–339, 1976

16. Orentreich N, Orentreich DS: "Cross-stitch" suture technique for hair transplantation. *J Dermatol Surg Oncol* 10:970–971, 1984

17. Deutsch HL, Orentreich N: Treatment of small external cancers of the nose. *Ann Plast Surg* 3:567–571, 1979

18. Orentreich N, Durr NP: Rehabilitation of acne scarring. *Dermatol Clin* 1:405–413, 1983

19. Orentreich DS, Orentreich N: Acne scar revision update, in *Advanced Dermatologic Surgery,* edited by PL Balin et al. Philadelphia, Saunders, 1987, pp 359–368

20. Dzubow LM: Scar revision by punch-graft transplants. *J Dermatol Surg Oncol* 11:1200–1202, 1985

21. Orentreich N, Selmanowitz VJ: Autograft repigmentation of leukoderma. *Arch Dermatol* 105:734–736, 1972

22. Falabella R: Repigmentation of stable leukoderma by autologous minigrafting. *J Dermatol Surg Oncol* 12:172–179, 1986

23. Falabella R: Repigmentation of segmental vitiligo by autologous minigrafting. *J Am Acad Dermatol* 9:514–521, 1983

24. Falabella R: Treatment of localized vitiligo by autologous minigrafting. *Arch Dermatol* 124:1649–1655, 1988

25. Johnson WC, Baker GK: Use of steel pins in hair transplantation. *J Dermatol Surg Oncol* 3:220–221, 1977

26. Orentreich DS, Orentreich N: Injectable fluid silicone, *Principles of Dermatologic Surgery,* edited by RK Roenigk, HH Roenigk. New York, Marcel Dekker, 1989

27. Orentreich DS, Orentreich N: Excision of epithelialized sinuses, in Surgical Gems in Dermatology Volume 2 edited by P. Robbins. New York Igaku-Shoin 1991, pp 33–34

28. Selmanowitz MD et al: Pigmentary correction of piebaldism by autografts, procedures and clinical findings. *J Dermatol Surg Oncol* **3:**615–622, 1977

29. Stough DB et al: Surgical improvement of cicatricial alopecia of diverse etiology. *Arch Dermatol* **97:**331–334, 1968

David E. Kent

25 Full-Thickness Skin Grafts

A *skin graft* may be defined as an intact piece of skin that has been completely separated from its donor site attachment and is transferred to a different recipient site. At this site, it reestablishes a new blood supply. A *full-thickness skin graft* (FTSG) by definition is an intact piece of integument consisting of the entire epidermis, complete thickness of dermis, with no connection to subcutaneous fat. A *split-thickness skin graft* (STSG) is defined as consisting of an entire thickness of epidermis, a varying thickness of dermis, and no connection to underlying subcutaneous fat. *Composite grafts* consist of intact skin, both epidermis and dermis, with an additional component such as fat or cartilage directly attached (e.g., ear wedge containing skin-cartilage-skin). *Autografts* are taken from one part of an individual and transplanted to a different site of the same individual. *Allografts* (homografts) are grafts obtained from one individual and transplanted to a different individual of the same species (e.g., human to human, rabbit to rabbit). *Xenografts* (heterografts) are grafts obtained from one individual of one species and transplanted to an individual of a different species (e.g., pig to human).

PHYSIOLOGY OF SKIN GRAFTS

Survival of transplanted skin is primarily dependent upon reestablishing blood supply to ischemic tissue. The relative success and ease with which this survival occurs has been referred to as skin graft *take*. Vascularization of skin grafts has been extensively studied.[1-4] This skin graft take has been divided into three phases. These phases are: (1) plasma imbibition, (2) inosculation, and (3) capillary ingrowth. The phase of serum imbibition occurs during the first 24 to 48 h after skin graft transplantation. During this time, the graft survives by taking up nutrients from the wound exudate. The graft be-

comes edematous and increases in weight while graft pH drops and becomes acidotic (pH = 6.3 to 6.8). This occurs during the initial hours. There is a shift from aerobic to anaerobic metabolic pathways. Serum imbibition may also serve to protect the graft from dessication and keep the graft vessels patent.[5,6] Initially, a layer of fibrin serves to adhere the graft to the recipient bed.[7] This fibrin glue may also serve as a protective layer against infection.[8]

The phases of inosculation and capillary ingrowth are characterized by the host endothelial buds' "hooking up" to existing arterioles and venules present within the graft. These vascular buds grow through the fibrin layer. Some investigators feel the original viable graft vessels are important in reestablishing blood flow.[9,10] Other investigators had determined that preexisting graft vasculature may serve as conduits or nonviable channels through which new vascular endothelium advances.[11,14] Thus the graft is revascularized from ingrowth of new vessels from the margin and base of the recipient bed. Converse and Rapaport[1] suggest that inosculation is a chance encounter between host endothelium and existing graft vessels. This chance hookup of vessels may be triggered by a vasoactive cytokine's release from anaerobically driven tissue.[15] In summary, the phase of serum imbibition, which lasts for 24 to 48 h, nourishes and protects the graft during the early phase of graft take. Inosculation and capillary ingrowth actually occur simultaneously. Traditionally, actual blood flow has been observed on day 5 to 7 postgrafting. The speed at which vascularization occurs is dependent primarily on the vascularity of the donor site (e.g., postauricular faster than lower extremity) and secondarily on graft thickness (thinner grafts before thicker grafts).

Lymphatic drainage is established by the seventh postgraft day, and, at this point, the graft weight decreases toward its baseline.[16] Sensory reinnervation in grafted skin is a slow process that begins at 2 to 3 months and may take years to complete.[17,18] Touch and two-point discrimination are thought to be reliable parameters of graft reinnervation.[19] Grafts reinnervate initially at the graft margin, then move toward the center. This is dependent upon access to neurolemmal sheaths from the invading neural fibers.

Contraction and shrinkage of skin grafts have been carefully reviewed.[19–22] *Primary contraction* of grafts refers to the immediate shrinkage that occurs once the graft has been severed from its donor site. This is probably due to the recoil of elastic fibers. *Secondary contraction* is the contraction that occurs once the graft has been transferred to its recipient site. FTSGs initially contract greater than STSGs. However, once transplanted, STSGs have a greater potential to contract unless the recipient bed is fixed to an underlying rigid structure such as bone or cartilage. Myofibroblasts and contractile proteins are in part responsible for wound contraction.[19] Skin grafting may shorten the life cycle of myofibroblasts as well as reduce collagen synthesis in wounds. This results in reduced wound contraction.

INDICATIONS FOR FULL-THICKNESS GRAFTS

Full-thickness skin grafting is a useful technique for resurfacing and reconstructing various surgical defects. Selection of a full-thickness graft to resurface a defect depends on various factors. Local factors such as large defect size, location, lack of adequate adjacent tissue, and mobility are key considerations. Tissue quality factors such as irradiated tissue, underlying medical disease, adjacent hair-bearing skin, and heavy smoking may all adversely affect local tissue transfer and favor a graft. Irradiated skin typically is of poor quality with compromised vasculature. Smoking causes arteriolar constriction and may compromise larger random skin flaps.

Nonlocal factors may favor graft coverage. Aggressive tumors and uncertain margin control may prompt graft placement instead of flaps. This permits closer observation for tumor recurrence. Grafts are safe repairs, especially when the risk of flap failure is high. This is true when a random skin flap is proposed in an area of previous surgery where an uncertain blood supply exists. In addition, in certain anatomic areas, grafts may provide a better cosmetic result than flaps. Sites frequently used for full-thickness grafts include the distal nose, ear, lower eyelid, and inner canthus.

ADVANTAGES AND DISADVANTAGES OF FULL-THICKNESS GRAFTS

Full-thickness grafts offer several advantages over split-thickness grafts. Full-thickness grafts have less tendency to contract, and there is less tendency to develop a smooth sheen and resist cosmetics. Their cosmetic appearance is generally better and improves with time; they are more durable. There is a better chance for texture and thickness match, and, finally, no special or costly instrumentation is required. There are also disadvantages to FTSGs. There is creation of a donor site defect that must be repaired, risk of graft failure, chance of unfavorable appearance, contracture along free margins, as well as potential surgical complications at two sites. A clean, well-vascularized recipient bed is also necessary for full-thickness grafts.

DONOR SITE SELECTION

A variety of donor areas exist for FTSGs. One tries to match qualities of donor skin for the surrounding recipient area. Texture, color, and actinic damage vary from donor site to recipient site and should be matched if at all possible. Donor skin typically retains its various qualities (adnexa, thickness) after transfer. Most full-thickness grafts are harvested from preauricular skin, postauricular skin, supraclavicular and clavicular areas, neck, upper eyelid, nasolabial folds, and inner upper arm areas. The groin, hypothenar area, and wrist are less frequently used.

Preauricular grafts provide good color, texture, and actinic qualities for many facial defects. Two centimeters is the maximum diameter obtainable for most of these grafts.[23] The resultant incision line can be placed in a preauricular crease, and any dog-ear produced may be removed in a periauricular location with standard dog-ear repair or W-plasties.

Postauricular sites may yield larger grafts that tend to be less actinically damaged. Incision lines are also well camouflaged. However, large grafts may result in a pinned-back appearance of the ear that can be persistently uncomfortable, especially with glasses.

Supraclavicular donor sites are useful for very large grafts. Clavicular and infraclavicular sites may produce visible scars that are readily seen on women. Clavicular and inner arm grafts are thicker and may be trimmed and sculpted to match the defect depth. Anterior and lateral neck donor sites have actinically damaged skin that is useful.

Upper eyelid skin is thin and ideal for lower eyelid defects. One must be prepared to modify the contralateral upper lid to maintain facial symmetry.

The nasolabial line has sebaceous skin that works well for distal nasal defects. Like the upper eyelid, harvesting in this area may create facial asymmetry as well as a visible midfacial scar. Generally speaking, graft harvesting should be on the ipsilateral side as the defect and any potential for facial asymmetry should be visibly reviewed with the patient. Drawing the resultant donor site incision may be helpful for the patient to visualize.

SURGICAL TECHNIQUE

Surgical technique for full-thickness grafts must be meticulous, from selecting and sizing the donor site through completing the dressing. The following is a step-by-step sequence for full-thickness grafts:

1. Selecting the appropriate donor site: This has been covered in the preceding section.
2. Appropriately sizing the donor site: It is absolutely vital to correctly measure and size the graft. This should include the depth of the defect. Failure to correctly measure the graft may result in a too-small graft which might necessitate harvesting additional tissue or suturing two grafts together. A template is ideal to ensure exact sizing. Templates may consist of nonstick pads (Telfa, Release, Adaptic pads), 4- by 4-in gauzes, or sterile glove paper. An imprint of the defect is easily made, cut out along the blood-tinged paper, and placed over the donor area for marking. Outlining the rim of the defect with a sterile skin marker may facilitate this step. If any doubt exists about whether the graft is adequate, drawing a larger template should prevent cutting too small of a graft.
3. Harvesting the graft: Removal of the donor graft is performed with standard surgical technique. After the graft is incised, a tip of the graft—typically the closest end—is grasped, and with sharp and blunt dissection the graft is removed. The graft is usually removed with its subcutaneous fat attached. The graft should be placed in sterile saline, either in a sterile basin with cool saline or in a saline-soaked gauze. If the graft is placed in a soaked gauze, an instrument should be placed over the sponge and the surgical assistant made aware of where the graft is located so the sponge will not inadvertently be used. Next, hemostasis is obtained and the donor site is repaired, typically with a layered closure. Sometimes a local skin flap or split-thickness graft is required to close the donor defect.
4. Defatting the graft: Defatting the graft requires meticulous technique, patience, sharp scissors, and adequate lighting. Loupe magnification may also prove beneficial. The basic technique involves draping the graft over the index finger of the nondominant hand with the subcutaneous tissue facing upward. Then, utilizing sharp scissors, one meticulously removes the subcutaneous fat. This is done in small fat globules to prevent cutting holes through the entire thickness of the graft. The graft should be frequently moistened with saline to prevent desiccation. Once the fat is removed, the dermis may be thinned as to sculpt the graft thickness to match the surrounding defect thickness.[24] If a small nick is inadvertently cut through the graft, it does not need to be repaired. If a large hole is created, it may require closure with a simple 6-0 or 7-0 suture. Scissor selection is a personal preference. One may use iris scissors or curved utility scissors with one serrated edge. The serrated edge prevents tissue slip while defatting takes place.
5. Preparing the donor site: If the graft is placed at the same time of tumor removal, little donor site preparation is required. Absolute hemostasis must be obtained and any de-

vitalized tissue should be removed. Care must be taken to avoid charring the wound bed with the electrosurgical unit or Bovie. Simple pressure with a moist gauze is highly successful. Should oozing persist, liquid thrombin may be helpful, especially for patients on aspirin-containing medications. Additional preparation will be necessary with delayed grafts. This will be discussed below in "Delayed Grafting."
6. The graft: Once the recipient bed is prepared, the moistened graft is placed over the bed. The graft is aligned into position by using blunt ends of Adson's pickups or moistended Q-Tips. All wrinkles or folds should be straightened. The graft is then trimmed and tailored to the defect. The graft edges must proximate the recipient bed margin exactly. If not, a suboptimal result will occur.

Meticulous precise suturing technique is required for full-thickness grafts. Initially "tacking" interrupted sutures may be placed to hold the graft in position at key anchoring points. Then, interrupted or simple running sutures may complete graft placement. If running sutures are used, they must not bunch or pull the graft from the recipient bed margin. Typically used is a 5-0 or 6-0 caliber suture. Fast absorbable sutures [mild chromic (Davis + Geck, Waynes, NJ) and fast-gut (Ethicon, Inc., Somerville, NJ)] eliminate the need for suture removal and thus disturbing the graft during the postoperative period. They generally dissolve in less than 7 days. The PC Prime (Ethicon, Inc.) needle of the fast-gut has excellent handling qualities and resists bending and breakage. Either suture must be removed carefully from its package to prevent suture breakage. Plain chromic suture, either 4-0, 5-0, or 6-0 caliber, may be used to secure larger grafts that require longer time to take. Basting sutures may be used to secure the graft at sites other than the periphery. They are especially helpful for irregularly contoured surfaces such as around the nose or ear. They are useful for larger grafts to help provide even contact across a large surface area. These will be discussed below in "Basting Sutures."
7. Securing the graft: The graft must be secured and protected from the outside environment to allow for take. The dressing should: (a) prevent shearing forces from disturbing the graft and (b) firmly hold the graft against the recipient bed to reduce the potential for hematoma and seroma formation. The graft is immediately covered with a thin layer of antibiotic ointment followed by a nonstick contact layer (Adaptic, Xeroform, N-terface, Aquaphor gauze, Vaseline gauze, etc.). Sterile cotton balls or eye pads are moistened in saline or Betadine and placed over the contact layer. When this dries it provides firm, even support against the graft. This is secured in place with either a tie-over or non-tie-over dressing design.

A non-tie-over dressing may be secured with special weaved tape that is slightly stretchy. Tie-over dressings consist of suture that is used to secure the contour layer.

The sutures may be placed directly into the graft margin as a tacking suture or a few millimeters away from the graft edge. Tie-over suture is generally a silk suture. Silk has excellent knot stability and handling qualities. Nurolon (Ethicon, Inc.) is a treated nylon suture that has the strength of nylon and handles more like silk. Tie-over sutures are paired—one on each side of the graft. Typically four to eight tie-over sutures are required for the larger grafts. The technique is as follows:

a. Opposite sutures are grasped, a double throw is placed, and the suture is pulled down firmly, holding the contour layer in place.

b. A hemostat or an Adson pickup is then used to press (not pinch) the knot until another throw can be made and securely placed on top of the first knot.

c. An additional knot or two is placed.

d. All paired sutures are likewise tied.

e. The suture lengths may then be evenly divided and tied to each other over the individual knots for additional security, then the excess is cut off.

f. A protective layer (such as Band-Aid, gauze, or Telfa and tape) may be placed on top of the bolster to prevent picking and keep the curious observer out. The donor area is then dressed with a standard dressing.

Site-specific dressing modifications may be necessary. Grafts involving the ear may require a protective mastoid dressing, especially during sleep. Periorbital and eyelid grafts may require patching the eye closed. If the eye is patched, sterile ophthalmic ointment should be used. A prepatch visual accuity test should always be documented. If the patient has had recent eye surgery (cataract) or has documented eye disease such as glaucoma, the patient's ophthalmologist should be contacted prior to patching the eye closed to ensure safety.

Figures 25-1a–j and 25-2a–k illustrate surgical technique for full-thickness skin graft placement.

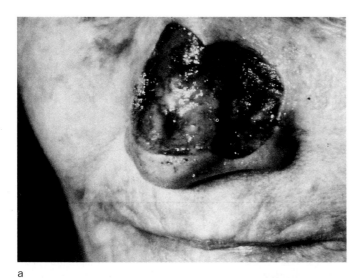

a

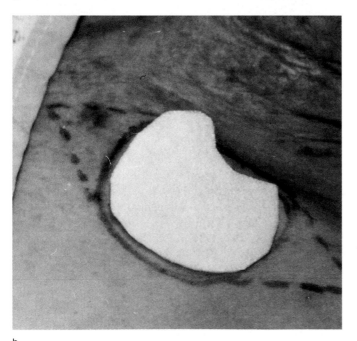

b

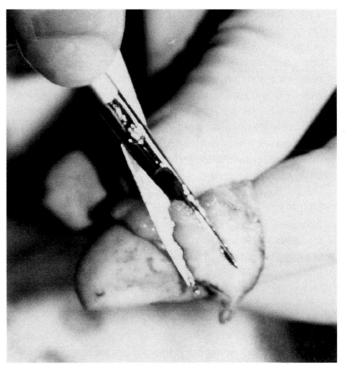

c

Figure 25-1 Surgical technique. *(a)* Surgical defect on nose; *(b)* template fashioned from Telfa pad and donor site selection; *(c)* defatting of graft (*Note:* graft draped fat side up over nondominant index finger). (*Continued*)

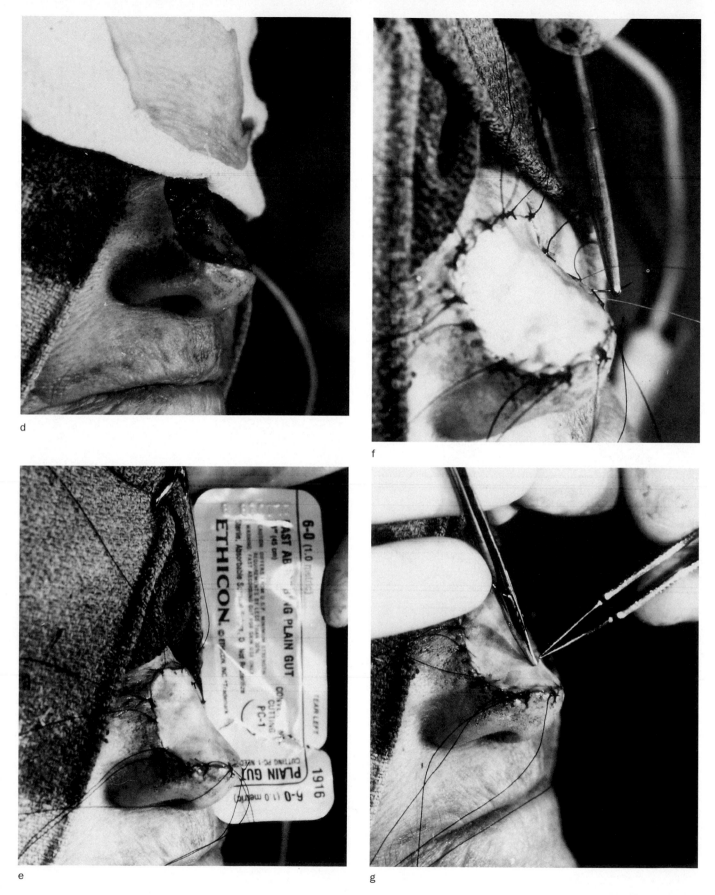

Figure 25-1 (*Cont.*)   (*d*) defatting of graft completed with deeper portion of dermis removed (*Note:* imprint of gauze through graft indicating a thin full-thickness graft); (*e*) graft trimmed to defect and secured in position by tie-over sutures prior to placement of running fast absorbable suture;   (*f*) running fast absorbable suture in place; (*g*) small nicks placed to allow for drainage and prevent fluid collection.

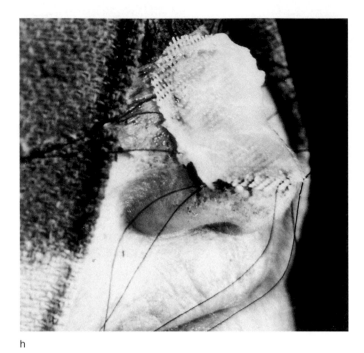

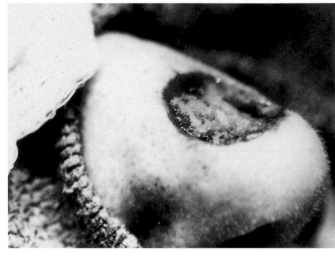

a

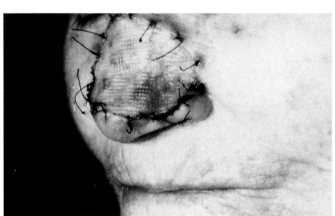

i

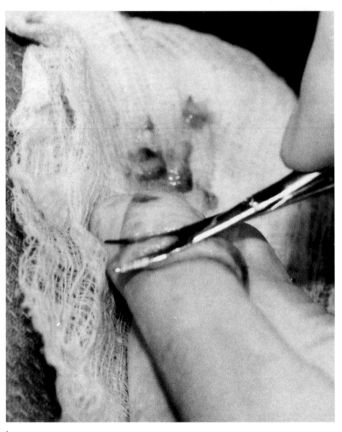

b

Figure 25-2 Surgical technique of full-thickness graft placement. (*a*) Defect on distal nose; (*b*) defatting of graft after donor site selection, sizing, removal, and repair. (*Continued*)

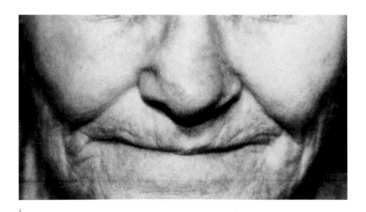

j

Figure 25-1 (*Cont.*) (*h*) antibiotic ointment placed on nonstick pad prior to securing tie-over dressing; (*i*) postoperative day 7 immediately upon removal of tie-over dressing (*Note:* temporary imprint of nonstick pad); (*j*) four weeks postoperatively (*Note:* no contour defect at site of drainage nick).

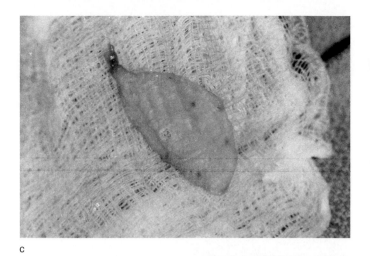

c

d

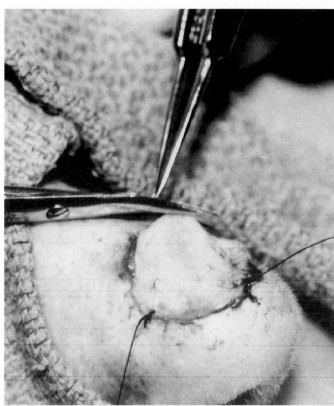

e

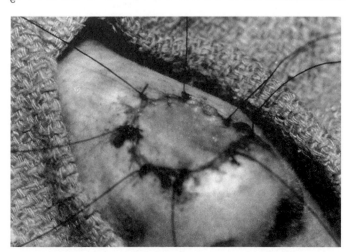

g

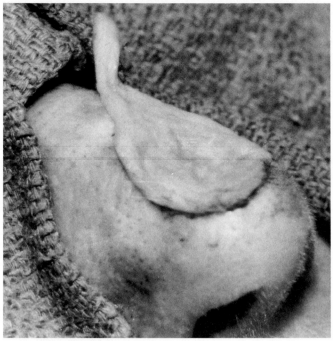

f

Figure 25-2 (*Cont.*)   *(c)* donor graft defatted (*Note:* inadvertent nick placement through and through in graft midportion); *(d)* graft placed over defect (*Note:* generous graft supply prior to trimming); *(e)* two tacking sutures placed and excess graft meticulously trimmed away; *(f)* hemostasis is checked with a sterile Q-Tip then spot-treated electrosurgically; *(g)* graft secured with tacking sutures.

303

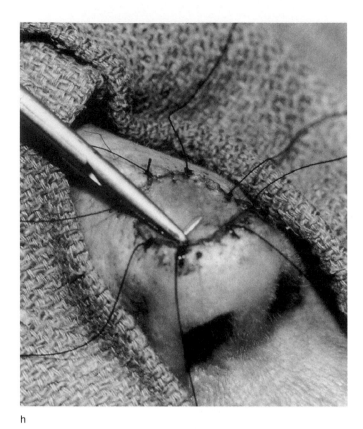

h

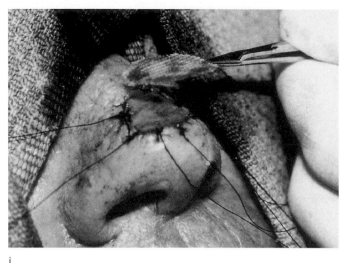

i

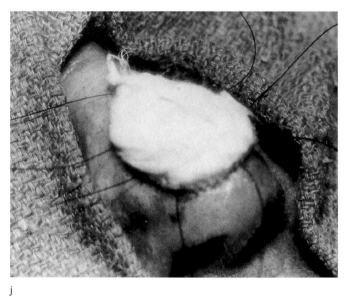

j

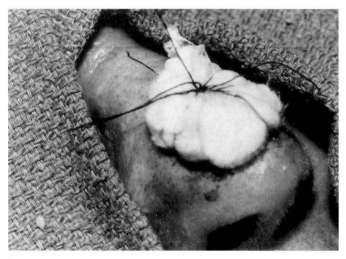

k

Figure 25-2 (*Cont.*) *(h)* running 6–0 fast absorbable suture being placed; *(i)* nonadherent dressing with antibiotic ointment being placed onto graft; *(j)* sterile cotton balls soaked in saline in place; *(k)* tie-over dressing completed prior to trimming excess suture.

PERIOPERATIVE MANAGEMENT

Specific instructions for postoperative care should be reviewed with each patient. These instructions should address:

1. Acceptable activity: Certain activity may be inappropriate for graft location. Extremities should be elevated with no dangling to help prevent swelling. The patient should avoid heavy lifting and vigorous activity to reduce perspi-

ration and increased humidity which favor bacterial infection.
2. Diet: If the lip or cheek is involved, the patient should avoid vigorous chewing. This might stimulate oozing under the graft.
3. Wound care: If the patient will be changing the dressing, demonstrating the procedure to the person responsible for care or the patient with the aid of a mirror may reduce confusion of care at home.

4. Cleaning technique:
   a. The periphery of the bolster where it contacts the skin may be cleansed of any dried serum by using cotton-tipped applicators (Q-Tips) and hydrogen peroxide in a gentle rolling motion.
   b. The excess peroxide is removed with another cotton-tipped applicator in a rolling motion.
   c. A thin film of antibiotic ointment is then applied at the bolster-skin junction, again by using a cotton-tipped applicator.
   d. The bolster is then covered with a Band-Aid or cut gauze and taped for additional protection.
5. Medications: Any postoperative medication such as pain medicine or antibiotics should be outlined, including potential side effects. Decisions when to restart any discontinued medications (e.g., aspirin, NSAIDs) should be reviewed.
6. Follow-up: Follow-up visits to inspect the graft and donor site should be scheduled. These will vary depending on distance from the facility for the patient, difficulty of the procedure, and individual patient setting. If the physician is concerned regarding a patient's ability to care for the operative site, frequent postoperative visits may be necessary. One should stress to the patient that his or her actions directly affect graft survival and ultimate appearance.
7. Removal of bolster dressing: Typically, this is done in 5 to 7 days. One easy technique includes:
   a. Moisten the cotton ball contour layer with hydrogen peroxide by using a syringe and an 18- to 21-gauge needle.
   b. Cut the tie-over sutures and peel them away from the graft edge.
   c. Using a moistened cotton-tipped applicator to stabilize the skin edge, gently elevate the edge of the bolster off the graft. If it sticks, soaking with normal saline or peroxide will help loosen the dressing off the graft.
8. Review graft appearance: Grafts take time to mature and completely take. Thus, the initial cosmetic appearance may be discolored and have contour irregularity. Reviewing the graft's color and contour and the future expectations of the patient is essential. Initially grafts may be pink, redish blue, or dusky. Darker colors may indicate superficial epidermal and dermal loss. However, the deeper papillary and reticular dermis may be viable. One must resist temptation and not debride these darker and sometimes mushy grafts. Even soupy, mushy grafts may "pink up" and should not be debrided. They should be managed conservatively with gentle cleaning, antibiotic ointment, and protection. Full-thickness loss of graft may be indicated by necrotic black tissue. Should a graft be lost, it is best not to debride away the necrotic tissue as this functions as an ideal biologic Band-Aid. Decisions regarding delayed grafting or revisions may be planned later. Finally, do not abandon patients with unfavorable outcomes. Frequent follow-up and a good patient-physician relationship with open communication will help to steady unfavorable results.

BASTING SUTURES

There are three techniques of placing basting sutures.

1. Blind placement: The suture is placed through the graft into the wound bed, then exits the graft in a single motion. While blind placement is technically the easiest, one risk is striking important neural or vascular structures in the wound bed with resultant bleeding. This may require removing the graft to effect hemostasis.
2. Direct visualization of needle placement using conventional suture:[25]
   Step a. The graft is trimmed and tailored for the defect.
   Step b. One side of the graft is secured using tacking or interrupted graft sutures. This ensures proper placement of basting sutures.
   Step c. The opposite side of the graft is elevated and basting suture sites in the wound are directly visualized.
   Step d. The needle is then passed through the graft into the wound bed under direct visualization and exits the wound bed. The suture is then completed by passing the needle back through the graft and the knot is secured. Regular fast-absorbing suture or nonabsorbable suture material may be used.
3. Double-armed basting suture placement:[26]
   Steps a and b are repeated.
   Step c. The graft is rotated on its hinged sutures away from the recipient bed.
   Step d. The basting suture site is then selected and a double-armed suture is placed in the recipient bed under direct visualization.
   Step e. The graft is then redraped over the wound, the needles are then strategically placed through the graft, and the knot is secured. Double-armed sutures yield precise placement; however, they are more costly and only one basting suture is available from each suture pack. Figure 25-3a–e illustrates placement of abasting suture under direct visualization.

DELAYED GRAFTING

Placement of a graft immediately after soft-tissue surgery may not be possible if exposed bone or cartilage is present. Intact undisturbed perichondrium or periosteum must be in place to supply vascularity to the graft. If exposed cartilage or bone exists, one may delay grafting until sufficient granulation tissue covers the exposed cartilage or bony surface.[27] This may take 2 weeks or longer, depending upon the size of the exposed surface. On ear defects with exposed cartilage, one may access granulation tissue from the opposite side of the ear by removing small 2- to 3-mm cylinders of cartilage

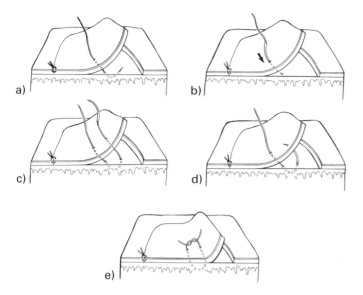

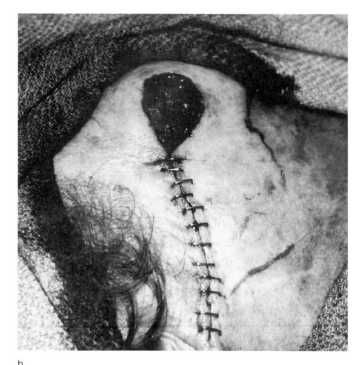

Figure 25-3 *(a)* FTSG placed over surgical defect with a tacking suture securing one end of the graft. Basting suture placement (under direct visualization) beginning with the basting suture needle passing first through graft, then wound. *(b)* Basting suture needle exiting wound bed. *(c)* Basting suture needle exiting wound bed and passing through graft. *(d)* Basting suture circuit completed. *(e)* Basting suture securely tied.

using a disposable skin biopsy punch. Care must be taken not to punch through the skin on the opposite side. The wound is then managed with daily cleaning, antibiotic ointment, and a nonstick dressing. The cartilage or bone must never be left uncovered without ointment as this will result in desiccation of the exposed tissue. When adequate granulation tissue is present, the wound is ready for grafting. At that time, devitalized tissue and any coagulum should be removed by light currettement. Also, a 1- to 2-mm margin at the periphery is excised away to expose well-vascularized tissue to facilitate capillary ingrowth.

BUROW'S GRAFTS

Burow's grafts are full-thickness grafts in which the donor area is immediately adjacent to the surgical defect. A thorough review of this topic has been well illustrated.[28] Burow's grafts are analogous to Burow's triangles excised as extra tissue protrusions (dog-ears). They have also been referred to as *island grafts*.[29] The advantages of Burow's grafts are that the improved color, texture, and actinic change match with the surrounding skin as compared with distant donor sites.

Surgical technique is not very different from that previously described. The donor site is selected immediately adja-

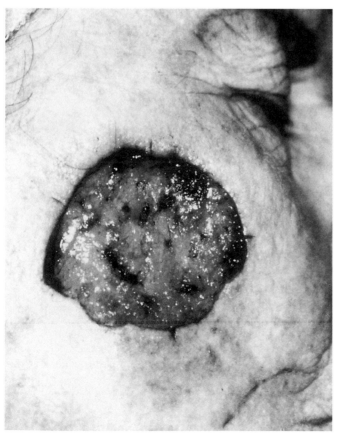

a

b

Figure 25-4 Burow's graft. *(a)* Defect right cheek (*Note:* gentian violet marking surgical scars on inferior portion of cheek, making blood supply for flaps uncertain). Donor site is lateral to surgical defect; *(b)* donor site removed, closed side to side, tension free with resulting defect smaller than initial defect. (*Continued*)

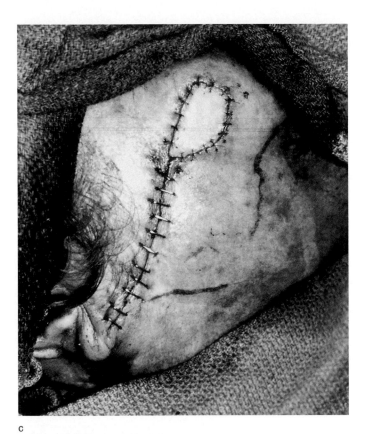

c

d

Figure 25-4 (*Cont.*) (*c*) graft secured into position; (*d*) appearance 2 months postoperatively.

cently to the surgical defect and preferably within the same cosmetic unit. The donor site should be of sufficient size and shape such that once harvested, the edge of the graft closest to the defect is advanced into the defect to coapt with the opposite side of the defect. The distal and midaspects of the graft are then moved proximally toward the defect. The donor site most distal to the graft is then closed in a side-to-side fashion, securing the fit. When performed on the mid- and

distal nose, the proximal aspect of the graft adjacent to the surgical defect should fan out slightly laterally to equal the diameter of the wound and not come off too narrowly. This compensates for the limited tissue mobility in the area. Figures 25-4*a–d* highlights Burrow's graft tissue movement.

GRAFT FAILURE

FTSG success rates should be very high. It is rare that a full-thickness graft fails to take on the head and neck area. The most frequent causes of graft failure are hematoma formation and graft-bed contact disruption or movement. Infection is an infrequent cause of full-thickness graft failure. Less than meticulous technique characterized by excessive necrotic debris left in the surgical wound, persistent oozing, folding of the graft, and desiccation of the graft prior to placement are causes that hopefully can be avoided.

COMPLICATIONS

Bleeding is a postoperative complication that must be evaluated immediately. It is difficult to quantitate the volume of blood the patient sees, as the bolster may absorb blood and the graft may float off the recipient bed. One must inspect the graft. If active bleeding exists, the graft should be taken off and hemostasis accomplished. This may require suture, spot electrodesiccation, pressure, liquid thrombin, or, if uncontrollable, inpatient management and appropriate consultation. Bleeding can be prevented by meticulous technique, use of liquid thrombin, and preoperative evaluation to eliminate any reversible potential causes (i.e., chronic aspirin use, coagulation problems, etc.). Milia and cyst formation are not infrequently seen and are treated with simple incision and drainage. Graft hypertrophy is managed with massage and intralesional steroids. Contour irregularity may be improved with spot dermabrasion of the graft and the immediate surrounding area. Pigmentation, scaling, and erythema may be concealed with cosmetics. Graft contraction may be improved with massage or if marked may require revision and placement of a second graft.

REFERENCES

1. Converse JM, Rapaport FT: The vascularization of skin autografts and homografts: An experimental study in man. *Ann Surg* **143**:306, 1956

2. Converse JM et al: Plasmic circulation in skin grafts. *Plast Reconstr Surg* **43**:495, 1969

3. Vistnes LM: Grafting of skin. *Surg Clin North Am* **57**:939, 1977

4. Smahel J: The healing of skin grafts. *Clin Plast Surg* **4**:409, 1977

5. Clemmesen T: The early circulation in split thickness grafts. *Acta Chir Scand* **124:**11, 1962

6. Clemmesen T: Experimental studies on the healing of free skin autogafts. *Dan Med Bull* **14**(suppl):11, 1967

7. Burleson R, Ersman B: Nature of the bond between partial thickness skin and wound granulation. *Am Surg* **177:**181, 1973

8. Teh BF: Why do skin grafts fail? *Plast Reconstr Surg* **63:**223, 1979

9. Birch J, Branemark PL: The vascularization of a free full thickness skin graft: A vital microscope study. *Scand J Plast Reconstr Surg* **3:**1, 1969

10. Holler JA, Billinghom RE: Studies of the origin of the vasculature in free skin grafts. *Ann Surg* **166:**896, 1967

11. Peer LA, Waller JC: The behavior of autogenous human tissue grafts. *Plast Reconstr Surg* **7:**6, 1951

12. Zarem HA et al: Development of microcirculation in full thickness autogenous skin grafts in mice. *Am J Physiol* **212:**1081, 1967

13. Ljungvist A, Almgard IE: The vascular reaction in the free skin allo and autografts. *Acta Pathol Microbiol Scand* **68:**553, 1966

14. Wolff K, Schellander FG: Enzyme histochemical studies on the healing process of split thickness skin grafts. *J Invest Dermatol* **45:**38, 1965

15. Converse JM et al: Vascularization of split thickness skin autografts in the Rat. *Transplantation* **3:**22, 1965

16. McGregor IA, Conway H: Development of lymph flow from autografts and homografts of skin. *Transplant Bull* **3:**46, 1956

17. Waris T et al: Reinnervation of human skin grafts: A histochemical study. *Plast Reconstr Surg* **72:**439, 1983

18. Fitzgerald MJT et al: Innervation of skin grafts. *Surg Gynecol Obstet* **124:**8080, 1967

19. Poten B: Grafted skin: Observation on innervation and other qualities. *Acta Chir Scand Suppl* **257:**1, 1960

20. Rudolph R: Imbibition of myofibroblasts by skin grafts. *Plast Reconstr Surg* **63:**473, 1979

21. Bertolami CN, Donoff RB: The effect of full thickness skin grafts on the actomyosin content of contracting wounds. *J Oral Surg* **37:**471, 1979

22. Bertolami CN, Donoff RB: The effect of skin grafting upon prolyl hydroxylase and hyaluronidase activities in mammalian wound repair. *J Surg Res* **27:**359, 1979

23. Breach, NM: Pre-auricular full-thickness skin grafts. *Br J Plast Surg* **31:**124, 1978

24. Hill TG: Enhancing the survival of full thickness grafts. *J Dermatol Surg Oncol* **10:**639, 1984

25. Adenot J, Salsche SJ: Visualized basting sutures in the application of full thickness skin grafts. *J Dermatol Surg Oncol* **13:**1236, 1987

26. Kent DE, Greenway H: *Double Armed Basting Suture for Precise Skin Graft Placement.* Presented at the Annual Meeting of the American College of Mohs Surgeons, Am Coll Mohs Surg, Castle Harbor, Bermuda, Apr 28, 1987

27. Ceilley RI et al: Delayed skin grafting. *J Dermatol Surg Oncol* **9:**288, 1983

28. Zitelli JA: Burow's grafts. *J Am Acad Dermatol* **17:**271, 1987

29. Chester EL Jr: Closure of a surgical defect in a nose using island grafts from the nose. *J Dermatol Surg Oncol* **8:**990, 1982

Roy C. Grekin

26 Flap Surgery

In 1991 the American Council on Graduate Medical Education (ACGME) officially recognized training in flap and graft surgery as part of the surgical curriculum in the standard dermatology residency. Dermatologists had long been training in and performing these procedures, backed by a solid foundation in the basic education apropos to these skills. These basics include but are not limited to knowledge of the anatomy of the skin and underlying soft tissues, wound-healing, complications and their management, cutaneous oncology, anesthesia techniques, and precautions against infections. These essential areas are covered in numerous dermatologic texts, including this one. This chapter will concern itself with a discussion of the fundamental concepts of cutaneous flap surgery. The basics of tissue movement will be described, relative to those flaps pertinent to dermatologic surgery, followed by an algorithmic approach to flap selection.

DEFINITIONS

A universally understood vocabulary is important in the discussion of any topic. In flap surgery there are definitions and terms which must be understood and uniformly applied for effective instruction, communication between physicians, and appropriate documentation.

A *primary defect* is the surgical wound created by excision of a lesion; it is the object of the closure.

The *secondary defect* is the wound resulting from moving surrounding tissue into a primary defect. Location of the secondary defect and the ability to close it are critical concepts in flap surgery. Closure of the secondary defect may be used to manipulate lines of tension in the surgical site.

Primary motion describes the type and direction of tissue movement by the skin flap necessary to cover the primary defect.

Secondary motion is the reaction of the surrounding skin to the primary motion of the flap. It is absolutely essential to understand and assess the effects of secondary motion on the position and function of nearby anatomic structures when choosing and designing a flap.

The *pedicle* connects the flap to the surrounding tissue; it is also called the *base* of the flap. Survival of the flap is dependent upon blood flow across the flap. Placement and size of the base must take into account local arterial blood flow into the flap as well as venous and lymphatic drainage.

The *key suture* is generally, though not always, the first suture placed when a flap is moved into position. It both aligns the flap over the primary defect and redirects the tension of the closure toward the secondary defect.

CLASSIFICATION

Flaps may be classified based on a number of systems. An understanding of these systems and adherence to a uniform and consistent nomenclature is important for documentation and communication purposes.

In the most general sense, flaps may be classified by location. Thus, flaps may be described as being local, distant, or free flaps. *Local* flaps come from within the same or an adjacent cosmetic unit. *Distant* flaps are recruited from nonadjacent skin. Because the skin of the flap is transposed over intervening skin of one or more cosmetic units, these flaps are executed in two or more stages. After a local blood supply is developed in the flap, the pedicle is severed and returned to its initial site. *Free* flaps represent a combination of characteristics between flaps and grafts. They are excised at a distant site along with a named (major) artery and completely severed from the skin as in harvesting a graft. The free skin is then sewn into the primary defect anastomosing the artery to a major artery in the surrounding skin. The transplanted skin thus carries its own blood supply analogous to flaps.

Flaps may also be classified according to their blood supply. *Axial* pattern flaps are based on a named (major) artery. Their advantage is that of a more secure blood supply. This allows the surgeon to harvest larger flaps with smaller width/length ratios. They are generally reserved for large defects or for performing distant repairs requiring long pedicled flaps. *Random* pattern flaps are not based on any specific artery. They are most successful in richly vascularized regions, particularly the head and neck, or when small flaps are performed in other areas. Because of the lack of a defined blood supply, there are restrictions on the size of the flap and on the width/length ratios considered safe for optimum flap survival. These will be discussed in detail below.

A final classification is based on the type of flap movement. *Advancement* flaps are slid in a linear fashion from adjacent skin into the primary defect. *Rotation* flaps are slid in an arcuate manner into the surgical defect. *Transposition* flaps are cut, elevated, and rotated over intervening tissue into the defect. Transposition flaps are sometimes moved more than one cosmetic unit away from their harvest site, essentially bridging over the intervening skin. These *staged flaps* or *pedicle flaps* require at least two steps. The first stage moves tissue into the primary defect, with the relatively bulky pedicle spanning over normal skin. In 3 to 4 weeks, an adequate local blood supply develops in the flap tip, and the pedicle is severed and discarded or replaced to its original position.

In dermatologic surgery the most commonly employed flaps are local, random pattern flaps that either are advanced, rotated, or transposed into the primary defect. The remainder of this chapter will focus on each of these flaps individually, stressing basic design concepts, surgical execution, and areas of specific utility supported by clinical examples. This discussion is intended to be foundational and cannot supplant the need for hands-on instruction and proctored experience.

ADVANCEMENT FLAPS

Advancement flaps are often considered the simplest flaps due to their linear, uncomplicated movement pattern; however, no flap should ever be thought of as "simple." Such underestimation can result in poor aesthetic results or flap failure due to design- and execution-related complications.

Advancement flaps are sliding flaps. They may also be thought of as pulling flaps as they are moved into the primary defect by a pulling motion. The direction of movement is linear (Fig. 26-1). As a result, the secondary motion or tension is also linear and opposite in direction to the primary movement. This is important to remember when working near free margins such as the eyelids, nasal alar rim, or lips. If a flap is advanced directly up to or down to such a margin in perpendicular fashion, the force of the secondary motion may pull down upon or elevate the cosmetically and functionally important

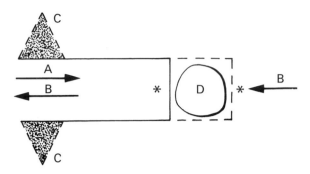

Figure 26-1 Schematic of advancement flap. (*A*) Primary motion; (*B*) secondary motion; (*C*) dog-ear removals; (*D*) primary defect; * = key suture.

margins. Advancement flaps are generally best moved across such anatomic features parallel to their long axis.

For random pattern advancement flaps, an adequate pedicle must be maintained to ensure the blood supply to the distal flap tip. In general, a 3:1 length/width ratio is considered safe. In areas of rich vascular supply, such as the helix of the ear or nasal dorsum, 4:1 length/width ratios are safely achieved. At times the length, configuration, and location of a defect and the elasticity and extensibility of surrounding tissue do not allow for adequate flap length to fill the defect. In these situations the defect can be widened to allow for a wider and therefore longer flap, or double advancement flaps may be employed as discussed below.

Once designed and cut, the flap is undermined in a mid-subcutaneous fatty plane (Fig. 26-2*b*). Enough fat must be maintained to protect the blood supply and fill the defect but not so much as to create a bulky or "pincushion" appearance. The undermining should be continued 1 to 2 cm beyond the base of the flap and around the edges to facilitate movement.

The key suture pulls the flap across and closes the primary defect. It is best placed in the center of the advancing distal flap margin and then into the far edge of the defect (Figs. 26-1 and 26-2*c*). Some texts will demonstrate key suture placement in the corners of the flap. Since the key suture is a tension-bearing stitch, corner placement may stress blood flow into these areas, resulting in tip necrosis.

Movement of the flap creates two wounds of unequal length along each side of the flap. The inside flap margin (base of flap to tip of flap) is shorter in length than the outside margin (base of flap to distal edge of defect). This creates a tissue redundancy and protrusion (i.e., dog-ear) along the outside margin on the sides of the closure. Besides creating aesthetic problems, it also inhibits flap movement, increasing tension on the distal wound. Removal of the dog-ears is accomplished by one or both of two methods. In larger wounds and in areas of greater tissue elasticity the excess tissue may be shared along the length of the wound. By employing the "rule of halves," the surgeon can "reef" redundant tissue along the outer wound edges, resulting in a smooth flat closure. This method does not facilitate flap movement.

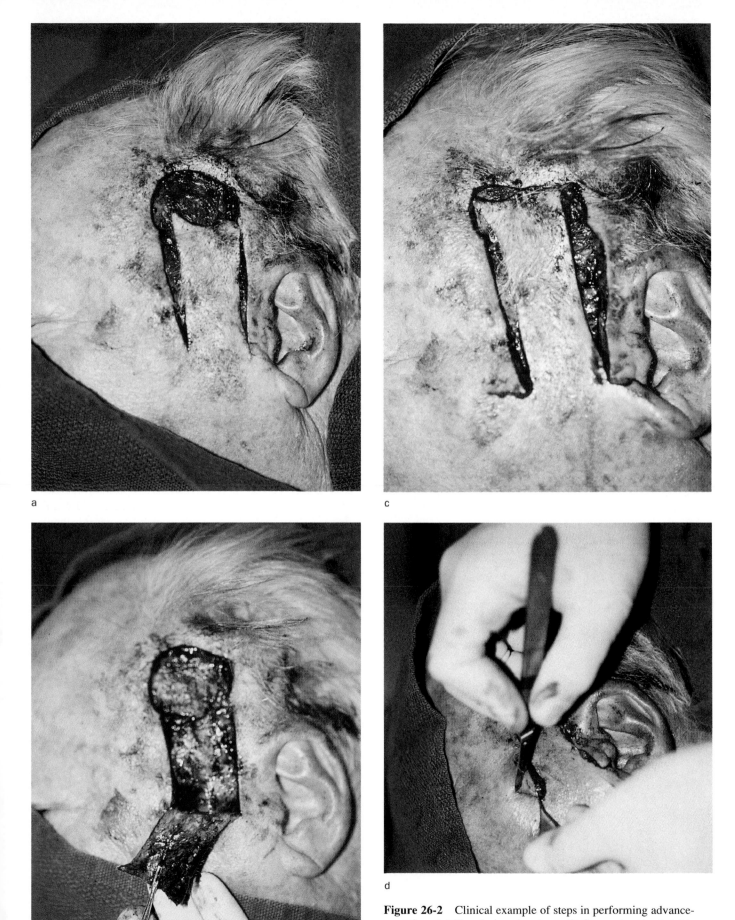

Figure 26-2 Clinical example of steps in performing advancement flap. (*a*) Flap designed and cut; (*b*) flap undermined; (*c*) key suture placed; (*d*) dog-ear removal;

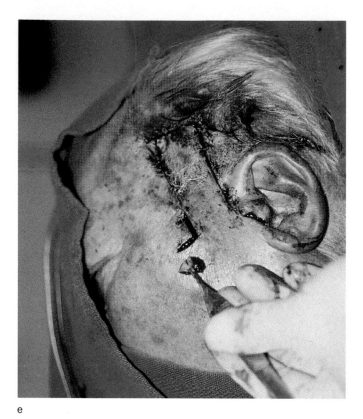

e

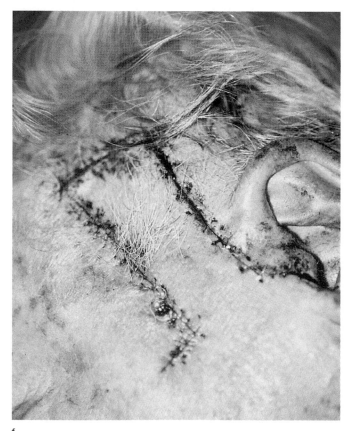

f

Figure 26-2   (continued) (*e*) dog-ear removal; (*f*) final closure appearance.

The second dog-ear repair method is to remove small triangles of tissue from the outer margin to shorten its length. The triangles may be excised from anywhere along the wound length and should be placed where best camouflaged in skin tension lines or anatomic borders. When placed at the base of the flap, the dog-ear repair has its greatest effect on improved flap movement (Figs. 26-1 and 26-2*d–e*). The first cut is best made right at the base of the flap and extended away from the flap creating an L-incision. With appropriate undermining, the skin along the side of the flap can be elevated and the excess outer edge skin will overlap the L-incision. Where the excess skin aligns with this *L* it is excised, completing the dog-ear repair.

Advancement flaps are most useful in areas of good tissue extensibility and elasticity. These include the cheek (Fig. 26-3), preauricular region, lips, and chin. They are also indicated in areas of pronounced linear skin tension lines or cosmetic borders. The forehead, nasal dorsum (Fig. 26-4), and helix of the ear represent such sites. There are several variations on the basic advancement flap design. These will be covered in greater detail in subsequent chapters covering regional repairs. These variations include the double advancement flap (H-plasty), single-arm advancement (Burow's wedge advancement), bilateral single-arm advancement flaps ("O-T" or "A-T"), and island pedicle advancement flaps.

H-plasty and O-T variations are used when a single flap cannot cover a defect without excessive tension or in areas of poor blood supply. They also have the advantage of limiting effects on surrounding structures as each flap cancels the secondary motion of the other by pulling in the opposite direction (Fig. 26-5). The H-plasty is therefore particularly useful around the eyebrows (Fig. 26-6) to maintain the precise location of these structures.

The single-arm (Burow's wedge) advancement and its doubled counterpart, the O-T closure, have the added advantage of improved cosmetic camouflage (Fig. 26-7). As only one incision is made, it is more easily hidden along cosmetic borders such as the nasolabial fold and supraalar crease for nasal sidewall repair (Fig. 26-8) and the vermilion border for upper lip repair (Fig. 26-9). The single-arm advancement flaps have a very broad base and are therefore extremely safe, well-vascularized flaps. The O-T double advancement flaps are useful to limit secondary motion effects or when one flap cannot cover the defect (Fig. 26-10).

The island pedicle flap is conceptually more difficult to grasp. Its advantage is that it is smaller than a standard advancement flap and when used in properly selected areas is more easily camouflaged. Unlike other advancement flaps, the island pedicle is not only pulled but also pushed into place over the primary defect by a V-Y closure of the secondary defect. This minimizes the effects of secondary motion on the tissues surrounding the primary defect. These flaps require a good underlying fat layer for both adequate movement and blood supply. They are most useful on the lateral upper lip, lateral malar prominences, and inferior nasal sidewall above

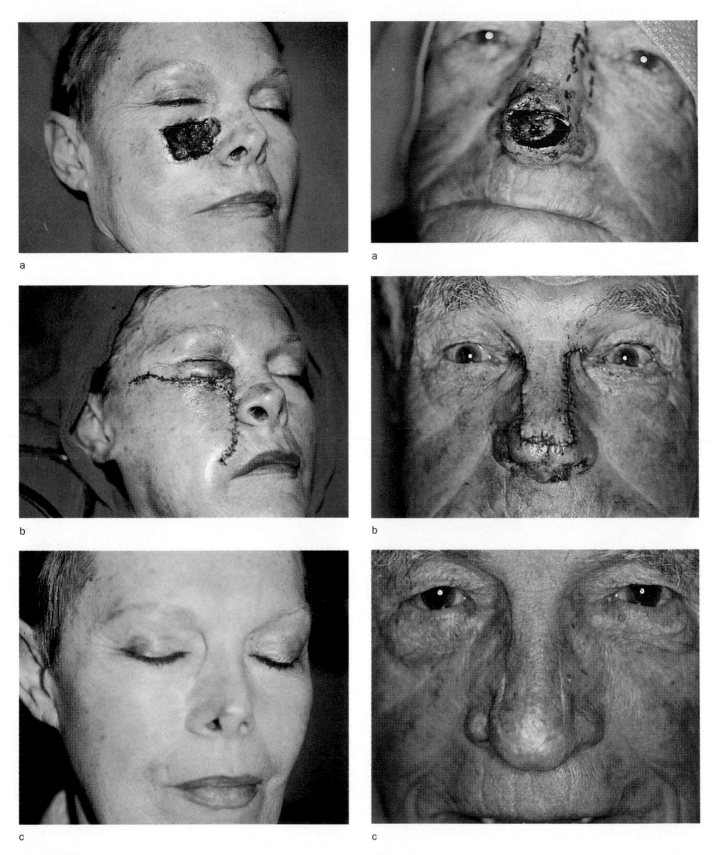

Figure 26-3 Clinical example of cheek advancement flap. (*a*) Defect; (*b*) flap sutured in place; (*c*) result at six months.

Figure 26-4 Clinical example of nasal dorsum advancement flap. (*a*) Defect with flap designed; (*b*) flap sutured in place; (*c*) result at six months.

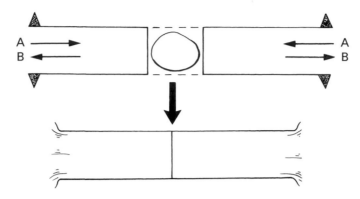

Figure 26-5 Schematic of H-plasty (double advancement flaps). (*A*) Primary motion; (*B*) secondary monion. Note that forces cancel each other.

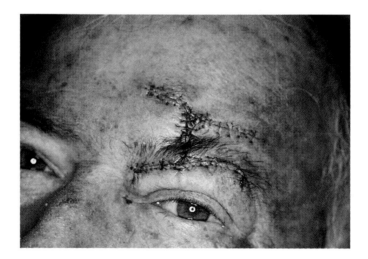

Figure 26-6 Clinical example of H-plasty involving eyebrow skin.

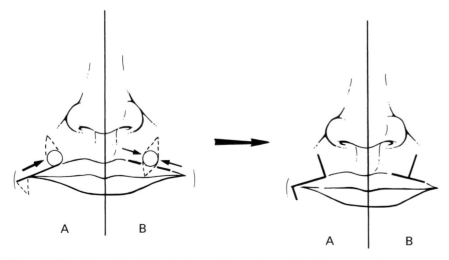

Figure 26-7 Schematic of (*A*) single-arm (Burrow's wedge) advancement flap, and (*B*) O-T double advancement flaps.

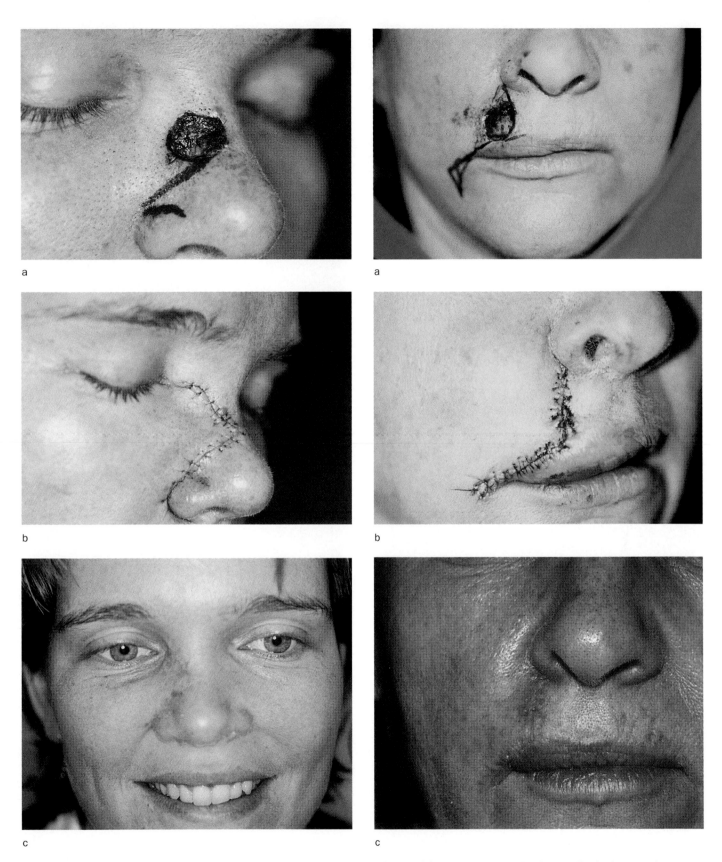

Figure 26-8 Clinical example of nasal single-arm advancement flap. (*a*) Defect with flap designed; (*b*) flap sutured in place; (*c*) result at one month.

Figure 26-9 Clinical example of upper lip single-arm advancement flap. (*a*) Defect with flap designed; (*b*) flap sutured in place; (*c*) result at three months.

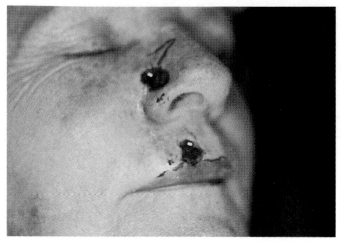

a

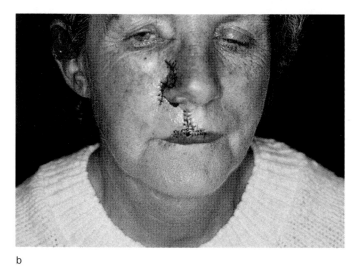

b

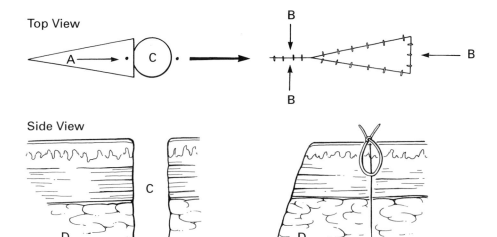

c

Figure 26-10   Clinical example of O-T double advancement flaps on upper lip. (*a*) Defect with flaps designed; (*b*) flaps sutured in place; (*c*) result at one month.

Figure 26-11   Schematic of island pedicle flap; top and side view. (*A*) Primary motion; (*B*) secondary motion; (*C*) primary defect; (*D*) fat columnar pedicle.

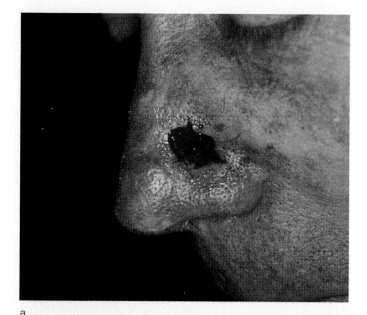

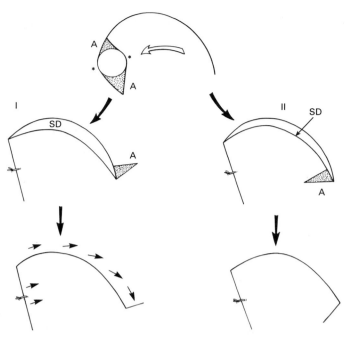

Figure 26-13   Schematic of rotation flap. Key: ⇒ = primary motion; * = key suture; A = dog-ear removals; SD = secondary defect; → = secondary motion; (I) classic flap and dog-ear removal; (II) backcut demonstrated (note narrowed base).

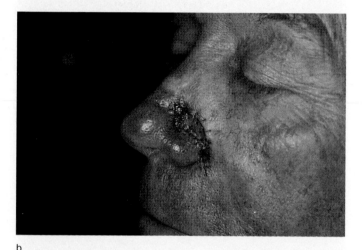

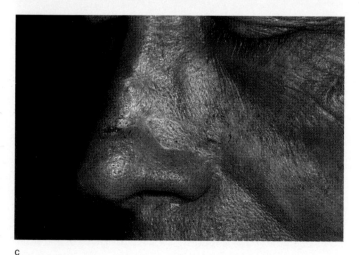

Figure 26-12   Clinical example of island pedicle flap on nasal sidewall. (*a*) Defect; (*b*) flap sutured in place; (*c*) result at three months.

the supraalar crease. On the surface they appear as a graft because the flaps are designed as triangular islands of skin, with their flat base being the lateral edge of the primary defect (Fig. 26-11). Unlike other flaps, the flap is not undermined. Rather, the incisions defining the flap are carried straight down through the fat to muscle fascia. This creates a pedicle or column of fat beneath the skin. The distal portion of the flap is tapered to a triangular point with an approximate 30° angle. The outer edges of this cut are sutured together side to side, forcing the triangular flap forward on its fatty pedicle into the primary defect (Fig. 26-12). Again, survival and movement depend on the volume and length of the fat pedicle, and therefore these flaps are restricted to areas with good fatty layers. The forehead and nasal dorsum are risky sites for this flap.

ROTATION FLAPS

The rotation flap is also a sliding flap that is pulled into position across the primary defect. It differs from the advancement flap in part by the direction of its primary motion and therefore by the forces of its secondary motion. The primary motion describes an arc of a circle as opposed to the straight line of a classic advancement flap. The secondary motion is directed tangentially along that arc of rotation away from the primary defect (Fig. 26-13).

Design of a rotation flap is slightly more complex than that

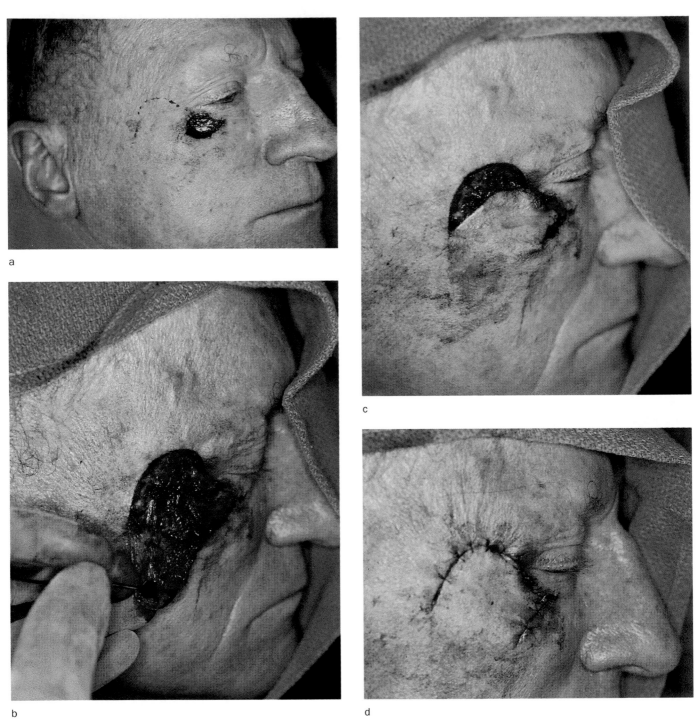

Figure 26-14 Clinical example of steps in performing a rotation flap. (*a*) Defect; (*b*) flap cut and undermined; (*c*) flap rotated into place, creating secondary defect; (*d*) closure complete.

of an advancement flap. As with all random pattern flaps, survival of a rotation flap depends in part on the adequacy of its pedicle. Another important consideration, however, is that the degree of force of the secondary motion is inversely proportional to the flap/defect size ratio. In other words, the larger the flap in relation to the defect, the less the stress will be on

tissue and structures surrounding the defect. For these two reasons, rotation flaps tend to be large, particularly around free margins (e.g., lower eyelids). In areas of lesser tissue extensibility they must also be cut large, such as on the forehead, scalp, or dorsal hands. A general rule of thumb when designing rotation flaps is to consider the flap and defect as a half circle (Fig. 26-13). The flap/defect size ratio should be 3:1 or 4:1 to ensure adequate blood supply across the pedicle and to limit stresses due to secondary motion. As expertise is gained, the surgeon will learn how to manipulate these ratios depending on the region involved and factors of differing elasticity, extensibility, and free margins.

The flap should be cut and undermined to a depth as previously described for advancement flaps. The undermining is carried beyond the base of the flap and around the edges of the flap and the primary defect for 1 to 2 cm (depending on size of the defect and local anatomy). The key suture is placed through the center of the leading edge of the flap and is anchored into the far edge of the primary defect, thus pulling the flap across the defect and closing it (Figs. 26-14b–d). Using the tip of the flap as depicted in some texts to place the key suture should be avoided to prevent strangulation and necrosis.

The flap may be envisioned as rotating around an axis located at the proximal base in relation to the primary defect. Its degree of movement and resulting tension of the secondary motion are in part determined by forces related to the distal base of the defect which exerts a tethering effect on the flap. Attachment of the flap at this point determines the limits of movement. If there is too much tension across either the primary or secondary defect, this may be relieved by one or more of several methods. The first is simply to undermine farther beyond the edges of the flap and defect in all directions. The second is to enlarge the flap by extending the arcuate excision from the distal base. The third is to perform a back cut. This technique involves cutting *into* the base of the flap at its tethering point [base of flap farthest from the primary defect (Fig. 26-13)]. A small cut is made first and then the flap is tested for improved movement. The back cut changes the tethering point, moving it closer to the primary defect. This is an effective maneuver but risks limiting blood supply to the flap by narrowing the base.

Once the flap is placed across the primary defect, the secondary defect becomes apparent along the outer arc of the flap. In general this will appear as a crescentic tissue gap (Fig. 26-14c). The rotation flap is designed such that the tension of the repair is transferred from the primary defect to closure of the secondary defect. The surgeon must take this into account for the design, location, and orientation of the defect.

In general, rotation flaps require two dog-ear repairs. The first tissue redundancy is along the outer edge of the crescentic secondary defect; this is a longer wound length than the inner edge. It may be sewn out by the rule of halves in some cases. More often the outer arc is shortened by removal of a triangle of tissue from anywhere along the outer arc, preferably in a site well camouflaged (Fig. 26-13).

The second tissue protrusion occurs at the base of the primary defect at the axis point of the rotating flap. Whenever tissue rotates about itself, a bunching effect occurs which inhibits rotation and outpouches, creating a poor aesthetic appearance. This excess tissue is removed by cutting a triangle or by M-plasty (Figs. 26-13 and 26-14c). It is important that the dog-ear repair be designed and cut directed away from the base of the flap so as not to compromise flap viability.

Rotation flaps are most useful in areas with arcuate cosmetic borders or arcing skin tension lines. These include the lateral forehead/temple regions (Fig. 26-15), cheeks, upper lip (Fig. 26-16), and chin. They are most easily employed in more elastic skin as they are pulling-type flaps. However, they are also useful in regions with very inelastic, nonextensible skin such as the scalp, nasal dorsum, and dorsal hands. In such skin, the flap must be cut large in comparison to the defect to minimize tension on the closure and facilitate closure of the secondary defect. Ratios exceeding 4:1 for flap/defect size are appropriate in such circumstances.

In some cases, tissue movement is not adequate even with large flap size/defect size ratios. In other instances (e.g., dorsal hand), there simply is not enough space to create a large flap to counteract poor tissue movement. And in still other situations, with a midline defect or defect bordering two cosmetic units, a single rotation flap may result in distortion of anatomic positioning of surrounding structures. In these cases, double rotation flaps may be used to effect closure while minimizing wound tension and preserving anatomic positioning. Double rotation flaps may follow the same arc of a circle—directly opposing one another or having their arcs extend from opposite poles of the defect—the so-called O-to-Z repair (Figs. 26-17 and 26-18). In both repairs, roughly half the wound is closed by each flap. They are smaller therefore than a single rotation flap used for the same defect. Their secondary motions counteract one another, negating effects on local anatomic positions. They may also aid in wound camouflage if designed well within skin tension lines or cosmetic borders.

TRANSPOSITION FLAPS

Transposition flaps are conceptually the most difficult of this group to design and execute. However, these efficient flaps offer a number of advantages to the surgeon performing facial repair. Transposition flaps are small compared to advancement and rotation flaps, generally equaling the size of the defect. They are pushed rather than pulled into the defect, which allows them to drape into place. This removes most forces of secondary movement from around the primary defect, transferring tension of the repair to the secondary defect. Thus they are ideal for use around free margins such as nasal alar rims and lower eyelids. Lastly, the geometric broken-line appearance of the incision lines may aid in the long-term camouflage of the wounds.

The primary motion of transposition flaps is one of rotation (Fig. 26-19). They differ from rotation flaps in that they are not sliding in nature; rather, they are cut, lifted, and then rotated over intervening tissue into the primary defect. As the flaps are essentially the same size as the defect, these flaps are

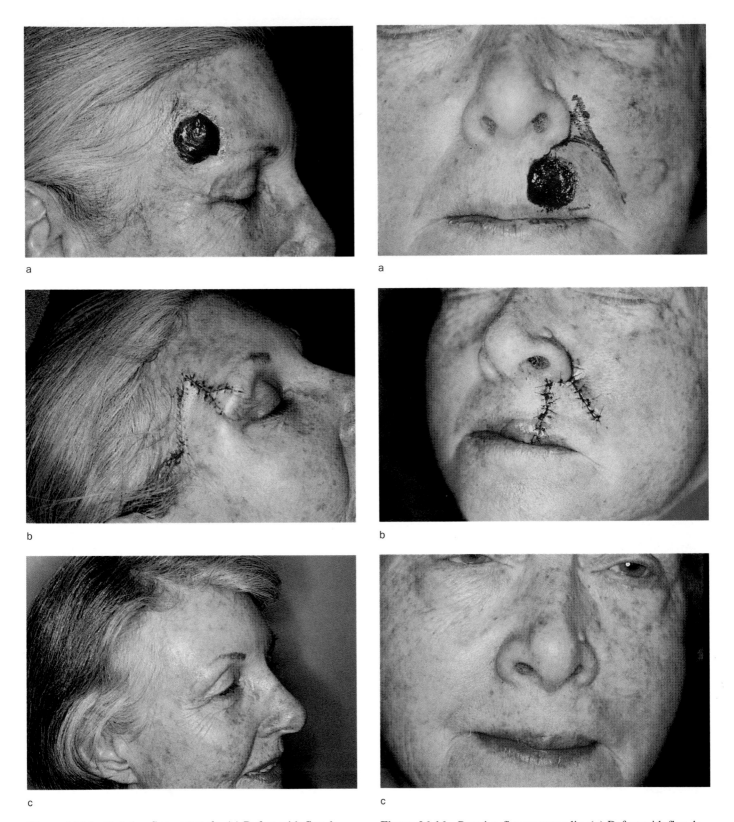

a

b

c

Figure 26-15 Rotation flap on temple. (*a*) Defect with flap designed; (*b*) flap rotated into place; (*c*) result at six months.

Figure 26-16 Rotation flap on upper lip. (*a*) Defect with flap designed; (*b*) flap rotated into place; (*c*) result at one year.

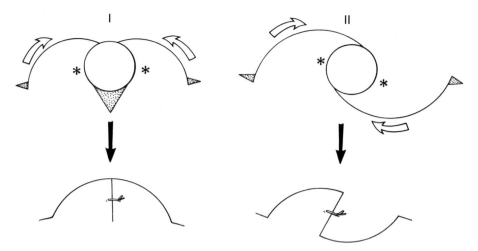

Figure 26-17   Schematics of (I) double rotation flaps and (II) O-Z double rotation flaps. ⇒ = Primary motion; * = key sutures; (shading) = dog-ear removals.

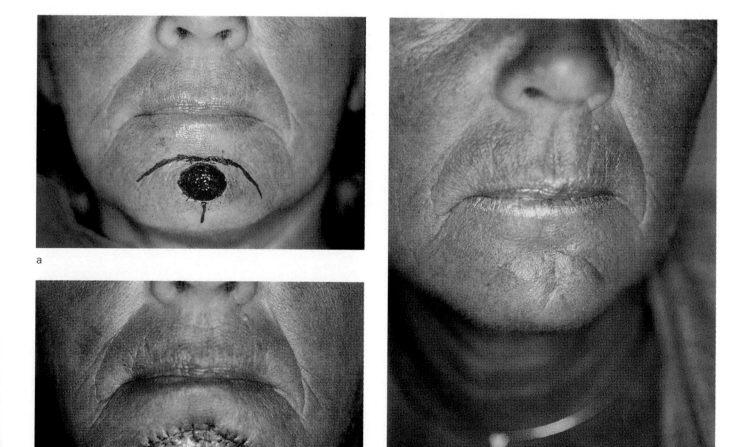

Figure 26-18   Double rotation flap on chin. (*a*) Defect with flap designed; (*b*) flaps rotated in place; (*c*) result at one month.

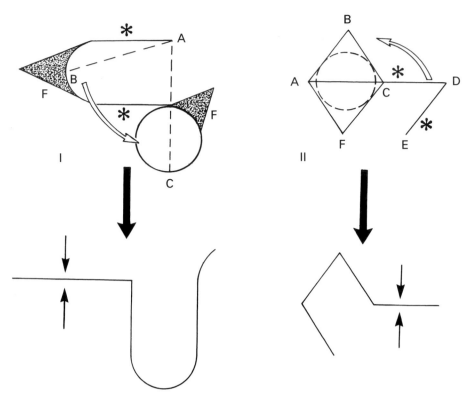

Figure 26-19 Schematic of transposition flap. (I) Banner flap. A-B = A-C. (II) Rhombic flap. A-B = C-D; ⇒ = Primary motion; * = key sutures; → = secondary motion; Shading = dog-ear removals.

economical in their tissue use and undermining when compared to the 3:1 and 4:1 flap/defect size ratios employed with advancement and rotation flaps. Transposition flaps also differ from advancement and rotation flaps in the forces behind their movement. Because of the 1:1 flap/defect size ratio, when the flap is elevated, the secondary defect thus created will equal the primary defect. The secondary defect will generally lie 45° to 90° from the main axis of the primary defect. The key suture in transposition flaps closes that secondary defect as opposed to sliding flaps where the key suture closes the primary defect. In so doing, the lifted flap is pushed into the primary defect and drapes across the wound. This draping action results in minimal to no tension about the primary defect. This renders these flaps ideal for use around free margins. The tension of these repairs, and therefore the secondary motion, occurs around the closure of the secondary defect. Placement of the secondary defect (i.e., harvesting of the flap) is a critical concept.

In determining from where to elevate a transposition flap, several factors must be considered. First, in dealing with noncircular wounds, the flap should always be designed off the short axis of the defect. Harvesting a transposition flap off the long axis results in a long narrow-pedicled flap. This configuration also requires excessive rotation of the flap, placing increased tension on the pedicle and further limiting blood supply. The next factor, and possibly the most important, is placement of the secondary defect in relation to surrounding anatomy. Since the tension of this repair, secondary motion, is across the secondary defect, the donor site must be situated such that the tensions of its closure parallel free margins (Fig. 26-20). The third factor is camouflage. The multiple geometric broken lines and the small flap size facilitate camouflage. However, this can be maximized by using cosmetic borders

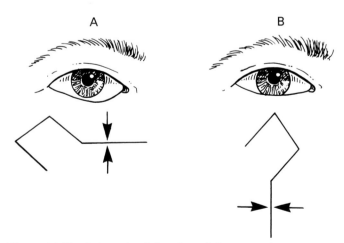

Figure 26-20 Schematic of direction of closure tension vectors for a rhombic transposition flap. (A) Incorrect location of secondary defect leads to secondary tension, which distorts the eyelid (ectropion). (B) Proper location of secondary defect results in secondary tension vectors that parallel lid margin.

and aligning these flaps as much as possible within skin tension lines. It is inherent in transposition flaps due to their 60° to 90° rotations that at least one closure line will cross rather than parallel the skin tension lines.

Once the key suture is placed closing the secondary defect and pushing the flap into the primary defect, the closure is essentially effected. Remaining work merely fine-tunes the flap to fit the defect, sutures the rest of the incision lines, and removes dog-ears. Dog-ears are somewhat variable and depend on the specific type of transposition flap used. There will always be one dog-ear at the point of rotation at the base of the primary defect. This should not be removed until the flap is in place. This redundant tissue created by rotation of the flap into the primary defect can be removed either by excision of a triangle of tissue or by M-plasty (Fig. 26-19). The second dog-ear at the secondary defect closure depends on the shape of the flap. Often it is designed into the flap when it is cut as in a nasolabial fold flap (Fig. 26-19).

Transposition flaps carry several different nominal designations. These are relative to their particular configuration or location and reflect on the efforts of surgeons to refine and improve transposition flap utilization. The classic banner-type transposition flap may therefore be termed a *glabellar turndown flap* or *nasolabial fold flap*. The rhombic flap is geometrically designed as a rhombus with 60° angles, while a 30° angle is half the size with angles facilitating easier closure of the secondary defect. The bilobed flap is a double-lobed flap allowing transfer of tissue from greater distances when required to reduce tension in closure of the secondary defect.

The banner flap is the classical design for transposition flaps (Figs. 26-19a and 26-21). It is a finger-shaped flap which generally rotates from 60° to 120° into the primary defect. Its width is the same as the primary defect; the length depends on the degree of rotation as flaps effectively shorten with greater rotational distances. Length can be determined by measuring the distance from the distal base of the flap to the far edge of the primary defect. It is wise to add a few millimeters to the length to make up for that lost due to rotation. Instead of designing a blunt-tipped flap, a 30° angle tip added will remove the need to repair a dog-ear at that closure point (Fig. 26-21). The flap should then be cut and undermined; this last step should be carried into tissues surrounding the flap margins. Undermining around the primary defect is controversial, but some believe it may lessen the problem of "pincushioning" of the flap (thickening). Following control of bleeders, the flap is elevated and the secondary defect closed side to side. This is the key suture in transposition flaps (with the exception of the bilobed flap for which the tertiary defect is closed first) and accounts for most of the secondary motion and tension in these closures. Closing the secondary defect pushes the flap across the primary defect. The flap is anchored in place, trimmed to fit, and then the dog-ear created at the axis of rotation removed in a fashion similar to that described for rotation flaps (Fig. 26-21b). These same closure steps apply to all transposition flaps.

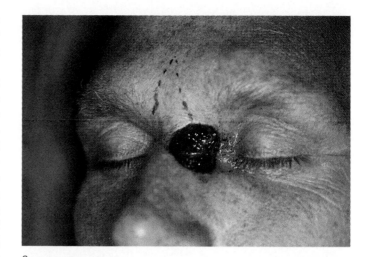

a

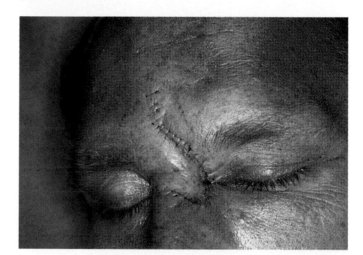

b

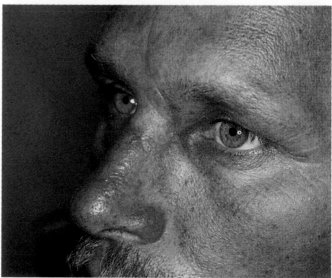

c

Figure 26-21 Clinical example of glabellar transposition flap. (*a*) Defect with flap designed; (*b*) flap sutured in place; (*c*) result at one month.

The rhombic and 30°-angle flaps are geometrically designed with well-defined sharp angles as compared to banner flaps. They are often shorter, and it is believed that their sharp angles and zigzagging lines create scars less well noticed by the human eye. The rhombic flap is designed by extending the short diameter of the defect through one obtuse angle of the rhombus (primary defect) for a distance equivalent to one side of the rhombus (Figs. 26-22a–b). A 60° angle is then made designing the far end of flap to parallel the near side of the rhombic defect in direction and length. After the surgeon cuts

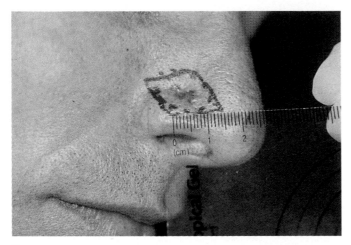

a

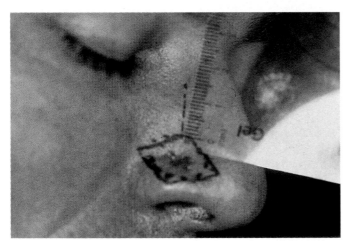

b

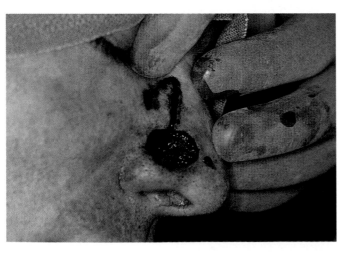

c

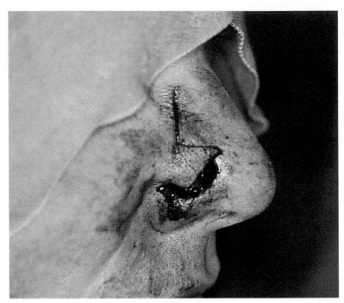

d

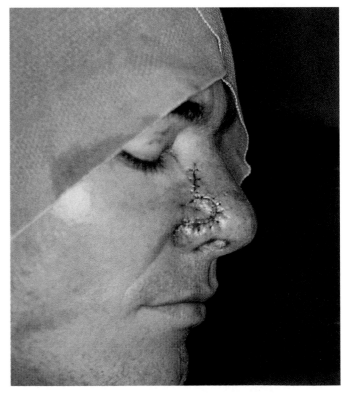

e

Figure 26-22 Clinical example of rhombic transposition flap. (*a*) Defect being measured; (*b*) flap measured; (*c*) flap cut; (*d*) key suture placed; (*e*) closure completed.

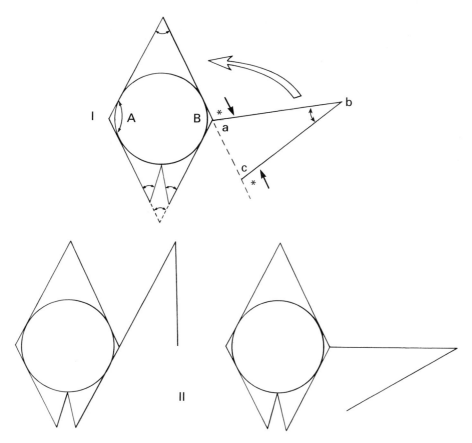

Figure 26-23 Schematic of 30°-angle transposition flap. (I) Correct design. * = key suture; ac = 1/2Aa; ab = AB; ⇒ = primary motion; → = secondary motion. (II) Incorrect design.

and undermines the defect, the key suture closes the secondary defect (Fig. 26-22*c–d*). Because 60° angles are not favorable closure angles, dog-ears will need repair at the tip of secondary defect and at the base of the rhombic primary defect. Circular defects can be closed with this flap by drawing the rhombus around, not within, the defect. Either the flap can be trimmed to fit the circular defect or the primary defect enlarged to accommodate the flap. Both options are acceptable and offer advantages relative to geometric broken-line camouflage versus tissue sparing.

The 30° angle flap was designed to provide more favorable closure angles. It is also predicated on partially closing the primary defect by side-to-side motion allowing for a smaller flap. The secondary motion is thus shared between the primary and secondary defect (Fig. 26-23*a*). A diamond-shaped primary defect is designed with 30° angles top and bottom and 150° obtuse side angles. A plumb line is drawn extending one side of the diamond through an obtuse angle. The flap is designed off this plumb line as its base. The width of the base of the flap equals one-half of the short diameter of the primary defect. The flap is designed as an isosceles triangle with each of its two long legs equal to a side of the primary defect. Because the base of the flap is only half as wide as the primary defect, it can only fill half of the defect. The remaining

closure is completed by side-to-side motion; therefore, this flap must be used in areas where such motion is possible and will not alter local anatomy and free margins negatively. Its advantages include a sharing of secondary motion which limits tissue distortion in any one area and the basic geometry which eliminates most dog-ear repairs. It is a particularly useful flap on cheek areas (Fig. 26-24).

A bilobed flap is considered when a transposition flap closure is desired but there is insufficient tissue movement to close the secondary defect. By adding a second lobe to the flap to bring tissue from a more distant site, the secondary defect can be closed (Fig. 26-25). This design spreads the tension of the closure over a wide area similar to a rotation flap. The bilobed flap is most useful on the nose. The first lobe is designed 75 to 100 percent of the size of the primary defect; the second lobe is one-half the size of the first. The lobes may be designed without or with 30° angle tips to obviate dog-ear repair. Each lobe must rotate the same number of the degrees but the overall rotation of the flap may vary from 90° to 180°. After the flap is cut, elevated, and undermined, the tertiary defect of the second lobe is closed first (Figs. 26-26). This pushes both lobes into their respective new locations. Once the primary lobe is anchored into the primary defect, the dog-ear created by the rotation may be excised by removing a tri-

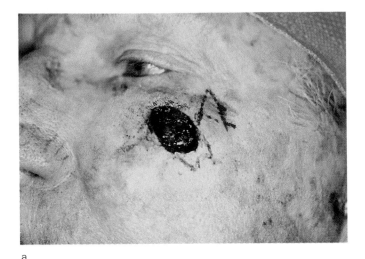

a

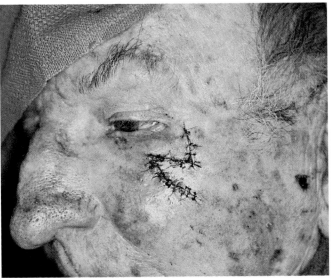

b

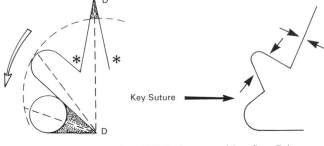

Figure 26-25 Schematic of bilobed transposition flap. Primary lobe is equal to primary defect in size. The secondary lobe is about half the size of the primary lobe. Both lobes must rotate through the same arc. * = key suture; ⇒ = primary motion; → = secondary motion; D = dog-ear removal.

Figure 26-24 Clinical example of a 30°-angle flap on left cheek. (*a*) Defect with flap designed; (*b*) flap sutured in place; (*c*) result at one month.

angle of tissue from the flap base. This author believes it is important with all flaps not to remove excess tissue until after the flap is in place. In this way only the tissue necessary to remove the dog-ear will be sacrificed, and compromise of the flap base and blood flow will be minimized.

Staged transposition or pedicle flaps follow the same design and movement principles. They are harvested more than one cosmetic unit away from the defect and transposed over that skin. The distal tip of the flap which will fill the primary defect must be cut to the size of the defect. It may require aggressive thinning to avoid pincushioning. The pedicle is not sutured into place but is left free with only moist dressings (e.g., Xeroform gauze) overlying the skin intervening between the donor site and primary defect. A blood supply develops into the distal tip of the flap from surrounding and underlying skin in 3 to 4 weeks. At that time the pedicle is clamped to ensure the integrity of that newly developed blood flow. If the blood flow is adequate, the pedicle is severed and suturing completed at the primary defect. The pedicle may be either discarded or returned to its donor region. Examples of staged flaps include the midline forehead and staged melolabial fold flaps to repair the nasal tip, as well as the staged rebuilding of helix and antihelical defects from retroauricular skin.

WHICH FLAP, WHEN, WHERE, AND WHY

Designing and executing a flap based on line drawings may seem rather simple when practicing on a foam rubber model, pig's foot, or cadaver. However, transferring these exercises to an actual facial defect can be difficult and fraught with possible complications. Many things must be considered to ensure a functionally and cosmetically successful procedure. Cosmetic units and borders, skin tension lines, blood and lymphatic flow, tissue elasticity, and local anatomy all play

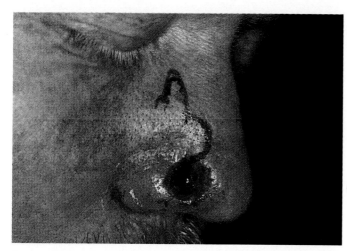

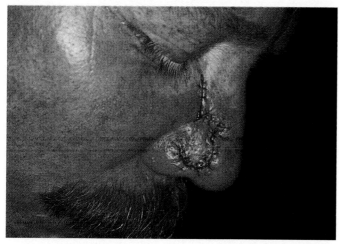

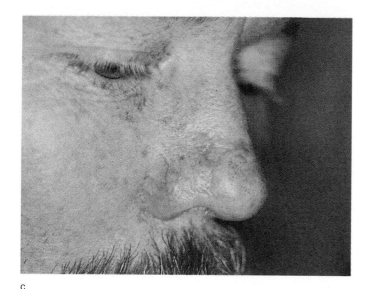

Figure 26-26 Clinical example of bilobed transposition flap. (*a*) Flap designed; (*b*) flap in place; (*c*) flap at two months.

roles in the final appearance of a flap along with technical execution. When dealing with a specific defect on a patient's face, how then do surgeons decide which flap will best repair the defect? What questions do we ask ourselves and answer in the decision-making process?

The author routinely goes through a mental checklist of six questions concerning the selection of a flap closure for any defect. If all the questions can be answered favorably, the flap under consideration will be a good, workable choice. It may not necessarily be the best choice, as one of several flaps may work well to repair a particular defect. One should always consider several flaps when planning any closure, working through the advantages and disadvantages of each. It is unwise to use, always by routine, a single flap in a given situation without considering all the possibilities in every case. Variations in local anatomy, defect size and depth, available tissue, prior surgeries, and patient factors such as smoking or diabetes may impact the appropriateness of a given flap in a given patient. It is a good exercise, especially early in one's career, to make a list of the following six points to go over for each flap until they become second nature:

1. Where is there excess tissue near the defect? For local random pattern flaps, tissue must necessarily be nearby for survival reasons. Regions of the face tend to have fairly standard reservoirs of tissue for repair. Examples include:
   a. forehead—glabella, temple
   b. nose—nasolabial fold, medial cheek, upper lateral nasal sidewall, glabella
   c. lip—nasolabial fold, cheek, lip, chin
   While these reservoirs are reproducible, they are not invariable. Available tissue must be manually determined by digital manipulation (pushing, pulling, pinching) for each individual case.

2. Can the tissue reach the defect without excessive tension? This depends in part on the amount of tissue in the reservoir and also the distance to the defect. Also, critical length/width ratios must be maintained to ensure flap viability. If a flap is unduly stretched to effect a repair, then blood flow will be compromised, leading to flap necrosis. Anatomic distortion may also occur.

3. Can the secondary defect be closed? This is mainly important for rotation and transposition flaps. In these flaps the design is such that tension is intended to be shifted from the primary defect, which cannot be closed primarily, to the secondary defect, which should be able to be closed primarily if properly designed. Except in special situations, it does not make much sense in dermatologic surgery to create a flap which results in a nonclosing secondary defect.

4. Is the pedicle wide enough and properly placed? The flap depends on blood flow in both directions across the base. Lymphatic drainage is also important. Normal blood flow patterns should be noted and taken advantage of where

possible. On the face it is not absolutely necessary to follow arterial patterns as the flap is not based on an artery (random versus axial pattern flap). However, it may help the survival and appearance of flaps if they are inferiorly and laterally based for both optimum blood flow in and out and lymphatic flow out. Impaired outward flow may play a role in flap thickening (pincushioning).

5. What will the flap's movement affect? Both primary and secondary motions can have deleterious effects on the position of surrounding anatomic structures. Downward or lateral pull on an eyelid, elevation of an alar rim or vermilion border, or alteration of a hairline can negate the benefits of any closure. Experience is the most important factor in determining what works where. However, understanding flap motion and manipulating the skin and local structures manually to simulate primary and secondary movements can help the surgeon get a feel for flap effect on local anatomy.

6. Can the incision lines be hidden? The ability to camouflage the incision lines is very important to the final outcome and has been well covered in a previous chapter. Skin tension lines, wrinkles, cosmetic borders, and the use of geometric broken lines must all be considered. The surgeon must be able to visualize, or draw on the patient, where all lines of closure will fall. Placement of incision lines within skin tension lines facilitates not only camouflage but also takes advantage of favorable skin elasticity and extensibility factors. Placing incisions within cosmetic borders aids camouflage. It is especially important not to cross cosmetic borders when possible as accentuated scarring may occur. While camouflage is aesthetically important, it must not override other considerations relative to flap survival and anatomic distortion.

SUMMARY

The use of skin flaps in dermatologic surgery is accepted practice. This does not exempt the dermatologic surgeon from the responsibilities of appropriate training, proctoring, and development of skills commensurate with those needed throughout the surgical disciplines. The proper respect for the complexity of flap surgery and associated risks must be maintained. Technical skills must be supported by knowledge of the basic science relative to skin anatomy and physiology, wound healing, and complications. Factors particular to the individual patient must be considered for each procedure. Only then can we satisfy the requirements of qualified flap surgeons as demanded by our patients and peers.

SUGGESTED READINGS

Jackson IT: *Local Flaps in Head and Neck Surgery.* St. Louis, Mosby, 1985

Moy RL: *Atlas of Cutaneous Facial Flaps and Grafts: A Differential Diagnosis of Wound Closures.* Philadelphia, Lea & Febiger, 1990

Salasche SJ, Grabski WJ: *Flaps of the Central Face.* New York, Churchill-Livingstone, 1990

Zitelli JA (ed): Local flaps (special issue). *J Dermatol Surg Oncol* **17:**101–208, 1991

Summers BK, Siegle RJ: Facial cutaneous reconstructive surgery: General anesthetic principles. *J Am Acad Dermatol* **29:**669–681, 1993

Summers BK, Siegle RJ: Facial cutaneous reconstructive surgery: Facial flaps. *J Am Acad Dermatol* **29:**917–941, 1993

Tromovitch TA et al: *Flaps and Grafts in Dermatologic Surgery.* Chicago, Year Book, 1989

Michael J. Fazio
John A. Zitelli

27 Lip Reconstruction

The lips are multifunctional folds of skin, mucosa, and muscle which consist of many small cosmetic subunits and naturally occurring landmarks. Their location, conspicuously and symmetrically suspended in the central facial region with a paucity of surrounding tissue laxity, renders reconstruction challenging for even the most experienced surgeons. Because there are no bony or cartilaginous supporting structures, the lips are capable of a wide range of motion and a multitude of functions. A competent oral aperture contributes to proper deglutition, verbal (phonation) and nonverbal (facial expressions) communication, oral continence, and maintenance of a stable intraoral milieu.[1,2] Thus, it is extremely important to consider functional integrity as well as the aesthetic outcome when planning reconstruction of defects involving the lip and perioral tissue.

In this chapter, the authors present a regional approach to reconstruction of both cutaneous and full-thickness defects of the lips.[3] Preoperative considerations require an expansive knowledge of perioral anatomy and cosmetic boundaries, vascular supply, and motor and sensory innervation, as well as an understanding of areas of tissue availability. Finally, proper postoperative care will optimize the aesthetic and functional outcome of the reconstructive procedure.

PREOPERATIVE CONSIDERATIONS

Topographic anatomy of the perioral region delineates the important landmarks, boundaries, and small cosmetic subunits of the lips.[4] The upper lip is composed of three cutaneous subunits and the upper vermilion (Fig. 27-1). The two lateral cutaneous subunits of the upper lip are bounded superiorly by the nose, laterally by the melolabial folds, and medially by the philtral crests. The philtrum is the central cutaneous subunit of the upper lip which consists of a variably sized depression between the philtral crests. The sole cutaneous component of the lower lip is bounded laterally by the inferior extension of the melolabial fold and inferiorly by the labiomental crease. The lateral commissure at the angles of the mouth separates the upper and lower lips. The vermilion of the upper and lower lip is a uniquely modified tissue separating the dry, cutaneous portion of the lips from the inner, moist mucosal membranes (Fig. 27-2). The wet-dry line or red line is demarcated by the point of contact of the upper and lower lips. A small protuberance of the orbicularis oris muscle forms the white roll at the vermilion-cutaneous junction. As discussed below, realignment of this structure is extremely important to prevent notching of the lip.

The favorable lines of closure lie within the relaxed skin tension lines, which are created by the cutaneous tension from the underlying facial musculature (Fig. 27-3). In the perioral region, these lines are usually perpendicular to the vermilion-cutaneous junction. During reconstruction of the lips, care should be taken to close the wound within the relaxed skin tension lines. Since the relaxed skin tension lines may not be readily apparent in the perioral region, especially on the lower lip and chin, asking the patient to perform several facial expressions may assist the surgeon in determining the favorable lines of wound closure. If possible, optimal cosmetic results are obtained by placing the incisions along the boundaries of the cosmetic units (i.e., infranasal crease, philtral crests, melolabial folds, labiomental crease, or vermilion-cutaneous junction).[5]

The orbicularis oris is a sphincter-type muscle suspended between a number of synergistic- and antagonistic-acting muscle groups. The lip elevators lift the angle of the mouth upward and posteriorly and form the melolabial fold. Stimu-

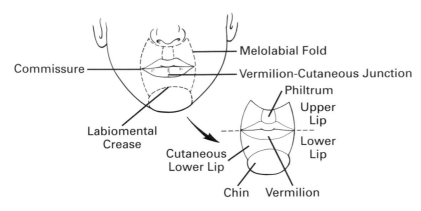

Figure 27-1   Topographic anatomy of the lips.

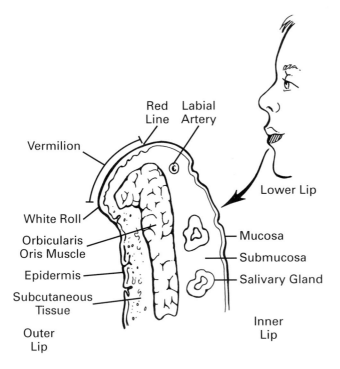

Figure 27-2   Cross-section of lower lip.

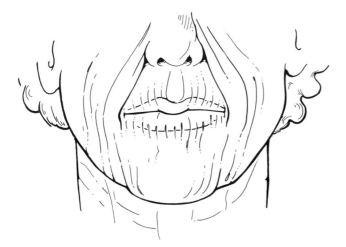

Figure 27-3   Radial relaxed skin tension lines of lip.

lation of the lip depressors leads to inferior and posterior movement of the angle of the mouth. The lip retractors converge laterally to the oral commissure to form the modiolus and contribute to lateral movement of the mouth. Together, the perioral musculature contributes to a complex range of motion and facilitates the many functions of a competent oral aperture.

Motor innervation for the muscles of facial expression is via branches of cranial nerve VII (facial nerve). The lip elevators and orbicularis oris musculature are innervated by the buccal branch, the lip depressors are innervated by the marginal mandibular branch, and the thin platysma muscle is innervated by the cervical branch of the facial nerve. Damage to the branches of the facial nerve, especially the marginal mandibular branch, may lead to severe cosmetic and functional deformity of the oral aperture.

Sensory innervation of the perioral region is via branches of cranial nerve V (trigeminal nerve). The infraorbital branch provides sensation to the upper lip and the mental branch innervates the lower lip. A thorough understanding of the sensory innervation, including topographic anatomy of the infraorbital and mental foramina, will aid the surgeon in obtaining relatively painless anesthesia of the perioral tissue by the use of nerve blocks (Fig. 27-4). Both the infraorbital and mental foramina can be approached from either a percutaneous or an intraoral route. The authors have found intraoral routes to infraorbital or mental nerve blocks to be the most effective and least painful, especially if combined with preoperative topical anesthesia.[6]

The intraoral approach to regional anesthesia of the infraorbital nerve is obtained by inserting the needle into the superior labial sulcus, above the upper canine, and directing the needle superiorly approximately 1 cm below the infraorbital rim in the midpupillary line. Regional anesthesia of the mental nerve is obtained by inserting the needle into the inferior labial sulcus, between the base of the first and second bicuspid teeth, and directing the needle inferiorly in a midpupillary line. Approximately 0.5 to 1.5 cc of 1 percent Xylocaine with epinephrine is infiltrated to the tissue surrounding the foramen. After the regional anesthesia has taken effect (approxi-

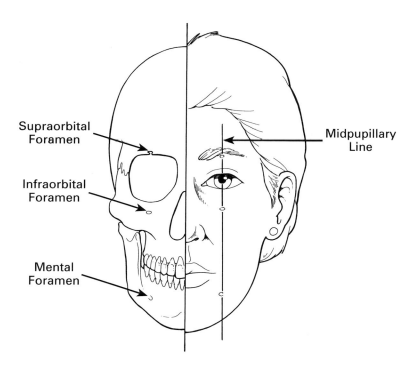

Figure 27-4   Topographic anatomy and foramen location for the main trigeminal nerve branches.

mately 10 min), a small amount of 1% Xylocaine with epinephrine should be infiltrated to the affected tissue in order to maximize hemostasis during the reconstructive procedure.

The vascular supply to the perioral region originates from the facial artery. Just laterally to the modiolus, the facial artery branches into the superior and inferior labial arteries. The labial arteries run in a submucosal plane immediately behind the orbicularis oris muscle (Fig. 27-2). Identification and ligation of the labial arteries are often necessary during reconstruction of full-thickness defects or wedge excisions.

Because of the higher incidence of nodal metastases of squamous cell carcinomas in the perioral region, understanding the pattern of lymphatic drainage from the lips and perioral tissue is extremely important. Drainage of the lower lip is primarily to the submental and submaxillary nodes. Drainage of the upper lip is more ambiguous, with primary drainage to the submaxillary, submental, buccal, and periparotid nodes. Although ipsilateral drainage is common, the potential for contralateral node drainage must always be considered during the metastatic workup.[7,8]

RECONSTRUCTION

The reconstructive modality of choice for repair of defects involving the lips and perioral tissue will largely depend on the location, size, and depth of the wound. Partial-thickness wounds may heal nicely by second intention, close primarily, or need local flaps. Occasionally, skin grafting can be used for reconstruction of superficial perioral wounds. Reconstruction

of full-thickness (into the oral cavity) wounds usually requires more extensive tissue rearrangement such as wedge repair, switch flaps, or full-thickness local flaps.[3,9–11]

Following a few basic principles will help optimize the final cosmetic outcome. Before undertaking any reconstructive procedure, one should clearly delineate and mark the cosmetic units and favorable lines of closure prior to local anesthesia. As outlined above, placing the incisions along the boundaries of the cosmetic subunits will optimize the final cosmetic result. Undermining of perioral tissue is ideally performed in the plane just above the muscular layer. This allows for a vascular-rich flap, minimizing the possibility of ischemic necrosis. Wide undermining around the defect and thinning of the flap will help minimize pincushioning (trapdoor formation). Because epinephrine causes vasodilation in the vascular tissue of muscle, diligent hemostasis prior to suturing is particularly important in the perioral tissue. Reconstruction of perioral defects requires a multilayered approach, carefully approximating the mucosal (chromic), submucosal, muscular, and subcutaneous tissues (Vicryl), followed by meticulous realignment and eversion of the vermilion border and cutaneous tissue (nylon) (Fig. 27-2).

Partial-Thickness Wounds

A recent study reviewed 200 cases for trends in reconstruction of partial-thickness lip defects.[3] Most of the partial-thickness wounds were repaired with local flaps, while second intention wound healing and skin grafting were not as commonly utilized. Although this study did not cover all defects or possible reconstructive procedures, it is useful as a reference to estab-

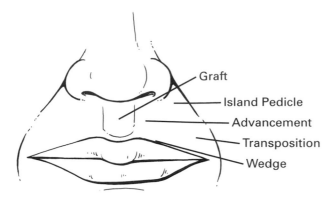

Figure 27-5 General guidelines for upper lip reconstruction.

lish an approach to reconstruction of partial-thickness lip wounds (Fig. 27-5).

Second intention wound healing has a limited use in management of lip and perioral wounds.[12] Because the lips have no bony attachment, the free margin of the lip may be unfavorably displaced during normal wound contracture, resulting in an eclabium formation and an incompetent oral aperture (Fig. 27-6). If the wound is very superficial, it will heal with mild contraction and a white scar. If the alternate choice of reconstruction would result in a high likelihood of lip distortion, then the small white scar may be a better choice. The only area where second intention healing may be the treatment of choice is a small wound around the alar crease and base of the nose [nasal sill (Fig. 27-7)]. Also, some wounds in the philtrum, where reconstruction is difficult without distortion, may heal better by secondary intention. Excellent cosmetic results are commonly seen after second intention wound healing of superficial wounds created by carbon dioxide laser vermilionectomy of the lower lip.

Skin grafts in the perioral region have a greater tendency to heal with a convex contour (pincushioning) than else-

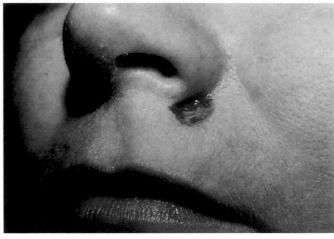

a

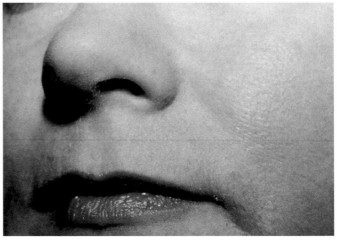

b

Figure 27-7 *(a)* Defect involving the nasal sill; *(b)* cosmetic results by secondary intention wound healing.

where, and thus they are infrequently used for lip repair. Also, graft color and texture match are usually poor in perioral tissue. An exception to this rule is use of Burow's full-thickness skin graft for repair of cutaneous philtral defects not involving the vermilion (Fig. 27-8).[13] In certain defects, the size and location of the wound preclude flap reconstruction and thus require skin grafting to minimize functional and cosmetic distortion of the lip. In these circumstances, optimal cosmetic outcome is achieved by replacing the entire cosmetic subunit [i.e., the philtrum (Fig. 27-9) or the lateral cutaneous lip (Fig. 27-10)].

Local skin flaps provide the most useful and diverse approach to achieving optimal cosmetic results when the surgeon is reconstructing wounds of the lips and perioral tissue. Since it is always preferable to use similar tissues when repairing wounds, local flaps adjacent to the wound provide superior thickness, color, and texture match. The process of wound contraction during wound healing is more active on

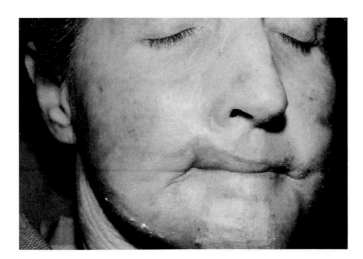

Figure 27-6 Eclabium of the upper lip resulting from secondary intention wound healing.

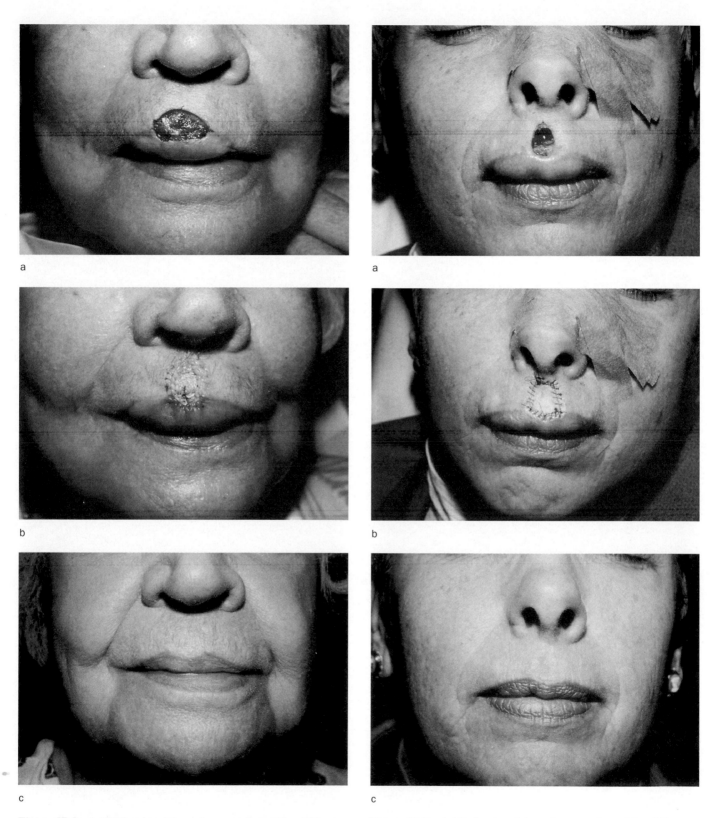

Figure 27-8 *(a)* Defect involving a large portion of the philtrum; *(b)* Burow's full-thickness skin graft; *(c)* result 6 months postoperatively.

Figure 27-9 *(a)* Defect involving a large portion of the philtrum; *(b)* full-thickness skin graft replacing the entire cosmetic subunit; *(c)* result 6 months postoperatively.

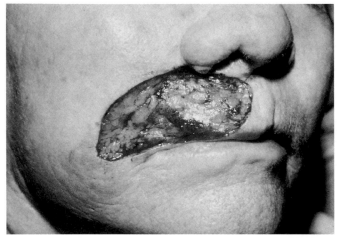

a

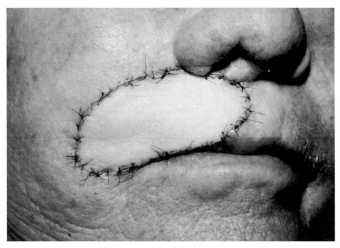

b

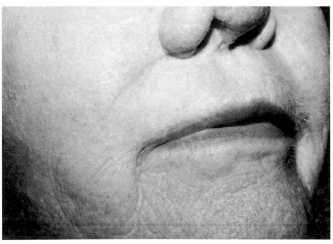

c

Figure 27-10 *(a)* Defect of entire lateral cutaneous subunit of upper lip; *(b)* full-thickness skin graft reconstruction; *(c)* result 6 months postoperatively.

the lip than other facial areas, which explains the high incidence of trapdooring with skin grafts; however, it also leads to a greater chance of retraction with local flaps. This is minimized but not completely prevented by meticulous hemostasis to avoid hematomas, adequate but not extensive undermining, and very careful instructions to the patient to avoid lip movement during the first 2 weeks after surgery. Intralesional steroids may be useful 1 month after surgery to control the frequent firmness in the treated area.

Because the lateral lip and cheek are the areas of greatest tissue availability, various forms of advancement flaps are able to utilize the redundant cheek tissue for wound repair. On the lip, a simple fusiform closure is performed by excising Burow's triangle superiorly and inferiorly to the defect to create a fusiform wound within the vertically oriented relaxed skin tension lines (Fig. 27-11). Fusiform closure results in lengthening of the wound and subsequent displacement of the free margin at the vermilion border. Fusiform closure of wounds less than 1 cm^2 in size commonly results in minimal displacement of the vermilion border, which usually returns to normal over several weeks. Primary closure of lip defects greater than 1 cm^2 usually results in permanent distortion of the vermilion border, and thus these wounds should be managed differently.

Contrary to popular belief, the vermilion border should not be considered an inviolable structure.[3] If the inferior portion of a fusiform repair extends onto the vermilion border, the excision should be lengthened through and around the vermilion to the mucosal portion inside the lip. Also, the inferior Burow's triangle should never be shortened to avoid crossing the vermilion border because this will cause greater displacement of the vermilion than a long triangle. Geometric variations of the fusiform closure, such as an M-plasty, A-to-L plasty (Fig. 27-12), or A-to-T plasty (Fig. 27-13), occasionally may be used to minimize displacement of the vermilion border. The A-to-T plasty is also useful in repairing wounds involving the nasal sill at the junction of the upper lip and nose.

Larger defects on the cutaneous portion of the lips are reconstructed with a more complex variation of the advancement flap. Complex advancement flaps require extensive undermining to release the redundant tissue of the lateral lip and cheek. Like the fusiform closure, tissue movement is in the horizontal direction; however, the superior and inferior Burow's triangles are displaced laterally into the melolabial fold. A releasing incision is commonly made at the lateral aspect of the defect, along the vermilion-cutaneous junction. Depending upon the size of the wound and tissue elasticity, Burow's triangles are removed superiorly (Fig. 27-14) or both superiorly and inferiorly (Fig. 27-15) along the melolabial fold. Because of the lateral tissue availability, there is usually only minimal displacement of the philtrum. Advancement of the wedge-shaped flap medially will tend to displace the vermilion border inferiorly; thus, the inferior edge of the flap may need to be trimmed for proper alignment of the vermil-

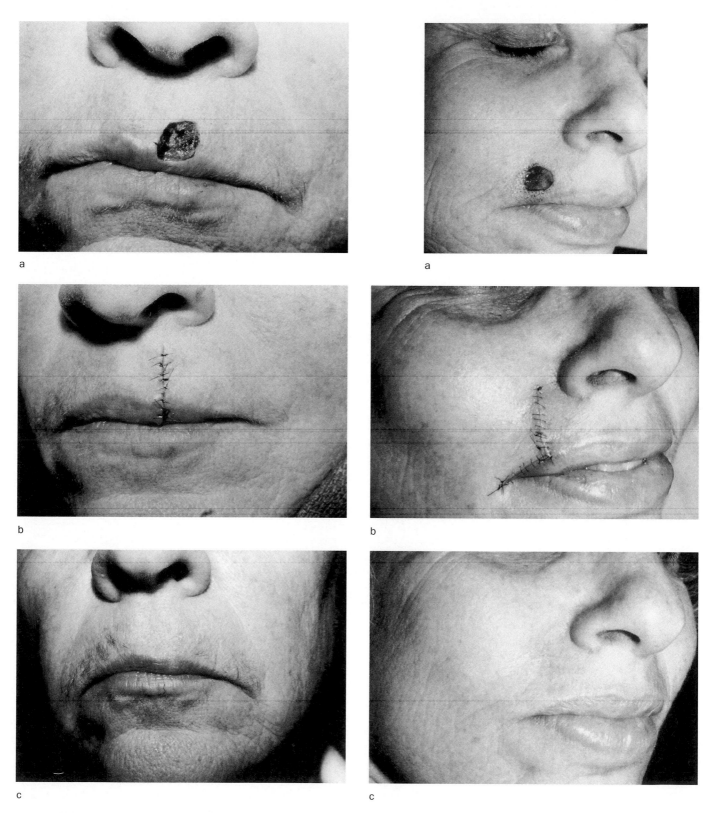

Figure 27-11 *(a)* Defect at the vermilion-cutaneous junction of the upper lip; *(b)* primary vertical closure extending through the vermilion; *(c)* result 6 months postoperatively.

Figure 27-12 *(a)* Defect of the upper lateral cutaneous lip; *(b)* vertical closure in the radial skin tension lines with a releasing incision at the lateral vermilion-cutaneous junction; *(c)* result 6 months postoperatively.

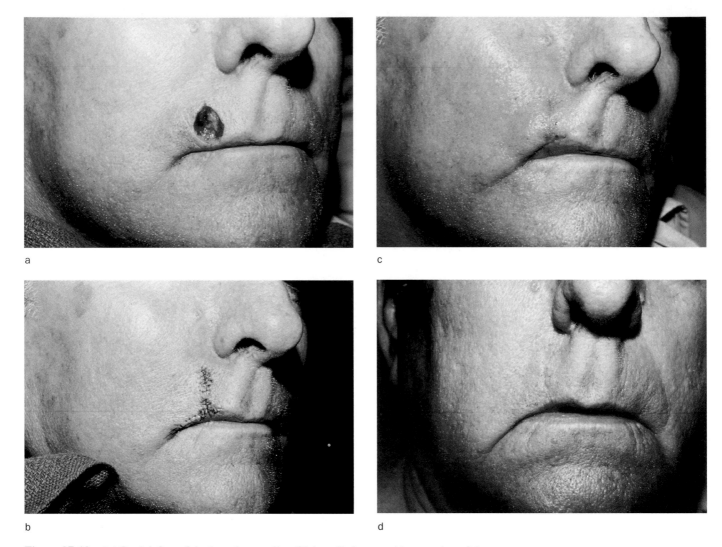

a

b

c

d

Figure 27-13 *(a)* Oval defect of the lateral upper lip; *(b)* A-to-T closure with extension of the lateral excision along the vermilion border; *(c)* induration of the operative site 1 week postoperatively; *(d)* result 6 months postoperatively.

ion. A common complication of any flap crossing the melolabial line is blunting of the melolabial fold. A properly placed periosteal suture, connecting the periosteum of the pyriform aperture of the maxilla to the dermis of the flap, will help restore the natural crevice of the superior portion of the melolabial fold as it approaches the nasal ala.[14] The periosteal tacking suture will also serve as a boundary to minimize medial displacement of the cheek fat pad and help maintain the normal contour of the cheek (Fig. 27-15).

Rotation flaps are infrequently used to repair wounds of the perioral tissue because it is difficult to place the incisions within the normal relaxed skin tension lines. Occasionally, oval defects of the upper lateral lip may be repaired by incising laterally of the defect in an arclike fashion within the melolabial fold and by removing a small Burow's triangle inferiorly of the defect within the radial relaxed skin tension lines (Fig. 27–16). Unfortunately, the rotation flap has a ten-

dency to pincushion and may displace the melolabial fold medially, resulting in an unnatural, asymmetric appearance. Reconstruction of larger wounds with a rotation flap may upwardly displace the lateral oral commissure. In the authors' experience, the island pedicle flap will usually give a superior cosmetic result for a defect in this location.

The island pedicle flap has several useful applications for repair of wounds in the perioral tissue.[3,15] As mentioned previously, defects of the upper lateral lip are ideally located for wound closure with an island pedicle flap. A variably sized triangular incision is made infralaterally of the defect, extending deeply into the subcutaneous tissue. Because of the abundant vascularity in the perioral tissue, a relatively small central subcutaneous pedicle will provide adequate blood supply and allow for maximum mobility of the flap. After the subcutaneous pedicle has been meticulously dissected, superficial undermining of the defect, flap, and donor skin (ap-

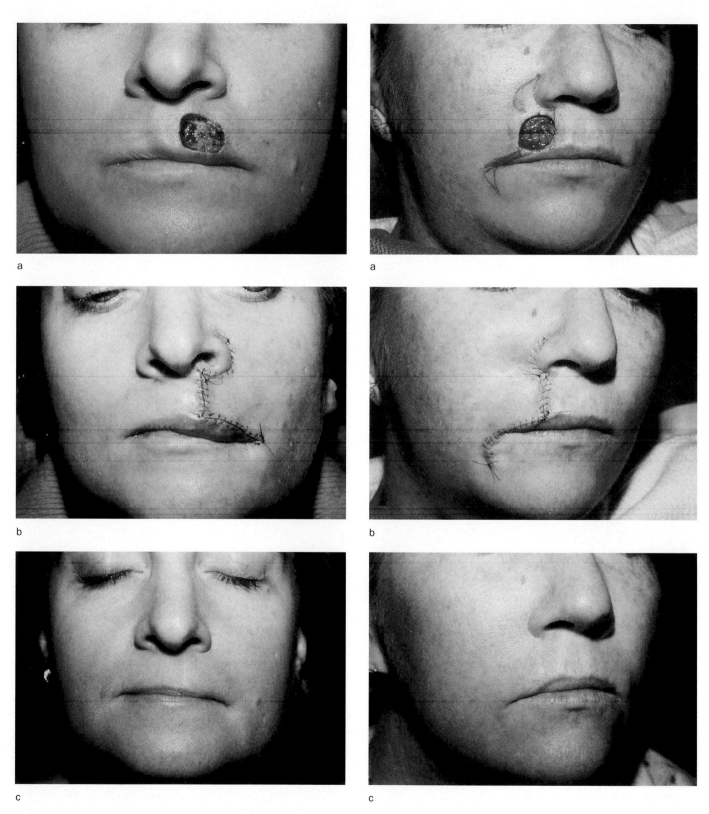

Figure 27-14   *(a)* Defect of lateral cutaneous lip extending to philtral crest; *(b)* perialar Burow's triangle superiorly and a releasing incision excised at the lateral aspect of the defect at the vermilion-cutaneous junction. A small wedge of tissue was removed from the inferior aspect of the flap to minimize downward displacement of the vermilion; *(c)* result 6 weeks postoperatively.

Figure 27-15   *(a)* Defect confined to lateral cutaneous subunit of upper lip; *(b)* perialar Burow's triangle, lateral releasing incision, and inferior Burow's triangle removed to facilitate cheek advancement; *(c)* result 6 weeks postoperatively (note the periosteal stitch at the superior aspect of the melolabial fold).

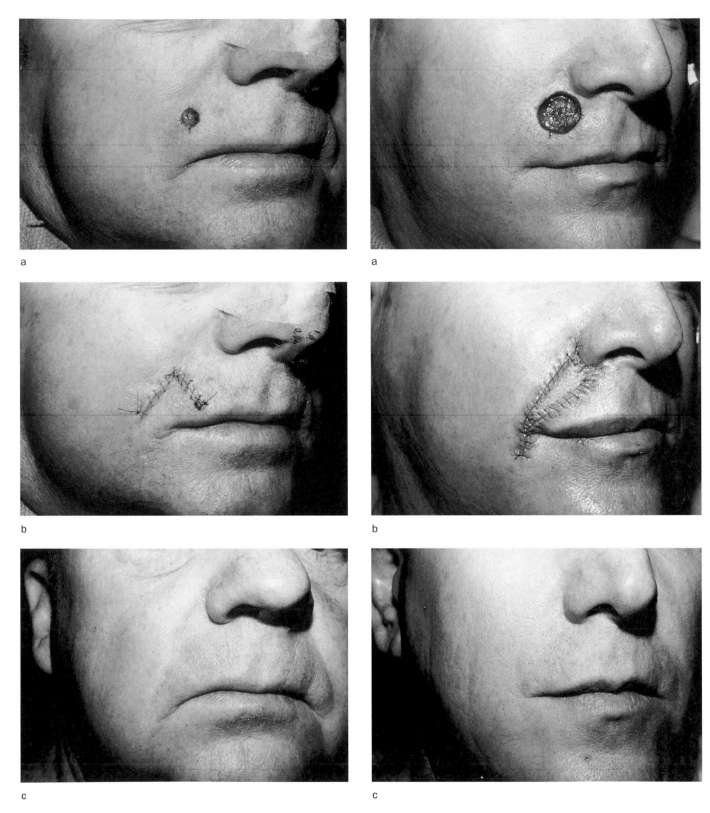

Figure 27-16 *(a)* Small defect of the lateral upper lip; *(b)* reconstruction with a rotation flap; *(c)* result 6 months postoperatively.

Figure 27-17 *(a)* Defect at the superior-lateral upper lip; *(b)* reconstruction of the wound with an island pedicle flap from the inferior melolabial fold; *(c)* result 6 months postoperatively.

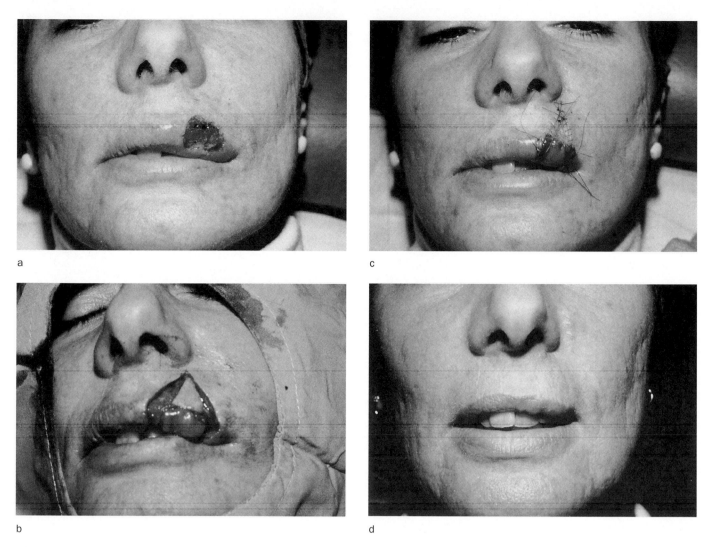

Figure 27-18 (a) Large defect involving both cutaneous and vermilion portion of the lateral upper lip; (b) bilateral cutaneous and mucosal island pedicle flaps (c) reforming the vermilion-cutaneous junction; (d) result 6 weeks postoperatively.

proximately 1 mm) will facilitate wound eversion during closure. To minimize pincushioning of the flap, the authors have found it useful to square off the circular defect prior to advancement of the triangular pedicle flap. After advancement of the triangular flap into the wound, the secondary defect is easily closed along the melolabial fold (see previous page).

A double island pedicle flap is useful in reconstruction of large defects of the upper lip which extend onto the mucosa.[3] Because of the unique shape and central location of the philtrum, wedge repairs or advancement flaps will tend to distort the natural-occurring landmarks and lead to an asymmetric appearance. The double island pedicle flap is created by incising triangular flaps superiorly of the defect extending toward the nose and inferiorly of the defect along the midline of the intraoral mucosa of the lip. The two island pedicle flaps are meticulously trimmed and advanced into the wound with special attention given to re-creating the vermilion (Fig. 27-

18). Another application of the double island pedicle flap is for repair of defects involving the cutaneous portion of the lower lip. Triangular incisions are made infralaterally of the defect and the flaps are meticulously dissected as outlined above. The flaps are advanced, rotated, and sutured together at the approximate midline of the wound. This flap leads to excellent functional and cosmetic results with minimal distortion of the labiomental crease (Fig. 27-19).

Transposition flaps are extremely useful in mobilizing local tissue on many areas of the face, especially the nose. Depending upon the size and location of the wound, the transposition flap can be inferiorly (Fig. 27-20) or superiorly (Fig. 27-21) based to harvest excess tissue from the melolabial fold. Unfortunately, in the perioral region, transposition of cheek tissue onto the lip will commonly result in pincushioning and blunting of the melolabial fold, and thus alternative forms of reconstruction are more commonly used.

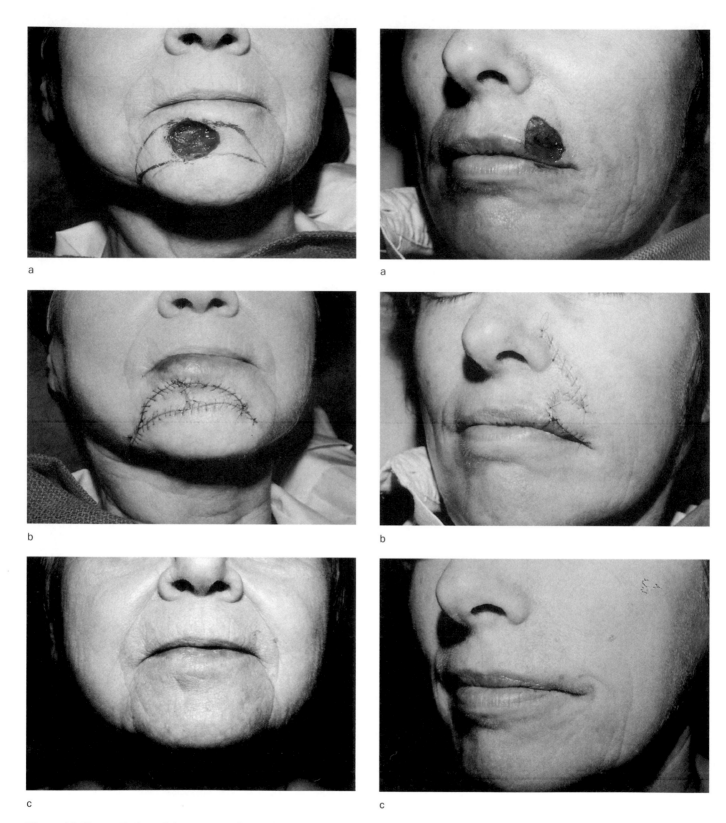

Figure 27-19 *(a)* Defect of the cutaneous lower lip; *(b)* reconstruction with bilateral island pedicle flaps; *(c)* result 6 months postoperatively.

Figure 27-20 *(a)* Defect of the lateral cutaneous lip extending across the vermilion-cutaneous junction; *(b)* reconstruction with an inferiorly based transposition flap; *(c)* result 6 months postoperatively.

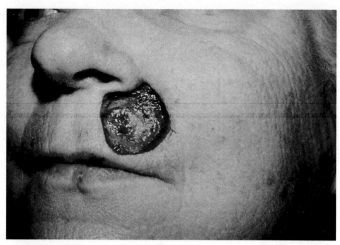

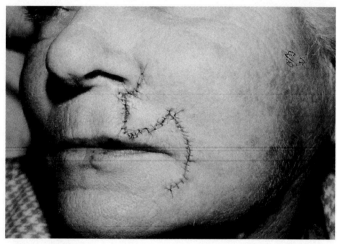

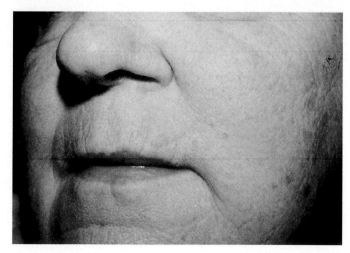

Figure 27-21 *(a)* Defect involving a large portion of the upper lateral cutaneous lip; *(b)* reconstruction with a superiorly based transposition flap; *(c)* result 6 weeks postoperatively (note mild pincushioning of the flap).

Although the carbon dioxide laser is commonly used for vermilionectomy of the actinically damaged lower lip, mucosal advancement flaps may be useful in certain circumstances. Removal of squamous cell carcinoma from the lower lip may occasionally result in wide wounds of the vermilion tissue, without significant involvement of hair-bearing skin. Since wedge repair of this type of wound would reduce the size of the oral aperture, mucosal advancement flaps can be used to minimize functional and cosmetic distortion (Fig. 27-22). Furthermore, most patients with squamous cell carcinoma of the lower lip have widespread actinic cheilitis which is also treated by vermilionectomy.

Complex wounds which involve several cosmetic subunits may require a combination of surgical techniques for adequate reconstruction. In Fig. 27-23, the wound involves the vermilion, cutaneous upper lip, and philtrum. A new philtrum was redesigned from the remaining portion and advanced inferiorly as an island pedicle flap. Special attention was given to re-creating Cupid's bow angles. The left side of the philtral crest was elongated and lowered with a Z-plasty. The remaining portion of the wound was repaired with a bilateral mucosal advancement flap.

Full-Thickness Wounds

Full-thickness wounds of the lips and perioral tissue extend through the mucosa into the oral cavity. In general, wedge repair of the upper lip is useful for small cutaneous defects on or near the vermilion as well as for full-thickness defects. Wedge repair of small defects does not distort the lip and, more importantly, the risk of complication is extremely low. Postoperative bleeding, lip retraction, and deformities are very rare in comparison to local flap closures for the same defect. On the other hand, wedge repair for larger defects (2 cm or greater) will result in distortion. Therefore, local flaps are more useful for these larger defects if the wound is cutaneous only and not full thickness. Usually, full-thickness lip defects of the upper lip which are less than one-third of the vermilion length (1.5 to 2 cm) can be closed primarily in a wedgelike fashion (Fig. 27-24).[16,17] Patients with excessive perioral tissue laxity may have lower lip defects of up to one-half of the vermilion length adequately reconstructed by primary closure (Fig. 27-25).[7] Various modifications of the wedge closure may be helpful to achieve optimal functional and cosmetic results. When the surgeon is reconstructing larger defects of the lower lip, a W-plasty modification is useful for limiting the extent of the surgical incision to the labiomental crease. Larger defects of the upper lip may benefit from removal of a crescent-shaped wedge of tissue, superior of the defect in the perialar region, to release the redundant cheek skin and preserve the functional integrity of the oral aperture.[10,18]

Full-thickness wounds which involve the lateral commissure present an added complexity to the reconstructive surgery. In Fig. 27-26, wedge resection would decrease the size of the oral aperture and adversely displace the lateral

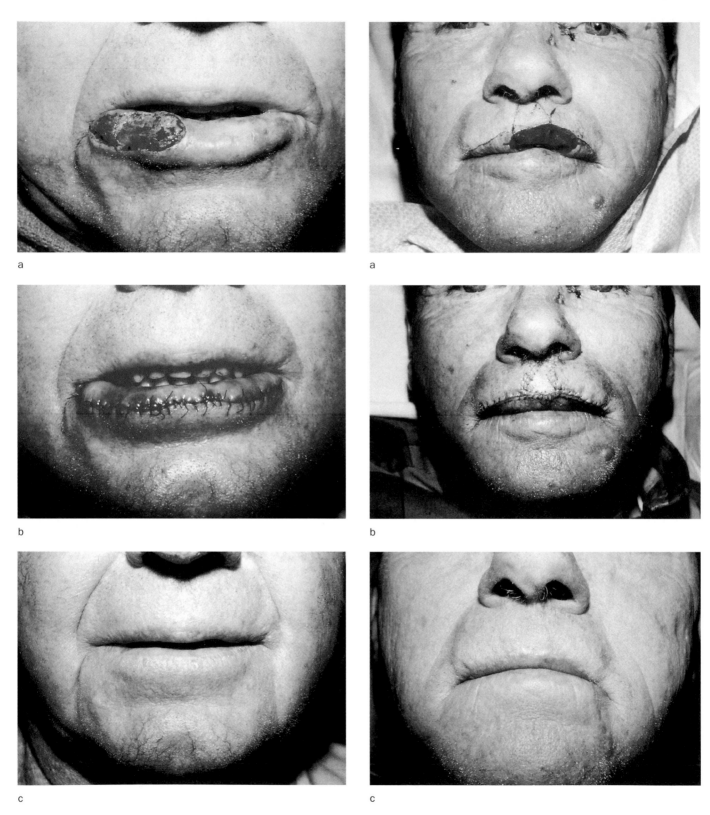

Figure 27-22 *(a)* Wide defect of the vermilion tissue and evidence of extensive actinic cheilitis on the lower lip; *(b)* vermilionectomy and mucosal advancement; *(c)* result 6 months postoperatively.

Figure 27-23 *(a)* Defect involving the vermilion, philtrum, and cutaneous lateral lip; *(b)* reconstruction with a combination island pedicle flap, Z-plasty, and mucosal advancement flaps; *(c)* result 6 months postoperatively.

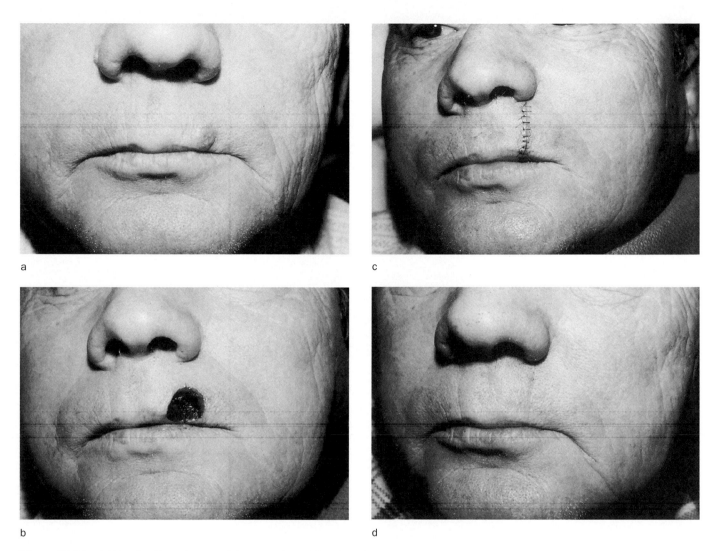

a

b

c

d

Figure 27-24   *(a)* Basal cell carcinoma of the upper lateral lip; *(b)* defect extending deeply to the orbicularis muscle; *(c)* wedge reconstruction; *(d)* result 6 weeks postoperatively.

commissure. The surgical goal was to enlarge the aperture and reform the commissure to prevent leakage of food and fluids. The wedge portion was standard by excising Burow's triangle inferiorly around the chin to minimize the dog-ear. Burow's triangle was removed from the left lateral aspect of the upper lip to facilitate a sliding myocutaneous flap. Finally, the vermilion of the upper lip was recreated by mucosal advancement.

Full-thickness defects greater than one-third of the vermilion length usually require more extensive tissue rearrangement. The Stein-Abbe-Estlander flap is a full-thickness, lip-switch flap which is pedicled on the labial artery.[9,10,19,20] These flaps are created by incising a wedge of tissue from the lip opposite the defect and rotating the full-thickness flap on its vascular pedicle into the defect. Once collateral circulation has been established (approximately 2 to 3 weeks), the pedicle is transected and the vermilion is carefully realigned.

For defects greater than one-half of the vermilion length,

recruitment of large amounts of local tissue can be accomplished by the Karapandzic technique.[21] This full-thickness flap can be used for defects of the upper lip or lower lip and has the distinct advantage of maintaining its own neurovascular supply; it thus facilitates restoration of the muscular integrity of the oral aperture (Figs. 27-27 and 27-28). Total reconstruction of the lower lip may require unilateral or bilateral cheiloplasty followed by medial advancement of the cheek tissue (Fig. 27-29).

POSTOPERATIVE CONSIDERATIONS

Immediately following wound repair, an antibiotic ointment is applied to the incision and the wound is covered with a simple pressure dressing. The pressure dressing is left in place for the first 24 h postoperatively. After the first day, the patient can remove the dressing and begin daily application of an-

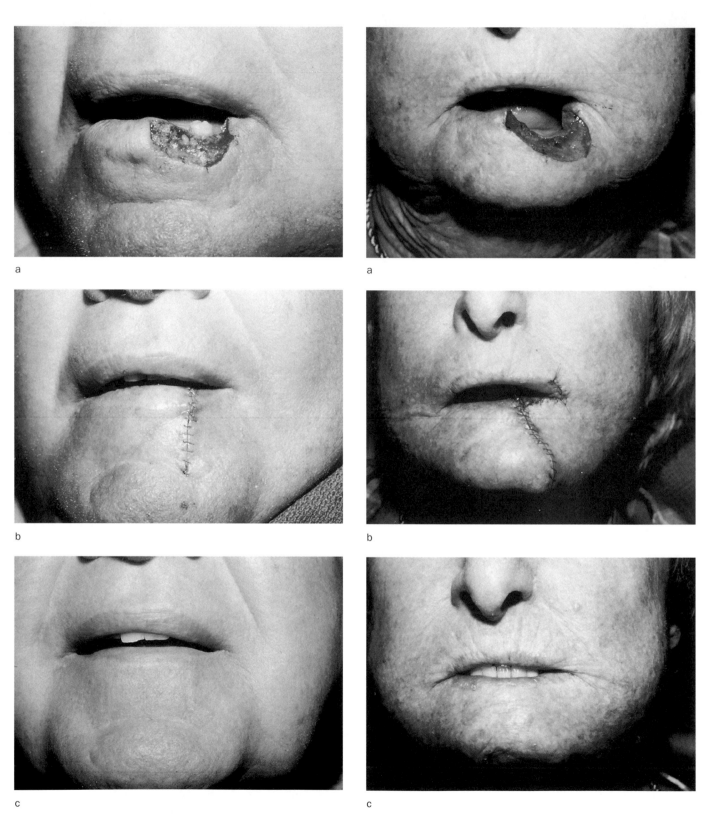

a

b

c

a

b

c

Figure 27-25 *(a)* Full-thickness defect involving approximately a third of the lower lip; *(b)* wedge reconstruction; *(c)* result 6 weeks postoperatively.

Figure 27-26 *(a)* Large full-thickness defect of lower lip; *(b)* reconstruction with a combination wedge inferiorly, myocutaneous flap, and mucosal advancement; *(c)* result 6 months postoperatively.

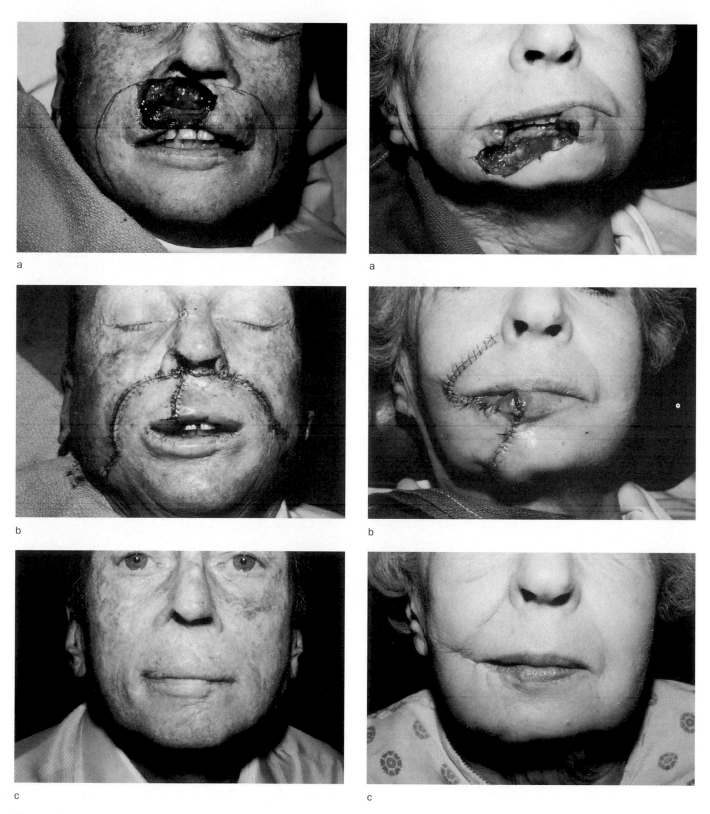

Figure 27-27   *(a)* Large full-thickness defect of middle upper lip; *(b)* reconstruction with a Karapandzic flap; *(c)* result 6 months postoperatively.

Figure 27-28   *(a)* Large full-thickness defect of lower lip; *(b)* reconstruction with a unilateral variation of a Karapandzic flap; *(c)* result 6 weeks postoperatively.

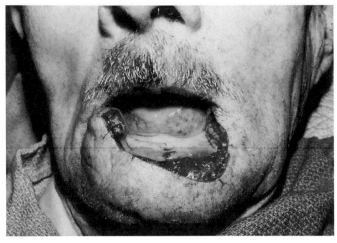

a

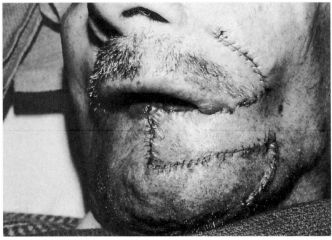

b

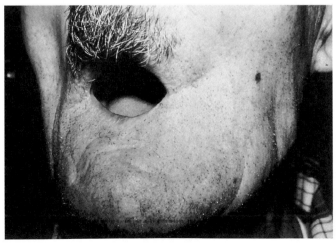

c

Figure 27-29 *(a)* Full-thickness defect involving majority of lower lip; *(b)* reconstruction with unilateral cheiloplasty, excision of Burow's triangles in the melolabial fold, followed by medial advancement of cheek tissue; *(c)* competent oral aperture 6 months postoperatively.

tibiotic ointment. It is extremely important to stress that the patient should minimize use of his or her lips, including chewing, talking, laughing, smiling, or frowning. Liquids and small bites of soft foods are highly recommended postoperatively. Patients who wear dentures should remove the dentures prior to the reconstructive procedure and not reinsert them until 1 to 2 weeks postoperatively. Alternatively, the patient may leave the dentures in place without removing them for 1 to 2 weeks. Informing the patient that his or her cooperation with the postoperative instructions will contribute to optimal cosmetic results tends to increase patient compliance. The cutaneous sutures are usually removed at 5 to 7 days postoperatively. Prophylactic antibiotics are not routinely used after reconstruction of clean cutaneous wounds. In extenuating circumstances where the initial tumor is grossly infected or the surgical wound extends into the oral cavity, a postoperative course of penicillin or a cephalosporin is prescribed.

REFERENCES

1. Stranc MF: Reconstructive surgery of the lips and chin, pt 2: Lip reconstruction, in *Plastic Surgery of the Head and Neck,* edited by RB Stark. New York, Churchill-Livingstone, 1987, pp 1243–1257

2. Stranc MF, Page RE: Functional aspects of the reconstructed lip. *Ann Plast Surg* **10:**103, 1983

3. Zitelli JA, Brodland DG: A regional approach to reconstruction of the lip. *J Dermatol Surg Oncol* **17:**143, 1991

4. Salasche SJ et al: Lips, in *Surgical Anatomy of the Skin,* edited by SJ Salasche et al. Norwalk, Conn, Appleton & Lange, 1988, pp 223–240

5. Burget GC, Menick FJ: Aesthetic restoration of one-half the upper lip. *Plast Reconstr Surg* **78:**583, 1986

6. Gormley DE: A simplified, painless method of anesthetizing the lower lip. *J Dermatol Surg Oncol* **7:**963, 1981

7. Goslen JB, Thomas JR: Cancer of the perioral region. *Dermatol Clin* **7:**733, 1989

8. Larson DL et al: Lymphatics of the upper and lower lips: A clinical and experimental study. *Am J Surg* **114:**525, 1967

9. Panje WR: Lip reconstruction. *Otolaryngol Clin North Am* **15:**169, 1982

10. Jackson IT: Lip reconstruction, in *Local Flaps in Head and Neck Reconstruction,* edited by IT Jackson. St. Louis, Mosby, 1985, pp 327–411

11. Davidson TM et al: Surgical excisions from and reconstruction of the oral lips. *J Dermatol Surg Oncol* **6:**133, 1980

12. Zitelli JA: Wound healing by second intention: A cosmetic appraisal. *J Am Acad Dermatol* **9:**407, 1983

13. Zitelli JA: Burow's grafts. *J Am Acad Dermatol* **17:**271, 1987

14. Zitelli JA: Tips for wound closure: Pearls for minimizing dogears and applications of periosteal sutures. *Dermatol Clin* **7:**123, 1989

15. Skouge JW: Upper lip repair: The subcutaneous island pedicle flap. *J Dermatol Surg Oncol* **16:**63, 1990

16. Sebben JE: Wedge resection of the lip: Minimizing problems. *J Dermatol Surg Oncol* **11:**60, 1985

17. Knowles WR: Wedge resection of the lower lip. *J Dermatol Surg Oncol* **2:**141, 1976

18. Webster JP: Crescentic peri-alar cheek excision for upper lip flap advancement with a short history of upper lip repair. *Plast Reconstr Surg* **16:**434, 1955

19. Abbe R: A new plastic operation for relief of deformity due to double hair lip. *Med Rec* **53:**447, 1898

20. Estlander JA: A method of reconstructing loss of substance in one lip from the other lip. *Plast Reconstr Surg* **42:**360, 1968

21. Karapandzic M: Reconstruction of lip defects by local arterial flaps. *Br J Plast Surg* **27:**93, 1974

Glenn D. Goldstein
Jemshed A. Khan

28 Reconstruction of the Forehead and Temple

FOREHEAD

The anatomic boundaries of the forehead extend superiorly to the normal anterior hairline, inferiorly to encompass the eyebrows and glabella, and are demarcated laterally by the temporal bony ridges associated with the origin of the temporalis muscle.[1]

The Cutaneous Forehead and Eyebrow

The most prominent feature of the forehead is the eyebrows. Morphologically, the eyebrows represent specialized appendages of the hair-bearing scalp rather than extensions of facial tissue.[2] Eyebrow positioning serves an important role in communicating and signaling gender, age, and emotional status. The eyebrows protect the eyelids and eyeball from mechanical injury, rivulets of forehead sweat, and radiant energy.[2]

The male eyebrow usually rests at the level of the superior orbital rim, whereas the female brow is more arched and rests slightly higher.[2] The head of the eyebrow overlies the frontal sinus and the tail is usually found in the region of the zygomaticofrontal suture.[3] The bulky skin of the eyebrow contains robust, deep hair follicles, which extend into the underlying subcutaneous fat, as well as abundant sweat and sebaceous glands.[2] The hairs of the male eyebrow are greater in number and more irregular than those of the female eyebrow.

Between the heads of the eyebrows lies a smooth and often hairless zone known as the glabella. The skin of the forehead and glabella is sebaceous and oily, and its subtle hues are not easily matched by skin grafts. Horizontal forehead creases and the borders of the eyebrows provide useful camouflage for incisions, provided that one does not induce noticeable asymmetries of eyebrow height. Vertical incisions in the glabella heal well.

Because forehead skin is often thick and relatively inelastic, closure of forehead defects often requires extensive undermining in either the subcutaneous or subgaleal plane. Regional nerve blocks of the supraorbital and supratrochlear neurovascular bundles can be employed for forehead surgery but do not provide the hemostasis of infiltrative anesthetic and epinephrine solutions.

The Subcutaneous Forehead and Eyebrow

The subcutaneous fat of the eyebrow and forehead cushions the bony skeleton from trauma and also facilitates the mobility of the eyebrow. Fibrous septa traverse the subcutaneous layer and connect the skin to the underlying superficial galea aponeurotica.[1] Blood vessels arriving from the superficial temporal fascia meander through the deep stratum of subcutaneous fat.[4] Supraorbital and supratrochlear neurovascular bundles emerge through the periosteal, galeal, and muscular layers of the eyebrow (Figs. 28-1 and 28-2) before entering the deepest stratum of the subcutaneous layer which they then follow superiorly into the scalp.[5]

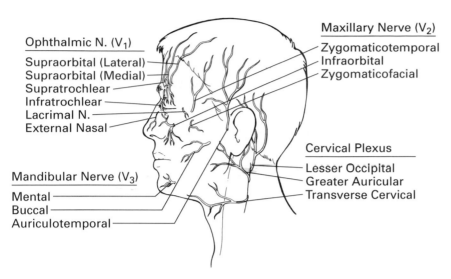

Figure 28-1 Cutaneous sensory nerve branches.

The Superficial Musculoaponeurotic System

Lying immediately deeply to the subcutaneous fatty tissues of the forehead are the galea aponeurotica and associated frontalis muscle. These layers of the forehead along with the superficial temporalis fascia of the temple and the occipitalis and galea of the scalp constitute an important portion of an anatomically continuous functional unit termed the *superficial musculoaponeurotic system* (SMAS).[1] The galea aponeurotica, occipitofrontalis muscle, superficial temporal fascia, and superficial periauricular muscles all lie within the same connected plane and are components of that portion of the SMAS which allows the scalp, temple, and forehead to glide easily over the skull (Fig. 28-3). In general, the superficial SMAS either contains or lies immediately deeply to the neurovascular bundles of the forehead, scalp, and temple. The

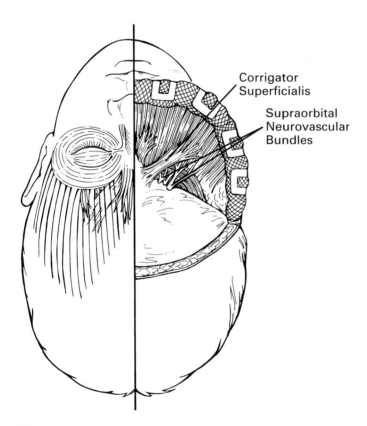

Figure 28-2 The supraorbital neurovascular bundles are closely associated with corrugator supercilii. (From Shore.[5])

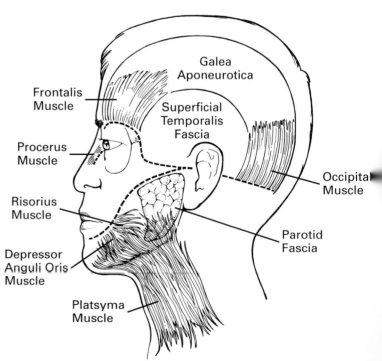

Figure 28-3 Suprazygomatic and infrazygomatic SMAS divisions.

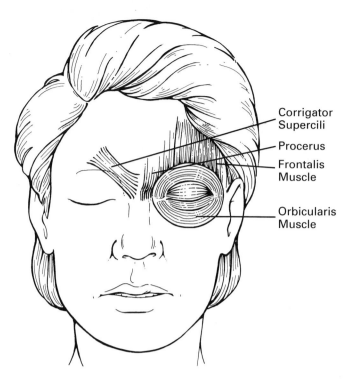

Figure 28-4 The corrugator supercilii, the procerus, and the orbital, preseptal, and part of the pretarsal obicularis oculi muscles are responsible for the forced eyelid closure and deep brow furrows; the frontalis muscle opposes the eyebrow protractors and does not participate in the forehead eyelid closure.

deep aspects of the SMAS generally contain the facial motor nerves.

The Superficial Galea Aponeurotica

The superficial galea aponeurotica is a diaphanous anterior leaflet of the galea aponeurotica which overlies the frontalis muscle and contains numerous attachments to the overlying skin and subcutaneous fat layer.[2] Development of a plane between the skin and superficial galea aponeurotica requires sharp dissection because of these attachments. These firm attachments are responsible for the transverse skin creases of the forehead. The proximity and the attachments of the anterior galea aponeurotica to the subcutaneous fatty layer render dissection in this area bloody and risk injury to sensory nerves. The inferior extents of the superficial galea aponeurotica and the frontalis muscle intermingle with the orbicularis oculi and other muscles of the eyebrow before inserting into the eyebrow skin.[3]

The Muscular Layer of the Eyebrow and Forehead

The frontalis muscle is one of four muscles contributing to the muscular layer of the eyebrow which lies deeply to the subcutaneous fat (Fig. 28-4). The frontalis, procerus, orbicularis oculi, and corrugator supercilii muscle fibers all interdigitate and are sometimes difficult to distinguish at their cutaneous

insertions.[2] The frontalis muscle elevates the eyebrow, whereas the procerus and the corrugator supercilii depress the head of the eyebrow. The corrugator supercilii also draw the head of the eyebrows closer together.

The Frontalis Muscle The sheetlike frontalis muscle is the major muscle of the forehead (Figs. 28-3 and 28-4). The frontalis muscle constitutes the anterior belly of the epicranius or occipitofrontalis muscle. If one takes into account its associated galeal aponeurosis, the frontalis is also the most complex forehead muscle. The vertically oriented muscle fibers of the paired frontalis muscles originate from the galea aponeurotica at about the level of the anterior hairline. Posteriorly, the galea aponeurotica is continuous with the occipital muscle. Anteriorly, the galea aponeurotica splits and envelops the frontalis, lining both the superficial and deep surfaces of the frontalis.

The Procerus Muscle The procerus muscles extend from the most medial and inferior aspect of each frontalis muscle and insert into the nasal bones (Figs. 28-3 and 28-4). Though the procerus appears to be an extension of the frontalis muscle, it is a distinct muscle with separate innervation from the infraorbital branch of the facial nerve. The action of the procerus muscle is to depress the heads of the eyebrows, resulting in transverse wrinkle lines at the root of the nose. Because of the truculent facial appearance created by procerus muscle contraction, Duchenne dubbed the procerus muscle the "muscle of aggression."

The Orbicularis Oculi Muscle The orbicularis oculi muscle is the most superficial of the eyebrow muscles.[2] Only the uppermost fibers of the orbital portion of the orbicularis oculi muscle contribute to the superficial muscular layer of the eyebrow (Figs. 28-3 and 28-4). These superior fibers intermingle with the lowermost aspect of the deeper lying frontalis muscle. Portions of the two muscles may be so intermeshed as to be surgically indistinguishable. The superior portion of the orbital orbicularis oculi muscle also melds with the overlying skin.

The Corrugator Supercilii Muscle The obliquely oriented corrugator supercilii muscles are the deepest-lying muscles of the muscular plane of the eyebrow (Figs. 28-3 and 28-4). The muscle fibers arise from the frontal bone medially to the supraorbital notch and then travel superiorly, anteriorly, and laterally for 2 to 3 cm, blending in with the orbicularis oculi and frontalis fibers before inserting into the skin of the medial half of the eyebrow.[3] The supraorbital and supratrochlear neurovascular bundles pass anteriorly through the lower border of the corrugator supercilii (Figs. 28-2 and 28-4).[5] Contraction of the corrugator supercilii muscles draws the heads of the eyebrows closer together and depresses them, thus creating a froward countenance and vertical glabellar skin folds.

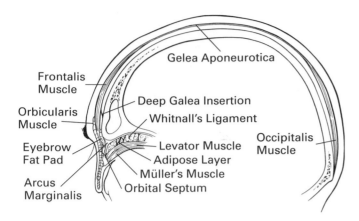

Figure 28-5 Parasagittal cross-section of the brow, forehead, and scalp.

The Deep Galea Aponeurotica

The deep galea aponeurotica is thick, well defined, and adherent to the undersurface of the frontalis muscle (Fig. 28-5).[1] Except for its insertion on the periosteum of the supraorbital rim, the deep galea aponeurotica is separated from the underlying periosteum of the frontal bone by an avascular plane of loose areolar tissue known as the *subgaleal space*.[1] Blunt dissection in this plane, which is continuous with the subgaleal plane of the scalp, allows easy peeling of the scalp and forehead tissue from the underlying periosteum (Fig. 28-6).

The Eyebrow Fat Pad

An inferior extension of the subgaleal space forms a specialized fat pad of the eyebrow which is located inferiorly to the deep galeal insertion and overlies a portion of the orbital septum (Fig. 28-5).[2] This fat pad of the eyebrow lies immediately deeply to the muscular plane of the eyebrow. Firm attachments between the superficial muscular layer and the eye-

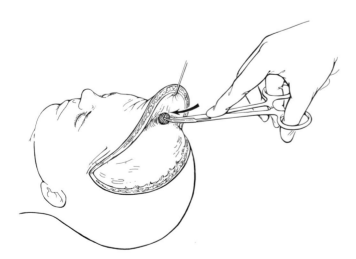

Figure 28-6 The forehead and scalp flap are easily dissected in the subgaleal plane. Bleeding is usually minimal in this plane.

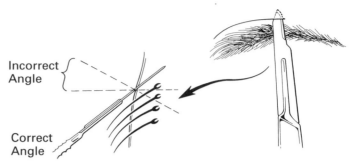

Figure 28-7 The scalpel blade should be angled parallel to the shafts of hair follicles to avoid hair loss.

brow fat pad are present medially and help to suspend the medial eyebrow. The eyebrow fat pad is known by many other terms, including the *adipose, cellulo adipose,* and *submuscular fibroadipose* layer of the eyebrow.[2] The eyebrow fat pad is most well developed laterally and contributes to eyebrow mobility.

The Subgaleal Space

The subgaleal space is located between the deep galea aponeurotica and the periosteum. This important surgical plane is relatively avascular and easily negotiated with blunt dissection.[1] The subgaleal plane is most often approached through a coronal or hairline incision (Fig. 28-6). Entering the subgaleal plane of the forehead usually requires dividing the galea and/or frontalis muscle. A surgical drain should be placed, and these structures should be repaired prior to skin closure in order to decrease wound gaping and hematoma.

Avoiding Complications

The major morbidities associated with subgaleal dissection can be avoided with appropriate attention to anatomic detail. When the cutaneous incision is made in a hair-bearing area, the blade angle should be beveled parallel to the hair shafts in order to avoid damage to follicles (Fig. 28-7).[6] Raney neurosurgical clips or Dandy hemostatic clamps may have to be placed to limit bleeding from the blood vessels which course deeply through the subcutaneous layer and just above the galea.[6]

The motor nerve supply to the frontalis muscle is especially vulnerable during forehead surgery (Fig. 28-8).[1,4] The temporal branch of the facial nerve courses obliquely over the periosteum of the proximal one-third of the zygomatic arch and then continues superiorly and anteriorly deeply in the superficial temporalis fascia until it penetrates the undersurface of the frontalis muscle not greater than 2 cm superiorly to the lateral eyebrow (Figs. 28-9, Fig. 28-10).[4,7] Hence, any lateral extension of the subgaleal dissection plane should be developed directly on the deep temporalis fascia, or deeper, in order to avoid injury to the overlying temporal branch of the fa-

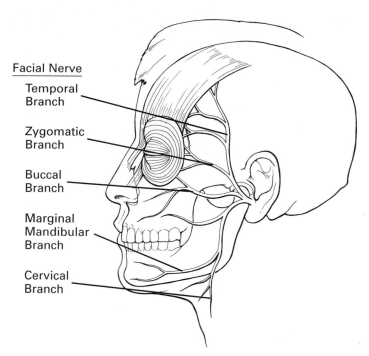

Facial Nerve
Temporal Branch
Zygomatic Branch
Buccal Branch
Marginal Mandibular Branch
Cervical Branch

Figure 28-8 The most vulnerable area of the temporal branch of the facial nerve is at the proximal zygomatic arch.

cial nerve. Inferolateral dissection onto the temple requires further precautions which are discussed below in "Temple."

During inferior dissection in the subgaleal space, care should be exercised in order to avoid injury to the supraorbital and supratrochlear sensory neurovascular bundles. These

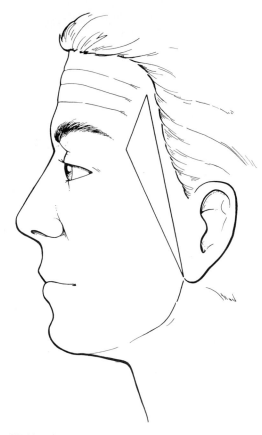

Figure 28-10 The area in which the temporal branch of the facial nerve may lie.

bundles traverse the subgaleal space after emerging from the orbit and passing through the inferior portion of the corrugator supercilii to lie eventually in the deep subcutaneous layer (Figs. 28-1, 28-2, 28-4, and 28-9).[4]

The Pericranium

The periosteum adherent to the outer table of the skull is termed the *pericranium*. Periosteal elevators are used to reflect this layer from the underlying bone. When the outer table of the skull is exposed and free skin grafts are employed, the surface of the outer table should be lightly burred to stimulate blood supply for the free graft.

RECONSTRUCTION OF THE FOREHEAD

The forehead comprises approximately one-third of the face. It is important, before planning any reconstruction of the forehead, to remember the anatomy discussed previously. The goal of dermatologic surgery in this area is to maintain the symmetry of the eyebrows, hairline, and periorbital structures by camouflaging the final scar lines into relaxed skin tension lines whenever possible as well as by hiding lines in hair-bearing areas.

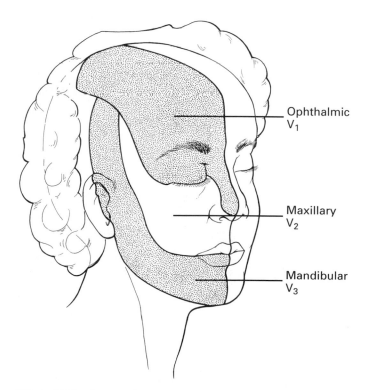

Ophthalmic V1

Maxillary V2

Mandibular V3

Figure 28-9 Sensory dermatomes of the trigeminal nerve.

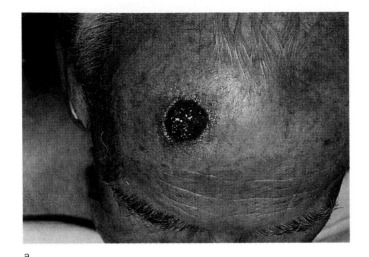

a

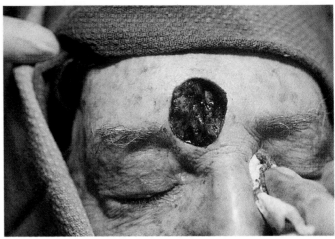

a

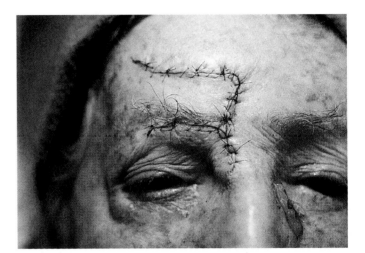

b

b

Figure 28-11 *(a–b)* Primary fusiform closure of an upper fore-head defect. Note horizontal closure lies in the relaxed skin tension lines of forehead.

Primary Fusiform Closure

Small defects or excisions on the forehead and temple can easily be repaired by primary fusiform closure. The relaxed skin tension lines which run perpendicularly to the vertical fibers of the frontalis muscle make an excellent camouflage area for scars (Figs. 28-11*a–b*). Vertical closures in the center of the forehead work well due to vertical lines present in the glabellar area and the reduced number of frontalis fibers in the midline. Occasionally, older patients who have deep furrows from sun exposure have some vertical lines which can also be used to hide scar lines.

Advancement Flaps

The suprabrow area lends itself well to unilateral (Figs. 28-12*a–c*) or bilateral horizontal advancement flaps (Figs. 28-13*a–c*), which maintain eyebrow symmetry, and takes advan-

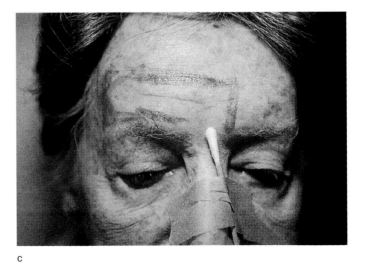

c

Figure 28-12 *(a–c)* A suprabrow and glabella defect closed by unilateral horizontal advancement flap. Note there is no eyebrow elevation and horizontal incisions are well camouflaged due to relaxed skin tension lines. The vertical incision is invisible due to lack of midline frontalis fibers.

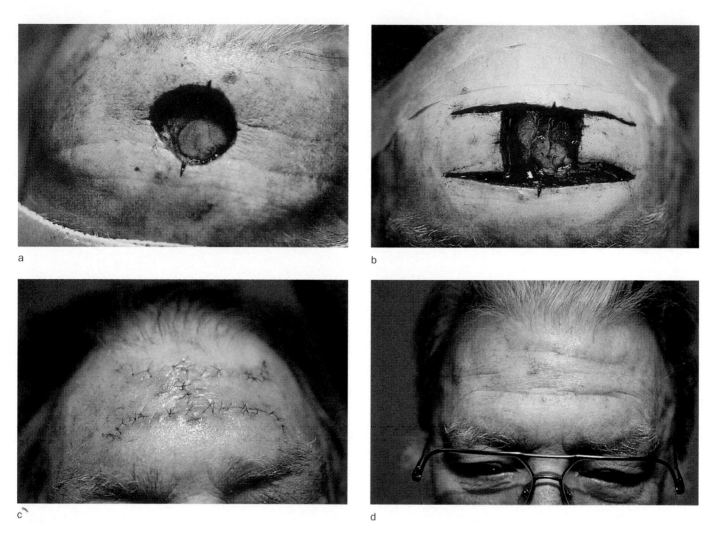

Figure 28-13   *(a–d)* A midline forhead defect closed by a bilateral horizontal frozen advancement flap. Note incision lines are well hidden in existing relaxed skin tension lines.

tage of the lateral skin movement. These flaps alleviate elevation of the eyebrow and result in no loss of hair-bearing areas. A subcutaneous tacking suture to the periosteum will help to prevent eyebrow elevation.[8] Sometimes, an eyebrow elevated as much as 5 to 10 mm will gradually return to a normal height due to gravity within 6 months.[1] Occasionally, A-to-T flaps for defects in the suprabrow area will prevent eyebrow elevation and will take advantage of lateral skin movement (Figs. 28-14*a–c*).

Island Pedicle Flaps

Island pedicle flaps alone or in combination with other flaps can be helpful in closing surgical defects on the forehead (Figs. 28-15*a–b*). These flaps have excellent blood supply since they are not severed from the underlying adipose tissue. Since forehead skin is often quite sebaceous and inelastic, island pedicle flaps can also utilize lateral skin movement and help maintain color and texture properties.

Rotation and Transposition Flaps

Rotation and transposition flaps are rarely used on the forehead due to the curvilinear lines resulting from tissue movement. These scar lines often run against relaxed skin tension lines and should be avoided whenever possible.

Tissue Expansion

Intraoperative tissue expansion or chronic tissue expansion may be helpful for large defects of the forehead. The use of a 30-mL Foley catheter can generate 1 to 2 cm of tissue in 20 min.[9]

Secondary Intention

Healing by secondary intention on the forehead for large defects rarely results in satisfactory cosmetic appearance. Defects close to the eyebrow may result in permanent asymme-

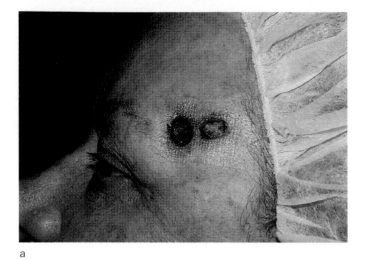

a

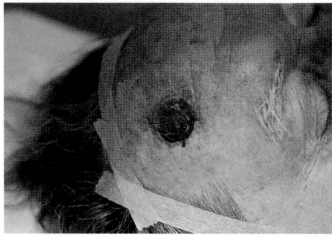

a

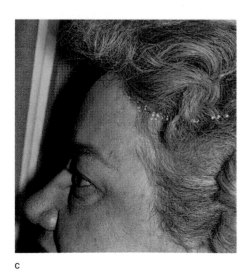

b

c

Figure 28-14 *(a–c)* A lateral suprabrow defect closed by an A-to-T advancement flap. Note there is no eyebrow displacement and horizontal incision is well camouflaged in eyebrow border.

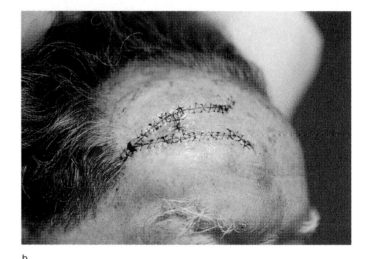

b

Figure 28-15 *(a–b)* An upper forehead defect repaired by a combination advancement and island pedicle flap. Note that island pedicle flap prevented advancement of hairline.

try of the eyebrow following contraction of the scar (Figs. 28-16*a–c*).

Skin Grafts

Occasionally, healing by secondary intention of the forehead followed by delayed full-thickness skin graft may result in an acceptable cosmetic result. Split-thickness skin grafts are usually used as a last resort or as a temporizing measure for massive forehead defects.

TEMPLE

For the purposes of this discussion, the cutaneous anatomic boundaries of the human temple are defined by the suprazygomatic extent of the temporalis muscle and deep temporal

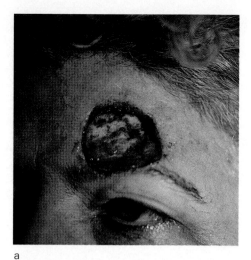

a

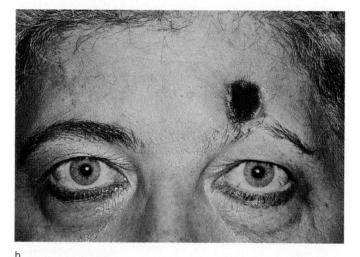

b

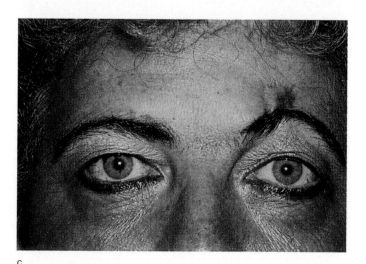

c

Figure 28-16 *(a)* Large suprabrow defect healed by secondary intention; *(b)* healing at 4 weeks' duration; *(c)* healing at 10 weeks' duration. Note undesirable elevation of eyebrow from secondary intention.

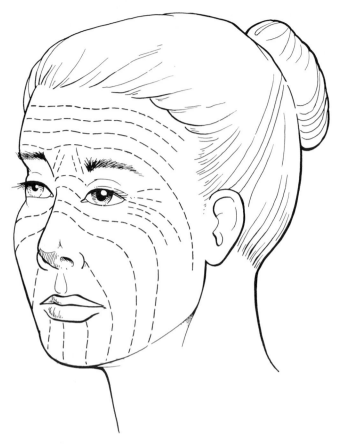

Figure 28-17   Relaxed skin tension lines of forehead and face.

fascia. Relaxed skin tension lines, useful for camouflaging incision, radiate from the lateral canthal angle as crow's feet or curve onto the temple as extensions of forehead creases (Fig. 28-17). The hairlines and junctures of the sideburns and temple also help to hide incisions.

Cutaneous Innervation

The main sensory nerve supply of the temple arises from the auriculotemporal branch of the mandibular nerve and the zygomaticotemporal branch of the maxillary nerve (Fig. 28-1).[1] These nerves are not readily accessible to nerve blocks; hence, infiltrative anethesia is usually employed for temple surgery.

Superficial Musculoaponeurotic System

Superficial Temporal Fascia

In the temple region, the muscular layer of the SMAS is less developed than that of the forehead and contains only a few lateral orbicularis fibers and strands of the anterior auricular muscle. The primary structure of the SMAS that is found in the temple is the superficial temporal fascia located immediately beneath the subcutaneous fatty layer (Fig. 28-3).[1] The

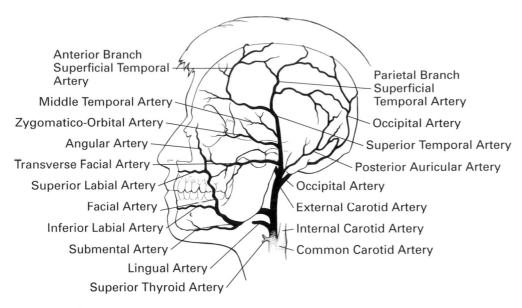

Figure 28-18 Arterial blood supply to temple and forehead.

adult superficial temporal fascia is 2- to 4-mm thick, highly vascularized, and rich in connective tissue. At boundary regions, the superficial temporal fascia blends with the adjacent scalp-galea and frontalis muscle, thus reflecting the anatomic and functional commonality of these SMAS components.

Superficial Temporal Artery and Auriculotemporal Nerve

Sensory nerves and large vessels, including the proximal superficial temporal artery and vein and auriculotemporal branch of the mandibular nerve, course through the superficial aspects of this fascia before eventually entering the deep subcutaneous layer (Figs. 28-1, 28-18, and 28-19).[4] The pulsations of the superficial temporal artery are palpable anteriorly to the tragus where it gives off the transverse facial artery. The superficial temporal artery ascends to the level of the superior attachment of the ear where it bifurcates into anterior (frontal) and posterior (parietal) branches (Fig. 28-18).[1] The bifurcation lies within the upper stratum of the superficial temporal fascia, and its corresponding vein lies in the deepest stratum of the overlying subcutaneous fat layer. As the superficial temporal artery ascends towards the scalp, however, it lies more superficially in the deepest stratum of the subcutaneous fat layer.

Adherence of Superficial Fascia and Skin   The superficial aspects of the superficial temporal fascia blend with the overlying subcutaneous layer and are connected to it and the dermis by vertically oriented fibrous strands.[1] Adherence be-

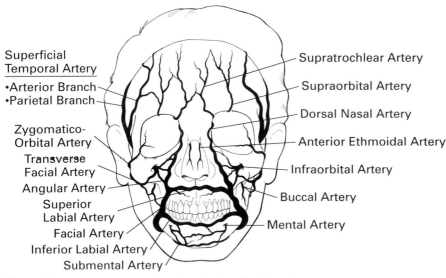

Figure 28-19 Arterial blood supply to forehead and temple.

tween the superficial temporal fascia and the overlying sub-cutaneous and dermal layers is slight at the level of the zygo-matic arch but increases rapidly superiorly near the scalp.[1]

Intertemporal-Fascial Plane

A loose avascular tissue lies beneath the superficial temporal fascia and separates it from the underlying deep temporal fas-cia.[1] This avascular areolar tissue allows the two fascial lay-ers to glide upon one another easily—this can be experienced by clenching the jaw while massaging the temples over the tight temporalis muscle. The two fasciae also peel apart eas-ily, thus providing a logical plane for lateral extension of the subgaleal forehead dissection. However, inferior dissection in this plane jeopardizes the temporal branch of the facial nerve.

Deep Temporal Fascia

The tough, milky-white, fan-shaped deep temporal fascia fuses with periosteum in all directions, blending with the mandible inferiorly and blending with the superior temporal line of the skull superiorly and laterally.[1] Inferiorly, the deep temporalis fascia splits into anterior and posterior leaflets which envelop the fat pad lying immediately superiorly to the zygomatic arch (Fig. 28-3).[4] The anterior leaflet fuses with the periosteum of the zygomatic arch over which runs the fas-cicles of the temporal branch of the facial nerve.[4] Therefore, in the area of the zygomatic arch, it is important not to dissect directly over the anterior leaflet of the deep temporal fascia

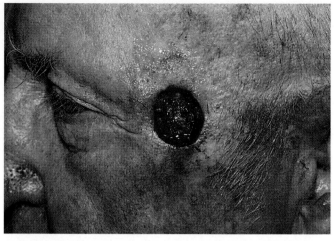

a

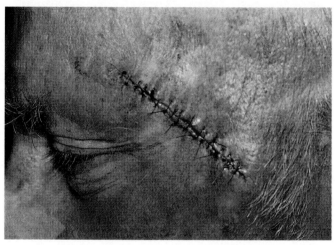

b

Figure 28-21 *(a–b)* Temporal defect reconstructed by primary fusiform closure.

since one jeopardizes the temporal nerve (Fig. 28-8). Dissec-tion planes beginning superiorly and extending inferiorly into this zone should lie deeply to the anterior leaflet of the deep temporal fascia. Dissection planes beginning laterally and ex-tending anteriorly into this zone (i.e., face-lift) should lie in the superficial stratum of the subcutaneous layer.

Temporalis Muscle

The fan-shaped temporalis muscle lies immediately beneath the deep temporal fascia (Fig. 28-20). The temporalis muscle originates from the periosteum of the temporalis fossa and then passes through the concavity of the zygomatic arch to in-sert into the coronoid process and anterior border of the mandibular ramus.[4] Its motor innervation comes from the an-terior deep temporal nerve (of the mandibular division of the trigeminal nerve) which ascends to penetrate the muscle on its undersurface.[1]

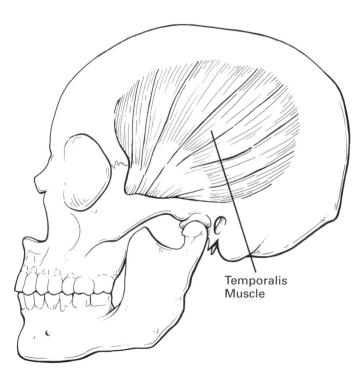

Temporalis
Muscle

Figure 28-20   Temporalis muscle.

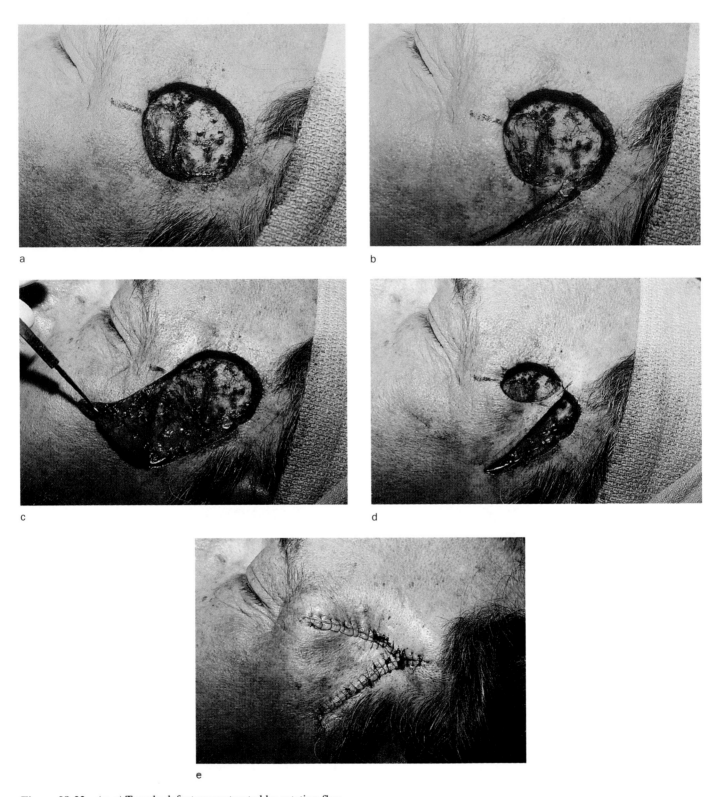

Figure 28-22   *(a–e)* Temple defect reconstructed by rotation flap.

RECONSTRUCTION OF THE TEMPLE

In dermatologic surgery of the temple, the most important structure is the temporal branch of the facial nerve. The temporal branch innervates the muscles of the eyebrow on their undersurface (i.e., frontalis, corrugator supercilii, procerus, and upper orbicularis oculi muscles) as well as the auricular muscles.[2] As mentioned previously, the nerve runs within the fascia of the temporalis muscle and is most vulnerable over the zygomatic arch. The best way to remember the pathway of the temporal branch is to draw a line from the ear lobe to the lateral eyebrow and from the ear lobe to the highest wrinkle on the forehead. The triangle formed by the hairline and these boundary lines should alert the surgeon to its pathway (Fig. 28-10). It is important to warn all patients that possible motor loss of the ipsilateral eyebrow and forehead can result if the nerve is injured.

Primary Fusiform Closure

Small defects of the temple can be camouflaged in the lateral periorbital lines best seen when the patient is asked to squint, in the extension of the relaxed skin tension lines of the forehead (Figs. 28-21a–b), or in the anterior temporal hairline.

Rotation and Transposition Flaps

Rotation flaps are most useful for medium and larger defects of the temple because of the reservoir of excess skin from the cheek. This skin can easily be rotated superiorly and medially to cover these areas, with excellent cosmetic results.

The incision lines of the flap can be hidden in the preauricular sulcus and anterior hair-bearing area of the temple (Figs. 28-22a–e). Movement of hair-bearing skin into hairless areas should be avoided. Transposition flaps can also take advantage of cheek laxity.

Secondary Intention

It is not uncommon to allow large defects of the temple and temporal hair-bearing areas to heal by secondary intention.

Results can be cosmetically pleasing and superior to full-thickness or split-thickness skin grafts.

CONCLUSION

Excellent outcome in forehead and temple reconstruction challenges the abilities of the dermatologic surgeon. Superior results in this area are achieved when the surgeon adheres to the three basic hierarchic principles of forehead and temple reconstruction: (1) Avoid iatrogenic facial nerve injury, (2) maintain symmetry of landmark structures, and (3) camouflage incision lines.

REFERENCES

1. Salasche SJ et al: *Surgical Anatomy of the Skin.* Norwalk, Conn, Appleton & Lange, 1988, pp 164–182

2. Whitnall SE: *Anatomy of the Human Orbit.* London, Henry Frowde & Hodder & Stoughton, 1921, pp 105–111

3. Doxanas MT, Anderson RL: *Clinical Orbital Anatomy.* Baltimore, Williams & Wilkins, 1984, pp 57–89

4. Zide B, Jelks G: *Surgical Anatomy of the Orbit.* New York, Raven Press, 1985, pp 13–19

5. Shore JW: Essential blepharospasm, in *Oculoplastic Surgery,* edited by CD McCord, M Tanenbaum. New York, Raven Press, 1987, pp 475–492

6. Tardy MD, Tom LW: Aesthetic correction of the ptotic brow, in *Cosmetic Oculoplastic Surgery,* edited by A Putterman. New York, Grune & Stratton, 1982, pp 147–176

7. Pitanguy I, Ramos AS: The frontal branch of the facial nerve: The importance of its variations in face lifting. *Plast Reconstr Surg* **38:**352–356, 1966

8. Dzubow LM: *Facial Flaps: Biomechanics and Regional Application.* Norwalk, Conn, Appleton & Lange, 1990, pp 102–113, 129–134

9. Siegle RJ: Forehead reconstruction. *J Dermatol Surg Oncol* **17:**200–204, 1991

J. Ramsey Mellette, Jr.

29 Reconstruction of the Ear

The external ear is an important functional and structural appendage. Although it is not usually praised for beauty, significant deformities can be distracting and distressing. Functional and aesthetic reconstruction can be simplified by a regional approach utilizing commonly known principles and techniques of surgical repair. In a step-by-step fashion, reconstructive options for the external ear are discussed in this chapter.

ANATOMY

A comprehensive and concise review of ear anatomy is available in Salache et al.'s excellent test.[1] The following discussion will deal primarily with anatomic considerations for reconstruction.

The external ear (Fig. 29-1) consists of thin skin, with very little subcutaneous tissue, supported by an irregular plate of cartilage. The cartilage is thickest at the concha, of medium thickness along the antihelix, and thinnest at the helical rim where, especially inferior to the auricular tubercle, it is more of a fibrocartilaginous structure. Passing inferiorly along the helix and antihelix, there is progressively more subcutaneous tissue with the lobule being devoid of cartilage. The abundance of skin and subcutaneous tissue in the lobule has special significance when planning reconstruction along the rim of the ear because of the mobility of the cartilaginous ear afforded by this adjacent noncartilaginous tissue.

The anterior auricular skin is tightly adherent to the underlying cartilage and contains little subcutaneous tissue. On the posterior ear, there is slightly more subcutaneous tissue, a rich blood supply, and more mobility of skin, especially inferiorly, close to the posterior auricular groove. When tumors have been removed from the anterior ear, exposing cartilage devoid of perichondrium, the cartilage can often be removed in its entirety to provide this richly vascularized tissue as a recipient site for a full-thickness graft.[2] In addition, this thicker, more mobile posterior skin can be mobilized as single or double transposition flaps, or as pedicle flaps, to cover helical and antihelical defects.

RECONSTRUCTION

Superior Helical Rim

Superior helical rim defects (Fig. 29-2) of sizes up to 3 cm in length can be repaired by either postauricular (Fig. 29-3) or preauricular transposition flaps, which can be quite long and broad. A pedicle with a 1:3 or 1:4 width/length ratio is planned but has been exceeded without difficulty, allowing coverage of the entire superior helical rim. This is illustrated in Figs. 29-4–29-10, indicating where it was necessary to remove intervening normal tissue (Fig. 29-5) to facilitate flap transfer. Small midsuperior helical defects can sometimes be repaired with a single (Figs. 29-11–29-13) or double (Figs. 29-14–29-17) transposition flap from the postauricular skin. In Figs. 29-14–29-17, an angular flap based on the bilobed principle was used. This "birhombic" design combines a 30° angle flap with a 40° angle flap to close a 60° angle rhombic defect.[3]

Helpful Hints

1. Measure carefully to ensure adequate flap length. It is better to err on the side of excess.
2. On the superior rim, place the first suture in the tip of the flap and secure this flap to the helix with a vertical mattress to provide wound eversion.

Posterior-Middle Helical Rim

Most defects of this area (Fig. 29-18) can be successfully closed by helical rim advancement flaps (Fig. 29-19). Defects

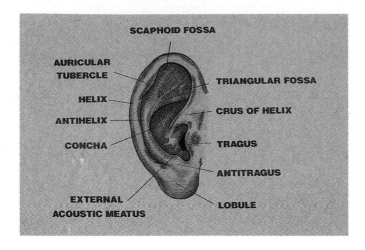

Figure 29-1

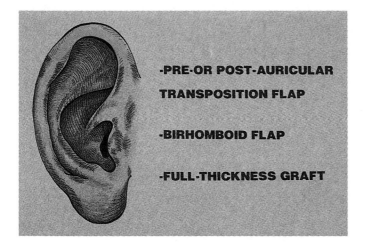

Figure 29-2

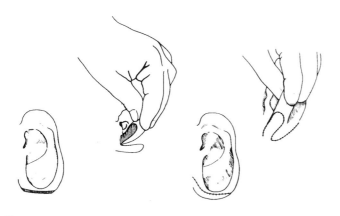

Figure 29-3

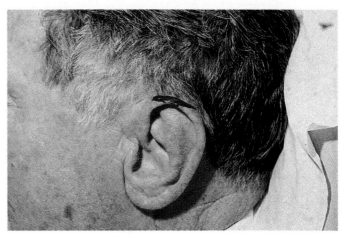

Figure 29-4

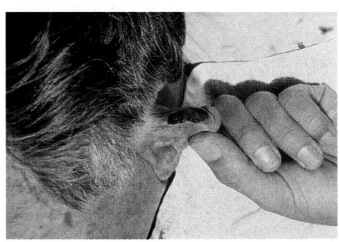

Figure 29-5

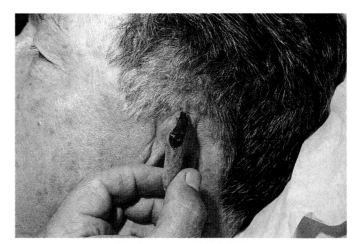

Figure 29-6

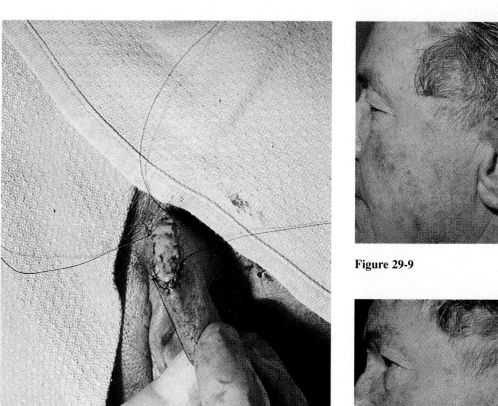

Figure 29-7

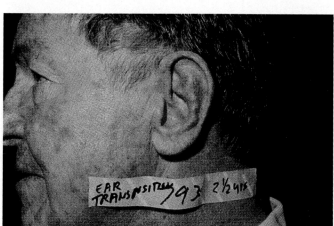

Figure 29-9

Figure 29-10

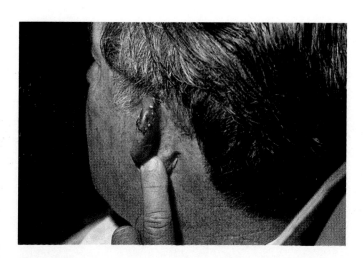

Figure 29-8

of up to 2.5 cm in length have been repaired with excellent cosmetic results (Figs. 29-20–29-25). As with the superior helical rim, smaller defects can often be repaired with a single or double transposition flap from the postauricular skin. For defects of greater magnitude, and those which include the superior as well as posterior-inferior rim, the chondrocutaneous advancement flap may be utilized.[4] With both flaps, the anterior-superior helix may also be mobilized to facilitate closure.

Helpful Hints

1. With the rim advancement flap, mark the intended incision line anteriorly and posteriorly. The incision is made from anterior to posterior and carved inferiorly *into the lobule* to obtain mobility. The success of this flap depends largely upon the laxity afforded by the lobule, so be bold with this incision (Figs. 29-19, 29-21–29-22).

2. The detached helical rim is advanced upward and secured

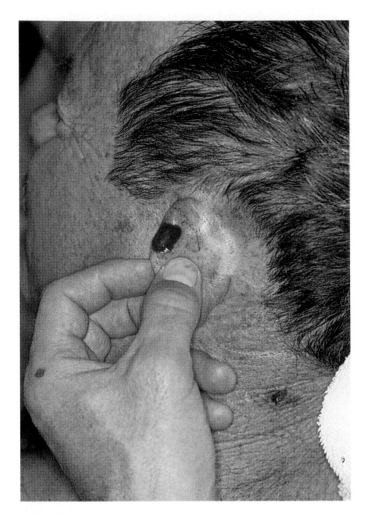

Figure 29-11

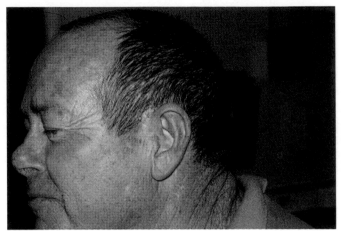

Figure 29-13

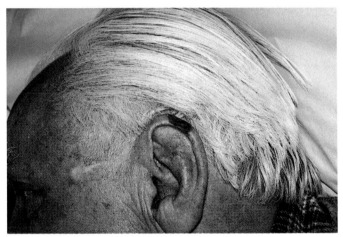

Figure 29-14

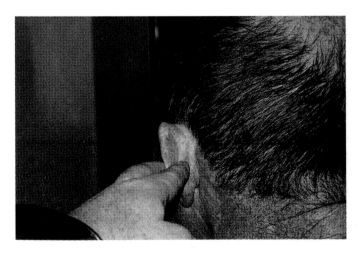

Figure 29-12

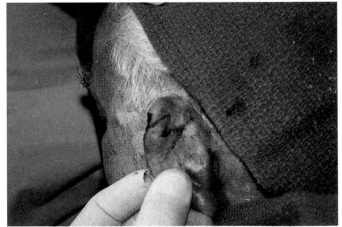

Figure 29-15

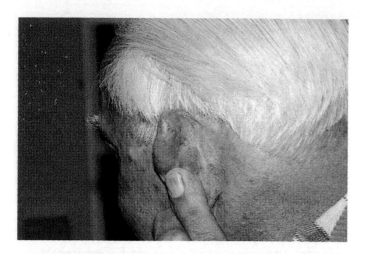

Figure 29-16

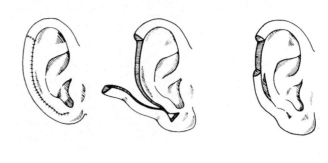

Figure 29-19

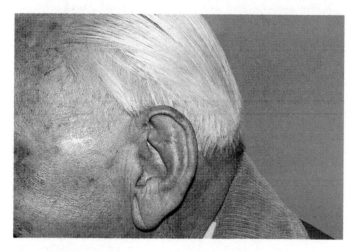

Figure 29-17

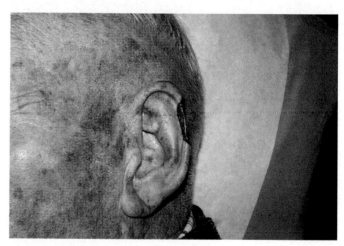

Figure 29-20

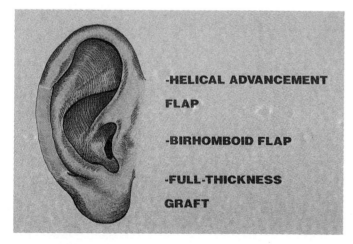

Figure 29-18

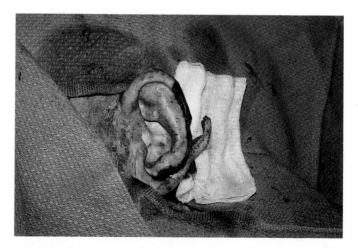

Figure 29-21

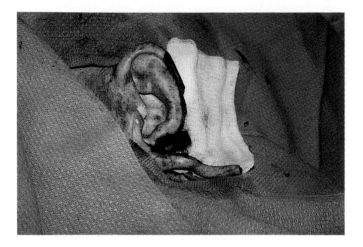

Figure 29-22

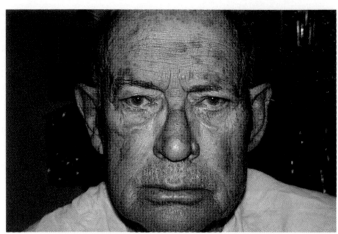

Figure 29-25

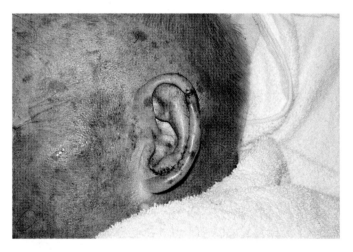

Figure 29-23

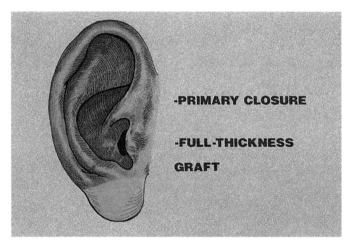

Figure 29-26

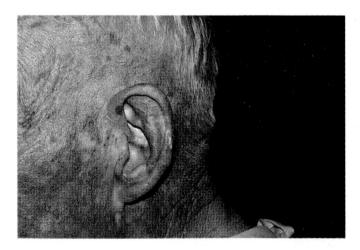

Figure 29-24

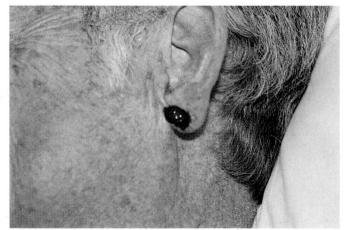

Figure 29-27

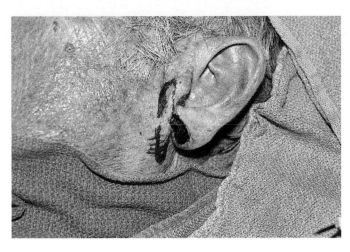

Figure 29-28

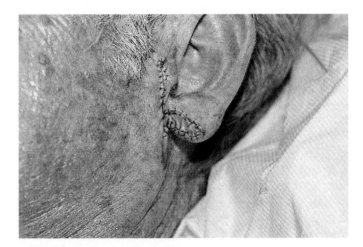

Figure 29-29

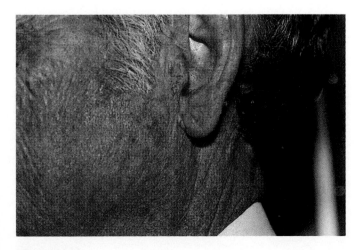

Figure 29-30

superiorly by a vertical mattress suture. The remainder of the flap is secured with interrupted sutures.

3. Some bunching of tissue will occur in the lobule. The unequal sides principle of halving the closure will usually obviate the need for a Burow's triangle.

Lobule

The lobule (Fig. 29-26) can be closed primarily, usually with a wedge-type excision. In order to avoid shortening or distorting of this lobule, transposition flaps such as the banner flap (Figs. 29-27–29-30) may be developed from adjacent cheek skin, preferably from the preauricular crease (Fig. 29-28). A lobule "rim advancement" flap may be utilized (Figs. 29-31–29-34). The lobule will accept a full-thickness graft.

Helpful Hints

1. The rim of the lobule is a continuation of the helical rim. If closure involves attachment of the lobule to the rim, a vertical mattress suture will help prevent notching.
2. Excessive loss of the lobule may result in noticeable asymmetry. Occasionally, a small wedge resection in the opposite lobule has been utilized to reestablish symmetry.

Tragus and Crus of Helix

Primary closure or a single rhombic transposition flap (Figs. 29-35–29-38) is most often employed in this area.

Scaphoid Fossa and Triangular Fossa of Antihelix

In this area (Fig. 29-39) with exposed cartilage (Fig. 29-40), application of a full-thickness graft from the skin inferior to the mastoid process after removal of underlying cartilage (Figs. 29-41–29-44) has been the preferred method of repair.[3] Grafting here has been unusually successful. It is important to note that the superior and inferior crura which form the triangular fossa are thought important for structural support. If the helical rim and inferior antihelical cartilage adjacent to the defect are preserved, most of this cartilage may be removed without structural compromise. Note that in Fig. 29-41 part of the anterior-inferior crus of the triangular fossa was left intact. With more extensive defects and/or in situations where it is deemed important to preserve cartilage (Fig. 29-45), this area can be repaired by a postauricular pedicle flap (Figs. 29-46 and 29-47). The leading edge of this flap is along the posterior aspect of the ear, approximating the posterior limits of the defect in the anterior surface (Fig. 29-46). The flap is designed as an advancement flap and is extensively undermined. An incision is made through the posterior skin and cartilage with a small ellipse of cartilage removed to prevent flap constriction. The skin is then advanced through the cartilage to cover the anterior ear defect (Fig. 29-48). The pedicle is divided, after 10 to 14 days, by incising it at the point of

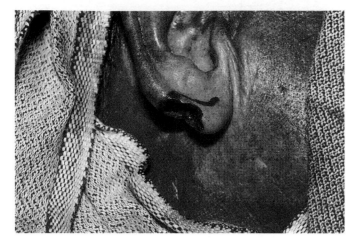

Figure 29-31

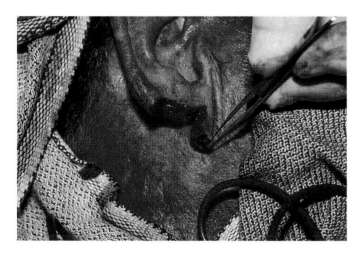

Figure 29-32

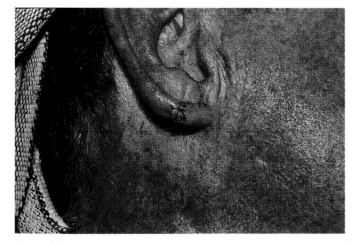

Figure 29-33

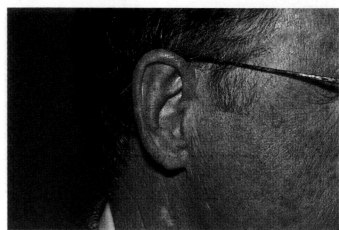

Figure 29-34

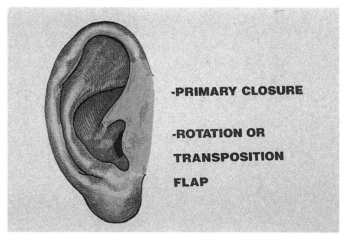

-PRIMARY CLOSURE

-ROTATION OR

TRANSPOSITION

FLAP

Figure 29-35

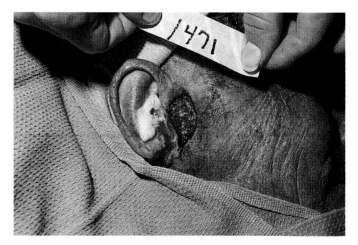

Figure 29-36

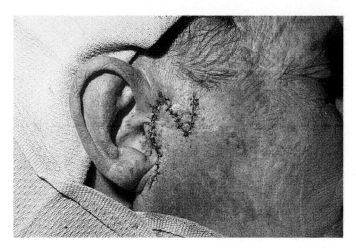

Figure 29-37

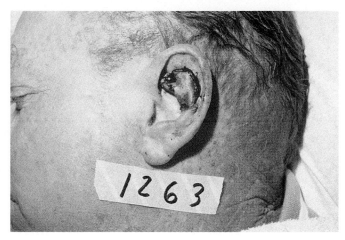

Figure 29-40

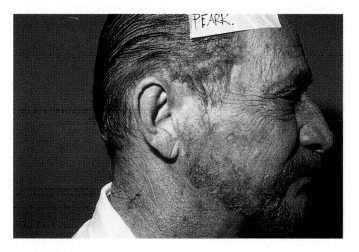

Figure 29-38

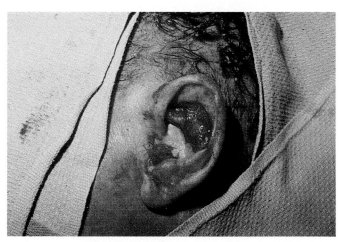

Figure 29-41

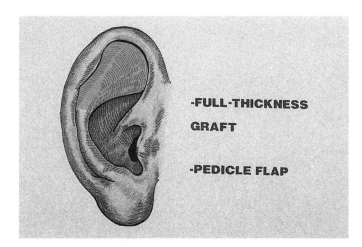

Figure 29-39

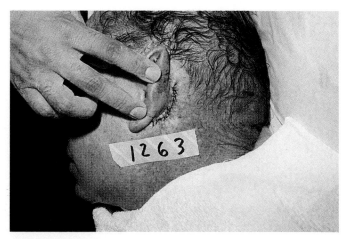

Figure 29-42

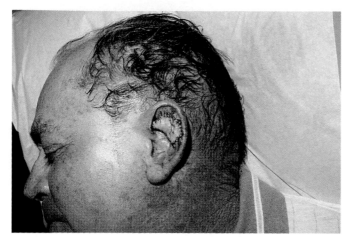

Figure 29-43

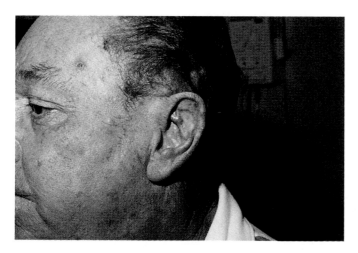

Figure 29-44

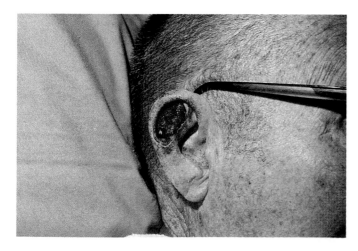

Figure 29-45

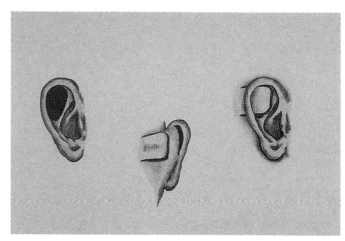

Figure 29-46

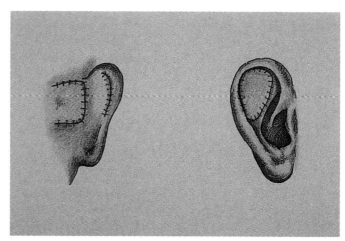

Figure 29-47

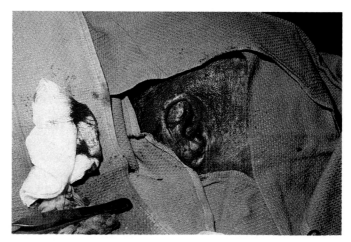

Figure 29-48

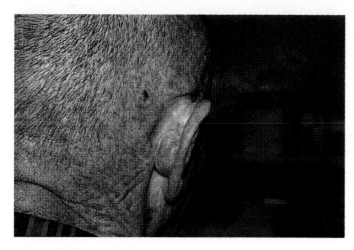

Figure 29-49

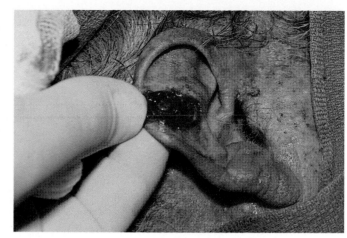

Figure 29-52

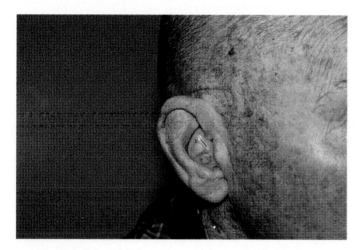

Figure 29-50

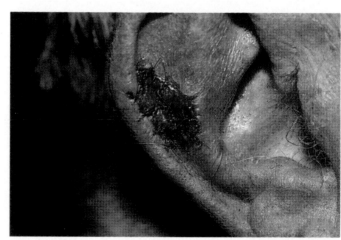

Figure 29-53

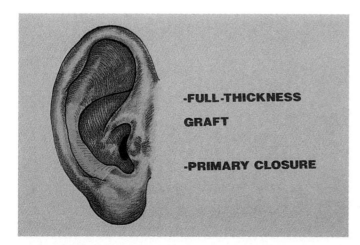

Figure 29-51

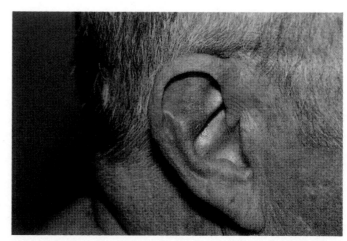

Figure 29-54

insertion into the anterior ear (Fig. 29-47). The long-term result is seen in Figs. 29-49–29-50. Variations of this flap may be utilized for other defects of the antihelix and concha.[5]

Helpful Hints

1. For full-thickness grafts, through-and-through basting sutures may prove to be more desirable than tie-over dressings.
2. A small Penrose drain may be used beneath the pedicle flap to facilitate cleaning of this area, usually with hydrogen peroxide and/or acetic acid. Gentamicin cream or ointment is usually applied.
3. The pedicle flap is divided, after 10 to 14 days, by incising it at the point of insertion into the anterior ear. Interrupted sutures or Steri-Strips will suffice for the closure of the insertion.

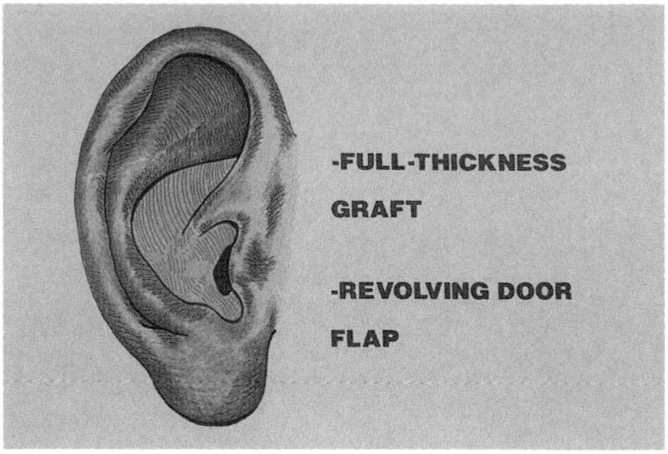

Lower Antihelix

In this area (Fig. 29-51), often the adjacent helix or concha is involved. Full-thickness grafts (Figs. 29-52–29-54) and primary closures have proved to be the most frequent closure here.

Concha

The entire conchal cartilage can be utilized for reconstruction of the contralateral ear and for nasal tip and ala reconstruction, so there is significant latitude for repairs in this area (Fig. 29-55). Flap techiques, including the "revolving door" island flap and those described by Gingross and Fickrell, may be utilized as well as full-thickness grafts in this area (Figs. 29-56–29-58).[5,6] The revolving door island flap is useful and clever but may result in pinning the ear too closely to the head. An alternative flap is a preauricular transposition or "finger" flap (Figs. 29-59–29-62); this may be superiorly or inferiorly based. In Figs. 29-63–29-66, the defect extended into the external meatus, and the tip of the flap was split to line the defect superiorly and inferiorly.

Helpful Hints

1. Carefully measure the flap pedicle to ensure adequate length. The undersurface should be trimmed to provide thinning of the flap to achieve good contour and wound apposition.
2. Partial removal of cartilage in this recipient area to expose the richly vascularized perichondrium of this reverse side may improve viability of flaps in this area.
3. To help prevent stenosis and to secure the flap, the meatus may be packed with Xeroform.

Combined Defects

Large defects involving both the convex and concave surfaces of the ear may be encountered (Fig. 29-67). Occasionally,

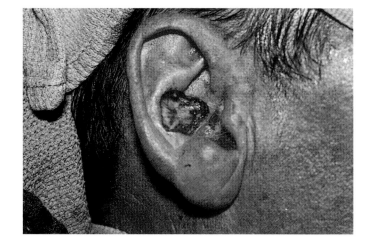

Figure 29-55

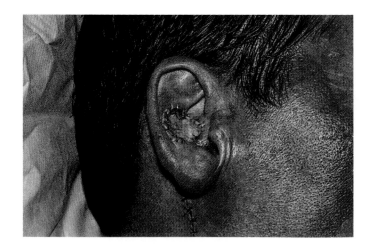

Figure 29-56

Figure 29-57

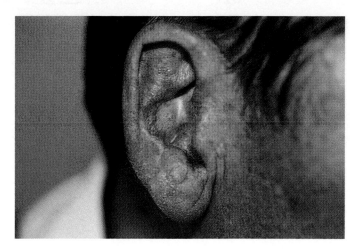

Figure 29-58

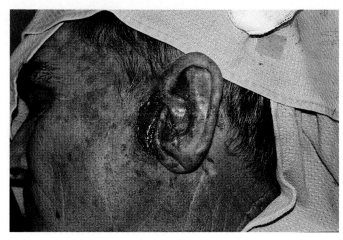

Figure 29-61

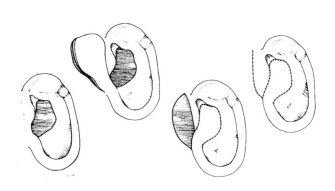

Figure 29-59

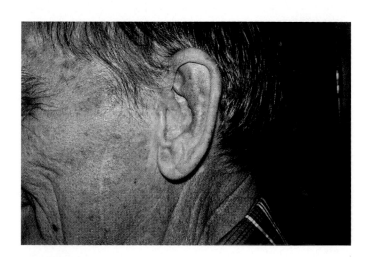

Figure 29-62

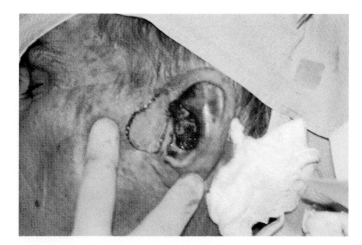

Figure 29-60

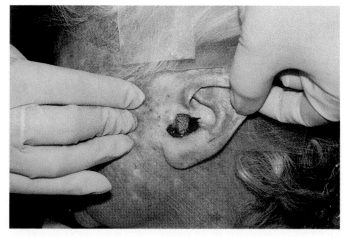

Figure 29-63

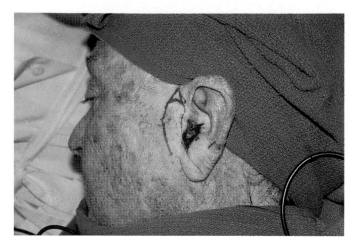

Figure 29-64

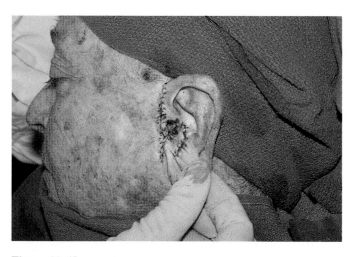

Figure 29-65

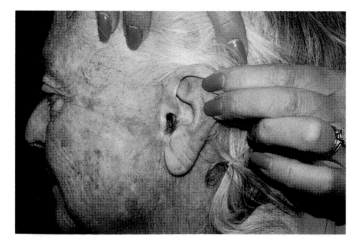

Figure 29-66

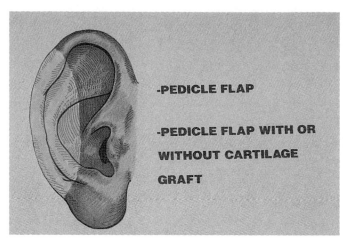

-PEDICLE FLAP

-PEDICLE FLAP WITH OR WITHOUT CARTILAGE GRAFT

Figure 29-67

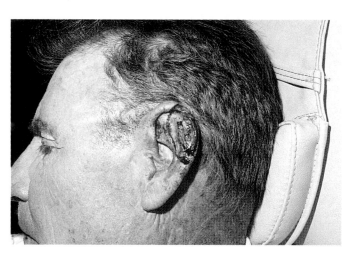

Figure 29-68

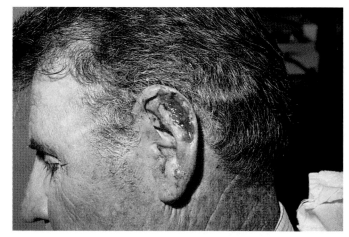

Figure 29-69

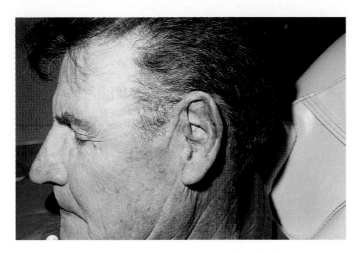

Figure 29-70

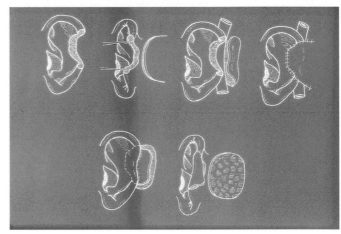

Figure 29-72

these can be allowed to heal secondarily by developing cartilaginous "windows" to provide granulation tissue from the postauricular subcutaneous tissue (Figs. 29-68–29-70). However, exposed cartilage is susceptible to infection and inflammation, and extensive destruction by unrelenting chondritis has been encountered.

When defects involve the full thickness of the ear (Fig. 29-71), an excellent repair can be provided by a postauricular pedicle flap. The flap is planned with the leading edge in the postauricular sulcus and is measured to provide sufficient length to replace the anterior and posterior defect (Fig. 29-72). The flap is advanced and sutured to the anterior surface of the ear (Fig. 29-73). A Penrose drain is placed, and, in 10 to 14 days, the flap is divided at its posterior attachment with this tissue then folded to cover the posterior aspect of the defect. This flap provides the necessary thickness to preclude support by a cartilage graft (Figs. 29-74 and 29-75). The defect created by mobilizing the defect is allowed to heal secondarily or repaired with a split- or full-thickness skin graft.

A large defect, which included loss of cartilage as well as extensive pre- and postauricular soft tissue, was encountered

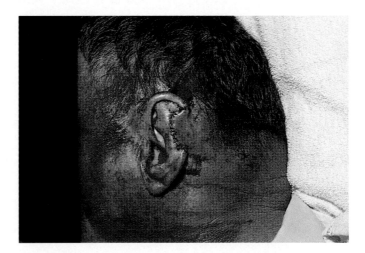

Figure 29-73

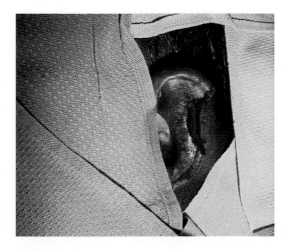

Figure 29-71

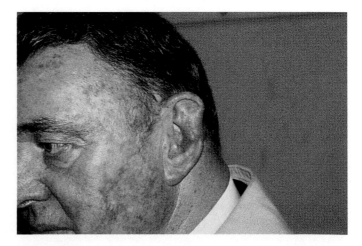

Figure 29-74

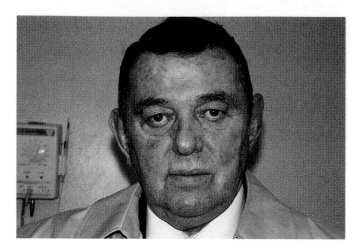

Figure 29-75

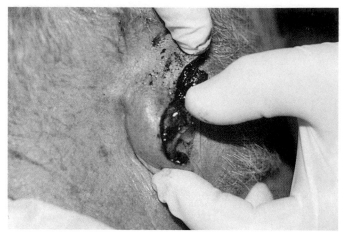

Figure 29-77

after Mohs surgery for a long-term recurrent basal cell carcinoma (Figs. 29-76 and 29-77). The remaining cartilage was essentially devoid of perichondrium. A large postauricular pedicle flap was developed (Fig. 29-78), and a few millimeters of uncovered triangular fossa cartilage were allowed to heal by secondary intention. The long-term result reveals complete healing with an acceptable cosmetic result (Figs. 29-79 and 29-80).

Helpful Hints

1. Few problems have been encountered with the pedicle flap. Some thinning and trimming may be necessary to ensure good contour.
2. The patient is allowed to shower and shampoo after the first 24 h. Daily cleaning with hydrogen peroxide and application of a Telfa dressing with an antibiotic ointment are recommended.
3. Prior to dividing the flap, pressure or a tourniquet is applied to the pedicle to ensure that an adequate blood supply has been established.

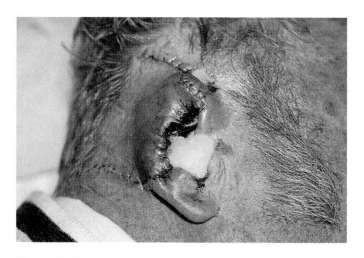

Figure 29-78

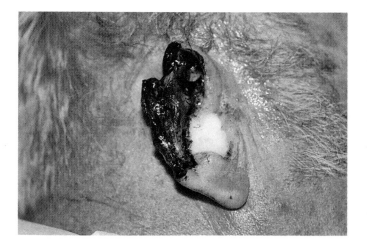

Figure 29-76

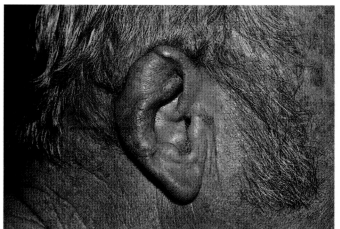

Figure 29-79

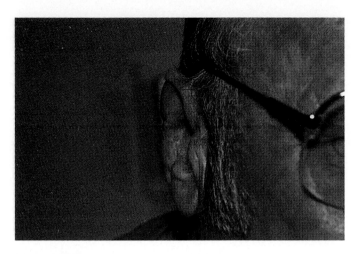

Figure 29-80

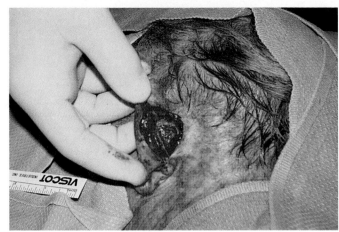

Figure 29-82

The Posterior Ear

Many of the techniques for anterior ear reconstruction can be utilized posteriorly (Fig. 29-81). Single transposition flaps may be utilized to close medial (near the postauricular sulcus) defects of varying sizes. A 5- by 3-cm defect was closed by a single 30° angle transposition flap (Figs. 29-82–29-84). Approximately 75 percent of the conchal cartilage was removed (Fig. 29-82) to facilitate this closure. When defects are encountered more laterally toward the postauricular rim, a double transposition flap (*bi-rhomboid*), as shown in Figs. 29-85–29-88, may be necessary.

Helpful Hints

1. As with most transposition flaps, extensive undermining is required. Laxity is provided by the skin of the postauricular sulcus and adjacent mastoid area.
2. As in the single rhombic transposition, the donor defects are closed first to relieve tension in the recipient bed.

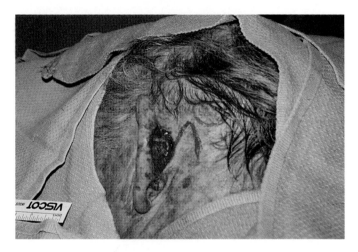

Figure 29-83

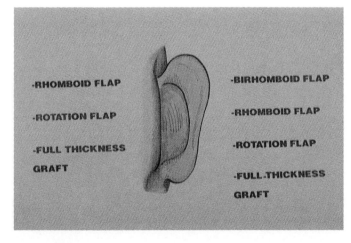

Figure 29-81

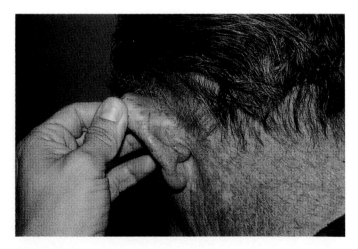

Figure 29-84

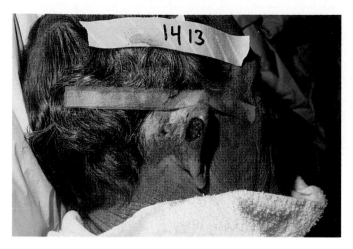

Figure 29-85

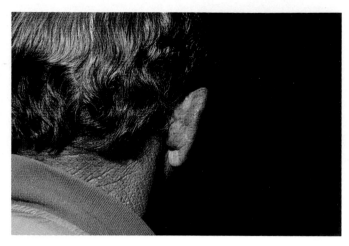

Figure 29-88

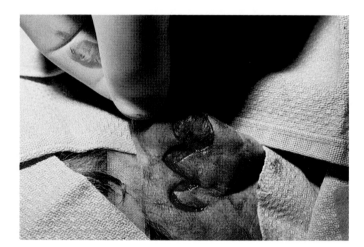

Figure 29-86

REFERENCES

1. Salache SJ et al: Regional anatomy, pt 3: The ear, in *Surgical Anatomy of the Skin.* Norwalk, Conn, Appleton & Lange, 1988, p 218

2. Mellette JR, Swinehart JM: Cartilage removal prior to skin grafting in the triangular fossa, antihelix, and concha of the ear. *J Dermatol Surg Oncol* **16:**1102–1105, 1990

3. Mellette JR: *Bi-rhombic Flap in Facial Reconstruction.* Presented at the Advanced Surgical Techniques Symposium 334, American Academy of Dermatology, Washington, D.C., Dec 7, 1988

4. Antia NH, Buch VI: Chondrocutaneous advancement flap for the marginal defect of the ear. *Plast Reconstr Surg* **39:**472, 1967

5. Jackson IT: Ear reconstruction, in *Local Flaps in Head and Neck Reconstruction.* St. Louis, Mosby, 1985, p 251

6. Gingross RP, Fickrell KL: Techniques for closure of conchal and external auditory canal defects. *Plast Reconstr Surg* **41:**568–571, 1968

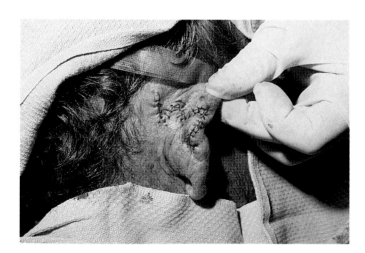

Figure 29-87

Nicholas R. Telfer
Ronald L. Moy

30 Nasal Reconstruction

Although nasal reconstruction is an ancient art[1,2], the complexities of nasal anatomy and physiology continue to make the repair of nasal defects one of the most challenging aspects of dermatologic surgery, especially as skin cancer (particularly basal cell carcinoma)[3–10] has a marked predilection for nasal skin, making the nose a common site for reconstructive surgery.[3] Nasal tumor excision and repair can be performed as a single procedure, usually involving wide excision with sacrifice of large amounts of normal tissue,[3,11–13] especially when dealing with recurrent or infiltrating tumors.[14] Highly accurate removal of skin cancer by Mohs micrographic surgery (MMS) results in both consistently high cure rates and the conservation of as much normal tissue as possible[3,4,8,15,16] and may be the treatment of choice for many primary and recurrent nasal carcinomas.[9] Nasal defects resulting from MMS can often be repaired without modification, although occasionally the sacrifice of a surrounding area of normal tissue may allow a more aesthetic reconstruction of an entire cosmetic unit.[17–19]

To produce optimal cosmetic and functional results, nasal repairs must be carefully planned and based upon a sound knowledge of the physiologic importance and anatomic complexity of the nose.[20,21]

NASAL ANATOMY

The nose is a respiratory and olfactory organ made up of skin and muscle overlying a skeleton of bone and cartilage which is lined with mucosa. The paired nasal bones support the thin skin of the upper nose, which is usually elastic and easily undermined. The underlying bony rigidity resists distortion and contributes to the successful outcome of many skin flaps on the upper nose. In contrast, the skin of the lower nose is generally thicker, more sebaceous, less elastic, and more tightly bound down—features which directly affect surgery in this area.[3] The lower nose is supported by the paired alar cartilages which articulate via fibrous bands with the superiorly placed paired lateral cartilages which, in turn, articulate with the single midline septal cartilage and the paired nasal bones (Fig. 30-1).[22] Each alar cartilage is shaped like a wishbone, with the apex supporting one side of the nasal tip (Fig. 30-2).

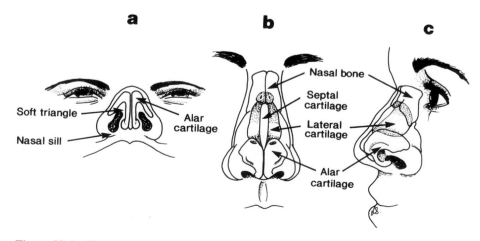

a   **b**   **c**

Soft triangle — Alar cartilage

Nasal sill

Nasal bone

Septal cartilage

Lateral cartilage

Alar cartilage

Figure 30-1   The supporting nasal structures: nasal bones and cartilage (see text.)

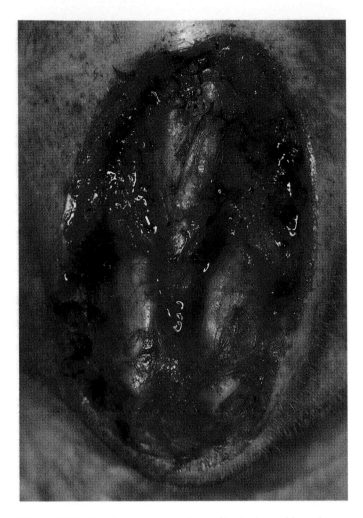

Figure 30-2   Nasal anatomy: portions of both alar and lateral nasal cartilage exposed during Mohs micrographic surgery.

The lateral crus passes obliquely laterally and upward, and the medial crus bends inferiorly to support one side of the columella.[23] Consequently, the majority of the ala is not supported by cartilage. Rather, it is supported by fibrofatty attachments and by the action of the nasalis muscle.[24,25] The nasal cartilages are highly mobile and do not resist distortion well. Consequently, many repairs have the potential to deviate the lower nose, either laterally or superiorly. In a similar fashion, the unsupported alar margin is susceptible to distortion, elevation, and notching following surgery.

COSMETIC SUBUNITS AND AESTHETIC ASPECTS

Figure 30-3 illustrates the surface anatomy and cosmetic units of the nose and surrounding areas.[17] The upper two-thirds of the nose consist of the sidewalls and dorsum.[26] Each sidewall merges with the inner canthus and the cheek. The lower third of the nose consists of the supratip and the lobule; the latter comprises the tip, alae, soft triangles, and the membranous septum.[9,24] The nasal sill is the entrance to the vestibular floor, and the soft triangle lies at the junction of the ala with the columella.[24] The soft triangles are the only parts of the nose where external skin lies directly on lining skin, with no intervening supporting structures, and are notoriously difficult to reconstruct.[24]

The principles of cosmetic subunit repair dictate that, whenever possible, incision lines should be placed within the nasal sulci and grooves or at the boundaries of subunits.[17,27–29] If a defect extends into more than one subunit, separate repair of each unit may be appropriate,[30] and, similarly, when a surgical defect involves most of a single cosmetic unit, a better aesthetic appearance may result if the remainder of the skin of that unit is sacrificed and the entire unit is reconstructed.[17–19,28,31,32] In this way, the junctions between transferred tissue and the remaining nasal skin can be made less noticeable.[25,31] In addition, should a pincushion deformity develop, the bulging of an entire cosmetic unit may be much less obvious than if only a part of the area was involved.[31]

PHYSIOLOGY

The internal (spiral) nasal valve is located at the junction of the vestibular skin with the nasal mucosa. It lies in the region between the septum and the junction between the lower margin of the upper lateral cartilage and the upper margin of the alar cartilage. It is the narrowest portion of the upper respiratory tract, and its patency depends upon the support of both the alar and lateral cartilages.[19,24]

Nasal surgery can result in loss of nasal cartilage, wound contraction, or scar formation, any of which may interfere with the normal function of the internal valve.[33–37] Forces which interfere with the free movement of the nasal cartilages

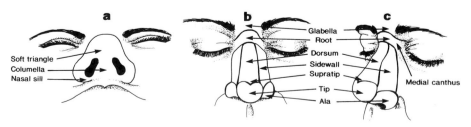

Figure 30-3   The major cosmetic subunits and surface anatomic features of the nose.

disturb airflow and can result in symptoms of nasal stuffiness, rhinitis, and obstruction.[34,38]

APPROACHES TO RECONSTRUCTION

There are no simple guidelines to nasal reconstruction, although a number of approaches to management,[21,39–41] reconstructive algorithms,[27,42] and classifications of nasal defects[11,41,43] have been proposed. However, one reasonable approach to the repair of soft-tissue defects is to consider more conservative options first.[20] Superficial wounds and wounds in certain anatomic areas may heal naturally with excellent cosmetic results,[44–47] and direct primary closure often works well on the upper nose.[26] Full-thickness skin graft repair often works well for nasal defects with an adequate subcutaneous bed, although the skin color and texture match may be poor, especially in males with thick sebaceous nasal skin. In general, local skin flaps offer a superior color and texture match for nasal skin and are the repairs of choice for deep nasal defects. Penetrating defects may require reconstruction of the nasal lining and provision of structural support. A vast array of local flaps exist for nasal soft-tissue reconstruction, and the final choice in any particular case depends not only on the location and size of the defect but also on the skill and experience of the surgeon.

SECONDARY INTENTION HEALING

Some nasal wounds can be allowed to heal completely by secondary intention, with the expectation of a good cosmetic and functional outcome.[44–48] Other advantages include an extremely low risk of infection, minimal discomfort, great ease and safety, and the avoidance of pain or scarring at a flap or graft donor site.[14,45,46] Disadvantages include longer healing times, the need for regular wound care and frequent dressing changes, deformity due to wound contraction, and the formation of hypertrophic scars.[14,44–46]

The cosmetic outcome of naturally healing nasal defects can be predicted with a reasonable degree of accuracy.[44,47] Superficial wounds (e.g., following one or two stages of MMS) will heal well in almost all areas of the nose, and some deeper wounds may heal with a satisfactory cosmetic result, especially on concave surfaces and in the nasal grooves and sulci.[44,46,47] With the notable exception of the inner canthal region, secondary intention healing of deep defects on the upper nose does not tend to give good cosmetic results, and such defects are best repaired surgically.[44,46] Natural healing can be useful for wounds on the lower nose, although deep wounds on convex surfaces are unlikely to yield a cosmetically acceptable result.[26,44] Natural healing of alar defects may result in alar elevation or notching, especially where the wound approaches or involves the alar rim.[46,48]

In selected cases, secondary intention healing can be used as an adjunct to, rather than replacing, wound reconstruction,[14] without significant morbidity.[49] A period of natural healing prior to skin grafting allows wounds to decrease in size by wound contraction and to fill partially with granulation tissue.[14] Similarly, a period of delayed healing may allow the closure of large nasal defects with a local flap when immediate reconstruction would have involved a larger flap or more extensive procedure.[14] Finally, secondary intention healing can result in a reasonable cosmetic result following the necrosis of nasal flaps or grafts.[14,45]

PRIMARY CLOSURE

The mobility of the thin upper nasal skin may allow direct primary closure of small deep wounds after suitable undermining.[3,13,26] The best direction for closure might be transverse, longitudinal, or oblique and can be found by undermining the defect and using skin hooks or by designing an ellipse parallel to the relaxed skin tension lines;[20,50] these lines lie across the nasal dorsum in a slightly falling horizontal array and turn vertically in the glabellar region.[20] Whenever possible, incision lines should be placed within natural nasal creases.[20] Midline defects of the nasal dorsum can be closed in a vertical direction, especially in patients with a wide nose and lax skin.[26] In this situation, extension of the superior end of the repair beyond the junction of the nasal bones and upper cartilages reduces the risk of a persistent and unsightly soft-tissue protrusion in this area.[26] Primary repair is less useful on the distal nose, where the closure of large defects can result in an unacceptable degree of nasal distortion.[27]

SKIN GRAFTS

Split-thickness Skin Grafts

In general, split-thickness skin grafts on the nose give a poor cosmetic result, and they are best avoided.[8,27,51] If most of the skin of the upper nose has been removed, the remaining skin can be sacrificed to resurface the entire upper nasal cosmetic units with a split-thickness graft. The cosmetic result can be acceptable, although the color match often remains poor.[19] Following the excision of large, recurrent, or invasive nasal tumors, reconstruction may be deliberately delayed and defects temporarily covered with thick split-thickness grafts to allow a period of observation.[3–5,8,9,51,52] If no tumor recurrence is evident after a suitable period, definitive reconstruction may then be performed.

Full-thickness Skin Grafts

Full-thickness skin grafts usually offer a better color and texture match than the best split-thickness graft and have less tendency to contract (Fig. 30-4).[52] They may be used to repair superficial nasal defects,[13,51,52] either immediately following tumor removal or following a period of secondary intention

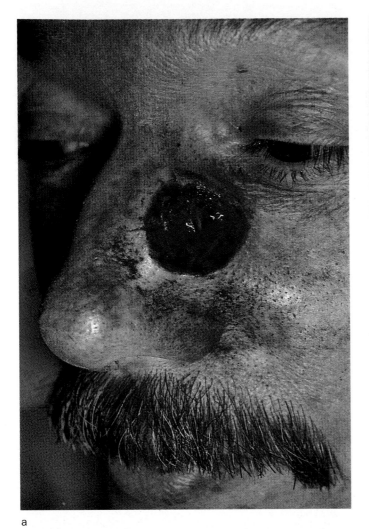

a

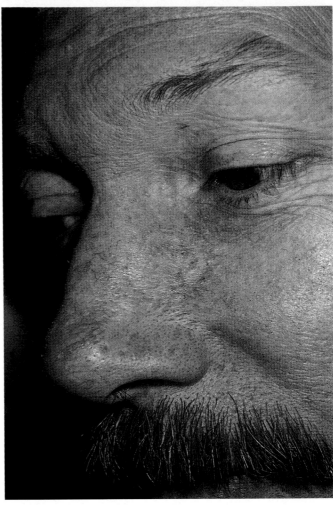

c

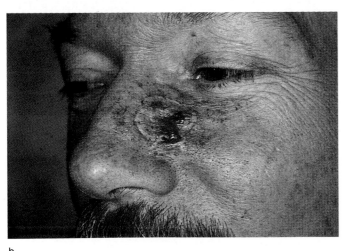

b

Figure 30-4 Full-thickness skin graft, supraclavicular donor site: (*a*) Upper lateral nasal sidewall defect; (*b*) skin graft repair at three weeks; (*c*) skin graft repair at two months (no revision).

during which the wound will contract and granulation tissue will begin to fill deep defects, possibly enhancing graft viability.[14] Composite grafts of skin and subcutaneous fat may occasionally be used for small deep defects,[8] although graft survival is likely to be poor.[53] The use of square or rectangu-

lar grafts, rather than round or oval shapes, may reduce the risk of puckered scarring at the wound edges.[52]

Advantages of full-thickness skin grafts include easy coverage of defects, minimal nasal distortion, and the prevention of wound contraction. Disadvantages include using donor skin that differs in color and texture from the recipient site and the creation of a second scar at the donor site. Hyperpigmentation of full-thickness skin grafts may be a significant problem in dark-skinned patients.[11]

Many potential donor sites exist, each offering one or more useful qualities such as an easily repaired or inconspicuous donor site or a reasonable match for nasal skin color, texture, and degree of actinic damage. The cosmetic result of skin graft repairs is often improved by dermabrasion.[31,54] Differences in skin texture and color may be camouflaged with the use of cosmetics and, much less commonly, by tattooing.[55] Among the most popular donor sites are adjacent nasal skin (Burow's graft, Fig. 30-5)[56,57] and the preauricular,

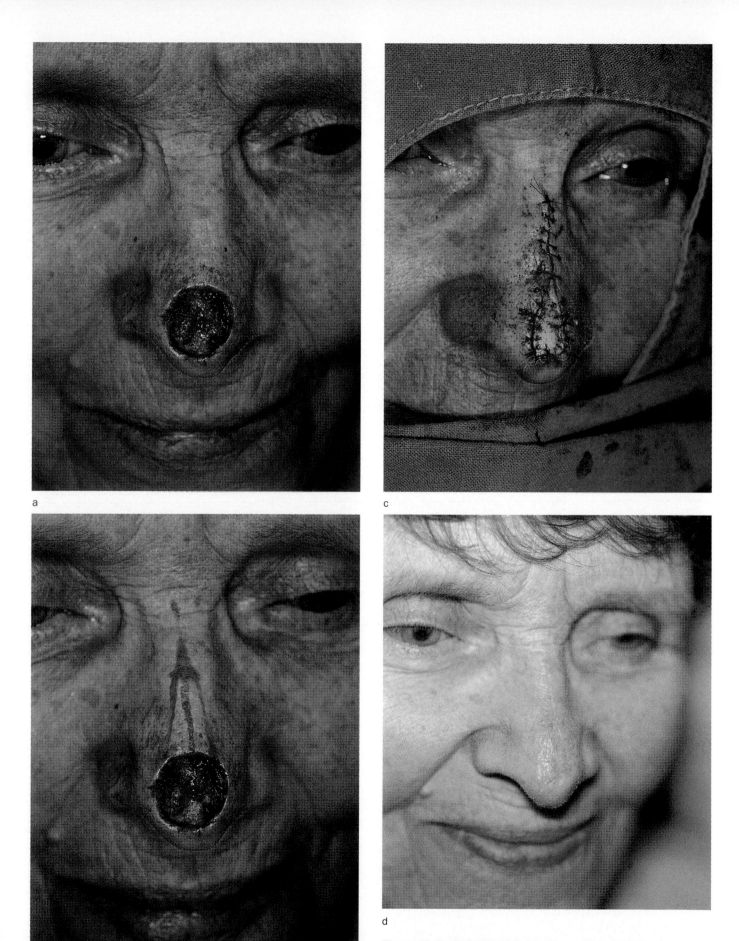

Figure 30-5 Burow's graft: (*a*) Nasal supratip defect; (*b*) graft design; (*c*) graft repair; (*d*) result at two months, frontal view (no revision). (*Continued*)

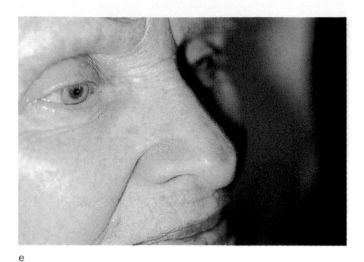

e

Figure 30-5 (*Cont.*) (*e*) result at two months, lateral view (no revision).

postauricular, and supraclavicular areas. The advantages and disadvantages of the most commonly reported donor sites are listed in Table 30-1. Less commonly used donor sites include the conchal bowl, alar crease,[58] glabella,[21] and submental region.[27]

Composite Grafts

Composite grafts consist of skin and other structures and include combinations of skin and fat,[8,53] skin and perichondrium,[59] and skin and cartilage.[60,61] Skin and cartilage composites may be used to repair deep defects of the lower nose,[10,13] columella,[21] and alar free margin.[8,11,13,21,51] The auricular helix, conchal bowl, and lobe are the most common donor sites,[24,27,61] and the donor defect can be closed in a variety of ways.[27] To allow for contraction, the graft can be designed slightly larger than the defect.[61] The graft is secured in place with a layer of sutures in both the internal and external skin, and a nasal pack can be used to form a temporary internal splint.[51]

Persistent redness[27] and a high failure rate[11,31,61] are the main complications associated with composite grafts.

Free Cartilage Grafts

Free cartilage grafts can be used to provide structural support for skin flaps and are most commonly harvested from the nasal septum,[62] conchal bowl,[62] auricular rim,[21] and occasionally from costal cartilage.[63] Cartilage grafts can be placed within nasolabial[3,4,11,51,64] or forehead flaps,[4,11,65] or a composite graft of skin, perichondrium, and cartilage may be used.[4,24] Free cartilage grafts require highly vascular tissue beds to ensure their survival,[31,62] and these grafts may curl with time.[11]

SKIN FLAPS

General Features

In general, the advantages of flaps over grafts are that they carry their own blood supply and provide both bulk and superior protection for underlying structures. A large number of

TABLE 30-1

Donor sites for full-thickness skin grafts for nasal reconstruction, with their advantages and disadvantages

Donor site	Advantages	Disadvantages
Postauricular[10,11,18,51]	Well-hidden scar; good match for upper nose	Little sun damage; persistent redness possible;[31] poor match for lower nose
Preauricular[10,31,51,131]	Sun damaged skin; good match for mid and lower nose	Limited size; visible scar
Upper eyelid[21,51]	Thin skin; good match for upper nose	Limited size; poor match for lower nasal skin
Burow's graft[56,57] (dog-ear or island grafts)	Best skin match; single wound	Limited size; donor site closure can produce distortion of the distal nose; increased risk of necrosis
Posterolateral neck[19]	Can give good match for sun damage	Visible scar
Supraclavicular[10,11,27,51] (Fig. 30-4)	Large grafts possible; fair texture match for lower nose	Sun damage is often minimal in males; visible scar; may become wrinkled and shiny;[31] color match may be poor
Nasolabial fold[21,132]	Good texture, color, and sun damage match; scar can be placed in nasolabial fold	Limited size; facial scar
Conchal bowl	Good texture and color match; donor site heals well	Donor site requires daily care
Perichondrial cutaneous graft[59] (conchal bowl skin, subcutaneous tissue, and perichondrium)	Good cosmetic result; no graft contraction	Donor site requires complex repair
Upper inner arm[8]	Less risk of edge hypertrophy (?)	Poor match for color and sun damage

skin flaps have been described for the repair of nasal defects. The majority take advantage of the reservoirs of skin in the upper nose, adjacent cheek, melolabial (nasolabial) fold, and the forehead.[11] The skin in all of these areas offers a reasonably good color and texture match for nasal skin.

Many facial flaps are random; that is, they rely on the generally rich facial blood supply and are not based on any defined blood vessels. However, some island pedicle flaps[66,67] and most forehead flaps are based upon a defined blood supply,[68] which must be carefully preserved during surgery. Local skin flaps tend to work best in patients with thin, loose nasal skin, as the thick and sebaceous skin of the nose often bleeds profusely and can be difficult to manipulate and evert.[26]

Surgical undermining is relatively simple on the upper nose and becomes increasingly more difficult toward the nasal tip. Undermining is usually performed below the muscles of the upper nose and above the perichondrium or periosteum in order to prevent vascular injury.[69,70] It is unclear whether flaps with rounded edges[20] or with sharply angled edges[26,71] give better cosmetic results on the nose, although the trapdoor and pincushion deformities may be more common in rounded flaps.[71] If thin flaps are sutured tightly across the nose, the underlying bone and cartilage skeleton can become accentuated and produce a sharp-looking or beaked appearance.[69] Similarly, excessive upward or lateral tension in distal nasal repairs may produce distortion of the nasal tip or alar margin. A minor degree of such distortion may be present immediately following repair and may be accentuated by the presence of both edema and local anesthetic. Fortunately, the elastic nature of the nasal cartilages will often allow a degree of relaxation with time.[69,72] It is important to achieve good eversion of nasal suture lines, particularly on the lower nose where the junctions between thick nasal dermis and transferred flap skin often tend to groove with healing, producing unsightly, depressed scars.[25] Finally, the cosmetic result of many nasal flap repairs may be improved by an early regional dermabrasion.[73]

Advancement Flaps

Skin laxity in the nasal root and glabella allows closure of upper nasal defects with relatively small advancement flaps.[21,42] Longer flaps can be used to repair more distal nasal defects, although this results in long incision lines,[26] a loss of the normal concavity of the nasal root, and possible elevation of the nasal tip.[69] A "pinch" modification of this flap converts the leading edge into two small rotation flaps and may permit the design of a wider and shorter flap.[74] In general, however, classic advancement flaps have only a limited role in nasal reconstruction.[26]

Sliding V-Y advancement flaps may be used to repair supratip defects[75] but can be difficult to mobilize, especially in young patients.[8,20] Defects of the nasal sidewall may be repaired by using a cheek advancement flap. This flap takes advantage of the laxity of cheek skin and moves either by true advancement or by a combination of advancement and rotation, depending on how far posteriorly the upper incision line is extended.[20] A common problem with this flap is blunting or obliteration of the nasofacial sulcus. To minimize this risk, buried sutures may be placed tacking the flap down to the maxillary periosteum.[76] The bipedicle flap[77] is another advancement flap variation that can be used to repair defects of the dorsum or supratip.[11] The skin of the nasal dorsum is undermined from the defect to the nasal root, where a transverse incision is made. The dorsal nasal skin is then advanced to fill the defect, and the upper nasal defect is repaired by direct primary closure or, occasionally, by a full-thickness skin graft.[52]

Rotation Flaps

Small rotation flaps are readily performed on the upper nose and are possible on the lower nose,[20,50,78,79] although transposition flaps may give better results.[26] Larger rotation flaps make use of the loose skin of the upper nose and glabella,[20] where a back cut may facilitate flap movement (Fig. 30-6). A rotation flap using most of the dorsal nasal skin was first described by Rieger[80] for the reconstruction of nasal tip defects, although it, or a variant based on one side of the nose,[78] can also be used to repair nasal sidewall defects.[16,78] Rieger's flap is also known as the *extended glabellar,* the *frontonasal,*[16,81] and, most commonly, the *dorsal nasal flap.*[82]

Problems associated with this flap include long incision lines which may leave noticeable scars[26] and permanent elevation of the nasal tip.[80] The flap can be brought low enough to replace a missing alar rim, but the upper nasal defect cannot then be closed directly and must be repaired with a skin graft.[83]

When designing and using the dorsal nasal flap, surgeons often use the following guidelines:

1. Limit the upper scar to the glabella and avoid extension onto the forehead.[16]
2. Elevate the flap subcutaneously along the lateral nose to avoid a step deformity.[16]
3. Plan the lateral incision low on the side of the nose, near the cheek.[81]
4. Carefully place the sutures along the lateral nose where skin of different thicknesses is brought together.

Transposition Flaps

The following are some of the most useful flaps in nasal reconstruction, including the rhombic, nasolabial, and bilobed flaps.

Rhombic Flap

Nasal defects may be modified to accept rhombic flap designs such as those described by Limberg, Dufourmental, and Webster, or these flaps may be rounded to fit the existing defects.

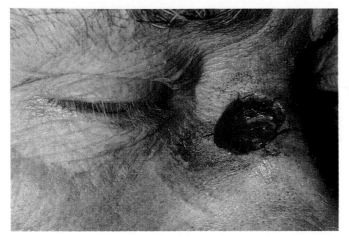

a

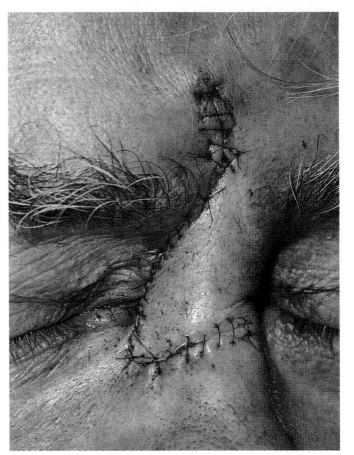

c

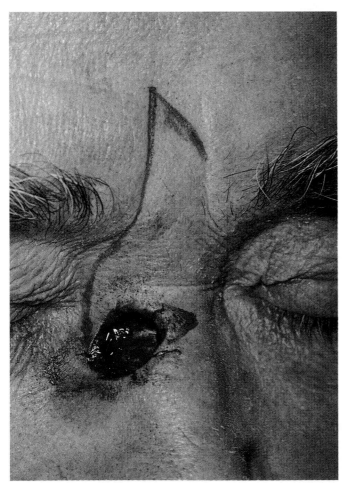

b

Figure 30-6 Glabellar rotation flap: (*a*) upper nasal defect;
(*b*) flap design; (*c*) flap repair; (*d*) result at one year (no revision).

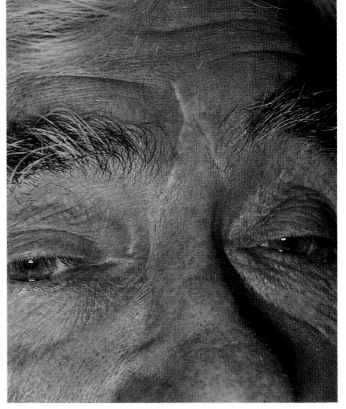

d

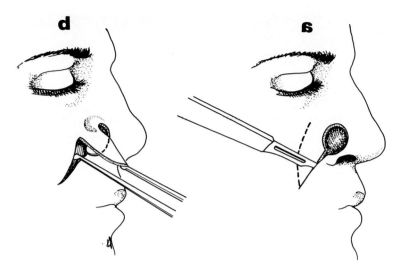

Figure 30-7 Classical nasolabial flap design. Note how large angle of transposition creates a superior bulge, often requiring a secondary revision (see text).

It is debatable whether sharply angled flaps[26,71,84] or rounded flaps[20] look more natural on the nose. Usually, these flaps move the looser skin of the upper and lateral nose to fill defects of the lower and more central areas and are of most value in the repair of upper and midnasal defects. A transposition flap taking skin from across the nasal dorsum and moving it to the lower nose has been called a *banner flap*.[72,85] This design allows closure of the donor site along the relaxed skin tension lines, which can elevate the nasal tip, an effect which can be useful if a degree of tip ptosis exists.[72] This illustrates the important fact that the maximum tension in a rhombic flap occurs at the closure of the secondary (donor) defect.[86]

Nasolabial Flap

Cheek skin lying adjacently to the melolabial crease (the name *nasolabial flap* is anatomically incorrect but widely accepted) provides a good match for the skin of the lower nose.[4] The highly vascular,[12] superiorly based nasolabial flap can safely be designed with a length/width ratio of up to 4:1[87] and can be used to repair large defects of the lower nose and ala.[4,10–12,26,51,87,88] The medial incision line lies in the melolabial fold and the lateral incision line lies on the cheek from where the flap is harvested. Following undermining of the cheek, the donor site is closed primarily. The resulting scar is well hidden,[20] and an early dermabrasion may further improve the cosmetic result.[4] In the traditional design, the flap must twist through a large angle of transposition (Fig. 30-7), leaving a medial tissue redundancy (dog-ear) requiring a second revisionary stage.[51] However, a simple modification makes the flap easier to move and gives superior cosmetic results: A triangle of skin (with a 30° apex pointing toward the inner canthus) is excised from the superior aspect of the surgical defect[88,89] or used as a turndown flap to replace any loss of nasal lining.[89] This allows the flap to reach the defect through a smaller angle of transposition as a one-stage procedure.[89] (Figs. 30-8 and 30-9). A two-stage, pedicled nasolabial flap can be used to repair full-thickness defects of the

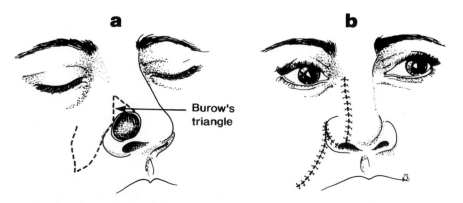

Figure 30-8 Modified (one-stage) nasolabial flap design. Note how use of Burow's triangle allows flap to slide–rather than twist–into position (see text).

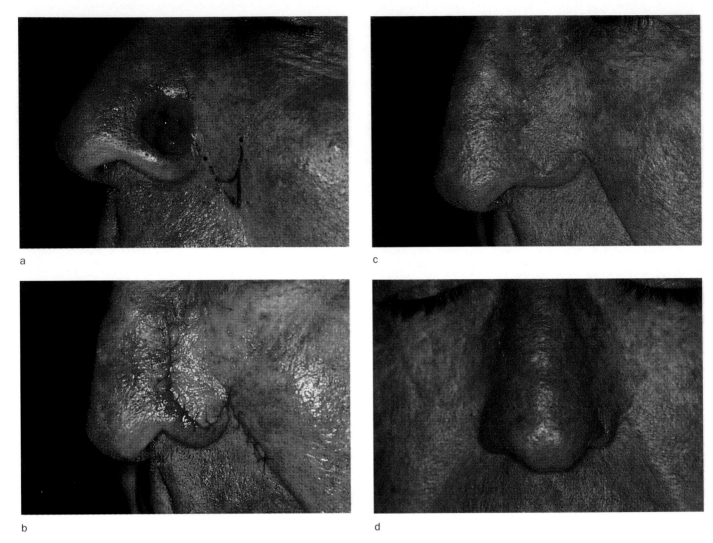

a

c

b

d

Figure 30-9 Nasolabial flap: (*a*) Nasal alar defect and flap design (note Burow's triangle at upper edge of defect); (*b*) flap repair; (*c*) result at three months, side view (no revision); (*d*) result at three months, frontal view (no revision).

tip,[13] ala,[90] and columella,[91] with a secondary procedure needed to divide the flap and return the pedicle to the cheek. It is also possible to tunnel nasolabial flaps inside the nose to reconstruct the nasal lining;[4,92] however, this procedure is associated, at least in theory, with a risk of occult skin cancer development in the transplanted sun-damaged skin.[31]

The nasolabial flap has certain recognized disadvantages:

1. Blunting or loss of the nasofacial (nasomaxillary) angle[20,51]
2. Trapdoor or pincushion deformity[8,93–95]
3. Persistent edema and bulkiness[11]

The use of suspension (tacking or pexing) sutures[76] to attach the undersurface of the flap to the maxillary periosteum may help preserve the nasofacial sulcus,[20,89] and careful thinning of the flap together with wide undermining of both the flap

and surgical defect may minimize flap bulkiness and trapdoor deformity.[89,93,94] Alternatively, a delayed second procedure may be performed to thin the flap and re-create the alar crease.[96]

Variations of the nasolabial flap can also be used to repair full-thickness alar defects:

1. When portions of the alar rim has been lost, the tip of the flap can be folded inside the nostril, re-creating the alar margin and providing an internal lining[3,4,10–12,51,88] (Fig. 30-10). A cartilage graft may be implanted within the flap to provide structural support.[3,4,11,51,64] The reconstructed ala is often bulky and may require secondary defatting procedures.[11,20,24,51]
2. A mirror image of this flap is the *reverse* nasolabial flap, which can be used to reconstruct the junction of the ala to the cheek and upper lip.[26,97] This is a large nasolabial hinge flap based on a vascular subcutaneous pedicle in the

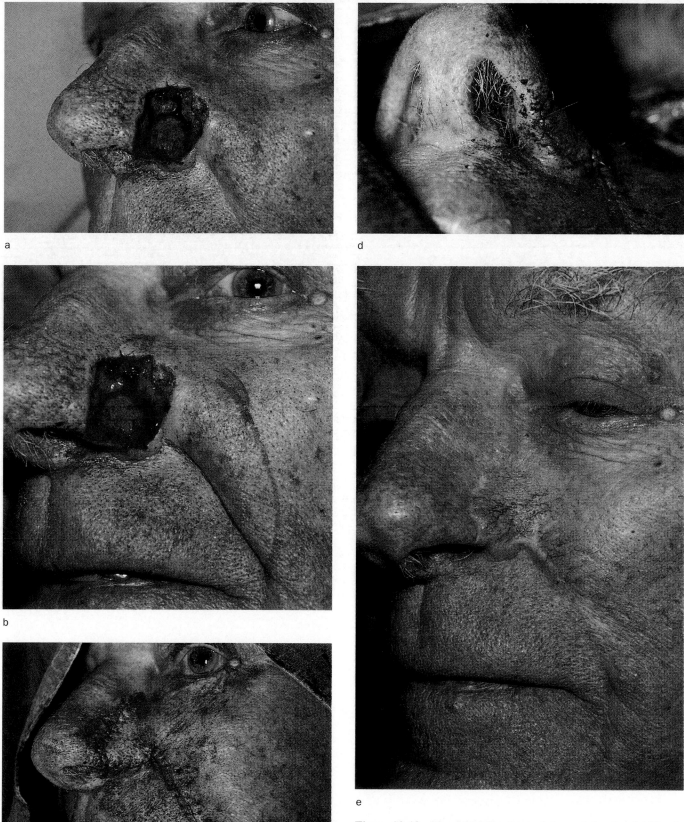

Figure 30-10   Nasolabial flap to repair loss of alar rim: (*a*) Nasal alar defect; (*b*) flap design (note Burow's triangle at upper edge of defect); (*c*) flap repair; (*d*) inferior view showing use of flap to recreate alar rim; (*e*) result at four months (no revision).

superior and lateral margin of the defect. It is flipped over so that the external skin re-creates the internal nasal lining and then turned over upon itself to re-create the ala and a more natural-appearing crease at the junction of the ala and the cheek.[26]

3. For full-thickness defects, the nasal lining can be reconstructed with a superiorly based hinge flap of nasal skin[42,89] and a nasolabial flap used to repair the remaining outer defect. Smaller defects of the nasal lining can be repaired by a nasolabial flap with its underside lined by a split-thickness skin graft. Single or paired nasolabial flaps with or without implanted cartilage grafts may be used to reconstruct the columella and anterior nasal septum.[3,4,87,91,92,98]

Bilobed Flap

The bilobed flap is a double transposition flap with a common pedicle,[99] which may be designed on the lower[70] or upper[100] nose. This flap allows the stepwise downward movement of loose upper nasal skin to facilitate closure of defects less than 1.5 cm in diameter[70] on the lower third of the nose. It is particularly useful for the repair of alar or tip defects where there is insufficient tissue laxity to fill the defect with a single transposition flap.[8,20,21,27,70,99,101] The leading, or primary, lobe fills the surgical defect, while the second lobe fills the defect left by the primary lobe; the defect left by the second lobe lies in an area of lax skin and is closed primarily (Figs. 30-11 and 30-12).[102]

Since the bilobed flap was originally described, several useful design modifications have been reported:

1. By reducing the angle of transposition of each lobe from the originally described 90° to 45°,[99,102] the movement of both lobes is facilitated.[70,101]
2. The initial excision of Burow's triangle of skin from the edge of the main defect at the point of rotation where a dog-ear would be formed facilitates movement of the primary lobe of the flap into the defect.[70]

3. The design of a primary lobe which is both slightly larger than the secondary lobe and slightly smaller than the surgical defect anticipates a degree of advancement closure of each wound, provided the flap is well undermined.[101]
4. The design of the secondary lobe from the skin overlying the nasal bones may reduce the risk of distal nasal distortion.[101] Advantages of the bilobed flap include the use of adjacent nasal skin, with a consequently ideal color and texture match[70,101] and absent or minimal nasal distortion.[70] Disadvantages include the creation of a complicated scar line,[101] the crossing of cosmetic unit boundaries, and a tendency to develop the trapdoor deformity. An early regional dermabrasion frequently improves the appearance of the repair,[70] and wide undermining together with thinning of the primary lobe[101] often improves the result and may reduce the risk of trapdoor deformity.[70]

The trilobed flap is a three-lobed variant of the bilobed flap[99,103] but is not commonly used. Although the bilobed flap is most frequently planned with rounded lobes, it can also be designed as a double rhomboid flap.[26,71]

Pedicle Flaps

Pedicle flaps include two-stage pedicle flaps such as forehead flaps and island flaps moving on pedicles of muscle or subcutaneous tissue.

Subcutaneous Island Pedicle Flaps

Island flaps based on subcutaneous tissue pedicles are sometimes useful in the repair of defects on the upper nose and lateral sidewall. However, the lack of subcutaneous fat makes island pedicle flaps more difficult to use on the distal nose.[69] Large subcutaneous V-Y pedicle flaps comprising most of the dorsal nasal skin can be used to repair supratip defects but will commonly elevate the nasal tip.[75,77] The limited movement of two small subcutaneous island pedicle flaps may be combined to repair small nasal tip defects.[104] Other island flaps that may be useful are nasolabial island flaps[66,105] and

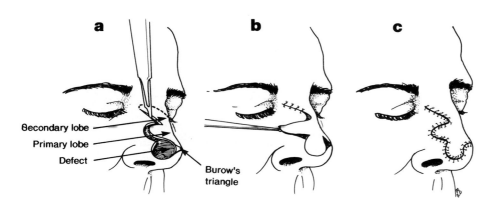

Figure 30-11 (*a*) Lateral nasal tip defect with flap designed and incised. Note Burow's triangle at edge of defect; (*b*) leading (primary) lobe of flap fills surgical defect, and secondary lobe defect is closed directly; (*c*) flap sutured in place (see Fig. 30-12).

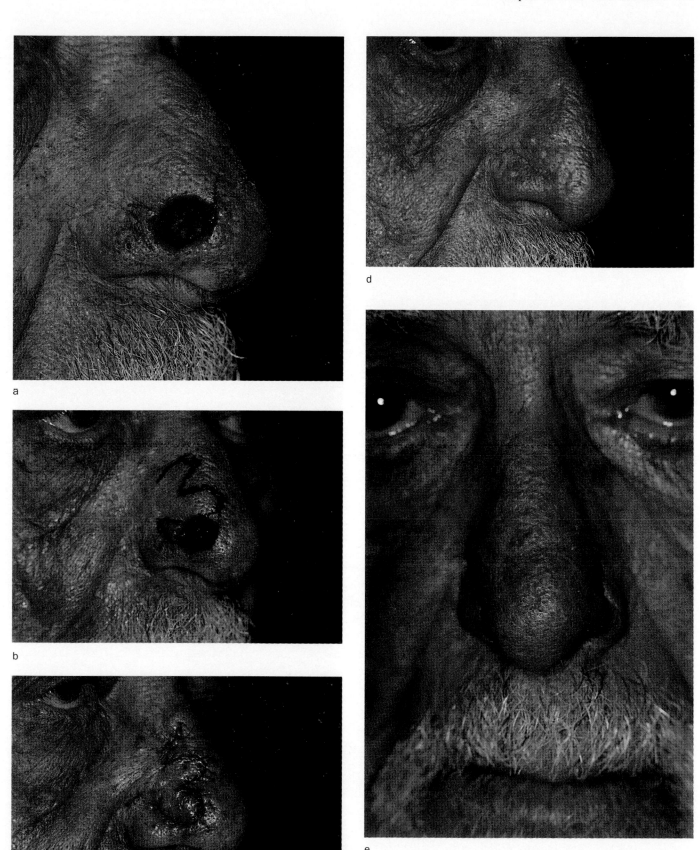

Figure 30-12   Bilobe flap: (*a*) Nasal tip defect; (*b*) flap design;
(*c*) flap repair; (*d*) result at four months, lateral view (no revision);
(*e*) result at four months, frontal view (no revision).

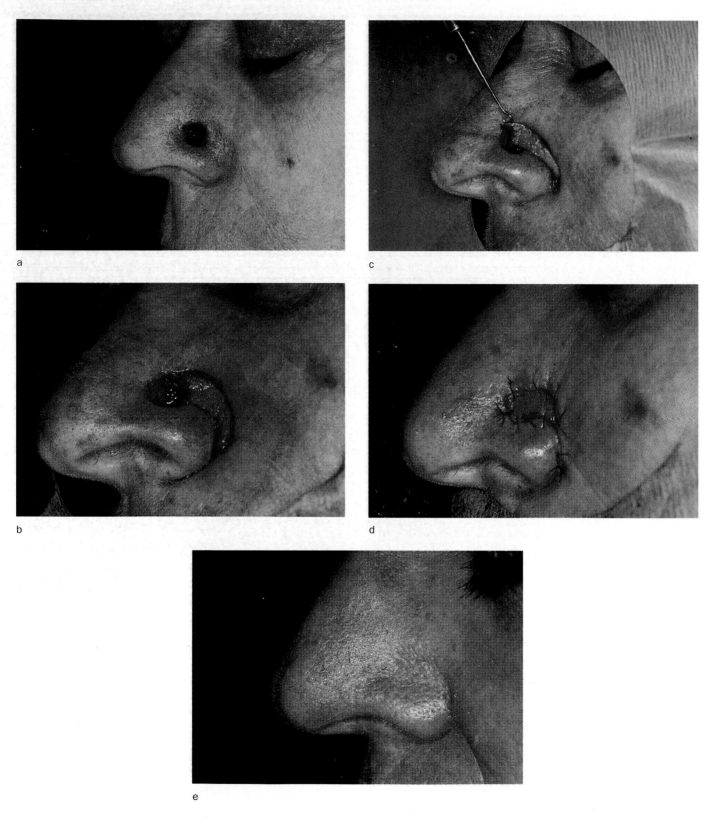

Figure 30-13   Nasalis myocutaneous flap: (*a*) Nasal alar defect: (*b*) flap designed and incised;
(*c*) flap movement; (*d*) flap repair; (*e*) result at four months (single dermabrasion).

the nasalis myocutaneous flap.[67,106,107] Buried subcutaneous island pedicle flaps can be moved from the cheek[108] or forehead[4] to the nose. Their main use is for filling deep defects in a single stage, but the buried pedicle often creates a noticeable subcutaneous bulging in the glabellar or nasal sidewall areas.[26]

Nasalis Myocutaneous Flap

This musculocutaneous island flap is useful in the repair of defects of the alar crease and lateral supratip.[67,106,107] An axial island flap, the nasal is myocutaneous flap is based upon the branches of the angular artery that supply the nasalis mus-

cle, and it moves on a pedicle of nasalis muscle which crosses the dorsum of the lower nose.[109] The flap is mobilized and advanced in a V-Y manner to fill the surgical defect. The best cosmetic results are obtained when the inferior incision line is hidden in the alar crease and when an early regional dermabrasion is performed (Fig. 30-13).

Forehead Flaps

Forehead flaps are axial pedicle flaps which can be used to reconstruct large nasal defects, especially of the distal nose and ala (Fig. 30-14).[2,3,10,11,20,42,110–112] Many different designs of

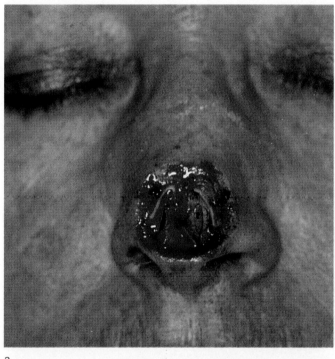

a

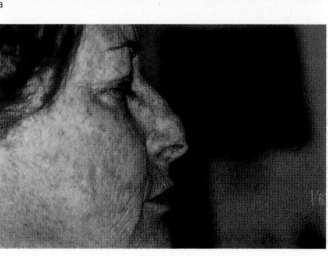

b

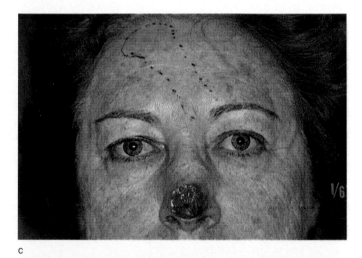

c

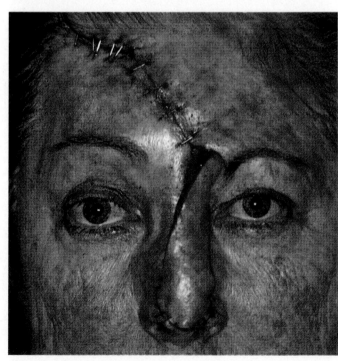

d

Figure 30-14 *(a)* Deep nasal defect into the nasal vestibule; *(b)* side view of nasal defect; *(c)* para-median forehead flap planned; *(d)* flap sutured. *(Continued)*

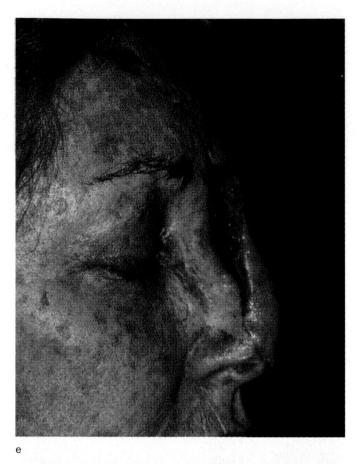

e

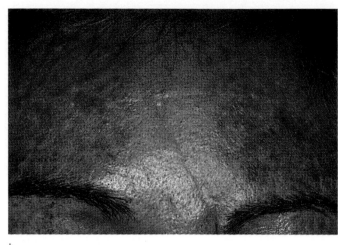

h

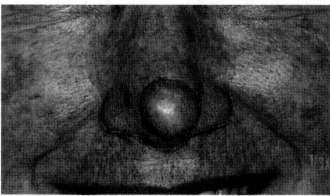

f

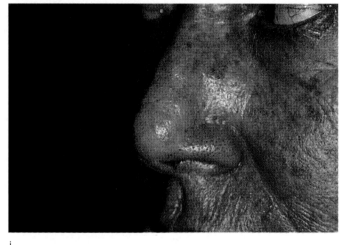

i

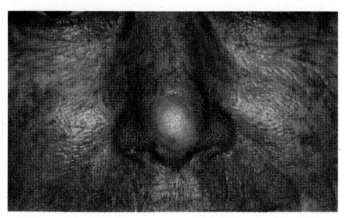

g

Figure 30-14 *(Cont.)*   *(e)* three weeks postoperative at the time of severing the pedicle; *(f)* trapdooring of flap, treatment with steriods and dermabrasion; *(g)* front view, six months postoperative; *(h)* forehead, six months postoperative; *(i)* side view at six months postoperative.

this two-stage flap have been described,[2,20,113] although the midline[110] or paramedian[2] flaps are most commonly used and may give the best overall results.[2,4,20] Compared with other forehead flap designs, including the scalping flap,[114,115] these flaps have the advantage of a donor site that can be directly closed.[110] The length of a midline forehead flap is limited in part by the anterior hairline;[51] other designs are longer and provide more tissue,[42,114,116] but their donor sites may require closure with split-thickness skin grafts.[42]

Midline flaps based on the supratrochlear vessels[20,31] and their anastomoses[68] can be designed either in or just off the midline. Positioning the flap to the side of the midline opposite the nasal defect facilitates rotation of the flap pedicle.[3,24] The great vascularity of the flap allows precise thinning and trimming of the tip.[112,117] The donor site can often be closed primarily,[110] although secondary intention healing or a skin graft may be necessary in the upper forehead.[51,117] Skin expansion before or after flap transfer may provide extra skin for reconstruction and may allow a low-tension forehead closure.[118,119] Between 10 and 21 days after flap movement, the pedicle is divided and may be returned to the forehead.[20,51,112] This procedure may be needed to return the eyebrows to their normal position[11,112] but may not be necessary if the base of the pedicle is kept quite narrow.[31]

Disadvantages of the midline flap include a tendency to thicken, the need for two stages,[16] and the fact that one or more surgical revisions are often required.[51] The main advantages are the amount of skin provided and its good color and texture match for nasal skin.

If a forehead flap is used to repair large penetrating defects of the nasal ala, an internal nasal lining and structural cartilage support can be provided directly as free grafts[117] or by placing a cartilage graft,[115] skin-cartilage graft,[114] or split-thickness skin graft under the skin of the forehead sometime before raising the flap.[13,24,65] Structural support of the upper nose and dorsum can be provided by skeletal rib or iliac crest bone grafts[11,120,121] anchored to the nasal process of the frontal bone and covered with a forehead flap.[3]

SECONDARY PROCEDURES AND SCAR REVISION

It is often wise to allow nasal tissue to soften and scars to relax for at least 4 months before secondary surgical procedures are performed.[8,31] The major exception is dermabrasion: The thick skin of the nose lends itself well to dermabrasion,[25] which may be most beneficial soon after surgery.[16,73] Dermabrasion of incisional scars may smooth out discrepancies of color and texture following flap[4,16,25] and skin graft[31,54] repairs.

Single or repeated injections of triamcinolone acetate in varying concentrations will produce softening and flattening of scars as well as reduce persistent nodularity of flaps.[8] Careful injection technique and the use of appropriate steroid con-

centrations significantly reduce the risk of skin or subcutaneous atrophy.[8]

Correction of the trapdoor (pincushion) deformity in flaps may involve steroid injections, defatting procedures, multiple Z-plasties,[93,94,122] or, in extreme cases, excision of the flap and replacement with a skin graft.[95]

Various techniques have been described to correct nasal valve dysfunction following nasal surgery, including Z-plasty, skin grafts, and auricular composite[103] or septal cartilage grafts to replace lost nasal structural support.[33]

It is often difficult for skin flaps to reconstruct the sharp angles found around the nose (e.g., where the ala meets the cheek), and, if such creases remain blunted, secondary procedures may be performed to divide flaps and re-create normal-appearing grooves.[24] Alae reconstructed by the use of two flaps, one for lining and one for skin cover, are often bulky and may require one or more defatting procedures.[24]

Although not widely practiced, it is possible to improve the color match of both flaps and grafts by the judicious use of tattooing.[55] Although secondary intention healing can give excellent cosmetic results in selected cases, a scar revision, dermabrasion, or steroid injections may be required if thickened scars develop.

PROSTHETICS

Partial or total nasal prostheses may be of value in both cosmetic and functional rehabilitation.[5,123] Extensive nasal tumors may be treated by total rhinectomy and the permanent use of a prosthetic nose.[52] Alternatively, a prosthesis can be used if delayed reconstruction is planned.[5,10,21] An accurate color match is essential and requires the services of an expert prosthetist. Patients must be able to clean and apply the prosthesis, which may be retained in place by a combination of adhesives and appliances such as those used for spectacles or dentures.[21,123]

REGIONAL APPROACH TO NASAL RECONSTRUCTION

Nasal Root/Glabella

Due to the local skin laxity, and the underlying rigidity of the nasal bones, a great many repairs work well in this area. Direct primary closure, rotation and transposition flaps, and full-thickness skin grafts may be used successfully.

Dorsum

The cosmetic results of secondary intention healing may not be ideal in this area. Small midline defects are readily repaired with either full-thickness grafts[27,42] or direct closure in a vertical direction.[26] Larger defects can be repaired by using rotation,[16,50,80,82] rhombic, or bilobed flaps. Very large or penetrating defects may require complex reconstruction of nasal lining, support, and external skin (see "Major Nasal Reconstruction").

Nasal Sidewall

Secondary intention healing and direct primary closure may be appropriate for certain defects in this area. Larger defects on the upper sidewall may be closed with either a rhombic or rotation flap by utilizing the laxity of the skin of the upper cheek or the nasal root and glabella. A cheek advancement flap may be useful for the closure of nasal sidewall defects, and cheek skin can be transferred to the nose either as a nasolabial flap[51] or as a subcutaneous island flap based on the lateral cheek.[25]

Tip and Supratip

The skin of the lower nose is usually tightly bound down, preventing extensive undermining and subsequent closure without distortion. Thin defects may heal well by secondary intention, but deeper defects on the convex surfaces of this area tend to heal with poor cosmetic results.[44,46] Deeper defects are commonly repaired with full-thickness skin grafts[9] or, occasionally, auricular composite grafts.[29] Larger and deeper defects requiring closure with a skin flap may be repaired with bilobed (Fig. 30-12),[70,101] dorsal nasal,[80,82] or bipedicle[77] flaps. The tendency of the nasobial flap to contract and bulge limits its use for reconstruction of the nasal tip.[31,94] Small, deep defects of the lateral supratip can be repaired with the nasalis myocutaneous flap (Fig. 30-14).[67,106] Extensive defects may require repair with a forehead flap.[4,5]

Ala

Selected defects of the nasal ala may heal well by secondary intention.[44,46] Direct primary closure of anything other than small defects may be difficult and may not be advisable. Full-thickness skin grafts and auricular composite grafts[9,31,61] may work well for slightly larger or full-thickness defects, respectively. Skin from the upper nose, adjacent cheek, nasolabial fold, or forehead provides the best color and texture match for lower nasal skin[11,24] and is one reason why the nasolabial,[3] bilobed,[70,101] and forehead flaps are frequently used to repair large alar efects.[3]

A superiorly based nasolabial flap is a common method for repairing larger alar defects.[88,91] The repair can be performed in stages;[96] however, if the alar base and free margin are intact and if the flap is carefully thinned, a single-stage repair can often be achieved (Figs. 30-9 and 30-10).[25,89] The tendency of this flap to contract and bulge may be an advantage, helping to re-create the natural fullness of the ala.[31]

Full-thickness defects require the reconstruction of the inner nasal lining as well as external coverage. This can be achieved in a number of ways:

1. Adjacent cheek[124] or nasal skin can be turned over in a turndown or hinged fashion.[3,24,103,125]
2. A nasolabial flap[3,9,12] or reverse nasolabial flap[97] can be folded on itself inside the nose. The reconstructed ala is often bulky and may require secondary defatting procedures.[24,31]
3. Flaps can be mobilized from the lateral nasal wall or septum.[3,31]

Skin flaps and scar tissue alone may not be sufficient to maintain fully either alar shape or nasal valve patency; cartilage grafts within a reconstructed ala may be necessary for a good long-term result.[24,25,64,65] Supporting cartilage can be provided by an auricular composite graft with the skin removed from one side. This graft can provide an internal lining and structural support, and a bilobed, rhomboid, nasolabial, or forehead flap can provide external coverage.[3] A number of intricate procedures have been described to mobilize septal cartilage[126] or remnants of alar cartilage to provide support for alar reconstruction.[31] These techniques illustrate the multidisciplinary approach that is often necessary to achieve the successful removal of nasal tumors and subsequent nasal reconstruction.[3,5,8,9]

Two complex flaps offer the combination of an internal and external nasal lining together with internal structural support:

1. A conchal cartilage graft can be implanted within a folded nasolabial flap.[64]
2. An auricular skin-cartilage composite graft is implanted beneath the skin of the forehead sometime before a forehead flap is raised. This composite flap contains auricular skin to provide internal nasal lining, cartilage for structural support, and forehead skin for aesthetic external coverage.[24,65] In contrast to the normal anatomic position of the lateral crus of the alar cartilage, implanted cartilage grafts are often placed along the free margin of the ala, from the tip to the alar base, in order to achieve a more predictable and natural-looking alar rim.[24]

Columella

Skin cancers in this area, although rare, can be aggressive and invade the nasal septum, upper nasal vestibules, nasal tip, and the upper lip.[3,4] Full-thickness skin grafts allow relatively simple reconstruction of purely cutaneous defects; however, some columella repairs can be difficult,[5,42] especially if some or all of the septum is lost.[11] Auricular composite grafts may be useful in the repair of partial defects.[3,11,21,42,61] Total columella reconstruction may require the use of a forehead flap[111,127] or paired nasolabial flaps,[3,4,42,91,92,98] either of which may require bone or cartilage grafts for support.[11]

MAJOR NASAL RECONSTRUCTION

Major nasal defects can involve the loss of any combination of skin, mucosa, and structural support; each of the lost nasal structures needs to be replaced,[11,18,29,62,120,128] and it may be difficult, and often unwise, to plan a one-stage reconstruction of a full-thickness defect with any one local flap.[9,20] Any such repair is likely to be followed by flap contraction due to granulation of the undersurface of the flap.[20] Defects of nasal mucosa or structural support must be repaired prior to replacing the missing skin, and these often complex procedures are a further illustration of the benefits of a multidisciplinary approach to nasal reconstruction.[3,5,8,9,43]

Reconstruction of the nasal lining may involve the following:

1. Split- or full-thickness skin grafts can be placed on the subcutaneous aspects of flaps.[20] These grafts may be placed at the time of flap repair or may be buried beneath the planned flap 1 or 2 weeks prior to flap transfer.[20]
2. Free mucosal grafts harvested from the buccal mucosa can be used.[20,129,130] The donor sites heal well by secondary intention.[20]
3. A hinge or turnover flap can be fashioned from the free margin of a full-thickness defect and freed from the surrounding skin except for a subcutaneous pedicle. The flap is then free to turn over into the defect, where the external skin replaces the nasal lining.[18,20,42,124,125] The external defect on the nose or cheek is made larger by this technique and is covered with a flap such as a nasolabial[125] or forehead flap[18,20] or is closed directly.[124]
4. A nasolabial or reverse nasolabial flap can be used to replace lost nasal lining with cheek skin.[63,97]
5. Pivoted mucosal flaps can be raised from intranasal donor sites (vestibule, vault, and septum). These flaps are thin and yet provide highly vascular beds for free bone or cartilage grafts.[117]

Reconstruction of missing nasal bone or cartilage is required to support skin flaps, maintain a normal nasal shape, and prevent nasal collapse. Support can be provided in a number of ways, such as the following:

1. A skin-cartilage composite graft together with a cutaneous flap can be used.[20]
2. Cartilage grafts may be placed within folded nasolabial flaps in the reconstruction of the nasal ala.[20] Alternatively, cartilage or bone grafts[20] can be buried beneath the tips of planned nasolabial or forehead flaps, and sometime later they are transferred to the nasal defect as an integral part of the flap.[20]
3. Sculpted bone or cartilage grafts can be assembled on a highly vascular, pivoted septal mucosal flap and covered with a thin forehead flap.[62,117]
4. Cartilage grafts can be inserted into skin flaps as a secondary procedure after the flaps have been allowed to es-

tablish a local blood supply,[20] although the results may be inferior to the primary placement of cartilage.[117]
5. Structural support of the upper nose and dorsum can be provided by skeletal rib or iliac crest cantilever bone grafts[11,114,120,121,128] anchored to the nasal process of the frontal bone and covered with a forehead flap.[3]

REFERENCES

1. Mazzola RF: History of nasal reconstruction: A brief review. *Handchir Mikrochir Plast Chir* **19:**4–6, 1987
2. Menick FJ: Aesthetic refinements in use of forehead for nasal reconstruction: The paramedian forehead flap. *Clin Plast Surg* **17:**607–622, 1990
3. Baker SR, Swanson NA: Management of nasal cutaneous malignant neoplasms: An interdisciplinary approach. *Arch Otolaryngol* **109:**473–479, 1983
4. Baker SR, Swanson NA: Regional and distant skin flaps in nasal reconstruction. *Facial Plastic Surgery* **2:**33–44, 1984
5. Baker SR et al: Mohs' surgical treatment and reconstruction of cutaneous malignancies of the nose. *Facial Plastic Surgery* **5:**29–47, 1987
6. Conley J: Cancer of the skin of the nose. *Arch Otolaryngol* **84:**55–60, 1966
7. Conte CC et al: Skin cancer of the nose: Options for reconstruction. *J Surg Oncol* **39:**1–7, 1988
8. Rudolph R, Miller SH: Reconstruction after Mohs cancer excision. *Clin Plast Surg* **20:**157–165, 1993
9. Siegle RJ, Schuller DE: Multidisciplinary surgical approach to the treatment of perinasal nonmelanoma skin cancer. *Dermatol Clin* **7:**711–731, 1989
10. Vieira RC: Reconstruction of the nose with malignant disease. *Clin Plast Surg* **8:**603–613, 1981
11. Antia NH, Daver BM: Reconstructive surgery for nasal defects. *Clin Plast Surg* **8:**535–563, 1981
12. Hagerty RF, Smith W: The nasolabial cheek flap. *Am Surg* **24:**506–510, 1958
13. MacFee WF: The surgical treatment of cancer of the nose, with emphasis on methods of repair. *Ann Surg* **140:**475–495, 1954
14. Panje WR et al: Secondary intention healing as an adjunct to the reconstruction of mid-facial defects. *Laryngoscope* **90:**1148–1154, 1980
15. Swanson NA et al: Mohs' surgery: Techniques, indications, and applications in head and neck surgery. *Head Neck Surg* **6:**683–692, 1983
16. Wee SS et al: The frontonasal flap: Utility for lateral nasal defects and technical refinements. *Br J Plast Surg* **44:**201–205, 1991
17. Burget GC, Menick FJ: The subunit principle in nasal reconstruction. *Plast Reconstr Surg* **76:**239–247, 1985
18. Lesavoy MA et al: Nasal reconstruction. In: Reconstruction

of the head and neck. Lesavoy MA (ed). Baltimore, Williams & Wilkins, 1981, pp 63–79.

19. Tromovitch TA et al: Nasal defects, in *Flaps and Grafts in Dermatologic Surgery,* edited by TA Tromovitch et al. Chicago, Year Book, 1989, pp 121–168

20. Renner G, Davis WE: Adjacent flaps for nasal reconstruction. *Facial Plastic Surgery* **2:**17–32, 1984

21. Thomas JR: Problem-specific analysis in nasal reconstruction. *Facial Plastic Surgery* **2:**1–8, 1984

22. Galindo SDL et al: Anatomical and functional account on the lateral nasal cartilages. *Acta Anat* **97:**393–399, 1977

23. Zelnik J, Gingrass RP: Anatomy of the alar cartilage. *Plast Reconstr Surg* **64:**650–653, 1979

24. Barton FE: Aesthetic aspects of partial nasal reconstruction. *Clin Plast Surg* **8:**177–191, 1981

25. Barton FE: Aesthetic aspects of nasal reconstruction. *Clin Plast Surg* **15:**155–165, 1988

26. Zitelli JA, Fazio MJ: Reconstruction of the nose with local flaps. *J Dermatol Surg Oncol* **17:**184–189, 1991

27. Manson PN et al: Algorithm for nasal reconstruction. *Am J Surg* **138:**528–532, 1979

28. Menick FJ: Artistry in aesthetic surgery: Aesthetic perception and the subunit principle. *Clin Plast Surg* **14:**723–735, 1987

29. Millard DR: Reconstructive rhinoplasty of the tip. *Clin Plast Surg* **8:**507–520, 1981

30. Dzubow LM, Zack L: The principle of cosmetic junctions as applied to reconstruction of defects following Mohs surgery. *J Dermatol Surg Oncol* **16:**353–355, 1990

31. Burget GC: Aesthetic restoration of the nose. *Clin Plast Surg* **12:**463–480, 1985

32. Gonzalez-Ulloa M: Restoration of the face covering by means of selected skin in regional aesthetic units. *Br J Plast Surg* **9:**212–221, 1956

33. Adamson JE: Constriction of the internal nasal valve in rhinoplasty: Treatment and prevention. *Ann Plast Surg* **18:**114–121, 1987

34. Cottle MH: Concepts of nasal physiology as related to corrective nasal surgery. *Arch Otolaryngol* **72:**11–20, 1960

35. Courtiss EH, Goldwyn RM: The effects of nasal surgery on airflow. *Plast Reconstr Surg* **72:**9–19, 1983

36. Robinson JK, Burget GC: Nasal valve malfunction resulting from resection of cancer. *Arch Otolaryngol Head Neck Surg* **116:**1419–1424, 1990

37. Stucker FJ, Smith TE: The nasal bony dorsum and cartilaginous vault: Pitfalls in management. *Arch Otolaryngol* **102:**695–698, 1976

38. Hinderer KH: Diagnosis of anatomic obstructions of the airways. *Arch Otolaryngol* **78:**660–662, 1963

39. Lupo G, Mazzola RF: Choices of techniques in nasal repairs. *Handchir Mikrochir Plast Chir* **19:**7–9, 1987

40. Maniglia AJ: Reconstructive rhinoplasty. *Laryngoscope* **99:**865–870, 1989

41. O'Quinn B et al: Classification of nasal defects: A practical guide for reconstruction. *Otolaryngol Head Neck Surg* **95:**5–9, 1986

42. Baker SR: Regional flaps in facial reconstruction. *Otolaryngol Clin North Am* **23:**925–946, 1990

43. Patton TJ, Thomas JR: Classification and etiology of nasal defects. *Facial Plastic Surgery* **2:**9–15, 1984

44. Becker GD et al: Nonsurgical repair of perinasal skin defects. *Plast Reconstr Surg* **88:**768–776, 1991

45. Goldwyn RM, Rueckert F: The value of healing by secondary intention for sizeable defects of the face. *Arch Surg* **112:**285–292, 1977

46. Zitelli JA: Secondary intention healing: An alternative to surgical repair. *Clin Dermatol* **2:**92–106, 1984

47. Zitelli JA: Wound healing by secondary intention: A cosmetic appraisal. *J Am Acad Dermatol* **9:**407–415, 1983

48. Diwan R et al: Secondary intention healing: The primary approach for management of selected wounds. *Arch Otolaryngol Head Neck Surg* **115:**1248–1249, 1989

49. Mordick TG et al: Delayed reconstruction following Mohs' chemosurgery for skin cancers of the head and neck. *Am J Surg* **160:**447–449, 1990

50. Borges AF: W-Plastic rotation flap to cover nasal defect. *Ann Plast Surg* **25:**303–305, 1990

51. Bennett JE: Reconstruction of lateral nasal defects. *Clin Plast Surg* **8:**587–598, 1981

52. Bennett JE, Thurston JB: Cancer of the nose: Ablation and repair. *Clin Plast Surg* **3:**461–469, 1976

53. Rees TD: The transfer of free composite grafts of skin and fat: A clinical study. *Plast Reconstr Surg* **25:**556–564, 1960

54. Robinson JK: Improvement in the appearance of full-thickness skin grafts with dermabrasion. *Arch Dermatol* **123:**1340–1343, 1987

55. Hance G et al: Color matching of skin grafts and flaps with permanent pigment injection. *Surg Gynecol Obstet* **44:**624–628, 1979

56. Zitelli JA: Burow's grafts. *J Am Acad Dermatol* **17:**271–279, 1987

57. Chester EC: The use of dog-ears as grafts. *J Dermatol Surg Oncol* **7:**956–959, 1981

58. Vecchione TR: The use of proximal nasal tissue in nasal reconstruction. *Aesthetic Plast Surg* **6:**177–178, 1982

59. Stucker FJ, Shaw GY: The perichondrial cutaneous graft: A 12-year clinical experience. *Arch Otolaryngol Head Neck Surg* **118:**287–292, 1992

60. McLaughlin CR: Composite ear grafts and their blood supply. *Br J Plast Surg* **7:**274–278, 1954

61. Tromovitch TA et al: Composite grafts, in *Flaps and Grafts in Dermatologic Surgery,* edited by TA Tromovitch et al. Chicago, Year Book, 1989, pp 65–67

62. Burget GC, Menick FJ: Nasal reconstruction: Seeking a fourth dimension. *Plast Reconstr Surg* **78:**145–157, 1986

63. Millard DR: Reconstructive rhinoplasty for the lower two-thirds of the nose. *Plast Reconstr Surg* **57:**722–728, 1976

64. Guerrerosantos J, Dicksheet S: Nasolabial flap with simultaneous cartilage graft in nasal alar reconstruction. *Clin Plast Surg* **8:**599–602, 1981

65. Gillies H: A new free graft applied to the reconstruction of the nostril. *Br J Surg* **30:**305–307, 1943

66. Hagan WE, Walker LB: The nasolabial musculocutaneous flap: Clinical and anatomical correlations. *Laryngoscope* **98:**341–346, 1988

67. Wee SS et al: Refinements of nasalis myocutaneous flap. *Ann Plast Surg* **25:**271–278, 1990

68. McCarthy JG et al: The median forehead flap revisited: The blood supply. *Plast Reconstr Surg* **76:**866–869, 1985

69. Dzubow LM: Nose, in *Facial Flaps: Biomechanics and Regional Application,* edited by LM Dzubow. Norwalk, Conn, Appleton & Lange, 1990, pp 69–101

70. Zitelli JA: The bilobed flap for nasal reconstruction. *Arch Dermatol* **125:**957–959, 1989

71. Dzubow LM, Miller SJ: The dual rhombic flap: A technique to utilize distant tissue laxity for reconstructive surgery. *Arch Dermatol* **127:**1772–1774, 1991

72. Masson JK, Mendelson BC: The banner flap. *Am J Surg* **134:**419–423, 1977

73. Yarborough JM: Ablation of facial scars by programmed dermabrasion. *J Dermatol Surg Oncol* **14:**292–294, 1988

74. Peng VT et al: "Pinch" modification of the linear advancement flap. *J Dermatol Surg Oncol* **13:**251–253, 1987

75. Hauben DJ: Subcutaneous V-Y advancement flap for closure of nasal tip defect. *Ann Plast Surg* **23:**239–244, 1989

76. Salasche SJ et al: The suspension suture. *J Dermatol Surg Oncol* **13:**973–978, 1987

77. Strauch B, Fox M: V-Y bipedicle flap for resurfacing the nasal supratip region. *Plast Reconstr Surg* **83:**899–903, 1989

78. Cronin TD: The V-Y rotational flap for nasal tip defects. *Ann Plast Surg* **11:**282–288, 1983

79. Snow SN et al: Nasal tip reconstruction: The horizontal "J" rotation flap using skin from the lower lateral bridge and cheek. *J Dermatol Surg Oncol* **16:**727–732, 1990

80. Rieger RA: A local flap for repair of the nasal tip. *Plast Reconstr Surg* **40:**147–149, 1967

81. Marchac D, Toth B: The axial frontonasal flap revisited. *Plast Reconstr Surg* **78:**686–694, 1985

82. Rigg BM: The dorsal nasal flap. *Plast Reconstr Surg* **52:**361–364, 1973

83. Hardin JC: Alar rim reconstruction by a dorsal nasal flap. *Plast Reconstr Surg* **66:**293–295, 1980

84. Monheit GD: The rhomboid transposition flap re-evaluated. *J Dermatol Surg Oncol* **6:**464–471, 1980

85. Elliott RA: Rotation flaps of the nose. *Plast Reconstr Surg* **44:**147–149, 1969

86. Becker FF: Rhomboid flap in facial reconstruction. *Arch Otolaryngol* **105:**569–573, 1979

87. Cameron RR et al: Reconstructions of the nose and upper lip with nasolabial flaps. *Plast Reconstr Surg* **52:**145–150, 1973

88. McLaren LR: Nasolabial flap repair for alar margin defects. *Br J Plast Surg* **16:**234–238, 1963

89. Zitelli JA: The nasolabial flap as a single-stage procedure. *Arch Dermatol* **126:**1445–1448, 1990

90. Climo MS: Nasolabial flap for alar defect. *Plast Reconstr Surg* **44:**303–304, 1969

91. Wesser DR, Burt GB: Nasolabial flap for losses of the nasal ala and columella: Case report. *Plast Reconstr Surg* **44:**300–302, 1969

92. DaSilva G: A new method of reconstructing the columella with a naso-labial flap. *Plast Reconstr Surg* **34:**63–65, 1964

93. Ausin A: The "trap-door" scar deformity. *Clin Plast Surg* **4:**255–261, 1977

94. Koranda FC, Webster RC: Trapdoor effect in nasolabial flaps: Causes and corrections. *Arch Otolaryngol* **111:**421–424, 1985

95. Walkinshaw MD, Caffee HH: The nasolabial flap: A problem and its correction. *Plast Reconstr Surg* **69:**30–34, 1982

96. Redman RD, Olshansky K: Anatomical alar reconstruction with staged nasolabial flap. *Ann Plast Surg* **20:**285–291, 1988

97. Spear SL et al: A new twist to the nasolabial flap for reconstruction of lateral alar defects. *Plast Reconstr Surg* **79:**915–920, 1987

98. Nicolai JPA: Reconstruction of the columella with nasolabial flaps. *Head Neck Surg* **4:**374–379, 1982

99. Zimany A: The bi-lobed flap. *Plast Reconstr Surg* **11:**424–434, 1953

100. Tardy ME et al: The bilobed flap in nasal repair. *Arch Otolaryngol* **95:**1–5, 1972

101. McGregor JC, Soutar DS: A critical assessment of the bilobed flap. *Br J Plast Surg* **34:**197–205, 1981

102. Morgan BL, Samiian MR: Advantages of the bilobed flap for closure of small defects of the face. *Plast Reconstr Surg* **52:**35–37, 1973

103. Meyer R: Aesthetic aspects in reconstructive surgery of the nose. *Aesthetic Plast Surg* **12:**195–201, 1988

104. Emmett AJJ: The closure of defects by using adjacent triangular flaps with subcutaneous pedicles. *Plast Reconstr Surg* **59:**45–52, 1977

105. Giebfried JW et al: Reconstruction of nasal defects with a nasolabial island flap. *Arch Otolaryngol Head Neck Surg* **113:**295–298, 1987

106. Rybka FJ: Reconstruction of the nasal tip using nasalis myocutaneous sliding flaps. *Plast Reconstr Surg* **71:**40–44, 1983

107. Constantine VS: Nasalis myocutaneous flap: Repair of nasal supratip defects. *J Dermatol Surg Oncol* **17:**439–444, 1991

108. Harahap M: Some useful flaps for covering some defects in the nose. *J Dermatol Surg Oncol* **8:**126–131, 1982

109. Zide BM: Nasal anatomy: The muscles and tip sensation. *Aesthetic Plast Surg* **9:**193–196, 1985

110. Kazanjian VH: The repair of nasal defects with the median forehead flap: Primary closure of forehead wound. *Surg Gynecol Obstet* **83:**37–49, 1946

111. Sawhney CP: Reconstruction of partial loss of nose. *Clin Plast Surg* **8:**521–534, 1981

112. Thomas JR et al: The precise midline forehead flap as a musculocutaneous flap. *Arch Otolaryngol Head Neck Surg* **114:**79–84, 1988

113. Figi FA, Moorman WL: The median forehead flap: Indications and limitations. *Plast Reconstr Surg* **24:**163–174, 1959

114. Converse JM: Clinical applications of the scalping flap in reconstruction of the nose. *Plast Reconstr Surg* **43:**247–259, 1969

115. Converse JM, McCarthy JG: The scalping forehead flap revisited. *Clin Plast Surg* **8:**413–434, 1981

116. Sawhney CP: A longer angular midline forehead flap for the reconstruction of nasal defects. *Plast Reconstr Surg* **58:**721–723, 1976

117. Burget GC, Menick FJ: Nasal support and lining: The marriage of beauty and blood supply. *Plast Reconstr Surg* **84:**189–203, 1989

118. Adamson JE: Nasal reconstruction with the expanded forehead flap. *Plast Reconstr Surg* **81:**12–20, 1988

119. Manders EK et al: Soft-tissue expansion: Concepts and complications. *Plast Reconstr Surg* **74:**493–507, 1984

120. Ortiz-Monasterio F, Olmedo A: Reconstruction of major nasal defects. *Clin Plast Surg* **8:**565–586, 1981

121. Wheeler ES et al: Bone grafts for nasal reconstruction. *Plast Reconstr Surg* **69:**9–18, 1982

122. Marino H: Levelling of linear scars with Z-plasties. *Clin Plast Surg* **4:**239–245, 1977

123. Holt GR, Parel SM: Prosthetics in nasal rehabilitation. *Facial Plastic Surgery* **2:**74–84, 1984

124. Hauben DJ, Sagi A: A simple method for alar rim reconstruction. *Plast Reconstr Surg* **80:**839–842, 1987

125. Bethea H: Closure of large nasal defects with double rotated pedicle flaps. *Am J Surg* **95:**299–300, 1958

126. Millard DR: Aesthetic reconstructive rhinoplasty. *Clin Plast Surg* **8:**169–175, 1981

127. Heanley C: The subcutaneous tissue pedicle in columella and other nasal reconstruction. *Br J Plast Surg* **8:**60–63, 1955

128. Millard DR: Total reconstructive rhinoplasty and a missing link. *Plast Reconstr Surg* **37:**167–183, 1966

129. Rayner CRW: Oral mucosal flaps in midfacial reconstruction. *Br J Plast Surg* **37:**43–47, 1984

130. Soutar DS et al: Buccal mucosal flaps in nasal reconstruction. *Br J Plast Surg* **43:**612–616, 1990

131. Field LM: The preauricular site for donor grafts of skin: Advantages, disadvantages, and caveats. *J Dermatol Surg Oncol* **6:**40–44, 1980

132. Hernandez-Perez E: A simplified method of grafting full-thickness skin onto defects on the nose. *J Dermatol Surg Oncol* **7:**80–81, 1981

David M. Duffy

31 Understanding Sclerotherapy

Sclerotherapy which employs injectable irritants to destroy vascular tissue is best divided into two therapeutic "camps" on the basis of vessel size and the presence or absence of varicosity, valvular incompetence, and other factors. For vessels over a certain size (approximately 3 mm), the indications for specific treatment regimens are pretty well accepted with some conflict as to the ideal *combination* of surgery and sclerotherapy. Excellent articles and textbooks are available detailing their treatment.[1–3] In marked contrast, there is a great deal more art than science regarding the best way to treat small varicose and nonvaricose vessels (under 2 mm) in size.

The object of this chapter is to acquaint the reader with some of the general principles underlying the broad variety of responses which occur in patients undergoing this treatment.[3,4] There are several cardinal principles which must be understood:

1. Individuals are amazingly variable. Treatment responses can be surprising, paradoxical, and unpredictable.
2. A large number of host factors, including the individual's ability to heal damaged vessels, have a great deal more to do with treatment outcome than any possible combination of therapeutic strategies.
3. Because of this innate treatment variability, which, when less than ideal, is often attributed to lack of proper technique, various experts on the subject will butt heads and publish diametrically opposing views as to the best way to carry out the treatment.[5]
4. Fortunately, at least 90 percent of treated patients are both satisfied with the results of treatment and grateful.[6] This popular technique is safe, effective, and becoming more widely accepted. It is definitely here to stay.

GENDER

Over 95 percent of the patients treated in one practice were women, most of whom could identify a family member with the same complaint.[6] This statistical preponderance is most likely related to the effect of estrogens and other uniquely feminine hormones upon the regulation of vessel growth.[7] Regarding this relationship, there is an appalling lack of knowledge to which feminists could point justifiably as another sign of masculine insensitivity. Judah Folkman, the vascular growth factor guru, sums up the current state of ignorance when he states, "estrogen tends to potentiate certain forms of neovascularization, but we have absolutely no idea what the biochemical link is."[8] Cutaneous blood vessels affecting the legs of women, which worsen with pregnancy, ovulation, or menstruation or appear after sclerotherapy, may provide clues to unlock the riddle of estrogen-mediated vessel growth in more ominous disease states, particularly hormonally mediated tumor angiogenesis (Fig. 31-1).

VASCULAR GROWTH DYNAMICS

Proliferation and Quiescence

Cells constituting the human vascular tree have the unique ability to be rapidly catapulted from a state of relative quiescence in which about 3 per 1000 are undergoing mitosis into an almost neoplastic hyperproliferative state in which entire cell populations duplicate every 24 h. Under conditions of physiologic/endocrinologic stress (menstruation, ovulation, placenta formation, and wound healing), this entire process begins and *stops* quickly with great precision. Uncontrolled

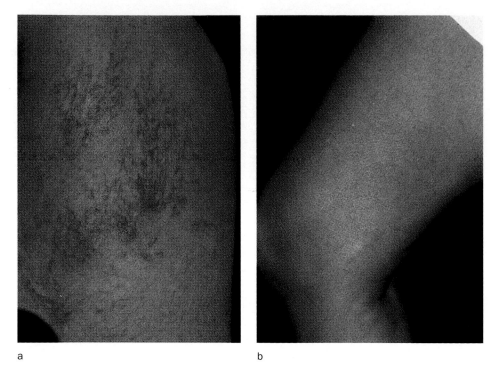

a   b

Figure 31-1   *(a)* Extensive telangiectasia and reticular vein hypertrophy at the 8th month of the first pregnancy. *(b)* Shows compete clearing without treatment 2 years post partum. With preceding pregnancies, these vessels often occur earlier and are more persistent.

and persistent vascular proliferation occurs in a broad variety of pathologic processes (inflammatory, infectious, neoplastic, and immunologic).[9]

Etiology/Taxonomy

The occurrence of spider and varicose veins probably belongs to a newly recognized category of diseases of blood vessel growth regulation—a concept suggested by Judah Folkman.[9]

SCLEROTHERAPEUTIC CRUDITY AND THE SPECTRUM OF POSTTREATMENT RESPONSE

In an era when obscenely expensive lasers can *confine* tissue damage with optical precision, a few dollars spent for a disposable syringe, needle, and sclerosant provide a cost-effective but relatively crude method of damaging cutaneous vasculature. This crudity takes the form of nonselective clinically apparent and *inapparent* vessel damage and *stimulation* of sclerosant-resistant proliferative new vessel growth. The "trauma" of sclerotherapy occurs not only to targeted vessels, but it also affects normal surrounding vasculature both superficial and deep.

Time Frame

The true spectrum of treatment responses is not always immediately apparent, taking in some cases months to years to become evident, often in the form of new vessel growth and unexpected variability and complications in response to repeated treatments. Moreover, repeated treatments can themselves produce persistent patterns of new vessel growth quite different from the vessels for which the patient originally sought treatment.

PATIENT EVALUATION

Host factors which suggest the use of substantially lower sclerosant concentrations include histories of spontaneous bleeding of the affected vessels, easy bruisability, and other conditions which could be expected to increase cutaneous and vascular fragility or thrombosis (i.e., advanced age, diabetes, the presence of underlying malignancies, immunologic disorders, and coagulation abnormalities). On physical examination, the most valuable indicator of extraordinary vascular fragility is the presence of dilated, tortuous, and elevated (varicose) vessels in the 0.75 mm to 2 mm range; often these are cyanotic or blue-green in color. These vessels may also be

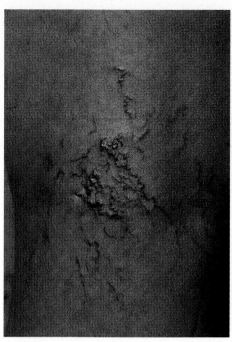 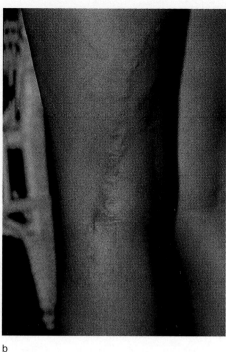

a   b

Figure 31-2 *(a)* Varicosities occurring in small vessels. Small varicose vessels can be extraordinarily fragile and are often treated with lower concentrations of sclerosants. *(b)* "Typical" varicose veins.

a visible indication of underlying venous hypertension and significant deep venous disease.

Host Factors Which Affect Treatment Outcome

Varicosity

Varicose veins are, by definition, elevated above the surface of the skin, dilated, and/or tortuous (Fig. 31-2).[10] Common usage has created the perception that varicose veins are large and green in color when, in fact, smaller vessels can also be varicose.

Fragility, Size, and Varicosity

Vessels of a certain size (0.6 mm to 1.5 mm) are often quite delicate, and varicose veins of all sizes are often thin-walled and quite fragile. Such vessels are sometimes explosively destroyed, often in association with severe and unintentional perivenular damage, even when very weak sclerosants are used.

Unpredictable Fragility

In contrast to varicose veins which often occur in elderly patients in association with other stigmata of cutaneous and vascular fragility (i.e., ecchymoses), some young individuals,

with no history of easy bruisability or bleeding disorders, present themselves with vessels which are small (0.5 mm or under), nonvaricose, but extraordinarily and unexpectedly fragile (Fig. 31-3). These vessels are also easily destroyed, often with a great deal of bruising, using ultralow concentrations of sclerosants. This inexplicable fragility has provoked endless disputes about the ideal concentration for use on small vessels.[11]

ANATOMY: DEEP/SUPERFICIAL

The second that any vessel comes in contact with a sclerosant, both the treated vessel and its deep and superficial tributaries can also be damaged, producing varying degrees of necrosis and neovascularization (repair). Unseen deeper vessels can be more fragile and subject to thrombosis or other complications than the vessels on the surface which are intentionally being treated. The treatment of a 2-mm superficial vein in an elderly patient could not be excluded as a cause of a nonfatal pulmonary embolus (Fig. 31-4).[6]

ELECTRON MICROSCOPY

Electron microscopic photographs of large and small varicose veins reveal atrophic areas in the vessel walls described as

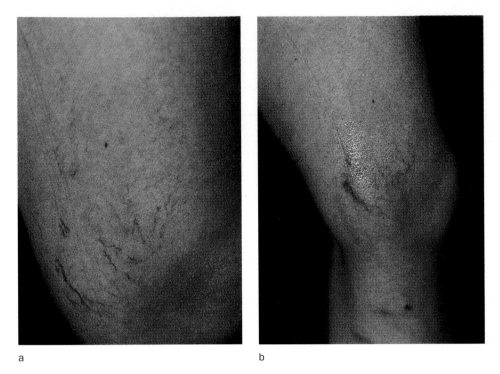

a   b

Figure 31-3 *(a)* Pretreatment photograph of a 31-year-old patient with a "varicose" spider vein. *(b)* Shows the effect of low concentration (0.5% Aethoxysklerol) sclerosant on this patient. This extraordinary fragility can't always be predicted and is seen more commonly in elderly patients.

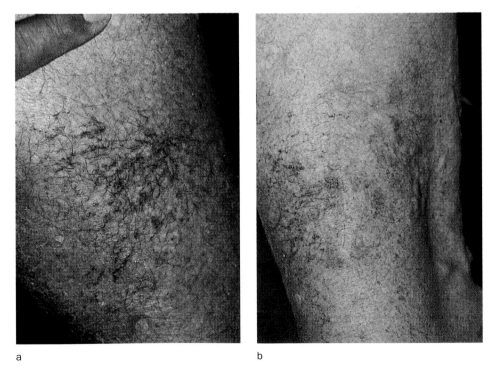

a   b

Figure 31-4 *(a)* Pretreatment photograph of 1–2 mm varicose vessels occurring in an 86-year-old man who developed a pulmonary embolus 2 weeks after treatment. *(b)* Taken 3 years post-treatment and suggests proximal venous obstruction. In this patient, an underlying malignancy had produced coagulation disorders which probably contributed to this pulmonary embolus via the propagation of a clot through an incompetent sapheno femoral valve.

fenestrations or gaps.[12] These gaps, which have also been observed in psoriatic vasculature,[13] result in nonuniform destruction of the vessel wall following treatment which becomes clinically apparent in the form of thrombi and pigment where the atrophic sections of the vessel walls are thrombosed and more severely damaged than intervening areas of relatively thick and resistant vessel wall.

VESSEL SIZE AND COLOR

Vessels 0.4 mm and smaller in size are almost always bright red; vessels between 0.5 mm and approximately 1.5 mm gradually become darker red, cyanotic, or blue-green in color; vessels larger than 2 mm are generally blue-green.

Factors which influence the color of blood vessels are (1) the color of intraluminal blood, (2) the thickness and color of overlying skin, (3) the thickness of the vessel wall, (4) the presence or absence of fascial gaps over which vessels appear to change color, and (5) the degree of vasodilation in surrounding vessels which reflect light.

SCLEROSANT INTERACTION: CLINICAL SETTING

Small red vessels can be either quiescent or proliferative. As a general rule, they occur in the quiescent state in previously untreated patients, responding predictably, by fading, to repeated treatments. When they occur in the proliferative state as a sequela of treatment or other traumas (neovascularization), they are often unresponsive or respond very slowly to high concentrations of sclerosants. The existence of red vessels suggests vascular immaturity and recent onset. Patients will describe the evolution of small vessels becoming larger and more cyanotic after repeated pregnancies or with the passage of time. Vessels between 0.6 mm and 1.5 mm can be proliferative, but they are generally quiescent, fragile, and occur most commonly in older patients. The presence of these larger spider veins, which are themselves varicose and associated with larger varicose veins, should suggest the possibility of venous hypertension. Extraordinarily low concentrations of sclerosants (0.25% to 0.06% Polidocanol or its equivalent) can produce quick and dramatic destruction.

PRE- AND POSTTREATMENT VESSEL POPULATIONS: A SPECTRUM OF RESPONSES

Posttraumatic Vessels

Since sclerotherapy can destroy or weaken treated vessels and stimulate new vessel growth (neovascularization), vessels remaining or appearing after treatment (proliferative, quiescent, and nonviable) can be viewed as constituting separate clinical entities, distinct in terms of predictable treatment responses from populations of vessels which existed before treatment.

Patterns of Response to Sclerotherapy

There are only three *visible* responses to sclerotherapy. All are usually associated immediately or later with some degree of neovascularization, thrombi, and/or hemosiderotic hyperpigmentation.

1. Sudden destruction (large vein varicose pattern): Usually, but not always accompanied by palpable thrombi and hemosiderotic hyperpigmentation, this process is common in *all* vessels, both varicose and nonvaricose, over 0.7 mm in size. Previously untreated (quiescent) vessels, between 0.2 mm and 0.5 mm in size, can occasionally disappear without a trace after one treatment. This event, usually heralded as a triumph of therapeutic judgment, is, in fact, a statistical quirk (Fig. 31-5).[14]
2. Gradual destruction (telangiectatic pattern cumulative sclerosis): Quiescent vessels about 0.45 mm and smaller usually exhibit a fading pattern with progressive diminution in size and lightening in color as they gradually fibrose and disappear with repeated treatments, usually without much thrombosis or hyperpigmentation except for areas where the needle has penetrated the skin and areas of microscopic vessel atrophy (Fig. 31-6).
3. Variable destruction: Vessels between 0.3 mm and 0.75 mm in size, particularly those remaining after treatment, can exhibit either the rapid or fading pattern on an individual basis, no matter what changes are made in treatment techniques (i.e., changes in sclerosant concentrations, compression, etc.). Occasionally, a vessel weakened but *appearing* unchanged by a previous treatment is suddenly destroyed following a second treatment and usually exhibits thrombi and/or pigmentation.

LOCATION

The location of treated small vessels will affect their response to treatment and the occurrence of complications. Important areas, all differing one from another, follow.

Lateral Thigh

The lateral thigh is routinely subjected to blows and falls. Neovascularization occurs commonly; ulcerations are less common here than on the inner knees.

Inner Knee

This area can be rendered partially avascular as a consequence of the patient's sleeping position. Patients who sleep on their sides will often develop vessels at the area of contact. In one psoriatic patient, Köebner's phenomenon was ob-

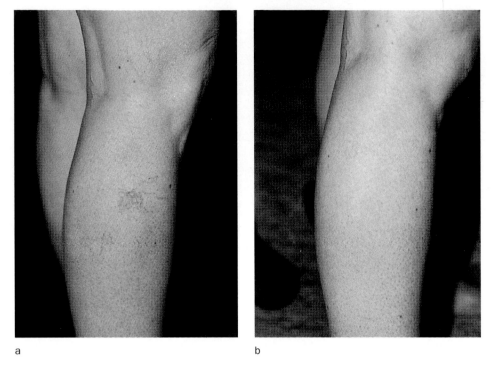

a   b

Figure 31-5 *(a)* Taken before treatment of a small patch of spider telangiectasia which responded quite dramatically to one treatment. *(b)* Results after one treatment. Generally speaking, patients with small clusters of vessels which are not numerous (low surface area) can expect this type of result, with or without compression.

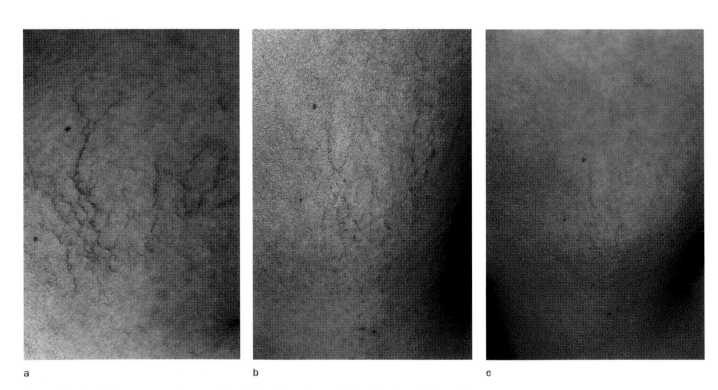

a   b   c

Figure 31-6 *(a)* Pretreatment photograph of telangiectasia, varying in size from 0.1 mm, bottom of the inner knee. *(b)* Reveals the effect of one treatment. Note this fading process in which vessels become smaller in diameter, the larger vessels often disappearing first, with minimal pigment in this case. *(c)* Taken 10 months after a second treatment. Note there is no visible pigmentation which is generally not seen following treatment of vessels under 0.4 mm. Higher concentrations of sclerosants might have caused a more rapid resolution of these vessels, but an increase in the occurrence of pigmentation and neovascularization is often associated with the use of higher concentrations.

served in this area; neovascularization and ulcerations are common here.[35]

Ankle/Feet

Hydrostatic pressure here is maximal. Healing can be slow, which intensifies the effect of sclerotherapy. Circulatory peculiarities make the area also more prone to posttreatment ulceration. Neovascularization is uncommon, but sclerosant pooling and thrombosis in vessels peripheral to those treated are common.

Buttocks and Hips

Hydrostatic pressure is low and damage is less sudden. Hemosiderotic hyperpigmentation is less common here in vessel types that produce it in more dependent areas. Vessels in the 2-mm or 3-mm range often disappear quickly without thrombosis or pigmentation.

Face

Telangiectasias here can be much less responsive to injections, and ulcerations are more common, even when very low concentrations of sclerosants are used. Larger vessels (over 1 mm) on the face may be dangerous to treat. Cautery or lasers are generally a better choice for facial telangiectasias under 0.3 mm. Vessels in the 0.4 mm to 0.5 mm range have responded well to treatment.

PREGNANCY

Pregnancy often results in the occurrence of proliferative (resistant to treatment) vessels. Many patients report that with each succeeding pregnancy vessels become more persistent, larger, and darker, in color. When advising patients who are or plan to become pregnant, the physician should defer any treatment during pregnancy unless symptomatology makes it important and should delay treatment after pregnancy for 3 to 6 months because often, at least after the first pregnancy or two, vessels which appear or worsen during pregnancy will involute with time. Injections are usually avoided during lactation. Light support hosiery is often recommended to minimize fatigue during pregnancy.

THE EFFECTS OF MULTIPLE TREATMENTS, PROGRESSIVE DAMAGE, AND RESISTANCE

Repeated treatments can act synergistically to potentiate tissue damage caused by previous treatments or paradoxically and more perversely to render vessels resistant to sclerosant concentrations which could have instantly destroyed them

had they been used at the first treatment. Moreover, repeated treatments routinely stimulate the growth of new and highly resistant vasculature (matting) blush areas.

Resistant Vessels

1. Primary resistance: This resistance is common in large vessels where sclerosant dilution occurs. These vessels which appear unchanged by previous treatments are, in fact, *resistant* to commonly used concentrations of sclerosants. This primary resistance occurs in less than 5 percent of all patients treated for small vessels.[6]
2. Neovascular vessels (matting, blush areas/proliferative vessels): This type of new vessel growth appears as a consequence of intense and protracted inflammatory neovascularization.[9] Vessels of this type, usually bright red in color, measuring 0.2 mm and smaller, are occasionally larger and darker. This process occurs to some degree in almost all patients following sclerotherapy, external trauma, surgery, or pregnancy. These vessels can be quite resistant to treatment within a certain time frame. With the passage of time (6 months to 2 years), perhaps when the proliferative phase is finally over, they again become sensitive to sclerotherapy. Patients are warned to cease treatment, at least for a time, when neovascular vessels appear.
3. Recurrence/cyclicity: Patients who present for the first time with small, less than 0.3 mm, but quiescent bright red vessels, particularly in areas of trauma, can develop a syndrome the author calls *come-and-go vessels* in which the treated vessels disappear quite nicely and then reappear, identical in size and distribution, several months to years later. These vessels often reveal a cyclic quality to their occurrence and resolution independently of treatment.

THE LASER

For resistant small vessels, copper vapor and/or dye lasers are occasionally reported to be of benefit. Pigmentation of some sort following their use is routine. The costs are high; time and delayed sclerotherapy are often better choices.[1]

SCLEROSANTS

General Rules

There is no perfect sclerosant. All can cause tissue necrosis (ulcerations), uncontrolled superficial and deep venous thrombosis, and occasional pulmonary emboli. Allergies and anaphylaxis can occur with all but pure hypertonic saline. Sclerosants can also cause damage, to some degree, to normal veins and surrounding tissues.

Sclerosant Choice

Every sclerosant has its devotees, and the choice of a particular sclerosant is influenced not only by the needs of the patient but by the experience of the individual practitioner and the availability and legal status of the sclerosant. In America, only two drugs are approved for the treatment of varicose veins of any size involving the legs, although another drug, ethanolamine, has been approved for the treatment of esophageal varices.[15] Sodium morrhuate, approved in 1930, and sodium sotradechol, approved in 1946 by the Food and Drug Administration (FDA), are far more toxic and no more effective for the treatment of small vessels (up to 6 mm in size) than hypertonic saline or polidocanol; the latter, it is hoped, soon will be sanctioned by the FDA for this purpose.[1,16] Also, see below: sotradecol/Sotradecol.

Commonly Used Sclerosants: Equivalent Concentrations

One percent Polidocanol (Aethoxysklerol, dihydroxypolyethoxydodecane) is the equivalent of 30% saline or about 0.33% Sotradecol. All of these figures are approximate. Each type of solution may exert more or less effect on vessels of a certain size and in certain clinical settings.

Selecting Sclerosant Concentrations

Several articles have appeared recently suggesting that certain concentrations of sclerosants are particularly appropriate for one vessel size or another.[11,17] In general, for vessels smaller than 2 mm, no concentration over 0.75% Polidocanol or its equivalent is necessary. Experienced sclerotherapists often select three concentrations: high (0.75% Polidocanol/23.4% saline/0.2 to 0.3% Sotradecol), medium (one-half of that concentration), and low (one-fourth of that concentration). For vessels 0.5 mm and smaller, quiescent or proliferative, 0.75% Polidocanol is generally employed. For vessels between 0.5 mm and 1.5 mm, the decision to use half- or quarter-strength sclerosants has to be made on an individual basis. For large vessels over 3 mm or 4 mm, where dilution plays some role, sometimes the evacuation of blood from the treated area achieved by elevating the extremity permits the use of substantially lower concentrations.

Hypertonic Saline

Hypertonic saline, available as an abortifacient in 23.4% concentration, is an excellent sclerosant for the treatment of small vessels. It has the disadvantage of being a weak sclerosant which, if extravasated, can produce contact ulcers in small volumes and is relatively painful for the patient, even when the physician uses good technique. It causes no allergies, although when combined with heparin (or Xylocaine) it loses that advantage.

Polidocanol, Hydroxypolyethoxydodecane (Aethoxysklerol) (Chemische Fabrik Kreussler & Co., Wiesbaden-Biebrich, Germany)

The most forgiving of all of sclerosing agents, polidocanol is painless for the patient, particularly when dilute, and does not produce tissue necrosis upon direct contact in high (3%) concentrations (Fig. 31-7).[18] It has the disadvantage of containing alcohol as a dispersant and should not be used on patients taking drugs such as disulfiram (Antabuse). It also has the disadvantage, along with all other sclerosants (other than hypertonic saline), of causing allergies. (The LD_{50} for Polidocanol is 1200 mg/kg in mice) and is every bit as effective as more powerful agents in the treatment of small vessels.

Sotradecol (Wyeth-Ayerst Laboratories, Philadelphia, PA)

The most potent of the three agents discussed, sotradecol is three to four times more powerful than Polidocanol and about 90 times more potent, on a percentage basis, than hypertonic saline. The LD_{50} for this agent in mice is reported to be 90 mg/kg (plus or minus 5 mg).[16] For large vessels, this potent agent is an excellent choice, producing predictable and uniform results. Sotradechol will produce contact necrosis in relatively low concentrations, and it will cause anaphylaxis and/or fatalities at a much higher rate than Polidocanol. In one recent case, a 55-year-old patient died after the administration of 0.5 cc of 0.5% Sotradecol.[1,16,19]

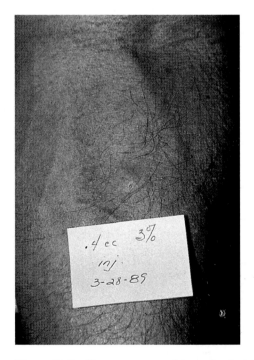

Figure 31-7   The appearance of the author's right volar forearm following the intradermal injection of 0.4 cc, 3% polidocanol. No ulceration occurred following this injection. However, ulcerations can occur with any sclerosant through as yet unspecified mechanisms.

High Concentrations of Sclerosants

The use of high concentrations of sclerosants can usually be expected to produce more rapid destruction of the treated vessels and more damage to the deeper system than lower concentrations. Complications related to this sudden destruction (hemosiderotic hyperpigmentation, palpable thrombi) are also more common, subject to a great deal of individual variability.

Low Concentrations of Sclerosants

The use of more dilute sclerosants generally, but by no means always, produces slower damage to the treated vessel with a sometimes lower incidence of thrombi and hyperpigmentation. Increased numbers of treatments are the rule and treatment failures are more common. In certain subsets of very fragile vessels, dramatic lowering of sclerosant concentrations will not prevent sudden destruction with a single treatment. Certain vessels may be benefited by the injection of low concentrations of sclerosants in surrounding larger "feeder" vessels (feeder injection).

COMMON COMPLICATIONS

Neovascular Vessels (matting)

Proliferation of new vessels can occur following treatment of vessels of all sizes using all concentrations and types of sclerosants. This complication is reported to occur between 5 and 40 percent of treated patients.[1,16,20]

These vessels—which are usually, but not always, smaller than those originally treated—are often bright red in color and measure between 0.05 and 0.15 mm in size. Larger (0.5 mm to 2 mm in size) vessels occasionally occur following treatment as well. One study suggests that matting is more common in patients receiving estrogen replacement therapy, patients heavier than established norms, and patients whose vessels have been present for many years.[21]

Typically, neovascular vessels can be seen immediately or several months after one or more treatments. Occasionally, they will occur within a week after the first treatment (Fig. 31-8).[22] Vessels which appear following treatment can be enormously resistant to high concentrations of sclerosants as compared to vessels of the same size which appear in previ-

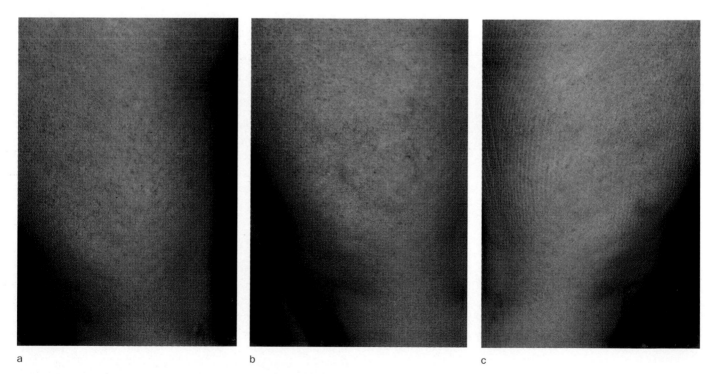

a   b   c

Figure 31-8 *(a)* A pretreatment photograph showing spider telangiectasia in the 0.3 mm to 0.5 mm range. *(b)* Neovascularization at 6 days posttreatment; an extremely rare event in previously untreated patients. *(c)* Almost complete resolution of neovascular vessels without treatment.

ously untreated patients. Often, the vessels at least partially involute without treatment or become responsive to future treatments after delays of 3 months to 2 years.

Pigmentation

Macular and reticular hyperpigmentation which, upon biopsy, proves to be hemosiderin occurs commonly following treatment of certain types and sizes of vessels, particularly those which are destroyed *suddenly*.[23] Certain ploys have been advocated to predict or minimize this complication, including measurement of serum ferritin levels,[24] the injection of feeder vessels, and the use of compression. Heparin has been added to hypertonic saline to minimize clotting and thus possibly lower the incidence of pigmentation.[25] Nevertheless, the occurrence of this complication is not completely avoidable but is relatively predictable. Treatment is generally tincture of time. Baker's solution and other exfoliants have been used with variable results.[6] Pigmentation is most common in small vessels between 0.6 mm and 2 mm and occurs routinely following treatment of vessels larger than 2 mm.

Thrombosis

Superficial thrombi are not of purely cosmetic importance because lawsuits have been filed by patients who are terribly distressed by their appearance. At about 3 to 4 weeks posttreatment, thromboses can easily be incised and drained, of-

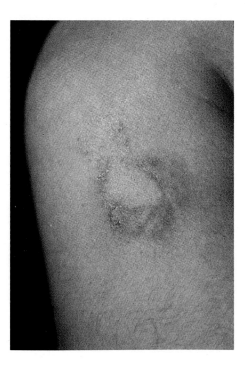

Figure 31-9 Prolonged, bone-white blanching of the skin following the injection of hypertonic saline. This is a premonitory sign of impending tissue necrosis and should be treated immediately with dilution therapy.

ten improving the appearance of the patient. Of more importance are uncontrolled propagating thrombi in the deep venous system which, fortunately, are uncommon.[1]

Thrombophlebitis

Superficial thrombophlebitis occurs with an incidence of 0.5 percent in the author's experience. Curiously enough, the author has not seen an increased incidence in patients taking progestational agents.

Pulmonary Emboli

Only one case of a pulmonary embolus following the treatment of small vessels has been reported in the American literature. A Mayo Clinic study suggests that emboli are a rare complication of large vessel sclerotherapy, occurring in 0.14 percent of patients, all of whom were over 50 years of age. In this study, no specific risk factors could be identified, but all the patients who developed emboli had had vessels present for more than 20 years. One had a history of system lupus erythematosus; another, a history of a previous deep venous thrombosis. Patients with histories of deep venous thrombosis should never be treated until adequate duplex evaluations are carried out.[26]

Extravasation Ulcers: Clinical Observations

Tissue necrosis, which is histologically thrombotic and infarctive, occurs because of several mechanisms.[1] In one study, the author was able to show that ulcerations occurred when 0.5 cc of 0.5% Sotradecol was injected directly into the dermis but did not occur when the same volume of 0.33% was employed.[18] Hypertonic saline, in this same study, regularly produced ulcerations in volumes over 0.3 cc and concentrations over 10%. Ulcerations occurred occasionally in lower than 10% concentrations. Polidocanol did not produce ulcerations when injected in 3% concentration into the author's forearm. The addition of phentolamine (Regitine) to sclerosants did not prove effective in reducing the incidence of such ulcers.[18]

Nonextravasation Ulcers

When ulcerations of vessels occur following treatment with solutions that will not produce necrosis upon direct contact with the skin, it is obvious that other mechanisms are at work. The tip-off to an impending ulceration is often the sudden occurrence of a large ecchymosis and profound or prolonged blanching in both the treated vessel and the skin around it (Fig. 31-9). In another group of patients, none of these premonitory events occur, but sometimes up to 6 weeks after treatment an ulceration will develop in the treated area, usually preceded by a crust or a blister. Biopsy-proven pyoderma gangrenosum occurred following the use of Polidocanol.[27]

The author's observations suggest that patients at risk for these ulcerations are (1) those with vessels on the feet, ankles, and face; (2) those with collagen vascular disease (systemic lupus erythematosus and Raynaud's phenomenon);[28] and (3) those who have had high concentrations of any sclerosant. It is important to understand that ulcerations can also occur with low concentrations of sclerosants, in the absence of risk factors.

The pathogenesis of the cryptogenic ulcer is largely speculated; however, histologically, it resembles ulcerations which occur following injections of Zyplast in the glabellar area.[29] Recent studies detailing the effect of leukocyte adhesion molecules upon thrombosis occurring after reperfusion injury may also shed some light upon this process.[30]

TREATMENT FOR EXTRAVASATION/IMPENDING TISSUE NECROSIS

Immediate dilution of extravasated ulcerogenic agents, such as hypertonic saline, with large volumes of normal saline (about ten times more than the extravasation assumed to occur) is employed. Horrific mistakes have occurred when improperly labeled sclerosants were used for dilutional purposes (Fig. 31-10). Accordingly, the use of a simple, gummed, colored sticker to identify sclerosants is advisable (Fig. 31-11). For those who practice sclerotherapy, a 10 cc syringe full of normal saline attached to a no. 25, 0.5-in needle should be

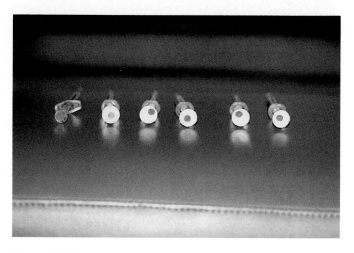

Figure 31-11 A simple way of avoiding ghastly mistakes. Gummed, colored labels attached to the piston of the syringe identifying sclerosants are a very useful method of avoiding mistakes. Normal saline should be kept in a 10 cc syringe with a 25-gauge needle to avoid any miscalculations.

readily at hand to cope with impending tissue necrosis. The author's limited investigation suggests that the deeper the extravasation occurred and the more quickly the diluents were used, the more successfully tissue necrosis was avoided.

INSURANCE

Whether or not small vessels are cosmetic (have no functional importance) or whether they do cause enough discomfort to be judged as a "medical disorder" is the subject of much debate. In one study, 40 percent of those responding noted a diminution in discomfort after treatment of small vessels.[6] For large vessels, insurance companies seem more anxious to pay for surgical procedures which are a great deal more expensive than sclerotherapy. In time, a certain degree of reason will apply, but, at this juncture, patients must be told that insurance companies often balk at paying for treatment.

PERVASIVE PUBLIC MISPERCEPTION AND MALPRACTICE

The fact that treatment formulas are empirical and no scientific consensus has been established adds even more spice to controversies surrounding this technique. A recent malpractice case demonstrates the ambivalence of some members of the surgical community toward the treatment of small vessels. In this case, a prominent vascular surgeon testified against an extremely experienced sclerotherapist dismissing both this particular physician's treatment and the treatment of small vessels in general as pure quackery and without value. This

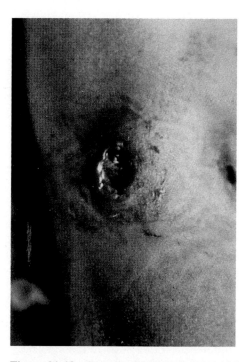

Figure 31-10 Reveals the kind of ulcer which occurs when mislabled hypertonic saline is substituted for normal saline in an attempt to head off such an ulcer.

surgeon, with impeccable credentials, testified in court that he had advised his patients to "use cosmetics" to conceal small vessels. He was completely unaware that thousands of patients have received safe and satisfactory treatment.[31]

Photography

For those who practice sclerotherapy, before and after photographs are a must. Patients will forget how they looked, and malpractice suits have been settled adversely against the physician on the basis of appearance, pigmentation, and vague symptomatology scientifically unrelated to the treatment performed by the physician but emotionally appealing to juries. Complicating the picture even further is the fact that, by far, the safest drugs for the treatment of small vessels are not FDA approved, so the physician who uses them is at a greater risk for legal action but the patient is being treated more safely.

As a general rule, it is important not to diminish the possibility of side effects when discussing this procedure with patients. Those who are contemplating adding the technique to their repertoire would be well advised to discuss their intentions with their malpractice insurer.

CONTROVERSIES

Compression

The use of compression hosiery, which exerts graduated pressure highest at the ankle and 40 percent less pressure above the knees, has been advocated following sclerotherapy for small vessels. Its use has been breathlessly heralded as a major breakthrough for treatment of all vessels.[32] In the case of larger (over 3 mm) vessels, the use of compression hosiery is routine and an integral part of the treatment process. For small vessels, its use is controversial. The author's clinical experience suggests that its routine use following treatment of small vessels is unnecessary. Hosiery and/or compression dressings are reserved for certain types of patients, particularly those who have masses of small vessels, discomfort, or lifestyles requiring prolonged standing or immobile sitting. For patients with small (under 2 mm) vessels, light compression hosiery is well tolerated and quite appreciated. Jobst sheer hosiery, 12 mm to 14 mm, is routinely used for these patients who almost all notice a reduction in fatigue and achiness when they use the hosiery, particularly at the time of menstruation. Jobst, Medi, and Sigvaris all provide excellent heavier (20 mm to 50 mm) hosiery for treatment of larger vessels. Like all garments, each type and manufacturer has sizes and designs more or less ideal and fitting better or worse for certain individuals.

Injecting Feeder Veins

"It is only after all varicose and feeder veins are treated that telangiectasias are treated. This order of treatment will best minimize posttreatment hyperpigmentation, telangiectatic matting and recanalization."[33] Vessels large and small often communicate with one another, but the analogy that one should "think of spider veins as the fingers and of the feeding varicose vein as the arm"[33] may present a false metaphor for the true relationship of large and small vessels. Large vessels which communicate with telangiectasias can be treated and disappear without any change in the appearance of the telangiectasias (Fig. 31-12). Conversely, telangiectasias which communicate freely with larger vessels can be treated and disappear with no change in the appearance of the larger vessel. The following facts also can be documented: (1) Blue-green feeder vessels, around 2 mm in size, are often more fragile and more rapidly destroyed than small (0.5 mm and smaller) vessels; (2) neovascularization occurs regularly when the larger vessels are injected as well; and (3) the injection of the feeders often does not reduce the number of treatments necessary or delay the recurrence of new vessels. One useful ploy may be the administration of a small (0.5 cc) volume of a low-concentration sclerosant (i.e., 0.5% Polidocanol or its equivalent) into larger vessels at the same time the spider vein is injected. Under certain circumstances, this small volume of sclerosant is gradually diluted and slowly squeezed into the superficial vessels through muscular action.[34]

Laboratory Procedures: Duplex Scanning and Doppler Examinations

The routine use of Doppler examinations has been advocated for all patients undergoing sclerotherapy. The author's studies indicate that asymptomatic patients with no visible varicose veins generally do not need a Doppler examination and that its use constitutes an added and unnecessary expense. For evaluating patients, symptomatology is most important. Individuals who have swelling of the legs or a great deal of pain, even in the absence of any visible varicosity, should undergo a careful duplex scanning. This noninvasive but expensive modality is quite dependent upon the skill of the person carrying it out. Those who would perform sclerotherapy would be well advised to find a good technician.

CLINICAL PROFILES

Although there is a great deal of variability in the outcome of sclerotherapy, a certain number of treatment scenarios occur with enough regularity to be discussed as prototypical treatment outcomes.

Patient #1:

This 25- to 45-year-old female with a positive family history of either large varicose veins or telangiectasia presents herself for treatment of six to ten clusters of small (0.25 to 0.5 mm) vessels involving the inner knees, lateral thighs, popliteal

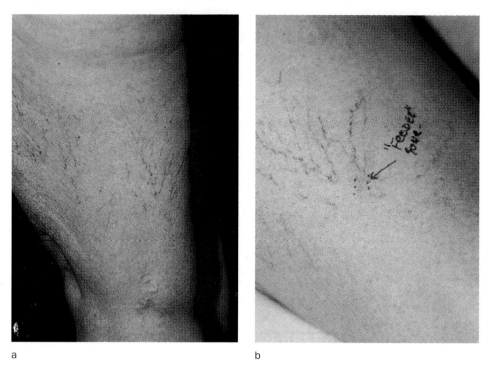

a   b

Figure 31-12 *(a)* Pretreatment photograph of a cluster of spider veins which was treated by injecting "feeders." *(b)* Reveals the "feeders gone, spiders remain" phenomenon (FGSR). Note that the larger vessels have thrombosed and the telangiectasia are still present but slightly faded.

fossa, and anterior tibial and gastrocnemius areas. She notes that these vessels, which were worsened particularly by the third pregnancy or with the passage of time, are mildly uncomfortable, but she has no symptomatology suggestive of deep venous disease. After three or four treatments with 0.75% Polidocanol, 23.4% hypertonic saline, or 0.2% to 0.3% Sotradecol, these vessels gradually fade with minimal pigmentation and neovascularization.

Long-Term Observations

When followed for 14 years, such patients are seen to develop new vessels requiring periodic treatment in the same areas. Occasionally, the same small vessel is seen to recur in contrast to large-vessel therapy in which the same vessel commonly recurs. Typically, new vessels, often smaller than those originally requiring treatment, slowly develop necessitating touch-up treatments. This phenomenon is seen most commonly in patients who have been treated for large numbers of vessels in certain locations (inner knees, gastrocnemious, lateral thighs) and is less common on the posterior legs (popliteal fossa and interior tibial areas).

Patient #2

This older (generally 55+) female presents herself with large numbers of darker, larger telangiectasias measuring between 0.5 mm and 1.5 mm. These are often varicose, and this patient may have symptomatology of deeper venous disease (pedal edema, aching, or fatigue). Despite the use of lower sclerosant concentrations (0.06 to 0.25% Polidocanol or its equivalent) and injection of her feeder veins, many of this patient's vessels are immediately destroyed resulting in hyperpigmentation and thrombosis, which are not of any major medical importance but can be distressing. Neovascularization, usually transient, often occurs following multiple treatments.

Fragile Vein Syndrome: A Case Report

This 68-year-old, white female is examined after one treatment with 1% Polidocanol, an agent which does not produce necrosis on tissue contact. Physical examination reveals numerous punched-out areas of cutaneous necrosis, some measuring several centimeters in size and extending to deep fascia. Her clinical course is prolonged, but the areas heal with some, but minimal, scarring. Measurement of the treated vessels, carried out the first visit, reveals that all of them were between 0.8 mm and 2 mm in size and described as varicose and bleeding easily with minimal tissue trauma.

The lessons to be learned from this patient are care in determining what concentration of solution to use and performance of two or three test areas with varying concentrations done at least twice to determine cumulative effects. The ul-

Arnold W. Klein
Gary D. Monheit
David M. Duffy

32 Soft-Tissue Augmentation in the Practice of Dermatology

INJECTABLE TISSUE AUGMENTATION

Many implantable substances have been used to augment soft-tissue defects and deformities. Some invariably produce cosmetic disasters. This was most certainly the case with impure paraffins and adulterated silicones.[1,2] Others, such as pure injectable-grade liquid silicone, while historically extremely useful in the skilled hands of certain physicians, have been declared illegal by the Food and Drug Administration (FDA) and are not available to the practitioner. For a substance to be useful, it must have both a high *use* potential producing pleasing cosmetic results and a minimum of untoward reactions. Furthermore it must have a low *abuse* potential such that widespread and possible incorrect or indiscriminate use should not result in significant morbidity.[3] Other desirable characteristics of a filling substance include reproducible implantation techniques that provide predictable persistent correction as well as ease in obtaining or fabricating the substance. Additionally, it should be noncarcinogenic, nonteratogenic, and nonmigratory. If the agent is not autologous, it must be FDA approved. FDA approval guarantees purity as well as accessibility to the agent and information regarding its use.

This chapter reviews two available FDA-approved filling substances, Fibrel and injectable bovine collagen (Zyderm

and Zyplast). It also highlights injectable medical-grade silicone. The use of injectable medical grade is currently illegal; nevertheless, a large body of information has been generated concerning its application by many distinguished and skilled investigators. Its exclusion from this chapter would be a serious academic error, but its inclusion should not be construed to indicate the advocacy or promotion of its use.

INJECTABLE BOVINE COLLAGEN

Injectable bovine collagen, Zyderm collagen (ZC) implant, has been in use since 1977 and received FDA approval in July 1981.[4] This became the first legally available product in the United States for soft-tissue augmentation. Its approval subsequently awakened interest in the entire field of filling agents. An estimated 800,000 individuals have received injectable collagen implants since this approval in 1981. Following the availability of Zyderm I (ZI) collagen, two additional forms, Zyderm and Zyplast have been released.

Formulations

ZC is derived from cowhide and is a purified suspension of dermal collagen. Processing of the material involves purification, pepsin digestion, and sterilization. Without disturbing the helical structure, the pepsin digestion removes the antigenic telopeptide regions and makes the product more immunologically acceptable to the human. ZC is 95 to 98 percent type I collagen, with the remainder being type III.[5] The collagen is suspended in phosphate-buffered physiologic saline containing 0.3% lidocaine. It is dispensed in syringes which are to be kept at a low temperature (4°C) so that the dispersed fibrils remain small and fluid. This will allow passage through a 30- or 32-gauge needle. Upon implantation and because of the higher temperature of the human body (37°C), larger fibrils are produced as intermolecular cross-linking occurs, with the implant ultimately assuming characteristics of a gel.

ZC is currently available in three forms, two of which differ only in concentration of material. These are ZI collagen (the original material), which is 3.5 percent by weight bovine collagen, and Zyderm II [ZII (introduced in 1983)], which is 6.5 percent by weight bovine collagen. Zyplast (ZP) implant, approved in 1985, is the third form. In this product, bovine dermal collagen is lightly cross-linked by the addition of 0.0075 glutaraldehyde. Glutaraldehyde produces covalent bridges between 10 percent of available lysine residues of the bovine collagen molecules. These bridges are intramolecular, intermolecular, and occur between fibrils themselves. Thus, ZP is in reality an injectable latticework of bovine collagen.[6] In contrast to ZC, this product is more resistant to proteolytic degradation and less immunogenic.[6–8] More importantly, the greater substantive nature of ZP makes it applicable for deeper contour defects not amenable to ZI or ZII collagen.[9,10]

Patient Selection and Skin Testing

Patient selection and proper skin testing are critical issues in the application of bovine collagen. Individuals with a history of an anaphylactoid event, lidocaine sensitivity, or previous sensitivity to bovine collagen are excluded from testing or treatment. Potential hypersensitivity is determined by intradermal testing. A test syringe containing 0.1 cc of ZI collagen is used to screen for allergy to ZI and ZP collagens. With only 0.1 cc of the collagen in the test syringe, a tuberculin-like test is performed in the volar forearm. The site is evaluated at 48 to 72 h and again at 4 weeks. Three to 3.5 percent of individuals have a positive skin test, 70 percent of which are manifest within 72 h.[11–13] Those reactions which occur within 48 to 72 h indicate a preexisting allergy to bovine collagen.[7,14] Swelling, induration, tenderness, or erythema that persists for 6 h or longer after implantation is the hallmark of a positive test. Certain individuals recommend a second test.[15–18] This is administered in the periphery of the face or the contralateral forearm. It is administered either 2 or 4 weeks after the initial test, with treatment commencing 2 weeks after the second test. In that most treatment-associated hypersensitive reactions occur at the first treatment session, this reduces the frequency of this most undesirable sequela by changing the first treatment exposure into a second test. Furthermore, treatment-associated hypersensitive reactions occurring after two negative tests are usually milder, indicating that the severely allergic individuals have been selected out. If an individual has not been treated for 1 year, a single retest is recommended.

Technique of Injection

Injection technique is a critical factor in the proper application of bovine collagen implants. ZI is the most versatile and forgiving, and technique-sensitive implantation factors include (1) lesion selection, (2) overcorrection, (3) tissue-plane placement, (4) position, (5) lighting, and (6) magnification. In regard to lesion selection, soft smooth-walled acne scars as

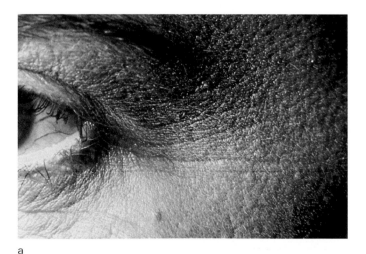

a

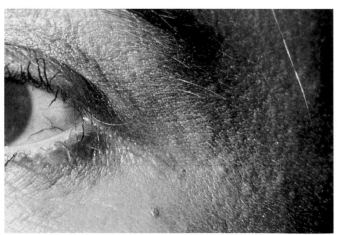

b

Figure 32-1 (*a*) Crows feet prior treatment with Zyderm I collagen. (*b*) Crows feet four weeks posttreatment with Zyderm I collagen.

well as mild age-related rhytides, such as glabellar frown lines, crow's feet, perioral lines, and the like, respond excellently to ZI (Figs. 32-1*a–b* and 32-2*a–b*). With ZI, one must deliberately overcorrect because only about 30 percent of the implanted volume remains after absorption of the saline vehicle. This overcorrection, however, should not be attempted over bony prominences (forehead) or in areas with an unusually thin dermis (crow's feet). At these sites, overcorrection may be unusually slow to resolve.

ZI is placed as superficially as possible with a 30-gauge needle. While the treatment site is held taut with the opposing hand, the needle tip is guided horizontally along the skin surface until it barely penetrates the skin. The needle, with the bevel down, is then gently elevated to tent up the skin, and the material is deposited in a tuberculin manner. Blanching and wheal formation are encouraged, and a flow is created in the skin by injecting at the advancing edge of each previously implanted volume. Magnification and good tangential lighting will improve one's ability to implant ZI. Finally, patients should remain seated during the procedure because certain soft-tissue defects disappear in the supine position.[19]

ZII leaves approximately 60 percent of the implanted material at the treatment sites. It requires greater force to inject and is useful for deeper acne scars, deep glabellar furrows, and other defects that are unresponsive to ZI. Techniques for injection with ZII are almost identical to those with ZI, save that one must respect its more concentrated form and realize that less overcorrection is required. It should not be utilized in areas such as crow's feet where overcorrection can be especially problematic.

ZP is a more robust form of bovine material. The absence of microfibrils in its composition and the presence of a rigid cross-linked product result in a material that resists superficial flow.[9] Furthermore, unlike ZI and ZII the material undergoes little condensation upon implantation. ZP works well for deep defects not amenable to correction with ZI or ZII. Deep nasolabial folds, deep distensible acne scars, deep drool grooves (marionette lines), and the like respond excellently to ZP (Fig. 32-3*a–b*); it should not be utilized in the glabellar region (see "Adverse Treatment Responses"). It works best when a flow is created with a 30-gauge needle in the mid-dermis, with minimal blanching and no beading. If the material is placed too superficially, unacceptable white ridging will occur. Proper placement of ZP is achieved by serially puncturing the skin to the level of the mid-dermis at a 20° to 90° angle depending on the practitioner's preference. Resistance of the dermal matrix should be felt upon injection because a lack of resistance would indicate the needle has penetrated the subdermal space. If this occurs, an unusually large volume of material will be used with a resultant minimal evanescent correction. As ZP flows into the dermis, the plane of the defect should rise only to the desired level of correction.

The value of molding or massage after ZP implantation has yet to be substantiated. Furthermore, it may force the material into the subdermal space where its ability to correct will be lost. Deliberate overcorrection with ZP is to be avoided. Excellent reviews on implantation techniques for bovine collagen include those by Klein,[9] Elson,[10] and Bailin and Bailin.[20]

Maintenance of Correction and Fate of Implant

Three treatment sessions are usually necessary to achieve maximum correction. While 70 percent of individuals require periodic touch-ups at 3- to 12-month intervals, a full 30 percent report correction for nearly 18 months before a touch-up is necessary. Acne scars and glabellar frowns appear to hold

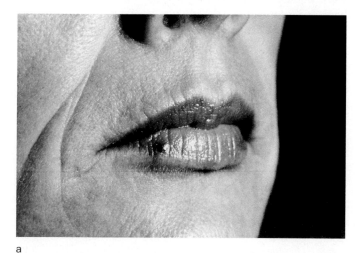

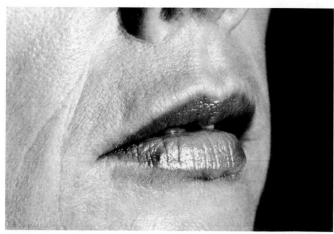

a

b

Figure 32-2   (*a*) Perioral lines, marionette lines, and nasolabial folds prior to treatment with Zyderm I collagen. (*b*) Perioral lines, marionette lines, and nasolabial folds, four weeks posttreatment with Zyderm I collagen.

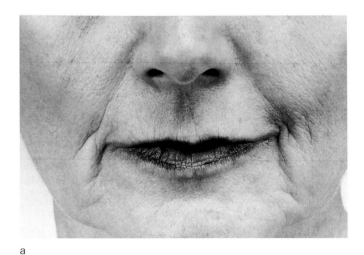
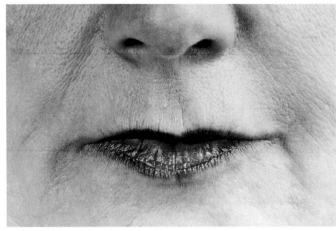

a   b

Figure 32-3   (*a*) Nasolabial folds and marionette grooves prior to treatment with Zyplast and Zyderm I collagen. (*b*) Nasolabial folds and marionette grooves, four weeks posttreatment with a combination of Zyplast and Zyderm I collagen.

correction the longest, while the mechanical stresses on other rhytides require touch-ups at 6- to 24-month intervals. Lesion location, active mechanical stresses, and personal response to implantation all play a part in longevity or correction.[12,21,22]

Multiple animal studies have evidenced gradual colonization of implanted bovine collagen by the recipient.[23,24] Furthermore, these studies reveal minimal inflammatory reactions and a high level of biocompatibility. In humans, histologic studies of ZP have also revealed deposition of host collagen.[25,26] Nevertheless, there is no convincing evidence in humans that this contributes to longevity of correction. Indeed, correction with all forms of bovine collagen appears to be lost as the material is displaced from its site of implantation in the dermis into the subcutaneous space.[27]

Adverse Treatment Responses

Adverse treatment responses to injectable bovine collagen can be divided into those that are either nonhypersensitive or hypersensitive in origin. Nonhypersensitive reactions include bruising from the mechanical trauma of injection. This can be decreased by the avoidance of aspirin and nonsteroidal antiinflammatory drugs in the recipient. Additionally, ice packs to the treatment sites 10 min prior to injection can lessen this effect. Also, slowing the speed of injection will lessen bruising.

Bacterial infection and reactivation of herpes simplex have been reported following ZC implantation. The latter can be addressed in susceptible individuals by suppressive doses of acyclovir prior to treatment.

Local necrosis with ZP, and rarely ZI and ZII, has been reported.[28] It is a *very* undesirable treatment sequela. It occurs at a rate of nine per 10,000 treated patients. Fifty-six percent of these events occur in the glabellar region, and physicians are cautioned against using ZP in that area. Histologically,

vascular interruption has been demonstrated as the etiology of these events. Physicians are cautioned that if severe blanching and pain occur on treatment they should immediately stop injecting. The value of massage, cool compresses, and/or nitroglycerin gel in this situation is unsubstantiated. With healing, severe scarring has been noted at these necrotic sites. Dermabrasion and/or ZI therapy have been advocated as treatments.

Two reports of partial vision loss after ZI injection have been noted. This is most probably the result of an occlusive event involving the retinal artery. This is a serious consequence of a cosmetic procedure, but it underscores the need to remember that the dermal site is the proper locale for implantation. Similar occlusive events have been described with the injection of many substances, including steroids into the head and neck region.[29]

Some individuals report intermittent swelling of treatment sites usually in response to precipitating agents such as alcohol, vitamin C, menses, and the like. At times, such intermittent reactions are associated with erythema and pruritus. Antibovine collagen antibodies have been demonstrated in some individuals who are "intermittent swellers." While these reactions usually last only a few hours, they can sometimes precede a full-blown hypersensitivity response. For this reason, further treatment of such individuals should proceed very cautiously.

Treatment-associated hypersensitivity reactions to ZC have been reported to occur in 1.3 to 6.2 percent of subjects following a single negative skin test.[11–13,30] The true incidence following one negative skin test is probably closer to 2 percent. Though they can occur at any time, the majority of treatment-associated hypersensitivity reactions occur after the first treatment session, lending further credence to the concept of double testing.[14] These reactions are almost always associated with circulating antibodies directed against bovine collagen, and, clinically, these reactions manifest as erythema, swelling, and edema at some or all of the treatment sites.[14,30] In most cases, at least 75 percent of the treatment sites react; nevertheless, less than 50 percent evidence a reaction at the test site. While 84 percent of such reactions subside in 11 months, some reactions have been reported to persist for more than 24 months. Humoral as well as cell-mediated immunity appears to be operative in these reactions, and the treatment and test site, if the latter is reactive, appear to be identical on histologic and immunologic analysis.[7,14,31]

The antibodies in individuals with these reactions are specific to bovine collagen, and no cross-reaction to human collagen has ever been demonstrated.[14,32,33] Furthermore, the response to bovine collagen determinants is heterogenous, with evidence of multiple antigenic targets being sites of recognition.[31,33] While anti-bovine antibodies have been demonstrated binding to the bovine collagen implants and infiltrating plasma cells, no binding of the surrounding host collagen has been seen.[34]

These reactions are frequently aggravated by factors such as sunlight and alcohol, and it must be remembered that these reactions are self-limited. Psychological support and watchful neglect are the best techniques in dealing with these time-limited events; nevertheless, if treatment is attempted, intralesional steroids (1 to 2.5 mg/cc) at 3 to 4 week intervals can cautiously be used.[18] The lack of available antigenic sites on the heavily cross-linked product or the deep dermal placement of ZP, where such reactions are less visible, accounts for the greater association of ZI and ZII with these hypersensitive reactions than ZP. Abcess formation is a rare severe hypersensitive response occuring at a rate of four per 10,000 treated individuals.[28] These reactions are usually associated with ZP and rarely ZI or ZII. Eighty-six percent of such individuals have associated anti-bovine collagen antibodies. Clinically, individuals develop painful indurated cysts at the sites of treatment. Incision and drainage as well as intralesional steroids (1 to 3 mg/cc) at 1- to 4-week intervals have been recommended. This is a long-lasting severe hypersensitive sequela which can last for more than 2 years. Analysis of extruded material from the abscesses has revealed bovine collagen implant.

Injectable Collagen Implant and Autoimmune Disease

The lay press as well as some physicians have speculated that injectable bovine collagen might induce autoimmune disease in the human host.[35] The possible precipitation of polymyositis/dermatomyositis (PM/DM) has been of particular concern. Xenogenic collagen has been used as hemostatic sponges, implantable sutures, and the like for decades with minimal adverse sequelae. There have been no reports of autoimmunity with their application.[14,34–39] Additionally, a panel of rheumatologists and immunologists found no supporting evidence

that bovine dermal collagen could induce autoimmune disease in the human host. One must remember that one to eight percent of the population evidence antibodies to bovine collagen prior to treatment or testing with ZC. This is possibly through dietary exposure, and these individuals are at no greater risk of developing autoimmune disease.[14,31] While some individuals have suggested that bovine collagen generates connective tissue disease by the production of cross-reacting antibodies to human collagen, no such antibodies have ever been demonstrated.[32] In regard specifically to PM/DM, as of August 30, 1990, 11 cases have been purported following injection with bovine collagen. Among the 500,000 individuals treated by that time, 12 to 23 cases would be expected by chance alone.[40] Additionally, a nationwide survey of 2341 rheumatologists and 322 PM/DM patients as well as a screening of the American Rheumatism Association Medical Information System (ARAMIS) data bank could reveal no case of PM/DM in the study period of 1985 to 1986 in which the individual received ZC prior to the onset of his or her symptons.[41] Thus, the existing scientific evidence would indicate that injectable bovine collagen is not an etiologic agent of autoimmune disease in humans.[42]

Injectable collagens (ZI, ZII, and ZP) are tools that provide the dermatologist with the means to treat contour irregularities. They provide a temporary, biocompatible solution in some but certainly not all cases. The adverse experiences, both allergic and nonallergic, are of an acceptable low level and only of local significance. The physician must develop an effective, reproducible technique of implantation to benefit from these assets.

FIBREL

The search for the ideal dermal filler has challenged investigators experimenting with wound healing and collagen synthesis. The ideal implant should be:

1. Physiologic
2. Safe
3. Permanent
4. Easily administered

The investigators searched for methods to stimulate collagen synthesis in scars and under rhytides. The use of substances such as oils and paraffins to create inflammation and, thus, lay down new collagen developed the basis for wound healing. Problems, though, developed such as prolonged inflammation and then scarring.[1,2] Silicone usage in microdroplet technique is designed to stimulate an encapsulating ring of collagen which later creates the scar correction. ZC implants were first thought to stimulate native collagen production, but later usage proved this theory wrong. Fibrel also stimulates production through reinjury and inflammation. Each of these techniques has attempted to re-create the body's own methods of repair for collagen synthesis and soft-tissue augmentation.

The safety of implants is an important yet controversial subject, with many of the implant materials under investigation for potential side effects and complications. Granulomatous reactions with scarring, allergy, infarction with tissue necrosis, and potential systemic disease have all been reported concerning implant material. Recently, emotional reports by the lay press have indicted implant material with little solid scientific data to back up the allegations.[42] None of the implant materials is permanent, and each has a particular longevity based on material used, location, and defect treated. A thorough understanding of each of these variables is necessary to master the use of these materials for skin contour correction.

The attempt to discover the ideal filling material has intrigued researchers as early as 1944 when Bailey and Ingraham published their results on the use of fibrin from pooled plasma to elevate cutaneous scars. The investigators theorized that the chemical agents in plasma initiated healing in collagen synthesis. It is this mechanism which attempted to produce excessive collagen under depressed scars and wrinkles and led to the development of Fibrel.

Spangler[43] first published his studies in 1957 on the use of fibrin to treat depressed scars. He treated more than 7000 cases with a product called *fibrin foam* with good results. Gottlieb[44] further refined the technique by formalizing the ingredients and technique. He named this the *GAP repair technique* because its recipe was a mixture of gelatin powder, aminocaproic acid, and plasma from the patient. This was injected under scars, and he reported contour improvement and lasting results in many depressed scars. The GAP technique was investigated further by Serono laboratories; the gelatin powder was lyophilized when mixed with aminocaproic acid and the fibrin moiety was added from the patient's serum. Clinical trials over 4 years resulted in FDA approval in 1985, and the product is now available for the treatment of depressed cutaneous scars and wrinkles.[45]

The Product and Its Mechanism

Fibrel utilizes the mechanisms of wound healing to re-create the necessary events for the production of collagen in a specific area. In review of wound healing, an injury to the skin damages tissue with the consequent release of platelets and thromboplastic and thrombolytic factors. Fibrinogen—through the release of thrombin—is changed to fibrin which then stimulates fibroblasts in and near capillaries to produce collagen.[46] During this same event, plasma profibrinolysin is produced in the resultant clot, producing fibrinolysin which inhibits or destroys the fibrin clot, thus curtailing further collagen production.

Fibrel provides the necessary ingredients to re-create this wound healing mechanism under scars and wrinkles. The absorbable gelatin powder provides a framework for the clot to form and remain stable under the scar. Plasma provides the necessary ingredients for collagen synthesis, and epsilon-aminocaproic acid (EACA) inhibits the production of fibrinolysin, allowing excessive collagen to be produced within the clot.[47] Thus, the treatment of skin depressions through Fibrel implantation will elevate the scar and produce a fibrin clot in which new collagen will be created that will give lasting elevation of the scar. The gelatin powder is a porcine derivative used widely as a hemostatic agent and is of low immunogenicity. It elevates the depression and provides a matrix to trap clotting factors for the deposition of new collagen (Fig. 32-4).

Fibrel is thus composed of a lyophilized mixture of 100 mg absorbable gelatin powder with 125 mg EACA. EACA has been shown to enhance collagen synthesis through a blockade of the fibrinolytic system.[47] Both the gelatin and EACA used in Fibrel are used routinely as hemostatic agents. Blood plasma provides a supplemental source of fibrinogen and other clotting factors that enhance the collagen matrix and add to the efficacy of Fibrel. Unlike collagen or silicone which remains as a foreign implant beneath the skin surface, Fibrel is absorbed as the new collagen is gradually incorporated into the skin. The gelatin substance in Fibrel provides a framework in which new tissue may grow. Histologic and preclinical data suggest that within 90 days the implant is colonized by the patient's own normal connective tissue as cells and blood vessels grow into the Fibrel implant.[48] Theoretically, Fibrel should be a physiologic implant with little chance of allergenicity or foreign body reaction. The gelatin powder elevates the depression and provides a matrix to enhance blood clotting by entrapping the necessary clotting factors and serves as a template for subsequent deposition of new extracellular matrix essential for wound healing. The antifibrinolytic action of EACA has a fibrin-stabilizing effect. In animals, it has been shown to enhance new collagen synthesis through blockage of the fibrinolytic system.[47]

The product Fibrel is a sterile kit that does not require refrigeration; it has a long shelf life and contains everything needed for treatment. The mixture of lyophilized gelatin powder and EACA is contained with a syringe in the kit, and it is reconstituted with 0.5 mL of the patient's serum and 0.5 mL of 0.9% normal saline. The syringe with the gelatin mixture is connected with an adapter to the saline serum syringe and the two are slowly mixed by making ten to 12 horizontal passes of the solution from one syringe to another. The suspension of Fibrel is then ready for injection.[49]

Indications and Technique

Fibrel is indicated as a dermal implant for the correction of depressed cutaneous scars and wrinkles. A thorough consultation and examination of the patient's defects should be performed prior to examination and those scars or wrinkles which will respond to filler substance are outlined. A skin test made by diluting 0.5 mL of the Fibrel suspension, 1:1000, with saline. It is placed in the patient's volar forearm. The test site is observed after 1 month to ensure that the patient is not allergic to the implant. A positive reaction would be induration and erythema that persists longer than 24 to 48 h.[45]

SOFT TISSUE AUGMENTATION

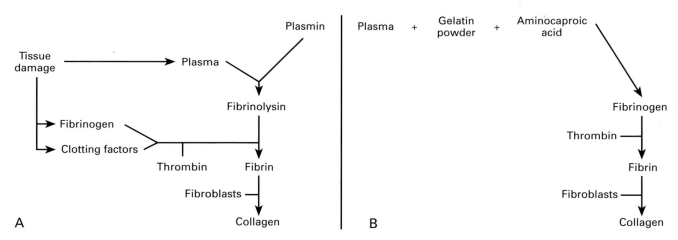

Figure 32-4   (*a*) Mechanism of normal wound healing after injury. (*b*) Effects of Fibrel in recreating the wound-healing mechanism.

Fibrel is used for depressed cutaneous scars which can be elevated by stretching the skin at the edges of the scar. The more fibrotic scars or ice-pick scars do not elevate well and require special treatment for elevation. Deeper creases, furrows, and grooves may also be treated with Fibrel as a dermal implant for elevation. Fine creases on the eyelids and lips and photoaging rhytides on facial skin do not respond as well to Fibrel injections because of the viscosity of the implant and the associated inflammation. During the consultation, lesions that will respond to the implant are identified, and a thorough explanation of the treatment technique, potential side effects, and morbidity, as well as complications, is given to the patient. Particular emphasis must be placed on the differences between this filling agent and ZC. Because Fibrel is a mechanism to create collagen through wound healing, an inflammatory reaction is a necessary component of the treatment. The patient should develop postoperative erythema, induration, and swelling which may last as long as 5 days. The patient must schedule the necessary postoperative recovery time.

Final collagen synthesis may take 6 weeks to 2 months. Patients must be informed of these differences so that they will understand the nature of healing and implant formation. Patients who should be excluded from Fibrel treatment are those with:

1. A history of keloid formation
2. Known sensitivity to gelatin and/or aminocaproic acid
3. Bleeding disorders
4. History of cardiac, renal, or hepatic disease
5. History of autoimmune disease
6. Pregnancy and/or lactation

After 1 month, the patient presents the skin test and, if negative, is available for treatment. The scar or wrinkle again is outlined and phlebotomy is performed to remove approximately 10 cc of the patient's blood. This is centrifuged for 10 to 15 min and clear serum is drawn into the mixing syringe. This is connected to the syringe with Gelfoam powder and the patient's plasma, and, with horizontal exchanges, the two are mixed together. The mixing exchanges should be performed slowly to avoid bubbling and frothing of the mixture. The process is concluded with Fibrel in the delivery syringe; air bubbles are expressed. The patient then is ready for injection.

The patient's scars are categorized into those which are distensible and those which are fibrotic and more bound down. The distensible scars can be injected with a 30-gauge needle by using the multiple puncture or fanning technique. These scars do not require preinjections of local anesthesia, and the injection is placed directly into the mid-to-upper dermis. The technique includes spreading the skin, entry of the needle at a 35° angle, an implant injection producing a peau d'orange and blanch. One hundred fifty percent correction is necessary due to equalization of serum and fluids during clot resorption. Care must be taken to avoid implant extrusion through pores or around the needle orifice or injection into the subcutaneous tissue. The direct puncture technique places the needle at the edge of the scar, advancing into the scar, and injection is made into the middle of the scar. The fanning technique, which is an adaptation of the single puncture, advances the needle in a circumferential pattern throughout the scar, introducing filler substance within the mid- and upper dermis of the entire scar. Common to all of these techniques is the placement of Fibrel within the mid-to-upper dermis and within the scar.

The approach to fibrotic scars utilizes a customized undermining needle available in the Fibrel kit. This device allows the cosmetic surgeon to create a dermal pocket for the injection of the filler substance. This will loosen the scar bonds, holding the scar downward, allowing the upper dermis and epidermis to elevate upward with the injection of the implant. One percent lidocaine is placed as a field block around the scar before the undermining is performed. The customized 18-gauge needle is advanced at a 35° angle within the dermis in multiple passes to sever collagen scar bonds and create a filling pocket. After undermining releases the upper portion of the scar and the pocket is complete, filling material is injected to elevate the scar. The implant is molded at the treatment site and ice packs are placed on the area after injection. Care must be taken to prevent extrusion of the implant from the needle site by direct pressure and by molding after the injection.

Wrinkle lines and furrows are treated in a similar fashion with the implant placed in the mid-to-upper dermis. Treatable wrinkles include glabellar furrows, forehead wrinkle lines, nasolabial and meilolabial wrinkles, and those at the lip commissure and cheek. The smaller fine lines on the lips themselves and crow's feet can produce overcorrected nodules with prolonged inflammation and thus have an increased morbidity with treatment. Most wrinkles are treated in a similar manner as distensible scars with a 30-gauge needle and intradermal filling. With the linear injection technique, the needle is placed in the base of the furrow and advanced intradermally along and under the groove. The implant is then injected under the groove with the resultant elevation producing a peau d'orange and blanching. The needle then is placed farther up the groove and injection continues until the full length of the crease is elevated upward. Immediate molding and compression are performed and an ice pack is placed over the treatment site. Postoperative erythema, inflammation, and induration occur following almost all Fibrel injections. These are necessary for scar correction, and the degree of inflammation is variable in all patients. Iced dressings placed over injection sites reduce, to some degree, the amount of inflammation, but anti-inflammatories should not be given as these would reduce collagen formation and the degree of scar correction. Inflammation and induration usually last 48 to 72 h, though occasionally the nodulation may be prolonged for 4 or 5 days.

Clinical studies on scar and wrinkle correction were performed over a 2-year period and also over a 5-year span. A multicenter study published in 1987 involved a total of 321 treated patients who were evaluated for degree of scar correction and longevity of correction. The patients were followed over 2 years using parameters of physician evaluation, patient evaluation, and photogrammetric analysis. The latter measurement uses a scar mold which is analyzed by computer to monitor volume correction of the scar. The results showed that 60 to 75 percent of the scars were correctable with Fibrel implant. Of those scars correctable after 2 months, 80 percent maintained correction at the end of 2 years. This was analyzed by all three parameters.[45] A further 5-year subjective analysis performed by Millikan[50] showed that 50 percent of this group maintained correction at the time. There is thus good objective evidence that Fibrel does have lasting scar correction over a greater period of time than ZC implants. These objective studies were not carried out for wrinkles, and objective results on these are not yet available.

Side Effects and Complications

Most side effects found with Fibrel have been localized and restricted to the trauma induced by local injection. These include pain upon injection, induration, erythema, inflammation, and purpura. The inflammatory response is a necessary part of the mechanism for collagen synthesis and should not be considered a side effect. Bruising and purpura can prolong the inflammatory response with nodules that may persist a week or two. Also reported are acne exacerbations at the site of injection and activation of herpes simplex virus infection.[51]

As Fibrel usage has become more common, rare unusual complications have been reported. A prolonged inflammatory response that has lasted as long as a month to 6 weeks has been noted in some patients.[52] This is not believed to be an allergic response but rather an idiosyncratic exaggeration of the inflammation and induration that normally resolve in 3 to 5 days. If the reaction in these patients is prolonged, symptomatic measures to reduce inflammation may be necessary. These patients have a negative skin test with no evidence of allergenicity; they have a similar response to the injection of serum alone in their skin. There appear to be no antecedent factors that indicate who will have this prolonged inflammatory reaction.[52] The inflammatory response, though, seems more reactive and prolonged upon injection of lips, glabella, and periorbital skin. It will resolve spontaneously, and the use of ice compresses and pressure seems to hasten its response. The patients need support and counseling during this postoperative period. Embolization with cutaneous necrosis has also been reported with Fibrel which is injected into the subcutaneous tissue. As with ZP collagen, the heavier suspension can cause infarction of larger subdermal vessels with resultant local tissue necrosis. A reported complication occurred as an injection of Fibrel to fill a rhinoplasty defect caused blanching over the nose with resultant infarction and loss of skin. Investigaton of the case revealed that the physician injected the material into subcutaneous tissue and fascia rather than skin.[53] Fibrel thus is a dermal filler substance and its use should be restricted to correction of skin defects. Special care also must be taken when the glabella or nose is treated.

There has been little evidence of true allergenicity to Fibrel, though potential allergy to porcine products in the gelatin should be considered. Thus far there have been few reported allergic problems in patients receiving Fibrel. Patients allergic to ZC have been successfully treated with Fibrel without allergic reaction; therefore, there seems to be no cross-reactivity between autoantibodies to collagen and allergic reactions to Fibrel. There has been no linkage of Fibrel to any systemic disease, autoimmune disease, or precipitation of systemic adverse reactions.

Fibrel is a device to create autologous collagen for the elevation of scars and wrinkles. It is physiologic and now appears to be safe. It is a bit more complicated in usage than ZC in that it requires the use of the patient's serum and, in some instances, a local anesthetic. There is an increased morbidity because postoperative inflammation is necessary for the creation of collagen. These differences must be understood by the patients for full appreciation of the implant used and successful compliance during healing. Fibrel has distinctive advantages, including prolonged longevity, little allergenicity, and associated techniques for superior scar elevation.

LIQUID SILICONE

In the early 1900s, a British chemist coined the term *silicone* to describe a large family of man-made polymers containing silica (SiO_2).[54] These compounds, whose viscosity is a functon of polymerization and cross-linkage, can exist as solids, gels, and liquids. Technologically advanced societies use all forms of silicones by the ton. They are ingested as antiflatulents (simethicone) and rubbed into the skin as cosmetics. Present in paint thinners, lubricants, and scar dressings, they are also injected into the human eye to stabilize the retina, wedged into hearts to serve as valve replacements, implanted as joints in fingers and hips, and used in contact lenses.

Silicone, in general, has been very beneficial to the progress of the human race. However, the use of liquid silicone to elevate scars and wrinkles has never achieved the status of an officially sanctioned therapeutic modality, and, for a variety of complicated scientific and political reasons, that status may never be achieved.

Physical Characteristics

The chemical name for liquid silicone is dimethylpolysiloxane fluid. This large molecule consists of repetitive units of ($-(CH_3)_2SiO-_x$). MDX4-4011, the silicone fluid used for FDA-approved investigations, is a refined derivative of Dow-Corning medical-grade 360 liquid silicone, the agent used ubiquitously as the needle, syringe, and intravenous (IV) tubing lubricant. This fluid is clear, colorless, odorless, unaffected by storage, will not support bacterial growth, and will remain in liquid form indefinitely. Its viscosity is 350 cSt, exactly the same as mineral oil.[55,56]

Animal Studies

Carcinogenesis

No convincing prospective data link silicone with carcinogenesis in human beings. Studies relating tumors in rats to silicone are very old and are proved to be related to a biopeculiarity of rodents (i.e., in these animals, cancerous changes can be induced by implanting *any* "smooth substances, including glass or metal balls"[57,58]).

Effect of Volume

Medical-grade silicone appears to be a nearly inert compound in small quantities.[59] When large volumes are employed, silicone physically can compromise vital structures.[60-63] Large

subcutaneous injections result in phagocytosis of silicone which is transferred through the reticuloendothelial system. Massive (20 g/kg) volumes of silicone can be ingested without systemic or local complications. Death occurs when large volumes of silicone are administered IV or interarterially.[60,64]

Immunogenicity

Although no antibodies to pure silicone liquid have ever been discovered, Kossovsky and Heggers have demonstrated immunologically mediated inflammatory reactions in ten guinea pigs sensitized with silicone and Freund's complete adjuvant.[65] They note in another study that the "data suggests that silicone protein complexes are potentially immunogenic."[65] Heggers' earlier work[66] demonstrated migration inhibition of peritoneal exudate cells from sensitized animals, and the author notes that the response is comparable to that elicited in purified protein derivative and may indicate that silicone acts as a hapten-like incomplete antigen. Further confirmation of this concept appears in several other articles.[67-69]

History of Liquid Silicone

Following its introduction in the 1940s for soft-tissue augmentation, liquid silicone, cheap, easy to use, and readily available, was criminally misused, particularly when employed in large volumes for breast augmentation. Horrific complications resulting from large volumes of liquid silicone deliberately adulterated (in a misguided attempt to hold such large volumes in place) led to legislation criminalizing its use in the state of Nevada. By 1964, the FDA declared silicone to be "a new drug." Its major American manufacturer, Dow-Corning, limited its access to a few officially sanctioned, experienced investigators.[54,56,59]

Clinical Experience

Despite its eclipse as a manufacturer-sponsored investigative drug, injectable silicone was used privately with great success in thousands of patients over a period of almost 40 years. Orentreich, Selmanowitz, Webster, Aronsohn, and Balkin reported excellent results in the treatment of well over 100,000 patients for scars, wrinkles, postrhinoplasty defects, podiatric problems (diabetic neurotrophic ulcers), plantar callosities, and decubitus ulcers.[59,60,70-78] (Figs. 32-5, 32-6, 32-7, 32-8)

Literature Review

Results of Officially Sanctioned Studies

Only two serious tissue reactions could be documented in a 20-year, FDA-approved study of MDX4-4011: migration of silicone following the use of large volumes in the leg of a polio patient and massive facial necrosis after 25 cc was implanted in the face of a woman with Weber-Christian disease, rheumatoid arthritis, and an atypical mycobacterial infection.[79,80]

Effect of Volume

In humans, small amounts of silicone injected into the subcutaneous space produce a small polymorphonuclear infiltrate followed by scant lymphocytic response.[81] A delicate, primarily fibrohistiocytic capsule forms, surrounding individual microdroplets of silicone.[81,82] When large volumes of silicone are implanted, this capsule becomes thicker (Fig. 32-9). Silicone is phagocytized by tissue histiocytes which carry it to other organs.[63,64,82,83] This process is not generally associated with adverse consequences and can be compared to the transport of tattoo pigments into the reticuloendothelial system.[54] Granulomas or "siliconomas" associated with foreign body giant cells and marked granulomatous response are extremely rare.[84] Most importantly, *none* of the major problems associated with implant mammary augmentation or high-volume injectable silicone mammary augmentation have been reported when silicone was used in small volumes.[59]

Reported Complications

Pneumonitis and acute respiratory distress syndrome have been reported, and sudden death following intravasclar injections of silicone has occurred.[85,86] Injection of large volumes of intentionally adulterated or contaminated silicone into the breasts has led to necrosis and ulcerations, sometimes secondary to pressure-induced vascular lymphatic compromise and/or the migration of fluids to distant sites.[54,55,87] Erysipelas-like reactions have been reported, and blindness and loss of neurologic function or death have occurred when liquid silicone was injected in ophthalmic and meningeal vessels.[86] Shedding or spallation of particulate silicone from damaged hemodialysis pump tubing has resulted in severe hepatitis and pancytopenia in patients undergoing hemodialysis.[88–90]

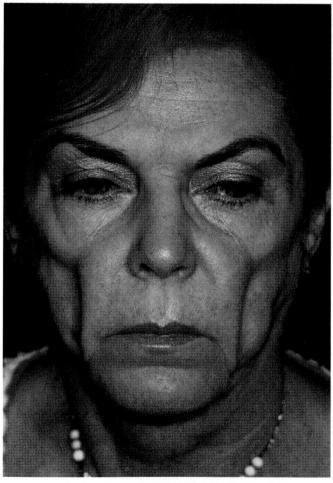

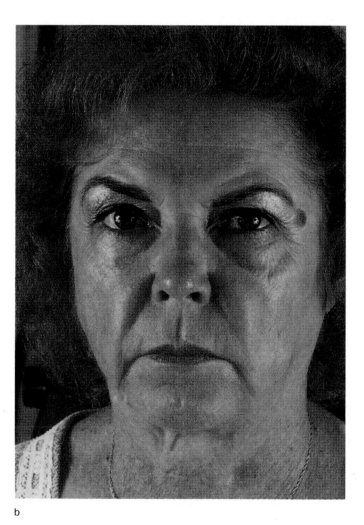

a   b

Figure 32-5   (*a*) Pretreatment. Patient suffered febrile illness associated with massive lipodystrophy on face and shoulders; (*b*) 8 years posttreatment with very satisfactory results.

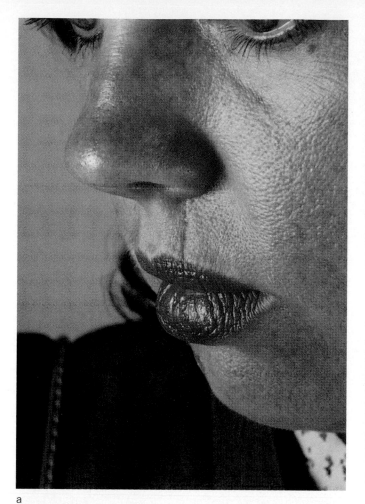

a

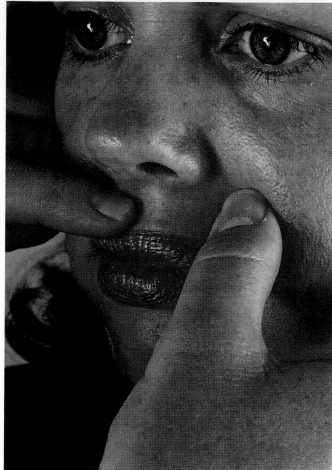

b

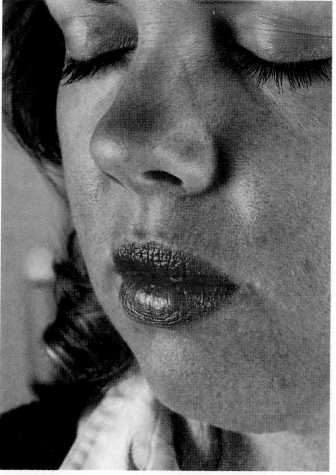

c

Figure 32-6   (*a*) Pretreatment scar resulting from laceration some 20 years earlier; (*b*) stretch test indicates that this pliable scar will respond well to silicone injections; (*c*) 10 years posttreatment (after two treatments).

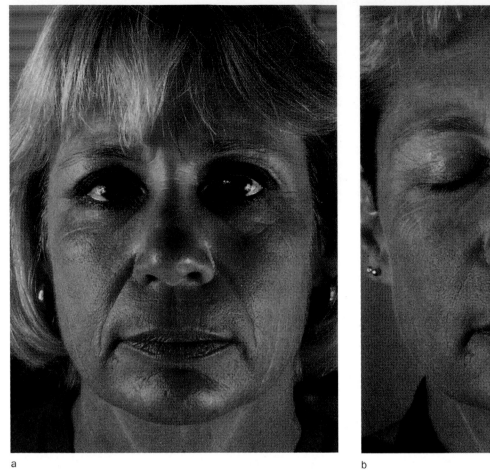
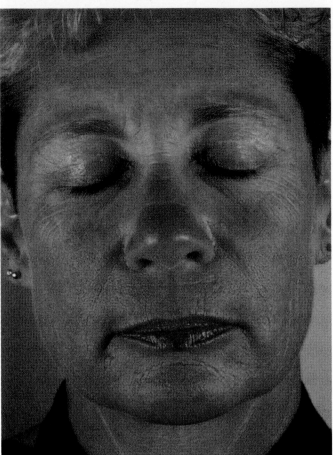

a   b

Figure 32-7 (*a*) Pretreatment nasolabial creases; (*b*) 7 years posttreatment.

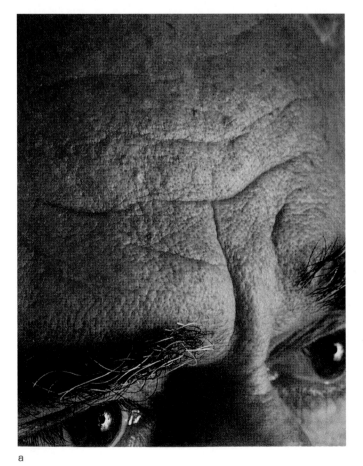
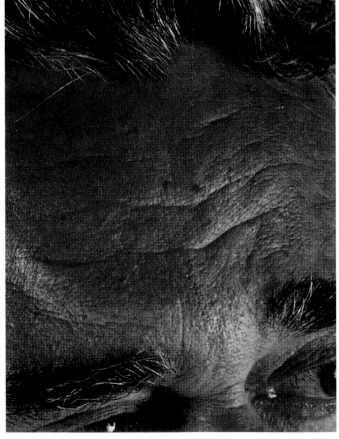

a   b

Figure 32-8 (*a*) Pretreatment glabellar creases; (*b*) 10 years posttreatment with silicone injections shows good results for glabellar creases.

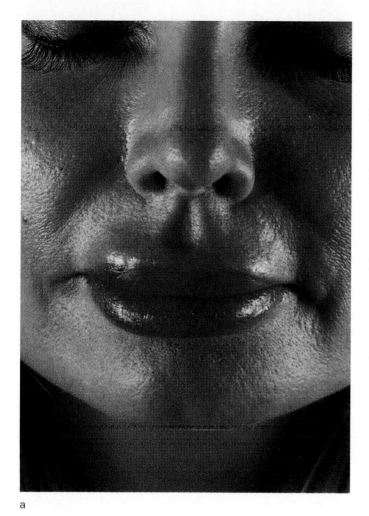
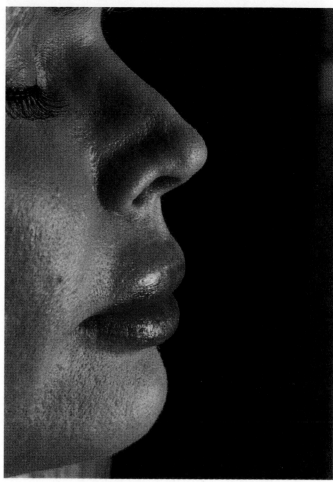

a

b

Figure 32-9   (*a*) Posttreatment results of the injudicious injection of extremely large volumes of silicone; (*b*) although asymptomatic, large volumes of silicone are disfiguring.

Breast Augmentation   Silicone fluids and gels used for implantation mammoplasty are combined with fillers and catalysts. Silicone breast implant shells contain both pure silicone liquid and 30 percent silicone dioxide filler. Particles of this filler are implicated in the development of adjuvant disease, a syndrome which includes fever, arthritis, and renal failure.[91,92] Scleroderma or eosinophilic fasciitis has occurred following breast augmentaton but has never occurred following the injection of small amounts of pure liquid silicone.[93,94]

Granulomas   This complication, which clinically takes the form of persistent or intermittent nodular swelling often associated with erythema, induration, or purple discoloration of the skin (Fig. 32-10), can be exacerbated by exercise, alcohol, allergies, and infections. Histologically, these granulomas resemble the diffuse granulomas occasionally seen following bovine collagen implantation, and, although foreign body giant cells and a marked granulomatous response have been reported, they are rare following pure liquid silicone, common

following liquid silicone to which adulterants are added, and much more commonly seen when solid silicone implants are employed (small-particle synovitis).[59,82,84,95–99] The incidence of granulomas from the use of pure liquid silicone is stated to be 1:10,000 patients.[55] Webster et al. reported no granulomas in 17,000 injections. Wilkie[101] reported granulomas in 13 of 92 patients injected with silicone of unspecified purity. One explanation for the association of granulomas with infectious processes becomes evident in the observation that capsule formation around silicone implants was accelerated by the presence of infection.[102]

Minor Complications Following Cutaneous Implantation of Small Volumes of Pure Liquid Silicone

Technique- and Non-technique-dependent Overcorrection (Nodularity Beading)   Overcorrection, clinically evidenced by the presence of firm nodules of silicone, appears in several settings. When silicone is deposited in the papillary dermis

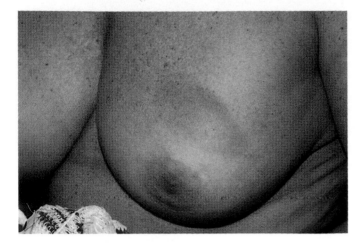

Figure 32-10 Granuloma resulting from injection of silicone of unknown purity some 20 years earlier.

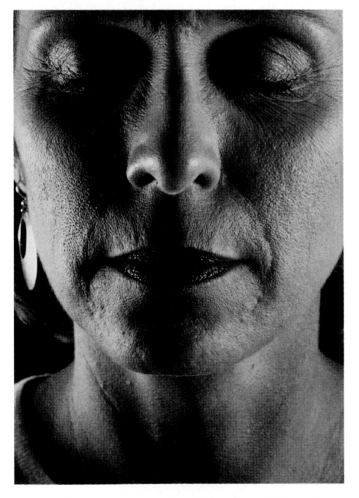

Figure 32-11 Posttreatment demonstrates effect of silicone injected too closely to surface, resulting in ridging, although this same process can occur even with good technique. Some individuals simply overreact to silicone in terms of collagen deposition.

rather than the reticular dermis at the level of subcutaneous fat, excessive fibrohistiocytic proliferation occurs, leading to the slow development of dermal nodules.[60] Inappropriate volumes of silicone implanted at any level can produce visible or palpable nodules. Scar tissue is prone to the development of keloidal nodularities which can occur years after treatment; these often respond to intralesional triamcinolone acetonide.[103]

A second type of overcorrection occurs, particularly in certain regions of the face such as the forehead, in which the injected silicone is displaced to the lateral aspects of the wrinkle, resulting in a beaded appearance (Fig. 32-11). Pitted, bound-down scars exhibit the same response as injected silicone is deflected to the scar perimeter, resulting in a doughnut-like, elevated collarette. Pliable scars can initially respond very well and over a period of time undergo excessive fibroplasia, increasing in volume-resulting elevations (Fig. 32-12). This process is not related to bad technique.

Erythema, ecchymosis, hyperpigmentation, and telangiectasia are also reported. Patients occasionally complain of textural changes in the skin or increased firmness of tissue where silicone was injected. Serious complications probably occur in 0.2 of 1 percent of all treated patients.[103–105]

CURRENT STATUS

Dr. David Kessler, the appointed commissioner of the FDA, may have sounded the death knell for liquid silicone when he told the media that the sale, shipment, distribution, manufacture, use and promotion of silicone are illegal.[105] In a letter to the president of the American Society for Dermatologic Surgery, Dr. Kessler notes that "this product is illegal except for one experimental opthalmologic protocol."[106]

COMMENTARY: THIS PRODUCT IS ILLEGAL

Although liquid silicone could benefit millions of people, there are at least three reasons why it may never receive official sanction:

1. Silicone has been grossly misused, has the potential for further misuse, and the public distrusts it. No manufacturer would be wlling to accept product liability for its misuse, a fact of life which forced the Dow-Corning Corporation to withdraw its advocacy for silicone some years ago.[56]
2. All of the good news concerning silicone is unofficial; all of the bad news is well documented. Bad news sells newspapers.
3. All forms of silicone are under attack, and, although about 98 percent of the population with specific problems would benefit from liquid silicone, fear of complications occurring in the other 2 percent has led to a negative attitude at the FDA.[107]

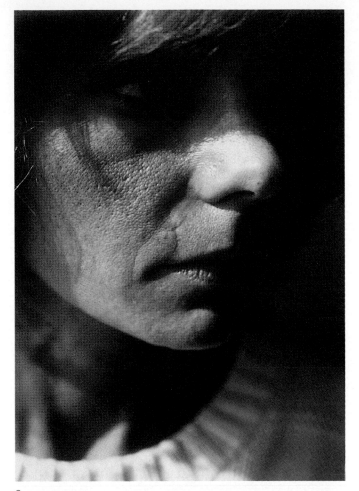

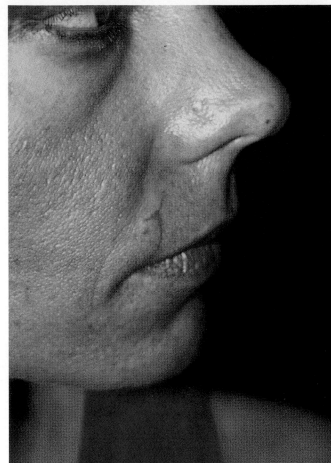

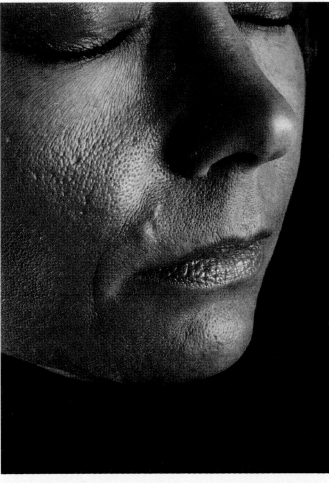

Figure 32-12 (*a*) Pretreatment notch-shaped scar following cancer surgery which occurred some 5 years earlier; (*b*) same scar 5 years later with some increase in scar bulk evident; (*c*) continuation of scarring process. This increase in scar bulk was successfully treated using Kenalog. Patient lost to follow-up.

REFERENCES

1. Urback et al: Generalized paraffinoma (sclerosing lipo granuloma). *Arch Dermatol* **103**:277–285, 1971

2. Klein JA et al: Paraffinomas of the scalp. *Arch Dermatol* **121**:382–385, 1985

3. Klein AW, Rish DC: Substances for the soft tissue augmentation: Collagen and silicone. *J Dermatol Surg Oncol* **11**:337, 1985

4. Knapp TR et al: Injectable collagen for soft tissue augmentation. *Plast Reconstr Surg* **60**:389, 1977

5. Wallace DG et al: Injectable collagen for tissue augmentation, in *Collagen, vol 3, Biotechnology,* edited by ME Nimni. Boca Raton, Fla, CRC Press, 1988, pp 117–144

6. McPherson JM et al: The preparation and physiochemical characterization of an injectable form of reconstituted, glutaraldehyde cross-linked, bovine corium collagen. *J Biomed Mater Res* **20**:79, 1986

7. DeLustro F et al: Reaction to injectable collagen in human subjects. *J Dermatol Surg Oncol* **14**(suppl 1):**49,** 1988

8. Elson JL: Clinical assessment of Zyplast implant: A year of experience for soft tissue contour correction. *J Am Acad Dermatol* **116**:707, 1988

9. Klein AW: Indications and implantation techniques for the various formulations of injectable collagen. *J Dermatol Surg Oncol* **14**(suppl 1):**49,** 1988

10. Elson ML: Corrections of dermal contour defects with the injectable collagens: Choosing and using these materials. *Semin Dermatol* **6**:77, 1987

11. Castrow FF II, Krull EA: Injectable collagen implant—update. *J Am Acad Dermatol* **9**:889, 1983

12. Cooperman LS et al: Injectable collagen: A six-year clinical investigation. *Aesthetic Plast Surg* **9**:145, 1985

13. Kamer FM, Churukian MM: The clinical use of injectable collagen: A three-year retrospective study. *Arch Otolaryngol* **110**:93, 1984

14. DeLustro F et al: Reaction to injectable collagen: Results in animal models and clinical use. *Plast Reconstr Surg* **79**:581, 1987

15. Klein AW, Rish DC: Injectable collagen: An adjunct to facial plastic surgery. *Facial Plastic Surgery* **4**:87, 1987

16. Klein AW: In favor of double testing. *J Dermatol Surg Oncol* **15**:263, 1989

17. Elson ML: The role of skin testing in the use of collagen injectable materials. *J Dermatol Surg Oncol* **15**:301, 1989

18. Klein AW, Rish DC: Injectable collagen update. *J Dermatol Surg Oncol* **10**:519, 1984

19. Klein AW: Implantation techniques for injectable collagen: Two-and-one half years of personal clinical experience. *J Am Acad Dermatol* **9**:224, 1983

20. Bailin PL, Bailin MD: Collagen implantation: Clinical applications and lesion selection. *J Dermatol Surg Oncol* **14**(suppl 1):**49,** 1988

21. Robinson JK, Hanke CW: Injectable collagen implant: Histopathologic identification and longevity of correction. *J Dermatol Surg Oncol* **11**:124, 1985

22. Bailin MD, Bailin PM: Case studies: Correction of surgical scars, acne scars, and rhytides with Zyderm and Zyplast Implants. *J Dermatol Surg Oncol* **14**(suppl 1):31, 1988

23. Armstrong R et al: Injectable collagen for soft tissue augmentation, in *Contemporary Clinical Applications, New Technology and Legal Aspects,* edited by JW Boretos, M Eden. Parkridge, NJ, Noyes Publications, 1984, pp 528–536

24. McPherson JM et al: An examination of the biologic response to injectable, glutaraldehyde cross-linked collagen implants. *J Biomed Mater Res* **20**:93, 1986

25. Kligman AM, Armstrong RC: Histologic response to intradermal Zyderm and Zyplast (glutaraldehyde cross-linked) collagen in humans. *J Dermatol Surg Oncol* **12**:351, 1986

26. Kligman AM: Histologic responses to collagen implants in human volunteers: Comparison of Zyderm collagen with Zyplast implant. *J Dermatol Surg Oncol* **14**(suppl 1):35, 1988

27. Stegman SJ et al: A light and electron microscopic evaluation of Zyderm collagen and Zyplast implants in aging human facial skin: A pilot study. *Arch Dermatol* **123**:1644, 1987

28. Hanke CW et al: Abscess formation and local necrosis after treatment with Zyderm or Zyplast collagen implant. *J Am Acad Dermatol* **25**:319–326, 1991

29. McGraw R et al: Sudden blindness secondary to injection of common drugs in the head and neck, pt 1: Clinical experiences. *Otolaryngology* **86**:147, 1978

30. Siegle RJ et al: Intradermal implantation of bovine collagen: Humoral responses associated with clinical reaction. *Arch Dermatol* **120**:183, 1984

31. McCoy JP et al: Characterization of the humoral immune response to bovine collagen implants. *Arch Dermatol* **121**:990, 1985

32. Cooperman LS, Michaeli D: The immunogenicity of injectable collagen, pt 2: A retrospective review of seventy-two tested and treated patients. *J Dermatol Surg Oncol* **10**:647, 1984

33. Ellingsworth LR et al: The human immune response to reconstituted bovine collagen. *J Immunol* **136**:877, 1986

34. DeLustro F et al: Immune response to allogeneic and xenogeneic implants of collagen and collagen derivatives. *Clin Orthop* 1990 Vol. 260, pp 263–279

35. Cohen IK et al: Zyderm (letter). *Plast Reconstr Surg* **73**:857, 1984

36. Chvapil M et al: Medical and surgical applications of collagen. *Int Rev Connect Tissue* **6**:1, 1973

37. Pachence JM et al: Collagen: Its place in the medical device industry. *Medical Devices and Diagnostic Letters Journal* **9**:49, 1987

38. DeLustro F et al: A comparative study of the biologic and immunologic response to medical devices derived from dermal collagen. *J Biomed Mater Res* **20**:109, 1986

39. Simpson RL: Collagen as a biomaterial, in *Biomaterials in Reconstructive Surgery,* edited by LR Rubin. St. Louis, Mosby, 1983, pp 109–117

40. *Hotline,* American College of Rheumatology, edited by R. Panush and R Thoburn, 8/26/91. Atlanta, Ga.

41. Lyon MG et al: Predisposing factors in polymyositis-dermatomyositis: Results of a nationwide survey. *J Rheumatol* **16:**1218, 1989

42. Klein AW: Bonfire of the wrinkles. *J Dermatol Surg Oncol* **17:**543–544, 1991

43. Spangler AS: Treatment of depressed scars with fibrin foam: Seventeen years of experience. *J Dermatol Surg Oncol* **1:**65–69, 1975

44. Gottlieb S: *Gap Repair Technique* (poster exhibit). Annual meeting of the American Academy of Dermatology, Dallas, Tex, Dec. 5, 1977

45. Milliken L et al: Treatment of depressed cutaneous scars with gelatin matrix implant: A multicenter study. *J Am Acad Dermatol* **16:**1155–1162, 1987

46. Clark RAF: Cutaneous tissue repair: Basic biologic considerations, pt 1. *J Am Acad Dermatol* **13:**701–725, 1985

47. Nilsson IM et al: Antifibrinolytic activity and metabolism of E-aminocaproic acid in man. *Lancet* **1:**1233–1236, 1960

48. Postlethwaite AE et al: Chemotactic reaction of human fibroblasts to type I, II, and III collagens and collagen-derived peptides. *Proc Natl Acad Sci USA* **75:**871–875, 1978

49. *Instruction Guide.* Fibrel Technique Workshop, MEDED program for Serono Corp, Boston, Mass, July 28, 1988

50. Millikan L: Long term safety and efficacy with Fibrel in the treatment of cutaneous scars. *J Dermatol Surg Oncol* **15**(8):837–844, 1989

51. Rosen T: Fibrel, a new implant material. *J Dermatol Surg Oncol* **16:**155–162, 1987

52. Personal communications with physicians reporting complications to the Mentor Corporation, Goleta, CA, 1990

53. Personal communications with physicians reporting complications to the Mentor Corporation, Goleta, CA, 1991

54. Orentreich NO: Soft-tissue augmentation with medical-grade fluid silicone, in *Biomaterials in Reconstructive Surgery,* edited by: Leonard R. Rubin, MD, St. Louis, Mosby, 1983, pp 859–881

55. Orentreich DS, Orentreich NO: *Injectable Fluid Silicone: Principles of Dermatologic Surgery.* New York, Marcel Dekker, 1988

56. *The Dermabrasion, Chemical Peel, Silicone and Collagen Symposium.* American Society for Dermatologic Surgery, Tulane University Medical School, New Orleans, July 4–8, 1984

57. Jose Otero: *Silicone Issues and Controversies.* Presented at Valley Medical Center Hospital Bulletin, vol. 16, no. 7, Fullerton, CA, July 15, 1991, pp 5–6

58. Ruffenach G: Study links silicone gel to cancer. *Wall Street Journal,* Nov 10, 1988, pp B–1

59. Clark DP et al: Dermal implants: Safety of products injected for soft tissue augmentation. *J Am Acad Dermatol* **21:**992–998, 1989

60. Selmanowitz VJ, Orentreich NO: Medical-grade fluid silicone: A monographic review. *J Dermatol Surg Oncol* **3:**597–611, 1977

61. Ben-Hur N et al: Local and systemic effects of dimethylpolysiloxane fluid in mice. *Plast Reconstr Surg* **39:**423–426, 1967

62. Nosanchuk JS: Injected dimethyl polysiloxane fluid: A study of antibody and histologic response. *Plast Reconstr Surg* **42:**562–566, 1968

63. Rees TD et al: Silicone fluid research; A follow-up summary. *Plast Reconstr Surg.* **46:**50–56, 1970

64. Ashley FL et al: The present status of silicone fluid in soft tissue augmentation. *Plast Reconstr Surg* **39:**411–419, 1967

65. Kossovsky N et al: Experimental demonstration of the immunogenicity of silicone protein complexes. *J Biomed Mater Res* **21:**1125–1133, 1987

66. Heggers JP: Biocompatability of silicone implants. *Ann Plast Surg* **11**(1):38–45, 1983

67. Kossovsky N et al: The bioreactivity of silicone. *Critical Reviews in Biocompatability* **3**(1):53–85, 1987

68. Kossovsky N et al: Ventricular shunt failure: Evidence of immunologic sensitization. *Surgical Forum* **34:**527, 1983

69. Heggers JP et al: Immunologic responses to silicone implants: Fact or fiction? *Plastic Surg Research Forum* **13:**13–18, 1990

70. Webster RCP et al: Injectable silicone for facial soft-tissue augmentation. *Arch Otolaryngol Head Neck Surg* **112:**290–296, 1986

71. Webster CP et al: Rhinoplastic revisions with injectable silicone. *Arch Otolaryngol Head Neck Surg* **112:**269–276, 1986

72. Webster RC et al: Injectable silicone: Its history and its current status. *Am J Cosmetic Surg* **3:**31–81, 1986, no 2

73. Aronsohn RB: A 22 year experience with the use of silicone injections. *Am J Cosmetic Surg* **1:**21–28, 1984

74. Balkin SW: Plantar keratoses: Treatment by injectable liquid silicone. *Clin Orthop* **87:**235–247, 1972

75. Balkin SW: Treatment of painful scars on soles and digits with injection of fluid silicone. *J Dermatol Surg Oncol* **3:**612–614, 1977

76. Balkin SW: *Fluid Silicone Augmentation in the Diabetic Foot: A Fifteen Year Study* (scientific exhibit). Presented at the 1979 annual meeting of the American Diabetes Association, Los Angeles, June 9–12, 1979

77. Balkin SW: The fluid silicone prosthesis. *Clin Podiatry* **1:**145–164, 1984

78. Balkin SW: Treatment of corns by injectable silicone. *Arch Dermatol* **3:**1143–1145, 1975

79. Blumenthal R: New York dermatologist is fighting with FDA over silicone injections. *The New York Times,* July 19, 1984, pp A–3

80. Achauer BM: A serious complication following medical-grade silicone injection of the face. *Plast Reconstr Surg* **71:**251–253, 1983

81. Nedelman CI: Oral and cutaneous tissue reactions to injected fluid silicones. *J Biomed Mater Res* **2:**131–143, 1968

82. Travis WD et al: Silicone granulomas: Report of three cases and review of the literature. *Hum Pathol* **16:**19–27, 1985

83. Hawthorne GA et al: Hematological effects of dimethylpolysiloxane fluid in rats. *J Reticuloendothel Soc* **7:**587–593, 1970

84. Rudolph R et al: Myofibroblasts and free silicone around breast implant. *Plast Reconstr Surg* **62:**195, 1978

85. Chastre J et al: Acute pneumonitis after subcutaneous injections of silicone in transsexual men. *N Engl J Med* **308:**764–767, 1983

86. Ellenbogen R, Rubin L: Injectable fluid silicone therapy: Human morbidity and mortality. *JAMA* **234:**308–309 1975

87. Kopf EH et al: Complication of silicone injections. *Rocky Mt Med Journal* **73:**77–80, 1976

88. Bommer J et al: Silicone storage disease in long-term hemodialysis patients. *Contrib Nephrol* **36:**115–126, 1983

89. Bommer J et al: Storage of silicone particles in macrophages: An iatrogenic complication in dialysis patients. *Artif Organs* **6:**330–333, 1982

90. Leong ASY et al: Spallation and migration of silicone from blood-pump tubing in patients on hemodialysis. *N Engl J Med* **306:**135–140, 1982

91. Sergott TJ et al: Human adjuvant disease, possible autoimmune disease after silicone implantation: A review of the literature, case studies, and speculation for the future. *Plast Reconstr Surg* **78:**104–114, 1986

92. Uratsky NF et al: Augmentation mammoplasty associated with severe systemic illness. *Ann Plast Surg* **3:**445–447, 1979

93. Spiera H: Scleroderma after silicone augmentation mammoplasty. *JAMA* **260:**236–238, 1988

94. Kumagai Y et al: Clinical spectrum of connective tissue disease after cosmetic surgery: Observations on 18 patients and a review of the Japanese literature. *Arthritis Rheum* **27:**1–12, 1984

95. Stegman SJ et al: Adverse reactions to bovine collagen implant: Clinical and histologic features. *J Dermatol Surg Oncol* **14**(suppl 1):39–48, 1988

96. Barr RJ et al: Necrobiotic granulomas associated with bovine collagen test site injections. *J Am Acad Dermatol* **6:**867–869, 1982

97. Barr RJ, Stegman SJ: Delayed skin test reaction to injectable collagen implant (Zyderm). *J Am Acad Dermatol* **10:**652–658, 1984

98. Brooks NA: Foreign body granuloma produced by an injectable collagen implant at a test site. *J Dermatol Surg Oncol* **8:**111–114, 1982

99. Ruiz-Esparza J et al: Necrobiotic granuloma formation at a collagen implant treatment site. *Cleve Clin Q* **50:**163–165, 1983

100. Webster RC et al: Injectable silicone: Report of 17,000 facial treatments since 1962. *American Journal of Cosmetic Surgery* **3:**41–48, 1986

101. Wilkie TF: Late development of granuloma after liquid silicone injections. *Plast Reconstr Surg* **60:**179–188, 1977

102. Heggers JP et al: Acceleration of capsule formation around silicone implants by injection in a guinea pig model. *Plast Reconstr Surg* **73:**9–98, 1984

103. Duffy DM: Silicone: A critical review. *Adv Dermatol* **5:**93–110, 1990

104. Greenberg JH: Information Postal Survey of Selected Physicians in Dermatology. Presented to American Academy of Dermatology, Dallas, Texas, Dec, 1991

105. Cinons M: FDA assails wrinkle treatment as illegal. *Los Angeles Times,* June 11, 1991, p 5

106. Letter to President, American Society for Dermatologic Surgery, from Commissioner, Food and Drug Administration, Rockville, MD, October 22, 1991

107. Zeckhauser RJ, Visusi WK: Risks within reason, (editorial). *Science* **248:**559–563, 1990

Richard G. Glogau
Seth L. Matarasso
Andrew C. Markey

33 Microlipoinjection: Autologous Fat Grafting

INJECTABLE SUBSTANCES FOR SOFT-TISSUE AUGMENTATION

The clinical need for injectable substances for soft-tissue augmentation remains undisputed. A variety of problems ranging in severity from hemifacial atrophy to early visibility of dynamic expression lines in photoaging suggest the need for a reproducible, safe, elegant, and widely applicable injectable which can address a range of anatomic contour defects from the dermis throughout the subcutaneous soft tissue. There are several materials in clinical use today, each with its own set of advantages and disadvantages. Zyderm (Collagen Corp., Palo Alto, California) is a highly purified bovine collagen implant which is the most widely used in skin surgery today.[1] The material can be injected through a fine 30-gauge, $1/2$-in needle, gives a temporary correction measured in weeks to months, and is well tolerated by all but a small percentage of patients who become sensitized and suffer local delayed hypersensitivity reactions.[2] The relatively short-lived effect and the cost of the material make its use in large contour defects impractical.

Fibrel (Mentor Corporation, Santa Barbara, California) is a commercial product, derived from collagen, which utilizes the patient's own serum combined with epsilon-aminocaproic acid to make a gelatinous protein complex which can also be injected through a fine-gauge needle into dermal pockets which are predissected.[3] While the lack of allergenicity is appealing,[4] the need for venipuncture, the morbidity of pretunneling the dermis with attendant bruising, edema, pain, and

the cost per milliliter of prepared material have limited the widespread use of this product.

Injectable liquid silicone had been used by some practitioners for years though generally in small amounts.[5,6] Utilizing serially placed microdroplets injected into the dermis, practitioners induced a controlled fibroplasia which produced a greater volume correction than that which is attributable to the injected substance itself. However, historical problems of misuse, such as improper placement of larger amounts of the material in the subcutaneous spaces particularly when injected into the female breast, gave rise to numerous complications, including granulomatous reactions, lymphatic migration, and exuberant fibroplasia with resultant scarring.[7]

The lack of a Food and Drug Administration (FDA)-approved commercial product for intradermal use and current concerns over long-term immunologic reactions to the gel forms of silicone used in breast implants make widespread adoption of injectable silicone unlikely in the near future. Indeed, in 1992, the FDA aggressively sought to stop use of microdroplet silicone in the United States, with resulting prohibition by malpractice carriers effectively eliminating its use in future practice for the foreseeable future.

HISTORICAL ATTEMPTS AT GRAFTING FAT

Lack of satisfaction with these materials for a variety of reasons has turned physicians' attentions to autologous fat as a potential source for augmentation, but the interest in fat is not limited to recent times.[8] The early attempts at autologous fat grafting were generally disappointing, though anecdotal reports encouraged further work. Most early surgical experiments involved the sharp dissection of bulk fat which was then placed in prepared pockets of subcutaneous tissue.[9] These rudimentary fat grafts then underwent ischemic necrosis, liquefaction, and absorption. Peer's studies[10] in the 1950s demonstrated that even small pieces, placed atraumatically, lost at least 50 percent of their volume over time. As interest in silicone grew, Peer's work was largely forgotten until the popular explosion of liposuction in the 1980s.

CURRENT CROSS-SPECIALTY EXPERIENCE

The desire for optimizing a viable technique for autologous fat grafting is not limited to dermatology and plastic surgery. Both neurosurgeons and orthopedic surgeons have experimented with free fat grafts in laminectomy procedures to minimize ingrowth of scar tissue and subsequent symptomatic compression of dorsal nerve roots.[11–18] Ophthalmologists have struggled with the problem of managing the postenucleation orbit and have examined the utility of fat grafts or dermal fat grafts.[19–24] Authors seem somewhat divided on the predictability of the individual techniques, yet clearly have documented long-term survival in many instances.[12,13,17,18,25] In fact, it is apparent that the long-term survival of the grafts may give rise to certain unwanted complications depending on the location and evolving histopathology of the graft.[24,26–29]

LIPOSUCTION AND THE FRENCH EXPERIENCE

Current cosmetic surgical interest in the phenomenon of autologous fat grafting is closely related to the development of liposuction surgery.[8] Illouz[30] published in the American literature in 1986 his experience with using injectable fat grafts to repair overzealous liposuction performed by another surgeon, although he had been working on methods to utilize the fat obtained during liposuction surgery as early as 1983. He reviewed his experience through 1988 and concluded the technique was useful.[31]

Fournier[32] focused attention on the reductionist model of autologous fat grafting utilizing common hand-held syringes to both harvest and reinject fat but published his work in the French literature. It is his work which has provided the primary stimulus for current techniques of fat grafting. In any event the renewed interest in fat as a material for potential grafting was heightened by the advent of liposuction surgery, which suddenly made large amounts of the tissue readily available.[33]

COSMETIC SURGICAL EXPERIENCE

Following the publications by Illouz and Fournier, the literature exploded with anecdotal reports relating experiences in autologous fat grafting in breast augmentation.[34–40] A fire storm of controversy erupted about the technique, and the literature suddenly filled with both strident warnings and enthusiastic endorsements.[41–51] Certainly an issue of concern yet to be adequately addressed was the presence and character of calcification that could be seen in the grafts.[52]

Other authors turned their attention to the correction of facial defects.[22,53–65] Interesting preliminary work on the treatment of the aging hands has also been presented.[66,67]

There seem to be two distinctly different patterns within this body of anecdotal literature. First is the group of surgeons who use macrotechniques of liposuction (cannula > 2 mm, machine vacuum, in-line traps, etc.) to obtain fat for grafting, usually as a procedure incidental to liposuction being undertaken for body contouring.[30,34,35,37–39,56,60,64,65,68–70] In contrast, a second group of surgeons favors microtechniques utilizing hand-held syringes, low-pressure vacuum, closed systems, and fat generally harvested specifically for the purposes of augmentation.[32,53,54,57,67,71,72]

Long-term evaluation of implanted grafts has been made possible with newer techniques of magnetic resonance imaging (MRI) and probably represents a standard for evaluation of graft survival though no comparison studies between the different techniques of fat grafting utilizing MRI have yet been published.[1,68,73]

ANIMAL MODELS AND BASIC RESEARCH

Some interesting work has been published on animal models for autologous fat grafting.[74–80] Some preliminary attention has been given to the effect of cannula or needle size, vacuum, and aqueous media to adipocyte morphology and survival,[81] but there are obviously large gaps in knowledge of the quality, makeup, and survival characteristics of harvested fat, as well as the extent to which variations in technique may affect the clinical outcome.

TECHNIQUES

At present, the authors use a method which is closely aligned with that described by Fournier.[32,82] The authors have consistently used the upper outer buttock area as a donor area of first choice and the abdomen as second choice. The upper outer buttock seems preferred for several reasons: (1) It is readily approachable for harvesting with the patient in a prone or sitting position, which is less threatening to the patient; (2) most individuals possess readily available amounts of subcutaneous fat in this area, even if they are thin, aesthetic individuals; (3) this area in both men and women appears to be more resistant to dietary fluctuation than other areas; and (4) it is a relatively insensitive area.

The authors prepare the site for harvesting by injecting the area with a dilute solution of lidocaine (Xylocaine) and epinephrine, similar in concentration to that which is used for liposuction with the exception of hyaluronidase (Wydase) and sodium bicarbonate, both of which are eliminated from the formula (see Table 33-1).

The solution is injected into the subcutaneous space in a ratio of approximately 3:1 of anesthesia to anticipated or desired yield of fat. For example, if one wishes to harvest approximately 20 cc of fat as a final yield, it would be reasonable to inject about 60 cc (or more) of the anesthetic solution into the donor subcutaneous area.

To minimize risks of bleeding, hematoma, and free blood in the harvested fat, it seems beneficial to wait a few minutes after introduction of the anesthetic solution into the subcutaneous space for the vasoconstrictive effect to become apparent. This is readily seen as clinical blanching of the overlying skin and will be readily familiar to those surgeons conversant with the *wet* or *tumescent* technique of liposuction surgery. In addition, patients are cautioned in their preoperative consultations to avoid aspirin and nonsteroidal anti-inflammatory agents for at least 10 days prior to surgery.

The overlying skin is then prepared with an antibacterial scrub such as Hibiclens and draped as appropriate to maintain a clean field. A small dermal wheal is then raised with the usual local anesthetic of choice, usually 0.5 cc of lidocaine 1% with epinephrine 1:200,000. A small stab incision, usually 2 to 3 mm, is made in the skin with a no. 11 scalpel blade.

The needle and syringe are then introduced to the subcutaneous space. The authors use a 12- or 13-gauge, single-hole distal beveled needle, $1^1/_2$- to 4-in length, with a Luer-Lok hub and the distal point beveled at a 45° angle. This needle tip is relatively blunt yet still provides some degree of cutting when moved with force along its long axis. The tip is therefore relatively atraumatic and less likely to sever vessels than a more conventional sharp-tipped needle.

The needle is mounted on a conventional hypodermic syringe, usually 20 cc capacity with a Luer-Lok-type hub. The syringe is always primed with 1 or 2 cc of sterile normal saline to remove all potential dead space from the syringe and needle before introducing the needle tip into the subcutaneous space. This last point is critical to the ease of harvesting and

TABLE 33-1

Components of local anesthesia for donor area

Sterile normal saline	500 mL
2% Lidocaine	24 mL
Epinephrine 1:1000 aq	0.25 mL

one for which surgeons are specifically indebted to Dr. Fournier for providing.

The syringe is held in the dominant hand while the nondominant hand grasps the skin and underlying fat surrounding the entry point and slightly elevates the tissue away from the underlying fascia. The syringe plunger is pulled back about halfway and held in position while the hand begins to move the syringe rapidly up and down in a vertical motion in an axis perpendicular to the skin plane and parallel to the long axis of the needle.

The fat will in a moment or two rapidly come into the syringe. If the needle's axis falls away from the perpendicular, the yield seems to drop off. After a number of strokes, the plunger needs to be pulled back farther to reapply the vacuum, and the strokes are repeated. Picking up and putting down the tissue with the nondominant hand in between bursts of vertical strokes of the syringe seems to bring fresh fat into the syringe and increase the yield.

If the fat coming into the syringe appears to be arriving with excess blood, the stroking is stopped, the syringe withdrawn, and the tissue rearranged with the nondominant hand. The needle is reintroduced and the process continues.

What comes into the syringe will be yellowish-white or pink-tinged slivers of fat with a mixture of tissue fluid and some anesthetic solution. When the syringe is about two-thirds to three-quarters full, the syringe is withdrawn, the 13-gauge needle removed in a sterile fashion, and the syringe recapped with the plastic hub that originated on the syringe. The syringe is then placed upright with the plunger at the top, and the contents of the syringe are allowed to layer out. In a matter of minutes, the fat quickly rises to the top, and the acellular infranatant can be readily discarded.

A few milliliters of sterile Ringer's lactate solution is then drawn up into the syringe and the contents agitated for a moment; the syringe is recapped and again allowed to stand for a couple of minutes. The effect is to remove the free blood from the fat, and the infranatant rapidly moves from red or pink to clear or barely tinged after just one or two washings.

The fat is then transferred in a sterile fashion using a Luer-Lok to Luer-Lok needle with a large gauge to the syringe that will be used to inject the fat, usually a 10-cc syringe. In this fashion, a number of 10-cc syringes can be filled in a matter of 10 min, cleaned, and ready to inject.

The recipient area, which has previously been photographed, marked, and cleaned, is readied for injection by raising a small wheal with local anesthesia at the point designated for the entry of the injection needle. It is not necessary to attempt to anesthetize the entire subcutaneous space where the fat is to be injected. Although there is some discomfort associated with the injection, it relates primarily to the sudden stretch and expansion of the subcutaneous space and is well tolerated by most patients. On a theoretical basis, it seems useful to avoid producing vasoconstriction in the recipient bed, if possible, so the authors have avoided anesthesia with epinephrine in the recipient bed.

For injections of fat into the subcutaneous space beneath the nasolabial folds, the authors commonly use an injection point within the nasolabial lines just lateral to the corner of the mouth and inject from 3 to 10 cc of fat per side. This injection point gives access to the upper and lower lip. The chin and marionette lines at the lower mouth can be accessed from injection points in the submental area, out of cosmetic view, and commonly receive between 3 and 5 cc of fat per side.

The authors usually inject the fat with an 18-gauge needle, although occasionally the particular quality of the fat harvested will require a larger 16 gauge. To avoid leaving needle marks at the injection site, the authors find that the needle should enter the skin almost parallel to the skin plane with the bevel facing upward. By so doing, the needle produces a tiny arcuate incision rather than a small circular punch which tends to heal as a small pitted scar.

Once the needle is in the subcutaneous plane, it is advanced to the farthest point of interest. The plunger is then drawn back to aspirate and make sure no vessel has been entered inadvertently. The fat is then injected as the needle is withdrawn to avoid intravascular injection. The fat will frequently seem to dissect along the subcutaneous plane on its own without the need to repeatedly advance and withdraw the needle. This is important because it allows the fat to be placed without inducing undesired subcutaneous hemorrhage.

After the fat is introduced, the needle is withdrawn and point pressure over the injection site is applied, while any molding can be undertaken by firm massage to encourage proper distribution of the fat in the subcutaneous plane. The fat resists attempts to displace it laterally, however, so attention must be paid during injection not to overinject a given area. In fact, overcorrection is probably not desirable since it is improbable that excessively large volumes can be sustained by passive diffusion from the recipient bed. Rapid revascularization of the inner portions of large volumes of grafted fat seems also unlikely.

The exception to the molding principle is the dorsal hand. About 7 to 10 cc of fat can be placed in the subcutaneous tissue over the dorsal wrist through a small injection site in the skin with the skin pinched up well away from underlying fascia, creating a little ball of fat. The needle is withdrawn and digital pressure put over the injection point as the patient then *tightly* clenches his or her fist. The fat is then readily massaged in an even distribution over the back of the hand, down to the finger webs, and into the dorsal proximal fingers.

After the injection of fat is completed, a small Steri-Strip dressing is applied to the injection site. Likewise, the donor site incision is closed with a small Steri-Strip dressing or one 5–0 nylon suture. The patient is usually instructed to use ice compresses intermittently for a few hours to minimize swelling and bruising, as well as instructed to avoid aspirin products. Patients are routinely given postoperative antibiotics, usually cephalexin (Keflex) 500 mg b.i.d. for 3 days.

CLINICAL RESULTS AND EVALUATION

Representative examples of treated sites are shown in the accompanying illustrations (Figs. 33-1–33-3). Long-term survival of the grafts will require further investigation with MRI and biopsy studies currently underway. Experience with patients suffering from idiopathic facial atrophy and with patients suffering from subcutaneous atrophy associated with linear morphea, scleroderma, coup de sabré, etc., clearly show sustained correction over time.[57,83] Results seem to depend on repeated injections of smaller amounts over time

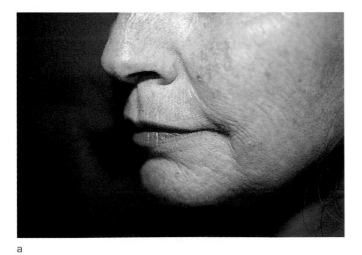

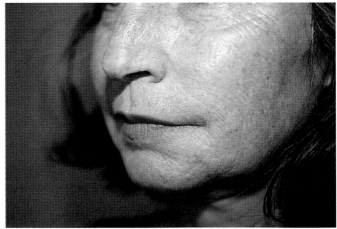

a   b

Figure 33-1 (*a*) Nasolabial folds were injected with approximately 7 cc of fat on each side and a repeat injection was made at 4 months; (*b*) follow-up picture is approximately 8 months later, 1 year after initiating treatment.

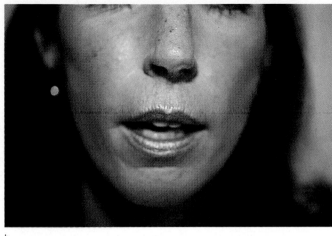
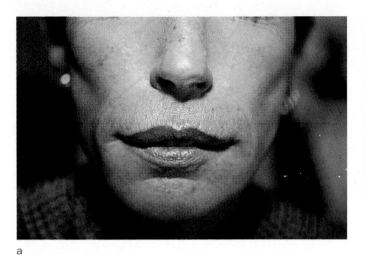

a   b

Figure 33-2 *(a)* Sunken areas just lateral to the nasolabial folds were injected with approximately 12 cc of fat on each side, twice over a 3-month period; *(b)* follow-up picture is 7 months after the second treatment, 10 months after beginning treatment.

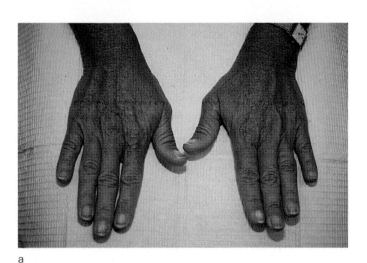
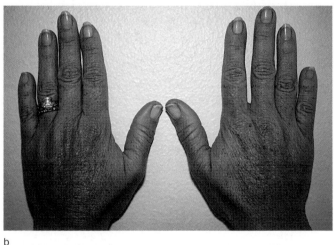

a   b

Figure 33-3 *(a)* Dorsal hands were injected once with approximately 8 cc of fat each; *(b)* follow-up picture is 1 month later.

rather than single injections of larger amounts which seem to be subject to lower take rates and higher volume resorption.

While no comparison studies as yet exist, the time interval for correction, even in cases where total resorption of the fat graft appears to occur, can be at least as long as other commercially available filler substances. The lack of predictability, however, remains a major problem for the acceptance of the technique. In some cases, correction appears to be sustained for remarkably long periods of time. In others, the effect is transient and may be substantially gone within weeks. The variables affecting graft survival have not yet been identified and may be as diverse as body type, gender, specific anatomic donor area, harvesting method (high versus low

vacuum, cannula versus syringe, "open" versus "closed" systems, etc.), composition of anesthesia, mobility of the recipient site, dietary influences (weight gain/loss), and so forth.

COMPLICATIONS

The complications with this technique have been relatively minor. The authors occasionally encounter bruising in some patients, but usually more in the donor site than the recipient site. The authors have observed one hematoma in the donor site of a patient who, following the procedure, reported for her usual aerobic workout because she "felt fine." There have been, in the authors' experience, no cases of infection, significant bleeding in the recipient site, hematoma in the recipient site, and dysthesia or abnormal sensation.

The edema which occurs in the recipient site can be cosmetically significant and lasts for several days. Under no circumstances should one imply to the patient that the treatment sites will be cosmetically unnoticed in the immediate postoperative period. Ice compresses appear to help with the degree of swelling that patients encounter, and the authors encourage its use for the first 24 to 48 h.

The fat in the recipient site can be temporarily uneven or lumpy, although in the authors' experience this fades over the first few days as the general edema subsides. The authors encounter this problem less frequently when there is slight undercorrection of the injection sites.

Surgeons need to be aware of two reports[84,85] of intravascular injection with catastrophic consequences resulting from injection in the glabellar area, mimicking previous reports of accidents following glabellar injection of Zyderm, triamcinolone acetonide, or any particulate matter. As a general course, the authors do not offer injection of the glabellar folds and creases to patients for this reason, preferring to pursue other treatment options. Indeed, animal models suggest the thrombogenic nature of fat introduced into vascular spaces.[86]

PROPOSED AREAS FOR RESEARCH

For research to move forward in this area, more biopsy and MRI studies need to be accomplished to quantify and qualify the nature of grafts over time. It is certainly the authors' clinical impression that serial injections over time offer the best chance of permanent correction, and clinical photographs may reinforce that impression, but better documentation of graft survival with objective criteria is needed.

More information about the nature of the preadipocyte and the components of the normal system which influence differentiation and maturation of this cell into the terminal lipocyte is necessary. More information on metabolic influences on the lipocyte and whether pharmacologic manipulation of the graft might enhance graft survival of the adipocytes would also be useful.

Can factors in the recipient bed be manipulated that would increase the vascularity of the recipient space and enhance graft survival? Do the grafted fat cells which survive retain their donor characteristics as do hair transplants? If so, does harvesting from areas which are relatively resistant to dietary restriction make sense? Or, should fat be utilized from more sensitive areas which could be encouraged to expand in the postgraft period by dietary manipulation? Are there growth factors present in lipomas which could be useful in preparing fat for transplantation?

Undoubtedly, further research will help define the limits of this promising technique. The readily available material, lack of allergenicity, low morbidity, and ability to generate large volumes over time seem to hold great promise if the variables of microlipoinjection can be defined.

REFERENCES

1. McPherson J et al: Development and biochemical characterization of injectable collagen. *J Dermatol Surg Oncol* **14**(suppl 1):13–20, 1988

2. Stegman S et al: *Cosmetic Dermatologic Surgery,* 2d ed. Chicago, Mosby-Year Book, 1990

3. Millikan L: Long-term safety and efficacy with Fibrel in the treatment of cutaneous scars: Results of a multicenter study. *J Dermatol Surg Oncol* **15**:837–842, 1989

4. Gottlieb SK: Soft tissue augmentation: The search for implantation materials and techniques. *Clin Dermatol* **5**:128–134, 1987

5. Klein AW, Rish DC: Substances for soft tissue augmentation: Collagen and silicone. *J Dermatol Surg Oncol* **11**:337–339, 1985

6. Webster RC et al: Injectable silicone for facial soft-tissue augmentation. *Arch Otolaryngol Head Neck Surg* **112**:290–296, 1986

7. Franz FP et al: Massive injection of liquid silicone for hemifacial atrophy. *Ann Plast Surg* **20**:140–145, 1988

8. Newman J, Ftaiha Z: The biographical history of fat transplant surgery. *Am J Cosm Surg* **4**:85–87, 1987

9. Billings EJ, May JJ: Historical review and present status of free fat graft autotransplantation in plastic and reconstructive surgery. *Plast Reconstr Surg* **83**:368–381, 1989

10. Peer LA: *Transplantation of Tissues: Transplantation of Fat,* ed. Baltimore, Williams & Wilkins, 1959

11. Bryant MS et al: Autogeneic fat transplants in the epidural space in routine lumbar spine surgery. *Neurosurgery* **13**:367–370, 1983

12. Deburge A et al: [The fate of fat grafts used in surgery of the lumbar spine] L'evolution des greffons graisseux utilises en chirurgie du rachis lombaire. *Rev Chir Orthop* **74**:238–242, 1988

13. Langenskiöld A, Valle M: Epidurally placed free fat grafts visualized by CT scanning 15–18 years after diskectomy. *Spine* **10**:97–98, 1985

14. Long DM: Free fat graft in laminectomy (letter). *J Neurosurg* **54**:711, 1981

15. Mayfield FH: Autologous fat transplants for the protection and repair of the spinal dura. *Clin Neurosurg* **27**:349–361, 1980

16. Sakamoto K: [Experimental study on pedicle fat grafts after laminectomy: Comparison of pedicle fat and free fat grafts]. *Nippon Seikeigeka Gakkai Zasshi* **61**:743–753, 1987

17. Weisz GM, Gal A: Long-term survival of a free fat graft in the spinal canal: A 40-month postlaminectomy case report. *Clin Orthop* 1986

18. Van AP et al: The fate of the free fat graft: A prospective clinical study using CT scanning. *Spine* **11**:501–504, 1986

19. Nunery WR, Hetzler KJ: Dermal-fat graft as a primary enucleation technique. *Ophthalmology* **92:**1256–1261, 1985

20. Martin PA et al: Dermis-fat graft: Evolution of a living prosthesis. *Aust N Z J Ophthalmol* **14:**161–165, 1986

21. Bullock JD: Autogenous dermis-fat "baseball" orbital implant. *Ophthalmic Surg* **18:**30–36, 1987

22. Kempf KK, Seyfer AE: Facial defect augmentation with a dermal-fat graft. *Oral Surg Oral Med Oral Pathol* **59:**340–343, 1985

23. Smith B et al: Dermis-fat orbital implantation: 118 cases. *Ophthalmic Surg* **14:**941–943, 1983

24. Wojno T, Tenzel RR: Pathology of an orbital dermis-fat graft. *Ophthalmic Surg* **16:**250–253, 1985

25. Martin FS: Failure of autologous fat grafts to prevent postoperative epidural fibrosis in surgery of the lumbar spine. *Neurosurgery* **24:**718–721, 1989

26. Cabezudo JM et al: Symptomatic root compression by a free fat transplant after hemilaminectomy: Case report. *J Neurosurg* **63:**633–635, 1985

27. Mayer PJ, Jacobsen FS: Cauda equina syndrome after surgical treatment of lumbar spinal stenosis with application of free autogenous fat graft: A report of two cases. *J Bone Joint Surg* [Am] **71:**1090–1093, 1989

28. Patrinely JR et al: Macrocystic enlargement of orbital dermis-fat grafts. *Ophthalmic Surg* **18:**498–502, 1987

29. Shore JW et al: Management of complications following dermis-fat grafting for anophthalmic socket reconstruction. *Ophthalmology* **92:**1342–1350, 1985

30. Illouz YG: The fat cell "graft": A new technique to fill depressions (letter). *Plast Reconstr Surg* **78:**122–123, 1986

31. Illouz YG: Present results of fat injection. *Aesthetic Plast Surg* **12:**175–181, 1988

32. Fournier PF: Microlipoextraction et microlipoinjection. *Rev Chir Esthet Lang Franc* **10:**40–45, 1985

33. Report on autologous fat transplantation: ASPRS Ad-Hoc Committee on New Procedures, September 30, 1987. *Plastic Surgical Nursing* **7:**140–141, 1987

34. Agris J: Autologous fat transplantation: A 3-year study. *Am J Cosm Surg* **4:**95–102, 1987

35. Bircoll M, Novack BH: Autologous fat transplantation employing liposuction techniques. *Ann Plast Surg* **18:**327–329, 1987

36. Bircoll M: Cosmetic breast augmentation utilizing autologous fat and liposuction techniques. *Plast Reconstr Surg* **79:**267–271, 1987

37. Grossman JA: Body contouring: Suction-assisted lipolysis and fat transplantation techniques. *AORN J* **48:**713–714, 1988

38. Johnson GW: Body contouring by macroinjection of autogenous fat. *Am J Cosm Surg* **4:**103–109, 1987

39. Krulig E: Lipo-injection. *Am J Cosm Surg* **4:**123–129, 1987

40. Chajchir A et al: [Comparative study on lipoinjection and other methods] Estudio comparativo de la lipoinyeccion con otros metodos. *Med Cutan Ibero Lat Am* **16:**489–496, 1988

41. Bircoll M: Reply (letter). *Plast Reconstr Surg* **80:**647, 1987

42. Bircoll M: Autologous fat transplantation to the breast (letter). *Plast Reconstr Surg* **82:**361–362, 1988

43. Bircoll M: Autologous fat tissue augmentation. *Am J Cosm Surg* **4:**141–149, 1987

44. Dixon PL: Autologous fat injection and breast augmentation (letter). *Med J Aust* **148:**537, 1988

45. Ettelson CD: Fat autografting (letter). *Plast Reconstr Surg* **80:**646, 1987

46. Fox BS: Autologous fat injection and breast augmentation (letter). *Med J Aust* **149:**284, 1988

47. Hartrampf CJ, Bennett GK: Autologous fat from liposuction for breast augmentation (letter). *Plast Reconstr Surg* **80:**646, 1987

48. Horl HW et al: [Autologous injection of fatty tissue following liposuction—not a method for breast augmentation] Autologe Fettgewebsinjektion nach Liposuktion—keine Methode zur Brustaugmentation. *Handchir Mikrochir Plast Chir* **21:**59–61, 1989

49. Linder RM: Fat autografting (letter). *Plast Reconstr Surg* **80:**646–647, 1987

50. Osterhout D: Breast augmentation by autologous fat injection (letter). *Plast Reconstr Surg* **80:**868–869, 1987

51. Pohl P, Uebel CO: Complications with homologous fat grafts in breast augmentation surgery. *Aesthetic Plast Surg* **9:**87–89, 1985

52. McLean NR, Sutherland AB: The mistaken diagnosis of calcification in a free dermis-fat graft on the chest wall (letter). *Br J Surg* **71:**479, 1984

53. Asken S: *Lipo-suction and Fat Transplantation under Local Anesthesia,* 2d ed. Westport, Conn, Med-Arts, 1987

54. Asken S: Facial liposuction and microlipoinjection. *J Dermatol Surg Oncol* **14:**297–305, 1988

55. Bisaccia E et al: Fat transfer: A "pinch" technique for accurate placement of donor tissue. *J Dermatol Surg Oncol* **15:**1072–1073, 1989

56. Chajchir A, Benzaquen I: Liposuction fat grafts in face wrinkles and hemifacial atrophy. *Aesthetic Plast Surg* **10:**115–117, 1986

57. Glogau RG: Microlipoinjection: Autologous fat grafting. *Arch Dermatol* **124:**1340–1343, 1988

58. Matsudo PK, Toledo LS: Experience of injected fat grafting. *Aesthetic Plast Surg* **12:**35–38, 1988

59. Moscona R et al: Free-fat injections for the correction of hemifacial atrophy. *Plast Reconstr Surg* **84:**501–509, 1989

60. Newman J: Preliminary report on "fat recycling" liposuction fat transfer implants for facial defects. *Am J Cosm Surg* **3:**67–69, 1986

61. Newman J, Levin J: Facial lipo-transplant surgery. *Am J Cosm Surg* **4:**131–140, 1987

62. Newman J, Tompkin E: Correction of the ptotic chin by lipo-transplants. *Am J Cosm Surg* **5:**279–281, 1988

63. Roenigk HJ, Rubenstein R: Combined scalp reduction and autologous fat implant treatment of localized soft tissue defects. *J Dermatol Surg Oncol* **14:**67–70, 1988

64. Teimourian B: Repair of soft-tissue contour deficit by means of semiliquid fat graft (letter). *Plast Reconstr Surg* **78:**123–124, 1986

65. Tobin HA, Middleton WG: Hemifacial atrophy: A case report of fat transplantation. *J Otolaryngol* **18:**125–127, 1989

66. Abergel RP, David LM: Aging hands: A technique of hand rejuvenation by laser resurfacing and autologous fat transfer. *J Dermatol Surg Oncol* **15:**725–728, 1989

67. Vida TV: Lipoinjection and aging hands: The combination of dermabrasion, chemical peel, and lipoinjection for the aesthetic improvement of aging hands. *Am J Cosmetic Surg* **6:**27–32, 1989

68. Horl HW et al: Technique for liposuction fat reimplantation and long-term volume evaluation by magnetic resonance imaging. *Ann Plast Surg* **26:**248–258, 1991

69. Lafontan M et al: [A new approach to reconstructive plastic surgery: Reimplantation of adipose tissue fragments obtained by liposuction] Reflexions sur une nouvelle approche de chirurgie plastique reparatrice: la reimplantation de fragments de tissu adipeux preleves par liposuccion. *Ann Chir Plast Esthet* **34:**77–81, 1989

70. Matarasso HA et al: A collection device for suction-assisted lipectomy and autologous fat transplantation. *Ann Plast Surg* **20:**492–493, 1988

71. Asken S: Autologous fat transplantation: Micro and macro techniques. *Am J Cosm Surg* **4:**111–121, 1987

72. Hin LC: Syringe liposuction with immediate lipotransplantation. *Am J Cosm Surg* **5:**243–248, 1988

73. Liang MD et al: Evaluation of facial fat distribution using magnetic resonance imaging. *Aesthetic Plast Surg* **15:**313–319, 1991

74. Bartynski J et al: Histopathologic evaluation of adipose autografts in a rabbit ear model. *Otolaryngol Head Neck Surg* **102:**314–321, 1990

75. Nguyen A et al: Comparative study of survival of autologous adipose tissue taken and transplanted by different techniques. *Plast Reconstr Surg* **85:**378–386, 1990

76. Pettersson P et al: Insulin binding in differentiating rat preadipocytes in culture. *J Lipid Res* **26:**1187–1195, 1985

77. Smahel J: Experimental implantation of adipose tissue fragments. *Br J Plast Surg* **42:**207–211, 1989

78. Smahel J: [Adipose tissue in plastic surgery] Problematik des Fettgewebes in der Plastischen Chirurgie. *Handchir Mikrochir Plast Chir* **16:**111–114, 1984

79. Smahel J: Adipose tissue in plastic surgery. *Ann Plast Surg* **16:**1986

80. Wexler DB et al: Phonosurgical studies: Fat-graft reconstruction of injured canine vocal cords. *Ann Otol Rhinol Laryngol* **98:**668–673, 1989

81. Campbell GL et al: The effect of mechanical stress on adipocyte morphology and metabolism. *Am J Cosm Surg* **4:**89–94, 1987

82. Fournier P: Chance and lipoextraction: Thoughts and progress in lipoplasty (reduction and augmentation). *Am J Cosm Surg* **5:**249–255, 1988

83. Pinski KS, Roenigk HJ: Autologous fat transplantation: Long-term follow-up. *J Dermatol Surg Oncol* **18:**179–184, 1992

84. Dreizen NG, Framm L: Sudden unilateral visual loss after autologous fat injection into the glabellar area. *Am J Ophthalmol* **107:**85–87, 1989

85. Teimourian B: Blindness following fat injections (letter). *Plast Reconstr Surg* 361–362, 1988

86. Sikorski JM: Venous thrombosis produced by the local injection of fat. *J Bone Joint Surg* [Br] **65:**340–345, 1983

Edward Glassberg
Kristin Walker
Gary Lask

34 Lasers in Dermatology

The first laser, a continous wave ruby laser, was developed over 30 years ago in 1959 by Maiman.[1] Shortly thereafter, Leon Goldman, a dermatologist and pioneer in the medical application of lasers, developed a laser laboratory at the University of Cincinnati to study laser-tissue interactions.[2] In the ensuing 30 years, the widespread availability and utilization of the carbon dioxide (CO_2) and argon lasers have placed dermatologists at the forefront of medical laser application and development. The more recent introduction of pulsed and tunable dye lasers specifically designed to interact with endogenous and exogenous chromophores has greatly advanced the specificity and usefulness of medical lasers, especially in the field of dermatology. This chapter details the indications for laser therapy and the medical and investigational lasers with applications in clinical dermatology (see Table 34-1). The general guidelines indicating which lesions are amenable to which type of laser therapy will be followed by a specific discussion of each laser type.

Laser is actually an acronym for *light amplification by stimulated emission of radiation*. There are three basic properties which distinguish laser light from natural light—namely, coherence, monochromaticity, and collimation. Coherence refers to the fact that the photons emitted are temporally and spatially in phase. Monochromaticity refers to the single-wavelength nature of (most) laser light, which, when visible, is of single pure color. Collimation refers to the nearly parallel direction of all emitted photons resulting in minimal beam divergence over a given distance.

Lasers traditionally emit in the ultraviolet (UV), visible, near, or far infrared parts of the electromagnetic spectrum, but can in fact consist of free electrons or even x-rays. The lasing medium, which is the substance stimulated to produce the coherent light, can be gas (as in CO_2, argon, or krypton lasers), liquid [as in tunable or pulsed dye lasers (PDLs)], or solid [as in ruby, alexandrite, or neodymium:yttrium-aluminum-garnet (Nd:YAG) lasers]. The excitation source can be an electric current, optical flash lamp, or another laser (as with argon-pumped tunable dye lasers). When a high enough percentage of the lasing medium molecules absorb the energy needed to elevate electrons from a ground to excited state, a population inversion takes place. When many electrons simultaneously return to ground state, synchronous monochromatic coherent photons are released and when reflected and focuscd by a scries of mirrors in the lasing chamber a laser beam is emitted. The final collimated beam which exits the laser may be delivered either without modification, through a series of modifying lenses, or through a fiber-optic or articulated arm delivery system.

Laser-tissue interactions may take on any of several characteristics, depending on the nature of the tissue, laser energy, wavelength, and output format. In addition, the use of exogenous photosensitizers can also define the nature of laser and tissue interaction. Thermal effects of varying degrees are the most apparent and significant for many lasers—especially relatively high-power cutting lasers such as the CO_2 or Nd:YAG lasers. This thermal effect can result in protein denaturation, coagulation, or vaporization and charring of tissue. Thermal effects probably play a role in most destructive applications of lasers; these effects can be targeted to specific natural chromophores (photothermolysis) such as hemoglobin or melanin and will be discussed later in this chapter.

Rapid absorption of microsecond or nanosecond pulsed laser energy can further result in acoustic or "shock wave"

TABLE   34-1

Lasers Used in Dermatology

Name	Mode	Wavelength(s)—nm
Carbon Dioxide	CW,[a] SP[b]	10,600
Argon	CW	488/514
Vascular Pulsed Dye	Pulsed	577/585
Copper Vapor	CW	578/511
Argon-Pumped Tunable Dye	CW	Variable (visible—infrared)
Gold Vapor	Pulsed	628
Q-Switched Ruby	QS[c] Pulsed	694
Pulsed Dye Pigment	Pulsed	510
Alexandrite	Pulsed, QS	720–800
ND:YAG[d]/KTP[e]	CW, or QS	1064/532
Helium-Neon	CW	632
Gallium-Arsenide	CW	904

a) CW = continuous wave
b) SP = superpulsed
c) QS = Q-switched
d) Nd:YAG = Neodymium: Aluminum-Yttrium-Garnet
e) KTP = Potassium Titanyl Phosphate

mechanical destruction of tissue by explosive expansion and vaporization, as with the 585 nm PDL for vascular lesions.[3,4] Purely biochemical or metabolic effects can be seen when exogenous photosensitizers are used to sensitize malignant tissue, as in photodynamic therapy. The laser light-photosensitizer interaction results in the generation of singlet oxygen and other highly reactive molecular species which then severely disrupt various cellular processes and interfere with cell membrane integrity. Other, less well-defined, subtle biochemical modifications can occur with low-energy [e.g., helium-neon (He-Ne)] laser light and can result in inhibition of immune function in lymphocytes[5] or modifications in collagen messenger ribonucleic acid (mRNA) or protein production of cells in vitro.[5,6] This area of low-energy laser stimulation remains somewhat controversial and will be discussed briefly toward the end of this chapter.

TYPES OF LESIONS TREATABLE BY LASER

The range of lesions and conditions treatable by laser therapy is quite vast (see Table 34–2). Many applications remain investigational, anecdotal, or as alternatives of convenience where conventional or non-laser therapy may be equally effective. There are many applications, however, in which lasers provide a superior result to other alternatives or, in some cases, are the only effective therapy available, and this will be the primary focus of this chapter.

As mentioned previously, the laser can be used as a primary cutting instrument (CO_2, Nd:YAG) and essentially can function as a "light scalpel." The potential advantages include effective continuous coagulation of small vessels 0.5 mm in diameter or less,[1] sealing of lymphatics and nerve endings (to diminish edema and possibly postprocedure pain), and extreme precision with the option to use computer-controlled preprogrammed scanning devices. Other forms of tissue destruction include coagulation and vaporization (e.g., UV excimer, CO_2, Nd:YAG). Hemostasis is generally achieved by defocusing a beam and decreasing the density of delivered energy. Vaporization can also be achieved with brief high-energy pulses and can literally remove a single cell layer at a time.[7] More laser-specific potential effects include photothermolysis (discussed below), photodynamic metabolic derangements, and biomodulation or biostimulation, which has been used in attempts to promote wound healing.[8]

Lesions treatable by laser therapy or surgery may be broadly grouped into four categories: (1) vascular lesions; (2) pigmented lesions (*a*) benign melanocytic/melanotic, (*b*) exogenous pigment; (3) benign lesions or neoplasms; and (4) malignant or premalignant lesions. Within each broad clinical category there are multiple options depending on the precise nature of the lesion.

Vascular Lesions

Vascular lesions are particularly amenable to laser therapy because of the presence of a natural and highly absorbent chromophore—oxyhemoglobin. Port-wine stains (PWSs), capillary and cavernous hemangiomas, telangiectasias, spider angiomas, pyogenic granulomas, senile angiomas, poikilodermas of Civatte, venous lakes, and many other benign vascular lesions are very effectively treated with various laser systems.[9] The argon laser used on hemoglobin (which has absorption peaks in the 410 to 420, 540, and 580 nm ranges), was the first laser to target this chromophore specifically. Since argon lasers emit primarily at 488 and 514.5 nm (blue and green light), they are not truly specific for hemoglobin but are significantly absorbed by this chromophore. The potential absorption of argon laser energy by melanin limits to some extent the usefulness of this laser, especially in darkly pigmented skin. In addition, argon laser thermal injury is limited to about 1 mm in depth and thus is primarily useful in superficial lesions (see "The Argon Laser" below).[2]

There are presently three more recently developed systems for treating vascular lesions, and each can very specifically target the longest wavelength absorption band of oxyhemoglobin at 577 nm. These include the flash lamp-pumped pulsed tunable dye laser emitting at 577 or 585 nm, the 578 nm copper vapor laser (CVL), and the argon laser-pumped tunable dye laser at 577 nm. Each system can be effective for various vascular lesions, but the most selective is the flash lamp-pumped PDL which has demonstrated excellent clearing of PWS, early hemangiomas, telangiectasias, and other le-

TABLE   34-2

Types of Lesions Treatable by Laser*

Vascular	Pigmented	Benign	Premalignant/Malignant
Port-wine stains	**Endogenous (Melanin)**	**Appendageal Tumors**	**Premalignant**
Capillary/strawberry	Lentigines	Syringoma	Actinic keratoses
hemangiomas	Ephelides	Trichoepithelioma	Actinic cheilitis
Telangiectasias	Melanocytic nevi	Adenoma sebaceum	Bowenoid papulosis
Spider angiomas	Nevi of Ito/Ota	**Nonmelanocytic Nevi**	**Malignant†**
Pyogenic granulomas	Melasma	Collagenoma	Basal cell carcinoma
Senile angiomas	Postinflammatory pigment	Elastoma	(especially superficial)
Poikiloderma of Civatte	Nevus spilus	**Hyperplasias**	Squamous cell carcinoma
Venous lakes	Becker's nevus	Sebaceous hyperplasia	Bowen's disease
Rosacea	Café au lait spots	Rhinophyma	Erythroplasia of Queyrat
Scar erythema	Mongolian spots	Keloids	**Typical Lasers Used**
Lymphangiomas	(± lentigo maligna	Xanthelasma	CO_2, Nd:YAG, argon, argon-
Angiokeratomas	or congenital nevi)	**Cystic lesions**	pumped dye laser for
Typical Lasers Used	**Exogenous**	Milia	photodynamic therapy
Argon, vascular pulsed dye,	Professional, amateur,	Digital cysts	
copper vapor, argon-	medical, and traumatic tattoos	**Infectious lesions**	
pumped tunable dye, Potassium	**Typical Lasers Used**	Verrucae	
Titanyl Phosphate (KTP)	Q-switched ruby, Q-switched	Mycotic nails	
Less common	Nd:YAG, pulsed dye pigment,	**Inflammatory Disease**	
CO_2, Nd:YAG	Q-switched alexandrite	Hidradenitis	
	Less Common	Hailey and Hailey disease	
	Copper vapor, KTP, CO_2, argon	Lichen sclerosus	
		Ulcerations	
		Nonmalignant	
		Typical Lasers Used	
		CO_2, Nd:YAG, argon, copper	
		vapor	
		Less Common	
		He-Ne, gallium arsenide	

* This list is merely a representative sampling of reported lesions and conditions treated by laser. The listing of a lesion indicates nothing about efficacy nor are lasers necessarily the accepted mode of treatment.

† Malignant lesions are not routinely treated by laser except for investigational trials of photodynamic therapy.

sions, with an extremely low incidence of scarring or permanent epidermal changes.[3,10] Each system and its merits are discussed in detail in "Laser Systems" below.

All of the above mentioned laser systems are limited in depth of penetration because of the high absorption by hemoglobin and the relatively short wavelength of the emitted laser light. For deep or bulky vascular lesions, such as large capillary or cavernous hemangiomas, a deeper penetrating infrared laser, like the CO_2 or Nd:YAG, can be used to excise or vaporize a lesion while maintaining reasonable hemostasis.[11] Some degree of fibrosis and clinical scarring is inevitable in these cases due to nonspecific thermal injury, but acceptable cosmetic results can be achieved in appropriately selected cases when the optimal techniques are employed.[11]

Pigmented Lesions

For the purposes of this chapter, benign pigmented cutaneous lesions may be divided into two basic categories: (1) endogenous (primarily melanotic/melanocytic in nature) and (2) exogenous (including professional, amateur, and traumatic tattoos). Many different laser systems have been employed to

near infrared Nd:YAG laser in its ability to inhibit fibroblast proliferation.[27] The authors have found that only earlobe keloids have significant cure rates with lasers, but this also is true with cold steel surgery.

Tattoos are also treated with CO_2 laser, but some hypertrophic scarring frequently results.[28] This scarring can be minimized by limiting postoperative physical activity, using pressure bandages, and using intralesional steroid injections. Improved results occur if the pigment is superficial and limited to the papillary dermis; pigment removal therefore can be more complete, which eliminates any "ghost" images caused by remaining pigment as seen in post-argon laser treatment. With the bloodless operative field, tattoo pigment may be visualized throughout the procedure.

Both the excisional and vaporizing actions of the CO_2 laser are employed when treating a hyperplastic condition such as rhinophyma. Using local anesthesia, the surgeon can excise the bulbous tissue masses bloodlessly. As the normal shape of the nose becomes more apparent, excision is replaced by lower irradiance vaporization to refine the surface contours. This is similar to dermabrasion but is bloodless, pain free with local anesthesia, and accurate, although some scarring can occur.

Recently, CO_2 laser abrasion for aged, sun-damaged facial skin has been demonstrated to be an effective modality with comparable or even fewer complications than chemical peels or dermabrasion. The cosmetic and therapeutic benefits appear to be significant and similar to those obtained from a chemical peel of these lesions.

There have been reports of less postoperative pain after CO_2 vaporization of onychomycotic nails, although this has not been the experience of the authors. Besides this possible benefit, CO_2 laser treatment is no more successful at curing a fungal infection than nail avulsion unless additional agents, such as antimycotics, are used.[27]

Malignant tumor excison with the CO_2 laser has been fairly extensively performed, with the main disadvantage being coagulation necrosis in the excised specimen, which may minimize the accurate evaluation of histologic margins. It has been postulated that since the laser seals lymphatics and blood vessels, it may be of value where metastatic spread may occur via these routes. Further studies need to be conducted to support this.

Technique

Unlike various other lasers, the CO_2 laser does not utilize a fiber-optic cable for laser energy delivery. Currently, the CO_2 laser requires an articulated arm with multiple mirrors, limiting to some extent the management of the unit in performing procedures. More recently, a flexible coated tubing and fibers have been developed which are relatively easy to manipulate. To assist the physician, a red He-Ne-aiming beam is needed to guide placement of the invisible CO_2 laser beam.[2] Clear glass or plastic protective eyewear should be worn by all present in the laser room.

The CO_2 laser is a continuous wave laser that can be used in a shuttered or superpulsed mode. Superpulsing delivers higher peak energies in briefer pulses than conventional shuttered pulsing, confining thermal injury to a narrower field during tissue cutting. With the superpulsed CO_2 laser mode, decreased hemostasis during excisional surgery occurs, possibly because of insufficient thermal diffusion to seal vessels.[1] Most CO_2 laser surgery is conducted under local anesthesia with the continuous mode either focused or defocused.

Two distinct therapeutic functions can be performed depending on whether the beam is focused or defocused. A focused CO_2 laser beam bloodlessly excises tissue, while a defocused beam vaporizes superficial lesions. To achieve the excisional or the vaporization functions of the CO_2 laser, the physician must vary the laser to skin distance. The beam is in the focused mode when the laser handpiece is closer to the skin, creating a small spot size generating high thermal temperatures for tissue excision. A beam diameter of 0.2 mm or smaller is used for tissue excision. By moving the handpiece farther from the skin, in the defocused mode, a larger spot size (2 to 8 mm) with lower power densities is produced, allowing vaporization of the superficial skin lesions. Minimal thermal damage occurs to surrounding tissues. Adequate vaporization often can be achieved with delivery of 4 to 5 W of power, but individual settings can vary from 1 to 10 W or more. Hyperkeratotic tissue such as verrucae may require an increase in power. Often, however, there is no need to adjust the power parameters when vaporizing with the CO_2 laser.

The CO_2 laser heats the water content of tissue up to 100°C, resulting in significant steam production.[1] A noxious laser plume of steam and cellular debris is also produced; therefore, an efficient suction and evacuation system must exist in the treatment area. One report suggests the possibility of viral particle spread in the laser plume following wart removal.[29] Again, this point emphasizes the requirement for highly effective smoke evacuators and filters. Also, extreme care must be exercised since burning or damaging surrounding tissue is a possibility. The use of safety goggles, wet drapes and sponges, nonreflective black coating on surgical instruments, and nonflammable materials is essential.[30]

Thermal damage following CO_2 laser excision results in decreased tensile strength for the first 3 weeks postoperatively. Theoretically, sutures are recommended to remain in place for a longer period of time compared with scalpel excision. The CO_2 laser has a reportedly lower incidence of postoperative pain and a potentially improved quality of resultant scarring compared with electrodesiccation, especially for treating deeper lesions, though results are highly variable with both modalities.

Complications and Contraindications

With the CO_2 laser, full-thickness epidermal destruction usually occurs. This destruction may also extend into the papillary or high reticular dermis.[31] Hypertrophic scarring is one condition which may result from this modality, especially following treatment of tattoos.[32] In one study, 64 percent of CO_2 laser users noted hypertrophic scarring in some patients, as well as keloid formation.[32,33] Hypertrophic scarring becomes more likely with the removal of deeper lesions which extend into the deep reticular dermis where this type of scar formation is expected. The arm, chest, and lip are noted as high-risk sites for scar formation.

Used as a vaporizing agent, the CO_2 laser can be controlled for depth and degree of tissue destruction by varying its power density. One study of scar formation revealed a linear relationship between scar formation and power densities in the range of 140 to 850 W/cm^2 or 10 to 60 W of power.[33] In the skin of rats, a statistically significant positive linear relationship between CO_2 laser power density delivered and the amount of scar formed at day 32 was found to be 0.3 μm of scar thickness per W/cm^2 of laser energy.[33] In all these experiments, a one-pass technique was performed, unlike the several passes needed for adequate vaporization of skin in clinical practice.

Low power densities may result in increased coagulation necrosis of surrounding tissues from increased thermal conduction. This is a consequence of an inadequate amount of power to immediately vaporize the target tissue.[33] A power density too high or too low may result in scar formation or further tissue damage.

Relative contraindications for treatment are similar to other laser modalities. The primary contraindications would be in patients prone to keloid formation. If the etiology of the lesion to be treated is uncertain, laser treatment is not advisable. Since it is a destructive modality, the tissue treated would not be preserved, making a diagnosis difficult when the destroyed lesion is viewed. Also, cosmetically sensitive areas need to be carefully evaluated prior to therapy.

The Argon Laser

Mode: Continuous wave (with ability for pulsed mode with a shuttering mechanism)
Wavelength: 80 percent of emission at 488 and 514.5 nm
Target chromophores: Hemoglobin and melanin
Medium: Gas (argon)

Background

Since about 1970, the argon laser has been used to treat various cutaneous disorders and has increased in therapeutic importance over the years. This laser is most beneficial when used for the treatment of vascular conditions, especially telangiectasias and PWS hemangiomas. The argon laser emits light between 480 and 520 nm in the blue-green visible light spectrum.[1] This laser is quite useful for both cutaneous vascular and pigmented lesions.

Many properties of the argon laser contribute to its value in treating various cutaneous lesions. Laser light penetrates the epidermis and is absorbed by either hemoglobin, melanin,

or other pigments in the dermis. This light is then converted to heat, resulting in thermal coagulation of blood vessels in the upper dermis. Other appendages in the dermis such as sweat glands and hair follicles are more resistant to the laser light, resulting in a relatively short time required for healing and re-epithelialization of the laser wound. Relative sparing of the uninvolved area also occurs. In studies of the histopathologic response to argon laser therapy, results have demonstrated some degree of destruction of vessels occurring up to a depth of 1 mm of dermis, replaced by a diffuse collagenous deposit with narrow vessels and reconstructed normal epidermis.[1,34] These changes have appeared to be stable and permanent as demonstrated by serial biopsies of lesions.[34]

Indications

The argon laser has been useful in many dermatologic conditions, especially for treating vascular lesions such as port-wine hemangiomas and telangiectasias among others, as well as some lesions containing melanin (see Table 34-4). Prior to the development of the PDL, the argon laser was the only consistently effective treatment for PWSs. The argon laser successfully lightens these lesions and flattens the nodular component arising in the mature PWS.[2] Children with port-wine hemangiomas require additional caution in choosing treatment options because of the potential for scarring, especially on the upper lip.[2] It has been shown that continuous wave argon laser can work well in children when small beam diameters and low energies are utilized.[35] However, most authors believe that the PDL is preferable to the argon laser for PWS treatment in children.[1]

TABLE 34-4

Some Lesions Treatable by Argon Laser*

Vascular	Pigmented	Miscellaneous
Port-wine stain	Lentigines	Tattoos
Telangiectasia	Ephelides	
Capillary hemangioma	Café au lait spots	
Venous lake	Seborrheic keratoses	
Spider angioma	Melasma	
Cherry angioma	Nevocellular nevi	
Angiokeratoma	Nevi of Ito/Ota	
Rosacea/rhinophyma		
Cavernous hemangioma		
Angiofibroma		
Glomus tumor		
Kaposi's sarcoma		
Pyogenic granuloma		
Superficial varicosity		

* This is only a partial list, not intended to be inclusive. Listing an entity does not imply laser is the optimum treatment modality.

The argon laser is still considered by many to be the treatment of choice for very hypertrophic PWSs or nodular areas within them. In adults with these lesions, laser testing with both argon and PDL may be performed to select the most effective treatment. Since the argon laser response depends upon fibrosis around the blood vessel wall, the test can only be evaluated for its full response approximately 4 to 12 months posttreatment. Postoperative wound care with dressing changes is required for 1 week to several weeks because of the usual epidermal disruptions.

One of the best uses for the argon laser is for treatment of low-flow hemangiomas, venous in origin. These results are especially pronounced in venous lakes of the lip and venous malformations of mucosal surfaces.[1] This laser has also been used in treating epidermal pigmented lesions because of the absorption of the argon laser light by melanin. Such lesions as lentigines and junctional nevi have been noted to lighten well with the argon laser. Deeper pigmented lesions have a greater potential for hypertrophic scarring. Other benign pigmented lesions—café au lait spots, seborrheic keratoses, and melasma, to name a few—may respond well to this therapy. Facial telangiectasias are particularly amenable to argon laser treatment; facial and neck telangiectasias are the most successful group of lesions treated in this manner.[36] In one study, 42 out of 50 patients treated experienced complete blanching without scar or recurrence after one laser application.[37] Superficial varicosities and lower extremity telangiectasias have been shown not to respond well to this therapy; however, hereditary hemorrhagic telangiectasias have proven amenable to argon laser therapy. Since this is a progressive disease, argon laser treatment is not a permanent cure; rather, it is a palliative procedure resulting in decreased frequency and severity of bleeding. Every 3 to 6 months, repeated treatments are needed.[34]

Tattoos have also been treated by the argon laser. In one study, 35 patients with tattoos of the face and extremities were treated with the argon laser.[38] Out of these patients, 21 had satisfactory removal of their tattoos.[37] However, now the Q-switched systems yield far superior results. A variety of miscellaneous vascular and melanotic/melanocytic lesions can be treated by the argon laser such as pyogenic granuloma and the telangiectatic component of acne rosacea to name a few.

Rhodamine-123 (Rh-123) is a mitochondria-specific dye that has recently been proven to be an effective tumor chemosensitizing agent for argon laser treatment of SCC cells and melanomas.[39] Rh-123 has not been tested in humans, but its effectiveness has been evaluated in mice. Complete tumor growth inhibition was observed, with tumor eradication occurring in nude mice sensitized with Rh-123 followed by argon laser treatment.[39] No local or systemic toxicity was demonstrated after a 3-week follow-up.[39] The argon laser can also be used to pump tunable dye lasers for similar therapies with other photosensitizers (see "Pumped Continuous Wave Tunable Dye Laser" below).

Technique

The argon laser light is delivered in a continuous wave, although a pulsed mode may be utilized with a shuttering mechanism. Gas is the lasing medium, and the beam is transmitted to tissue through a flexible fiber-optic cable. As with virtually all lasers, the appropriate protective eyewear must be worn by all personnel and patients present. Epidermal melanin can absorb a great amount of the argon laser light prior to deeper penetration; this prevents significant absorption of hemoglobin in tanned or darkly pigmented skin.

Patients with port-wine hemangiomas are often treated with local or general anesthesia. Broad lesions such as PWSs can be treated by using a computer scanner for the laser, providing a more uniform and controlled procedure and eliminating some human error when a lesion is "painted." For facial telangiectasias, the beam diameter can be adjusted to 0.5 to 1.0 mm, which is similar to the size of these lesions. This procedure may be conducted without local anesthesia and the pulse duration limited to less than 0.1 s, minimizing patient discomfort. Minimal crusting occurs post-laser treatment, and a dressing can be used according to the epidermal reaction.

Complications and Contraindications

The depth of penetration of the argon laser is one of its limiting factors. The induced thermal injury is limited to the upper 1 mm of the dermis.[1] Thus, this laser is most effective for lesions confined to the superficial papillary dermis or epidermis. As with other lasers, hypertrophic scarring is the main complication of the laser therapy. Sixty-nine percent of argon laser users reported at least one case of hypertrophic scarring.[32] In patients treated for port-wine hemangiomas, permanent loss of pigmentation has been reported in 20 percent of patients and hypertrophic scarring in approximately 5 percent.[32] In one report, undesirable pigmentary change was noted by 43 percent of physicians.[33] Deeply pigmented lesions also have an increased probability for hypertrophic scarring.

Certain relative contraindications exist for the argon laser. PWSs located on the upper lip or jaw as well as lesions on children younger than 17 years of age (although scarring potential may be related more to the color of the PWS rather than age) are relative contraindications to argon laser treatment. Lesions on the lower extremities also fall into this category. As with other modalities, extra caution should be taken in performing argon laser treatment on individuals who are susceptible to hypertrophic or keloid scarring. Since several lasers are available for treatment of vascular lesions, testing a site with the argon laser before treatment helps to prevent unnecessary complications.

The 577/585-nm Pulsed Dye Laser

Mode: Pulsed (450 µs)
Wavelength: 577 nm originally (subsequently converted to 585 nm)

Target chromophores: Primarily hemoglobin (melanin to a
   lesser extent)
Medium: Liquid, rhodamine-based organic dye

Background

The PDL was the first in a series of new laser systems designed to target specific chromophores and to treat specific lesions. The concept of photothermolysis was developed by Anderson and Parish[4] at Harvard in the early 1980s and was
subsequently applied in the development of this laser. Two
basic concepts are important in understanding photothermolysis: (1) the thermal relaxation time and (2) the absorption
spectrum. The PDL was designed to emit a brief high-energy
pulse of laser light, which should be shorter in length than the
thermal relaxation time of the target structure. The thermal relaxation time is the amount of time needed for the absorbed
heat energy to lose 50 percent of its initial value. If the pulse
is shorter than this thermal relaxation time, then the majority
of absorbed energy is retained by the target structure and nonspecific thermal damage is minimized. In the case of the PDL
at 577 or 585 nm, the target structures are superficial (usually
ectatic) dermal blood vessels found in various benign vascular lesions.

   The other key element in target specificity is the absorption spectrum of the target chromophore. Hemoglobin (in
most cases oxyhemoglobin) is the absorbing chromophore in
blood vessels and has a multipeak absorption spectrum with
peaks around 410 to 429 nm, 540 nm, and 577 nm. The original laser wavelength was set at 577 nm to match the longest
wavelength peak and to get maximum absorption of energy.
Empirical studies on pigskin later showed that by using 585-
nm laser light significantly deeper penetration of thicker lesions was achieved, and no loss in target specificity occurred.[40] Numerous clinical and histologic studies on the use
of this laser have established the remarkable specificity and
capacity to destroy target blood vessels with minimal damage
to surrounding structures and overlying epidermis.[3,4,41–43]

   One consideration in using the laser is the competing absorption of laser energy by overlying melanin in the epidermis.
Melanin absorption decreases with increasing wavelength
through the visible range, hence the reason for choosing the
577-nm absorption peak of hemoglobin, although the shorter
wavelength peaks are actually stronger (larger). For skin types
I to IV (the Fitzpatrick classification) on untanned skin, this
absorption by melanin generally is not significant enough to
cause any problems. On more deeply pigmented skin, however, the laser begins to lose its specificity, and nonspecific absorption in the epidermis diminishes its effectiveness and increases the rate of clinical complications.

Indications

The original indication for the flash lamp-pumped PDL was
the PWS or nevus flammeus, a congenital vascular birthmark
consisting of ectatic superficial venules in the dermis. Much

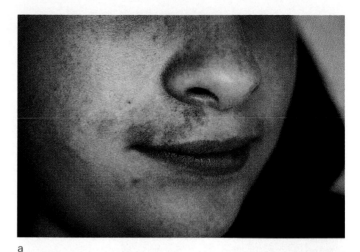

a

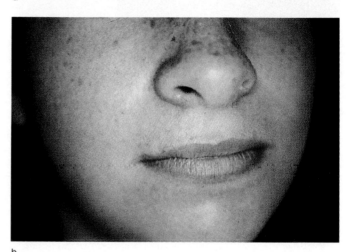

b

Figure 34-1   (*a*) Port-wine stain skin right upper lip; (*b*) after two
treatments with the 585nm pulsed dye laser.

of the early clinical work was done with PWSs on various
anatomic locations in adults and children.[3,4,41–44] Hundreds of
reported cases have documented a high success rate of approximately 75 percent of patients showing 50 percent or
greater lightening, with 30 to 40 percent showing complete or
nearly complete eradication of their lesion.[3,4,41,43] The incidence of scarring has been less than 1 percent overall, which
compares very favorably with the argon laser demonstrating
around 5 percent scarring.[32] In particular, lesions in children
(Fig. 34-1) (including infants) as well as lesions below the
head and neck have shown excellent results with minimal
complications (Fig. 34-2).[3,44]

   Facial telangiectasias are also particularly amenable to
PDL therapy, with a very high response rate.[3,43,45] Ectatic leg
veins, however, appear to be considerably less responsive,
and laser treatment is not equivalent to sclerotherapy. The diffuse telangiectatic matting which sometimes occurs as a complication of leg vein sclerotherapy does, however, respond
fairly well to PDL therapy.

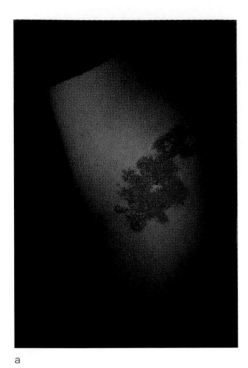

a

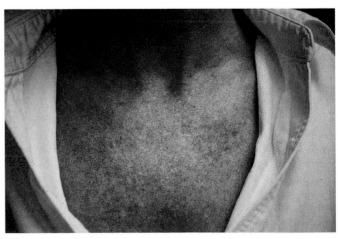

b

Figure 34-2 (*a*) Port-wine stain left posterior thigh; (*b*) after eight treatments with the 585nm pulsed dye laser.

Certain capillary (or strawberry) hemangiomas can also be treated by PDL. In particular, very early, evolving lesions during the first few weeks of life, which are predominantly macular, can be effectively aborted with minimal to no sequelae.[46] Once the lesion has matured or thickened beyond a few millimeters in depth, the laser light cannot penetrate deeply enough for effective therapy, as significant amounts of energy only penetrate 1 to 2 mm of depth.[4,47] This can be partly overcome by using a glass slide to compress the lesion prior to lasering or by using serial treatments. Too much compression can remove the target chromophore. Telangiectatic sequelae

of resolved or resolving hemangiomas can also be treated successfully. Cavernous or mixed hemangiomas do not respond well to the PDL as the vascular channels tend to be too large and deep to be effectively eradicated.

Other lesions which can respond well to the PDL include poikiloderma of Civatte (Fig. 34-3), venous lakes, cherry (senile) angiomas, small angiokeratomas, spider angiomas, and essential or rosacea-related telangiectasias.[1,45] In general, benign vascular ectasias or neoplasias which are predominantly macular or sessile and involve small vessels (venules or capillaries) will probably respond to the 577/585-nm PDL.

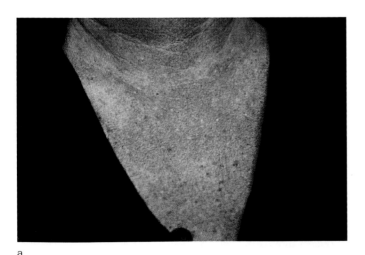

a

b

Figure 34-3 (*a*) Poikiloderma of Civate of chest; (*b*) after five treatments with the 585nm pulsed dye laser.

Technique

The operation of the 577/585-nm PDL is fairly straightforward. The beam is emitted with a 5-mm diameter at the focal point, which is indicated by a fixed-distance handpiece guide at the end of the fiber-optic delivery cable (a 2 mm and 3 mm diameter handpiece is also available for limited or narrow-diameter lesions). A green He-Ne, low-power-aiming beam is emitted through the same fiber-optic system to aid in beam placement. The laser is operated with a foot switch or hand switch depending on the model. Protective eyewear specific to this wavelength must be worn by the operator and all laser room personnel, as the brief pulsed beam is very intense and even reflected light can cause retinal damage. The patient must also wear protective plastic goggles, opaque goggles, or, if eyelid or periorbital lesions are being treated, protective eye shields. If general anesthesia is being used, care must be taken to avoid laser beam exposure to the plastic tubing of intravenous lines or endotracheal tubes, as these are combustible.[48] Also, hair needs to be moistened to prevent ignition.

The energy density is indicated in joules per square centimeter, and treatment parameters generally range from 5 to 7.5 J/cm^2. The lowest effective energy density which will clear the lesion should be employed. In a larger lesion such as a PWS, three to four different energy densities can be tested and evaluated at about 8 weeks for degree of response. The remainder of the lesion can be treated at the appropriate energy level. In general, lesions in children, pink-to-light-red lesions, and those of the neck or eyelids, may be treated with somewhat lower energies. Darker red-to-purplish lesions, or slightly raised areas, may require higher densities.

Pulses can be placed adjacent to one another or with a small (less than 10 percent) degree of overlap; greater overlap than this may result in greater nonspecific damage and an increased likelihood of scarring.[49] The reticular bridging pattern which results is eliminated by treating the interstices between pulses in another 6 to 8 weeks. The immediate clinical response within approximately 1 to 30 s is a blue-gray purpura developing at the site of the laser pulse. Pain is moderate but quite bearable in older children and adult patients. Younger children and infants may be anesthetized or sedated with oral, intravenous, or intramuscular agents. The topical anesthetic Eutectic Mixture of Local Anesthetics (EMLA) can also diminish the pain of laser pulse impact when applied 30 to 90 min prior to treatment.

A given lesion usually requires about two to five complete passes with the laser at about 2-month intervals to achieve maximal lightening or complete fading of facial PWSs. PWSs of the trunk or extremities may require more than ten treatments. Facial telangiectasias usually require only one or two treatments. These general guidelines apply to most lesions that can be treated with the PDL.

Wound care is minimal, as epidermal integrity is generally preserved after treatment. Topical application of an antibiotic ointment is reasonable, and gently cleansing with soap and water is acceptable. Occasionally, some degree of weeping or crusting may occur posttreatment, but healing proceeds regardless over 5 to 14 days.

Complications and Contraindications

Complications with the PDL are quite infrequent. The most common complication, posttreatment hyperpigmentation, which occurs in approximately 10 to 15 percent of patients, is usually focal within a treatment area and usually resolves within 2 to 3 months.[3] Hyperpigmentation is more likely in more darkly pigmented patients and when higher energy levels are used. Hydroquinone can be tried to hasten the resolution of the hyperpigmentation. Hypopigmentation is much less frequent (less than 5 percent) and also usually resolves within months. Scarring occurs at a very low rate of less than 1 percent of treated patients and also is focal within a treatment area when it occurs.[3,43,44] High energy levels as well as extensive overlapping of adjacent pulses may predispose the patient to scarring, which is generally atrophic in nature. Infections are also extremely rare (less than 1 percent) and usually result from inadequate routine posttreatment care.

Contraindications to treatment are few. The primary relative contraindication would be in patients with heavily pigmented skin, although the authors have personally noted partial responses in hispanic patients with type V skin (unpublished data). Patients who have demonstrated prior scarring or nonresolving hyperpigmentation should probably not be treated further unless it can be attributed to high energy levels or extensive overlapping. There are no age restrictions, as infants as young as 6 days old have been treated without complication.[46] Lower extremity lesions below the knee may have a lower response rate but treatment can be attempted.[3] Lesions composed of relatively large vessels, those with deep dermal components, or those thicker than 2 to 3 mm probably will not respond well. Any vascular lesion of questionable origin should be biopsied first and not treated if it is malignant. Lesions previously treated by other modalities (e.g., argon laser, cryotherapy, x-rays) with resultant scarring may appear more atrophic or notably hypopigmented after PDL therapy removes the residual erythema, and such lesions should be judiciously spot tested prior to attempting complete treatment of the lesion.

The Copper Vapor Laser

Mode: Effectively continuous wave (output is via a 6- to 15-kHz train of 30- to 50-ns pulses)
Wavelength: 578 nm (can also emit at 511 nm)
Target chromophores: Primarily hemoglobin (melanin secondarily)
Medium: Gas (copper vapor)

Background

The CVL is one of a number of heavy metal vapor lasers recently developed for industry which are being utilized for medical applications. Initially it was used for fingerprint identification and for military applications.[50] Presently it is being used to treat vascular lesions such as PWSs and telangiectasias and has similar indications to the 585 nm PDL.

Since the CVL laser emits at the same wavelength as the long wavelength absorption peak of oxyhemoglobin, it also can take advantage of the specific absorption of energy by the target chromophore. This laser differs from the PDL in its mode of power output, emitting light in 30- to 50-ns pulses between 6000 and 15,000 times per second, effectively behaving like a continuous wave laser. Clinical reports on the CVL are generally lacking, and comparative studies have focused on the histologic response of CVL versus 577/578-nm PDL. Walker et al.[51] showed that selective damage to PWS ectatic blood vessels occurred with the CVL and that damage to nonvascular structures was minimal. Epidermal damage occurred with a subepidermal blister within 24 h but scarring or histologic fibrosis was not significant.[51] Energy levels of 11 to 15 J/cm^2 produced fairly specific ectatic blood vessel necrosis.

In another study by Tan et al.,[52] reported in 1990, a direct comparison of PDL and CVL was performed on pigskin. Much greater fluences were needed with the CVL than with the PDL to get a clinical end point of purpura (34 versus 7.5 J/cm^2).[52] Also, blood vessel damage from the CVL only extended 0.2 to 0.3 mm versus 0.5 to 0.8 mm from the dermal-epidermal junction with the PDL. If clinical blanching or whitening was used as an end point, the CVL produced more severe damage than the PDL, including papillary dermal collagen injury.[52]

Indications

The indications for the CVL are rather poorly defined in view of the lack of significant numbers of clinical cases reported. It has been used with some success on PWSs as well as telangiectasias with little scarring reported.[50,51] Degree of clinical efficacy has not been reported in meaningful numbers at present. It is reasonable to assume that benign vascular ectasias of the type treatable by PDL (see "The 577/585-nm Pulsed Dye Laser" above) could be treated using the CVL. Decisive comparative clinical studies are needed, but histologic evidence and theoretical considerations indicate a possible greater overall efficacy using the PDL. One preliminary study showed comparable efficacy of the CVL and argon-pumped tunable dye laser.[53]

Technique

The CVL is used as a continuous wave laser, with spot sizes ranging from 1 to 3 mm in diameter delivered via a quartz fiber-optic delivery system.[51,52] Power settings of 0.30 to 3.6 W have been used with incident energy densities up to 11 to 25 J/cm^2 with a scanning rate of about 6 to 9 s/cm^2 over the lesion—generally a PWS.[50,51] The clinical end point is a blanching or whitening of the vascular red lesion, similar to the argon laser end point. Lesions are treated by a hand-held manually directed handpiece or alternatively by a computer-controlled scanning device, which may be more precise. Local or general anesthesia can be used depending on the size of the lesion and patient preference. Re-treatment, if it is attempted, is usually done several months after initial therapy. Since epidermal disruption and weeping posttreatment are very common, antibiotic ointment and a nonocclusive dressing are indicated. As with most lasers, protective eyewear must be used by the patient and all laser room personnel.

Complications and Contraindications

Since no significant series of cases have been reported in detail as of the time of this writing, little conclusive or concrete details or numbers can be given regarding complications. Hyperpigmentation occurs posttreatment but with uncertain frequency. Infections may be more likely with the CVL than with the PDL since epidermal disruption is more frequent; this, however, should be preventable with judicious, conscientious posttreatment wound care. Scarring does occur and probably with a greater frequency than with the PDL. Contraindications are similar to those described in "The 577/585-nm Pulsed Dye Laser" above.

The Argon Pumped Continuous Wave Tunable Dye Laser

Mode: Continuous wave

Wavelength: Variable (commonly 630 to 700 nm for photodynamic therapy and 577 nm for treatment of vascular lesions)

Target chromophores: Exogenous photosensitizers such as hematoporphyrins, rhodamine, and phthalocyanines for photodynamic therapy; hemoglobin for vascular lesions

Medium: The pumping source is a (gas) continuous wave argon laser (see "The Argon Laser" above). The emitting laser uses various organic dyes, each of which can cover an expected range of about 50 to 100 nm. The resulting light is filtered through a precisely machined prism or tuning wedge which allows passage of only a narrow band of monochromatic light of the desired wavelength.

Background

The argon laser-pumped continuous wave tunable dye laser is a very adaptable laser source capable of emitting coherent light of virtually any wavelength from visible blue light to the near infrared range. Currently the two primary medical applications for this laser include (1) treatment of vascular lesions by using low power and a small spot size at 577 nm[35] and (2) treatment of malignant tumors by using photodynamic therapy at various wavelengths such as 630, 675, or 690 nm depending on the particular photosensitizer used.

The use of the tunable dye laser to treat vascular lesions at 577 nm has been reported.[34,35] The technique involves using a lower power 0.1-mm beam, with 577-nm yellow light, and a relatively low power output but high resultant energy density (due to the small spot size). Superior results to argon laser therapy are reported, with comparable or superior results to the PDL at 577 nm.[35,54] Theoretical advantages of the 577-nm wavelength are discussed in "The 577/585-nm Pulsed Dye Laser" above and include deeper penetration with less competing melanin absorption. The narrow spot size of 0.1 mm is well suited to treating individual vessels of facial telangiectasias or PWSs as it fairly closely approximates the diameter of the target vessels.[35,54]

Indications

Generally speaking, benign vascular lesions which contain individually identifiable (with magnification) ectatic vessels of a caliber from roughly 30 to 300 μm should be amenable to the tunable dye laser therapy at 577 nm. Reported lesions previously treated with success include PWSs (a series of 82 patients),[35] as well as facial telangiectasias, hemangiomas, an angiofibroma, and vascular rhinophyma (a total of 25 patients in another study).[54] One study specifically addressed the use of the tunable dye laser for the treatment of PWSs in 92 children.[55] In two studies covering 174 adults and children, 89 percent of adults and 65 percent of children showed 60 percent or greater removal of ectatic PWS vessels, with several showing 80 to 100 percent clearing.[35,54,55]

Technique

The techniques that have been described vary in some respects, but overall follow general procedures. Test areas are treated initially to determine the lowest effective energy that can be used then are evaluated at 4 to 6 weeks. A 100-μm focused spot is used at 577 nm and individual vessels are traced and magnified three to eight times with the use of magnifying binoculars. One technique describes a continuous-pass trace of vessels moving at about $1/2$ cm per s at 80 to 800 mW, while another uses 0.05- to 0.10-s pulses at 700 to 1000 mW sequentially during the treatment of vessels. Resulting irradiances range from about 6000 to 52,000 W/cm². Clinical disappearance or blanching of the vessel is the end point, without graying, charring, or shriveling of the epidermis.[35,54,55] Treatment is generally tolerable without anesthesia, although local (1 percent lidocaine without epinephrine) anesthesia can be used, or heavy sedation or light general anesthesia can be used for younger children.[55] Sessions last 45 to 60 min and can cover 8 to 10 cm².

Posttreatment care may involve topical antibiotics with or without a dressing. Vessels turn brown-red in 2 to 3 days and then disappear in 5 to 10 days with epidermal blistering sometimes occurring.[35,54,55] Posttreatment pain is moderate and similar to a mild sunburn. Re-treatment can be attempted 2 to 3 months after initial therapy, with potential added clinical benefit. Mean number of treatments for maximal clearing averaged about two per lesion.[35,54,55]

Complications and Contraindications

Some epidermal blistering or weeping may occur posttreatment within the first 24 h but will usually not be siginificant. No infections, hypertrophic scarring, abnormal pigmentation, cutaneous depression, or atrophy has been reported.[34,54,55] The procedure is rather slow, tedious, and time consuming, especially when compared with the PDL. The technique is impractical for large lesions. Also, the erythema that results during the treatment makes visibility difficult after several minutes. A good deal of laser experience is important in performing the procedure correctly. Young children and those who are at particular risk when heavy sedation or general anesthesia is used are probably not good candidates unless they can tolerate local anesthesia.

Photodynamic Therapy with the Tunable Dye Laser

Background

As previously mentioned, photodynamic therapy is a relatively new antineoplastic modality using photosensitive compounds which are taken up by tumor tissue and targeted by laser or other light sources to initiate a phototoxic reaction. There is generation of toxic oxygen radicals which go on to destroy the tumors.[56] Relatively low energies are used, avoiding thermal effects and relying on the toxic metabolites to incur damage. The tunable dye laser is one of the primary light sources used in photodynamic therapy because its variable wavelength is entirely adaptable to peak absorption wavelengths of numerous photosensitizer dyes. Many, if not most, have absorption peaks in the 600- to 700-nm range, which is also among the best wavelengths for deep-tissue penetration. Hematoporphyrin derivative (HPD) and its more purified newer derivative dihematoporphyrin ether (DHE) are among the few photosensitizers approved for clinical trials and contain an absorption peak arond 630 nm. Other experimental dyes being investigated include benzoporphyrin derivative (BPD), Rh-123, chlorin e⁶, tetraphenylporphinsulfonate (TPPS), and various phthalocyanines, all of which can be activated with the tunable dye laser.[57–59] Clinically, photodynamic therapy has been used for palliation of lung, esophageal, and genitourinary carcinomas. In addition, this therapy has been used for palliation of cutaneous metastases of breast cancer as well as treatment of primary cutaneous cancers, including BCC, SCC, and malignant melanomas.[60–61]

Indications

Because it is such a new modality, with no real volume of comparative studies, it is impossible to recommend photodynamic therapy as primary therapy, save in exceptional situations. Good results have been obtained for small BCCs by using systemic HPD, but recurrence rates can be high, ranging from 11 percent in basal cell nevus syndrome to greater than 40 percent.[61-63] Topical agents such as TPPS were able to effect a cure in two out of three thin BCCs (less than 2 mm thick), but clinical follow-up was short.[62] In situ SCC (Bowen's) as well as advanced head and neck SCC have been successfully treated with DHE yielding complete to partial response and regression.[62] Phthalocyanines have shown promising results with SCC and melanoma cells in cultures.[57,64] Patients with countless BCCs or Bowen's lesions, with basal cell nevus syndrome or arsenic toxicity, may benefit from wide-field photodynamic therapy as an alternative to more destructive surgical procedures.

Technique

The primary clinical experience has been with HPD and DHE, with the photosensitizer being given intravenously as a bolus injection (about 3 to 4 mg HPD/kg body weight and 1.5 to 2 mg DHE/kg body weight), though actual doses vary depending on the protocol.[63] A period of 24 to 72 h is allowed to elapse before irradiation of the tumor. This seems to allow a possible differential accumulation or retention of photosensitizer within the tumor tissue. Power output typically ranges from 500 mW to about 3 W from the tunable dye laser, with irradiance being highly variable, depending on the size of the lesion, ranging as low as 5 to 10 mW/cm² on larger lesions. Total energy dose in Buchanan et al.'s study[63] ranged from 25 to 200 J/cm². A few patients developed moderate to severe pain during treatment.

With low-energy doses such as 25 J/cm² (for Bowen's), non-tumor-bearing skin was preserved. At greater densities, eschars generally develop and persist for several weeks after with resultant scarring.[63] With HPD or DHE, such exquisite cutaneous photosensitivity occurs that patients must stay out of sunlight for 3 to 4 weeks lest severe phototoxicity develop.

Complications and Contraindications

The most notable adverse effect of clinical photodynamic therapy as it is now administered is the prolonged cutaneous photosensitivity which can last 1 to 2 months.[65] HPD and DHE can also accumulate in visceral organs such as the liver and the spleen and potential long-term effects have not been identified. Newer generation photosensitizers, such as the phthalocyanines, may avert the potential complications of photosensitivity and visceral organ accumulation.[57,64]

As the selectivity of photodynamic therapy for tumor tissue is far from perfect, destruction of overlying and surrounding tissue is common, and scarring or contractures can occur during healing.[63] Recurrences and treatment failures are also still common with photodynamic therapy as recalcitrant, often terminal tumors are commonly being treated.[61-63] Much of the problems of tumor specificity may eventually be overcome with the use of monoclonal antibody photosensitizer conjugates used to target specific tumor antigens.[66,67]

The Gold Vapor Laser

Mode: Pulsed
Wavelength: 628 nm
Target chromophores: Exogenous photosensitizers such as HPD, DHE
Medium: Gas (gold vapor)

Background

The GVL, because of its output near 630 nm, has also been used recently as a light source for photodynamic therapy, not only for cutaneous malignancies but also for benign laryngeal papillomas.[63,68,69] The desired energy is emitted with a brief pulse rather than slowly with continuous wave (as with the tunable dye laser). The results have been comparable in many instances, but some differences between the GVL and tunable dye laser have emerged.[70] In terms of clinical efficacy, two studies found the GVL and argon-pumped tunable dye laser comparable in final results of photodynamic therapy, and one animal study of cutaneous warts found the GVL somewhat superior.[68-70]

Indications

Currently the primary indication for the GVL is in conjunction with photodynamic therapy, specifically with photosensitizers such as HPD or DHE which absorb efficiently in the 630-nm range. As with the argon-pumped tunable dye laser, photodynamic therapy remains primarily an investigational modality and generally is not a first-line therapy for cutaneous malignancies. It has, however, proven successful in treating thin BCCs, Bowen's disease, lesions of basal cell nevus syndrome, and in palliation for cutaneous metastasis of breast cancer.[61-63] Laryngeal papillomas have also been successfully treated.[68] The GVL is probably equivalent to the tunable dye laser in photodynamic therapy, involving such chromophores as HPD or DHE which absorb well at 630 nm, but may become less useful if newer photosensitizers such as BPD (which absorbs maximally around 690 nm) come into widespread clinical application.

Technique

In photodynamic therapy with the GVL, the photosensitizer is given intravenously, exactly as described in "Technique" in "Photodynamic Therapy" above. The targeted tumor is irradiated with the light, often all at once, or section by section if it is particularly large (greater than 100 cm²). Dosage varies with the nature and thickness of the tumor. Delivered energy densities range from 10 to 200 J/cm², with powers ranging from 500 to 1500 mW.

Complications and Contraindications

The hazards and caveats inherent in photodynamic therapy are essentially the same regardless of the stimulating light source; hence, the reader is referred to "Complications and

Contraindications" in "Photodynamic Therapy" above for the clinically relevant complications and warnings.

The Q-Switched Ruby Laser

Mode: Pulsed, Q-switched, 28 to 100 ns
Wavelength: 694 nm
Target chromophores: Melanin and exogenous tattoo pigments
Medium: Solid (ruby crystal)

Background

The continuous wave ruby laser was the first laser developed and used in clinical medicine but was fairly quickly usurped by the CO_2 and argon lasers. Modifications of the basic ruby laser by Q-switching have changed it to a pulsed mode with corresponding new applications. The technique of Q-switching was reported by Goldman et al.[71] in 1965, and as early as 1967 to 1968 Yules et al.[72,73] reported its use on dermal pigment. Reid et al.[74] reported excellent results on tattoos in 1983 and recently reported a 9-year experience.[13] Other recent reports have documented successful treatment of tattoos and pigmented lesions.[75,76]

The term *Q-switched* refers to a change in the quality of the optical resonating structures of the laser so that light is emitted in ultrabrief high-energy pulses, often in the nanosecond range.[7] Thermal destruction is minimal and spatially confined to the absorbing chromophore. Much of the resulting destruction is due to an almost instantaneous vaporization of tissues and water at the target chromophore site, resulting in a shockwave effect mechanically disrupting the target, dispensing pigment and presumably allowing further phagocytosis and clearing. Some thermally mediated chemical changes may also occur in tattoo pigment molecules, resulting in changes in optical properties and subsequent clinical lightening.

Indications

The primary indications for the Q-switched ruby laser include treatment of tattoos—professional, amateur, traumatic, and medical—as well as benign pigmented lesions containing epidermal or dermal melanin. In 1990, Taylor et al.[76] reported treatment of 35 amateur and 22 professional tattoos. After three to four treatments, 78 percent of the amateur and 23 percent of the professional tattoos showed a 75 to 100 percent clearing of the lesions, with an extremely low incidence of scarring (Fig. 34-4). Blue/black pigment responds best; red, green, and yellow intermediate pigment responds much less dramatically.[76] Treatment of 101 amateur and 62 professional tattoos was reported in 1990 with very similar results, showing a superior response with amateur tattoos and only about one-third of professional tattoos responding.[75] Reid et al.[13] in Scotland reported a 9-year cumulative experience with 418 patients with very comparable results. Ashinoff and Geronemus[77] reported a small series of traumatic and medical (radiation portal) tattoos successfully treated without scarring or pigmentary changes.

Treatment of benign pigmented lesions with the Q-switched ruby laser has been fairly successful as well, according to a number of recent reports and presentations. Excellent results in treating café au lait spots, lentigines (including labial), nevus of Ota (Fig. 34-5), and Becker's nevus have been reported from groups in New York and Boston.[78–80] Fairly comparable results on superficial lesions were obtained comparing the Q-switched ruby laser with the other pigmented lesion lasers, including the CVL at 511 nm and pulsed laser at 510 nm.[81,82]

Technique

The beam of the Q-switched ruby laser is typically emitted in a 5- or 6.5-mm spot with a 28-ns pulse (up to 100 ns). Energy densities from about 1 to 10 J/cm^2 are used. Typical tattoo

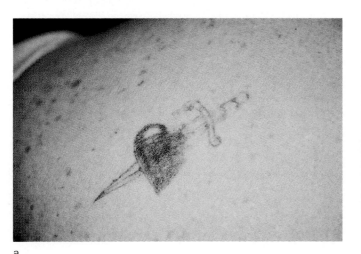
a

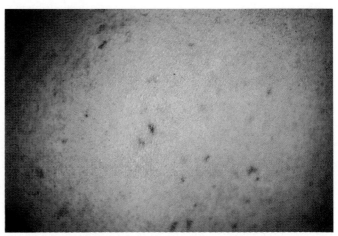
b

Figure 34-4   (*a*) Blue-black tattoo of right back; (*b*) after four treatments with the Q-switched ruby laser.

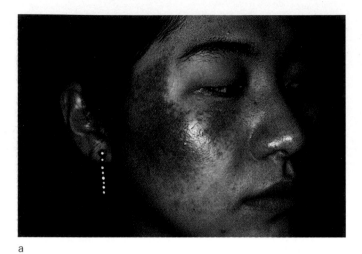
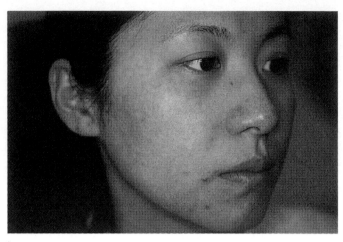

a   b

Figure 34-5   (*a*) Nevus of Ota right side of face; (*b*) after five treatments with the Q-switched ruby laser.

treatment energy densities range from 3 to 8 J/cm², with densities of 3 to 10 J/cm² for benign pigmented lesions. There is typically a 10- to 20-min transient gray-white color appearing on the skin immediately after the pulse, as well as some erythema and edema. A scale-crust usually forms during the 2 weeks postexposure, sometimes containing pigment;[76] occasional vesiculation also occurs. Pain is moderate and generally well tolerated without anesthesia, although some patients may elect for 1 percent lidocaine with epinephrine for local anesthesia, or EMLA cream. Patients may be re-treated at 8-week intervals, although continued fading of lesions may persist for up to several months.[75] Decreased incidence of persistent hypopigmentation has been noted by some physicians when the time between treatments is increased. Often, one to ten treatments of a given lesion are required for optimal fading. In the event of an exudate or vesiculated wound, hydrogen peroxide cleansing followed by antibiotic ointment is indicated. Otherwise, simple soap and water cleansing of a dry treatment site is adequate.

Complications and Contraindications

Complications are relatively few and minor with the Q-switched ruby laser. Scarring seems to be rare at or below 4 J/cm² and none has been reported.[13,75,76] A single case (out of 57 patients) of localized scarring (2 cm²) in a professional tattoo treated at 7 J/cm² has been reported.[76] No scarring has been reported to date in the treatment of benign pigmented lesions.[78–80] The most common reported complication is transient or prolonged confetti-like hypopigmentation at the treatment site. In one study, 39 percent treated at or below 4 J/cm² and 46 percent at or above 5 J/cm² demonstrated this side effect at 1 month posttreatment.[76] Although hypopigmentation tends to normalize or lessen over 4 to 12 months, up to 40 percent of patients may show some degree of hypopigmentation even after a year.[76] Hyperpigmentation is seen much less

commonly, in only 2 to 3 percent of the patients, and may be more frequent in darkly pigmented patients.[13,76] No posttreatment infections have been reported.

Expected transient changes include localized whitening, erythema, edema, occasional vesiculation, and superficial erosions at higher energies. Posttreatment pain is reportedly mild and likened to a mild sunburn.

There are no clear-cut absolute contraindications to Q-switched ruby laser treatment, but there are a number of relevant considerations. Patient compliance is very important as frequently five, six, or even more treatments may be needed to obtain maximal clearing of a given lesion (especially tattoos). Very dark-skinned patients can and have been treated successfully, but greater epidermal damage and slower or less complete fading of the lesions may be a problem.[75] Predominantly red, professional tattoos tend to respond poorly in general. Good results with red tattoos can be achieved with the 510-nm PDL and the Q-switched Nd:YAG laser at 532 nm.[83] Yellow or green pigment is intermediate in response, with blue-black responding best. Finally, in terms of melanotic pigmented lesions, a preliminary report has shown relatively poor response when the Q-switched ruby laser is used on melasma or postinflammatory hyperpigmentation. Use of the laser on these lesions, however, still requires further investigation.[79]

The Q-switched Alexandrite Laser and Pulsed (Dye) Pigment Laser

Mode: Q-switched, 100 to 120 ns (alexandrite laser); pulsed, 300 ns (dye laser)

Wavelength: 755 nm (alexandrite laser); 510 nm fixed (dye laser)

Target chromophores: Melanin (alexandrite or dye laser); exogenous pigments (primarily alexandrite; some respond to dye laser)

Medium: Alexandrite crystal [755 nm (alexandrite laser)]; organic dye [510 nm (dye laser)]

Background

These lasers are used for treating endogenous and exogenous pigmented lesions. The alexandrite laser, with a far red-near infrared output, and the so-called pigmented lesion dye laser (PLDL), with 510-nm output, are available separately but also are housed in a single modified unit for comprehensive treatment of pigmented lesions.

Quite similar in wavelength and pulse width to the Q-switched ruby laser, the alexandrite laser may be slightly more flexible, with a range from 720 to 800 nm and greater tissue penetration.[84] In general, preliminary results on tattoos have been comparable to the Q-switched ruby laser.[84–86] The 510-nm PDL has also shown promising initial results on benign pigmented lesions and may have an advantage over the Q-switched ruby laser for epidermal lesions as melanin has better absorption at 510 nm than 694 nm.[87–89] For deep dermal pigment, the Q-switched ruby laser theoretically has enhanced penetration due to its longer wavelength.

Indications

The alexandrite laser is used primarily for removing tattoo pigment. Black and blue pigments respond best, just as with the Q-switched ruby laser; green and yellow, to some extent; and red, least of all. With the use of red wavelengths (720 nm), some lentiginous lesions responded well in a pigskin model.[84] Several sessions were needed at 720 nm for tattoo treatments, with about 25 percent clearing after each session.[85] Tan and Lizek,[86] in a preliminary report, described 39 subjects with black and blue tattoos treated at 760 nm which responded well after serial treatments, without scarring.[86]

The PLDL at 510 nm is used primarily to clear benign pig-mented lesions but has also shown some success in clearing red tattoo pigment as well.[84,85] Lesions treated have included café au lait macules (Fig. 34-6), lentigines, postinflammatory hyperpigmentation, ephelides, melasma, seborrheic keratoses, and nevus spilus.[87–89] Results are variable and detailed studies are lacking at this time, but lentigines and freckles appear to do fairly well, often with complete clearing after one to four treatments.[87–89] Lip and hand lentigines are reportedly cleared up to 75 percent of the time with one or two treatments.[88]

Technique

The Q-switched alexandrite laser is commercially available with a wavelength at 755 nm. Pulse width on most machines is about 100 ns, with a 3-mm spot size and energy densities ranging up to 8 J/cm^2.[85,86] Typical energies used on tattoos range from 3 to 7 J/cm^2. Much like the Q-switched ruby laser, a transient (10 to 20 min) whitening occurs on the treated site immediately after laser impact. Erythema and edema usually manifest, with purpura sometimes developing.[85] The epidermis generally remains intact, though some crusting can occur at treatment sites. Lesions can be treated at 4- to 6-week intervals to allow time for healing and clinical lightening.[86] About four to seven treatments may be required to clear a tattoo lesion (black and blue do best) or get maximal fading.

The PLDL at 510 nm has a pulse width of 300 ns and a delivered energy density range of 2 to 4 J/cm^2, with a spot size of 5 mm.[87] Typical therapeutic energy densities range from 2 to 3.5 J/cm^2 depending on the response to various test spots at 0.25-J/cm^2 intervals.[89] Treating at too low (or high) energy can result in paradoxical hyperpigmentation.[88] Pain is moderate and anesthesia is usually not needed. Posttreatment transient whitening and/or purpura are very common, with crusting and vesiculation occurring at higher fluences.[87,88]

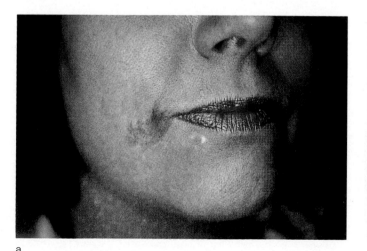 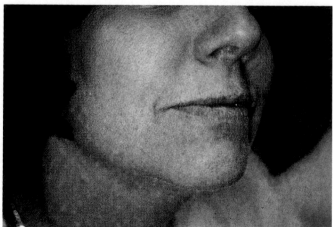

a

b

Figure 34-6   (*a*) Cafe au lait macule right cheek; (*b*) after four treatments with the 510nm pulsed dye laser.

Dressings are sometimes used to protect the treatment site, with healing over 10 to 14 days. Multiple treatments, from two to five or six at 4- to 6-week intervals, may be needed to clear a given pigmented lesion such as a café au lait macule. Lentigines usually require only one or two treatments.

Complications and Contraindications

The alexandrite laser virtually has the same potential side effects and precautionary warnings as the Q-switched ruby laser, and the reader is referred to "Complications and Contraindications" in "The Q-Switched Ruby Laser" for recommendations. Though published reports on scarring are lacking, no scarring has yet been described with the alexandrite laser in preliminary presentations.[84–86] Transient hypopigmentation is the primary side effect thus far described.[85]

The PLDL routinely results in purpura at treatment sites, and sometimes vesicles result, though infections have not been reported. Hyperpigmentation and hypopigmentation can occur and are usually transient but may persist for several months or longer. The incidence of scarring is apparently very low, but local atrophic areas can result from higher fluences, especially at sites below the neck. Caution should be used when more darkly pigmented patients are treated, along with judicious testing for hyperpigmentation. Lesions such as café au lait macules can recur, especially if undertreated.

The Neodymium:Yttrium-Aluminum-Garnet Laser

Mode: Continous wave (pulsed and Q-switching available with 10-ns pulse)
Wavelength: 1064 nm; 532 nm (frequency doubled)
Target chromophores: Tissue proteins
Medium: Solid (Nd:YAG crystal)

Background

The Nd:YAG laser is used in dermatology primarily for deep vascular lesions, though it has been applied to keloids, skin cancer, and various benign growths such as condylomata. The laser is absorbed primarily by tissue proteins, including hemoglobin, and has minimal absorption by water. These properties allow depth of penetration to 4 to 6 mm and coagulation of large vessels up to 4 mm in diameter.[7] Lesions can be "cooked" or coagulated in situ without cutting or vaporizing, as with the CO_2 laser.

The Nd:YAG laser can be used as a cutting tool, especially when contact probes of synthetic sapphire or ceramics are used; the latter mode allows shallower penetration (0.5 to 1 mm) and better control when cutting.[7]

More recent variations on the Nd:YAG include frequency doubling, which uses a potassium titanyl phosphate crystal (KTP) to halve the wavelength, creating a 532-nm beam with characteristics similar to the argon laser. This can be used to treat superficial vascular lesions or as a cutting tool.[90] Use of a Q-switched 1064- and 532-nm Nd:YAG laser is very effective for treating tattoos and pigmented lesions.[83] A 1.32-µm Nd:YAG laser is also available with greater water absorption, better cutting properties, and less thermal spread.[7]

Indications

As previously mentioned, the Nd:YAG laser's role in dermatology has revolved primarily around the treatment of deep benign vascular lesions. Several reports have described successful ablation of carefully selected cavernous and capillary hemangiomas and thick, mature, nodular PWSs, vascular macrocheilia, arteriovenous malformations, and lymphangiomas.[11,91–95] Some scarring is fairly common, but cosmetic results are generally good and superior to the appearance of the original lesion.

In 1984, Abergel et al.[96,97] reported suppression of collagen synthesis in keloid fibroblasts in culture by using the Nd:YAG laser. This was followed by clinical tests in 1984 and 1988 which showed notable flattening and softening of large keloids following treatment with the 1064-nm continuous wave Nd:YAG laser.[96,97] In the authors' experience, long-term follow-up has revealed frequent recurrences.

The Q-switched Nd:YAG laser at 1064-nm has been reported to be useful in the treatment of both professional and amateur tattoos.[83] In particular, 28 tattoos with mostly black ink, which were not responding to the Q-switched ruby laser, were treated with the Q-switched Nd:YAG. Over 50 percent lightening after a single treatment and no scarring or pigmentary changes were reported (Fig. 34-7).[83] Red tattoo ink was similarly treated with the frequency-doubled, 532-nm Nd:YAG, yielding good results in a preliminary report (Fig. 34-8).[83]

Technique

Treatment of vascular lesions with the Nd:YAG laser is typically performed under local anesthesia, but general anesthesia can be used for young children and very large lesions. The roughly 2-mm diameter beam is delivered via a fiber-optic system in 0.1- to 1-s pulses, at powers ranging from 10 to 70 Watts, with energy densities ranging from roughly 400 to 1000 J/cm^2.[11,93,94] Lesions are usually "dotted" but can also be treated with a continuous-stripe technique.[94] The clinical end point is initial blanching and clinical shrinking of the lesion. Compressible lesions can be blanched with a glass slide and lasered through the glass to enhance depth of penetration.[11,94] Edema and serosanguineous exudate are expected, and routine topical wound care is in order. Good to excellent final results were reported for nearly 72 percent of the cases in a study of 26 capillary hemangioma patients.[93]

Similar parameters to those mentioned above are used in keloid treatments, though energy densities may be as low as 60 J/cm^2, with nearly 12 laser exposures at separate intervals.[96] One study of 20 patients, with 17 follow-ups, described very significant to complete flattening in 8 of 17

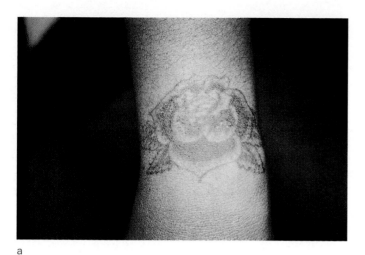
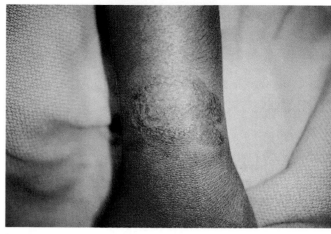

a
b

Figure 34-7   (*a*) Blue-black tattoo of right wrist; (*b*) after four treatments with the Q-switched Nd:YAG laser at 1064nm.

keloids treated.[98] The ultimate usefulness and longevity of this treatment modality remains to be elucidated.

In treating tattoos and pigmented lesions with the Q-switched Nd:YAG laser the energy levels vary depending on the spot size used.

Complications and Contraindications

Some degree of fibrosis is to be expected with most continuous wave Nd:YAG laser treatments, with clinically significant scarring reported in 10 to 30 percent of large vascular lesions.[93,94] Other reported complications include a small incidence of delayed healing, pigmentary changes (hypo- or hyperpigmentation), and postoperative bleeding, ranging from 3 to 8 percent.[93,94] Recurrent telangiectasias as well as treatment failures with lymphangiomas and keloids have also been reported.[94,98]

Caution should be used in treating any capillary or mixed cavernous hemangiomas in young children as they most often spontaneously regress, very often with good cosmetic results. Lesions causing physical or functional impairment or not resolving after 5 to 7 years of age are more appropriate treatment targets.[9] The 585-nm PDL is preferable when treating early capillary hemangiomas as they respond well with minimal or no resulting texture damage. As with any laser, lesions of unclear etiology should not be treated until a diagnosis is established. Also, because of the deep coagulation potential of the Nd:YAG laser, underlying and adjacent anatomic structures must be taken into account prior to surgery and potential benefits weighed against potential risks.

Complications such as scarring and pigmentary alterations, although rare, can occur with the Q-switched Nd:YAG laser.

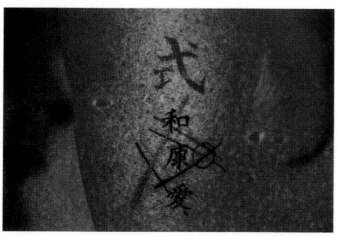
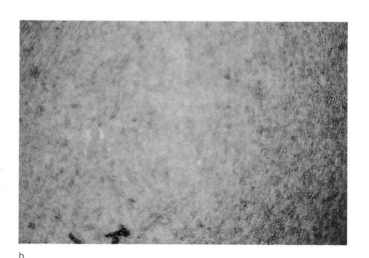

a
b

Figure 34-8   (*a*) Red tattoo of right arm; (*b*) after four treatments with the Q-switched Nd:YAG at 532n.

Low-Energy Laser Systems: Helium-Neon and Gallium-Arsenide Lasers

Mode: Continuous wave (He-Ne); pulsed, 200 ns 100 to 500 Hz (gallium-arsenide)

Wavelength: 632.8 nm (He-Ne); 904 nm (gallium-arsenide)

Target chromophores: Variable (not fully elucidated to date)

Medium: Gas (He-Ne); solid (gallium-arsenide diode)

Background

The application of low-energy laser systems to clinical dermatology remains a controversial and difficult-to-evaluate form of therapy.[8] Most studies revolve around low-energy doses of He-Ne and gallium-arsenide lasers for wound healing and limited immune system modulation. Studies range from well-controlled basic science investigations to poorly controlled, partially described animal and human trials. Much of the wound-healing studies derive from Europe, with a large series of articles published by Mester et al.[5,17,18,99–105] from Hungary, spanning the 1970s. Mester et al. reported significant laser stimulation of wound healing in persistent leg ulcers as well as in animal models. More recently reported and better documented effects include stimulation of collagen synthesis by fibroblasts in vitro and in vivo in various animal models and increased tensile strength in irradiated healing wounds.[6,104–111] A minority of basic studies found no such effects.[112–114] Immune modulatory effects include stimulation of monocytes to release growth factors and monokines, as well as inhibition of lymphocyte function and skin allograft rejection.[5,19,115,116]

Indications

As no low-energy lasers are currently approved by the Food and Drug Administration for clinical therapy, no recommendations along these lines are currently in order. As an investigational tool, however, the potential for the stimulation of ulcer or surgical wound healing cannot be entirely ignored with such a diverse (and sometimes controversial) body of evidence. Some potential for immune modulation of various lesions or skin grafts may also exist. Clearly, well-controlled, large prospective trials are needed to assess these potentials.

Technique

No general guidelines for treatment can be given because experimentally effective fluences range from fractions of a millijoule per centimeter to several joules per square centimeter for various applications.[19,109] Power outputs are typically in the milliwatt range, and wound-healing fluences often approach 1 J/cm^2. The entire field is irradiated at low fluences in sections or all at once, usually with neglible thermal changes.

Complications and Contraindications

To date, no adverse effects have been reported with the low-energy lasers described. Thermal damage is generally nonexistent, and these wavelengths are nonmutagenic as far as has been established. Lesions or debilitating conditions should generally not be treated with low-energy laser, experimental protocols where establed primary therapies remain to be tried.

THE FUTURE OF LASERS IN DERMATOLOGY

Many laser systems and their applications have been described in the preceding pages, and, notably, more than half have been developed in some form over the past 10 years. The explosion of new lasers and new applications of existing lasers within the field of dermatology reflects a rapidly increasing understanding of laser-tissue-chromophore interactions at the molecular, tissue, and organism levels. Increasingly target-specific modalities and wavelength combinations will continue to refine and expand the application of lasers to an increasing number of conditions. The continued use and characterization of exogenous chromophores will also increase the number of laser-treatable conditions and render therapy more effective, with a probable increase for photodynamic therapy in the treatment of neoplastic disease.

Laser therapy can and should be a dynamic part of every dermatologist's therapetic armamentarium, whether by direct use or referral to appropriate centers, when indicated. The fact that knowledge of, and familiarity with, relevant laser systems is now a part of the core curriculum of all accredited dermatology residences is an indication of the degree of legitimacy which laser therapy has achieved in recent years. As lasers become more accessible and perhaps affordable (with the advent of inexpensive portable, and powerful diode lasers), they will become yet more prevalent in the everyday practice of dermatology. Despite the hyperbole and glitz sometimes surrounding lasers, it is the authors' hope that this chapter has presented a reasonable overview of the potential uses and inherent limitations of medical lasers and a realistic approach to their application. Extensive training, more detailed and specific references, and a thorough familiarity with laser safety techniques are urged before the reader attempts medical and surgical therapy as outlined in these pages.

REFERENCES

1. Garden JM, Geronemus RG: Dermatologic laser surgery. *J Dermatol Surg Oncol* **16:**156, 1990

2. Hanke CW: Lasers in dermatology. *Indiana Med* **June:**394, 1990

3. Glassberg E et al: The flashlamp pumped 577nm tunable dye laser: Clinical efficacy and in vitro studies. *J Dermatol Surg Oncol* **14:**1200, 1988

4. Anderson RR, Parish JA: Microvasculature can be selectively

damaged using dye lasers: A basic therapy and experimental evidence in human skin. *Lasers Surg Med* **1:**263, 1981

5. Namenyi J et al: Effect of laser irradiation and immunosuppressive treatment on survival of mouse skin allotransplants. *Acta Chir Acad Sci Hung* **16:**327, 1975

6. Abergel RA et al: Biostimulation of wound healing by lasers: Experimental approaches in animal models and in fibroblast cultures. *J Dermatol Surg Oncol* **13:**127, 1987

7. Lipow M: *Laser Physics Made Simple.* Chicago, Year Book, 1986

8. Basford JR: Low energy laser therapy: Controversies and new research findings. *Lasers Surg Med* **9:**1, 1989

9. Glassberg E et al: Hemangiomas and other vascular malformations, in *Aesthetic Dermatology,* edited by LC Parrish, GP Lask. New York, McGraw-Hill, 1990, pp 50–57

10. Garden JM et al: The pulsed dye laser: Its use at 577nm wavelength. *J Dermatol Surg Oncol* **12:**134, 1987

11. Landthaler M et al: Neodymium-YAG laser therapy for vascular lesions. *J Am Acad Dermatol* **14:**107, 1986

12. David LM et al: CO_2 laser abrasion for cosmetic and therapeutic treatment of facial actinic damage. *Cutis* **43:**583, 1989

13. Reid WH et al: Q-switched ruby laser treatment of tattoos: A nine year experience. *Br J Plast Surg* **43:**663, 1990

14. Bailin PL et al: Removal of tattoos by CO_2 laser. *J Dermatol Surg Oncol* **6:**997, 1980

15. Olbricht SM et al: Complications of cutaneous laser surgery. *Arch Dermatol* **123:**345, 1987

16. Groot DW, Johnson PA: Lasers and advanced dermatologic instrumentation. *Australas J Dermatol* **28:**77, 1987

17. Mester E et al: Effect of laser rays on wound healing. *Am J Surg* **122:**532, 1971

18. Mester E et al: Stimulation of wound healing by laser rays. *Acta Chir Acad Sci Hung* **13:**315, 1972

19. Ohta A et al: Laser modulation of human immune system: Inhibition of lymphocyte proliferation by a gallium-arsenide laser at low energy. *Lasers Surg Med* **7:**199, 1987

20. Stanley RJ, Roenigk RK: Actinic cheilitis: Treatment with the carbon dioxide laser. *Mayo Clin Proc* **63:**230, 1988

21. Bailin PL et al: CO_2 laser modification of Mohs surgery. *J Dermatol Surg Oncol* **7:**621, 1981

22. Dougherty TJ: Photoradiation therapy for cutaneous and subcutaneous malignancies. *J Invest Dermatol* **77:**122, 1981

23. Schweitzer VG: Photodynamic therapy for treatment of head and neck cancer. *Otolaryngol Head Neck Surg* **102:**225, 1990

24. Bailin PL, Ratz JL: Use of the CO_2 laser in dermatologic surgery, in *Lasers in Cutaneous Medicine and Surgery,* edited by JL Ratz. Chicago, Year Book, 1985, pp 73–104

25. Ratz JL: Laser therapy update, *Current Issues in Dermatology,* edited by JP Callen. Boston, GK Hall, 1984, pp 244–251

26. Cotterill JA: The use of lasers in dermatology. *Practitioner* **228:**1033, 1984

27. Bailin PL et al: Laser therapy of the skin: A review of principles and applications. *Otolaryngol Clin North Am* **23:**123, 1990

28. Ratz JL et al: CO_2 laser treatment of port-wine stains: A preliminary report. *J Dermatol Surg Oncol* **8:**1039, 1982

29. Garden JM et al: Papillomavirus in the vapor of carbon dioxide laser treated verrucae. *JAMA* **259:**1199, 1988

30. Lunegan D: Practical laser safety, in *Surgical Applications of Lasers,* 2d ed, edited by JA Dixon. Chicago, Year Book, 1987, pp 79–94

31. Ratz JL, Bailin PL: The case for use of the carbon dioxide laser in the treatment of port-wine stains. *Arch Dermatol* **123:**74, 1987

32. Ratz JL et al: Post-treatment complications of the argon laser. *Arch Dermatol* **121:**714, 1985

33. Dobry MM et al: Carbon dioxide laser vaporization: Relationship of scar formation to power density. *J Invest Dermatol* **93:**75, 1989

34. Apfelberg DB et al: Expanded role of the argon laser in plastic surgery. *J Dermatol Surg Oncol* **9:**145, 1983

35. Scheibner A, Wheeland RG: Argon-pumped tunable dye laser therapy for facial port-wine stain hemangiomas in adults: A new technique using small spot size and minimal power. *J Dermatol Surg Oncol* **15:**277, 1989

36. Apfelberg DB et al: Treatment of nevus araneus by means of an argon laser. *J Dermatol Surg Oncol* **4:**172, 1978

37. Apfelberg DB et al: The argon laser for cutaneous lesions. *JAMA* **245:**2073, 1981

38. Apfelberg DB et al: Argon laser treatment of decorative tattoos. *Br J Plast Surg* **32:**232, 1979

39. Catro DJ et al: Rhodamine-123 as a new laser dye: In vivo study of dye effects on murine metabolism, histology and ultrastructure. *Laryngoscope* **99:**1057, 1989

40. Tan OT et al: Action spectrum of vascular specific injury using pulsed irradiation. *J Invest Dermatol* **92:**868, 1989

41. Garden JM et al: The treatment of port-wine stains by the pulsed dye laser: Analysis of pulse duration and long-term therapy. *Arch Dermatol* **124:**889, 1988

42. Glassberg E et al: Cellular effects of the pulsed tunable dye laser at 577nm on human endothelial cells, fibroblasts and erythrocytes: An in vitro study. *Lasers Surg Med* **8:**567, 1988

43. Polla LL et al: tunable pulsed dye laser for the treatment of benign vascular ectasias. *Dermatologica* **174:**11, 1987

44. Tan OT, Gilchrest BA: Laser therapy for selected cutaneous vascular lesions in the pediatric population: A review. *Pediatrics* **82:**652, 1988

45. Gonzalez E et al: Treatment of telangiectasias and other benign vascular lesions with the 577 nm pulsed dye laser. *J Am Acad Dermatol* **27:**220, 1992

46. Glassberg E et al: Capillary hemangiomas: Case study of a novel laser treatment and a review of therapeutic options. *J Dermatol Surg Oncol* **15:**1214, 1989

47. Garden JM et al: Effect of dye laser pulse duration on selective vascular cutaneous injury. *J Invest Dermatol* **87:**653, 1986

48. Epstein RH et al: Incendiary potential of the flashlamp pumped 585 nm tunable dye laser. *Anesth Analg* **71:**171, 1990

49. Kurban AK et al: Effect of single versus multiple pulse on cutaneous vasculature (abstract). *Lasers Surg Med* (suppl 1):44, 1989

50. Goldman L et al: New developments with the heavy metal vapor lasers for the dermatologist. *J Dermatol Surg Oncol* **13:**163, 1987

51. Walker EP et al: Histology of port-wine stains after copper vapour laser treatment. *Br J Dermatol* **121:**217, 1989

52. Tan OT et al: Histologic comparison of the pulsed dye laser and copper vapor laser effects on pig skin. *Lasers Surg Med* **10:**551, 1990

53. Schliftman AB, Brauner G: The comparative tissue effects of copper vapor laser (578nm) OSC on vascular lesions (abstract). *Lasers Surg Med* **8:**188, 1988

54. Orenstein A, Nelson JS: Treatment of facial vascular lesions with a 100u spot 577nm pulsed continuous wave dye laser. *Ann Plast Surg* **23:**310, 1989

55. Scheibner A, Wheeland RG: Use of argon-pumped tunable dye laser for port-wine stains in children. *J Dermatol Surg Oncol* **17:**735, 1991

56. Dougherty TJ: Photodynamic therapy, in *Methods in Porphyrin Photosensitization,* edited by D Kessel. New York, Plenum, 1985, pp 313–328

57. Glassberg E et al: Laser-induced photodynamic therapy with aluminum phthalocyanine tetrasulfonate as the photosensitizer: Differential phototoxicity in normal and malignant human cell lines in vitro. *J Invest Dermatol* **94:**604, 1990

58. Sacchini V et al: Preliminary clinical studies with PDT by topical TPPS administration in neoplastic skin lesions. *Lasers Surg Med* **7:**6, 1987

59. Castro DJ et al: Rhodamine 123 as a chemosensitizing agent for argon laser therapy. *Arch Otolaryngol Head Neck Surg* **113:**1176, 1987

60. Glassberg E et al: Skin cancer meets "star wars": Photodynamic therapy. *Int J Dermatol* (In Press)

61. Dougherty TJ: Photoradiation therapy for cutaneous and subcutaneous malignancies. *J Invest Dermatol* **77:**122, 1981

62. Tse DT et al: Hematoporphyrin derivative photoradiation therapy in managing nevoid basal cell carcinoma syndrome. *Arch Ophthalmol* **102:**990, 1984

63. Buchanan RB et al: Photodynamic therapy in the treatment of malignant tumors of the skin and head and neck. *Eur J Surg Oncol* **15:**400, 1989

64. Glassberg E et al: Hyperthermia potentiates the effects of aluminum phthalocyanine tetrasulfonate-mediated photodynamic toxicity in human malignant and normal cell lines. *Lasers Surg Med* **11:**432, 1991

65. Gregory RO, Goldman L: Application of photodynamic therapy in plastic surgery. *Lasers Surg Med* **6:**62, 1986

66. Singer CRJ et al: Differential phthalocyanine photosensitization of acute myeloblastic leukaemia progenitor cells: A potential purging technique for autologous bone marrow transplantation. *Br J Haematol* **68:**417, 1988

67. Singer CRJ et al: Phthalocyanine photosensitization for in vitro elimination of residual acute non-lymphoblastic leukaemia: Preliminary evaluation. *Photochem Photobiol* **46:**745, 1987

68. Shikowitz MJ: Comparison of pulsed and continuous wave light in photodynamic therapy of papillomas: An experimental study. *Laryngoscope* **102:**300, 1992

69. Go P et al: Laser photodynamic therapy for papilloma viral lesions. *Arch Otolaryngol Head Neck Surg* **116:**1177, 1990

70. McKenzie AL, Carruth JAS: A comparison of gold vapour and dye lasers for photodynamic therapy. *Lasers Surg Med* **1:**117, 1986

71. Goldman L et al: Radiation from a Q-switched ruby laser. *J Invest Dermatol* **44:**69, 1965

72. Yules RB et al: The effect of Q-switched ruby laser radiation on dermal tattoo pigment in man. *Arch Surg* **95:**179, 1967

73. Laub DR et al: Preliminary histopathological observation of Q-switched ruby laser radiation on dermal tattoo pigment in man. *J Surg Res* **8:**220, 1968

74. Reid WH et al: Q-switched ruby laser treatment of black tattoos. *Br J Plast Surg* **36:**455, 1983

75. Scheibner A et al: A superior method of tattoo removal using the Q-switched ruby laser. *J Dermatol Surg Oncol* **16:**1091, 1990

76. Taylor CR et al: Treatment of tattoos by Q-switched ruby laser. *Arch Dermatol* **126:**893, 1990

77. Ashinoff R, Geronemus RG: Rapid response of traumatic tattoos to treatment with the Q-switched ruby laser (abstract). *Lasers Surg Med* (suppl 4):71, 1992

78. Ashinoff R, Geronemus RG: Q-switched ruby laser treatment of benign epidermal pigmented lesions (abstract). *Lasers Surg Med* (suppl 4):73, 1992

79. Grevelink JM et al: Update on the treatment of benign pigmented lesions with the Q-switched ruby laser (abstract). *Lasers Surg Med* (suppl 4):73, 1992

80. Geronemus RG, Ashinoff R: Q-switched ruby laser therapy of nevus of Ota (abstract). *Lasers Surg Med* (suppl 4):74, 1992

81. McMeekin TO, Goodwin D: Comparison of Q-switched ruby, pigmented lesion dye laser and copper vapor laser treatment of benign pigmented lesions of the skin (abstract). *Lasers Surg Med* (suppl 4):74, 1992

82. Goldberg DJ: Benign pigmented lesions of the skin: Treatment with Q-switched ruby laser, copper vapor, and pigmented lesion laser (abstract). *Lasers Surg Med* (suppl 4):72, 1992

83. Kilmer SL et al: Q-switched Nd:YAG laser (1064nm) effectively treats Q-switched ruby laser resistant tattoos (abstract). *Lasers Surg Med* (suppl 4):72, 1992

84. Brauner GJ, Schliftman AB: Treatment of pigmented lesions of the skin with alexandrite laser (abstract). *Lasers Surg Med* (suppl 4):72, 1992

85. Fitzpatrick RE et al: The alexandrite laser for tattoos: A preliminary report (abstract). *Lasers Surg Med* (suppl 4):72, 1992

86. Tan OT, Lizek R: Alexandrite (760nm) laser treatment of tattoos (abstract). *Lasers Surg Med* (suppl 4):72, 1992

87. Ruiz-Esparza J et al: Selective melanothermolysis: A histologic study of the Candela 510nm pulsed dye laser for pigmented lesions (abstract). *Lasers Surg Med* (suppl 4):73, 1992

88. Fitzpatrick RE et al: Treatment of benign pigmented lesions with the Candela 510nm pulsed laser (abstract). *Lasers Surg Med* (suppl 4):73, 1992

89. Brauner GJ, Scliftman AB: Treatment of pigmented lesions with the flashlamp pumped PLDL ("brown spot") laser (abstract). *Lasers Surg Med* (suppl 4):73, 1992

90. Keller G et al: Use of the KTP for cosmetic facial surgery (abstract). *Lasers Surg Med* (suppl 4):71, 1992

91. Rosenfeld H et al: The treatment of cutaneous vascular lesions with the Nd:YAG laser. *Ann Plast Surg* 21:223, 1988

92. Landthaler M, Hohenleutner U: Laser treatment of congenital vascular malformations. *Int Angiol* 9:208, 1990

93. Achauer BM, VanderKamm VM: Capillary hemangioma (strawberry mark) of infancy: Comparison of argon and Nd:YAG laser treatment. *Plast Reconstr Surg* 84:60, 1989

94. Rosenfeld H, Sherman R: Treatment of cutaneous and deep vascular lesions with the Nd:YAG laser. *Lasers Surg Med* 6:20, 1986

95. Dixon JA, Gilbertson JJ: Argon and neodymium YAG laser therapy of dark nodular port wine stains in older patients. *Lasers Surg Med* 6:5, 1986

96. Abergel RP et al: Laser treatment of keloids: A clinical trial and an in vitro study with Nd:YAG laser. *Lasers Surg Med* 4:291, 1984

97. Abergel RP et al: Control of connective tissue metabolism by lasers: Recent developments and future prospects. *J Am Acad Dermatol* 11:1142, 1984

98. Sherman R, Rosenfeld H: Experience with the Nd:YAG laser in the treatment of keloid scars. *Ann Plast Surg* 21:231, 1988

99. Mester E et al: Stimulation of wound healing by means of laser rays. *Acta Chir Acad Sci Hung* 14:347, 1973

100. Kovacs I et al: Stimulation of wound healing by laser rays as estimated by means of rabbit ear chamber method. *Acta Chir Acad Sci Hung* 15:427, 1974

101. Mester E et al: Laser stimulation of wound healing. *Acta Chir Acad Sci Hung* 15:203, 1974

102. Mester E et al: Laser stimulation of wound healing. *Acta Chir Acad Sci Hung* 17:49, 1976

103. Mester E et al: Stimulation of wound healing by means of laser rays. *Acta Chir Acad Sci Hung* 19:163, 1978

104. Lyons RF et al: Biostimulation of wound healing in vivo by a helium-neon laser. *Ann Plast Surg* 18:47, 1987

105. Saperia D et al: Demonstration of elevated type I and type III procollagen mRNA levels in cutaneous wounds treated with the helium-neon laser: Proposed mechanism for enhanced wound healing. *Biochem Biophys Res Commun* 138:1123, 1986

106. Bosatra M et al: In vitro fibroblast and dermis fibroblast activation by laser irradiation at low energy. *Dermatologica* 168:157, 1984

107. Kana JS et al: Effect of low power density laser radiation on healing of open skin wounds in rats. *Arch Surg* 116:293, 1984

108. Braverman B et al: Effect of helium-neon and infrared laser irradiation on wound healing in rabbits. *Lasers Surg Med* 9:50, 1989

109. Enwemeka CS: Laser biostimulation of healing wounds: Specific effects and mechanisms of action. *J Orthop Sports Phys Ther* 9:333, 1988

110. Van Breugel HHFI, Bar PR: Power density and exposure time of He-Ne laser irradiation are more important than total energy dose in photo-biomodulation of human fibroblasts in vitro (abstract). *Lasers Surg Med* (suppl 4):10, 1992

111. Lievens P: Infrared laser therapy and bedsores (abstract). *Lasers Surg Med* (suppl 4):12, 1992

112. Hunter J et al: Effects of low energy laser on wound healing in a porcine model. *Lasers Surg Med* 3:285, 1988

113. Hallman HO et al: Does low energy helium-neon laser irradiation alter "in vitro" replication of human fibroblasts? *Lasers Surg Med* 8:125, 1988

114. Anneroth G et al: The effect of low-energy infrared laser radiation on wound healing in rats. *Br J Oral Maxillofac Surg* 26:12, 1988

115. Shields TD et al: The effect of laser irradiation upon human mononuclear leukocytes in vitro (abstract). *Lasers Surg Med* (suppl 4):11, 1992

116. Ghali LR, Dyson M: Comparison of the effect of light irradiation on the process of angiogenesis in vivo. *Lasers Surg Med* (suppl 4):12, 1992

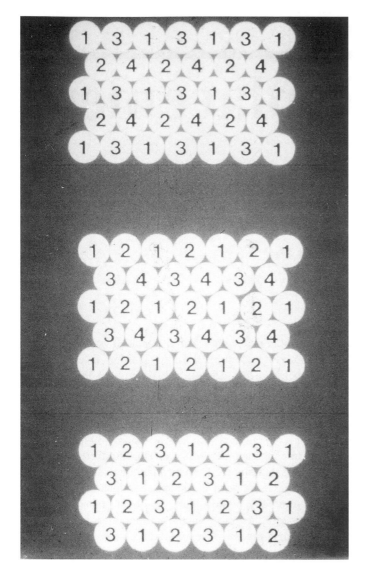

Figure 35-1 Any area of alopecia can be solidly filled in using one of three ways. The method shown in the superior part of this figure is the usual four-stage approach. In the middle of the figure, still-hairbearing areas are treated as shown. The approach at bottom is the three-stage filling described by the Orentriechs.

MINIGRAFTING

Minigrafting, a term first coined by Bradshaw, has been increasingly incorporated into hair transplanting in the last 5 to 10 years.[4–12] Minigrafting can be further classified into three subtypes:

1. Micrografting: Round grafts or strips of donor hair are very carefully sliced into small pieces containing one to three hairs each and placed into holes made with a no. 16-gauge hypodermic needle. These grafts are used anterior to the hairline to "soften" it and thereby make it less abrupt and more natural as well as to fill small hairless spaces be-

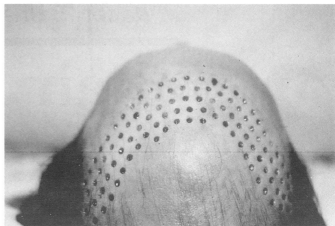

Figure 35-2 The basic pattern for the first (and second) session is a four- or five-row "U"-shaped recipient area.

tween grafts and within an individual graft where hair has not grown evenly across its surface. The terms *unigrafts* and *Mmunigrafts* have been used to describe single hair grafts obtained, inserted, and utilized in the same way.[7]

2. Round minigrafting: Grafts as small as 1.0 mm are obtained by using very small trephines, or, alternately, strips of donor tissue, or grafts of various sizes—usually 3.25- to 5-mm in diameter—are cut into sections containing approximately three or four and five or six hairs, respectively. These are inserted into small round holes prepared with a 1- to 2.5-mm diameter trephine. They too are used to fill small hairless spaces between or within previously transplanted grafts. In addition, they are employed extensively in females undergoing the procedure, as women characteristically have small hairless spaces interspersed between areas of diffuse, though sparse, hair growth.[8] They are also used exclusively by some operators to transplant entire areas in an effort to minimize the transitional "clumpiness" seen with punch grafting in sparse or bald areas.[9]

3. Slit grafting: Grafts similar to that described for round minigrafting are inserted into slits usually made by a no. 15 or no. 15A scalpel blade, rather than into round holes.[10–12] They are used for the same purpose described for round minigrafts but in the author's opinion are more successful in minimizing transitional clumpiness and in addition are especially useful in thickening areas of diffuse thinning in females as well as males in whom the objective is less dense filling (see "The Recipient Area" below). They are now used almost exclusively by the authors for transplanting the vertex where they produce a very natural look with only two or three sessions, and in combination with micrografts for the anterior 2–3 cm of the hairline when some sparseness in this zone is acceptable or even preferred. An added advantage of slit grafting is that because the incisions can be made between existing hairs,

few or none of them are eliminated when one is operating in still hair-bearing areas. One can thereby avoid the temporary thinning previously seen with early hair transplanting and in hair transplanting in females.

While the grafts for round minigrafting and slit grafting are frequently obtained by quartering a 4.5-mm round graft or bisecting a 3.75-mm round graft, the author tries try to avoid the terms *quarter graft* and *bisected graft*. Sometimes, for example, one can only trisect a 4.5-mm round graft if seeking three to four hairs per section as the hair in that graft is not dense enough, and, as alluded to earlier, the size of the round graft may vary to compensate for this. The meaning of quarter graft therefore is a vague one, requiring further definition of the size of the graft that was its source. On other occasions, one obtains the three- to four-hair and five- to six-hair sections by dividing a strip of hair-bearing skin instead of a round graft. Thus, the author prefers to utilize terms such as *"small"* (3–4 hair) and *"large"* (5–6 hair) slit grafts and *"small"* and *"large"* round minigrafts that explain more precisely the number of hairs that are being transferred and into what type of recipient site than do terms such as *minigrafting* or *quarter grafting* and *bisected grafts* whose meanings are less precise and in addition will vary from author to author.

All the types of minigrafts shed their crusts earlier and are therefore easier to camouflage postoperatively, are faster healing, and grow hair earlier (at approximately 2 months) than standard-sized round grafts. Their most important disadvantages are initially increased cost; compression of too much hair into narrow slits, producing artificially dense lines of hair in some individuals, and overall decreased density in the area being treated (see "The Recipient Area" below). The latter occurs because when slit grafts are utilized, no bald or potentially bald areas are actually being replaced with permanently hair-bearing ones as occurs with round grafting. Hair is only

being added to the area of alopecia or future alopecia. Sessions of minigrafting or a combination of minigrafting and standard round grafting (see "The Recipient Area") are done within the same time intervals described previously for standard round grafting.

Patients are in a prone position on their stomach for operations on the donor area and on their back with the head of the bed raised to a 45° angle for operations on the recipient area, except if the vertex is the recipient site, in which case the patient is usually placed in a sitting position. A prone pillow is especially useful when the occipital area is the donor site (Fig. 35-3). This pillow allows the patient to breathe easily with his or her face directed straight into the operating table. Hand punches are usually used in the recipient area but specially designed power punches are employed in the donor area.[13]

PLANNING

Choosing the hairline pattern begins with an estimate of where one expects the anterior-superiormost points of permanent temporal hair to be. These points are marked, and a third point is chosen anteriorly in the midline, to which a line can be drawn, joining the two temporal points and producing a natural-looking ovoid or slightly bell-shaped hairline (Fig. 35-4). The positioning of this midline point involves many factors, including the length of the face, patient objectives, and number of grafts available, but Norwood[14] has rightly pointed out that the hairline, when viewed laterally, should be more or less horizontal or the effect will be aesthetically unsatisfactory.

Whenever ARs are contemplated during the course of treatment, allowances must be made for how they will affect the chosen hairlines and part line. In addition, grafts should not be put into areas that could be excised instead. ARs not only decrease the size of the bald area, which thereby can be satisfactorily transplanted with fewer grafts, they also raise the superiormost border of the permanent fringe moving the future "part," which must almost always go through the untransplanted permanent fringe, to a cosmetically more acceptable level (Fig. 35-5).[15] ARs are discussed in greater detail elsewhere in this text. Some idea of the number of grafts used to cover given areas can be gleaned from Figs. 35-6–35-9.

In general, the lighter the color and the finer the texture of hair, the better. White or salt-and-pepper-colored hair is ideal (Fig. 35-6), with the second best being blonde (Fig. 35-7). The exception to these general rules is a patient with very coarse and curly Negroid-type hair. These latter characteristics produce an appearance of greater than actual density, and one can adequately transplant any given recipient site with fewer grafts than would be required in a straight-haired Caucasian (Fig. 35-8). The subject of transplanting in black patients has been covered in detail elsewhere.[16] Orientals tend to require significantly fewer grafts than the average Caucasian

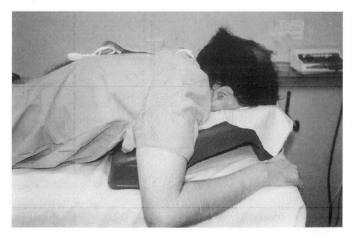

Figure 35-3 A "prone pillow" is especially useful when the occipital area is the donor site. It allows the patient to face directly down, optimally presenting the occipital area, while receiving fresh air laterally.

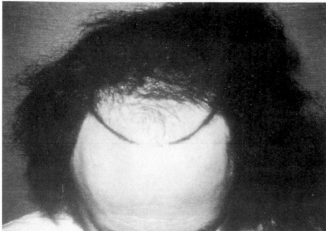

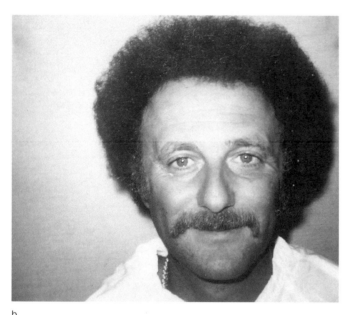

Figure 35-8 (*a*) Before transplanting. (*b*) After three transplanting sessions (290 grafts). This patient's curly, kinky, Negroid hair looks much thicker than it actually is, providing a good result with fewer grafts and sessions. His hair is cut relatively short so it curls on itself and styles easily with a "messing" action after hair is washed.

latter problem. It cannot be overemphasized that punch transplanting in patients who are not yet bald should only be carried out by physicians who have considerable experience. When punch transplanting is done properly, however, the effects are very gratifing (Figs. 35-9*a–e*).

All of the above comments relating to early transplanting apply equally to operating on women. In addition, of course one should be certain that a female patient has good prospects for maintaining a "male pattern" of androgenic alopecia (i.e., maintaining a relatively dense donor rim while thinning centrally). Some variations in approach are recommended in fe-

males. The most important are the treatment of only the left or right side of the recipient site at any given session and the use of smaller sessions, for example, 50 to 60 grafts per session.[18] Both allow for easier postsurgical camouflage. Smaller sessions also require lower doses of local anesthetic. Women, because of their smaller size, are more prone to show signs of lidocaine toxicity if larger sessions are employed. Lastly, transplanting only the left or right side of any given area of thinning allows for accurate assessment of the results

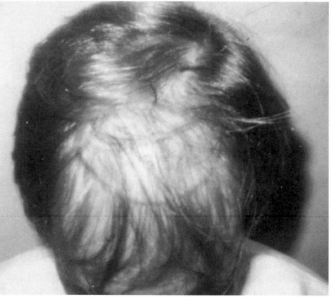

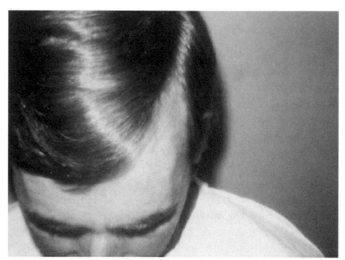

Figure 35-9 (*a*) Before transplanting. This patient chose to begin treatment before the recipient area was totally alopecic and while there was sufficient adjacent hair to comb over and completely camouflage the surgery once the hair was washed postoperatively. (*b*) Six months after the second transplanting session (200 grafts). The patient was able to postpone further treatment for over two years as hair density remained satisfactory from his two sessions.

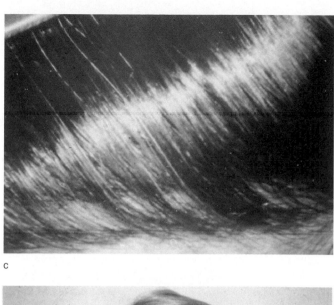

c

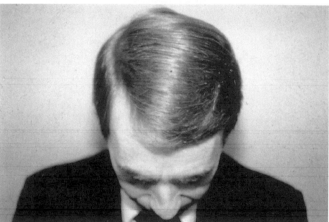

d

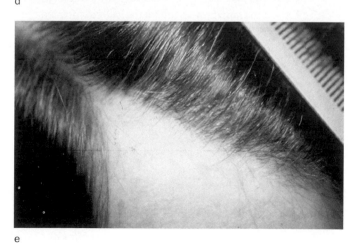

e

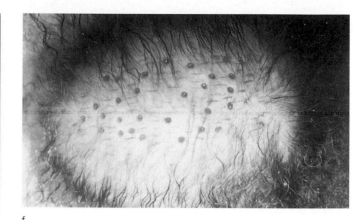

f

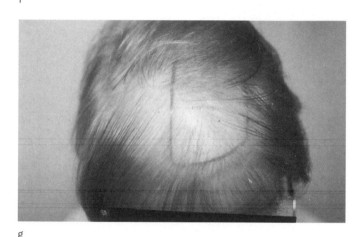

g

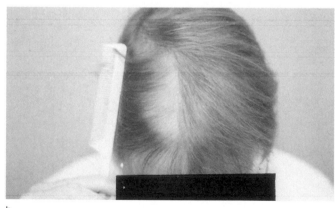

h

Figure 35-9 (*c*) Close-up of hairline combed back for critical evaluation (same date as *b*). Note alternating transplanted and non-transplanted lines. (*d*) After five sessions and 472 grafts. In addition to the frontal area, some grafts had been transplanted to the mid-scalp to increase density there. (*e*) Close-up of completed hairline with hair combed back for critical evaluation. These results were achieved with properly chosen round grafts and micrografting.

Figure 35-9 (*f*) Female patients generally have diffuse thinning sprinkled over a small, relatively round area of total alopecia. Slit grafts are used in the areas of diffuse thinning while totally bare sites are concomitantly punched out with trephines whose size conforms best to their diameter (2–4.5 mm). (The patient shown above had more large totally alopecic area than most women, and consequently had fewer small round grafts utilized than usually would be employed in combination with standard-sized round and slit grafts.) (*g*) Before transplanting. The area to be treated on the right side of this patient's recipient area has been delineated with a black crayon. (*h*) Six months after the first session of 60 standard-sized grafts, some of which were divided to produce round grafts of various sizes and some of which were sectioned to obtain "slit" grafts.

of that session by using the untreated side as a "control." Extensive use of slit grafts (in areas of diffuse thinning) and round minigrafts (for small areas of total alopecia) has become an integral part of transplanting in female patients (Figs. 35-9*f–h*).[8]

Age is not a contraindication to punch transplanting as long as health is satisfactory. The author has operated on a number of patients in their seventies with results as good as or better than those in younger individuals. On the other hand, in general, the author tries to avoid transplanting in those who are younger than 21 years old because of the increased difficulty in estimating the eventual extent of alopecia and long-term patient motivation. Exceptions to this general rule are made to accommodate those who are seriously emotionally affected by their premature hair loss.

Patients who use hairpieces are advised that they should not be worn for a week after any transplant session and as little as possible for an additional week. The same applies for hats, though they can be worn for short intervals if they have holes allowing for the circulation of air. Hairpieces and hats produce some warmth and moisture which are conducive to infection. Individuals who work in occupations or who have hobbies that expose them to dirt or debris are advised to avoid these circumstances for 1 week postoperatively.

PREOPERATIVE INSTRUCTIONS AND ANESTHESIA

Patients are advised to let their hair grow long enough prior to surgery to allow for camouflage of the donor site postoperatively. In addition, some patients prefer to change their hairstyle (e.g., growing one portion of their hair longer so that they can comb over the recipient area and thereby camouflage it as well). They are asked to start erythromycin (PCE) 333 mg three times a day beginning the night prior to or 2 hours before surgery. Antibiotics are discontinued 5 days postoperatively. Acetylsalicylic acid-containing drugs and vitamin E are avoided for 3 weeks prior to surgery to minimize surgical as well as postsurgical bleeding. No alcohol should be consumed for 1 week preoperatively for the same reason.

A personal and family general medical history is taken to rule out any contraindication to surgery. Where indicated, further laboratory tests or consultations with other physicians are ordered. Unless the patient objects, the author routinely notifies the family physician and dentist and inquires about any factors they believe the author should be aware of. All of the author's patients have a complete blood count (CBC), Venereal Disease Research Laboratories (VDRL) test, routine urinalysis, and testing for hepatitis antigen and HIV infection before treatment begins. These are repeated yearly should the course of treatment extend more than a 12-month period. The author also uses gloves, masks, and protective glasses during surgery.

Diazepam 20 mg is administered orally 30 min prior to surgery, both for its sedative effects and for minimizing lidocaine toxicity. A solution composed of equal parts of 2 percent lidocaine with 1:100,000 epinephrine and 0.5 percent bupivacaine is used to produce a field block in the donor area, while 2 percent lidocaine with 1:100,000 epinephrine is usually used as a field block for the recipient site. The use of a 30-gauge needle as well as preoperative diazepam minimizes the psychological and physical trauma of the anesthetic technique. In addition, the author generally will inject five or six spots along the proposed line of the field block and wait for the areas to be totally anesthetized before finishing the field block by injecting through the already anesthetized sites. In this manner, the patient only feels approximately six injections in each of the donor and recipient areas. A 1/200,000 solution of epinephrine is used superior to the field blocks to minimize bleeding. Some operators employ nerve blocks in addition to the field blocks while others use a Dermojet instead of needles.[19] The author has tried both of these variations and has not found either of them advantageous. Occasionally patients require stronger solutions of anesthesia—for example 3% or 4% lidocaine—in the recipient area. In the author's experience these individuals are often those with a Celtic background or with a past history of alcohol or drug abuse. Using sodium bicarbonate to buffer the ph of the lidocaine as suggested by McKay et al.[20] in order to minimize the pain of injections, results in increased bleeding. It has recently been employed only to produce less painful field blocks. Tumescent anesthethic techniques, in which dilute solutions of buffered lidocaine and epinephrine (0.1% and 1:250,000 respectively) are injected in large quantities, are now also routinely used by the author in the donor area.[21]

Pre-mixed nitrous oxide 50% with oxygen 50% (Entonox) is often used to minimize the pain and anxiety associated with local anesthesia, sometimes converting this aspect of the procedure into a pleasant experience.

Complications of anesthesia can be minimized by preparing the donor site and recipient site separately, rather than at the same time. The management of complications that may occur secondarily to local anesthesia has been described elsewhere.[22] Significant problems are vary rare.

THE DONOR SITE

Donor grafts are removed from areas that have reasonable prospects for maintaining hair growth for the life of the patient.[23] (Fig. 35-10*a*) The scalp is examined carefully with hair wet to aid in delineating areas of future thinning. As mentioned earlier a family history is also taken. If a patient is young it is wise to leave an extra 2.5–5 cm beyond any areas of forecasted hair loss as a margin of safety before the most superior line of donor grafts is harvested.

Curved scissors are used to clip the hair to approximately a 2 mm length in bands approximately 4.5–8 mm wide in the temporal area and approximately 6–10 mm wide in the occip-

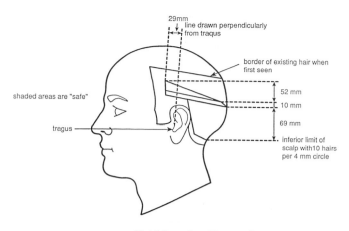

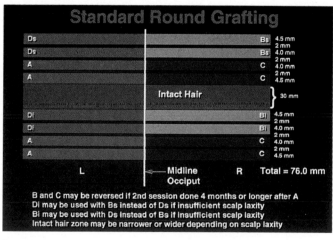

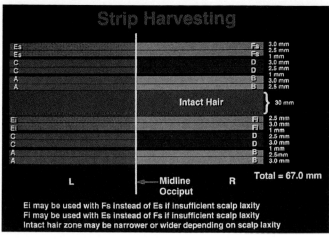

Figure 35-10 (*b*) Occipital donor area planning for standard round grafting: Sessions A, B, C, and D are 1st, 2nd, 3rd, and 4th sessions, respectively. As single row of round grafts will also be harvested from the temporal area on the same side of the head at the same time. (B) and (C) may be reversed if the second session to the same area is done four months or longer after session A. Note: (1) The superior border of the inferior rows A (first session, left side) and the inferior border of the superior rows A are 50.5 mm apart. This is true for the first session rows on the right side also. (2) The intact zone may be wider or narrower, depending on less or more scalp laxity, respectively. Alternately, and more and more frequently, inferior A on left side may be combined with superior C on right side, instead of superior A. (*c*) Occipital donor area planning for strip harvesting: A single or double strip is also harvested from the temporal area on the same side of the head at the same time. Sessions A, B, C, and so on, are 1st, 2nd, 3rd, and so on session, respectively. Note: (1) The superior border of the inferior rows A (first session on left side) are 43 mm from the inferior border of the superior rows A. This is also true for rows B (first session on right side). (2) A total of 67.0 mm of donor area will often yield enough grafts and 5–80 micrografts. The intact zone may be wider or narrower, depending on less or more scalp laxity, respectively. Also, now more frequently, the superior donor zone is taken from the contralateral side of the occipital area; for example, inferior E on left side may be combined with superior F on right side, instead of superior E.

ital area. In the temporal area a single zone is prepared, as *superiorly as appropriate donor hair is expected to survive permanently.* Subsequent temporal area harvesting will be carried out progressively more inferiorly. If round grafts are being used, a *single* row of 3.5–4.5 mm round grafts will be taken. If slit grafts or minigrafts are being used, 1–3 strips of tissue will be excised (at most, one 3 mm wide, and two 2.5 mm wide, or three 2.5 mm wide). Hair in the temporal area is often very susceptible to postoperative telogen effluvium and unacceptably wide scars are more prone to occur here than in the occipital area. Hence a single temporal donor zone is preferred over the double zones that are used in the occipital area (see below).

In the occipital area, an inferior donor zone is chosen so as

to obtain the finest textured *permanent* hair with appropriate density at this site. If round grafts are being used this zone will be approximately 10 mm wide (for two rows of 4 mm grafts) or 11 mm wide (for up to two rows of 4.5 mm grafts). A gap of intact hair will be left superior to the zone, and is often approximately 42 mm wide, though it will vary somewhat depending on what is viewed as the width of the "safe" donor area, scalp laxity and hair density, color, texture and wave. A second donor zone, similar to the first, is then clipped short just superior to the band of intact hair. Donor areas will be superior to each of these zones in future sessions (Fig. 34-10*b*).

It is important that excision of the scar from the previous harvesting be a component of each of the later sessions. Not only does this result in less scar tissue being left in the donor

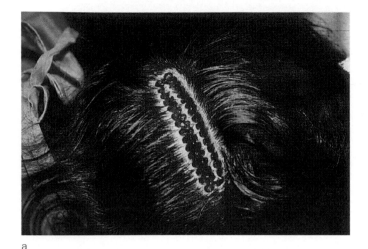

a

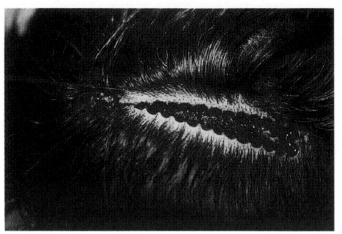

b

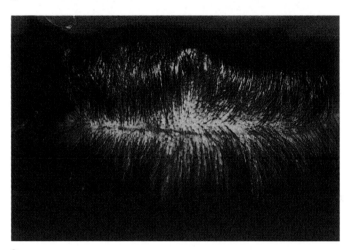

c

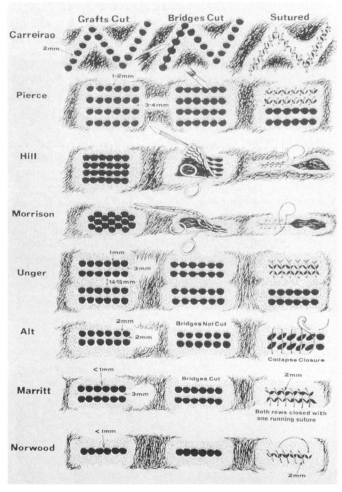

d

Figure 35-11 (*a*) Two rows of standard-sized round grafts are punched out, leaving an intact zone approximately 2.0 mm wide between them. The grafts are removed and the bridges between the graft sites are cut, leaving the intact zone "floating" in the middle of the donor site. (*b*) A running 2-0 Supramid suture is used to close the defect after the central bridge has been removed. Care is taken to have triangular convexities on one side of the wound fit into concavities on the opposite edge. (*c*) Four months postoperatively, the scar is usually no more than 1 mm wide and is barely visible even with lifting the hair and close inspection. It will be reexcised as part of any donor area taken immediately superior to it in subsequent sessions. (*d*) The various methods of donor site harvesting (reprinted with permission from O'Tar Norwood from Hair Transplant Forum).

area, it also results in "virginal" tissue on *both* sides of the suture line and no nearby scar interrupting the blood supply coming from inferiorly. Perhaps most importantly no matter how many times the donor area is used, only two narrow scars will be left in the occipital area and one in the temporal area.

If strip harvesting is being used for slit grafts or minigrafts, the clipped sections will be 3 mm or more narrower than those described above for round grafts (Fig. 34-10*c*). In the case of round grafts the clipped zones must allow for no less than a 2 mm wide space between the two rows of round grafts (see below). With strip grafting, not only are these gaps of intact hair unnecessary, but the donor strips themselves are narrower than the usual diameter of standard round grafts (4–4.5 mm). For both these reasons one is usually able to obtain 12 donor strips 2.5–3 mm wide from a smaller area than that required for 8 rows of standard sized round grafts. Put another way, a smaller donor area than that required for two sessions (and 8 rows) of round grafts will allow for three sessions (and 12 rows) of 2.5–3 mm wide strips. (These numbers will of course vary somewhat depending on hair characteristics and on the width of the scar produced subsequent to each harvesting.) Thus a "safe" donor area no more than 7.6 cm wide (less than one can expect in most patients) will yield more than 12 strips or 8 rows of standard round grafts with a 30 mm wide zone of intact hair left between the final inferior and superior donor scars. This is enough for 3 or 2 sessions respectively on each side of the midline. It is also *far* better than can be expected when total excision together with re-excision of previous scars is not employed.

After the hair is clipped, the area is rubbed with alcohol, and Povidine Iodine or Chlorhexidine Gluconate (Hibitane or Hibiclens) is applied and left in place to provide continuing antibacterial activity. Anesthesia is then carried out as described previously.

Saline is injected into donor lines immediately before harvesting, whether round grafts or strips will be taken. Enough should be used to produce good tissue turgor. Instrument sharpness is also extremely important in minimizing loss of hair matrices adjacent to incision lines. Our punches are kept razor-sharp. We also use Persona Plus blades for strip-harvesting as we have found them sharper than most.

Round grafts are cut angling the punch in the same direction as the hair at that site. The author generally begins with the most inferior occipital donor zone and cuts 15 sites, moving from the midline anteriorly. They almost touch each other on any given row. A second row of round grafts are then prepared in a similar fashion leaving a gap of intact skin approximately 2 mm wide between the superior and the inferior rows. Grafts in the inferior row are all removed before moving to those in the superior row. The intact band of hairbearing skin between these rows is then carefully excised and will be used to produce small slit grafts and micrografts (Fig. 34-11).[24] A Hyfrecator set at unipolar delivery and 80–100 is employed to cauterize any larger blood vessels and the edges of the wounds are sewn together with 2.0 Supramid on a CL30 needle using a continuous suture. If there is any tension on this closure, the edges of the wound will be undermined *and, if necessary, galeal sutures will also be employed* (2–0 Dexon or Vicryl). A Plume Master ESU smoke evacuator system is used in our office to vacuum up the fumes produced during electro-cautery of blood vessels. These fumes have been shown to contain carcinogens and chemicals that cause nasal polyps. We then move to the superior donor zone and treat it in a similar fashion. If undue closure tension is expected in the second zone, donor tissue will be taken from the side contralateral to the inferior zone (Figs. 34-10b and 10c).

The patient's head is removed from the prone pillow and is placed on its side. At this point, if I am treating the frontal aspect of the area of MPB, I will harvest a single line of round grafts in the temporal area (or, as noted earlier, up to 3 strips). Grafts are taken from the most posterior aspects first and we then move anteriorly. The grafts from the inferior occipital and temporal areas generally contain finer and sparser hair that is especially suitable for producing natural-looking hairlines.[15] In addition those from the temporal area will grey as the patient ages at about the same time as this is occurring in the remaining temporal area, thus producing a natural color change in the frontal recipient site. It is worthwhile emphasizing that when the hairline is being completed, during session three, in previously bald sites, or session two in still hairbearing recipient sites, round grafts will be taken from similar but contralateral sites in order to produce a uniform density and quality of hair in the hairline zone.

During the second session, if it is done six weeks after the first, similar paired rows are taken from contralateral and more superior sites in the occipital area and from somewhat more inferiorly in the temporal area. As has already been noted, if it is done after the first session has started growing (three and a half months or more), the second session is taken from the *same* level as the first, on the contralateral side. Third and fourth sessions are taken in the remaining intact donor area as shown in Figs. 10b and 10c, also generally employing pairs of rows.

While the author has found the above technique very advantageous, other operators use single long rows[25] or excise the entire donor area without leaving intact gaps of hair between round grafts.[26] Fig. 34-12 schematically summarizes the various techniques utilized. Many physicians continue to use round punches to obtain donor material, but an increasing number of surgeons use parallel scalpel blades to excise strips of hair-bearing skin that are then subdivided for minigrafting or, less often, square grafting.[27] (Figs. 13a–c). More will be said about strip harvesting below. Sutured single rows of round donor grafts produce uniformly excellent scars and are recommended by the author for smaller sessions. Unfortunately, such an approach will limit the session to 60–80 grafts and the latter will go from one anterior temporal area to the other, making it uncomfortable for the patient to sleep on either side of his head. Lines of anesthesia for field blocks are of course also longer, resulting in this aspect of the procedure being more uncomfortable as well. One can use *two* single lines of grafts instead of one, separating them by a reasonably wide intact donor area in order to leave temporal areas untouched, or to increase the number of grafts harvested, but once again the patient will "pay" for this with more numerous injections for anesthesia. Alt[13] and others minimize this problem by harvesting long rows of *paired* lines of donor grafts (Fig. 12a). This results in no more anesthetic discomfort than the technique I use and is advantageous in individuals with relatively tight scalps. The disadvantages of having both the right and left side of the donor area operated on, and therefore no comfortable side to sleep on, remains a problem however. In addition, as will be pointed out when the recipient area is

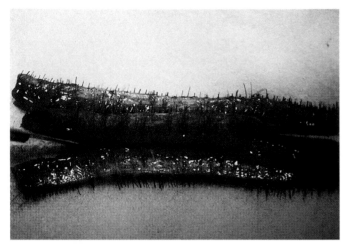

a

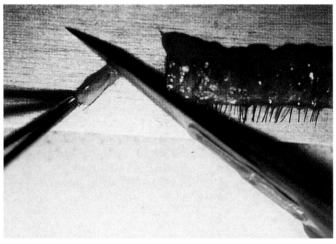

b

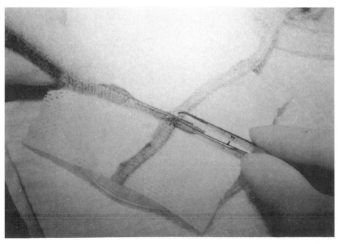

c

Figure 35-12 (*a*) Each strip of tissue is separated by exposing and cutting the joined tissue using the scalpel with a #11 blade. (*b*) The slit graft is laid on the tongue depressor and any excess fatty tissue is trimmed from the base of the graft, to within 1 mm of the deepest hair matrix.

discussed, I often require both temporal and relatively short inferior occipital donor lines to get enough grafts with the right combination of texture and density to use for the anterior $2–2\frac{1}{2}$ cm of the hairline: hence my preference for two pairs of donor lines in the occipital area in most sessions—one pair from inferiorly and one pair containing denser and coarser-haired grafts from more superiorly.

Parallel scalpel blades for excising strips of donor hair are used by the author whenever slit grafts are being prepared. Once again, I begin strip harvesting with the inferior donor zone. A power-punch with a 4–4.5 mm trephine is used to cut three holes on either end of the proposed lines, to produce the shape of a triangle (Fig. 13*a*) and thus a tapering of the ends of the strips. The round grafts are removed as described earlier and a 3 or 4 bladed scalpel is inserted at the edge of one triangular defect and drawn evenly across the donor zone to meet the triangular defect on the other end of the area (Fig. 13*b*). Just as with punch harvesting, care is taken to angle the blades in the direction of hair at that site and to go deep enough to include the hair matrices and some subcutaneous tissue in the strips that will be removed.

The strips are lifted by the assistant and small sharp scissors or a number 15 scalpel blade is used to separate them from their underlying bed. Bleeding can occasionally be quite brisk with strip harvesting, however with practice one becomes expert at controlling it with appropriately applied pressure. Larger bleeders are then cauterized and the wound is sutured closed in a similar fashion to that described for round grafting. The superior donor zone is then harvested and the patient's head is removed from the prone pillow and placed on its side for removal of 1–3 adjacent strips of donor hair from the temporal area—if additional grafts are needed or if one is treating the anterior third to half of the area of MPB. During subsequent sessions an additional blade and 1–2 mm wide spacer can be added to the multi-bladed scalpel handle. This extra tract is added to excise the scar from the previous harvesting at the same time as the new strips are being removed.

The author routinely takes two strips from each donor zone, however if scalp laxity is sufficient and if one is not intending to also harvest the temporal area, three strips may be obtained from either the inferior or superior donor zone or both. The objective with strip harvesting for slit grafting is usually 350–400 slit grafts and 70–80 micrografts per session, and the number and length of strips that will be taken is aimed at producing this number of grafts. The 2.5 mm wide strips will generally be used to produce 3–4 hair grafts and micrografts while the 3 mm wide strips will produce 5–6 hair grafts. The width of the strips will also be varied according to hair characteristics such as density, color, wave, and caliber. The denser the hair, the darker the color, the coarser the caliber, the fizzier the texture, and the more curl, the narrower the strip and vice versa.

Estimating the appropriate length of strips to produce the desired number of grafts is difficult. I routinely note on the

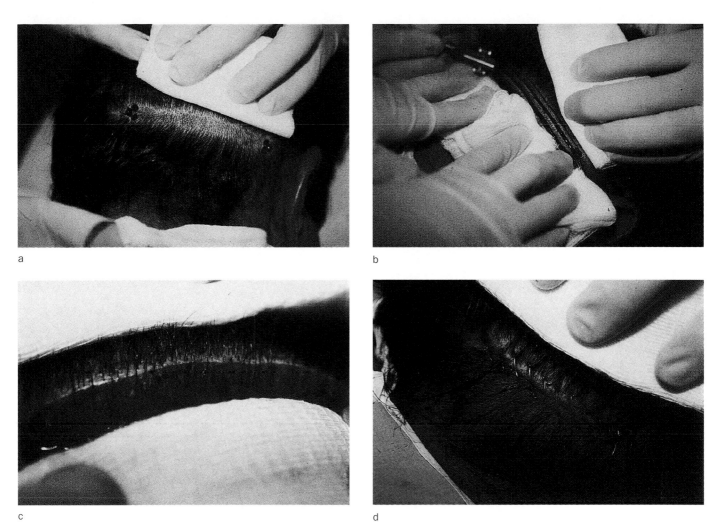

Figure 35-13   (*a*) Three holes are produced with a 4–4.5 mm trephine on either end of the proposed harvest, to produce the shape of a triangle, and thus a tapering of the end of the strips. The round grafts are removed and the bridges between them cut. (*b*) The donor zone is infiltrated with normal saline, to produce good turgor and a triple- or quadruple-bladed knife is inserted at the edge of the medial or lateral triangular defect. It is drawn evenly across the donor zone to meet the triangular defect at the other end of the area. Just as with punch grafting, care is taken to angle the blades in the direction of hair at that site and to go deep enough to include hair matrices. (*c*) The strip is carefully lifted from its bed using small scissors or a #15 scalpel blade; larger blood vessels are cauterized and a running 2-0 Supramid suture is used to close the defect. Undermining to the wound edges or placement of galeal sutures is used only if there will be any tension at the suture line without such use. Note how well one is able to match the angle of adjacent hair with scalpel incisions. (*d*) Donor site sutured.

first session the length and width of strips taken, and the number of grafts produced per centimeter. This is then used as a guide for future sessions. The choice of areas used for donor tissue are governed by the same principles as those previously described for harvesting round grafts.

Although excising strips of donor tissue with parallel scalpel blades will nearly always result in additional bleeding, the operator can far more easily find bleeders and cauterize them with a hyfrecator than when round grafts are being harvested. One quickly obtains expertise so that the time required

and the amount of bleeding encountered is not significantly different whether one uses parallel scalpel blades or round grafts. In addition, the preparation time for slit grafts will usually be significantly reduced if parallel scalpel blades are being used, and grafts prepared this way fit better into incisional slits. Lastly, and most importantly, the total excision techniques (T.E.T.) described above for both round graft harvesting and slit graft strip harvesting, result in less scarring and the most efficient use of donor areas. *The author has estimated at least a 50% increase in the number of grafts that can*

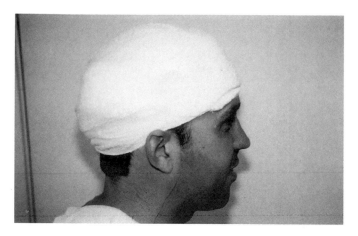

Figure 35-22 A somewhat modified turban type bandage that does not cover the ears is more comfortable than the standard one shown in Fig. 20. It is more liable to get dislodged or slip upwards, for example during sleep, and should therefore be secured for sleeping by some gauze going over the top of the bandage and tied under the chin.

The use of alkyl-2 cyanoacrylate to "glue" the grafts in place has been advocated as a way to avoid overnight bandaging.[31] Unfortunately, the glue also tends to mat surrounding hair and fixes the crust in place, significantly delaying its shedding. Orentreich and Orentreich[32] have described suturing grafts in place in order to avoid bandaging. This is useful if relatively small numbers of round grafts are being transplanted but even then results in a foreign body (the sutures) being left in the nonsterile recipient area, thus increasing the possibility of infection at that site. On the other hand, the Orentreichs have used it extensively for several years now and they and their patients remain enthusiastic.

Dr. Pierre Pouteaux has for many years used no cyanoacrylate, sutures, or overnight bandage. He asks patients to stay in his office for the full working day. Gauze soaked lightly with saline is applied to recipient and donor areas, and a tensor-like bandage is used to apply pressure and keep the gauze in place. The dressing is changed periodically and at the end of the day is removed entirely before the patient is sent home. Dr. Pouteaux reports that he has never had a graft fall out or been called because of overnight bleeding, as any potential problems make themselves known during the day and have been attended to before the patient leaves the office.[33]

For the past 8 years, the author has been applying a solution of 2 percent Minoxidil in an alcohol base just after the recipient area has been cleaned.[34] In addition, patients have been asked to continue twice daily applications of this solution for a period of 5 weeks. Most patients, though not all, note a later effluvium of hair from the transplanted grafts and a more rapid regrowth of hair than occurred before Minoxidil was used. Claims that the temporary effluvium seen with punch grafting can be avoided completely if Minoxidil is employed are greatly exaggerated in the author's opinion.

Intramuscular betamethasone sodium phosphate and betamethasone acetate (Celestone Soluspan) 12 mg and/or a 1-week course of prednisone are offered to patients after their first session as well as to those who are anxious about postoperative edema because of previous problems with it.[35] The usual contraindications to corticosteroids are respected.

A single intramuscular injection of ketorolac tromethamine (Toradol) 30 to 60 mg at the conclusion of surgery has dramatically decreased the need for postoperative oral analgesics in the authors' patients. It is, however, not offered to patients who prefer prednisone, who are bleeding more than the average patient during surgery, or who have a history of asthma. When required, acetaminophen with 30 mg of codeine, Percocet, oral Toradol, or meperidine may be used.

POSTOPERATIVE COMPLICATIONS

This subject has been covered in detail in a prevous publication[35] and includes the following:

1. Mild pruritus occurs in less than 5 percent of patients for a period of a few days to a few weeks. A combination corticosteroid and antibacterial preparation such as Valisone-G cream applied one to three times per day and as required for pruritus will usually control it with little difficulty.

2. Edema occurs in most though not all patients, beginning usually between 1 to 3 days after surgery and lasting for 7 to 10 days. Most often the edema is mild and disappears within a few days, but occasionally it will cause ecchymosis around the eyes resulting in discoloration that might last as long as 2 weeks. Oral and/or intramuscular corticosteroids as described previously, nonsteroidal anti-inflammatories such as ketorolac tromethamine (Toradol) or ibuprofen (Motrin), reclining at a 45° angle rather than lying flat for sleep, and frequent cold compresses to the forehead in the first few days after surgery all help to minimize the incidence and severity of edema.

3. Discoloration of grafts that are either mildly erythematous to violaceous is a temporary problem that cannot be foreseen. Usually there is only slight discoloration and a water-based makeup may be used to camouflage it. Most patients simply ignore it, and it disappears in usually 2 to 4 weeks.

4. Graft elevation may occur either because of an inappropriate donor graft/recipient-hole size ratio, insufficient trimming of subcutaneous fat from grafts, or excessive postoperative bleeding. It occurs in less than 5 percent of patients if correct technique has been employed and in all cases should be mild enough that simple hyfrecation of the elevated grafts will result in their complete flattening. This can be done, for example, during subsequent hair transplant sessions. A Hyfrecator set at no more than 50, unipolar delivery, will cause no damage to hairs and will flatten the grafts without any subsequent scarring or discoloration.

5. Hypoesthesia may result from the severing of nerves in the

11. Brad

12. Stoug
    Onco

13. Alt T
    W, N
    145–

14. Norw
    2(3):5

15. Ungei
    nizatic
    W, Nc
    1051–

16. Unger
    male,
    Pierce

17. Unger
    planta
    Marce

18. Unger
    tation,
    Dekke

19. Monhe
    W, Noi
    133–14

20. McKay
    infiltra
    Analg (

21. Unger
    Unger
    165–18

22. Abadir
    tol Surg

23. Cohen
    Dermat

24. Unger
    Unger
    pp 211–

25. Norwoo
    Transpl

26. Hill TG:
    cluster t

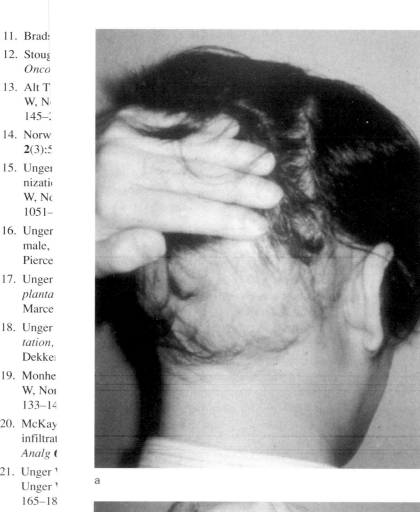

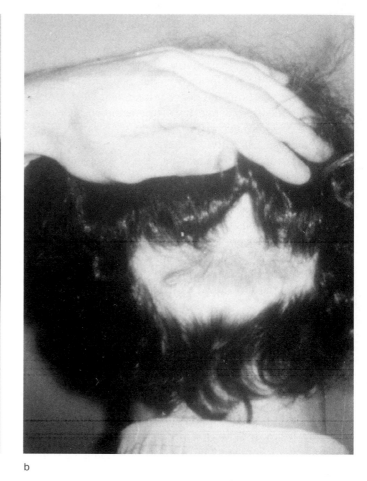

a

b

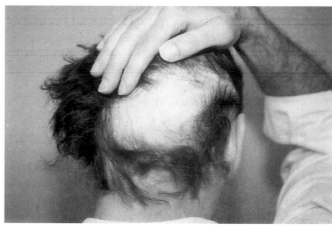

c

d

Figure 35-23 (*a*) A large area of cicatricial alopecia which developed as a complication of a "BOP" flap. The patient was referred to us for possible correction of the defect. (*b*) A large area of cicatricial alopecia which developed as a complication of a BOP flap. The patient was referred to us for possible correction of the defect.

donor or recipient area. Normally such decreased sensitivity will correct itself within a matter of a few weeks to a few months; however, if a larger branch of a nerve has been cut, hypoesthesia may last as long as 18 months. Rarely, a major-sized nerve will be involved and produces a *permanent* slight hypoesthesia. The latter should occur in less than 0.1 percent of surgeries.

6. A hematoma may develop postoperatively; however, in over 20,000 operative sessions, the author has never had this happen.

7. Hy
als
0.0
tie
wa
vo
sic
3.3
suc
8. An
eit
inc
pei
sol
the
fis
ing
off

More

1. Ke
if a
tiei
If t
his
be
pla
cea
on
kel
2. Inf
pat
tib
25(
tur
tib
occ
is e
the
ora
pre
otic
3. Ost
lite
4. Pos
all
ing
all
ori

To put
are rai
and ca
Alt
cuss A

sion were of sufficient size to allow for access to, and retention by, mucosal and pulmonary surfaces. Furthermore, their study indicated that commonly used personal protection standards such as operatory masks, goggles, and scatter shields do not prevent the respiration of these particles. In addition, the settling velocities of such small particles may extend the exposure for many hours after the procedure has been performed, thereby endangering personnel not directly involved in the procedure itself. The AIDS virus may be difficult to detect if a patient is in a latent period between infection and positive antibody test. There is also the legal implication of refusing a patient who had a positive blood test. It is quite clear that a risk to the physician, his or her assistants, and other personnel does exist. There is also certainly an increased risk to the AIDS-infected patient. Dermabrasion certainly should not be performed without the thorough history of high-risk behavior; protection of gloves, masks, and goggles; and the awareness that even with such protective devices a certain degree of risk remains.

Increasingly, aging skin is an indication for dermabrasion, especially that which has been actinically damaged and shows pathology such as premalignant solar keratoses. Dermabrasion has been shown to be as effective, if not more so, than topically applied 5-fluorouracil (5-FU) in the management of precancerous skin lesions.[15] In a study of half-face planing of actinically damaged skin, Burke et al.[16] showed that precancerous lesions were substantially reduced and their future development was retarded over a 5-year period. In addition, dramatic improvement in rhagades is seen in dermabrasion patients, making dermabrasion a viable modality in the treatment of aging skin (Figs. 36-3 and 36-4).

Yarborough[17] demonstrated that dermabrasions performed on traumatic or surgical scars approximately 6 weeks postinjury often result in a complete disappearance of the scars (Figs. 36-5 and 36-6). In fact, in the author's experience, surgical scars responded so well to dermabrasion that most patients who have had excisional surgery are told that it is likely they may have a dermabrasion 6 weeks postoperatively. Al-

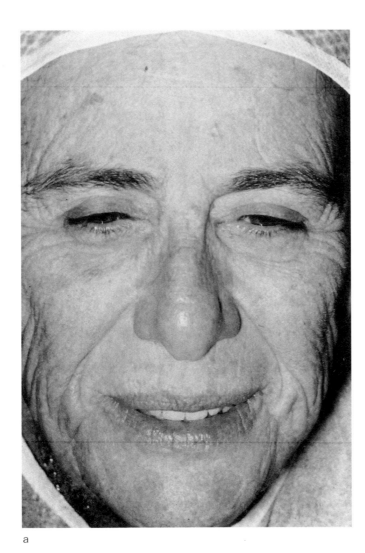

a

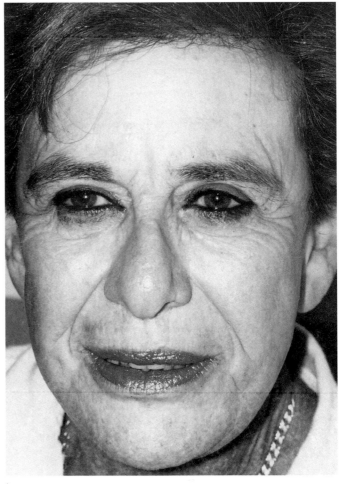

b

Figure 36-4 (a) Predermabrasion for wrinkles; (b) postdermabrasion for wrinkles.

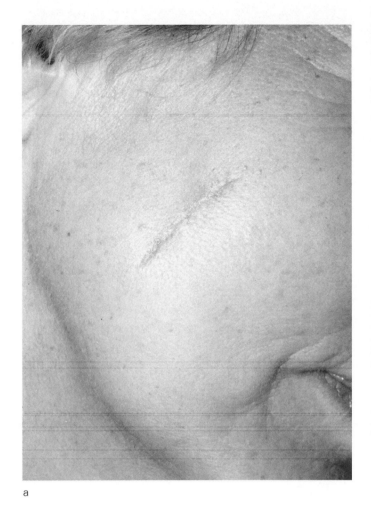

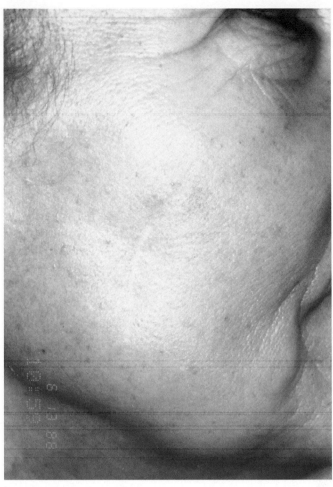

a

b

Figure 36-5 *(a)* Predermabrasion of 6-week-old surgical scar; *(b)* postdermabrasion of 6-week-old surgical scar.

though this is usually not necessary, its anticipation by the patient eases introduction when necessary. This is especially true in patients who have very sebaceous skin or in facial areas such as the nose where improvement following dermabrasion is most dramatic. The improvement in scars following dermabrasion is further enhanced by the postoperative use of biosynthetic dressings which have been demonstrated to significantly effect collagen synthesis resulting in cosmetic improvement in the surgical scar (Fig. 36-7).[8] Varicella scars have been especially responsive to dermabrasion 6 weeks after healing.

Removal of tattoos can be accomplished with superficial dermabrasion followed by application of 1 percent gentian violet and a Vaseline gauze dressing changed daily for 10 days. The gentian violet delays healing, causing some pigment to leach out into the dressing and creating continued inflammation which causes phagocytosis of additional pigment. Caution to abrade only the very upper papillary dermis will avoid scarring. Do not attempt to remove the pigment by abrasion. Professional tattoos are more responsive than amateur or trau-

matic tattoos, but all can be improved. Usually 50 percent resolution can be achieved with one procedure, which can be repeated every 2 to 3 months until the desired result is achieved. Tattoos are a very good training procedure for the novice in dermabrasion.

Benign tumors such as adenoma sebaceum and syringomas may be successfully dermabraded with marked cosmetic improvement, especially when combined with electrodesiccation of individual lesions, but gradal recurrence is the rule. Dramatic improvement may be achieved with rhinophyma when dermabrasion is combined with electrofulguration (Fig. 36-8).

INSTRUMENTATION

A wide variety of abrading instruments are commercially available. They vary from hand engines to cable-driven power sources and battery-operated units. The important consideration in terms of the power source is that it has the torque nec-

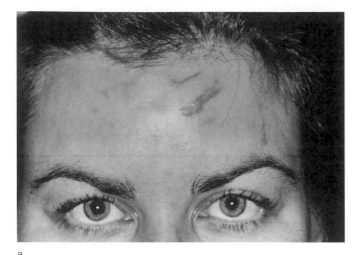

a

b

Figure 36-6   *(a)* Predermabrasion of 6-week-old traumatic scar; *(b)* postdermabrasion of 6-week-old traumatic scar.

essary to continue a sustained and even drive of the abrading surface, either a wire brush or diamond fraise. Excellent reviews by Yarborogh[18] and Alt[19] of the wire brush and diamond fraise dermabrasive techniques require little elaboration. It cannot be overemphasized, however, that no article can be substituted for thorough hands-on experience in a preceptorship environment where the student is able to watch and assist someone experienced in the art of dermabrasion. Most authors agree that the wire-brush technique requires more skill and runs a higher risk of potential injury, as it is able to cut much deeper and much more quickly than the diamond fraise. It is this author's opinion that, with the exception of the extra-coarse diamond fraise, superior results are achieved with the wire brush.

One of the current controversies surrounding dermabrasion surgery is the use of preabrasive chilling of the skin. A clinical work reviewing various cryesthetic materials available to chill the skin prior to sanding have shown that the materials, which freeze the skin below −30°C and especially below −60°C, have the risk of causing substantial tissue necrosis and subsequent scarring.[20–22] It is necessary to freeze the skin prior to dermabrasion in order to have a rigid surface

which will abrade evenly and to preserve anatomic markings which might otherwise be distorted when the tissue is thawed and stretched. Since thermal injury may result in excessive scarring, caution would suggest that using cryesthetic agents that do not freeze below −30°C is prudent and is as effective as those which freeze deeper.

TECHNIQUE

Preoperative staged analgesia has made dermabrasion a feasible technique for an outpatient setting. Diazepam, administered approximately 45 min to 1 h preoperatively, in conjunction with 0.4 mg of atropine intramuscularly (IM) as an amnestic and antivagal agent tends to make the patient more comfortable and less anxious. Prior to administering regional block anesthesia with a lidocaine-bupivacaine mixture, 1 cc of intravenously administered fentanyl gives the patient a great sense of euphoria while relieving the discomfort associated with injection of regional anesthesia. Fentanyl offers the advantage of being rapid in onset and very short in duration, thus allowing most patients to recover completely from its ef-

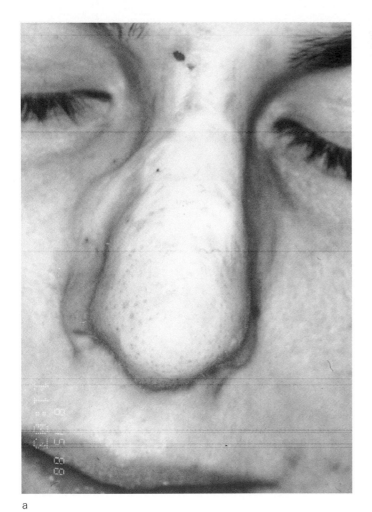

a

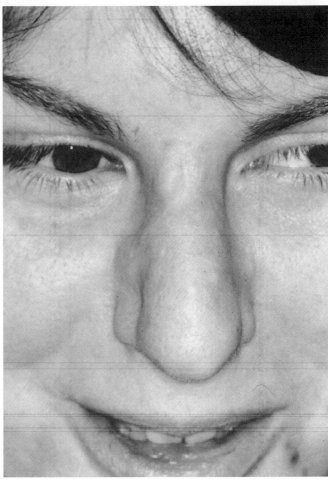

b

Figure 36-7 *(a)* Scar preabrasion; *(b)* postabrasion and biosynthetic dressings.

fect within 30 to 45 min. Once fentanyl has taken effect, the administration of the regional anesthesia to the supraorbital, infraorbital, and mental foramina usually results in anesthesia of 60 to 70 percent of the entire face. When this is coupled with the use of the refrigerant spray, most patients can be dermabraded without pain. The use of nitrous oxide analgesia to supplement anesthesia if the patient becomes uncomfortable during the procedure allows the procedure to progress without interruption.

Once the skin has been rendered solid by the refrigerant spray, the sanding procedure begins in areas no larger than that which can be abraded in approximately 10 s or approximately 1-in² areas. The dermabrasion instrument, which should be grasped firmly in the hand, should be pulled only in the direction of the handle and perpendiclarly to the plane of rotation. Back and forth or circular movements may gouge the skin. The wire brush particularly requires almost no pressure and produces multiple microlacerations which are a sign of the adequacy of the depth of the procedure. Adequate depth is recognized by several landmarks as one progresses through the skin. The removal of the

skin pigmentation signifies passage through the basal layer of the epidermis. As one advances into the papillary dermis, the small capillary loops of the papillary plexus are identified as the tissues thaw and punctate bleeding results. As the papillary dermis is entered farther, faintly visible, small, parallel strands of collagen become apparent. It is the fraying of these parallel strands that signifies that dermabrasion is carried to the correct level. Going farther may result in scarring.

Many authors suggest using cotton towels or cotton gloves as absorbent material for blotting instead of using gauze which may become ensnared in the dermabrading instruments. The entanglement of gauze in the instruments results in a loud flapping which frightens the patient and may often compromise the function of the instrument itself.

In this author's experience, it is easiest to begin the dermabrasion centrally beside the nose and work outwardly, as these are usually the areas of greatest disfigurement and also greatest anesthesia, thus allowing the patient the least discomfort and giving the physician the most time to proceed. Special attention must be paid to fixation by traction when dermabrading the lip, which can be ensnared in the machine

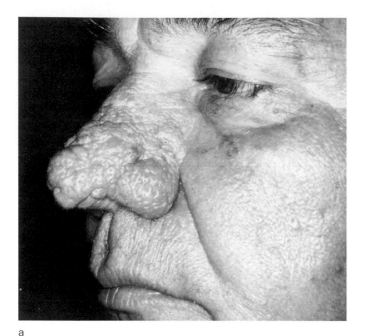

a

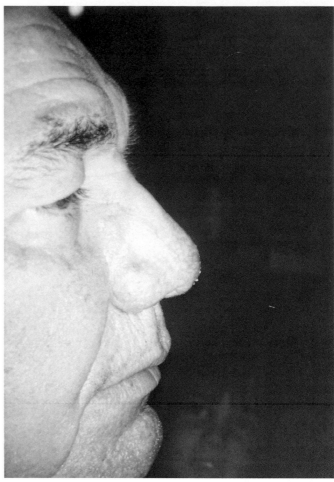

b

Figure 36-8 *(a)* Predermabrasion for rhinophyma; *(b)* postdermabrasion for rhinophyma.

causing significant laceration. Staying constantly parallel to the surface is essential, especially in areas of complex curvature such as the chin and malar eminences. Dermabrasion should always be carried out within the facial units to avoid demarcation by pigmentation when and if possible. Dermabrading to just beneath the jaw line, out to the preauriclar area, and up to the suborbital areas ensures that a uniform texture and appearance will be achieved. Fifty percent trichloroacetic acid can be applied to any unabraded skin, the eyebrows, and the first few centimeters of the hairline to blend pigmentation even better.

Immediately following the procedure, any excessive bleeding may be controlled by the application of topical thrombin. Pain relief is achieved as soon as biosynthetic dressings are applied at the end of the procedure. Postoperatively, patients are put on prednisone 40 mg a day for 4 days, which greatly reduces postoperative edema and discomfort. One of the most important recent advances has been the use of acyclovir in patients who have had a history of herpes simplex. Acyclovir is begun 24 h preoperatively at a dose of 400 mg tid and continued for 5 days; no patients on this regimen have developed postoperative herpes simplex, even those who have a preexisting history of that problem.

Most patients re-epithelialize completely between 5 and 7 days postoperatively when biosynthetic dressings have been used. Some of the dressings, such as Vigilon, must be changed daily. Others, such as Omiderm, may be applied at the time of dermabrasion and left intact until they peel off spontaneously at about 5 to 7 days. Both of the biosynthetic dressings mentioned need to be covered initially with gauze held in place by flexible surgical netting. After the skin has re-epithelialized, the patients are usually restarted on topical tretinoin by the seventh to tenth postoperative day. If the patients have a previous history of pigmentary problems, such as melasma, they are also started on topical hydroquinone at the same time as the tretinoin. If by the tenth to fourteenth day the patient shows signs of disproportionate erythema, a topical 1 percent hydrocortisone is begun. The patients are cautioned prior to surgery that it will take at least a month for their skin to be normal in its appearance. Most patients, however, are able to return to work within 7 to 10 days of surgery if light makeup is applied. The compulsive daily application of sunscreens is essential for at least several months postoperatively.

COMPLICATIONS

Milia are one of the most common complications of dermabrasion and usually appear 3 to 4 weeks postsurgery. If tretinoin has been utilized postoperatively, milia are rarely encountered, and when they do occur they will usually resolve with continued tretinoin. Acne flares are another common complication in patients who are prone to acne. If the patient has had active acne in proximity to the dermabrasion, the acne flare can often be prevented by starting tetracycline in the immediate postoperative period. When acne does occur, tetracycline institution will usually cause its prompt resolution. Although erythema is expected following dermabrasion, persistent or unusually severe erythema after 2 to 4 weeks should be treated promptly with topical steroids to avoid hypertrophic scarring. If hyperpigmentation begins to appear several weeks postsurgery, the institution of topical hydroquinone and tretinoin causes its resolution.

While infrequent, postoperative infection can occur as the result of dermabrasion. The most common organisms are *Staphylococcus aureus,* herpes simplex, and *Candida.* Staphylococcus infection usually manifests itself within 48 to 72 h of dermabrasion with unusual facial swelling and honey crusting as well as systemic symptoms such as fever. Herpes simplex infections may result, if the patient was not pretreated with acyclovir, and are recognized by severe disproportionate pain usually 48 to 78 h postsurgery. *Candida* infections usually result in delayed healing and are recognized somewhat later at 5 to 7 days, with exudation and facial swelling as clinical symptoms. Appropriate treatment with staphylocidal antibiotics, acyclovir, or ketoconazole usually results in resolution of the infections without sequelae.

REFERENCES

1. Kurtin A: Corrective surgical planing of skin. *Arch Dermatol Syphilol* **68:**389, 1953

2. Kronmayer E: Die Heilung der Akne Durch ein Neves Narben Lases Operations ver Faren: Das Stranzen. *Ilustr Monatsscehr Aerztl Poly Tech* **27:**101, 1905

3. Burke J: *Wire Brush Surgery.* Springfield, Ill, Charles C Thomas, 1956

4. Mandy SH: Tretinoin in the pre and post operative management of dermabrasion. *J Am Acad Dermatol* **115:**878, 1986

5. Hang VC et al: Topical tretinoin and epithelial wound healing. *Arch Dermatol* **125:**65–69, 1989

6. Maibach H, Rovee D: *Epidermal Wound Healing.* Chiago, Year Book, 1972

7. Mandy SH: A new primary wound dressing made of polyethylene oxide gel. *J Dermatol Surg Oncol* **9:**153, 1983

8. Alvarez OM et al: The effect of occlusive dressings on collagen synthesis in the superficial wounds. *J Surg Res* **35:**142, 1983

9. Roenigk HH Jr et al: Acne retinoids and dermabrasion. *J Dermatol Surg Oncol* **11:**396–398, 1985

10. Rubenstein R, Roenigk HH Jr: A typical keloids after dermabrasion of patient's taking isotretinoin. *J Am Acad Dermatol* **15:**280–285, 1986

11. Moy R et al: Effects of systemic 13 cis-retinoic acid on wound healing in vivo Exhibit ADD, poster presentation at Am. Academy of Derm Annual meeting, December, 1987

12. Moy R et al: Effect of 13 cis-retinoic on dermal wound healing (abstract) *J Invest Dermatol* **88:**508, 1987

13. Dzubow CM, Miller WH Jr: The effect of 13 cis-retinoic acid on wound healing in dogs. *J Dermatol Surg Oncol* **13:**265, 1987

14. Wentzell J et al: Physical Properties of Aerosols Produced by Dermabrasion. *Arch Dermatol* **125:**1637–1643

15. Field L: Dermabrasion versus 5 fluorouracil in the management of actinic keratoses, in *Controversies in Dermatology,* edited by I Epstein. Saunders, Philadelphia 1984, pp 62–102

16. Burke J et al: Half-face planing of precancerous skin after five years. *Arch Dermatol* **88:**140, 1963

17. Yarborough JM: Dermabrasive surgery state of the art. *Clin Dermatol* **5:**75, 1987

18. Yarborough JM: Dermabrasion by wire brush. *J Dermatol Surg Oncol* **13:**610, 1987

19. Alt T: Facial dermabrasion: advantages of the diamond fraise technique. *J Dermatol Surg Oncol* **13:**618, 1987

20. Hanke CW et al: Laboratory evaluation of skin refrigerants used in dermabrasion. *J Dermatol Surg Oncol* **11:**45–49, 1985

21. Dzubow LM: Survey of refrigerant and surgical techniques used for facial dermabrasion. *J Am Acad Dermatol* **13:**287–292, 1985

22. Hanke CW et al: Complications of dermabrasion resulting from excessively cold skin refrigeration. *J Dermatol Surg Oncol* **11:**896–900, 1985

used from which the product can be applied. Phenol chemical peels are deep peels that are often indicated for wrinkles and coarse skin resulting from photodamage. Phenol peels have been used and histologically studied for many years by a number of well-known physicians.[29,30,31] Although deep photodamage is the major indication, acne scars and other deep skin problems can be treated and improved with phenol peels.

TECHNIQUE

Planning the Peel: Considerations Before the Procedure

Before beginning a peel on a patient, it is important to assess possible factors or exposures that may affect the outcome of the peel. For instance, a history of topical retinoic acid, gly-colic acid, or recently used topical 5-Fluorouracil may sensi-tize a patient's skin, as well as certain oral medications such as 13-*cis*-retinoic acid. There is possible increased potential for scarring postdermabrasion for patients previously treated with 13-*cis*-retinoic acid. It is not clear whether oral or sys-temic retinoids increase the risk of scarring in chemical peels.[32] Other medications such as photosensitizing drugs or oral contraceptives may increase the risk of pigmentary prob-lems. It has been speculated that previous dermabrasions or previous deep peels may increase the potential for scarring.[2] Caution should be used if the patient has had either procedure. One article states that patients with atopy and fair skin may be more sensitive than others to superficial peels.[33]

Physical characteristics of skin are also very important. Those who tolerate stronger peeling agents tend to be older patients with more chronic sun exposure, solar lentigines, and deep wrinkles. The possible mechanism for this increased tol-erance may be that the penetration of the peeling agent is par-tially blocked by the accumulation of solar elastosis in the up-per papillary dermis. Ruddy telangiectatic skin and skin with actinic keratoses can be less tolerant, depending on how much erythema is associated with the actinic keratoses.

Thicker, more sebaceous-quality skin may tolerate more stringent superficial peels than thinner, less sebaceous skin.[26] Part of the resistance to peels may be the quantity of seba-ceous oils that is extruded on the surface of the skin of seba-ceous skin. Skin preparation with alcohol and acetone needs to be more vigorous, and areas such as the nose may require more scrubbing to achieve an even, proper peel.

When considering deeper peels, it is important to consider the Fitzpatrick skin type of the patient. The darker skin types will have a tendency to hyperpigment. Ideal patients for the phenol Baker-Gordon chemical peels are blond-haired, blue-eyed Caucasians because the skin will manifest minimal to no color change in most of these patients after the peel.

It is prudent to document the peeling process.[18] Documen-tation is very important in procedures for consistency of tech-nique. The skin condition being treated and skin characteris-tics that may affect the peel should be noted. A record sheet for superficial peels helps to keep track of variations in tech-nique (Table 37-5). Records should emphasize skin prepara-tion method, duration of the peel, and the type and concentra-tion of the agent. Photos can be difficult to take consistently from the same angle and same lighting but can be very im-portant for records. Uniform pictures can be taken even with-out a special photography room. Taking a side-angle view, one can always line the top of the ear horizontally with the lat-eral canthus of the eye and line the tip of the nose vertically with the edge of the contralateral cheek.

Pretreatment with daily topical retinoic acid or AHA may additively increase the efficacy of the peel.[3,5] In the author's office, patients are given 10% glycolic acid to apply daily for 2 weeks prior to a peel.

Skin Preparation

The patient is instructed to clean off any makeup or sun-screen. This is followed by a skin preparation with chlorhex-idine, acetone, or Jessners' (Table 37-6) solution. The purpose of the preparation is to remove debris and a variable amount of stratum corneum evenly, depending on the preparatory ma-terial and the extent of scrubbing which can enhance the peel effect. Jessners' solution removes most of the stratum corneum. Acetone is thought to remove some of the stratum corneum, and chlorhexidine probably only removes surface

TABLE 37-5

Factors Affecting the Efficacy of Chemical Peeling Agents

Severity of the skin preparation

Cleaning agent to prepare the skin

Type of peeling agent

Concentration of the peel

Time in contact with the peeling agent

Amount of peeling agent applied

Degree of rubbing

Reapplication requirements

Extent of neutralization

TABLE 37-6

Jessners' Solution

14 g Resorcinol

14 g Salicylic acid

14 cc Lactic acid

100 cc Ethanol (qs)

debris and oils. Often, two cleanings are performed to remove surface oils, makeup, and debris evenly. Degreasing is important because even small amounts of oils from the skin will cause increased surface tension and allow less penetration of the peeling agent. Many factors in the skin can cause irregular peeling effects if not cleaned evenly. If erythema occurs on sensitive skin after cleaning with acetone, lower concentration peels or shorter application of the peels in these specific areas is recommended. Some dermatologists will gently scrub with alcohol and acetone until the dark film (probably keratin debris) appearing on the gauze disappears.[28] A study showed that skin preparation with acetone scrubbing will cause a much deeper peel than gentle cleaning with a chlorhexidine solution.[34]

Applying the Glycolic Acid Peel

The glycolic acid is applied with a fan-shaped brush. A simple tray is set up to do the peel. The fan brush ideally coats the skin surface with an even amount of the glycolic acid gel while minimizing trauma to the skin. Additionally, the brush allows application of the peel in very close proximity to the eyes with no problems. The glycolic acid is carefully applied to one cosmetic unit at a time to ensure even coverage. One hand is used to stretch out furrows and creases, while the other hand applies the glycolic acid, ensuring coverage in the area. Often, with a cotton applicator or the same brush, more of the glycolic acid will be firmly rubbed into furrows or finely creased areas, such as the nasolabial folds or perioral creases, to enhance the effect in that area. Some keratotic areas will not respond as well and require firm rubbing to react properly. Because the 50% and 70% glycolic acid is a gellike substance, some of the peeling agent may collect more on certain areas slightly; however, unlike TCA, glycolic acid does not react more in areas with more peeling agent on it. The areas around the eyes have to be treated separately, by using a semimoist cotton applicator, to ensure that the peeling agent does not get into the eyes. The patient is instructed to keep the eyes closed to minimize tearing. Tears are wiped dry to avoid capillary movement of the chemical agent into the eye. The application is within a few millimeters from the eyelid ciliary margin. All types of peels should be feathered below the jaw and into the hairline to minimize a line of demarcation.[28] The glycolic acid is left on the skin for a set amount of time measured with a stopwatch. A timer is set at the time of initial contact of the glycolic acid. The skin is then neutralized very carefully with a water-soaked gauze and a buffered neutralizer. Caution should be taken when sodium bicarbonate is used for neutralization because the glycolic acid and sodium bicarbonate form an entropic reaction which creates heat. This heat could intensify or damage the peeled skin. The patient is then told to rinse the skin under cool running water. Occasionally, a patient will complain of stinging of the eyes, even if no glycolic acid has actually entered them, but it will resolve after the peel has been neutralized. A water-soaked gauze can be used to wipe the eyes gently, or a squeeze bottle with water can be kept at hand to rinse the eyes if needed. Patients with moderate to severe erythema are given a mild corticosteroid cream to apply twice daily to affected areas for 2 days.

Superficial chemical peels need to be repeated to have maximal benefit.[33] The initial application is usually 50% solution and is left on for a carefully timed 3 min. If the patient has repeated peels every 2 to 4 weeks, the time is increased by 30 s or the concentration of the glycolic acid is increased to 70%. If the patient has very sensitive skin, the peel may be started at 2 to 2.5 min. Eventually, some patients will tolerate peels lasting for up to 10 min, especially if they have severe chronic sun damage. For acne, it appears that the peeling agent will penetrate the pores and plugs more readily than the epidermis. When glycolic acid is used to treat acne, it is usually left on only 1 to 2 min.

Applying the TCA Peel

TCA peels are applied in a similar manner as the glycolic acid peels, although some differences are noted. Small variations in technique can cause larger variations in depths of peeling and possible scarring.[26] Variations in technique are evident in articles describing work with TCA. Any of the procedures, when used consistently, can be safely and effectively used. Preparation of the skin is the same to remove oils and excess keratin debris. TCA is also applied evenly with several cotton applicators or cotton balls. The same basic pattern of starting on the forehead, proceeding down one cheek, and proceeding around the face to the other cheek is recommended. TCA can be reapplied into furrows in a similar manner as glycolic acid. In addition, keratotic lesions can be re-treated with a cotton applicator and TCA since keratoses can be more resistant to frosting. The TCA should be drained at the side of the bottle to decrease the chances of dripping. Unlike glycolic acid, TCA elicits erythema very quickly, and frosting appears within 1 to 2 min. It is important not to let the TCA drip or collect in a pool to prevent overreaction in areas. The discomfort from TCA can be more severe than that from glycolic acid, and having patients fan their skin will cause some relief. If the discomfort is too great, the peel can be stopped for several minutes before proceeding so that the patient can rest. As mentioned, reapplication may deepen the peeling effect.

Some physicians may apply TCA once evenly, and others may apply it until frosting is achieved. Usually, neutralization is performed with water or a 5% bicarbonate solution. Neutralization for superficial peels of TCA should be done immediately within 60 to 90 s or soon after frosting appears, although the skin itself may neutralize the peel; therefore, many peel specialists do not neutralize.[28] Probably, neutralization after frosting is not very helpful because the TCA reaction has already reached its end point.

Usually, the first application should be light and the agent should not be reapplied to any areas. One approach is to apply a trial of 10% or 15% TCA for 1 min before neutralizing. The timer is started at initiation of TCA application. An erythema or mild frosting is achieved. At the end of 1 min, the area is rinsed or wiped with water. The process is repeated once a week or biweekly and the time increased by 30 s to a maximum of 2 min. The TCA concentration will then be increased by 5% up to 25% or 30%. When TCA concentration is increased, the time of peeling before neutralization is started at 1 min again.

Another technique is to use a 30% to 35% solution, without progressing to higher concentration peels. After skin preparation, TCA is applied into all the peel areas. Without reapplication of the TCA, the skin is allowed to frost or blanch.[26,35] The area is then neutralized immediately after blanching, although neutralization may have a limited effect at this time. Often, it is easier to section the face into anatomic units to apply the TCA, and then neutralize before moving on to the next facial area.

Different factors may affect the strength of the superficial peel (Table 37-7). The most important difference between applying TCA or glycolic acid is that glycolic acid reactivity is very dependent on the length of time that the glycolic acid stays on the skin. The amount of glycolic acid applied is not as critical as with TCA peels. On the other hand, TCA is very dependent on the concentration, on the amount of TCA used, and on the application pressure. If a lower concentration of TCA is continuously applied several times or reapplied after a frost appears, the peel will be deeper and be equivalent to a higher concentration. The time of neutralization makes a difference in the peel reaction only if the peel is neutralized from 1 to 2 min before frosting occurs.[26]

Applying the Phenol Peel

Because of the risk of systemic toxicity that is possible with phenol peels, a more thorough history and exam is required. Cardiac, renal, and liver systems should be cleared before the peel is given.[36] Prepeel sedation and analgesics are required to control the pain during the procedure.

The Baker-Gordon phenol should be made fresh for each patient being peeled. The ingredients need to be continuously

T A B L E 3 7 - 7

Superficial Resorcin Peel

24% Sulfur

24% Resorcin

0.5% Carboxymethylcellulose

1.0% Aluminum-magnesium silicate

2.5% Sorbitol

2.5% Glycerin

45.5% Deionized water

stirred well to create an even peel (Table 37-4).[37] As with TCA, a single applicator is used to brush the phenol in broad strokes across the skin. Firm, broad strokes should be used. A strong white frosting occurs rapidly. Because of the systemic absorption, the phenol is applied in stages across the face. The application should be in small anatomic sections so that the phenol absorption in the bloodstream is minimized. Taping is often used after the application of the phenol to increase the absorption of the peel. Pieces of tape are applied in short 2- to 4-cm strips of overlapping layers.[36,38] After the tape is removed in 2 days, drying agents are used to dry off the crust and exudate that accumulate under the peel. More recently, the Baker-Gordon chemical peel has been performed without taping, with effective results.[39]

Combination Peels

Retinoic acid has been used as a daily topical agent.[32] Several studies have indicated the use of topical retinoic acid for the treatment of actinic keratoses, wrinkles, and pigmentation. Further investigations are still needed to evaluate its effectiveness. Topical retinoic acid as a prepeel treatment 2 weeks before dermabrasions will reduce healing time and decrease complications postdermabrasions.[40] "Retinizing" the skin before procedures is thought to improve wound healing and speed epithelialization. Topical retinoic acid can be used in conjunction with a superficial peel to enhance the effects of the peel. Studies focusing on the use of the two modalities together have not been done, although it is commonly advocated.[26] The precaution for using retinoic acid is that it also deepens the effect of peels, probably by thinning the upper portion of the epidermis (stratum corneum and upper stratum malpighian).

An alternative to topical retinoic acids as a prepeel agent is 10% glycolic acid, which can be used for 2 weeks before any superficial peel (glycolic or TCA).[7] Although further studies are warranted, prepeel 10% glycolic acid may enhance penetration of superficial peels as topical tretinoin does.

Combination peels have been used to some extent in different variations. The principles behind combining peels is that one agent can enhance the penetration of the other agent while decreasing some of the toxic risk and morbidity of deeper peels. TCA 35%, alone, does not consistently penetrate deeper than the papillary dermis. However, 45% to 60% concentrations of TCA have a significant risk of pigmentary alteration and scarring.[41] TCA at 50% to 70% has even higher risk of uneven hypopigmentation and persistent erythema. Recently, a study showed that solid carbon dioxide (CO_2) applied before 35% TCA is effective and shows histologically a wound depth similar to phenol, without the risks of higher strength TCA.[42] Solid CO_2 blocks are dipped into a 3:1 solution of acetone and alcohol and then applied directly to the skin for 3 to 10 s before several coats of TCA. The use of Jessners' solution before 35% TCA has been applied has proved also beneficial. One article suggested that using Jessners' solution with 35% TCA reduces the significant scarring risk of higher concentrations of TCA.[3] Jessners' solution is applied with moist cotton applicators and allowed to frost lightly. After several minutes, 35% TCA is applied evenly with several cotton applicators. Neither the CO_2 of Jessners' solution with TCA is described with neutralization. These two combination peels are rated as medium-depth peeling procedures. As designed, both peels are a substitute for deep phenol peels in improving deep wrinkles and deeper hyperpigmentation with limited side effects.

Jessners' or 20% TCA can enhance 50% and 70% glycolic acid. These combinations allow for more accelerated peeling while only producing mild erythema and only focal mild crusting. As with other superficial peels, these combinations can be repeated regularly in 2 to 4 weeks. Preliminary histologic studies suggest that the depth of penetration is enhanced when combinations with glycolic acid are used.[43]

The procedure for applying a prepeel agent before glycolic acid is similar to the regular peel procedure described for TCA. Jessners' solution is applied thinly and allowed to dry on the face for 2 min. Some clinicians will firmly rub the Jessners' solution on or apply three even coats. Next, the glycolic acid is put on and neutralized as described previously.[3,45] The skin is likely to have more erythema and, on occasion, more sloughing of epidermis with resulting crusting than with glycolic acid by itself.

Other Peeling Agents

Jessners' solution is composed of resorcinol, salicylic acid, lactic acid, and ethanol (Table 37-7). It is one of the light peels that have been used in facial salons as well as physicians' offices over the years.[33] By itself, Jessners' solution is applied lightly with a soaked cotton ball or soaked cotton applicator. The solution is allowed to dry without neutralization. Several layers can be applied to achieve a deeper penetration.[42] Histological studies have not been done to determine the skin depths from layering the solution on, although rubbing the solution more vigorously can deepen the peel. Improvement in pigmentation and fine wrinkles can be seen from treatment with Jessners' solution. There have been reports of systemic toxicity. Therefore, the use of Jessners' solution is often limited to the face. Jessners' may enhance the effects of TCA and glycolic acid by allowing a more even and deeper penetration.[3] More articles on Jessner's formula now describe its use in conjunction with other peeling agents.

Resorcin has been used since first introduced in 1882 and is a derivative of phenol.[44] It has been shown to separate the epidermis at the stratum granulosum while causing a deep inflammation. Histology shows that resorcin can cause an increase in glycosaminoglycans, elastic fibers, fibroblasts, and a thickened papillary dermal band[25] and can be effective for fine wrinkles, actinic damage, pigmentation, and other problems which are also indications for light peels.[44] Formulations

vary from 10% to 50%. One recommended formulation for superficial peeling is listed in Table 37-7.

The rescorcin paste is applied as a mask layer across the face by using a tongue blade or small brush. After the paste is removed in 5 to 10 min, a "resorcin membrane" remains, which persists for 4 to 5 days. Fresh skin appears when the damaged skin desquamates off. Complications are minimal, with hyperpigmentation reported to be less than 1% in a Hispanic population.[44]

POSTPEEL

Patients are warned about crusting and erythema for 3 to 7 days after any peel. Discomfort usually occurs only during the procedure and is a combination of stinging and pruritis. No oral analgesia or oral steroids are usually required after the peel procedure.

As mentioned, mild cortisone cream can be given if the inflammation and erythema are uncomfortable. Later, after 30 to 60 min, makeup can be used to cover the treated areas. The face can be rinsed, but the patient is told not to scrub. A noncleansing soap lotion can be provided. For crusting, an antibiotic ointment is applied, and the crust is not to be mechanically removed.[2] Patients are advised not to apply AHAs or topical retinoic acid for at least 4 to 5 days after the peel to avoid deepening the reaction of the peel.[26] Protection from sun exposure is strongly recommended for at least 2 weeks, especially when pigmentation problems are treated. A written sheet informing patients of discomfort, crusting, and erythema is important with instructions on general care of the skin.

INDICATIONS FOR CHEMICAL PEELS

Chemical peels are very effective for many skin conditions (Table 37-2). Listed below are the most common conditions treated with superficial peels.

Wrinkles

Wrinkled, sun-exposed skin shows accumulation of the elastotic material. This elastotic deposition is thought to lack structural support quality leading to a sagging, nonelastic, wrinkled skin. Some patients will have many fine wrinkles across the cheeks and around the eyes and mouth. On occasion, patients will have wrinkles that crosshatch. The reason for the elastotic deposition is not understood. One theory is that the fibroblasts are damaged by ultraviolet radiation and produce altered collagen and elastin.[45]

The improvement of photoaged skin by chemical peels involves new collagen deposition either on top of or in place of the upper papillary zone of elastotic-damaged deposits.[5,11] Medium and deep peels are thought to function histologically like dermabrasions by causing a similar scar formation in the upper papillary dermis.[13] Superficial peels may achieve satisfactory results by repeatedly stimulating the skin and stimulating new collagen growth, without causing the deeper wound healing of deep chemical peels.

For wrinkles, the glycolic acid or TCA peel penetration is enhanced by using stronger skin preparations and increasing the strength of the peel. Repeated 70% glycolic acid (Fig. 37-1) and 35% TCA can be used; however, glycolic acid and TCA will need to be pretreated with another chemical agent. Jessners' solution or solid CO_2 slush are used with regular peeling agents (TCA or glycolic acid) as combination peels to increase significantly the depth of peel penetration.[2]

The Baker-Gordon phenol peel is the most consistent in the treatment of moderate to deep rhytids.[37,38] A single phenol peel will give very positive benefits beyond some of the repeated chemical peels with other agents.

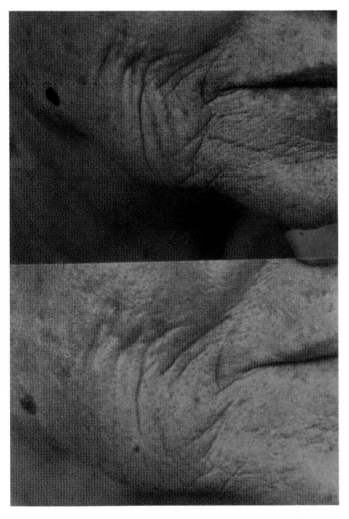

Figure 37-1 (*a*) Deep creases on an elderly woman. (*b*) After two months of peels, the creases were beginning to smooth. (Courtesy of Dr. Romulo Mene)

Actinic Keratoses

Chemical peels can be used to treat actinic keratoses that are not excessively hyperkeratotic. The result can be beneficial by decreasing the formation of skin cancers and also in clearing a number of actinic keratoses to even the blotchy appearance of the skin. There is a tendency to produce hypopigmentation scars when treating individual actinic keratoses lesions with spot liquid nitrogen or electrocautery. 5-Fluorouracil can effectively remove multiple lesions but is very uncomfortable and cosmetically noticeable for a longer period of time than a superficial chemical peel. Many patients will not be compliant with such a harsh therapeutic regimen. Topical retinoic acid has been reported to be only minimally effective as a solitary agent for actinic keratoses, although it can complement the penetration of 5-Fluorouracil for patients with thicker hyperkeratotic lesions.

Seventy percent glycolic acid causes increased epidermolysis and discohesiveness of the cells, thus thinning actinic keratoses.[12] Patients will actually have resolution of most of their actinic keratoses. If some of the thicker actinic keratoses do not resolve, the lesions are always thinner, thus making them easier to treat with 5-Fluorouracil or other modalities. The advantage of pretreating a patient with chemical peels before 5-Fluoraouracil is the decreased discomfort and time required for application of the 5-Fluorouracil.[20]

TCA at 30% or 35% has also been found to be effective to treat actinic keratoses.[47] TCA will work better in removing lentigines and wrinkles than 5-Fluorouracil cream yet will be as effective in removing actinic keratoses. TCA can also be applied locally to specific lesions; however, thicker actinic keratoses may still require liquid nitrogen or other therapy.

Another variation for actinic keratoses treatment is 5-Fluorouracil for only 2 weeks to bring out many previously subclinical lesions,[48] followed by a peel of glycolic acid or TCA localized to the remaining inflamed lesions. Using repeated peels at this point may prevent or retard the appearance of further actinic keratoses.

Acne

Although acne is not usually treated with superficial peels, the peeling agent may effectively reduce comedones and pustules.[1] Glycolic acid has been reported to penetrate into open and closed comedones very readily.[46] TCA is used successfully as an acne exfoliant for active acne lesions and improving acne scarring.[1,48]

The use of glycolic acid or TCA for acne and acne scarring should be at a more superficial depth and should produce less reaction than other glycolic acid peels. Thus, 50% glycolic acid can be applied for only 1 to 2 min over the entire face. Often, no redness is seen at the time of neutralizing the glycolic acid. After one or two of these light peels, the acne can be the same or look worse; new comedones come to the surface after several peels. After three to five peels repeated

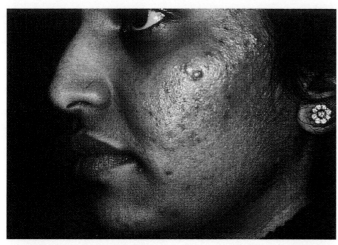

a

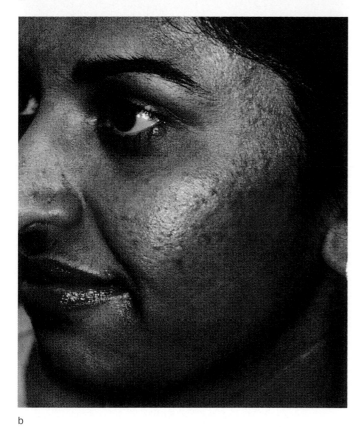

b

Figure 37-2 (*a*) Young girl with acne and acne scars. (*b*) After several months of glycolic acid peels and daily glycolic acid lotions, the acne cleared and the surface contours were smooth on her cheeks.

every 3 weeks, a majority of comedones and pustules are gone (Fig. 37-2). If the 10% glycolic acid is used thereafter, the peel effect may be maintained for at least 6 months. TCA at concentrations of 15% to 20% is applied for 30 to 45 s and thoroughly neutralized right away. After a number of these very light peels, acne scars and acne are also thought to be im-

proved;[33] however, the actual improvement has not been subjected to well-controlled comparison studies. These peeling agents can be more potent keratolytic and comedolytic acne treatments than retinoic acid for certain acne cases.

For acne, superficial, not deep, peels are recommended. For acne scarring, superficial and deeper peels can be very beneficial. Deeper peeling with phenol and high concentrations of TCA will restructure sufficient amounts of collagen in the dermis to smooth layers of scarring. Even repeated glycolic acid 70% chemical peels will improve scarring if the peel is allowed to penetrate into the dermis.

Melasma

Melasma is a blotchy, irregular melanin hyperpigmentation that classically appears on areas of the face.[8,49] Most notably, melasma appears on the forehead, upper cheeks, and upper lip, although other areas of the face can also show the hyperpigmentation. Estrogens and progesterone are thought to be partially responsible for melasma, especially during pregnancy or with use of oral contraceptives.

Much of the difficulty in treating melasma is that patients prone to having melasma also have a tendency for postinflammatory hyperpigmentation. Dermabrasions and deeper peels have been used, but the results are not consistent and have a higher incidence of side effects than superficial chemical peels.[6]

Patients can apply a mixture lotion of 10% glycolic acid and 2% hydroquinone or topical tretinoin, 4% hydroquinone, and mild corticosteroids.[49] The lotions are applied twice a day before and after a series of peels (Figs. 37-3–37-4). Fifty percent glycolic acid chemical peels or 15% to 25% TCA peels are used, although TCA peels may cause more problems than glycolic peels. Crusting should be minimized because of the risk of hyperpigmentation on darker skin. A regimen of four to five peel treatments is recommended to the patient before very clear improvements are clinically made (Fig. 37-4). It is recommended to repeat the peel every 3 to 4 weeks. A sunscreen with maximum UVA and UVB coverage is strongly recommended to the patient to prevent further darkening.[2,5,6]

The mechanism by which glycolic acid and TCA works on hyperpigmentation is not known. Glycolic acid, as with other AHAs, is closely related chemically to ascorbic acid.[46] There are studies suggesting that ascorbic acid has a direct effect on melanocytes by inhibiting melanocyte activity.[22] Another possible effect of glycolic acid and TCA light peels is that they allow better penetration of the hydroquinone to the melanocytes in the epidermal basal layer or upper papillary dermis or directly damage and decrease the number of the melanocytes.

Lentigines

Lentigines are flat brown macules appearing on the sunexposed areas of the skin such as the temples and upper

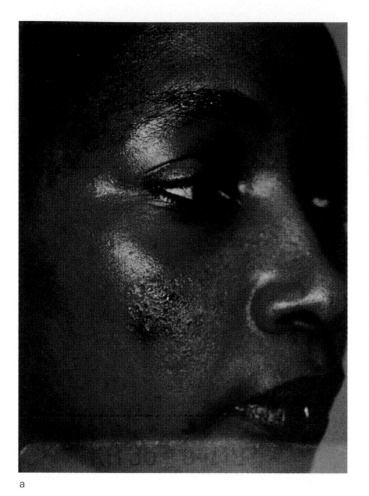

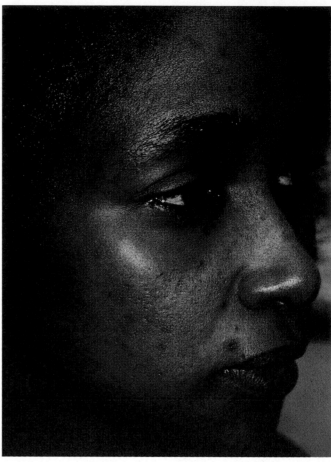

a

b

Figure 37-3   (*a*) Black female with hyperpigmentation on the middle of her cheek. (*b*) Repeated 70% glycolic acid peels were applied locally to the area, lightening the lesion after three months.

cheeks. Lentigines are due to an increase of melanocytes and melanocytic activity at the epidermal basal layer. Some dermatologists now believe that lentigines also have a keratotic component along with the hypermelanization component. These lesions have been called *keratoses simplex*.[46] Much of the aging that occurs on the hands is a function of the number of these lentigines lesions.

Peels can be very effective in the treatment of lentigines. By repeating light peels of glycolic acid (Fig. 37-5) or 20% to 35% TCA (Fig. 37-5). In the author's experience, the chemical peel must penetrate through the lentigo lesion to the papillary dermal layer to be effective. On some patients, Jessners' formulation may allow the glycolic acid to penetrate deeply enough to remove the lesions. Deeper peels are also very effective when applied locally to each lesion and are well tolerated on the hands, chest, and back. Jessners' formula is a good prepeel adjunct to enhance penetration of the peel.[3] It is recommended to the patient to apply 10% glycolic acid or topical retinoic acid before and after the superficial chemical peels when lentigines are treated.

COMPLICATIONS

Hyperpigmentation is probably the most common side effect caused by chemical peels. Usually, the deeper peels are more susceptible to postinflammatory hyperpigmentation. For instance, pigmentation problems occur in 67 percent of phenol peels.[50] Many believe that color outcome cannot be fully predicted for peels. Medium-pigmented or olive-skinned patients (Asians, Hispanics, Mediterraneans) can have irregular pigmentation.[10,51] If patients experience persistent hyperpigmentation 2 weeks after a peel, they can apply glycolic acid 10% with 2% hydroquinone lotion or 4% hydroquinone alone to lighten areas. With TCA, even at 10% to 35%, hyperpigmentation can occur and be persistent. Glycolic acid has not caused permanent hyperpigmentation in any patient at this time. Even deeper peels of CO_2 and 35% TCA (medium peels) have caused very few complications. Theoretically, the skin in a darker person can result in a line of demarcation, which is why the edge of anatomic areas such as under the angle of the jaw, around the eyebrows, and in the hairline should

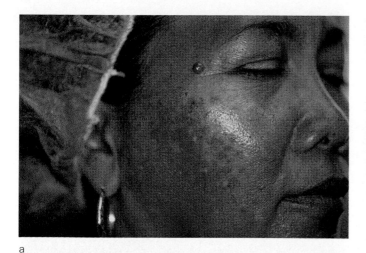

a

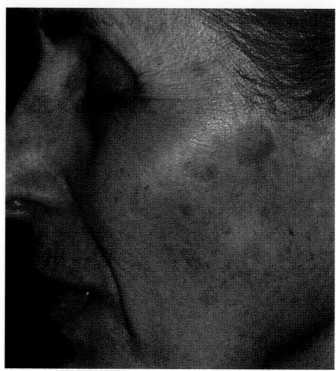

a

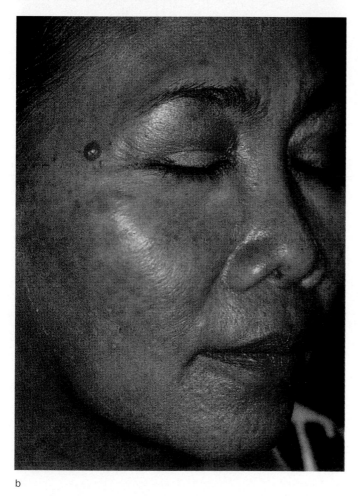

b

Figure 37-4   (*a*) Asian patient with melasma. (*b*) Daily glycolic acid lotions for two months improved pigmentation.

be feathered. Postpeel factors can enhance postinflammatory hyperpigmentation, including oral contraceptives, pregnancy, prolonged sun exposure, and photosensitizing drugs. One should restrict these factors for 2 to 4 weeks after the peel. Deeper peels need to be watched for 6 weeks to 6 months.

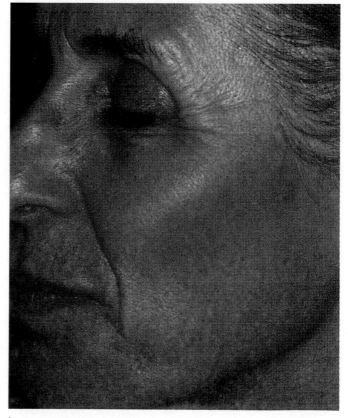

b

Figure 37-5   (*a*) This female patient had marked lentigines. (*b*) After a TCA 30% chemical peel, the lentigines were markedly improved. (Courtesy of Ron Moy)

Some anatomic areas are more susceptible to hyperpigmentation, including the jawline and around the mouth.

Persistent erythema occurs uncommonly with superficial peels.[2] Erythema should not last longer than 2 to 3 months; the majority of cases resolve within 2 to 3 weeks. Mild hydrocortisone ointment is applied for 2 days after the peel for patients with severe erythema. Erythema may be a sensitivity to the peel, with persistent inflammatory reaction. TCA tends to cause more erythema than glycolic acid.

Infections have not been a problem with superficial peels. The skin preparation agents and peeling agents themselves are bactericidal, although the crust may harbor and colonize skin and cause infections. The crust resulting from superficial peels is thinner and less adherent. It is recommended that patients use triple antibiotic ointment to wash the face gently. The crust usually washes off in 2 to 3 days.

Herpes simplex outbreak has occurred in light-peel patients, and hyperpigmentation and hypertrophic scarring also are potential hazards.[8] Patients should be questioned about history of herpetic outbreaks and incipient causes. Even though patients may not have had herpetic outbreaks for years, they can develop postoperative scarring and herpetic flares due to chemical peels.[52] Susceptible patients are put on acyclovir 200 mg orally three times a day.[2]

Hypertrophic scarring is very rare in superficial peels since this type of scarring may be a function of the depth of injury to the skin. Low-dose interlesional steroid shots are recommended. With deeper peels of phenol and TCA, certain facial areas appear to be prone to thick, overhealed scars. The perioral areas and along the length of the jaw are common areas of hypertrophic scarring involvement. Intralesional injections are often needed to soften the scars and alleviate the condition.

No allergies have been reported for patients treated with TCA or with glycolic acid. Renal hepatic or cardiac toxicities are associated with phenol but appear to be minimized when the peel is delayed between applications to facial segments.

CONCLUSION

Chemical peels can be safe and effective procedures for treating a variety of skin problems. Newer peels, such as glycolic acid and pyruvic acid, make peeling easier to be performed by more dermatologists and allow for a wider selection of patients to tolerate the procedure. Recently, histologic studies have furthered dermatologists' understanding of chemical peels by comparing different peeling agents. Future studies will encourage the increased use of chemical peels in treating a wider variety of skin conditions.

References

1. Monheit GD: Chemexfoliation: A review. *Cosmetic Dermatology* **1**:16–19, 1988

2. Brody HJ: Complications of chemical peeling. *J Dermatol Surg Oncol* **15**:1010–1019, 1989

3. Monheit GD: The Jessner's and TCA peel: A medium-depth chemical peel. *J Dermatol Surg Oncol* **15**:945–950, 1989

4. Murad H: Something old, something new. *Dermascope* April, 1989

5. Stegman SJ, Tromovitch TA: Chemical peels in cosmetic dermatologic surgery, in *Cosmetic Dermatologic Surgery,* edited by SS Stegman et al. Chicago, Year Book, 1984, pp 27–46

6. Townshend R: Skin peeling: A master's tool in skin care. *Aesthetics World* **12**:16–22, 1984

7. Brody HJ: The art of chemical peeling. *J Dermatol Surg Oncol* **15**:918–921, 1989

8. Collins PS: The chemical peel. *Clin Dermatol* **5**:57–74, 1987

9. Truppman ES, Ellenberg JD: Major electrocardiographic changes during chemical face peeling. *Plast Reconstr Surg* **63**:44–48, 1979

10. Goldman PM, Freed MI: Aesthetic problems in chemical peeling. *J Dermatol Surg Oncol* **15**:1020–1024, 1989

11. Ayres S III: Superficial chemosurgery: Its current status and its relation to dermabrasion. *Arch Dermatol* **89**:395–403, 1964

12. Spira M et al: Chemosurgery: A histological study. *Plast Reconstr Surg* **45**:247–253, 1970

13. Ayres S III: Dermal changes following application of chemical cauterants to aging skin. *Arch Dermatol* **82**:578, 1960

14. Rees RD: Chemabrasion with special reference to rehabilitation of the aging face. *Geriatrics* **20**:1039–1047, 1965

15. Stegman SJ: A comparative histologic study of the effects of three peeling agents and dermabrasion on normal and sun damaged skin. *Aesthetic Plast Surg* **6**:123–135, 1982

16. Baker TJ, Gordon HL: Chemical face peeling and dermabrasion. *Surg Clin North Am* **51**:387–401, 1971

17. Kligman AM et al: Long-term histologic follow-up of phenol face peels. *Plast Reconstr Surg* **75**:652–659, 1985

18. Behin F et al: Comparative histological study of mini pig skin after chemical peel and dermabrasion. *Arch Otolaryngol* **103**:271–277, 1977

19. Stegman SJ: A study of dermabrasion and chemical peels in an animal model. *J Dermatol Surg Oncol* **6**:490–497, 1980

20. Brodland DG et al: Depths of chemexfoliation induced by various concentrations and application techniques of trichloroacetic acid in a porcine model. *J Dermatol Surg Oncol* **15**:967–971, 1989

21. Van Scott EJ, Yu RJ: Hyperkeratinization, corneocyte cohesion, and alpha hydroxy acids. *J Am Acad Dermatol* **5**:867–879, 1984

22. Haas JE: The effect of ascorbic acid and potassium ferricyanide as melanogenesis inhibitors on the development of pigmentation in Mexican axolotols. *American Osteopathic* **73**:674, 1974

23. Lotter AM: Human pigment factors relative to chemical face peeling. *Ann Plast Surg* **3**:231–239, 1979

24. Moy LS et al: Effect of glycolic acid on collagen production

by human skin fibroblasts. Submitted, Journal Derm Surgery, 1995.

25. Letessier SM: Chemical peel with resorcin, in *Dermatologic Surgery,* edited by RK Roenigk, HH Roenigk. New York, Marcel Dekker, 1989, pp 1017–1024

26. Collins PS: Trichloroacetic acid peels revisited. *J Dermatol Surg Oncol* **15:**933–940, 1989

27. Spinowitz A, Rumsfield J: Stability time profile of trichloroacetic acid at various concentrations and storage time conditions. *J Dermatol Surg Oncol* **15:**974–975, 1989

28. Greenbaum SS, Lask GP: Facial peeling: A trichloroacetic acid, in *Asethetic Dermatology,* edited by LC Parish, GP Lask. New York, McGraw-Hill, 1991, pp 139–143

29. Brody HJ: Medium depth peeling of the skin. *J Dermatol Surg Oncol* **12:**1268–1275, 1986

30. Brown AM et al: Phenol-induced histological skin changes: Hazards, technique and uses. *Br J Plast Surg* **13:**158, 1960

31. McCullough EG, Langsdon PR: *Dermabrasion and Chemical Peel: A Guide for Facial Plastic Surgeons.* New York, Thieme, 1988, pp 53–112

32. Moy RL et al: Effects of systemic 13-cis-retinoic acid on dermal wound healing in rabbit ears in vivo. *J Dermatol Surg Oncol* 1990 August, 16(5):721–723

33. Stagnone JJ: Superficial peeling. *J Dermatol Surg Oncol* **15:**924–930, 1989

34. Stegman SJ: Chemical face peeling (editorial). *J Dermatol Surg Oncol* **12:**432, 1986

35. Roenigk HH et al: Acne, retinoids, and dermabrasion. *J Dermatol Surg Oncol* **11:**396–398, 1985

36. Alt TH: Occluded Baker-Gordon chemical peel: Review and update *J Dermatol* **15:**980–992, 1989

37. Baker TJ, Gordon HL: Chemical peel with phenol, in *Skin Surgery,* edited by E Epstein, E Epstein Jr. Philadelphia, Saunders, 1987, pp 423–438

38. Baker TJ, et al: Long-term histological study of skin after chemical face peeling. *Plast Reconstr Surg* **53:**522–525, 1974

39. Beeson WH, McCough EG: Chemical face peeling without taping. *J Dermatol Surg Oncol* **11:**985–990, 1985

40. Mandy SH: Tretinoin in preoperative and postoperative management of dermabrasion. *J Am Acad Dermatol* **15:**878–879, 1986

41. Resnick SS: Chemical peeling with trichloroacetic acid. *J Dermatol Surg Oncol* **10:**549–550, 1984

42. Brody HJ, Hailey CW: Variations and comparisons in medium-depth chemical peeling. *J Dermatol Surg Oncol* **15:**953–963, 1989

43. Moy LS et al: Epidermal and dermal histologic effects of different peeling agents on the skin of guinea pigs and minipigs. Submitted, Journal Derm Surgery, 1995.

44. Perez EH: Different grades of chemical peels. *American Journal of Cosmetic Surgery* **7:**67–60, 1990

45. Uitto J et al: Cutaneous aging: Molecular alterations in elastic fibers. *J Cut Aging and Cosm Dermatol* **1:**13–26, 1988

46. Van Scott EJ, Yu RJ: Alpha hydroxy acids: Procedures for use in clinical practice. *Cutis* **43:**222–229, 1989

47. Brodland DG, Reenigk RK: Trichloroacetic acid chemoexfoliation (chemical peel) for extensive premalignant actinic damage of the face and scalp. *Mayo Clinic Proc* **63:**887–897, 1988

48. Van Scott EJ: Personal communication, August, 1990.

49. Kligman AM, Willis I: A new formula for depigmenting human skin. *Arch Dermatol* **111:**40, 1975

50. Litton C, Trinidad G: Complications of chemical face peeling as evaluated by a questionnaire. *Plast Reconstr Surg* **67:**739–743, 1981

51. Pierce HE, Brown LA: Laminar dermal reticulotomy and chemical face peeling in a black patient. *J Dermatol Surg Oncol* **12:**69–73, 1986

52. Rappaport MJ, Kamer F: Exacerbation of facial herpes simplex after phenolic face peels. *J Dermatol Surg Oncol* **10:**57–58, 1984

John W. Skouge

38 Split-Thickness

A *split-thickness skin graft* (STSG) can be defined as a piece of skin that consists of the epidermis and a partial thickness of dermis. This is in contrast to a full-thickness skin graft that consists of the epidermis and the full thickness of dermis.

STSGs are classified by the relative thickness of dermis that is included with the epidermis. They are usually divided into thin, medium, and thick grafts (8- to 12-, 12- to 18-, and 18- to 30-in thickness, respectively) (Fig. 38-1). While thin and thick grafts have had their advocates in the past, and there may be a couple of specific reasons for their use, the most commonly used split graft is the medium, thickness graft of approximately 0.015 in.

The dermal blood vessels arborize as they rise within the dermis toward the epidermis. A thin graft, the exposed undersurface of which is at a higher plane within the dermis, would be expected to have a finer capillary network exposed. This exposure should allow for a more rapid connection between the capillaries of the graft and the recipient bed. In addition, a thin graft has a smaller volume of tissue that requires revascularization which, in theory, should permit faster and more complete survival than would occur with a thicker graft. These characteristics of thin grafts become particularly important when considering grafting a wound whose vascular supply is compromised.

A thick STSG has several advantages over thin grafts. The qualities of skin that give it its specific color and texture include factors of dermal thickness, extent of vascular supply, and the number and types of adnexal structures contained within the dermis. A thick graft will contain more of these elements, and therefore a better cosmetic result can be expected. Thick grafts, by virtue of the thickness of dermis included in the graft, can withstand traumatic injury better than thin grafts. The greater amount of dermis contained within thicker grafts acts like a cushion to minimize breakdown after minor trauma. The only real disadvantage of thick grafts relates to the deeper injury at the donor site that results from its harvest. Such donor sites take a longer time to heal, and the postoperative morbidity is increased.

It is for these reasons that the medium-thickness graft often serves as a compromise between grafts that are thinner or thicker. The cosmetic result, the rapidity of revascularization, and the degree of injury to the donor site lie between those of the thin and the thick grafts.

INDICATIONS FOR SPLIT-THICKNESS GRAFTS

The healed STSG almost always appears white and contracted, often with overlying scale which is usually in marked contrast with the color and texture of the surrounding skin. Because of their nearly uniformly poor cosmetic appearance, these grafts are relegated to the role of functional repair only. Therefore, there are no absolute indications for STSGs, only relative ones. In cutaneous surgery, STSGs are most often used in the setting of skin cancer removal, for the repair of large defects, and for attempted repair of ulcers whose bases contain a compromised vascular supply.

The most common reason for STSG placement is for the repair of large defects that are either located in an area that is impractical to repair with full-thickness skin or is simply too large. It is important to consider the health, age, and cosmetic needs of the patient when making this decision. When cosmetic needs dominate the reconstruction picture, it may be necessary to undertake the extraordinary measures that may be needed to transfer a large amount of full-thickness skin. This may involve extensive dissection for a large local flap, the movement of a distant or microvascular flap, or the placement of a large full-thickness graft.

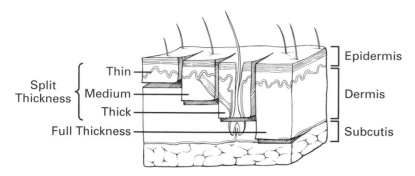

Figure 38-1 Classification of split-thickness skin grafts.

STSGs are frequently used in the setting of skin cancer surgery when the surgeon is concerned about the cleanness of the surgical margins. A definitive repair with full-thickness skin for such a wound may result in delayed recognition of a deep tumor recurrence. The nearly transparent covering provided by a split-thickness graft allows the surgeon to observe the area, thereby permitting earlier recognition of a recurrence. These concerns certainly override the cosmetic limitations that split-thickness grafts provide. At some later time, 6 months or even years after grafting, when the risk of recurrence has decreased, the graft can be removed and a more cosmetic repair can be performed. In the author's experience, when offered the choice, most patients will choose to keep the graft, as they have grown accustomed to the appearance.

There are several other relative indications for split grafts. A split graft can be used as a temporary coverage in order to prevent infection when definitive reconstruction is delayed by several days or a week. Split grafts are used to cover wounds whose vascular supply is compromised on which a full-thickness graft would not survive.

CHOOSING A DONOR SITE

A number of factors must be considered when choosing the donor site for split-thickness grafting. Unlike local flap reconstruction, the harvesting of the graft generates a second and distant iatrogenic wound that not only requires care during the initial healing process, but also generates a scar that can be quite visible. In fact, the donor wound usually causes more morbidity during the immediate postoperative period than does the grafted site, with more pain and significant wound care requirements.

As has been mentioned, it is the expectation that an STSG will heal with a poor cosmetic result. It has been suggested that grafts harvested from above the neck, the so-called blush zone, will give an improved cosmetic result for the repair of facial defects. The scalp has, on occasion, served this purpose. Since the depth of incision is above the level of the hair follicles, the hair will regrow, thereby covering the donor site. For obvious cosmetic reasons, patients are reluctant to agree to having their heads shaved, which would be required for harvesting from this location. For the purposes of dermatologic surgery, there are generally many other potential donor sites. In addition, the improvement in cosmetic appearance of a graft harvested from the scalp is, at best, only slight.

In choosing a prospective donor site, the local anatomy must be considered. Skin thickness varies with both anatomic location and age. In general, a male's skin is thicker than a female's, and an adult's skin is thicker than a child's. Additionally, skin atrophies with age, under the influence of certain medications, and with debilitating disease. These factors are important so that one does not accidentally find that a split-thickness wound has turned into a full-thickness one.

Anatomic location is an important consideration when harvesting large grafts with either one of the large hand-held knives or the power dermatomes. In order to obtain an evenly cut graft, a flat, supported surface is required. The body sites that are best suited for such grafts include the thigh (anterior, lateral, and medial), the buttock, and the abdomen (Fig. 38-2). The thighs are well supported by underlying bone and muscle, the buttock is supported by the gluteal musculature, and the abdomen is usually fairly well supported by the underlying abdominal muscles.

The resultant donor site scar can be cosmetically disfiguring. Not only does it have the appearance of a burn scar, but it is square or rectangular in shape and therefore quite obviously visible. For these reasons, when cosmesis is of critical importance, the buttock is the preferred donor site since the scar can be hidden beneath clothing—even a bathing suit.

The postoperative wound care requirements for the donor site may dictate the site that is chosen for harvesting. This is especially important for elderly patients operated on in an outpatient setting and whose wound care will be managed by family. In such situations, wound care needs may take precedence over the final cosmetic appearance of the donor scar. The anterior and lateral thigh are the preferred donor sites is these situations. These sites are readily accessible to the surgeon, dressings are easily applied by staff, and wounds in these locations are easily cared for by family and patient. In addition, these locations permit relatively free ambulation since they do not interfere with sleeping, bending, or sitting.

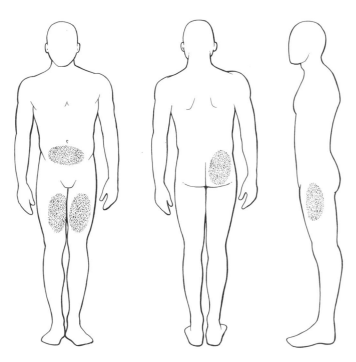

Figure 38-2 The preferred donor sites for grafting with the Padgett, Brown, and Zimmer dermatomes shown.

The donor site operative wound requires separate discussion. In the past, donor defects were simply covered with dry gauze and debrided of the dried serosanguineous material intermittently in the postoperative period by tearing off the gauze. The pain associated with this type of care was extraordinary and was a major reason for hospitalization and narcotic analgesia. While there are a number of reasonable ways of dealing with such wounds, the use of OpSite and other semipermeable and occlusive membranes has revolutionized wound care for such partial-thickness wounds. Coverage with one of these dressings not only decreases or even eliminates the pain, but the dressing keeps the wound surface moist and retains over the wound the serous drainage which contains growth factors that significantly decrease healing time. The serous drainage will build up over the first several days after surgery, and therefore the dressing should be changed at that time in order to minimize the sudden release of fluid from one edge of the dressing.

ANESTHESIA

The choice of anesthesia used depends upon several factors, including the health of the patient, the choice of the surgeon and the patient, and certain surgical considerations. While these factors always must be considered, in the ambulatory surgical setting, local anesthesia with or without sedation is nearly always sufficient to operate safely and comfortably. While the author nearly always uses 1% lidocaine with epi-

nephrine, in the situations where it is desirable to minimize drug amounts, the donor site can be completely numbed using the tumescent technique and 0.1% lidocaine with 1:1 million epinephrine. One percent lidocaine injected intradermally will produce immediate anesthesia.

Tumescent anesthesia involves the instillation of local anesthetics subcutaneously. Since the anesthetic must penetrate the fibrous sheath surrounding the cutaneous nerves as they pass through the subcutis and into the dermis, anesthesia is delayed by approximately 10 min. There are, however, several advantages to the tumescent approach. There are very few free nerve endings in the subcutaneous space, and therefore the passage of the needle through the fat and the actual injection of the anesthetic is nearly painless. In addition, very small total amounts of anesthetic are required to numb a large area of skin completely. For example, 30 to 60 cc of 0.1% lidocaine with epinephrine 1:1 million is sufficient to numb an area that measures 6 by 8 cm. This is the equivalent of only 3 to 6 cc of a 1% lidocaine solution. Since the vascular absorption rate of local anesthetics from the subcutaneous compartment is measured in hours, the risk of systemic complications in patients at even the highest cardiac risk is extremely low.

STERILE TECHNIQUE

Sterile technique must be maintained during the grafting procedure. The risk of infection at the donor site is negligible, especially when OpSite or another membrane is used for wound coverage. At the grafted site, on the other hand, the risk of infection is small but of critical importance. Infection risk is increased because the split-thickness graft consists of avascular tissue that remains avascular for several days after surgery until vascular connections reform, and this puts the tissue at particular risk during that critical time.

While the risk of infection must always be considered, antibiotic coverage is not required for all grafting procedures. Antibiotics are recommended for any wound that is felt to be contaminated and in at-risk patients. Chronic leg ulcers always present a difficult problem since they are usually contaminated by both gram-positive and gram-negative organisms. Culture and sensitivity studies are routinely indicated in such patients before grafting.

SURGICAL TECHNIQUES

Preparations for Surgery

The preparation for STSG is rather simple. The donor site must, of course, be chosen. The donor site is then shaved of all hair. When OpSite is used to cover the donor site, it is important to shave the entire surface area that will be covered by the dressing in order to allow better adherence of the dressing. The donor site is then carefully marked with a surgical marking pen and infiltrated with local anesthesia. The site is then prepared and draped in the usual manner.

The necessary equipment includes the following:

- The harvesting instrument
- Petri dish containing sterile saline-soaked gauze
- Basic surgical instruments and drapes
- Staples or suture materials
- Dressing materials for donor and recipient sites

Instrumentation

There are many tools, both manual and automatic, that have been developed for harvesting of split-thickness grafts. Generally, these instruments either cut very small grafts or very large ones. While no one device is clearly superior to any other, it is important to be comfortable with at least two techniques, one for harvesting large grafts and one for harvesting small ones. Various methods will be described below and the advantages and disadvantages of each will be described.

Razor Blade

The simplest freehand grafting tool is the double-edged razor blade. It is extremely sharp and inexpensive. When purchased, most blades come from the manufacturer clean but not sterile. Since they cannot be steam autoclaved, the blades must be prepared for surgery by gas or wet sterilization. The blade is used whole or it may be split in half. Because of its size, only small, postage stamp-sized, irregularly edged grafts can be harvested. The disadvantages of cutting split-thickness grafts with the razor blade are the limitation of the small size and the fact that its extreme sharpness can result in a deeper injury than anticipated.

In order to harvest a graft, the razor blade is held between the thumb and index or third finger and is placed parallel to the skin surface. The surgeon and the assistant apply tension across the donor site during harvesting. Only gentle forward and downward pressure is necessary while a gentle back-and-forth motion is applied to the blade.

Bard-Parker No. 15 Blade

The Bard-Parker no. 15 blade can be used to harvest small- to medium-sized split-thickness grafts. With significant practice, medium-thickness grafts up to 3 cm or more can be harvested with great reliability. This technique has certain advantages over the razor blade method. A graft of the exact dimensions required for the recipient defect can be cut, unlike all other methods which cut square or rectangular grafts, thereby sacrificing more skin than is necessary.

The lateral upper arm or thigh is the preferred donor site, although almost any anatomic site may be used. The exact size of the graft needed is marked. With the blade held perpendicularly to the epidermal surface, the initial cut scores the skin only and includes the entire perimeter of the graft. The depth of the incision is so superficial that the weight of the

scalpel itself is sufficient to achieve the desired depth. An assistant is absolutely necessary when harvesting. The assistant applies multidirectional countertension around the graft while the surgeon also applies tension. With the blade held parallel to the skin surface, the blade tip is inserted at one side of the scored perimeter. The graft is cut by gently pulling the blade from one side of the graft to the other, slowly increasing the amount of the graft that is cut with each pass. Pickups may be needed toward the end of grafting in order to minimize folding of the graft, which may interfere with the last few cuts necessary to free the graft.

This method is preferred by the author for the harvesting of small grafts. Such grafts are sometimes used to repair auricular skin cancer defects. The arm is the preferred donor site since the sterile field can be limited to one area and donor site wound care is very simple.

Weck Knife

The Weck knife is one of several freehand knives specifically designed for cutting split-thickness grafts. It comes with a handle, disposable blades, and several templates that control the thickness of the graft. The advantages of the Weck knife system is the low investment cost and the ease of use.

The knife is used in the following manner: (1) The blade is slid onto the handle, and the template is attached; (2) the knife is then placed parallel to the skin; and (3) with an assistant applying tension, a back-and-forth sawing motion is used while the knife is advanced through the skin. Moderate downward pressure and only slight forward pressure are required to advance the knife. The thickness of the graft is determined by the template that is used and to a lesser extent by the degree of downward pressure utilized.

The Weck knife is simple to use and very inexpensive. Because of the sawing action required of such a manual instrument, the resultant graft has saw-toothed lateral edges that therefore limit the real usable amount of graft harvested.

Pinch Grafts

Pinch grafts have been used by surgeons for many years. Because the harvesting technique is so simple and alluring, pinch grafts have had many advocates. Unfortunately, the cosmetic results are often unacceptable and therefore, with few exceptions, the technique should be relegated to the annals of surgery. However, because the technique is still in widespread use, it will be described.

The term *pinch* comes from the fact that a small fragment of skin is pinched and elevated by pickups. With the skin so elevated, a sharp iris scissors is used to snip off the fragment of skin (i.e., the graft) (Fig. 38-3). The graft that is generated is obviously very small and has some interesting characteristics. Because of the manner in which the graft is cut, the graft thickness varies from epidermis only at the edges to sometimes full-thickness dermis at the center. It is the irregularity of the grafts that also represents their severe limitations. The

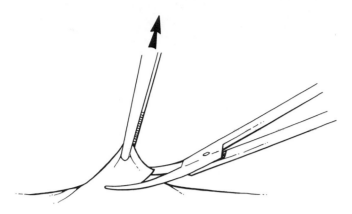

Figure 38-3 Pinch Grafting: A small fragment of skin is elevated with a pick-ups and snipped off with a small, sharp scissors.

healed donor sites have a pockmarked appearance, while the healed grafts appear as small hillocks. With the ease of harvesting small grafts by using the razor blade, no. 15 blade, or the small Davol dermatome, pinch grafts should have limited use in surgery.

Electric Dermatomes

There are several electric dermatomes that are available for the harvesting of split-thickness grafts. The only small unit is the Davol dermatome. There are, however, three dermatomes that permit the harvesting of large grafts, including the Brown, the Padgett, and the Zimmer. These units replace the sawing motion required when harvesting grafts by hand, thereby allowing the formation of grafts that are more even in thickness and width.

Davol Dermatome

This dermatome is a battery-powered unit that cuts small postage-sized grafts. The advantage of this unit is its simple design and use, while the disadvantage is the small size of the graft that is generated.

The Davol dermatome looks very much like a portable toothbrush with its rechargeable handle and charging base. Neither the handle nor the base can be sterilized. The sterile kit that accompanies the unit contains a single-use sterile grafting head with blade attached and a sterile plastic bag.

The parameters of the Davol unit are fixed. The thickness of the graft is fixed at 0.015 in and the width is 3 cm. The dermatome is put together in the following manner: (1) The contents of the disposable kit are placed on a sterile tray, (2) the nonsterile handle is carefully dropped into the sterile plastic bag, (3) the twist then secures the end of the bag, and (4) the cutting head is then clicked into place over the bag and onto the end of the handle. This completes the assembly and the sterile dermatome is ready for use.

The cutting side of the dermatome is then placed against the skin with only moderate downward pressure applied; the unit is then turned on. Slight forward pressure applied to the unit will advance the dermatome, thereby harvesting the graft. The blade is not particularly sharp, and therefore only small lengths of graft can be harvested.

Brown, Padgett, and Zimmer Dermatomes

The large electric dermatomes that are in use include the Brown, the Padgett, and the Zimmer. Recently, the Brown dermatome was taken off the market and was replaced with the newly designed and high-tech-looking Zimmer dermatome. The Zimmer Co. (Dover, Ohio), will no longer sell the Brown dermatome, nor will it repair existing units, but will continue to sell blades for it. Fortunately, there are still several small companies that will continue to repair the Brown.

The advantage of the Brown over the Padgett was that it was steam autoclavable while the Padgett was not. This made the Brown an ideal dermatome for use in an office setting where gas sterilization was not available. The Zimmer dermatome is also steam autoclavable and will undoubtedly replace the Brown unit in the office setting. When considering purchasing either the Padgett or the Zimmer, surgeons must assess availability of gas sterilization for a unit of this size. Because of liability issues, many hospitals will not permit access to their large gas sterilization units by office-based physicians for their personal dermatomes. This regulation may limit the choice for office surgeons to the Zimmer.

There are differences between the three dermatomes described. The Zimmer has been in use for only a year or two, and so its long-term reliability is uncertain. Its design is similar to that of the Padgett, and the author expects it would have a similar reliability pattern. The Padgett is a very sturdy instrument with fewer moving parts than the Brown; it, therefore, requires fewer repairs. Because of this reliability, the Padgett is more often found in hospital operating rooms where instruments often receive greater abuse. The Brown is a much more fragile instrument and must be handled carefully. Even with such careful maintenance, however, intermittent repairs are required. The Padgett and Zimmer units can be purchased as either electrically powered or nitrogen driven.

The difference in reliability relates to the design differences of the units. One of the apparent advantages of the Brown is that incremental differences of graft width can be set. This feature differs from the Padgett and Zimmer units, which come with 3 templates (2-, 4-, and 6-in widths) for choosing the desired width of a proposed graft. While the greater choices that the Brown offers mean that a more exact-sized graft can be cut, the disadvantage is that this design has more moving parts that serve as a source for more frequent repairs. The mechanism that sets graft thickness is also much more cumbersome on the Brown than on either the Zimmer or the Padgett. The thickness dials can easily go out of alignment—probably the most common reason for repair of the Brown. The mechanisms for the Zimmer and the Padgett seem much simpler, and, while the Padgett certainly has a history of reliability, the author expects the similar design features of the Zimmer also would demonstrate long-term reliability.

Dermatome Grafting Technique

The technique for grafting is similar for each instrument. Each dermatome comes with disposable, single-use blades. The blades are attached, and either the appropriate template is secured for the Padgett or the Zimmer, or the width is set on the Brown. The desired graft thickness is then set for thin, medium, or thick grafts. The Brown is calibrated only in thousandths of an inch, while the other two units show both thickness in thousandths of an inch and in millimeters.

A small amount of lubricant is then applied to the blade and to the skin to be grafted. While sterile mineral oil is the traditional lubricant of the operating room, any of the easily available sterile and water soluble lubricants (such as Surgilube) will suffice. An assistant then applies tension with one hand, a block of wood, or tongue depressor at the distal end of the proposed graft, while the surgeon places the nondominant hand behind the dermatome, applying countertension to the skin. The dermatome is then placed flat to the skin and the unit is engaged. Moderate downward pressure and slow but even forward pressure will result in a graft of even thickness and width. At the end of grafting, the advancing tip of the dermatome is moved away from the skin surface as if it were an airplane taking off. This action will generally separate the graft from the donor site. Special attention must be paid at this point: If the graft does not easily separate, the dermatome must be turned off and the graft not lifted any farther. This will avoid damage to the graft. The graft can then be separated with a scalpel or scissors. The graft is then placed on sterile, saline-soaked gauze in a petri dish or placed directly onto the recipient defect. The donor site is then covered with a dressing.

The graft is then placed over the recipient defect. Recall that these dermatomes always cut grafts that are square to rectangular, and therefore they will need to be trimmed in order to fit the size of the defect. During trimming, the author recommends that one edge of the graft be placed at the edge of the defect and secured with a suture or staple. To be sure that the graft is not miscut, the author recommends trimming the graft of redundant skin in quadrants, securing the graft edges as the procedure progresses. A serrated scissors will grasp the skin much more easily and will facilitate this process (Fig. 38-4).

Securing the Graft

In theory, if a graft could be draped over its recipient defect, without hematoma, seroma, or infection occurring, the graft

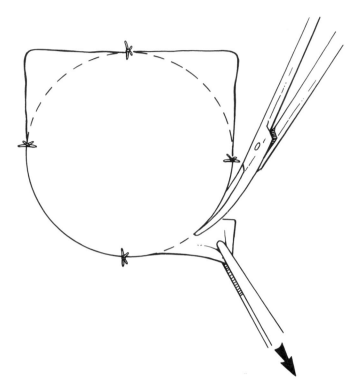

Figure 38-4   After the rectangular/square graft is placed over the defect, it is secured in four quadrants. The excess graft is then carefully excised so that the graft exactly fits the defect.

could be left without support or suture and it would survive. Unfortunately, since nearly all dermatologic surgical patients are ambulatory, it is obligatory that the graft be carefully secured and efforts made to prevent those factors that will interfere with the survival of that graft.

The nutritional support and future blood supply to the graft does not come from the edges of the defect but rather from the floor of of the defect. It is therefore necessary for the graft to be held firmly to the defect floor as well as secured at the perimeter.

The perimeter of the graft is generally secured with sutures or staples (Figs. 38-5 and 38-6). Occasionally, very small grafts may be left without perimeter support. Unlike full-thickness grafts for which precise approximation of the edges is necessary, such exact suturing technique is not critical. If a small portion of the edge of the graft overlaps the surrounding skin, it will simply necrose and separate, without adverse effect on the viable portions of the graft. The only disadvantage of leaving more than a thin layer of overlapping skin in place is that after suture removal, that edge will dehydrate and tend to catch on dressings, sometimes causing bleeding and slight separation of the adjacent attached graft.

While simple, interrupted sutures are sufficient for smaller grafts, their application is extremely time consuming and offers no advantages over a faster placed over-and-over running suture. The author generally recommends the placement of interrupted sutures at the four quadrants around the graft. These

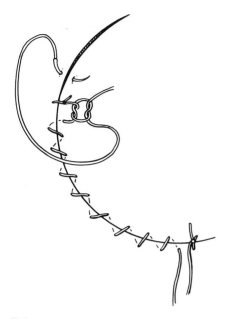

Figure 38-5 A running stitch is used to secure the perimeter of the graft.

are placed before the running suture is begun and assist in orienting the graft while the surgeon trims it. They are left long so that the running stitch can be tied to them in order to prevent complete unraveling should a portion of the running stitch break.

Ideally, there should be no tension on the wound. Therefore, the caliber of the suture material is relatively unimportant at least with regard to the security of the wound. Generally, the smaller the caliber of suture used, the easier it is to manipulate

and tie. The author uses 5-0 or 6-0 suture for this purpose. Any of the nonabsorbable, synthetic suture materials work well, although one of the rapidly absorbing chromic gut sutures, which dissolve in a week or less, will simplify suture removal. Gut suture has a high degree of friction when passing through tissues and therefore can take a bit more time to place.

As has been mentioned, the graft itself must be held tightly to the base of the defect to allow imbibition of nutrients immediately after surgery and for revascularization of the graft. Proper central support will also aid in preventing or at least minimizing the development of hematomas or seromas. This is accomplished with either suture or support dressing or a combination of both.

Centrally placed stitches are referred to as *basting sutures*. The sutures are placed in a manner that includes a portion of the graft and the subjacent wound bed. Individual interrupted sutures with 5-0 or 6-0 material may be used to secure small or large grafts. The author prefers to use a running basting suture technique for large grafts that was described by Glogau (Fig. 38-7). This method uses an over-and-over technique that permits the securing of the graft in many spots very rapidly. An advantage of basting sutures, aside from the obvious purpose of holding the graft to the defect bed, is that should a hematoma or seroma develop, the sutures will tend to loculate the fluid, thereby limiting dissection of the fluid between the graft, with greater survival of the graft.

A small but important detail of suturing must be mentioned. Most surgical defects that are to be grafted have a vertical dimension as well as the obvious horizontal one. There are sidewalls to the defect that must be addressed. When planning the graft and when securing it in place, the surgeon must drape the graft down the vertical sidewalls as well as over the

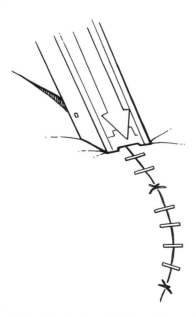

Figure 38-6 Alternatively, the perimeter of the graft may be secured with staples.

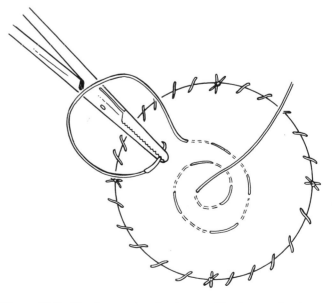

Figure 38-7 If a tie-over dressing is not utilized, a running basting-suturing technique may be utilized to secure the central portion of the graft to the defect floor.

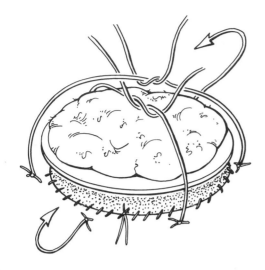

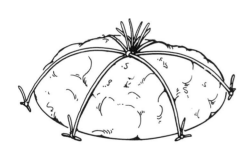

Figure 38-8 The tie-over stent minimizes the risks of hematoma and seroma formation, as well as holds the graft to the underlying bed thereby increasing the potential for graft survival.

horizontal defect floor in order to avoid tenting of the graft over that concavity, which will result in loss of that portion of the graft.

SURGICAL DRESSINGS

A dressing consisting of an antibiotic ointment applied to the suture line, covered with a nonstick layer, such as Telfa or Xeroform, which is then secured with pressure, may be adequate for small grafts or those large grafts having a firm base or covering convex surfaces such as the scalp. This type of dressing allows for observation of the wound, which may be necessary for wounds that are potentially contaminated or are creating a great deal of drainage.

Otherwise, the preferred dressing is the tie-over dressing. This dressing is placed at the time of grafting and generally remains in place until suture removal. The advantages of this dressing include (1) it completely isolates the wound from the outside environment; (2) it immobilizes the graft by providing even pressure over the graft, thereby keeping the graft in constant contact with the wound bed; (3) it minimizes the risk of hematoma or seroma formation; and (4) it minimizes wound care for the patient and family since the dressing remains in place until suture removal.

The dressing is placed in the following manner: Interrupted 3-0 to 5-0 sutures are placed in pairs opposite each other across the graft. The sutures are left long so that they can be tied to each other. Two to four pairs of sutures are generally placed, depending upon the size and shape of the graft. A layered dressing is applied to the graft. This dressing, generally consists of an antibiotic ointment applied to the sutures, followed by a nonstick layer. Above this layer, material must be placed that provides bulk and molds to the contours of the graft and recipient bed. This bulky layer may consist of Vaseline-impregnated gauze, Xeroform gauze, or simply cotton balls that have been moistened, wrung out, and then pressed into place. The cotton will conform to the shape of the graft and defect, will dry out, and create a hard castlike mold. The sutures are then tied over the entire dressing, with each suture tied to its pair from the opposite side of the graft (Fig. 38-8).

The only real disadvantage of the tie-over dressing is that the graft cannot be observed through the healing process without destroying the integrity of the dressing. In theory, should a hematoma, seroma, or infection occur, such a problem might go unnoticed, or recognition would at least be delayed until a portion or all of the graft might be lost. In reality, these complications are rare enough that the benefits of the tie-over dressing nearly always outweigh the risks.

POSTOPERATIVE EXPECTATIONS AND COMPLICATIONS

Split-thickness grafting can be difficult for many patients. There are two wounds that must be dealt with, and pain can be a problem. The discomfort arises from the donor site but can be alleviated with acetaminophen or a mild narcotic analgesic. The semipermeable wound dressings, such as OpSite, that cover the donor site significantly decrease the pain associated with these partial-thickness wounds.

Infection is always a concern, but, as long as the grafted wound is one that has been surgically generated, antibiotic coverage is rarely necessary. Contaminated wounds, on the other hand, require special consideration and antibiotic coverage as determined by the appropriate bacterial culture and sensitivity studies.

The expectation for split-thickness grafting is for 100 percent survival of the graft. This goal cannot always be achieved, but it is worthwhile evaluating all aspects of the procedure to determine the causes of graft failure. Graft take (i.e., revascularization) occurs in 3 to 5 days. While initial graft survival is ensured by this time, the new vascular connections are fragile and easily broken. Therefore, sutures, staples, or dressings are usually left in place for several days longer.

Complications are divided into early and late complications. Early complications relate to the initial failure of graft survival, and late complications generally relate to aesthetic and functional deficits.

Early Complications

Technical Considerations

Technical considerations are very important in the ultimate survival of split-thickness grafts. As has been discussed, adequate immobilization of the graft is of critical importance in graft survival. An additional technical point is to be sure not to place the graft upside down. While this seems trivial, the distinction between dermal side and epidermal side can be blurred, especially when the graft is sitting in sterile saline and when a lubricant has been used. In general, the dermal side of the graft has a more glistening appearance which will help to distinguish sides. More importantly, a split-thickness graft will always curl slightly onto itself, and that curling always occurs toward the dermal side.

Hematomas and Seromas

Hematoma and seroma formation will elevate a portion or all of a graft, thereby resulting in failure of that portion of the graft. Most often, these risks can be anticipated and therefore prevented. The initial decision point arises at the time of grafting. A wound that is draining profusely may not be ready for grafting or may require further preparation before a graft can be placed. Meticulous hemostasis and the appropriate pressure dressings will aid in prevention of these problems. Wound elevation and minimizing patient activity during the initial postoperative period also will help to prevent problems. At the time of grafting, small slits can be placed through the graft, especially at dependent sites, so that any fluid that forms will drain from beneath the graft rather than elevate the graft. Basting sutures will also help in at least loculating a collection of blood serum, thereby minimizing the degree of graft loss. In the extreme situation, meshing of the graft may permit attachment of a graft while allowing significant drainage of fluid.

Infection

Infection at the donor site is a rare complication. Sterile technique and appropriate wound care will minimize this concern. The risk of infection at the graft site depends upon the nature of the original defect. Fresh surgical wounds may be grafted without antibiotic coverage. Particularly large surgical wounds and those that have remained open for many hours may require coverage with the appropriate antibiotic(s).

Chronic ulcers are frequently infected and are almost universally contaminated with bacteria. Such wounds require special consideration with regard to preparing the wound as well as taking frequent culture and sensitivity studies preoperatively to determine the appropriate antibiotic coverage necessary. Thin split grafts may survive over some contaminated wounds for which thick grafts would not. Meshed grafts must always be considered when surgeons graft contaminated wounds.

Movement

During the first days after grafting, any shearing motion of the graft over the underlying defect bed will prevent revascularization or at the very least will cause separation of the very fragile vascular connections that must develop for graft survival. When shearing occurs after the first 24 h, graft failure will likely result. Graft movement is usually preventable at the time of grafting with proper suturing technique and use of support dressings. Despite these technical considerations, excessive ambulation after surgery may result in graft separation and subsequent failure. Thorough instructions given to the patient and family are therefore critical if the patient is to be treated at home. Occasionally, hospitalization is necessary since this may be the only place where movement restrictions may be adhered to by the patient.

Late Complications

Functional Complications

It is estimated that split-thickness grafts may contract as much as 70 percent. This is in marked contrast to full-thickness grafts and local flaps for which wound contraction is considered to be only a minor consideration. The contraction that occurs with split grafts arguably arises either within the substance of the graft or at the level just below the graft where a plate of fibrous tissue develops. While the overlying graft may take on a wrinkled appearance, the major concern is not cosmetic but rather functional. The forces of wound contraction can be very powerful, resulting in joint contractures when a graft is placed over that joint. Such contractile forces become important to the dermatologic surgeon when facial defects are grafted, especially when a graft is placed in proximity to the free margins of the vermilion, nasal ala, or eyelid. Wound contraction in these situations may pull these important structures away from their normal anatomic locations. This contraction may occur even when the graft is placed some distance away from a free margin. Distortion of these anatomic sites is certainly cosmetically disfiguring and may also be of significant functional concern, especially when ectropion formation is the result.

Grafts that are placed over defects that have little underlying soft tissue support, such as over a bony prominence or the skull, or which have marginal vascular supplies, such as lower leg ulcerations in the setting of vascular insufficiency, are subject to traumatic injury. Such grafts are very fragile and may be subject to frequent breakdown and secondary ulceration. Patients must be educated about ways to protect such grafts. Long-term protection of the grafts is necessary as is regular application of moisturizers which aid in keeping the grafts supple and therefore less susceptible to injury.

Cosmetic Considerations

On rare occasion, a split-thickness graft will heal with a very good color and texture match with the surrounding skin. In the author's experience, this has been seen in patients who have had large, shallow defects of the forehead and temple whose skin is white. Aside from these specific instances, split-thickness grafts heal with markedly contrasting color and texture to the surrounding unaffected skin. There is, in addition, at least some final depression to the healed graft, and the surface may be uneven or wavy.

These split-thickness grafts do not retain any adnexal structures, including hair and eccrine glands. Therefore, their surface is usually dry and susceptible to scaling and a dirty appearance unless carefully cleaned. The lack of hair-bearing potential is particularly noticeable when a graft is placed on an area that was previously hair bearing.

SUMMARY

Split-thickness skin grafting is an important surgical modality that must be in the arsenal of therapeutic tools available to the dermatologic surgeon. Despite the cosmetic limitations that such grafts exhibit, there are reasons why these grafts must be placed. The techniques of split-thickness skin grafting are relatively simple to learn and master, and their ease of placement in the ambulatory surgical setting puts their use squarely in the hands of the dermatologic surgeon.

Jeffery A. Klein

39 Tumescent Liposuction with Local Anesthesia

Liposuction totally by local anesthesia is a dermatologic surgical technique for sculpturing the body by removing localized accumulations of subcutaneous fat. Invented and developed by dermatologists, the tumescent technique for liposuction totally by local anesthesia has revolutionized liposuction worldwide.

Localized accumulations of fat, which are often inherited and frequently prove impossible to eliminate simply by exercise or dieting, can be removed permanently by liposuction surgery. A small stainless steel tube, called a cannula (from the Latin word for reed, tube, or cane), is the surgical instrument used to extract fat with the aid of a powerful vacuum pump.

Fat is removed as tunnels are created within the fatty tissue when the cannula is moved radially from a small skin incision. As the cannula is advanced and retracted through adipose tissue, fat is aspirated and then transported via a plastic hose into a collection canister. With the healing process, these tiny tunnels collapse, resulting in an improved body contour.

AREAS TREATED BY LIPOSUCTION

The areas of the body that are most frequently treated by liposuction include the abdomen, thighs, knees, hips, waist, legs, submental chin and jowls, calves, ankles, arms, and male breasts. Men typically comprise approximately 20 to 30 percent of liposuction patients.

TUMESCENT TECHNIQUE

The tumescent technique permits regional local anesthesia of the skin and subcutaneous tissue by direct infiltration. Large volumes of a dilute anesthetic solution of lidocaine and epinephrine in physiologic saline are infiltrated directly into the targeted fatty areas which become swollen and firm or tumescent. The tumescent technique permits liposuction of large volumes of fat totally by local anesthesia, without intravenous (IV) sedation, narcotic analgesia, or general anesthesia.

As a result of the widespread capillary vasoconstriction caused by the epinephrine in the anesthetic solution, there is minimal bleeding during and after surgery. The tumescent technique permits liposuction of large volumes of fat, with about 8.5 mL whole blood is suctioned for each liter of extracted fat.

In addition, the subcutaneous infiltration of large volumes of physiologic saline permits liposuction of more than 3 L of pure fat with virtually no IV fluid replacement.

The mechanical effects of the technique permit improved surgical results. Liposuction is more accurate, and irregularities of the skin are minimized. The tumescent technique separates subcutaneous fatty tissue from subjacent nerves and blood vessels, minimizing the risk of inadvertent injury of these structures by a cannula. Tumescence reduces the chance of inadvertently passing the cannula too closely to the dermis, creating unwanted depressions or surgical irregularities of the skin.

IMPROVED SAFETY WITH LOCAL ANESTHESIA

Liposuction with general anesthesia was originally developed in Europe around 1980. By 1982, American surgeons, including dermatologists, were beginning to popularize this procedure. Initially, liposuction with general anesthesia was rather unsophisticated, being associated with significant bleeding, pain, prolonged healing times, and aesthetic imperfections.

Dermatologists were the first to develop a technique that permitted liposuction totally by local anesthesia, without sedation, narcotic analgesics, or general anesthesia. This development was motivated by several factors: (1) Dermatologic surgeons traditionally prefer local anesthesia over general anesthesia for any sort of cutaneous surgery; (2) few dermatologic surgeons had hospital privileges for performing liposuction with general anesthesia, thereby influencing their use of local anesthesia; and (3) local anesthesia is safer and permits superior aesthetic results. This third factor was the ultimate reason for the preference of local anesthesia over general anesthesia. More specifically, there are advantages to the tumescent technique with local anesthesia rather than other techniques that rely on general anesthesia, including greater safety, elimination of surgical blood loss, elimination of the risks of general anesthesia, elimination of heavy IV sedation and narcotics, elimination of the unpleasant side effects of general anesthesia, minimal postoperative recovery time, and minimal postoperative pain and inflammation. Furthermore, with the tumescent technique there is a reduced risk of infection and fewer risks of surgically induced irregularities of the skin.

Because of the additional time required to infiltrate the local anesthesia, liposuction by the tumescent technique takes more time than general anesthesia. This is the only apparent advantage of general anesthesia, while the greatest risks of liposuction surgery are the dangers of anesthetic agents and excessive bleeding.[1]

DIFFERENCES BETWEEN SURGICAL SPECIALTIES

Plastic surgery and dermatology literature differ greatly in the use of either general or local anesthesia for liposuction. Plastic surgery literature focuses on the use of general anesthesia for liposuction surgery.[2-6] The use of local anesthesia for liposuction is well described in the dermatology literature.[7-16] Recently, plastic surgeons have begun to advocate the tumescent technique, in conjunction with general anesthesia, because of its ability to minimize bleeding, minimize postoperative pain, and optimize aesthetic results.[17]

There is also considerable variation between specialties in the use of vasoconstrictive solutions to maximize hemostasis. Plastic surgeons traditionally use either the dry or wet technique for liposuction. The dry technique uses general anesthesia without infiltration of dilute epinephrine to the sites targeted for liposuction. With the dry technique, it is estimated that 20 to 45 percent of the aspirate is blood, and the hematocrit drops 11.2 percent for each 1000 mL of aspirate.[18-21] The official guidelines of the American Academy of Dermatology state that "Because of the availability of safer methods, the dry technique is now rarely indicated."[22]

GOOD CANDIDATES FOR LIPOSUCTION

A liposuction surgery is a success when the patient is happy with the results. As with any cosmetic surgery, the ultimate success depends upon judicious patient selection as much as upon surgical skills. The best candidates for liposuction are in good health and have realistic expectations of liposuction. There are no definite age limits or weight limits. Most patients have localized accumulations of fat; however, some of the happiest patients have been somewhat obese. It is important to emphasize that liposuction is not a treatment for general obesity. An overweight person whose weight has been stable for many years and who has certain problem areas of fat may be an excellent candidate for liposuction.

LOCAL VERSUS GENERAL ANESTHESIA

Although the tumescent technique can be used in conjunction with general anesthesia or with deep IV sedation, large-volume liposuction can be done routinely with absolutely no sedation. Local anesthesia is safer than general anesthesia.[23,24] Many of the deaths associated with general anesthesia have occurred in healthy young patients, are the result of human error, and are considered preventable.[25,26] Deaths due to anesthesia are believed to occur at least once in every 2500 to 10,000 administrations of general anesthesia.[27-29] Life-threatening complications of general anesthesia are the most dangerous aspects of liposuction surgery.[1] Because the tumescent technique for liposuction surgery can be done totally with local anesthesia, without sedation, the high-risk drugs associated with general anesthesia are simply not used.

Complications are fewer and less catastrophic with local anesthesia than with general anesthesia.[24] For example, regional anesthesia is associated with a lower incidence of postoperative thromboembolism.[30] There is a reduction of intraoperative blood loss with the use of regional anesthesia for colon, gynecologic, hip, and prostate surgery.[31] In a study of dental anesthetic mortality in England from 1970 to 1979, general anesthesia was associated with 110 deaths, compared to only 10 deaths associated with local anesthesia.[24] This difference is all the more remarkable because local anesthetics were used far more frequently than general anesthesia.

When nitrous oxide, sedatives, and narcotic analgesics are

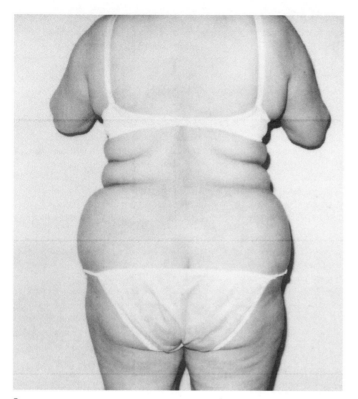
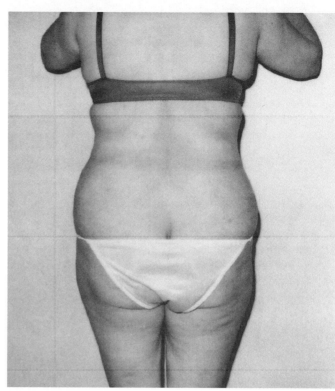

a

b

Figure 39-1   Female showing local focal collections of fat on hips, waist and flanks. Liposuction totally by anesthesia without sedation resulted in significant degree of cosmetic and functional improvement as illustrated by photograph taken three months after surgery. Note the residual excision site hyperpigmentation which usually disappears within 6 to 12 months.

given in sufficient doses that potentially cause respiratory depression, they are in fact general anesthetics.[32] More than 80 deaths have occurred after the use of midazolam, often in combination with narcotic analgesics; all but three occurred in patients unattended by anesthesia personnel.[33] Employing anesthetic techniques which avoid drugs that cause respiratory depression eliminates one of the most significant risks of anesthesia. The author suggests that patients who feel anxiety prior to surgery take 30 mg of flurazepam (Dalmane) an hour or two before surgery. Fewer than 5% of patients will require a small dose of midazolam. The use of parenteral sedation requires careful pulse oximetry.

MECHANICAL ADVANTAGES OF TUMESCENCE

The fluid mechanical distention of the targeted tissues provides benefits that are not available with simple general anesthesia or regional nerve blocks. Although the tumescent technique does change the dimensions of the areas targeted for liposuction, this alteration is not a disadvantage. With careful attention to uniform infiltration, the targeted fatty compartment becomes magnified without distortion. This magnification permits more precise removal of fat and minimizes skin surface irregularities.[17] Because the cross-sectional area of any fatty deposit is magnified, the fat can be suctioned with greater accuracy and uniformity. Magnification also assures the surgeon that the deeper layers of fat will be adequately removed. If a focus of tumescent fat has been missed, it is more easily detected both visually and by palpation. In the hands of an experienced surgeon, the use of small cannulas and the tumescent technique has virtually eliminated the risk of irregularities and undesirable aesthetic results.

PREOPERATIVE CONSIDERATIONS

Prior to liposuction, patients should be given written instructions for both preoperative and postoperative care (see Tables 39-1 and 39-2). Patients are told not to take aspirin or ibuprofen for 2 weeks before surgery. These drugs can promote bleeding by inhibiting platelet function.

Diet

Patients are asked not to take any solid food by mouth for at least 6 hours prior to surgery. After surgery, there are no di-

TABLE 39-1

Instructions for Care Before Liposuction*

The patient is responsible for the following before surgery:

1. Please read all the information in the *Liposuction Instruction & Information Booklet*. Do not hesitate to telephone to ask any questions that may occur to you after you have left our office.

2. Do not take aspirin (Anacin or Bufferin) or ibuprofen (Advil, Motrin, or Nuprin), or any medications containing these drugs, for 2 weeks before surgery; these will promote bleeding and bruising. It is OK to take Tylenol.

3. Do not drive home. Arrange to have someone drive you home after surgery. It is suggested that you arrange to have someone stay with you after surgery, although this is not strictly necessary.

4. Wear appropriate clothing on the day of surgery. There is usually quite a lot of drainage of slightly blood-tinged anesthetic solution after surgery. Since this drainage might stain clothing, we suggest that you chose your clothing with this in mind. Because we will apply elastic support garments on top of some bulky absorbent gauze padding, your clothing should be loose and comfortable.

Women: Please wear a comfortable bra that you would not mind getting stained from the blue ink that is used to mark the surgical areas.

Men: Please wear Jockey-type underpants or Speedo-type swim trunks. It is not as convenient to wear boxer-type underwear.

5. Bring a towel, and perhaps a plastic sheet, upon which to sit in the car while being driven home in order to prevent any drainage from staining a car seat.

6. Protect your bed, chairs, and carpets from drainage stains by covering them with towels placed over a plastic sheet such as a clean trash can liner.

7. Avoid solid food and caffeine before surgery. If your surgery is scheduled for the morning, do not eat solid food after midnight prior to surgery. If your surgery is scheduled for the afternoon, you may have a light breakfast, but only clear liquid for lunch. Please avoid caffeine just before surgery. We will provide you with a snack as soon as surgery is completed.

8. Please wear no unnecessary jewelry, no perfume (deodorant is OK), only the minimum of cosmetics (survival rations only), and no body moisturizers on the day of surgery.

9. Bring warm socks to prevent cold toes during surgery. If you tend to get cold hands, you are welcome to bring mittens to wear during the surgery. The operating room is kept relatively warm, about 75°F.

10. Bring your favorite soothing music. Patients usually enjoy listening to soothing quiet music during surgery. We have a large selection of compact discs (CDs). If you have any favorite CDs which you would like to share with us on the day of the surgery, you are welcome to bring them with you. Please label the little plastic case that holds your CD so that we will know to whom it belongs. Thank you.

*Information given to author's patient.

etary restrictions. Drinking generous amounts of liquids, such as fruit juices, is encouraged.

Prophylactic Antibiotics

Lidocaine is bactericidal for many pathogens commonly found on the skin.[34] Because the tumescent technique infiltrates lidocaine throughout the area to be treated by liposuction, the technique provides a measure of protection against surgical wound infection.

TABLE 39-2

Instructions for Care After Liposuction*

1. Driving: You should not plan to drive yourself home. It is recommended but not essential that you have a responsible adult with you on the day of surgery.

2. Activities: Quiet rest is recommended immediately after surgery. Later in the day or evening, you are welcome to take a short walk if desired. The day after liposuction surgery, you should feel well enough to drive your car and engage in light to moderate physical activities. You may carefully resume exercise and vigorous physical activity to 3 to 4 days after surgery. It is suggested that you begin with 25 percent of your normal workout and increase your activity daily as tolerated. Most people can return to a desk job within 1 to 2 days after surgery, although you must expect to be sore and easily fatigued for several days.

3. Elastic support garments: After liposuction surgery, a pair of elastic support garments is worn to prevent accumulation of fluid within the tunnels created by the removal of fat. Patients are required to wear these elastic girdles continuously for at least 24 h after the drainage has stopped. Most patients will wear their elastic garments for about 4 to 5 days. Because of the comfort these garments provide, some may choose to wear them for longer periods. Beginning the day after surgery, the elastic garments are removed daily to permit the patient to take a shower and to wash and dry the elastic garments. Wearing the garments for only a few days does not affect the ultimate outcome of the procedure. Wearing the garments longer tends to decrease swelling sooner.

4. Sound care: A large amount of drainage from the small incisions is normal during the first 24 to 48 h following liposuction by the tumescent technique. The slightly blood-tinged fluid is residual anesthetic solution. Large amounts of drainage can be expected when a large amount of fat is removed. In general, the more drainage there is, the less bruising and swelling there will be. During the first 48 h, you should sit or lie on towels. When there is a large amount of drainage, it is advisable to place a plastic sheet beneath the towel. Although it is not necessary, patients may choose to place additional gauze dressing over the drainage sites to absorb continuing drainage. Beginning the day after surgery, wash the incisions with soap and water and apply bacitracin antibiotic ointment twice daily. Please leave the incision sites open to the air rather than covering the incision with Band-Aids. Finish all antibiotics.

5. Discomfort and bruising: The soreness is worst 24 h after surgery and then improves almost daily. For relief of soreness and inflammation, take two Extra-Strength Tylenol every 4 h, while awake, for the first 48 h. Do not take aspirin or ibuprofen or medications that contain these drugs, such as Bufferin, Anacin, Advil, or Nuprin, for 5 days after surgery; these can promote bleeding. With the tumescent technique, most patients experience remarkably little bruising. Nevertheless, the more extensive the liposuction surgery, the more bruising you can expect.

6. Bathing: When showering, you may briefly get the incision sites wet. Afterward, pat them dry gently. Do not soak in a bath, swimming pool, or the ocean for 7 days after surgery.

7. Diet: After surgery, drinking generous amounts of fruit juices or soft drinks will prevent dehydration. A light meal is recommended for the first meal after surgery (sorry, no alcohol). You should resume your usual diet 4 h after surgery.

8. Follow-up appointment: Please call our office to schedule your follow-up appointment. You are welcome to return to our office for follow-up visits at no charge as often as you like. Please make an appointment for 2 to 4 weeks after surgery.

*Information given to author's patient.

The prophylactic administration of antibiotics reduces the risk of surgical wound infection.[35] Good operating room technique also minimizes surgical wound infection.[36] The incidence of surgical wound infection for liposuction with general anesthesia but without the tumescent technique has been estimated to be 1:1000 cases.[2] To the best of the author's knowledge, there has never been a serious infection with liposuction by the tumescent technique.

In the United States, perioperative prophylactic use of antibiotics is considered the standard of care. Patients are typically prescribed oral antibiotics such as cefadroxil 500 mg or doxycycline 100 mg taken twice daily beginning the day before surgery and continuing for a total of 5 days. It is explained to patients that there is no strong scientific proof that this regimen is necessary but that it is a clinical tradition that the surgeon would prefer to continue.

INTRAOPERATIVE CONSIDERATIONS

In light of the fact that the patient is fully alert during tumescent liposuction with local anesthesia, the standard operating room technique must be modified. Special consideration must be given to the patient's modesty, anxiety, and physical comfort.

The temperature of the operating room is usually kept between 72° to 76°F. Sensitivity to the patient's feelings about modesty is important. Female patients wear disposable cloth panties. Plastic sheeting and burgundy-colored terry cloth towels are draped over the operating room surgical table to absorb the copious drainage associated with tumescent liposuction. Patients must be afforded the opportunity to leave the operating room to use the toilet when necessary.

The quality of nursing care is an important factor in alleviating the patient's anxiety. A nurse who can provide a comforting hand to hold or distract the patient with conversation is a vital asset to treating patients who are fully alert and unsedated.

Formulation of Anesthetic Solution

Exposing sufficient lengths of sensory nerves to minimal concentrations of lidocaine can anesthetize large volumes of subcutaneous fat.[37] This effect is augmented and prolonged by the vasoconstrictive effects of epinephrine.[38]

For liposuction, the formulation for the anesthetic solution used in the tumescent technique continues to evolve since it was first published in 1987.[39] The traditional formula consists of lidocaine 0.05% to 0.01%, epinephrine 1:1,000,000, and sodium bicarbonate 12.5 mEq/L in physiologic saline.

The recipe should be varied depending on the clinical situation. A number of factors determine the minimal sufficient concentration of lidocaine. Although 0.05% lidocaine is sufficient for liposuction in fat with a minimal fibrous component, a concentration of 0.075% or 0.1% is required in the

more fibrous areas (see Table 39-3). The more fibrous the fatty tissue and the larger the cannulas, the more discomfort associated with liposuction by local anesthesia. The abdomen, male flanks, and male breasts are particularly fibrous and often require a 0.1% lidocaine concentration. The minimal effective epinephrine concentration is 0.5 mg/L (1:2,000,000). Recently, a 0.65 mg (1:1,500,000) concentration of epinephrine has become the standard. Sodium bicarbonate, $NaHCO_3$, by neutralizing the pH of the anesthetic solution, decreases the burning pain upon infiltration.[40–44] A bicarbonate concentration of 10 mEq/L is convenient and effective.

For patient comfort, the IV bags containing the anesthetic solution in physiologic saline are warmed to 40°C. Using chilled saline or cryoanesthesia causes patient discomfort without improving hemostasis and obligates the surgeon to monitor core body temperature.

Lidocaine Pharmacokinetics

Pharmacokinetics is the study of the rate of drug absorption, distribution, and elimination. In order to administer lidocaine optimally, it is necessary to have an understanding of how the dose, route, and rate of administration relates to the therapeutic effect and potential toxicity.

Factors which determine the rate of systemic absorption of lidocaine include vascularity of the site of injection, the use of a vasoconstrictive drug such as epinephrine, the concentration of lidocaine, and the rate of infiltration.[45,46] When a given dose of lidocaine is rapidly absorbed, the peak plasma concentration will be quite high. When an identical dose is absorbed much more slowly, such as when the tumescent technique is used, the peak plasma concentration is significantly lower.[47]

Lidocaine absorption is dramatically delayed when infiltrated with dilute epinephrine into relatively avascular tissue such as fat. Peak plasma lidocaine levels occur approximately 12 h after the initial infiltration. This gradual absorption explains the safety of large doses of dilute lidocaine, 35 mg/kg, in the tumescent technique for liposuction.[45] The safety of

TABLE 39-3

Recipe for the Tumescent Liposuction Anesthetic Solution

Lidocaine	Epinephrine
500 mg (0.05%)	with 0.5 mg (1:2,000,000) or
750 mg (0.75%)	with 0.75 mg (1:1,500,000) or
1000 mg (0.1%)	with 0.75 mg (1:1,500,000)
Sodium bicarbonate	10 mEq (10 mL of 8.4% of $NaHCO_3$)
Triamcinolone	10 mg (an optional ingredient)
Physiologic saline	1000 mL of 0.9% NaCl

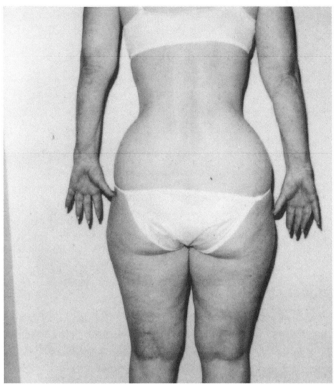
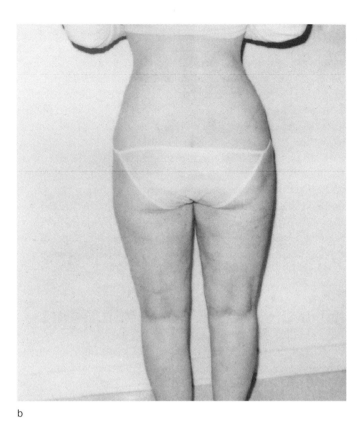

a   b

Figure 39-2   Photo of woman with a common form of lipodysmorphia with excessive accumulation of fat on hips, thighs and knees. Preoperative and three month postoperative photographs of this 72kg patient who had 21.7ml of whole blood removed during liposuction totally by local anesthesia using the tumescent technique without sedation. A total of 2,800ml of supranatant fat was removed from the hips, inner thighs, outer thighs and knees.

these large doses of lidocaine is not the result of removing lidocaine from the body by aspiration as has been previously assumed.[48,49] The lower the concentration of lidocaine in an anesthetic solution containing epinephrine, the slower its rate of absorption.[50] Rapid injection of a local anesthetic is associated with rapid systemic absorption.[51] Slow methodical injection of lidocaine is associated with slow, safer absorption.

What Is a Safe Lidocaine Dose?

The package insert for Xylocaine (lidocaine hydrochloride) and the *1992 Physicians' Desk Reference* (PDR) states, "For normal healthy adults, the individual maximum safe dose of lidocaine HCl with epinephrine should not exceed 7 mg/kg (3.5 mg/lb) of body weight and in general it is recommended that the maximum total dose not exceed 500 mg."[52] Neither Astra Pharmaceutical Products, Inc. (Westboro, Massachusetts), the manufacturer, nor the United States Food and Drug Administration (FDA) has any data to support this standard dose limitation.[53,54] In its 1948 application to the FDA for permission to market lidocaine, the manufacturer simply stated that the maximum safe dose of lidocaine is "probably the same as for procaine."[54]

The standard lidocaine dose limitation of 7 mg/kg is appropriate when lidocaine at 1% or 2% concentration with epinephrine is infiltrated rapidly or into highly vascular tissue. However, higher doses are safe when dilute lidocaine (0.05% or 0.1%) with epinephrine is infiltrated more slowly into relatively avascular subcutaneous fat. The current estimate for a safe maximum lidocaine dose for liposuction by the tumescent technique is 35 mg/kg.[45]

Local Anesthetic Toxicity

Lidocaine is the drug of choice for liposuction by local anesthesia because of its minimal toxicity compared to longer acting anesthetics which are more cardiotoxic.[55–59] Cardiovascular collapse from longer acting local anesthetics is often resistant to resuscitation.[60] Because the anesthetic effects of lidocaine last for several hours when infiltrated into subcutaneous fat during the tumescent technique, there is no clinical justification for using longer acting and potentially more cardiotoxic local anesthetics (see Table 39-4).

The toxicity of a local anesthetic is a function of its peak plasma concentration. Peak plasma concentration depends as much on its rate of systemic absorption as on its total

TABLE 39-4

Plasma Lidocaine Concentration and Toxicity

Concentration	Toxicity
3–6 µg/mL	Subjective pharmacologic effects
5–9 µg/mL	Objective toxicity
8–12 µg/mL	Seizures, cardiac depression
12 µg/mL	Coma
20 µg/mL	Respiratory arrest
26 µg/mL	Cardiac arrest

milligram-per-kilogram dose.[61] The rapid infiltration of 2500 mg of lidocaine for a face-lift can be fatal.[62] In contrast, the slow lidocaine absorption associated with the tumescent technique safely permits doses of 35 mg/kg of lidocaine because systemic absorption occurs over 18 to 36 h.[45]

Hemostasis

The degree to which infiltration with vasoconstrictive local anesthetic solutions is used in liposuction varies widely between different techniques. At one end of the spectrum is the *dry technique* which uses general anesthesia and no infiltration of a vasoconstrictive solution, it is the liposuction technique that causes the greatest degree of blood loss.[63] Approximately 20 to 45 percent of the volume of the aspirate obtained by the dry technique is whole blood.[20,21,64] Dermatologists have found that the dry technique is associated with such an unacceptably large blood loss that it is now widely considered below the standard of care for dermatologic surgery.[22] The *wet technique* also relies on the use of general anesthesia and is intermediate with respect to the degree of hemostasis that can be obtained in liposuction. The tumescent technique uses the greatest volume of vasoconstrictive subcutaneous infiltration and produces such exquisite hemostasis that most patients lose more blood during their routine presurgical laboratory studies than during liposuction. Hemostasis with the tumescent technique is so complete that only 8.5 mL blood is lost for every 1000 mL of fat that is aspirated.[65] The

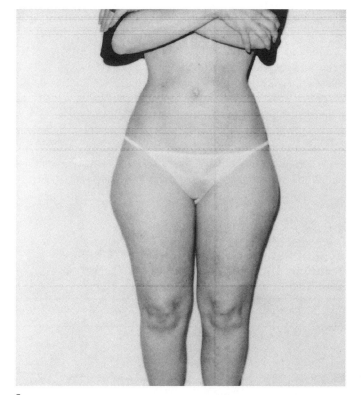
a

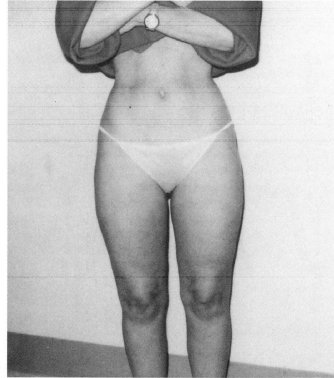
b

Figure 39-3 Photograph showing results of liposuction on a 56kg patient before and four months after surgery which removed 2,100ml of supranatant fat from outer thighs, anterior thighs, medial thighs and knees, using tumescent technique and micro-cannulas. Total of 20.1ml of whole blood were removed during this procedure attesting to the remarkable hemostasis provided by the tumescent techinique.

tumescent technique is the only technique that permits large-volume liposuction totally by local anesthesia without sedation or narcotic analgesics.

Excessive blood loss is frequently cited as one of the most worrisome complications of liposuction surgery by general anesthesia.[66,67] The dry technique, relying on general anesthesia, is associated with a 1 percent drop in the hematocrit for every 150 mL of tissue extracted by liposuction.[67] With the tumescent technique, patients can expect the hematocrit to decrease 1 percent for every 1000 mL of supernatant fat.

The wet technique uses general anesthesia as well as the infiltration of dilute epinephrine (1:100,000 to 1:400,000) with lidocaine (0.2% to 0.5%) in relatively small volumes (approximately 100 mL infiltrated for each 1000 mL of expected aspirate) prior to liposuction in order to promote hemostasis. With the wet technique, it is estimated that 15 to 30 percent of the aspirate is blood, and the hematocrit drops 7.3 percent for each 1000 mL of aspirate.[68–70] Even with the wet technique, surgical blood loss is so great that transfusion of autologous blood is recommended as a standard procedure for large-volume (greater than or equal to 1500 mL) liposuction.[71]

In contrast, in the tumescent technique for liposuction, about 2000 mL of dilute anesthetic solution (epinephrine 1:1,000,000 to 1:2,000,000, lidocaine 0.05% to 0.1%, and sodium bicarbonate 10 mEq/L in physiologic saline) is infiltrated for each 1000 mL of fat that is aspirated. With the tumescent technique, less than 1 percent of the aspirate is blood, and the hematocrit changes by less than 1 percent for each 1000 mL of aspirated fat.[17]

Intravascular Fluid Status

There was no clinical evidence of intravascular volume depletion despite minimal IV infusion of physiologic saline in 112 patients who had liposuction of more than 1500 mL of fat.[17] The injection of large volumes of fluids into subcutaneous tissues with the tumescent technique delivers fluids to the exact site where tissue injury will be induced by liposuction. It is an efficient method of preventing both third spacing at the site of injury and any associated intravascular fluid deficits.

Infiltration Technique

When the infiltration is done with care and skill, it is virtually painless. Once the infiltration is complete, there is minimal discomfort with the liposuction procedure. Because the local anesthetic remains in the affected tissues for over 12 h after the surgery, there is no immediate postoperative pain.

It is essential to begin the infiltration deeply throughout the targeted area. If one were to begin infiltrating in a superficial plane of adipose tissue, it would become difficult to palpate deeper layers accurately, and would preclude a precise and complete infiltration of deeper tissue (see Table 39-5).

The original description of the tumescent technique described the use of a hand-held syringe to accomplish the infiltration.[39] Subsequently, other methods for infiltration of large volumes of local anesthetic solutions have been described.[72] An efficient method uses a peristaltic pump to force the anesthetic solution from an IV bag reservoir through a sterile IV line and out through an attached needle or infiltrating cannula. To initiate the infiltration, a 30-gauge needle is used for an intradermal injection of small blebs of the dilute anesthetic solution at sites of percutaneous penetrations of larger needles used for subcutaneous infiltration or at incision sites for passing the liposuction cannulas.

The bulk of the infiltration is accomplished using 25-gauge (7.6-cm long) and 20-gauge spinal needles (8.9-cm long). For areas that are especially sensitive, using a thin 25-gauge spinal needle will minimize or eliminate the pain of infiltration. When the infiltration is done carefully, there is minimal discomfort, and there is no need for concomitant parenteral analgesia. An 18-gauge intradiscal needle (15-cm long) can be used after an area has been initially infiltrated using smaller spinal needles. The larger intradiscal needle allows more rapid and more uniform infiltration, but may cause more discomfort than a thinner needle. This larger needle is useful for both infiltration and for checking that the infiltration is complete and that no areas have been missed.

Finally, to test for completeness of the anesthesia, one can pass a 22-cm long, blunt-tipped cannula (14 or 12 gauge) throughout the targeted fatty compartment and infiltrate extra solution where discomfort is encountered. While one hand advances the infiltrating needle, the fingers and thumb of the other hand palpate both the deeper muscle plane as well as the expanding bolus of the fluid as the needle is advanced. In this way, one can infiltrate deeply with assurance that the needle tip will remain within adipose tissue.

When the tumescent technique is used for the leg, caution should be exercised so as to avoid an iatrogenic compartment

TABLE 39-5

Typical Range of Volumes of Dilute Anesthetic Solutions Used with the Tumescent Technique for Infiltration into Various Areas

Area	Range
Abdomen, upper and lower	(800–2000 mL)
Hip (flank or love handle), each side	(400–1000 mL)
Lateral thigh, each side	(500–1200 mL)
Anterior thigh, each side	(600–1200 mL)
Proximal medial thigh, each side	(250–700 mL)
Knee	(200–500 mL)
Male breast, each side	(300–800 mL)
Submental chin	(100–200 mL)

syndrome. Although I am not aware of an iatrogenic compartment syndrome ever having been caused by the tumescent technique, infiltration of the lower leg should be done with caution.

Liposuction Cannulas

Micro-cannulas are an absolute requirement for liposuction using the tumescent technique without sedation. The recommended cannulas are made from full hard-tempered stainless steel hypodermic needle stock in 14, 12, and 10 gauge. The inside diameter (ID) of these cannulas are as follows:

16 gauge = 1.2 mm (ID)
14 gauge = 1.6 mm (ID)
12 gauge = 2.2 mm (ID)
10 gauge = 2.7 mm (ID)

The advantage of using these micro-cannulas are (1) decreased pain, (2) smaller incisions with essentially invisible scars, (3) greater accuracy with minimal risks of postsurgical irregularities or depressions of the skin, and (4) surprising efficiency for removing large volumes of fat.

Ten-centimeter long, 16-gauge and 14-gauge cannulas are used sequentially for submental chin and jowl liposuction. The 12- and 10-gauge cannulas are used for body liposuction. Larger cannulas can remove fat more rapidly, but the small cannulas can remove fat more completely and more uniformly. Larger cannulas predispose the patient to contour irregularities and undesirable aesthetic defects. Larger cannulas cause more pain and necessitate higher concentrations of lidocaine or the concomitant use of IV narcotic analgesics.

Liposuction Technique

Just as it is essential to begin deeply when infiltrating the anesthetic solution, it is equally essential that the initial stages of liposuction be accomplished deeply. If liposuction by the tumescent technique is begun too superficially, it becomes difficult to palpate accurately the deeper tissue planes and to detect the interface between fat and fascia, and deeper layers of fat may not be adequately suctioned.

Body Liposuction is initiated with the narrow, 14-gauge cannulas. This allows the surgeon to control accurately the initial depth and direction of the cannula, and, if an incompletely anesthetized area is encountered, the discomfort will be minimal. By penetrating the fibrous septae of an entire area with a narrow cannula, subsequent use of larger cannulas will cause minimal discomfort. By following the tunnels already created by the narrow cannulas, wider cannulas can be used to remove residual fat more efficiently while being inserted with minimal resistance and optimal accuracy.

The 12-gauge cannula is sufficiently small so as not to remove fat too rapidly. This minimizes the risks of postsurgical irregularities. This safety factor permits the surgeon to direct the cannula superficially toward the dermis with minimal

risks of removing excess amounts of fat or creating depressions of the skin. For relatively thin patients, and for those who demand near-perfect results such as professional models, the 14-gauge cannula is often used for the entire case. Although using such a small cannula requires a little more time, this approach minimizes scars and optimizes aesthetic results. Typically, 14-gauge cannulas are used to remove approximately 25 percent to 75 percent of the fat in any particular area, with the 12 or 10-gauge cannulas used to remove the remainder of the fat.

Small cannulas permit incisions that are so small that sutures are not required. In fact, these incisions heal best without sutures, becoming virtually invisible. Small incisions can be placed anywhere. Placing incisions at the inferior or dependent margin of the area treated by liposuction promotes drainage of the blood-tinged anesthetic solution and more rapid resolution of postoperative bruising and edema.

POSTOPERATIVE CONSIDERATIONS

One of the greatest advantages of the tumescent technique without sedation is that postoperative recovery and care are dramatically simplified. With surgery totally by local anesthesia, there is no postoperative nausea, no vomiting, no orthostatic hypotension, no hypothermia, no postoperative shivering, and no lingering unpleasant side effects of potent systemic narcotics, sedatives, and general anesthesia. Drugs that depress respiration, such as narcotics and sedatives, are the leading causes of anesthesia-related morbidity and mortality.[73]

With the tumescent technique, patients are discharged ambulatory 30 min after the liposuction procedure is completed. If only one area has been treated, some patients are permitted to drive themselves home.

Bruising

With the tumescent technique, bruising is minimized. About 50 percent of patients have no bruises 7 days after surgery. The more extensive the liposuction surgery, the more bruising one can expect.

Placing incisions for cannula access at dependent site on the margin of targeted fatty compartment will facilitate postoperative drainage of blood-tinged anesthetic solution. This will markedly reduce the degree of postoperative bruising, swelling and soreness.

Reduced Pain

Immediately after liposuction surgery, there is surprisingly little discomfort when the tumescent technique has been used. Residual local anesthetic solution provides patients with prolonged postoperative local anesthesia for hours after surgery. Thus, patients require no narcotic analgesics. Because of its

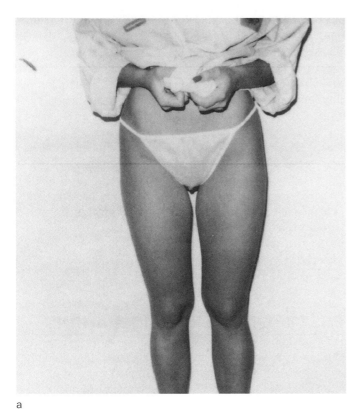
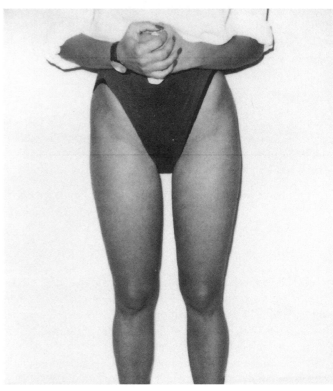

a   b

Figure 39-4   Before and after photographs depicting the results of tumescent liposuction on medial thighs and medial knees using micro-cannulas for maximum smoothness and minimal risk of post surgical irregularities.

anti-inflammatory effects on postoperative trauma, acetaminophen is recommended (1000 mg 3 to 4 times daily for 1 week).[74,75] Most patients do not require anything more potent for pain relief.

Some patients describe their soreness after liposuction as being very similar to what they feel after having exercised quite vigorously. The soreness is worst 24 h after surgery and then improves almost daily. Virtually every patient who has had liposuction under general anesthesia and then has had liposuction by the tumescent technique has found the latter to be much less painful.

Written Aftercare Instructions

Postoperative care begins with a complete set of written instructions which are provided to the patient twice: first at the time of the preoperative examination and also immediately after the surgery (see Table 39-2). Some preparations for the aftercare, for example, arrangements for the patient's transportation home after surgery, must be made well in advance of the surgery.

Because there is often a considerable postoperative drainage of very dilute, slightly blood-tinged anesthetic solution containing 1% whole blood, it is suggested that loose, comfortable clothing be worn for the trip home after the

surgery. Bringing a towel and a plastic sheet such as a plastic trash can liner to sit upon in the car while being driven home is also advised.

Immediate Postoperative Recovery

Although postoperative problems are uncommon, it is important to monitor pulse rate and blood pressure and to be observant for any orthostatic hypotension. Patients are observed for 30 min, with a registered nurse or physician constantly in attendance until the patient is discharged.

Because sedatives and narcotics are usually not necessary with the tumescent technique, patients may be discharged home as soon as they put on their absorptive dressings and elastic support garments. Employing anesthetic techniques that do not cause respiratory depression eliminates one of the most significant risks of anesthesia. When such drugs are used during surgery, patients must be monitored by recovery personnel well trained in providing emergency respiratory assistance if it should be required.

Drainage

Liposuction removes only a fraction of the anesthetic solution injected with the tumescent technique. Some of the anesthetic fluid drains out during surgery, requiring the use of numerous gauze sponges to soak up the solution. Following the surgery, there will be drainage of blood-tinged anesthetic solution from the small (3 mm to 5 mm) incision sites that accommodated the cannulas. Warning patients to expect copious postoperative drainage of a blood-tinged anesthetic solution, containing approximately 1% whole blood, will reduce their anxieties. Patients' attitudes toward this drainage become more positive when they understand that maximizing drainage will minimize postoperative bruising and swelling.

The patient has the option of either changing or ignoring the gauze pads once they become soaked. The patient should prepare for this copious drainage by using a plastic sheet and soft towels to cover and protect the sofa or bed for the first 24 to 48 h. Patients should take precautions to avoid having drainage stain a carpet. When there is voluminous drainage, it may be necessary for the patient to change gauze pads several times over the first 24 to 48 h postoperatively. If there is not a large amount of drainage postoperatively, the excess fluid will be excreted by urination over the next 24 h.

Elastic Support Garments

The marked diminution of bleeding associated with liposuction by the tumescent technique has simplified the requirements for postoperative care.

After liposuction surgery, two tumescent liposuction compression garments is worn to prevent accumulation of fluid within the tunnels in the subcutaneous fat created by the cannula. With the tumescent technique, there is minimal residual blood in these tunnels. Most of the postoperative drainage of the blood-tinged anesthetic solution typically ceases within 24 to 48 h. With the roof and the floor of the tunnels in direct apposition, fibroblast proliferation and closure of these tunnels probably occur almost immediately.

With older liposuction techniques, there is a considerable amount of interoperative bleeding and a significant amount of residual blood remaining in the tunnels after surgery. This necessitates weeks of prolonged postoperative use of elastic support garments or elastic tape. However, with the tumescent technique, using microcannulas, the tumescent liposuction compression garments are only briefly required. For facial or neck liposuction, an elastic binder is required overnight, which is less than 24 h following the surgery. For body liposuction, patients are asked to wear the elastic support garment postoperatively for 24 h beyond the day when all drainage ceases, usually 3 to 6 days. However, many patients, because of the comfort and security, prefer to wear their girdles for at least 1 week.

Patients are provided two pairs of comfortably snug elastic garments. Wearing two garments provides twice as much compression as one garment. The crotch of the pants is sewn with an opening provided to allow normal bodily functions without having to remove the garment. The sizes of the two garments are not necessarily the same. Bulky absorbent gauze

or pads are routinely taped onto the patient before the postoperative elastic support garments can be worn. The larger of the two garments, which is easier to pull on over the gauze pads, is the first to be put in place. The garments are worn inside out so that the seams do not irritate the patient's skin. The smaller and tighter of the two garments, the last to be placed on the patient, then slides on easily over the first garment.

Wound Care and Bathing

No sutures are used to close the small incision sites. The incisions are simply covered with bacitracin ointment and large bulky absorbent sterile gauze pads. The open incisions promote drainage of residual blood-tinged anesthetic solution, dramatically reducing postoperative swelling and bruising. Furthermore, unsutured small incision wounds heal with less inflammation and less scarring.

A word of caution is advisable for the morning after surgery when the patient removes the garments and dressings and takes a shower. Because of decompression orthostatic hypotension, an occasional patient will experience vasovagal light-headedness or syncope when the blood-tinged dressings and elastic garments are first removed. Patients are advised to have someone help them change their garments.

Patients are instructed to shower daily beginning the day after surgery. Incisions are washed with soap and water, gently dried, and the bacitracin antibiotic ointment is applied. Absorbent gauze pads are placed over any incision site that continues to drain.

While the elastic garment is being laundered, the patient may relax quietly until the garments are dry enough to be worn. Explicit instructions are given not to apply occlusive plastic bandages to the incision sites as these tend to promote inflammation. The elastic garment may be worn directly over the incisional wounds.

Physical Activity

Walking is encouraged as soon as possible after surgery. Most people feel well enough to go for a short walk in the evening of the same day as the surgery. The day following the surgery, all patients should be able to drive a car, take the children to school, or go to the market to do some light shopping. Progressly more vigorous physical activity may begin as soon as it is tolerated. Although some patients do return to work the day after surgery, most patients wait 48 h before returning to work. There is no restriction on sexual activity, with the caveat that common sense and gentleness be employed.

Inflammation

There are two types of postliposuction inflammation. The common type affects most patients to some degree. This inflammation presents as a mild to moderate soreness, tenderness, and subcutaneous lumpiness that resolve gradually without treatment 4 to 10 weeks after surgery.

A distinct and more unusual form of inflammation, termed *postliposuction panniculitis,* typically has its onset 10 to 20 days after the surgery. Panniculitis is a descriptive term referring to inflammatory nodules of subcutaneous fat.[76] Fewer than 4 percent of patients develop this more inflammatory condition characterized by a subacute onset 2 to 4 weeks postoperatively of painful palpable firm subcutaneous nodules that usually affect only a portion of the area treated by liposuction. Usually there is no visible change in the overlying skin; however, in some patients, one can observe focal pinkness or induration. To the clinician's fingers, these nodules feel warmer than the surrounding skin. Palpation elicits exquisite tenderness. A biopsy of affected subcutaneous fat has shown a histologic picture consistent with panniculitis. Special stains have shown no evidence of bacterial infection. Antibiotics have had no apparent clinical benefit. However, a brief course of prednisone, 20 mg per day for 7 to 10 days, is effective treatment.

Recently, formulation of the anesthetic solution for the tumescent technique has been modified to include 10 mg of triamcinolone per liter of solution. Triamcinolone is an anti-inflammatory corticosteroid with poor solubility in water. Since the addition of triamcinolone to the anesthetic solution for the tumescent technique, the incidence of postliposuction panniculitis has decreased to fewer than 2 percent of all patients. Furthermore, there has been an apparent decrease in the qualitative soreness experienced by otherwise unaffected patients.

DISADVANTAGES OF TUMESCENT TECHNIQUE

The only significant disadvantage of the tumescent technique for liposuction is the additional time required for the infiltration. If a nurse does the infiltration, then duration of the actual liposuction procedure is the same as when the tumescent technique is not employed. Achieving less than complete anesthesia necessitates the use of potent IV sedatives and narcotics with their associated risks and unpleasant side effects.

COMPLICATIONS OF LIPOSUCTION

To the best of the author's knowledge, the most serious complications of liposuction have always been associated with the use of general anesthesia. Cardiac arrest, pulmonary arrest, pulmonary thromboembolism, excessive bleeding, hypotension and shock, a delayed diagnosis of a perforated abdominal viscus, and infections are all more likely with general anesthesia.

The incidence of clinically apparent seromas and hematomas is extremely low with liposuction by local anesthesia and micro-cannulas. Nerve damage is rare when liposuction is carried out in a typical area of symmetric subcutaneous fat accumulation. Nerve damage is far more likely when liposuction is utilized in an anatomic area with superficial nerves such as the face and neck. Special care in this regard is necessary when treating a cervical lipoma. The tumescent technique may reduce the risk of liposuction of the face and neck by elevating the fatty tissue away from subjacent nerves.

Tachycardia as the result of an unrecognized predisposition for supraventricular tachycardia, or subclinical hyperthyroidism, or excessive sensitivity to epinephrine is a plausible complication associated with local anesthesia. Using a low concentration of epinephrine, such as 0.50 mg to 0.75 mg of epinephrine in 1 L of normal saline provides excellent hemostasis.

CONCLUSION

Tumescent liposuction is a surgical procedure invented and developed by dermatologists. It permits liposuction which is safer and less painful, with more rapid recovery and better aesthetic results, when compared to older techniques that rely on the use of general anesthesia, narcotic analgesia, or IV sedatives.

REFERENCES

1. Dillerud E: Suction lipectomy: A report on complications, undesired results, and patient satisfaction based on 3511 procedures. *Plast Reconstr Surg* **88:**239–246, 1991

2. Teimourian B, Rogers WB III: A national survey of complications associated with suction lipectomy: A comparative study. *Plast Reconstr Surg* **84:**628–631, 1989

3. Mladick RA: Lipoplasty. *Clin Plast Surg* **16:**1–403, 1989

4. Braunstein MC: Anesthesia, in *Lipoplasty: The Theory and Practice of Blunt Suction Lipectomy,* edited by GP Hetter. Boston, Little, Brown, 1990, pp 133–142

5. Rohrich RJ, Mathes SJ: Suction lipectomy, in *Plastic Surgery Principles and Practice,* edited by MJ Jurkiewicz et al. St. Louis, Mosby, 1990, p 1559

6. Grazier FM ed: *Atlas of Suction Assisted Lipectomy in Body Sculpture.* New York, Churchill-Livingstone, 1992

7. Field LM: The dermatologic surgeon and liposculpturing, in *Liposculpture the Syringe Technique,* edited by PF Fournier. Paris, Arnette Blackwell, 1991, pp 265–266

8. Coleman WP: The history of dermatologic liposuction. *Dermatol Clin* **8:**381–383, 1990

9. Narins RS: Liposuction and anesthesia. *Dermatol Clin* **8:**421–424, 1990

10. Klein JA: The tumescent technique: Anesthesia and modified liposuction technique. *Dermatol Clin* **8:**425–437, 1990

11. Lillis PJ: The tumescent technique for liposuction surgery. *Dermatol Clin* **8**:439–450, 1990

12. Replogle SL: The "standard technique" of liposuction: Viewpoint from a plastic surgeon. *Dermatol Clin* **8**:451–455, 1990

13. Stegman SJ: Technique variations in liposuction surgery. *Dermatol Clin* **8**:457–461, 1990

14. Hanke CW et al: The safety of dermatologic liposuction surgery. *Dermatol Clin* **8**:563–568, 1990

15. Fournier PF ed: *Liposculpture the Syringe Technique.* Paris, Arnette Blackwell, 1991, p 163

16. Klein JA: Anesthesia for dermatologic cosmetic surgery, in *Cosmetic Surgery of the Skin: Principles and Techniques,* edited by WP Coleman et al. Philadelphia, Decker, 1991, pp 39–45

17. Pitman GH: Refinements in liposuction, in *Liposuction and Aesthetic Surgery.* St. Louis, Quality Medical, 1993, pp 87–108

18. Courtiss EH et al: Large-volume suction lipectomy: An analysis of 108 patients. *Plast Reconstr Surg* **89**:1068–1079, 1992

19. Hetter GP: Blood and fluid replacement for lipoplasty procedures. *Clin Plast Surg* **16**:245–248, 1989

20. Goodpasture JC, Bunkis J: Quantitative analysis of blood and fat in suction lipectomy aspirate. *Plast Reconstr Surg* **78**:765–769, 1986

21. Gargan TJ, Courtiss EH: The risks of suction lipectomy: Their prevention and treatment. *Clin Plast Surg* **11**:457–463, 1988

22. Committee on Guidelines of Care. Guidelines of care for liposuction. *J Am Acad Dermatol* **24**:489–494, 1991

23. Kallar SK et al: Complications of anesthesia, in *Complications in Surgery and Trauma,* 2d ed, edited by LJ Greenfield. Philadelphia, Lippincott, 1990, pp 231–247

24. Coplans MP, Curson I: Deaths associated with dentistry. *Br Dent J* **153**:357–362, 1982

25. Tinker JH et al: Role of monitoring devices in prevention of anesthetic mishaps: A closed claims analysis. *Anesthesiology* **71**:541–546, 1989

26. Taylor G et al: Unexpected cardiac arrest during anesthesia and surgery. *JAMA* **236**:2758–2760, 1976

27. Epstein RM: Morbidity and mortality from anesthesia: A continuing problem. *Anesthesiology* **49**:388–389, 1978

28. Forrest JB et al: Multicenter study of general anesthesia, pt 2: Results. *Anesthesiology* **72**:262–268, 1990

29. Keats AS: Anesthesia mortality in perspective. *Anesth Analg* **71**:113, 1990

30. Modig J et al: Thromboembolism after total hip replacement: The role of epidural and general anesthesia. *Anesth Analg* **62**:174–180, 1983

31. Modig J: Regional anesthesia and blood loss. *Acta Anaesthesiol Scand* **89**:44–48, 1988

32. Moller JT et al: Hypoxemia in the postanesthesia care unit: An observer study. *Anesthesiology* **73**:890, 1990

33. Bailey PL et al: Frequent hypoxemia and apnea after sedation with midazolam and fentanyl. *Anesthesiology* **75**:826, 1990

34. Miller MA, Shelly WB: Antibacterial properties of lidocaine on bacteria isolated from dermal lesions. *Arch Dermatol* **121**:1157, 1985

35. Classen DC et al: The timing of prophylactic administration of antibiotics and the risk of surgical-wound infection. *N Engl J Med* **326**:281, 1992

36. Atkinson LJ: *Berry & Kohn's Operating Room Technique,* 7th ed. St. Louis, Mosby-Year Book, 1992

37. Raymond SA et al: The role of length of nerve exposed to local anesthetics in impulse blocking action. *Anesth Analg* **68**:563–570, 1989

38. Myers RR, Heckman HM: Effects of local anesthesia on nerve blood flow: Studies using lidocaine with and without epinephrine. *Anesthesiology* **71**:757, 1989

39. Klein JA: The tumescent technique for liposuction surgery. *Am J Cosmetic Surg* **4**:263–267, 1987

40. Stewart JH et al: Neutralized lidocaine with epinephrine for local anesthesia, pt 2. *J Dermatol Surg Oncol* **16**:842–845, 1990

41. McKay W et al: Sodium bicarbonate attenuates pain on skin infiltration with lidocaine, with or without epinephrine. *Anesth Analg* **66**:572–574, 1987

42. Stewart JH et al: Neutralized lidocaine with epinephrine for local anesthesia. *J Dermatol Surg Oncol* **15**:1081–1083, 1989

43. Larson PO et al: Stability of buffered lidocaine and epinephrine used for local anesthesia. *J Dermatol Surg Oncol* **17**:411–414, 1991

44. Klein JA: Anesthesia for liposuction in dermatologic surgery. *J Dermatol Surg Oncol* **14**:1124–1132, 1988

45. Klein JA: Tumescent technique for regional anesthesia permits lidocaine doses of 35 mg/kg for liposuction. *J Dermatol Surg Oncol* **16**:248–263, 1990

46. de Jong RH, Bonin JD: Local anesthetics: Injection route alters relative toxicity of bupivacaine. *Anesth Analg* **59**:925–928, 1980

47. Rowland M, Tozer TN: *Clinical Pharmacokinetics: Concepts and Applications,* 2d ed, Philadelphia, Lea & Febiger, 1989, pp 35–37

48. Asken S: *Liposuction Surgery and Autologous Fat Transplantation.* Norwalk, Conn, Appleton & Lange, 1988, p 63

49. Illouz YG, de Villers YT: Body sculpturing by lipoplasty. Edinburgh, Scot, Churchill-Livingstone, 1989, p 115

50. Gordh T: Xylocaine: A new local anesthetic. *Anaesthesia* **4**:4–9, 21, 1949

51. Scott DB: Evaluation of clinical tolerance of local anesthetic agents. *Br J Anaesth* **47**:328–333, 1975

52. Physicians' Desk Reference 1992, 46th ed. Montvale, NJ, Medical Economics, 1992, pp 637–639

53. Name of contact: Personal communication, month, day, year

54. The US Food and Drug Administration: Personal communication, month, day, year

55. Feldman HS et al: Comparative systemic toxicity of convulsant and supraconvulsant doses of ropivacaine, bupivacaine, and lidocaine in the conscious dog. *Anesth Analg* **vol**:794, 1989

tle since the 1980s. Various modifications in design and instrumentation have occurred, but, as of this time, the most commonly utilized reductions are still the midline, Y, and paramedian. Dramatic change has occurred with the advent of more extensive reductions such as the lateral reductions described by Marzola[11] and the extensive bilateral reductions or scalp-lifting procedures introduced by Bradshaw and Brandy.[12] The recent introduction of *scalp extenders* has been a breakthrough in basic scalp reduction technique. These scalp extenders can be placed under the galea prior to a midline reduction and enhance the stretch from the lateral aspects of the scalp, allowing for more scalp to be removed.

PATIENT SELECTION

Ideally the patient should have Hamilton[13] or Norwood[14] type III to type VI alopecia (Fig. 40-1) with good scalp laxity. Scalp laxity is the key to being able to remove the greatest amount of bald scalp. Usually, if the physician can firmly push both sides of the crown area medially and elicit three or more "wrinkles" of scalp, then the patient should have adequate mobility for a scalp reduction and expect that a signifi-

cant portion of scalp can be excised. Patients with less laxity can still be good candidates for reductions but the area excised will accordingly be less. In individuals with extremely tight scalps the area removed with scalp reduction can be marginal. These patients may need to have more than the usual number of scalp reductions to remove substantial amounts of scalp. It should be noted that in some instances scalp reduction may not be advisable. For example, a patient with type VI alopecia and a sparse donor area who undergoes reduction may find that the sides and back have thinned excessively due to stretching. This would be an unacceptable result to most patients. Similarly, a reduction should not be undertaken if the resultant scar cannot ultimately be adequately camouflaged. To perform a midline reduction and leave a scar running down the crown because there are not enough donor hairs to cover the scar is generally inappropriate.

As with any surgical procedure, there are sequelae and adverse reactions that can occur. The patient must be adequately informed. In deciding whether the patient is a good candidate for reduction, the physician should also take into account the patient's general physical condition. A physical exam may be in order for medical clearance. Routine complete blood count (CBC), Chemistry Screen (chem screen) 24, Prothrombin

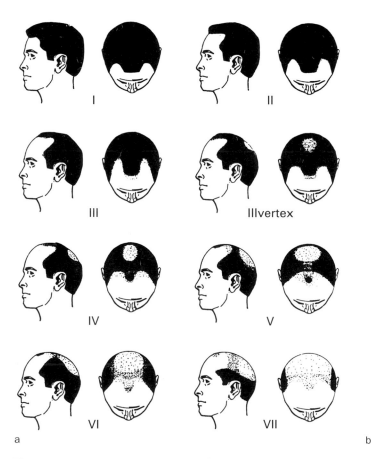

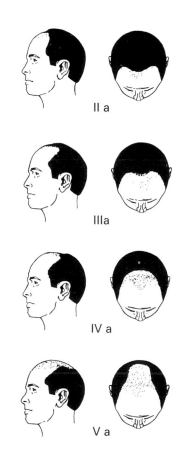

Figure 40-1 Norwood classification of types of male pattern baldness. From Norwood, O.T. and Shiell R. *Hair Transplantation*. 2nd ed. 1984. Permission obtained from the author and Charles C. Thomas, Publisher, Springfield, Illinois.

Time, Partial Thromboplastin Time (PT/PTT), hepatitis profile, and HIV status are recommended. Patients should be queried regarding any problems with bleeding, prior surgeries, or trauma which might provide information regarding a coagulopathy or alteration of the blood supply of the scalp. This information is especially important in planning an extensive scalp-lift which requires interruption of the occipital arteries. As reported, patients who have undergone prior hair transplantation should not be considered candidates for bilateral occipital parietal flaps (scalp-lifts).[15]

The patient's mental status should also be examined. Can the patient withstand a prolonged procedure? Can the patient accept a scar[s] and the ramifications of having the scar[s]? These and other psychological aspects may require inquiry. Patients who elect to have scalp reduction surgery should be convinced by themselves that they have significant areas of alopecia that need to be removed. Some patients who clearly have a type VI pattern but who still have some hair in the crown and vertex do not consider themselves bald enough to benefit from a scalp reduction. Many a patient has not made a close examination of the area of balding scalp. A Polaroid photo can be helpful in demonstrating to the patient the true extent of alopecia.

With regard to age, there are no absolute contraindications per se, but, as with hair transplantation, the physician must be cognizant of the patient's future pattern of alopecia and how visible scars may be at a later date.

Debate exists regarding whether to perform reductions prior to or after hair transplantation. In favor of the argument to perform reduction initially, one can better plan the overall outcome and the physician is better able to utilize donor hair more wisely. For instance, the "part" can be raised to an appropriate level at the outset rather than having it perhaps too low. If scalp reduction is performed first, the hairline can be properly designed. One risks the hairline being placed excessively low or broad if hair transplants are placed initially. When transplants are placed first, the extent of the reduction may necessitate removal of a portion of these grafts. Some of these can be reimplanted, but at times this is not possible. Carrying out the reduction first will stretch the hair-bearing scalp, thereby decreasing density in the future donor area. This can be compensated for in later hair transplant sessions by placing more grafts. Conversely, one could have difficulty harvesting grafts initially and subsequently performing a reduction, as the donor scalp density may then appear too sparse. Patients who elect to have extensive scalp-lifting procedures such as the bilateral occipital parietal (BOP) flap should without question have the flap surgery prior to any hair transplantation.

Those who advocate transplantation initially cite the fact that patients see new hair growth shortly after transplantation and observe a marked change in appearance after one session of grafts. Patients soon have a sense of satisfaction and accomplishment. The author believes that there is some truth to this because some patients who have undergone reductions may feel that only minimal improvement has occurred. These patients need to be shown their before-and-after photos to substantiate the improvement.

TYPES OF SCALP REDUCTION

There are numerous types and variations of scalp reductions; this chapter will review the techniques for the most commonly performed reductions (Fig. 40-2).

1. Midline reduction
2. Y or Mercedes pattern
3. Paramedian or lateral pattern
4. Extensive scalp lifting BOP, bitemporal parietal (BP), lateral lift, and circumferential reduction

Midline Reduction

The midline scalp reduction is the most commonly utilized reduction. It is a simple elliptical design which is easily performed by physicians with even modest surgical expertise. In patients with excellent scalp laxity, large amounts of bald

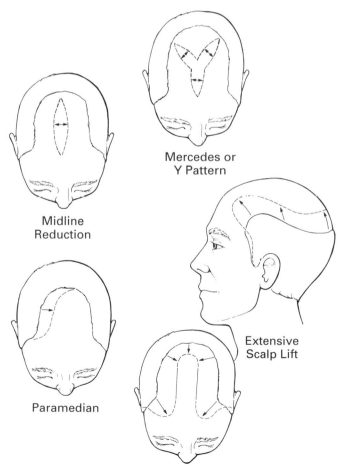

Figure 40-2 Patterns of common scalp reductions and the extensive scalp lift.

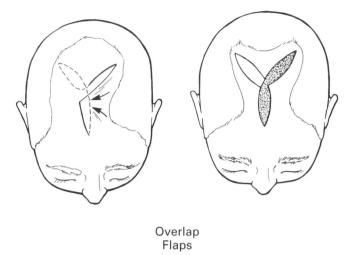

Overlap
Flaps

a

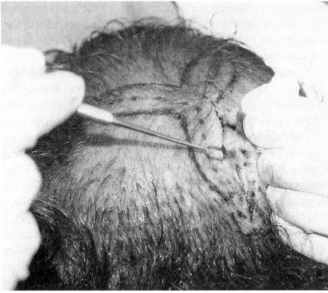

b

Figure 40-5 One flap is superimposed over the other to assess the portion of scalp that can be removed.

tern, though to a lesser degree, the occipital area is elevated. There is excellent visibility in undermining laterally, but one can encounter some difficulty medially.

The advantage of having the scar in the hair-bearing fringe can be a disadvantage if the patient continues to lose hair from the sides. The surgeon must carefully assess the patient's pattern of hair loss to determine whether the hair loss will extend farther down the sides. Continued hair loss could make the scar highly visible, necessitating refinement at a later time. The paramedian reduction raises the hair bearing scalp on one side, leaving one side higher than the other but this is rarely a concern. In fact subsequent reductions if required are usually carried out along the original incision to avoid placing another scar on the opposite side.

Preoperative Considerations

The usual preoperative measures are taken as discussed previously. Photographs are obtained in the immediate preoperative period. The area to be excised is marked off utilizing a wax pencil. The marking should be made just medially to the hair-bearing fringe to avoid a sharp demarcation between the bald scalp and the hair-bearing scalp. The design is a "lazy S," and the width of the design is (usually) maximal at the middle, tapering off sharply at the ends. Posteriorly, the flap is designed to extend just beyond the midline, while anteriorly it extends approximately to an imaginary line perpendicular to the lateral orbital rim and intersecting slightly posterior to the lateral margin of the appropriate frontal hairline. Once the design is completed, it is marked over with a Pilot marker. One can expect to remove approximately 3 to 4 cm in width of bald scalp, but this can of course vary as a function of scalp laxity. Alt has written that his average width of excision is 4.5 to 6 cm.

Basic Instrumentation

No. 10 Bard-Parker blade
Scalpel
Curved Metzenbaum or Mayo scissors
Hemostats
Adson-Brown forceps
Towel clamps or D'Assumpco clamp
Needle-holders

Anesthesia

Xylocaine 1% to 2% with epinephrine 1:100,000 or 1:200,000 is administered as a pericephalic block. The patient may be given sedatives per os and/or pain medication if desired. IM steroids can be utilized.

Technique

After being marked, the patient is brought into the operating area and prepared with Betadine or other suitable antiseptic preparation. The patient is placed in a Pron-Pillow. The surgeon and assistants are gowned appropriately. An incision is made at the lateral aspect of the marking. The incision is begun at the posterior point and extended anteriorly. It is carried down to the galeal-periosteal plane. Utilizing skin hooks, the surgeon elevates the lateral aspect of the flap and partially undermines with curved Metzenbaum or other suitable scissor as described previously. The bleeders at the edge of the flap are then cauterized. Undermining is continued to the attachment of the auricle laterally and to the insertion of the occipitalis muscle posteriorly. The medial portion of the flap is then undermined. Due to the design of the flap, undermining here can be limited by the curvature of the skull. Once undermined, the lateral portion of the flap is pulled over the medial portion, and a bloodstain mark or other mark is made. The portion of excess skin is then excised. One should always be conservative in removing the skin so as to avoid having to attempt the closure under extreme tension.

The closure is accomplished by first suturing the galeal layer, which can withstand considerable tension. Closure can be accomplished with interrupted or running suture such as 0-PDS II. The skin is closed with a nonabsorbable suture such as 4–0 Prolene, and the wound is dressed as discussed in "Midline Reduction" above. Postoperative instructions are given regarding wound care and follow-up visit for suture removal.

Extensive Scalp-Lifting

Extensive scalp-lifting or reduction differs from traditional reductions in that significantly more tissue is undermined. The undermining is carried past the *superior* nuchal ridge and subsequently to the *inferior hairline* at the nape of the neck. Additionally, the incision is extended anteriorly into the temple area and down into the sideburn, allowing the scalp to be moved anteriorly and medially to improve the temporal recession.

The technique is based on the work of Dr. Mario Marzola who developed a "lateral lift" in which one side of the scalp was raised and subsequently the other. Dr. Bradshaw then proposed performing the operation bilaterally and this was further refined by Dr. Dominic Brandy who coined the terms *BOP flap* or *scalp-lift*. Dr. Brandy has made several variations of this flap, including the BT[16] and modified Bitemporal flap (BT).[17]

There are several advantages to the scalp-lifting procedure over traditional reductions. The design of the flap allows for a substantially greater segment of scalp to be removed in a single session, thus expediting final results for the patient. Similarly, because the ultimate number of procedures is reduced, the monetary expenditure by the patient is less. There is no slot formation with extensive scalp-lifts, and the scars are in a cosmetically favorable location. Also, because the entire scalp is elevated and stretched, all hairs contribute to the final result, thus providing density far superior to transplants.

As noted previously, the scalp-lift aids in alleviating the areas of temporal recession. It is extremely difficult to provide excellent cosmesis in these areas by using hair transplants. Stretch-back is minimized with the lift, as the hair-bearing skin is sutured to bald scalp and any remaining bald scalp remains adhered to the skull—it is not undermined. Furthermore, the skin edges are closed under minimal or no tension, which also reduces stretch-back.

One must be cautious in assessing patients for the lift procedure.[15] As with other reductions, the surgeon must be cognizant of the patient's future hair pattern. The patients may need to be advised that should they continue to lose hair from the sides, the scar may be more noticeable and transplants may be required to camouflage the area. Patients with type VII baldness often are not good candidates. This may even be

true for some with type VI alopecia. Individuals who have a hairline set far off from the ear may be unhappy with the stretching of this area from the procedure, and those with thin hair in the occipital region may find that the stretching excessively thins out the remaining hair. Patients need to be informed that they may need to grow their hair longer for adequate cosmesis.

One disadvantage of the scalp-lift is hypesthesia at the crown secondary to the required transection of the occipital nerves. Localized necrosis is possible primarily in the area of the nuchal ridge; this complication rarely occurs when the occipital arteries have been previously ligated.[18] In the past, critics of the technique have cited necrosis as a major problem and their experiences have indicated a far higher rate than reported. It should be noted that these cases of necrosis occurred in patients who had not undergone prior ligation.[19,20] In some instances necrosis may have resulted from dissecting in the wrong plane. Necrosis may also have occurred because of the patient's head being improperly positioned at the time of moving the flap forward to mark the excision of excess scalp. This gives the false impression that more tissue can be excised than should be. With the patient's head extended the closure can be made, but when the patient attempts to flex the neck post operatively he is unable to adequately do so. There is too much tension on the flap in this situation. Additionally, the procedure may have been performed in patients who have previously had hair transplants. These patients have had alterations of the vasculature and should not be considered candidates for the bilateral lift; rather, these patients should undergo two successive lateral lifts separated by approximately 3 months.

Another disadvantage of the extensive scalp-lift is that it requires considerable surgical skill. There is substantially more undermining with the lift procedure as compared to other scalp reductions, and the undermining is in different planes. The surgeon must also be prepared to manage considerable bleeding and work quickly to avoid blood loss requiring transfusion.

Unless the patient has previously undergone hair transplantation which would compromise the scalp circulation, extensive scalp-lifting is carried out in two procedures. At times, a third procedure, carried out 3 months after the BOP flap, may be in order to remove any remaining bald scalp. This can often be performed as a simple midline reduction. A conservative BOP or BT flap may also be used (Fig. 40-6).

The initial procedure is the ligation or cauterization of the occipital arteries and the accompanying neurovascular bundles.[21] Ligating the occipital arteries and waiting several weeks prior to scalp-lifting enhances blood flow and the viability of the flaps created. This procedure is performed approximately 2-6 weeks prior to the actual lifting procedure. The patient must be advised preoperatively that there will be an area of hypesthesia at the crown which can be permanent, and this is an expected sequela of the procedure. The technique for ligation is described below.

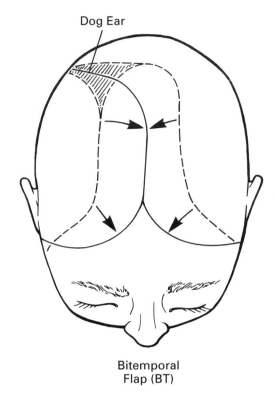

Figure 40-6 Schematic of the Bitemporal flap.

Technique for Ligation/Cauterization of the Occipital Arteries

Preoperative Considerations

The patient has been instructed to shampoo with Betadine or similar agent the night before and day of the procedure. A cephalosporin or other suitable antibiotic is prescribed for 3 days, starting the morning of the ligation. A sedative per os such as diazepam 5 to 10 mg and/or pain medication such as oxycodone and acetaminophen can be administered 30 to 60 min prior to the procedure.

With the patient sitting up, the occipital arteries are palpated just inferiorly to the nuchal ridge and marked with a wax pencil. Typically, the arteries can be found approximately 4.5 to 5 cm medially to the beginning of the postauricular hairline. Once the area of the occipital arteries is identified, a Doppler such as the Huntleigh Pocket Doppler* set at 8 MHz is employed to further delineate the artery on each side. The Doppler must be moved in all directions, and the point where the echo is loudest is marked. An X is drawn through this point. Marks such as dots are made around the X at the 3 o'clock, 6 o'clock, 9 o'clock, and 12 o'clock points, which will serve as sites for instilling the anesthetic. After both sides are marked, it is a good idea to recheck the X points and make sure that they are symmetrically placed in relation to one another (Fig 40-7). At times, a branch of the artery may be er-

*Huntleigh Healthcare, Manalapan, N.J. 07726

roneously identified instead of the main vessel. A Pilot marker is then used to mark over the various points.

Basic Instrumentation

No. 15 scalpel
5-in Weitlander retractor
Mosquito hemostats
Curved Metzenbaum scissors
Skin hooks

Anesthesia

Xylocaine 2% with epinephrine 1:100,000 is administered with a 30-gauge needle. The anesthetic solution is injected around the X. The needle is advanced until the skull is felt, and the needle is slowly withdrawn as the anesthetic solution is injected. Care is taken to avoid infusing the anesthetic into the artery. Using a 23-gauge needle, the physician injects the anesthetic solution between the dots. The same procedure is carried out on the other side.

Technique

The patient is brought into the operating suite and the area at the occiput is prepared with Betadine. The surgeon and staff are appropriately gowned and the patient placed in prone position. The patient's head is placed in a Pron-Pillow and the site is draped. Using a no. 15 blade, the surgeon makes a vertical incision approximately 2 to 2.5 cm in length over the center of the X on one side. This incision should extend into the fat and just to the fascia. Hemostasis is obtained with cautery. Once the fascia is identified, the Weitlander retractor is placed in the incision and opened. A Metzenbaum scissors can then be utilized to spread the fascia apart. This is best accomplished by opening and closing the scissors in line with the vertical incision. It can also be helpful to dissect the tissue by spreading the tissue perpendicularly to the incision. Electrocautery can be utilized to partially break through the fascia. During the dissection, in order to keep the surgical field clear, it is advised that suction be employed. As the tissue is spread, the surgeon will often feel the tissue "give" and the scissors will seem to sink into the area of the neurovascular bundle. The surgeon will observe the red-blue hue of the neurovascular bundle. At this point, the tissue is carefully dissected and the main branch identified as well as the medial and lateral branches (Fig. 40-8). The same process is then carried out on

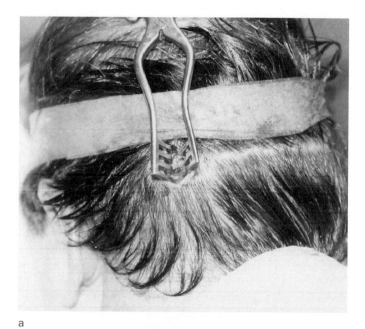

a

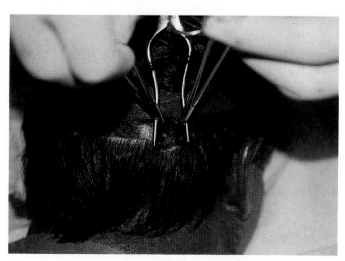

b

Figure 40-8 The occipital neurovascular bundles are demonstrated.

the other branches. The branches are then cut through the area of desiccation down to periosteum and the stumps checked for any bleeding. It is important to be certain that all of the branches, are identified. There should be a Y-shaped segment removed. The area is then examined for any bleeding and cauterized as required. The retractor is removed and again the incision is inspected for any bleeding. Once adequate hemostasis is achieved, the incision is closed in two layers with absorbable suture. The process is then carried out on the opposite side.

Polysporin is used as a dressing. The patient is advised to avoid strenuous exercise for 7 to 10 days. Patients may be given pain medication per os postoperatively as some patients actually complain of hyperesthesia initially. Patients are advised that they may experience an altered sensation at the crown for some time and there may be permanent loss of sensation in this area.

Scalp Lift Technique

Preoperative Considerations

Preoperatively, the patient is prescribed an antibiotic such as a cephalosporin to begin 1 to 2 days prior to surgery and to continue for 5 days. The patient is also given prescriptions for furosemide (40 mg b.i.d.) and potassium chloride (8 mEq b.i.d.) to begin the day following surgery and to continue for 5 days postoperatively. Prior to surgery, the patient is advised to take vitamin C, 2 g per day, and vitamin K (5 mg b.i.d.) which is begun 1 week prior to surgery. Compazine suppositories 25 mg are prescribed for nausea following the surgery if required. An analgesic medication such as hydrocodone with acetaminophen is prescribed to be taken following surgery. Oral steroids may be started prior to surgery or alternatively the patient may be given IM or intravenous (IV) steroids such as Celestone the day of surgery. Betadine shampoo is prescribed for the evening before surgery and the morning of surgery. The patient is requested to purchase a cervical collar and three Ace wraps to be used for the dressing after the surgery. As with other procedures, a CBC, PT/PTT, hepatitis profile, HIV assay, and ECG are obtained. Photographs are taken the day of surgery.

On the day of surgery, the patient is given Dramamine 200 mg po, Valium 10 mg, Tagamet 300 mg, and Reglan 10 mg. Decadron 8 mg is administered IM. Once the informed consent and photographs have been obtained, the patient is ready to be marked. With a wax pencil a line is drawn in the sideburn, anteriorly to the superficial temporal artery, beginning at the level of the midsideburn. A Doppler can be used to ascertain the position of the superficial temporal artery. The line is then extended along the fringe of balding scalp posteriorly and then directed along a similar course on the opposite side, ending at the midsideburn. The area of bald scalp to be removed is then marked off. One can usually expect to move the occipital area anteriorly approximately 3 to 4 cm, the sides medially approximately 3 to 4 cm, and the temporal recession areas anteriorly approximately 4 cm. It can be advantageous to make marks at these distances and then connect them as the lines are drawn. It is recommended that a midline sagittal line be drawn to ensure symmetry of design. The line delineating the area of bald scalp to be excised should start anteriorly at the point where the promontory of hair at the temple exists. After completing the design with the wax pencil, a Pilot marker is used over the lines drawn. The Pilot marker is also utilized to mark off the points where anesthesia is to be placed.

Basic Instrumentation

No. 10 Bard-Parker blade and scalpel
Lahey clamp
Poole suction
Double skin hooks
Straight and curved hemostats
*Brandy Suction-Elevator
*Brandy retractor
Rhytidectomy scissors
Curved Metzenbaum scissors
Needle-holders
Forceps

Anesthesia

Xylocaine 1% with 1:100,000 epinephrine is used to form a ring block. The line of anesthesia follows the hairline and extends from the anterior hairline, along the temple and preauricular area, around the ear down to the nape of the neck on one side, and then to the other side in similar fashion. The injections are made approximately 1-cm apart. A line of anesthesia, is also made across the nuchal ridge. Between the points injected with the 1% solution, $\frac{1}{4}$ % Xylocaine with epinephrine 1:400,000 is placed. The $\frac{1}{4}$ % solution is also infiltrated in the rectangular area delineated by the nuchal ridge, the lateral borders of the hairline posteriorly, and the inferior extent of the hairline. It is advised to inject across the area rather than pointing the needle straight down into the tissue. A 30-gauge needle is used for the 1% solution and a 27-gauge for the $\frac{1}{4}$ % solution. It is also advised that one use caution when injecting the preauricular area so as not to injure the superficial temporal artery. As noted previously, this artery should be palpated and/or found with the Doppler and its position marked. Damage to this artery can jeopardize the flap.

Along with local anesthesia, IV sedation should be utilized. Patients are usually given Versed (Midazolam) and fentanyl. These drugs should generally be administered by a qualified individual such as a nurse anesthetist or anesthesiologist. Patients should have appropriate monitoring such as pulse oximetry, ECG, and blood pressure monitoring. During

the procedure, a unit of Hespan (Hetastarch) is infused as a volume expander.

Technique

The patient is brought into the operating room and the local anaesthesia is administered. Betadine or similar solution is used as a surgical preparation, and the patient is placed in the prone position on a Prōn-Pillō. Oxygen is supplied via a cannula inserted through the Prōn-Pillō. The patient is draped, and the surgeon and staff are gowned.

The patient's head is turned to the left and the hair is wetted with sterile water. This aids in managing the hair and provides better visualization for the incision. The incision should originate at the midsideburn with a no. 10 scalpel and is extended to the midline of the occipital area. Contrary to the usual manner of moving the scalpel, the scalpel is pushed rather than pulled on the first pass. This allows the surgeon better visualization in staying along the desired path. In performing this maneuver, the surgeon inserts the scalpel only partially into the skin. The tip of the blade must remain above the skin to allow it to move smoothly. After incising to the occipital area, the scalpel is then pulled back along the same line. The depth of the incision should be down to periosteum except in the area of the temporalis muscle where it is actually taken down to deep temporalis fascia. With the incision on the left side completed, each assistant utilizes a double skin hook to begin to elevate the flap. Care must be taken in elevating the flap so as not to injure the temporal artery, which should lie within the flap. If the temporal artery is damaged, necrosis can occur.

The surgeon can use sharp or blunt dissection in the plane underneath the galea to elevate the flap approximately halfway down to the ear (Fig. 40-9). The physician should then stop and cauterize the bleeders carefully on the hair-bearing side. One can be very aggressive in using the cautery on the non-hair-bearing side of the incision as this tissue will be removed later in the procedure. Undermining is then continued down to the ear. The undermining can be facilitated by having one assistant hold the patient's head down with one hand while elevating the flap with the other. The second assistant uses both hands to keep the flap elevated as well (Fig. 40-10). Once the dissection is completed down to the ear, the patient's head is turned and the same process carried out on the right side.

After the parietal area dissection is accomplished, undermining in the occipital region is initiated. Sharp dissection is employed and the dissection proceeds until the occipitalis muscle is exposed. The assistants maintain upward tension on the flap to aid in the dissection. Attention is then directed back to the left side. With an assistant applying countertraction, a tunnel is made just posteriorly to the ear with a curved Metzenbaum or rhytidectomy scissors. The scissors can be held with both hands then opened, closed, and turned on its vertical axis to expedite undermining the postauricular skin. This skin can be extremely thin and adherent to the underlying tis-

* Robbins Instruments, Chatham, N.J.

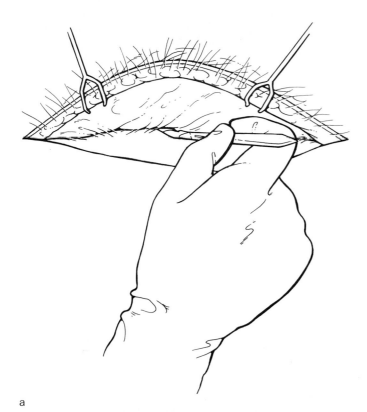

a

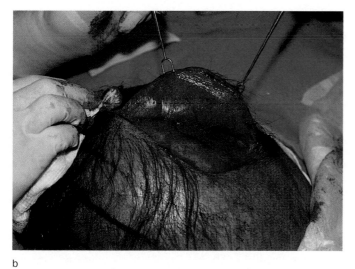

b

Figure 40-9 Illustration showing the elevation of the flap. Having the assistants utilize double skin hooks facilitates the dissection.

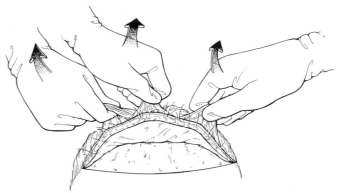

Figure 40-10 IIllustration showing the proper placement of the assistant's hands. The patient's head is turned to the side.

sue. One should be cautious so as to prevent puncturing the skin if possible. After making the tunnel, the surgeon returns to the occipital area and the occipitalis muscle is cut at the point of attachment to the periosteum. The surgery becomes more complex at this point as the surgeon must now undermine from the superficial plane behind the ear to the deeper plane at the occiput. To accomplish this, the assistants should elevate the flap as described previously. The surgeon initially dissects superficially, exposing some fat at the lateral portion

of the flap, but as the dissection moves farther posteriorly toward the occiput, the undermining must become deeper, ultimately splitting the trapezius fascia posteriorly. Upon completion of the lateral area, the patient's head is placed straight into the Pron-Pillow and the dissection continued toward the center of the occiput. It should again be emphasized that as the dissection proceeds toward the midline, the undermining must be in a deeper plane. No fat should be exposed as the hair follicles lie in the fat. Should fat be observed, the surgeon must move to a deeper plane. It is very helpful to utilize the Brandy Suction-Elevator while performing this part of the procedure (Fig. 40-11). The tip of the instrument is held against the flap while the surgeon simultaneously exerts an upward force. Apart from providing suction, it thus helps to support the flap and place it under tension, aiding the dissection. This phase of the procedure is completed when the undermining reaches the midline of the occipital area halfway down the nape of the neck. The patient's head is turned and the same steps taken on the right side.

The patient's head is then placed straight into the Pron-Pillow and the undermining is continued in the occipital region to a level approximately halfway between the nuchal ridge and the hairline of the nape. The goal in this area should be to divide the trapezius fascia. This will guarantee that the dissection is in the correct plane and no hair follicles are disturbed or transected. Should the surgeon go too deeply, one feels the scissors fall into a space. Simply aim more superficially to correct this problem. Apart from damaging hair follicles, the surgeon has little to fear in this area as there are no major vessels or nerves to damage. The undermining is again aided by using the Brandy Suction-Elevator instrument.

After dissection to the appropriate level in the occiput, the patient's head is turned to the left and the skin and its attachments are freed from the posterior ear sulcus. Again the surgeon forms a tunnel by holding a face-lift scissors in the manner described above. This should connect to the previously undermined skin at the posterior ear region. The surgeon then returns to the occipital area and completes the undermining

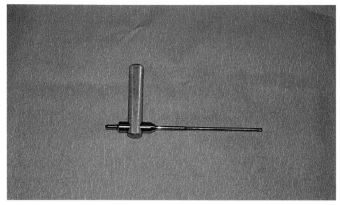

a

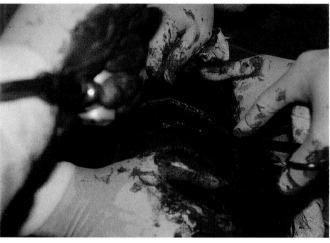

b

Figure 40-11   The Brandy Suction-Elevator is especially helpful in dissecting in the occipital area and keeping the area free of blood which aids in visualization.

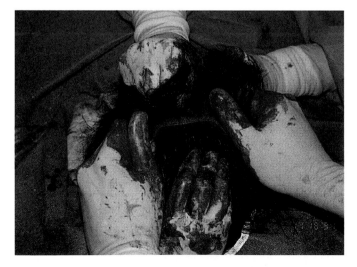

Figure 40-12   Photograph demonstrating the initial movement of the flap anteriorly and medially to demarcate the area to be excised. It is crucial that the patient's head be in a neutral position.

on the left side to the hairline of the nape of the neck. It is important not to undermine farther than the hairline as this would result in elevating the hairline when the flap is advanced. Next, the head is turned to the right, the right posterior ear sulcus is released, and the occipital area is undermined to the hairline of the nape. At this time, the postauricular muscles on the left and right can be divided to permit further movement from this area. The muscles should be left intact if it is felt that an excessive amount of supraauricular skin would be exposed when the skin is ultimately stretched.

The entire flap should now be completely free of attachments to the underlying tissue. The surgeon should examine the flap by feeling with a hand for attachments which would restrict the movement of the flap; any attachments should be released. It is imperative that the flap be undermined uniformly and, if necessary, further undermining should be carried out.

The surgeon is now ready to advance the flap and make the markings to excise the area of bald scalp from the occipital area. The patient's head is placed in a neutral position in the Pron-Pillow. This is crucial as having the head extended will cause the surgeon to excise too much scalp and place the flap on excessive tension upon closure. The surgeon grasps the flap with both hands and advances it anteriorly and medially (Fig. 40-12). The bald peninsula is overlapped to leave a bloodstain impression which will delineate the area to be excised. This marking may be less or more than the original estimate initially indicated; therefore, one must be able to adjust as required and not force the movement of the flap.

At the midline point of the bald peninsula, a Lahey clamp is applied by the surgeon. Forceps held by the assistants are placed laterally and tension is applied. The area indicated by the bloodstain is then excised and cautery is used as needed along the peninsula. The scalp flap is elevated with the Brandy hook retractor and irrigated with approximately 60 cc of saline per side. Suction is then used to collect the saline and the flap is inspected for any bleeders. Stab incisions are then made at the postauricular sulci bilaterally at the level of the ear lobes. Penrose drains are subsequently placed through these incisions and sutured into place with absorbable suture such as 4–0 chromic. Once this manuever is completed, the surgeon again inspects the flap for any bleeders and cauterizes them as required. The flap is now irrigated with a solution of thrombin (2.5 cc of 5000 U of thrombin with 5.0 cc of saline).

At this point, approximately 2 cm of the tip of the peninsula of bald scalp is elevated by sharp dissection just above the periosteum. With the patient's head in a neutral position, the flap is advanced. A pulley stitch is placed with 0-PDS II from the midline point of the flap, into the periosteum, then into the galea of the elevated bald peninsula, and back to the flap (Fig. 40-13).

The surgeon now advances the sides of the flap medially. This maneuver must be performed by moving both sides simultaneously (Fig. 40-14). The physician grasps the hair on both sides and pulls toward the center so the flaps overlap the

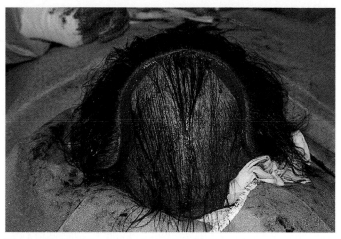

Figure 40-13 The flap is sutured to the remaining bald peninsula.

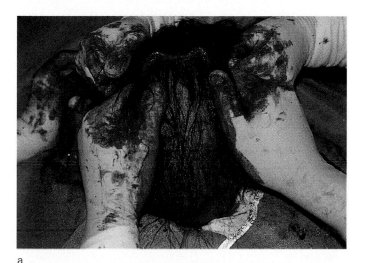

a

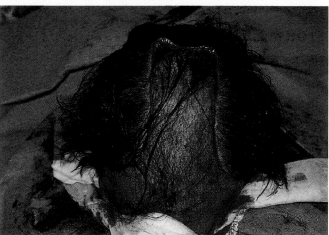

b

Figure 40-14 The two sides of the scalp flap are positioned to mark off the area to be excised. Both sides are moved simultaneously to avoid taking an unequal amount of scalp from one side. In performing this maneuver the patient's head should be in a neutral position.

bald skin and again leave a bloodstain impression. If the impression is not to the original line marked in ink, the surgeon should be certain to reinscribe the new lines symmetrically to ensure that equal amounts of bald scalp will be excised from each side. Once the marks are made, one may want to score the skin at several points to serve as reference points if the marks are accidentally obliterated.

The patient's head is then turned to the left. The flap is held at the temporal area with a Lahey clamp held by the surgeon. The assistants hold the tissue with forceps placed off to the sides of the Lahey clamp. Tension is exerted on the flap and the area marked off is excised. A suture is placed at the temporal recession area by using 0-PDS II in a pulley stitch. The same process is duplicated on the opposite side.

The flap is now in place. Next a tunnel is created with a Metzenbaum or other suitable scissors, at the level of the galeal-periosteal interface through the peninsula of bald skin. The tunnel is placed approximately 3 to 4 cm from the tip of the peninsula. A suture is then passed as a horizontal mattress through the galea on the left side, then through the tunnel created, and through the galea on the right, and finally back to the left. 0-PDS II is then placed as required along the flap to allow for good approximation of the skin edges. There should be little or no tension on the flap (Fig. 40-15).

Starting at the midline occipital area, a running suture of 4–0 PDS is used to suture the skin edge. The suture is run posteriorly to anteriorly to approximately the temple. A Penrose drain is next placed at the inferior aspect of the incision in the sideburn. The drain is sutured in place with 5–0 PDS. A 5–0 PDS is then placed just superiorly to the drain and continued to the point at the temple where the 4–0 PDS was ended. The same steps are carried out on the right side.

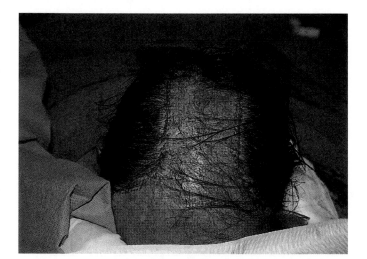

Figure 40-15 Photograph demonstrating closure of the flap. The surgeon should be able to close the skin edge under minimal tension. Since the surgeon has sutured hair bearing skin to bald skin that has not been undermined and because it is closed under minimal tension, stretch-back is nil.

Upon completion of the surgery, the head is washed with hydrogen peroxide and Johnson & Johnson's No More Tangles is used to aid in combing through the hair. K-Y jelly is then applied along the suture lines and the dressing applied. Two 4- by 4-in gauze sponges are placed lengthwise behind each ear. Two gynecologic pads are then placed across the nuchal ridge area and a third pad is placed overlapping the first two pads. A stack of sponges is placed over each ear partially covering the drains to absorb the drainage. A 6-in Ace wrap is placed around the head for several wraps. More 4-in by 4-in sponges are secured at the inferior aspect of the drains and the wrap is fastened. The remaining area of scalp is then covered with gynecologic pads and a circumferential wrap is made with two Ace bandages. As one assistant places the wrap around the scalp, the other assistant crosses the first assistant's wrap by moving from one side to the other in a posterior to anterior direction. A cervical collar is also placed to prevent the patient from flexing the neck for three to four days.

Once the dressing is completed, the patient is monitored for some time and given instructions as to follow-up and care. The patient is instructed to return the next day at which time the dressing is removed and the hair is shampooed, conditioned, and styled. Sutures are to be removed in 7 to 10 days.

Circumferential Reduction

Circumferential scalp reduction[22] is a variation of a modified major[23] reduction and extensive scalp lifting. It is well suited for patients with limited hair density at the sides and occiput. The design is essentially the same as an extensive scalp lift but there is less medial and anterior movement. The operative technique differs from lifting in that the undermining is carried out posteriorly only to the nuchal ridge or insertion of the occipitalis muscle. As stated above, the amount of advancement is diminished from that of a scalp-lift, but there is significant movement and the operative technique is simpler. If the surgeon desires more advancement, the occipital and periauricular muscles can be incised and the surgeon can undermine more aggressively medial and lateral to the occipital neurovascular bundles. Ligation of the occipital arteries is not required preoperatively, and it is not necessary to place drains. An advantage of this technique over standard reductions is that the scar remains in the hair-bearing fringe and hair direction is maintained. There is also the added advantage of anteriomedial movement in the temporal recessions and stretch-back is also diminished.

ADJUNCTS TO SCALP REDUCTIONS

Carbon Dioxide Laser

The CO_2 laser can be used for scalp reduction and extensive scalp lifting.[24,25] The CO_2 laser provides excellent hemostasis and cutting ability. The disadvantages include thermal damage, the expense, the space required, and the fact that it is sometimes awkward to use. Special precautions must also be taken to ensure protection from fire and laser plume inhalation. The laser tends to be slow to work with but this is primarily a result of power limitations. The *Ultrapulse CO_2 laser may provide more efficient cutting with decreased thermal damage.

Scalp Extenders

Recently, discussion has been raised regarding implanting devices which are attached to the galea for the purpose of stretching the scalp. Dr. Patrick Frechet[26] has presented his work on the use of a Silastic band which is attached to the galea by means of a row of hooks at each end. The procedure is performed under local anesthesia as part of a midline scalp reduction. Prior to closing the reduction, the device is inserted across the midline with a specially designed instrument that aids in attaching the band. Once the band is secured, the skin is closed. The band is left in place approximately 28 days at which time it is removed and a second reduction is performed. Hopefully enough bald scalp can be removed to provide adequate hair in the crown. At times, multiple placements of the device and subsequent reductions are required to achieve removal of all of the bald scalp. Dr. Frechet has apparently been successful in treating patients with type VI alopecia by using this method. A disadvantage of the procedure is the cost of the device which is not reusable but because fewer scalp reductions are required to reach the final point, the overall cost is less. Complications reported with extenders include seromas, hematomas, and infection.

Drs. Dominic Brandy[27] and James Bridenstine[28] have also developed a device which can be utilized to stretch the scalp. This device is a single band of Silastic to which Dacron is attached at the ends. As with the Frechet device, this band is attached to the galea but it is sutured into place. The amount of movement is similar to the Frechet device. The cost of the device is much less than the Frechet extender but it is not a ready made device. It must be constructed from the various components prior to use and sterilized.

Galeotomy

On occasion, it may be necessary to obtain extra stretch from a flap to facilitate adequate closure. A galeotomy can be performed by incising the galea superficially in an anterior to posterior direction, just to the point where it appears to open up and fat is observed. Because of the vasculature just above the galea, significant bleeding may occur. It is recommended that no more than three galeotomy incisions be made per side. Galeotomies should not be performed with extensive scalp-lifting as the temporal vessel may be injured, jeopardizing the flap.

COMPLICATIONS

Complications are rarely encountered with scalp reductions. The most common complications relate to suture reactions or reactions to wound dressings such as contact dermatitis. These problems are easily managed by removing the offending agent and treating the site with topical steroids. Infection is rather unusual, but should it occur it should be managed with the appropriate antibiotic.

On occasion, a hematoma may develop. Hematomas can be treated in the early stages by aspirating the hematoma with a large-bore needle and syringe. If the hematoma has begun to coalesce and the patient is experiencing pain, it may be necessary to open the area to evacuate the hematoma; otherwise, it can be managed with pressure dressings and pain management.

Necrosis can be a complication of scalp reduction. It is most often associated with attempting closure under marked skin tension. It also can be associated with damaging a vessel supplying the primary source of blood to a flap. This can occur with scalp-lifting if the temporal vessels are damaged. Necrosis can result from performing the BOP flap or similar flaps in people who have previously undergone hair transplantation. An area of necrosis can sometimes occur at the tip of the occipital flap created by a Mercedes or Y flap. The best way to prevent necrosis is to close the wound under minimal tension and avoid injuring important vessels.

At the first signs of diminished blood flow in an area, one can apply nitroglycerin ointment to the area several times per day. One may consider prescribing pentoxifylline (Trental) to promote oxygen delivery. If necrosis actually occurs, one should treat the area as any other open wound. The patient should be followed closely for signs of infection and treated appropriately. Usually, these areas of necrosis are ultimately rather small and are often amenable later to surgical revision. If necrosis occurs in the occipital area, it is often easy to include the scar revision as part of harvesting grafts for transplantation.

Excessive bleeding can be a problem even with routine scalp reduction. It is best controlled by maintaining meticulous hemostasis during the procedure. Injecting the incision lines with epinephrine 1:100,000 or 1:200,000 prior to starting the procedure can be helpful.

In performing a reduction other than an extensive scalp-lift and undermining in the occipital area, the surgeon must be careful not to injure the occipital arteries. If these vessels are disturbed, there can be profuse and rapid bleeding. It is sometimes necessary to further dissect the tissue and employ suction to achieve adequate visualization of these vessels to permit cauterization or ligation. Passing a suture through the scalp in an effort to stop the bleeding can be attempted. On occasion perforators from the skull can be difficult to coagulate. Bone wax can be used to aid in achieving hemostasis.

With extensive scalp-lifting, the bleeding can be severe. This is especially true when the surgeon is a novice in this procedure. It is imperative that the physician perform the procedure in a systematic fashion, a section at a time. One must be aggressive in utilizing cautery on the non-hair-bearing portions and cauterize as required as one progresses with the undermining. Once the flap is elevated it should be examined for bleeding sites. Thrombin should be used as described. It is also suggested that a unit of Hespan be infused for volume replacement. The surgeon may also consider having the patient supply a unit of autologous blood that can be infused if necessary. After the procedure, a hemoglobin/hematocrit may be in order to assess the patient's status.

Another complication of reductions can be facial edema. This problem can usually be alleviated by providing systemic steroids preoperatively and advising the patient to use cold packs. Should the problem occur despite the preoperative steroids, one can increase the dosage and prolong the course of steroids in an effort to diminish the edema. Diuretics may also aid in alleviating this problem. The patient should be assured that the problem is temporary and will resolve shortly.

On occasion, a foreign body reaction can occur which results in a cyst, sterile abscess, or suture granuloma. Upon closure of any reduction, the wound should be assessed for hair and other foreign matter. Irrigating the wound can help diminish the problem. When cysts develop, they can easily be removed by excision. If a suture begins to spit, the suture should be promptly removed.

After a scalp reduction, patients may experience telogen effluvium. The patient should be reassured that this is temporary and the hair will return. Rogaine may speed the patient's recovery.

A midline reduction or reduction that produces such a scar can produce a slot deformity. A remedy for the slot deformity has been devised by Dr. Frechet.[29] The Frechet flap consists of three transposition flaps which when completed produce a restoration of the swirl pattern in the occipital region.

Stretch-back

Norwood et al[10] described the phenomenon where, after a scalp reduction, the bald area remaining "reexpands" to some degree. The average cited by Norwood was 30 percent. Studies by Nordstrom[30] indicate that stretch-back occurs because of tension on the wound. Conversely Dr. Martin Unger[31] has reported that stretch-back is clinically insignificant if closure is made under minimal tension.

SUMMARY

Scalp reduction is an excellent procedure when the right design is selected for the right patient. It affords the patient a dramatic result in a minimum amount of time and is extremely safe. It can also save the patient considerable expense when compared to transplantation alone and can benefit those who might otherwise be poor candidates for hair replacement.

REFERENCES

1. Blanchard G, Blanchard B: Obliteration of alopecia by hair lifting: A New concept and technique. *J. Nat. Med. Assoc.* **69:**639–641, 1977

2. Unger MG: *Alopecia Reduction in Hair Transplantation,* ed. 2, Unger, WP and Nordstrom, REA ed. Marcel Dekker, Inc., New York, New York 1988, pp. 435–518

3. Unger MG, Unger WP: Personal communication, 1994

4. Sparkuhl K: Scalp reduction: Serial excision of the scalp with flap advancement. International hair Transplant Symposium, Lucernne, Switzerland, February 4, 1978

5. Stough DB, Webster RC: Esthetics and refinements of hair transplantation. International Hair Transplant Symposium, Lucerne, Switzerland, February 4, 1978

6. Unger MG, Unger WP: Management of alopecia of the scalp by a combination of excisions and transplantations. *J Dermatol Surg Oncol* **4:**620–672, 1978

7. Bosley LL, Hope CR, Montroy RE: Male Pattern Reduction (MPR) for surgical reduction of male pattern baldness. *Curr Ther Res* **25:**281–287, 1979

8. Schultz BC, Roenigk Jr, HH: Scalp reduction for alopecia. *J Dermatol Surg Oncol* **5:**808–811, 1979

9. Alt TH: Scalp reduction as an adjunct to hair transplantation. Review of relevant literature and presentation of an improved technique. *J Dermatol Surg Oncol* **6:**101–1018, 1980

10. Norwood OT, Shiell R, Morrison ID: Complications of Scalp Reductions. *J Dermatol Surg Oncol* 9:828–835, 1983

11. Marzola M: An alternative hair replacement method, in: *Hair Transplant Surgery,* 2nd ed. Norwood, OT and Schiell R, eds. Springield: Charles C. Thomas, 1984:314–324

12. Brandy, DA: The bilateral occipito-parietal flap. *J Dermatol Surg Oncol* **10:**1062–1066, 1986

13. Hamilton, JB: Patterned loss of hair in man: Types and incidence. *Ann NY Acad Sci* **53:**708–728, 1951

14. Norwood OT, Shiell RC: *Hair Transplant Surgery*, 2nd Ed. Charles C. Thomas, Springfield, Illinois, 1984, pp 5–10

15. Brandy, DA: Pitfalls and Pearls of Extensive Scalp-Lifting. *Am J Cosm Surg* **4(3):**217–223, 1987

16. Brandy DA: The Brandy bitemporal flap. *Am J Cosm Surg* **3(1):**11–15, 1986

17. Brandy DA: The modified bitemporal flap for the treatment of bitemporal recessions. *Aesth Plast Surg* **13:**203–207, 1989

18. Brandy DA: The effectiveness of occipital artery ligations as a priming procedure for extensive scalp lifting. *J Dermatol Surg Oncol* **17:**946–949, 1991

19. Unger MG: Postoperative necrosis following bilateral scalp reduction. *J Dermatol Surg Oncol* **14:**541–543, 1988

20. Unger MG: Counterpoint, the risks of the bilateral scalp reduction. *J Dermatol Surg Oncol* **14:**353–354, 1988

21. Brandy DA: A technique for occipital artery ligation (A priming procedure for extensive scalp lifting). *Am J Cosm Surg* **7(4):**261–267, 1990

22. Brandy DA: Circumferential Scalp Reduction. *J Dermatol Surg Oncol* **20:**277–284, 1994

23. Unger MG: The Modified Major Scalp Reduction. *J Dermatol Surg Oncol* **14:**180–84

24. Wheeland RG, Bailin PL: Scalp Reduction Surgery with the Carbon Dioxide Laser. *J Dermatol Surg Oncol* 1984: **10:**7 565–569

25. Rose PT: Extensive Scalp Lifting Utilizing the Carbon Dioxide Laser. Presented at The Third International Symposium on Cosmetic Laser Surgery, January 15–17, 1994 Marina del Rey, California

26. Frechet P: Presented at the 10th Annual Scientific Meeting of the American Academy of Cosmetic Surgery, January 21–24, 1994, Rancho Mirage, California

27. Brandy DA: Presented at the 10th Annual Scientific Meeting of the American Academy of Cosmetic Surgery, January 21–24, 1994, Rancho Mirage, California

28. Bridenstine J: Presented at the 10th Annual Scientific Meeting of the American Academy of Cosmetic Surgery, January 21–24, 1994, Rancho Mirage, California

29. Frechet P: A new method for correction of the vertical scar observed following scalp reduction for extensive baldness. *J Dermatol Surg Oncol* 1990; **16:**640–644

30. Nordstrom REA: "Stretch-back" in scalp reductions for male pattern baldness. *Plast Reconstr Surg* **73:**422–426, 1984

31. Unger MG: Stretch-back—Results in 56 patients. Presented at The World Congress of Hair Replacement Surgery, April 13–15, 1990, Dallas, Texas

Paul O. Larson
Stephen N. Snow
Frederic E. Mohs

41 Mohs Micrographic Surgery

Mohs micrographic surgery is a method of cancer extirpation in which cancerous tissue is removed by a saucerization excision then examined microscopically to graph out areas where there is remaining tumor. Positive areas are reexcised and the process repeated until a tumor-free plane is reached. It is considered the treatment of choice for skin cancers which are recurrent, ill defined, or where tissue sparing is important. Implicit in Mohs surgery is microscopic examination of 100 percent of the excised tissue margin. This permits maximum preservation of normal tissue and maximum assurance of cure.

HISTORY

Dr. Frederic Mohs developed the concept of micrographic surgery while a medical student at the University of Wisconsin.[1] He first used the Mohs surgery technique for cancer removal in 1936. As originally developed, zinc chloride fixative paste was applied to fix tumor cells prior to layered surgical excision. Dr. Mohs coined the word *chemosurgery* to describe the technique.

The first use of the fresh tissue technique came about in 1953 when Dr. Mohs was filming the fixed tissue excision of a basal cell carcinoma of the eyelid.[2] As the hour was late and the photographer had to leave, Dr. Mohs used local anesthetic without fixative to complete the final layers of excision. As the procedure was rapid and the outcome was good, he used the fresh tissue technique on all subsequent eyelid cancers. In 1969, he presented a series of 60 eyelid cancers excised using the fresh tissue technique with a 5-year cure rate of 100 percent. After Dr. Mohs was comfortable that the cure rate from use of the fresh tissue technique was acceptable, he extended its use to cancers in other locations. The use of the fresh tissue technique expanded rapidly after the publishing of Tromovitch and Stegman's[3] series in 1974 and Dr. Mohs[4] series in 1976. This technique became known as chemosurgery fresh tissue technique. At the present time, almost all Mohs surgery is done using the fresh tissue technique. In 1986, the procedure was renamed Mohs micrographic surgery to describe the technique more clearly.[5]

FRESH TISSUE TECHNIQUE

Excision

Local Anesthesia

Mohs surgery is generally performed in an outpatient setting, with local anesthesia. The skin surrounding the area to be excised is cleansed with standard antimicrobial agents, such as povidone-iodine, chlorhexidine gluconate, or alcohol. The skin is anesthetized with a local anesthetic, generally lidocaine 1% or 2% with epinephrine, by using a 30-gauge needle. The needle should not be introduced into the skin through the tumor, as there is a possibility that tumor might be implanted beyond the margins of the excision.[6] This is especially important when dealing with squamous cell carcinoma or malignant melanomas where the risk of implantation is greatest. Although the onset of anesthesia takes only several seconds with lidocaine, the full vasoconstriction from the epinephrine requires 10 to 15 min.

The anesthetic solution may be buffered with sodium bicarbonate to reduce the pain of infiltration.[7,8] Pain can also be reduced by low pressure infiltration of the anesthetic. EMLA Cream® (lidocaine 2.5% and prilocane 2.5%) Astra Pharmaceutical Products, Inc. Wesbovough. MA., a eutectic anesthetic mixture, shows some promise for topical anesthesia but requires application 1 h prior to surgery, and additional infiltration may also be required to achieve full anesthesia.[9,10] Application of topical lidocaine after excision of Mohs layers has been recommended; however, absorption characteristics for this method are not reported.[11]

Topical anesthesia of the conjunctiva can be achieved with anesthetics such as Opthaine. Cocaine is an excellent topical anesthetic for mucosal surfaces and periosteum and also causes vasoconstriction. The major disadvantage is the necessity to keep cocaine under lock and key and the need to report all usage.

Debulking Excision

The initial layer of excision is a debulking layer. Gross tumor is removed by a saucerizing excision and a portion is sent for diagnostic examination (Figs. 41-1a–b). The margins of the debulking excision are curetted to remove remaining gross tumor.[12,13]

Saucerizing Excision

The tumor is then removed by thin-layer saucerization (Figs. 41-1c–d), the outer edge of which will be examined for microscopic evidence of cancer. A key to successful Mohs micrographic surgery is the ability to harvest a thin, smooth layer of tissue without perforations, tears, or notched edges. A smooth unbroken specimen provides the most reliable specimen for examination. Although excision of a Mohs layer may appear simple, it requires skill and practice.

Premarking the margins of the proposed excision may be helpful, especially for the novice or where bleeding may obscure the intended margins. The margins may be marked with a surgical marking pen, Mercurochrome, or the tip of the scalpel.

Three-point or four-point evenly distributed traction is applied to the skin by the surgical assistant to provide counterforce to the pressure of the scalpel. This also helps with hemostasis. The angle of approach is generally at 45°, with the blade pointed toward the center of the defect. This permits flattening of the skin edge to a flat plane without missing skin edges. A plane of excision is developed by smooth, sweeping strokes with the belly of the scalpel. These sweeping strokes

are continued until a complete saucerized layer of tissue is harvested. An ideal Mohs layer is smooth, of even thickness, and without perforations or notching at the edges.

Mohs layers can also be excised using a surgical scissors. Scissors excision is helpful where the skin is very thin (i.e., eyelid) or where even traction on the skin is difficult (i.e., neck). It is particularly useful after a tissue plane has been established and the intent is to stay in the tissue plane. Scalpel excision is more useful for crossing tissue planes.

Hemostasis

Hemostasis following Mohs surgery excisions can be accomplished with a variety of hemostatics.[14] Arterial bleeding requires suture ligature. Arteriole bleeding may require only simple spot electrofulguration. Excessive electrofulguration or electrodesiccation is destructive to the wound bed and may only serve to delay healing and increase scarring. Capillary bleeding is usually best controlled with nondestructive hemostatic agents, such as oxidized cellulose (Oxycel or Surgicel) or Gelfoam, along with pressure. Other very effective hemostatics include microfibrillar collagen (Instat or Helistat). An advantage of microfibrillar collagen is that, when removed from a Mohs surgery wound, the wound bed is very clean and ready for repair of grafting. Thrombin solution is especially appropriate for hemostasis at the time of grafting, as there is no particulate material which would separate the graft from the graft bed. Aluminum chloride is useful for hemostasis in hair-bearing areas but creates a zone of eschar, which delays wound healing.

Mapping

The excised tissue must be reduced to a size which can be processed for microscopic examination [about 1 by 1 cm to 2 by 2 cm (Fig. 41-2a)]. This requires orienting, numbering, and labeling of each specimen; microscopic examination of each specimen; and construction of a map of the positive areas.[13,15,16]

Orienting

Accurate orientation of the surgical specimens is critical in Mohs surgery. The Mohs surgeon must be able to return to the exact areas which are positive for tumor and reexcise these microscopically positive areas. Various methods have been devised to help in this mapping and orientation. The simplest method of orientation is to map in relationship to standard planar anatomic position. The 12 o'clock position of a specimen is in the cephalad position, and the 6 o'clock position is the caudal position. Anatomic landmarks are also important in orienting. Reference to scars; folds; and anatomic markers, such as the ala, helix, antihelix, lip margin, eyelid margin, puncta, moles, or even skin tension lines, can be very useful

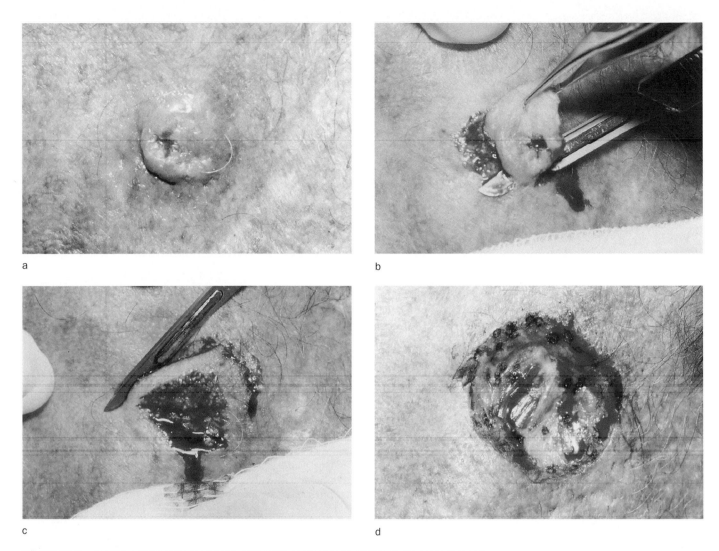

a

b

c

d

Figure 41-1 *(a)* Squamous cell carcinoma of the left neck prior to excision; *(b)* gross tumor is removed by debulking excision. Vertical sections are processed from this specimen for histologic diagnosis; *(c)* first Mohs layer is removed by thin saucerizing excision; *(d)* surgical defect after reaching a tumor-free plane using Mohs surgery.

in orienting a specimen. These markers do not move and are therefore more reliable than global orientation.

In excisions where precise orientation is critical, such as around the eye, the specimen may be oriented by creating a reference point or a landmark. Notching of the skin with the scalpel is commonly done. Placement of a staple is also very quick and will not disappear if there is some delay between layers.[17]

Tissue Marking

Marking specimens with tissue dyes allows precise orientation of excised tissue (Fig. 41-2*b*). This can be done more quickly and gives much more precise information than a suture marker used in general surgery. Tissue dyes stay on through the tissue-staining process, whereas a suture must be

removed from the specimen prior to cutting with the microtome. Thus, precise orientation may be maintained with the dyes.

The traditional dyes used for Mohs surgery include a red [20% merbromin (Mercurochrome)], blue (Prussian blue as in concentrated laundry bluing), and black (india ink).[5] These dyes must be concentrated to attain the proper color density. Commercial dye kits are also available (e.g., Davidson Marking System). The Davidson Marking System utilizes a series of up to five dyes. Pipe cleaner swabs are used for marking the standard dyes on the tissue specimens. The pipe cleaners act as a dye reservoir and also prevent drip formation on the end of the marker. Drips on the tip of the marker jump to the tissue to be marked, resulting in poorly localized dye markings. Methods of tissue orientation without dyes have also

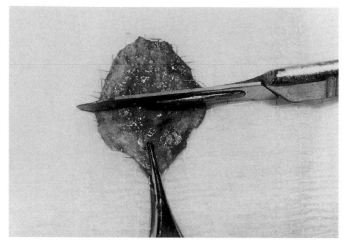

a

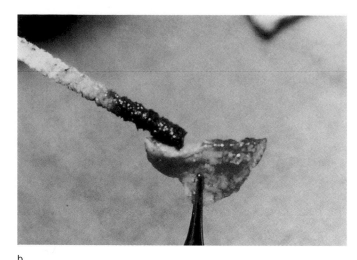

b

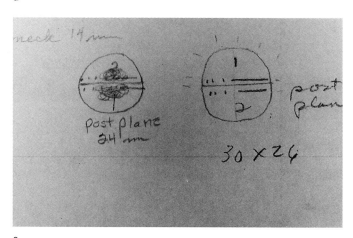

c

Figure 41-2 *(a)* Mohs surgery specimen is divided to a size which can be processed for frozen sections; *(b)* cut edges of specimen are marked with dyes which stay on the tissue through the sectioning and staining process; *(c)* tissue maps are drawn, showing the orientation and color markings of each specimen.

been proposed.[18] This may be a faster method but carries a greater potential for misorientation, especially for inexperienced technicians.

Mapmaking

The function of the map in Mohs surgery excisions is to record the tissue size, position, orientation, and color coding of the specimen so that the Mohs surgeon can return to a given spot and reexcise areas of residual cancer if necessary (Fig. 41-2c).

Standard mapping requires only paper and a pencil. The specimen is drawn as closely as possible to actual size, with orienting anatomic features drawn into place. Reference marks on the map must match the reference marks on the patient. The color codes on the map must match the colors on the tissue. The standard key for Mohs surgery specimens is shown in Fig. 41-3a.

Standard mapping practices are simple and straightforward. A routine marking system saves time and reduces error. The standard map patterns shown in Fig. 41-3b represent a large percentage of the simple excisions. Maps are generally marked with a vertical or horizontal axis. If the natural axis of

the lesion is at an angle, the axes may be rotated to fit the defect.

Other aides have been used for mapping Mohs specimens. Transparent overlays have been proposed for complicated lesions.[3] Polaroid photos can also be very helpful for general orientation.[19]

Laboratory Processing

Laboratory Setup

The Mohs laboratory is an integral part of the Mohs surgery procedure.[13,20] In order to maintain tight specimen control, it is standard procedure to maintain the laboratory in conjunction with the Mohs surgery clinic. This also facilitates rapid turnaround of tissue as large numbers of specimens may be processed daily. Specimens must be processed with the critical margin (the outermost margin of the excised specimen) mounted as a flat plane (Figs. 41-4–5a). The tissue block is frozen, then the critical margin is shaved off by microtome (Fig. 41-5b). The ribbon of tissue is mounted on a slide, stained, and coverslipped (Fig. 41-5c). Although most sec-

key to maps

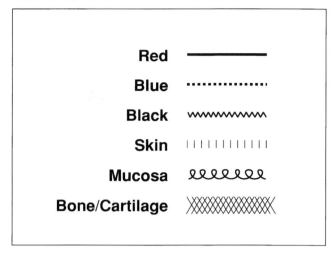

a

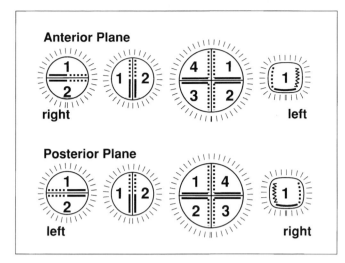

b

Figure 41-3 *(a)* Standard color and tissue keys used in Mohs micrographic surgery (from Mohs[5]); *(b)* routine mapping system used in Mohs micrographic surgery is sufficient for a large percentage of smaller excisions. Similar routines are used for larger lesions.

tions are processed by frozen sectioning, paraffin sections are occasionally requested to provide slides with the least distortion.[21] Tissue staining is usually done with routine hema-

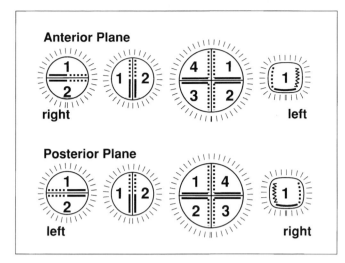

Figure 41-4 The *critical margin* is a useful term describing the outermost or most peripheral margin of the Mohs layer which is to be examined microscopically. Solid arrows point to the critical margin.

toxylin and eosin stains. Toluidine blue has a number of strong devotees, especially because of the rapid processing time. Special stains are being increasingly used for delineation of certain cancers such as dermatofibrosarcoma protuberans (DFSP) or perineural squamous cell carcinoma.[22]

Microscopic Examination

Microscopic examination of Mohs surgical specimens is done by the Mohs surgeon. The advantage of the Mohs surgeon acting as the pathologist is the very tight control of specimens attained by the Mohs surgeon. If skin edges or portions of a tissue block are missing on the prepared slide, the Mohs surgeon can easily have the tissue block recut or, if necessary, reexcise tissue from the missing area from the patient. An outside laboratory can process tissue that is received but cannot maintain the tight control over the orientation.

The Mohs surgeon examines each of the stained, horizontally prepared specimens or *flats*. Each microscopic section is examined in a routine gridlike pattern. Areas of residual cancer are marked with red pencil in the corresponding section of the surgical map. A full picture of any remaining areas positive for cancer is seen after examination and marking of each individual specimen. This map is then used to locate and excise any positive areas. The entire process is repeated until the entire peripheral and deep margins are at a tumor-free plane.

A great deal of attention has been focused on the ability of a Mohs surgeon to interpret Mohs surgery specimens in comparison to the pathologist. Grabski et al.[23] showed excellent correlation between Mohs surgeons and pathologists, with inconsistencies usually being resolved in favor of the Mohs surgeon. Rapini[24] has suggested that comprehensive exami-

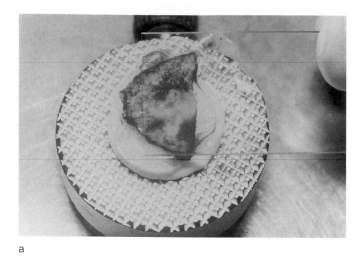

a

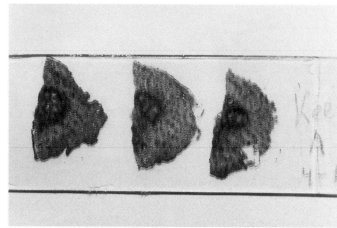

c

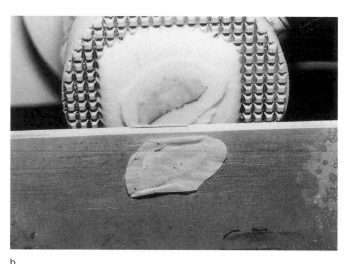

b

Figure 41-5 *(a)* The Mohs tissue layer is mounted top side down onto the cryostat chuck, with the flattened critical margin facing up; *(b)* a thin ribbon of tissue is removed from the critical margin of the tissue, transferred to a glass slide, and stained for tissue examination; *(c)* the microscope slide has been stained with hematoxylin and eosin for microscopic examination. Residual cancer can be seen grossly in the center of the tissue specimen.

nation of tumor margins by a dermatopathologist can be just as reliable in ensuring a tumor-free plane as the Mohs surgery technique. It may be possible for a compulsive dematopathologist to examine tissue margins adequately; however, it is unlikely that this can be accomplished as timely, efficiently, or cost effectively as routine Mohs micrographic surgery.

Wound Management

Mohs micrographic surgery is a method of tumor extirpation. Strictly speaking, the Mohs surgery technique implies nothing with regard to closure. In practice, a major part of Mohs surgery deals with wound management. Mohs surgery with the fixed tissue technique necessitated healing by secondary intention or delayed closure after separation of the final eschar. Since 1974, practically all Mohs surgery has been done with the fresh tissue technique. As a result, early primary closure became an important addition to the management of Mohs surgery defects.

Primary Closure

Primary closure for Mohs surgery defects has increased tremendously since the advent of the fresh tissue technique. The frequency of primary closures ranges widely from practice to practice. Informal questioning suggests a closure rate as low as 10 percent to as high as 90 percent. This great diversity in practice may be a result of differences in size and location of the wounds, referral practice, and patient expectations in different parts of the country. The advantage of early primary closure is that wounds are closed in a predictable fashion with rapid healing and simple wound care. Primary closures, however, require an additional procedure, potentially conceal outlying foci of residual tumor, and add to expense of the procedure.

Simple closures are easy to conceive and result in few complications. Skin edges in low-risk defects can be undermined sparingly to free up the skin edges. Dog-ears generally need to be removed to prevent puckering at the wound edges. Use of subcutaneous sutures depends on the degree of tension. Closures where cosmesis is important may be done with running subcuticular polypropylene or fine nylon. Defects where a quick functional closure is needed may be closed with staples. High-risk cancers where it is necessary to close to maintain function are best managed with simple closures without undermining.

Skin flaps may be necessary to close Mohs surgery defects when skin cannot be mobilized to close simply. Flaps have the advantage of generally having matching skin texture and color, as they are taken from adjacent skin. Flaps should be avoided, however, in defects resulting from multiply recurrent cancers or highly aggressive cancers where recurrence of a cancer may be hidden by the flap. Undermining the flap creates new tissue planes which allow rapid spread of any residual cancer.

Delayed Primary Closure

Delayed primary closure (tertiary or third intention healing) is a closure which is not done on the day the wound is created.[25] Simple closures, flaps, or grafts may all be done in a delayed primary fashion.

Delayed primary closure can be a very powerful option. Delayed closure permits the wound to granulate partially. This is particularly important when grafting over deep defects, as the granulation will reduce the depth of the wound. In patients who have inadvertently been on aspirin, a delay in closure allows return to normal platelet activity prior to closing. Delay also allows contaminated wounds which have been worked on for several days to clean up before closure. In addition, delay allows for orderly scheduling of the closure. It is best not to close immediately if the closure is rushed or ill conceived. Finally, a delay in closure allows for initial testing of healing by second intention—wounds with marginal indications for closure may be allowed to heal by second intention after a delayed inspection. Patients who require closure after a delay are generally much happier with the final closure, as they have had to see the defect for several days prior to closure.

Second Intention

Second intention healing of a wound is healing by spontaneous granulation and re-epithelialization without surgical intervention. Healing by second intention can be a very powerful tool for Mohs surgery defects.[26–29] The Mohs surgery wound is cleaned, treated with antibacterial agents, and sterile dressings are applied until healing is completed (Figs. 41-6a–d). Many defects can heal very well by second intention, with little scarring, no surgical risk, and low cost. Unfortunately, second intention healing can also result in unpredictable scarring, webbing, stricture, or distortion.

The ideal areas for second intention healing have been listed by Dr. Zitelli.[26] These are generally concave surfaces. Wounds which result from excision of multiply recurrent can-

cers may be treated most safely by allowing second intention healing. Second intention healing over dermis, muscle, and fat requires simple and meticulous cleaning, antisepsis, and coverage of the wound. A moist environment stimulates granulation tissue.

If perichondrium and periosteum are not destroyed, special care is taken to prevent desiccation of these tissues. If the perichondrium or periosteum is destroyed, granulation must be stimulated to cover these areas.[13,30] Cartilage can be perforated or excised to permit granulation from the perichondrium on the reverse side of the cartilage. Bone can be chiseled or burred until small bleeding points are seen.[30] Granulations will arise from these bleeding points and will eventually cover the entire defect. Small defects (less than 1 cm^2) may granulate without special intervention. Problem areas for second intention healing are those areas around free skin margins, such as the eyelids and lips and the nostril and ear canal. Closure in these areas may be necessary to prevent functional problems or distortion.

Partial Closure

Partial closure is closure of a portion of a wound, with the remainder left to heal by second intention.[31] A partial closure is used when the wound cannot be completely closed without excessively complicating the closure. Partial closures can be used to prevent or reduce distortion around movable areas such as the lips or eyelids.[32] With a partial closure, tissue is pushed in the direction of the closure axis, helping to prevent notching or ectropion. As partial closures provide open drainage, these wounds rarely develop wound infection or hematomas. There is, however, more potential for scarring than with complete closure.

Revision

Mohs surgery defects, like any other surgical defects, may need to be revised. Simple revision, such as scar abrasion, may be done as soon as 4 to 8 weeks after surgery.[33] Since scars mature and soften with time, complicated revisions should usually be delayed for about 6 to 12 months. The timing of each revision must be judged individually. It is best to inform the patient of the possibility of revision prior to surgery so that revision is not construed as something being done to correct a mistake. Complicated revisions may require the aid of a plastic surgeon, oculoplastic surgeon, or otolaryngologist.

Multidisciplinary Approach

At times, the Mohs surgeon must deal with problems which are best handled by a multidisciplinary approach, utilizing the expertise of a plastic surgeon, oculoplastic surgeon, otolaryngologist, orthopedist, neurosurgeon, oncologist or radiotherapist, and the patient's referring physician.[34,35] Clear channels

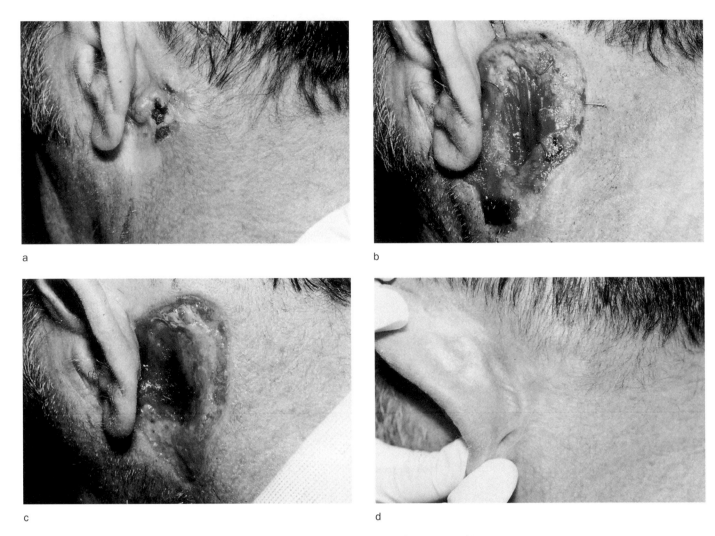

Figure 41-6 *(a)* Basal cell carcinoma of left postauricular region prior to Mohs surgery; *(b)* surgical defect after final layer of Mohs surgery. Note exposed sternocleidomastoid muscle fibers as center of defect. Staples used for orienting purposes were removed after surgery was completed; *(c)* granulating wound 9 days after surgery; *(d)* fully healed defect 6 months after surgery at the time of a routine examination.

of communication and understanding are important in developing these working relationships. Unfortunately, many specialists do not really know what Mohs surgery is. Surgeons utilizing the operating rooms may be unable to wait for specimens while the patient is under general anesthesia. They may also have difficulty in dealing with patients with large defects who end up on their doorstep with no advance warning. Advance planning and coordination should be done with ancillary services as much as possible. The multidisciplinary approach can be a valuable tool in the overall management of difficult skin cancers.

Results

The results of treating skin cancers with Mohs surgery have been excellent, as might be presumed with a method where 100 percent of the margin is examined. This is especially true for basal cell carcinomas where there is contiguous spread of tumor. The results are not as good when a tumor spreads in a noncontiguous fashion as in melanoma, Merkel's cell carcinoma, or in multiply recurrent lesions. The value of Mohs surgery can be appreciated by examining the treatment results for different cancers.

Basal Cell Carcinoma

Basal cell carcinoma is by far the most common cancer treated with Mohs surgery. Collective data compiled by Rowe et al.[36] indicate a cure rate of 99 percent in all primary basal cell carcinomas. The cure rate for recurrent basal cell carcinoma was 94.4 percent (Table 41-1).[37]

Squamous Cell Carcinoma

Squamous cell carcinoma may spread by contiguous spread or by metastasis. Dr. Mohs' overall cure rate for the excision

TABLE 41-1

Cure Rates (5 Year) of Basal Cell Cancers Treated with Mohs Micrographic Surgery*

	Excision	EDC†	XRT‡	Cryo§	Mohs
Primary	89.9%	92.3%	91.3%	92.5%	99.0%
Recurrent	82.6%	60.0%	90.2%	NA	94.4%

* Compiled data adapted and reprinted by permission of the publisher from long-term recurrence rates in previously untreated (primary) basal cell carcinoma: Implications for patient follow-up, Rowe et al, *J Dermatol Surg Oncol* 15:315–328 and from Mohs surgery is the treatment of choice for recurrent (previously treated) basal cell carcinoma, Rowe et al, *J Dermatol Surg Oncol* 15:424–431. Copyright 1989 by Elsevier Science Publishing Co., Inc.
† EDC = Electrodesiccation and Curettage.
‡ XRT = X-ray Therapy.
§ Cryo = Cryosurgery.

of squamous cell carcinomas of the head and neck in 3949 determinate patients was 95 percent (unpublished data). The 5-year cure rate was 97.5 percent in 3324 determinate cases with no previous treatment and 81.9 percent of 625 determinate cases with previous treatment.

Malignant Melanoma

Malignant melanoma has been treated with Mohs surgery by using both the fixed and fresh tissue techniques. Dr. Mohs reported using the fixed tissue technique in 200 patients with an overall 5-year cure rate of 65.2 percent (Table 41-2). Zitelli et al.[38] reported 26 determinate cases of malignant melanoma treated with the fresh tissue technique with a 5-year survival of 96.2 percent (Table 41-3). Comparison of this data is difficult as a large percentage of Dr. Mohs' patients had thick melanomas, whereas a large percentage of Zitelli's patients had thin melanomas.

Other Cancers

Mohs surgery has been used for a variety of other cancers, including DFSP, Bowen's disease, verrucous carcinoma, atypi-

TABLE 41-2

Cure Rates (5 Year) of 155 Determinate Cases of Stage I Malignant Melanoma Treated with Mohs Surgery Fixed Tissue Technique*

	Determinate	Success	%
Clark II	36	32	89
Clark III	34	30	88
Clark IV	27	17	63
Clark V	58	22	38
Total	155	101	65.2

* From Zitelli et al.[38]

TABLE 41-3

Survival Rates (5 Year) of 26 Determinate Cases of Stage I Malignant Melanoma Treated with Mohs Surgery Fresh Tissue Technique*

	Determinate	Survival	%
In situ	6	6	100
< 0.85 mm	10	10	100
0.86–1.69 mm	4	3	75
1.70–3.64 mm	4	4	100
> 3.87 mm	2	2	100
Total	26	25	96.2

* From Zitelli et al.[38]

cal fibroxanthoma, malignant fibrous histiocytoma, extramammary Paget's disease, lentigo maligna, Merkel's cell carcinoma, sebaceous carcinoma, leiomyosarcoma, hemangiosarcoma, sweat gland carcinoma, keratoacanthoma, and carcinoma of the larynx and parotid glands.[13,39,40] Other tumors will no doubt be added to this list.

Primary versus Recurrent

Cure rates for primary cancers treated with Mohs surgery are higher than those for recurrent cancers. Previously treated cancers may have discontinuous foci, as demonstrated by Wagner and Cottel.[41] Wagner and Cottel showed that of eight recurrent cancers treated initially with electrodesiccation and curettage, 50 percent had multiple foci of recurrent tumor. Excision of clinically apparent recurrent cancers with Mohs surgery may miss discontinuous, inapparent foci. The cure rates for treatment of recurrent cancers reflect the risk of multiple foci. The overall 5-year cure rate after treating a recurrent basal cell carcinoma is 94.4 percent versus 99 percent for a primary basal cell carcinoma according to data compiled by Rowe et al.[37]

Location

In most cases, the location of a skin cancer has little effect on the cure rate when Mohs surgery is used. There are several important exceptions. Dr. Mohs has compiled extensive data on cure rates at various treatment sites.[13] The lowest cure rates were in the ear canal (59.1 percent), nasal septum (84.9 percent), and outer canthus (91 percent). Dr. Robins[42] reported his lowest cure rate at the inner canthus. Although several published articles question the theory of tumor extension along embryonic clefts, these anatomic areas are clearly at high risk for recurrence.[43]

Indications

Commonly stated indications for Mohs surgery are listed in Table 41-4. Although small basal and squamous cell carcino-

TABLE 41-4

Primary Indications for Mohs Surgery*

1. Recurrent basal or squamous cell cancers
2. Ill-defined cancers (i.e., morpheaform, previously treated, or partially treated cancers; DFSP)
3. Embryonic fusion planes of the face (i.e., alar groove, ear canal, outer and inner canthi)
4. Maximum preservation of tissue (i.e., eyelids, nose, ear, genitalia)
5. Aggressive growth pattern cancers (i.e., basosquamous cell carcinoma, perineural or perivascular growth)
6. Large or deeply penetrating tumors

* From Mohs,[13] Snow,[16] and Lang and Osguthorpe.[39]

mas are often not on the indication list for Mohs surgery, it seems to make little sense to exclude the most effective and reliable method for treating these cancers.[13] The only real argument against Mohs surgery for small, uncomplicated cancers is the cost of Mohs surgery. This may be the fault of the reimbursement system for small, uncomplicated Mohs excisions rather than the Mohs procedure itself.

Advantages

Mohs micrographic surgery provides several major advantages (Table 41-5) for treatment of most skin cancers.[13] The high cure rates for skin cancers that spread by contiguous extension has been previously mentioned. Bumsted and Ceilley[44] studied the degree of tissue sparing in Mohs surgery. They found that conventional surgery would have resulted in a defect larger than the actual Mohs defect. The excess tissue excised by conventional surgery averaged 180 percent larger than the actual defect in primary lesions and 347 percent larger in recurrent lesions.

One of the clear advantages of Mohs surgery is the rapid processing time. Standard paraffin processing of tissue may

TABLE 41-5

Advantages of Mohs Surgery

1. High cure rate
2. Maximum preservation of tissue
3. Specimen processing/reading more rapid than standard processing
4. Low operative risk (less risk of cardiac or pulmonary complications with local anesthesia)
5. Extension of operability to patients considered inoperable by other methods
6. Outpatient procedure
7. Cost effective when compared to inpatient surgery

* From Mohs[13] and Lang and Osguthorpe.[39]

take 1 to 10 days for results to return. Mohs surgery can usually be completed within several hours to 1 day. In addition, Mohs surgery is generally done on an outpatient basis. This markedly reduces the cost of surgical excisions. It also allows for more rapid turnaround of specimens and ease in scheduling excision and closure.

Disadvantages

Although Mohs surgery is an excellent form of treatment for skin cancers, there are a few disadvantages, as with any other form of treatment.[45] Mohs surgery does not have a perfect record in treatment of cancers. The recurrence rate when Mohs surgery is used is very low for contiguously spreading tumors, but it may miss noncontiguous areas as may other forms of treatment.[41] The patient may have to undergo several sets of excisions before the surgeon reaches a tumor-free plane. This requires the patient to wait for the tissue examination, multiple injections, and if necessary, a closure procedure. Although the results are ready in 1 to 2 h in most cases, large lesions with many subsections may take 3 or 4 h to prepare. This makes the multidisciplinary approach to treating large or complicated cancers in the operating room very cumbersome.

FIXED TISSUE TECHNIQUE

The fixed tissue technique was the method of Mohs surgery used almost exclusively from its inception in 1936 until the 1970s when the fresh tissue technique became established. The fixed tissue technique is still used for treatment of melanoma and penile cancers, and occasionally for deeply invasive or vascular tumors and gangrene, although many Mohs surgeons are no longer familiar with its use.[13,38,46–48]

Zinc chloride paste is applied to the cancer to fix the cancer cells in place, so the tumor can be removed without dislodging the cells during surgery. The fixative paste is applied in a thin layer, then covered with an airtight dressing, and left in place for 12 to 24 h. Pain medication is generally prescribed. The patient returns to the clinic the following day, the dressing and fixative are removed, and the layer of fixed tissue is removed by a saucerizing excision. As the fixed tissue is devitalized, the excision is not painful, and the surgical field is bloodless. The specimens are oriented, marked, mapped, processed, and examined in the typical Mohs fashion. If there are outlying areas positive for cancer, the zinc chloride paste is reapplied and the whole procedure repeated until a tumor-free margin is achieved. The excision site is generally left to heal by second intention. A final zone of fixed eschar separates sharply from the underlying viable tissue and sloughs off in 5 to 14 days, leaving a pink, highly vascularized granulating bed. The wound then heals by routine granulation. The resulting scar is generally flush with the surrounding skin, uniform, supple, and resilient.

The results of treating skin cancers with the fixed tissue technique are well established. Dr. Mohs' overall cure rate for treating 10,531 determinate basal cell carcinomas by using the fixed tissue technique was 98.9 percent and for treating 2844 determinate squamous cell carcinomas was 93.7 percent.

There are several advantages to using the fixed tissue techniques of Mohs surgery. As with the fresh tissue technique, the fixed tissue technique allows examination of 100 percent of the surgical margin. Also, the fixed tissue technique provides a completely bloodless surgical field, enabling treatment of areas such as the penis.[46,47] Excision in a bloodless field may also allow safer treatment of patients who are HIV positive.[49] In addition, preoperative fixation may prevent intraoperative metastasis of highly implantable cancers such as malignant melanoma.[13] Finally, fixed tissue can also be used to treat bone, and scar tissue resulting from fixed tissue excision is surprisingly soft and supple.

There are disadvantages to treating skin cancer with the fixed tissue technique. Fixed tissue technique is more time consuming. The fixative paste generally must be left in place for 12 to 24 h before harvesting each layer. Excising several layers may take several days. In addition, there is pain and swelling associated with chemical fixation. This is usually of moderate degree and relieved with acetaminophen and/or codeine. Also, the quality of tissue sections can be variable. Although many fixed tissue specimens provide histology sections with excellent quality, other specimens can be friable, resulting in sections of poor quality. Finally, the fixed tissue technique is not well understood by patients or other physicians. Treatment with the fixed tissue technique requires a great deal of patient education. Referring physicians generally do not know how to take care of fixed tissue excisions.

In summary, the fixed technique has been largely replaced by the fresh tissue method of excision. It still has application in malignant melanoma, large or vascular tumors, and in penile cancers.

MOHS SURGERY FOR SPECIAL FACIAL SITES

Although a subsection on the practical aspects of Mohs surgery is not ordinarily included within a chapter on its general principles, this section highlights some time-tested techniques that improve surgical procedures and maximize tissue conservation for tumors in difficult facial sites. This section focuses on the responsibilities of the Mohs or dermatologic surgical assistant (SA) to help stabilize the operative site, ensuring the excision of high-quality flat tissue layers. Having a well-orchestrated, semiautonomous procedure that integrates excision with laboratory tissue processing is important to maximize safety and productivity. Over the years, the authors have found these techniques to be most satisfactory because they are simple, reliable, and inexpensive.

Lower Eyelid Tumors

Midline lesions that involve the lid margin are usually excised with the use of a chalazion clamp.[50] This forceps acts as a clamp to provide (1) a bloodless operative field, (2) a platform for cutting layers, and (3) a physical barrier to protect the eyeball. Eyelid surgery is preferably performed with two assistants: an SA to hold the lid-chalazion unit and another SA to pass cotton applicators to the surgeon, one by one, for hemostasis (Figs. 41-7 and 41-8).

Proper use of the forceps entails a coordinated effort between the Mohs surgeon who clamps the tumor and the SA

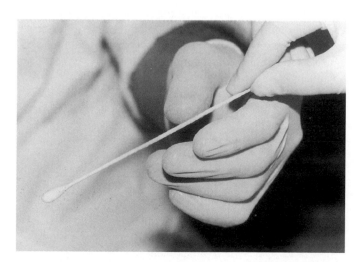

Figure 41-7 Hand-in-hand transfer of no. 6 cotton-tipped applicator to surgeon's fingertips for rapid hemostasis. This technique allows the surgeon to maintain direct sight of the operative field while performing surgery under magnification.

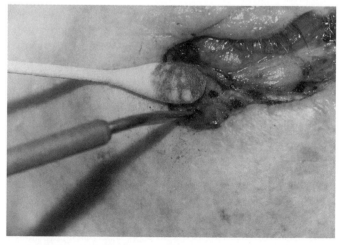

Figure 41-8 Cotton applicator technique for precise electrocautery. The applicator is rolled over bleeders, closely followed by electrofulguration tip. Precise hemostasis minimizes tissue necrosis and electroartifacts observed in Mohs microscopic sections.

who holds the clamp away from the eyeball during surgery. The authors' procedure for eyelid lesions consists of the following steps:

1. Two to three gtt of 0.5% tetracaine hydrochloride local anesthetic are administered onto the conjunctiva, followed by injection of buffered lidocaine with epinephrine perilesionally.
2. The patient is then asked to gaze up and away, while the lower lid is retracted inferiorly, exposing the fornix. The chalazion is inserted over the palpebral margin, with the open ring completely surrounding the tumor.
3. The forceps is pinched while the round nut is tightened until tissue is blanched.
4. The upper lid is closed to protect the cornea.
5. The clamp is then passed to the assistant, handle first.
6. To remove the chalazion, the lower lid is retracted while the round nut is unscrewed so that the lid does not snap back against the cornea when tension is released (Figs. 41-9a–d).

Before the clamp is grasped with the fingers, the SA's hand position is stabilized by resting the hypothenar eminence of the hand on the patient's forehead. Just enough pressure is placed on the forehead for stabilization so that if the patient inadvertently moves, the clamp and patient move in tandem. For lower lid surgery, the forceps is held about 1 cm away from the brow ridge instead of resting on it.

After the chalazion is removed, the surgical site is cleansed with 5% boric acid to wash away microcinders of coagulated debris that might irritate the cornea. Next, a very thin lacelike layer of Oxycel cotton cellulose (Deseret, Sandy, Utah) is delicately spread evenly over the operative site followed by copious amount of ophthalmic antibiotic ointment. The patient is asked to close the upper lid, and light pressure is applied by the patient over two to three layers of a folded Telfa (Kendall Co., Boston, Massachusetts) nonstick pad which has been moistened with boric acid. About 5 min later, the wound is checked for proper hemostasis. If hemostasis is achieved, the patient may be discharged with only a small Band-Aid that has been cut to the curvature of the lid for looks and to adsorb normal light tearing and discharge (Figs. 41-9e–f). The wound is cleansed daily with tap water or eye irrigating solution, but generally the patient's own tears provide sufficient cleansing of the wound site.

When the chalazion clamp is clamped, it distorts the eyelid by ballooning the tissue within the open ring while compressing the eyelid tissue under the ring, making it more likely to cut deeply into the eyelid at the lateral and inferior margins. The Mohs layer should be adjusted accordingly to preserve as much of the tarsal plate as possible. Preservation of the tarsal plate permits simpler repairs by partial closure or grafting rather than complicated flaps. During surgery, the screw may be tightened to improve hemostasis or loosened periodically to permit bleeding points to be identified and coagulated. As the screw is loosened, the tension on the hand

that is holding the clamp is gently relaxed so that the eyelid tissue does not slip out of the clamp before the desired level of hemostasis is achieved.

For tumors of the eyelids, the lid that is not operated upon serves as a shield to cover the eyeball during surgery. To protect the eye, either lid may be pulled obliquely in a lateral or medial direction while the patient looks away from the operative site. Voluntary closure of the eye causes the eyeball to rotate superiorly, further protecting the cornea. It is helpful to prewarn the patient to expect blood in the eye which will cause some temporary minor irritation and blurring of vision. If Gelfoam (Upjohn, Kalamazoo, Michigan) is used for hemostasis, it should be softened with boric acid solution or sterile normal saline before application to prevent corneal abrasion by its rough dry surface. Although Oxycel is fibrous when moistened, the diameter of individual microfibers is about 10 μm and does not appear to irritate the cornea.

The chalazion clamp has been used to facilitate excision of ear, lip, and tongue lesions. The main advantage is hemostasis. Using the chalazion in these areas also gives the SA practice and experience in handling this instrument so that when the chalazion is needed in more delicate eye surgery the SA is familiar with its use.[51] Eyelid surgery and postoperative wound care may be enhanced with the use of special instrumentation, corneal shields, lacrimal canaliculus stents, and ophthalmologic moisture chambers, whose discussion is beyond the scope of this section.[52–54]

Ear Tumors

Mohs surgery for ear tumors presents several problems: (1) surgical excision problems when the tumors involve the conchal bowl or external auditory canal, (2) laboratory processing of irregularly contoured ear cartilage, and (3) special open wound management considerations because of exposed cartilage. Local anesthetic is usually introduced on both sides of the ear because of the likelihood of entering the anterior or posterior ear surface when the cartilage is fenestrated during excision. Likewise, carefully coordinated dissection is necessary when removing cartilage to avoid injury to the SA's fingers.

Surgical excision of ear tumors is improved when the SA flattens the natural ear contours during surgery. This is accomplished by placing the second and third fingers behind the ear, while the thumb bends the ear backward against the fingers. Because of the convexity of the conchal area and the conic shape of the canal, the angled Beaver blade (Figs. 41-10a–b) permits the Mohs surgeon to remove a complete layer of tissue without significant nicks or notches. The dermal-cartilage layer, however, often has a bowl configuration which is difficult to process (Fig. 41-10c).

There are two general methods to flatten cartilage for laboratory processing. Excess cartilage may be trimmed with the scalpel, or the cartilage may be scored or divided on its top surface to improve flattening of the tissue by the technician (Fig. 41-10d). Alternatively, the technician may prefer to flat-

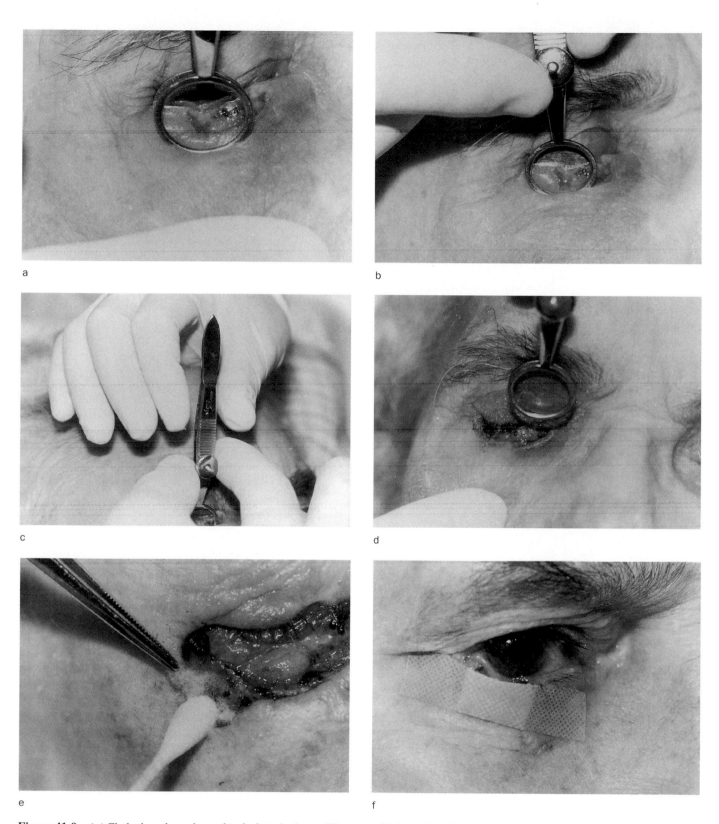

Figure 41-9 *(a)* Chalazion clamp is used to isolate the lower lid tumor; *(b)* tightening of screw by surgeon to cause tissue blanching. Note closure of upper eyelid for protection of eyeball; *(c)* correct method of passing chalazion clamp to assistant; *(d)* when the chalazion is removed, the lower lid is retracted to prevent lid whiplash; *(e)* application of a lacelike layer of Oxycel cotton, using forceps and applicator; *(f)* appearance of wound after Band-Aid is trimmed to cover lower lid defect.

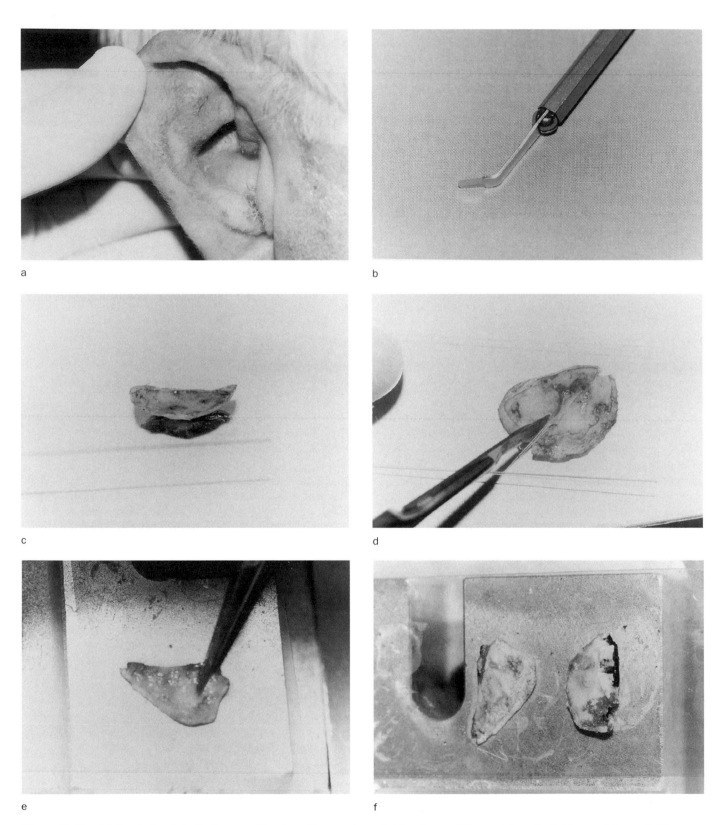

Figure 41-10 *(a)* Surgical assistant's finger and hand position evert conchal bowl, permitting excision of a flat layer of tissue; *(b)* Beaver blade no. 69B with hexagonal handle (Rudolph Beaver, Belmont, Massachusetts) used for acute angle surgery such as the ear canal and inner canthus; *(c)* appearance of bowl-shaped layer of skin and cartilage taken from the helix of the ear; *(d)* scoring cartilage at apex of convexity to permit specimen flattening; *(e)* room temperature dermal-cartilage unit immediately adheres to frozen x-ray film in cryostat when tissue is touched against it; *(f)* top view of completely flattened ear tissue against x-ray film (left); appearance of flattened undersurface of specimen after it is flipped over to show its bottom (right); *(g)* Merocel (Merocel Corp., Mystic, Connecticut) tampon in canal for hemostasis and hearing. The tampon is saturated with local anesthetic; *(h)* open ring curette to shave off protruding ear cartilage.

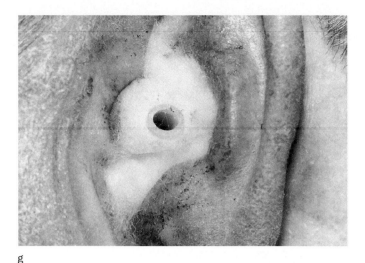

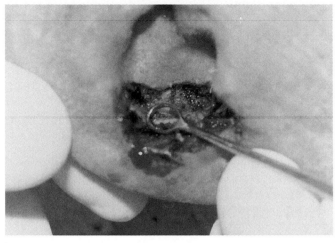

g

h

Figure 41-10   *(countinued)*

ten the tissue against a layer of Optimum Cutting Temperature (OCT) embedding compound (Miles Diagnostic Division, Elkhart, Indiana). The skin edge is cold fixed first, then the cartilage is flattened against a layer of OCT (Figs. 41-10*e–f*). In the ear canal, bleeding may be controlled with a Merocel tampon (Fig. 41-10*g*) that provides mild pressure and allows hearing.

Wound management of ear defects concentrates on preserving viable cartilage and removing excessively exposed cartilage before it becomes devitalized (Fig. 41-10*h*). Ear skin is thin overlying the antihelix and relatively thick over the concha, helix, and posterior surface of the ear. If cartilage is removed along with the Mohs layer, and wound management is expected to be by second intention healing, it is sometimes better immediately to trim back the cartilage about 1 mm from adjacent skin edge during the same operation to save time and avoid scheduling another operative session.

When second intention healing is the desired method of wound management, excess exposed cartilage may become devitalized about 1 week postoperatively. It is characterized by being soft and yellow. In order to stimulate wound healing and avoid chondritis, this cartilage must be cut back until firm white cartilage is reached, usually undercutting the overriding skin edge.[55]

Fresh cartilage is kept moist with antibiotic ointment, while Oxycel cotton cellulose is used only at the skin margins where bleeding occurs. Hemostatic agents placed over naked cartilage desiccate it and are unnecessary since cartilage does not bleed. Blood vessel competence determines the rate of wound healing over cartilage. It takes about 1 week for granulations to cover about 1 mm and 3 mm of exposed cartilage on the anterior and posterior ear surfaces, respectively. Split grafts can survive over approximately 1 cm of naked cartilage.

Lower Lip Tumors

Lip tumors present the problem of tissue stability during the cutting of a thin Mohs layer. The simplest method of tissue

stabilization and hemostasis is to pinch the lip between the fingers. To prevent slipping of the tissue, the lip is grasped with cotton gauze, with a cotton "flap" that flips up to absorb blood. If the labial arteries are transected, bleeding is usually controlled with electrocautery. Ligatures are generally not necessary.

Tumors of the Alar Groove and Nasolabial Groove

Mohs surgery on the alar groove and nasolabial groove is difficult because the tissue concavity prevents excision of a flat layer of tissue. Two steps that correct this situation are: (1) exposure of the concave groove by spreading the nasal tip and nasolabial fold between the fingers and (2) pressing the tip of a cotton applicator against the nostril to raise the alar groove depression thereby flattening the skin for surgical excision (Fig. 41-11). In doing so, the nostril skin becomes thinner and

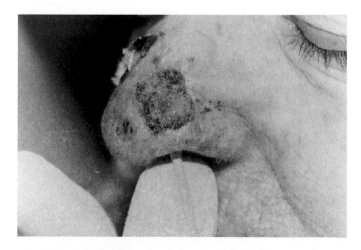

Figure 41-11   Applicator to elevate alar groove depression during Mohs layers. Note position of index finger supporting cotton tip to prevent the stick from breaking.

Mohs layers are proportionately thicker. Nasal perforations may be caused by aggressive electrocautery.

The aforementioned techniques typify the authors' style of Mohs surgery for the excision of small- to medium-size tumors in selected sites. These methods should serve as a brief guide for tumor excision. In any dermatologic surgery unit, one may want to experiment with these and other new ideas while continuously improving those that are proven. This attitude spurs productivity and often leads to greater patient satisfaction and to results greater than expected.

FACILITIES, INSTRUMENTS, AND THE HISTOPATHOLOGY LABORATORY

Facilities

The Mohs surgery facility is an unusual blend of ambulatory surgery facility and histopathology laboratory. The complexity of equipment needed parallels the level of surgical complexity being done in the facility. One of the unique features of a Mohs surgery facility is that it must deal with all areas of the superficial anatomy. The tables and chairs should be very versatile to allow proper positioning of the patient from head to toe. Lighting must be freely movable to allow proper illumination of all areas. This can be done with overhead lighting on tracks or headlamps with rechargeable battery packs.

Instruments

The instruments used for Mohs surgery are relatively simple. The skills used to practice Mohs surgery are more complex. The proper choice of instrument, however, is important to smooth technique.

The most basic Mohs surgery instruments include a standard scalpel handle, a Bard-Parker no. 15 blade, and a forceps of the surgeon's choice. Some Mohs surgeons like the Siegel handle, which is rounded, weighted, and rotated easily in the hand. Occasionally, it is necessary to use an angled scalpel blade, such as the angled Beaver blade. An excellent choice of forceps is a fine-toothed Adson with a suture platform. Delicate tissue (i.e., periocular tissue) is best handled with fine instruments such as a Westcott tenotomy scissors and a Bishop-Harmon or Roerster iris forceps, along with a delicate Castroviejo spring-loaded needle-holder. A fine-tissue scissors, such as a strabismus or small Mayo scissors, a bandage scissors for suture material, and needle-holder are essential. Other commonly used instruments include the chalazion clamp, periosteal elevator, a variety of curettes, bone rongeur, nail nipper, splinter forceps, Spencer scissors for suture removal, small osteotome, and small mallet. Other specialized instruments will no doubt be added to this list of instruments; however, most excisions can be managed with these instruments.

Histopathology Laboratory

The heart of the Mohs surgery clinic is the histopathology laboratory. The cryostats necessary for preparation of Mohs surgery specimens are expensive and require skill to operate properly. There are a variety of cryostats available, with each having advantages and disadvantages.[56,57] Equipment for manual or automatic tissue staining is required. In addition, microscopes for tissue examination and slide filing systems are necessary, along with routine laboratory equipment. The Mohs surgery laboratory must meet federal Occupational Safety and Health Administration (OSHA) standards and are subject to the Clinical Laboratory Improvement Act (CLIA) regulations.

FUTURE OF MOHS MICROGRAPHIC SURGERY

The underlying principle of Mohs micrographic surgery cannot be refuted—examination of 100 percent of the excised margin ensures cancer removal, with maximum preservation of normal tissue. The future direction of Mohs surgery must inevitably extend this principle into other fields of tumor extirpation. Recognition that full examination of tumor margins is important is reflected in articles from various surgical fields. Even authors more critical of Mohs surgery agree with the principle of full margin examination.[24] Methods must be developed to process large tissue specimens to allow rapid margin examination in an operating room setting. In addition, specific tumor recognition by use of immune antibody stains will allow more secure examination of tumors such as DFSP, squamous cell carcinomas, and melanoma. Other tools will be developed to aid in the evolution of Mohs surgery. Mohs surgery is an exciting field, with a basic principle which is simple but revolutionary, and will surely continue to grow with time.

REFERENCES

1. Mohs FE: Frederic E. Mohs, M.D. *J Am Acad Dermatol* **9**:806–814, 1983

2. Mohs FE: Mohs micrographic surgery: A historical perspective. *Dermatol Clin* **7**:609–611, 1989

3. Tromovitch TA, Stegman SJ: Microscopically controlled excision of skin tumors. *Arch Dermatol* **110**:231–232, 1974

4. Mohs FE: Chemosurgery for skin cancer: Fixed tissue and fresh tissue techniques. *Arch Dermatol* **112**:211–215, 1976

5. Mohs FE: Origin and progress of Mohs micrographic surgery, in *Mohs Micrographic Surgery,* edited by GR Mikhail. Philadelphia, Saunders, 1991, p 1

6. Salzman RS et al: Cutaneous implantation metastasis complicating a superficial temporal-middle cerebral artery anastomosis. *Neurosurgery* **11**:268–270, 1982

7. Christoph RA et al: Pain reduction in local anesthetic administration through pH buffering. *Ann Emerg Med* **17:**117–120, 1988

8. Larson PO et al: Stability of buffered lidocaine and epinephrine used for local anesthesia. *J Dermatol Surg Oncol* **17:**411–414, 1991

9. McCafferty DF et al: In vivo assessment of percutaneous local anaesthetic preparations. *Br J Anaesth* **62:**17–21, 1989

10. Ehrenstrom Reiz G et al: Topical anaesthesia with EMLA, a new lidocaine-prilocaine cream and the Cusum technique for detection of minimal application time. *Acta Anaesthesiol Scand* **27:**510–512, 1983

11. Robins P, Ashinoff R: Prolongation of anesthesia in Mohs micrographic surgery with 2% lidocaine jelly. *J Dermatol Surg Oncol* **17:**649–652, 1991

12. Phelan JT: The use of the Mohs' chemosurgery technic in the treatment of basal cell carcinoma. *Ann Surg* **168:**1023–1029, 1968

13. Mohs FE: *Chemosurgery: Microscopically Controlled Surgery for Skin Cancer.* Springfield, Ill, Charles C Thomas, 1978

14. Larson PO: Topical hemostatic agents for dermatologic surgery. *J Dermatol Surg Oncol* **14:**623–632, 1988

15. Lang PG Jr: Mohs micrographic surgery: Fresh-tissue technique. *Dermatol Clin* **7:**613–626, 1989

16. Snow SN: Techniques and indications for Mohs micrographic surgery, in *Mohs Micrographic Surgery,* edited by GR Mikhail. Philadelphia, Saunders, 1991, p 11

17. Larson PO: Staple and double-staple method of tissue orientation in Mohs micrographic surgery. *J Dermatol Surg Oncol* **13:**732–734, 1987

18. Grabski WJ, Salasche SJ: Mapping and orienting tissue during Mohs micrographic surgery: An alternate approach. *J Dermatol Surg Oncol* **17:**865–868, 1991

19. Koranda FC et al: Photo-mapping for microscopically controlled surgery. *J Dermatol Surg Oncol* **8:**463–465, 1982

20. Selak LS: The Mohs laboratory, in *Mohs Micrographic Surgery,* edited by GR Mikhail. Philadelphia, Saunders, 1991, p 299

21. Dhawan SS et al: Lentigo maligna: The use of rush permanent sections in therapy. *Arch Dermatol* **126:**928–930, 1990

22. Robinson JK, Gottschalk R: Immunofluorescent and immunoperoxidase staining of antibodies to fibrous keratin: Improved sensitivity for detecting epidermal cancer cells. *Arch Dermatol* **120:**199–203, 1984

23. Grabski WJ et al: Interpretation of Mohs micrographic frozen sections: A peer review comparison study. *J Am Acad Dermatol* **20:**670–674, 1989

24. Rapini RP: Comparison of methods for checking surgical margins. *J Am Acad Dermatol* **23:**288–294, 1990

25. Bennett RG: *Fundamentals of Cutaneous Surgery.* St. Louis, Mosby, 1988

26. Zitelli JA: Secondary intention healing: An alternative to surgical repair. *Clin Dermatol* **2:**92–106, 1984

27. Greenway HT, Breisch EA: Anatomy of the head and neck, in *Mohs Micrographic Surgery,* edited by GR Mikhail. Philadelphia, Saunders, 1991, p 150

28. Howe NR, Lang PG Jr: Daily observations during healing of a full-thickness human surgical wound by second intention. *J Dermatol Surg Oncol* **17:**933–935, 1991

29. Balle MR, Mikhail GR: Wound healing, in *Mohs Micrographic Surgery,* edited by GR Mikhail. Philadelphia, Saunders, 1991, p 222

30. Latenser J et al: Power drills to fenestrate exposed bone to stimulate wound healing. *J Dermatol Surg Oncol* **17:**265–270, 1991

31. Lang PG Jr: The partial closure. *J Dermatol Surg Oncol* **11:**966–969, 1985

32. Albright SD III: Placement of "guiding sutures" to counteract undesirable retraction of tissues in and around functionally and cosmetically important structures. *J Dermatol Surg Oncol* **7:**446–449, 1981

33. Katz BE, Oca AG: A controlled study of the effectiveness of spot dermabrasion ("scarabrasion") on the appearance of surgical scars. *J Am Acad Dermatol* **24:**462–466, 1991

34. Peters CR et al: The combined multidisciplinary approach to invasive basal cell tumors of the scalp. *Ann Plast Surg* **4:**199–204, 1980

35. Siegle RJ, Schuller DE: Multidisciplinary surgical approach to the treatment of perinasal nonmelanoma skin cancer. *Dermatol Clin* **7:**711–731, 1991

36. Rowe DE et al: Long-term recurrence rates in previously untreated (primary) basal cell carcinoma: Implications for patient follow-up. *J Dermatol Surg Oncol* **15:**315–328, 1989

37. Rowe DE et al: Mohs surgery is the treatment of choice for recurrent (previously treated) basal cell carcinoma. *J Dermatol Surg Oncol* **15:**424–431, 1989

38. Zitelli JA et al: Mohs micrographic surgery for melanoma. *Dermatol Clin* **7:**833–843, 1989

39. Lang PG Jr, Osguthorpe JD: Indications and limitations of Mohs micrographic surgery. *Dermatol Clin* **7:**627–644, 1989

40. Hanke WC, Melissa WL: Treatment of rare malignancies, in *Mohs Micrographic Surgery,* edited by GR Mikhail. Philadelphia, Saunders, 1991, p 261

41. Wagner RF Jr, Cottel WI: Multifocal recurrent basal cell carcinoma following primary tumor treatment by electrodesiccation and curettage. *J Am Acad Dermatol* **17:**1047–1049, 1987

42. Robins P: Chemosurgery: My 15 years of experience. *J Dermatol Surg Oncol* **7:**779–789, 1981

43. Wentzell JM, Robinson JK: Embryologic fusion planes and the spread of cutaneous carcinoma: A review and reassessment. *J Dermatol Surg Oncol* **16:**1000–1006, 1990

44. Bumsted RM, Ceilley RI: Auricular malignant neoplasms: Identification of high-risk lesions and selection of method of reconstruction. *Arch Otolaryngol* **108:**225–231, 1982

45. Rapini RP: Pitfalls of Mohs micrographic surgery. *J Am Acad Dermatol* **22:**681–686, 1990

46. Mohs FE et al: Microscopically controlled surgery in the treatment of carcinoma of the penis. *J Urol* **133:**961–966, 1985

47. Mikhail GR: Squamous-cell carcinoma of the penis. *J Dermatol Surg* **2:**406–408, 1976

48. Mikhail GR ed: The use of the zinc chloride fixative, in *Mohs Micrographic Surgery.* Philadelphia, Saunders, 1991, p 289

49. Hruza GJ, Snow SN: Basal cell carcinoma in a patient with acquired immunodeficiency syndrome: Treatment with Mohs micrographic surgery fixed-tissue technique. *J Dermatol Surg Oncol* **15:**545–551, 1989

50. Albom MJ: The use of a chalazion clamp in surgical procedures on eyelids. *J Dermatol Surg Oncol* **2:**284–285, 1976

51. Mikhail GR: Practical pointers, in *Mohs Micrographic Surgery,* edited by GR Mikhail. Philadelphia, Saunders, 1991, p 343

52. Bernstein G: Instrumentation for Mohs surgery, in *Mohs Micrographic Surgery,* edited by GR Mikhail. Philadelphia, Saunders, 1991, p 61

53. Rabinovitz HS, Epstein G: The corneal shield. *J Dermatol Surg Oncol* **11:**207–208, 1985

54. Larson PO: Surgical complications, in *Mohs Micrographic Surgery,* edited by GR Mikhail. Philadelphia, Saunders, 1991, p 193

55. Larson PO et al: Excision of exposed cartilage for management of Mohs surgery defects of the ear. *J Dermatol Surg Oncol* **17:**749–752, 1991

56. Hanke CW: Cryostats in chemosurgery. *J Dermatol Surg Oncol* **8:**346–347, 1982

57. Hanke CW, Lee MW: Cryostat use and tissue processing in Mohs micrographic surgery. *J Dermatol Surg Oncol* **15:**29–32, 1989

Deborah H. Atkin
Gary P. Lask

42 Ear Piercing and Surgical Repair of the Earlobe

Ear malformations may be the result of congenital anomalies as well as acquired or traumatic events. Disfigurement may result from cancerous lesions or subsequent surgical treatment. Absence of the ear or lobe is rare in comparison to accidental mutilation. Deliberate amputation or mutilation may be a form of punishment, for infidelity or immorality, in certain areas of the world such as in India. Congenital defects result from a failure of the normal development of the external ear, elements of which are derived from the hyoid arch. Failure of the ventral hillock may result in congenital absence of the lobe.[1]

Cosmetic aspects of reconstruction are of primary importance as the form and symmetry of the ears are important aspects of one's appearance. However, it has been suggested that an ear will appear as such as long as three curved lines appearing as a tragus, antitragus and concha, and helix are maintained.[2] In addition, many individuals choose to attract further attention to their ears by adorning them, often after ear piercing. Of obvious importance in the consideration of any surgical treatment or reconstructive process is the maintenance of hearing and the function of the external, middle, and inner ear.

EAR PIERCING

Earlobe piercing may be performed manually, with the aid of a needle, or by an automatic ear-piercing gun. The first step in piercing should be marking of the precise location to be pierced as well as careful consideration of position and symmetry, if desired, on the contralateral ear. It is important to have the patient review the proposed piercing sites prior to proceeding. The lobules are then cleansed with alcohol, and the site can be anesthetized with lidocaine if desired.

The manual method should be approached from the posterior aspect of the ear, with a 16- or 18-gauge needle advanced through the marked location on the anterior aspect of the lobe. The post of the earring is inserted in the needle and the tip is pulled back through the ear. The clasp is then placed on the posterior post. It is essential that the lobules, as well as the earring post and clasp, be cleaned with alcohol prior to the procedure. Piercing performed with the aid of a piercing gun "shoots" the earring through the selected location from an anterior approach. Slow, steady pressure is necessary for optimal placement when this method is utilized.

Earrings should remain in place for approximately 2 weeks to allow for healing of the ostium. The patient should clean the site with alcohol or hydrogen peroxide daily and apply Polysporin Ointment to the posts without removing them. Complications of piercing may include keloid formation, misplaced ostium, allergic reaction, or infection. History of keloid formation should be elicited prior to the procedure and, if positive, is an absolute contraindication to piercing. Allergic reactions can be minimized by avoidance of earrings containing nickel, the cause of many such reactions. Earrings of 24-kt gold have nearly no nickel, whereas most gold-plated and gold-filled earrings may contain amounts of nickel significant enough to pose a problem. Allergic reactions can be treated with topical steroids along with the switch to 24-kt gold or stainless steel earrings. Localized infections, which

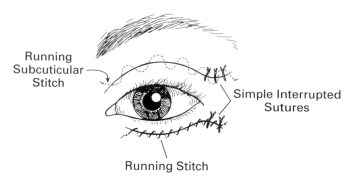

Figure 43-12   For the upper eyelid, a running subcuticular closure with 6–0 Prolene virtually eliminates milia formation; 2–3 simple interrupted sutures are used to reinforce the lateral component; sutures can be left up to 4 or 5 days. For the lower eyelid use a simple running closure with 6.0 Proline or fast obsorbing gut.

sionally cause milia or a mild inflammatory reaction. Tissue glue has also been used, and in the opinion of most surgeons just about any closure will ultimately yield an acceptable scar.

Supratarsal Fixation   This technique is advocated by certain authors (Flowers,[12] Sheen,[21] Bayliss,[10] and others) to create a very sharp, well-defined upper lid crease. It was first developed and remains often used to westernize the Asian upper lid. It involves placing sutures through the levator aponeurosis and attaching it to the overlying septum, orbicularis, and skin. The more complicated fixation techniques advocated by Flowers[12] and Sheen[21] seem a little more risky and are best reserved for the most experienced surgeons. Bayliss[10] advocates a simpler technique also described by Millard[28] that involves a single suture that closes the skin with a deep bite all the way through the levator aponeurosis. With any supratarsal fixation techniques, even in experienced hands, temporary ptosis, mild asymmetry, and occasionally a radically different "look" are the chief drawbacks. Permanent levator dysfunction and marked asymmetry are potential complications. Many surgeons, including Reese,[19] Reese et al.[20] Baker,[7] Baker et al.,[8] and others (with whom the author concurs), believe that a well-defined crease can be achieved with moderate to aggressive excision of orbicularis muscle. Gentle cautery of the entire inferior edge of the muscle excision can also be used. In effect, surgical trauma induces fibrosis, and "spontaneous" supratarsal fixation occurs without placing any sutures through the levator.

Male Blephraoplasty   The following modifications are incorporated to achieve the goals of a lower, less sharply defined crease. Unless there are well-defined existing creases, the lower segment of the incision is marked lower, only 9 to 10 mm above the lash line at its apex. The lateral segment is not carried out as far past the lateral canthus since a scar, though rare, cannot be readily camouflaged with makeup. The

orbicularis muscle excision is far more conservative. A 3- to 4-mm strip near the superior segment of the incision is largely sufficient and provides good exposure of the septum, which is incised along its length. Fat excision is aggressive, and closure is carried out in the same manner. In men, even more often than in women, brow ptosis and even marked asymmetry secondary to brow ptosis can be quite noticeable preoperatively and should be pointed out and discussed with the patient.

Asian Blephroplasty   The cosmetic surgeon is likely to encounter two types of requests for blepharoplasty from patients with oriental eyelids. One is the aging patient complaining of heavy eyelids and excess skin folds, and the other is the young patient requesting creation of an upper lid crease. For the aging Asian patient, if the oriental aspect is to be preserved, the same general concepts of male blepharoplasty are followed, with little or no muscle excision and moderate to liberal excision of fat. If a "double eyelid," meaning creation of a crease is desired, the placement and definition of the crease are critical to patient satisfaction and need to be discussed at length preoperatively. Sometimes it is useful to review with the patient photographs of models, Asian calendars, or magazines. These are often good sources to determine the type of crease desired.

The author prefers a conservative, relatively low, soft crease that both preserves and enhances the appearance of the oriental upper eyelid. The author best achieves these results with a skin incision started medially about 3 mm above the lash line, arching slowly to 7 to 8 mm at the midpupillary line, and then lowered only slightly toward the lateral canthus. Excess skin is excised as needed, though always conservatively. A 3- to 5-mm strip of muscle is excised to the level of the lower segment of the skin incision. A thin strip of septum is excised, and all of the fat that can be readily prolapsed is clamped and excised. Cautery is applied to the lower edge of the muscle incision and underlying septum. The wound is closed with running subcuticular and a few deeper interrupted 6–0 Prolene sutures. No attempt is made to incorporate the levator aponeurosis into the closure.

A standard blepharoplasty procedure with reasonable excision of muscle, septum, and fat, as previously described (regardless of age and amount of skin excised), will almost always result in a permanent crease (Figs. 43-13*a–d*). Supratarsal fixation, however, remains by far the most widely advocated and commonly used technique to create an upper lid crease in young Asian women. It has the advantage of predictability, ensures symmetry, and can be performed quite rapidly after a simple skin incision. For best results, in addition to supratarsal fixation, it is often necessary to remove a significant amount of fat even in the young Asian patient. For an even more radical change, the epicanthal fold can be obliterated by means of a Z-plasty.[17] This type of procedure is best left to those surgeons most experienced with Asian blepharoplasty.

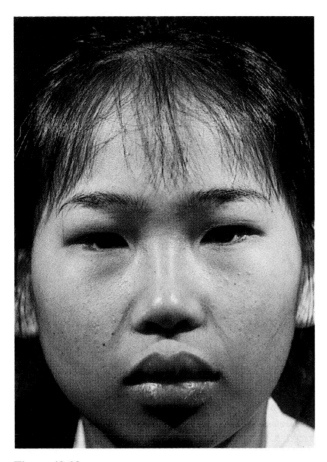

Figure 43-13a

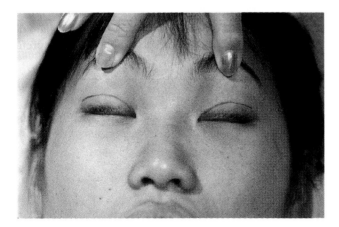

Figure 43-13b

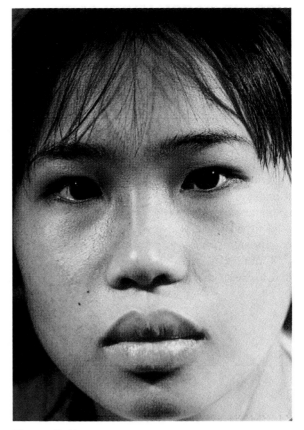

Figure 43-13c

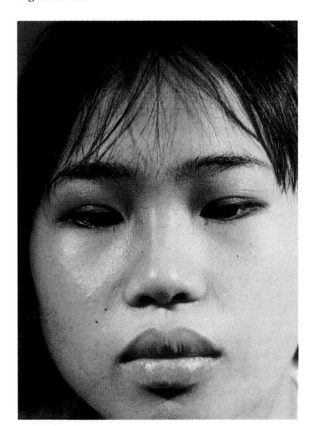

Figure 43-13d

Figure 43-13 Oriental blepharoplasty in a 19-year-old patient. A soft, relatively low crease combined with aggressive fat excision has created a more open, aesthetically pleasing look, while preserving a natural, oriental appearance to the eyelids. (*a*) Preoperative photos demonstrate lack of a crease and fullness of the upper lid resulting in a less desirable, closed, slit like appearance of the eye. (*b*) Outline of the proposed incision; in the young Asian patient no skin is excised. (*c*) Postoperative result in neutral gaze after excision of a strip of orbicularis musle and moderately aggressive fat resection. (*d*) Postoperative result in down gaze demonstrates well formed crease.

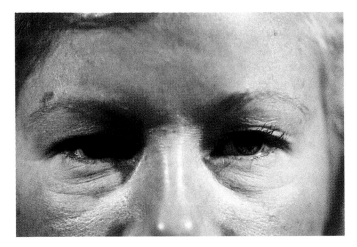

Figure 43-23c

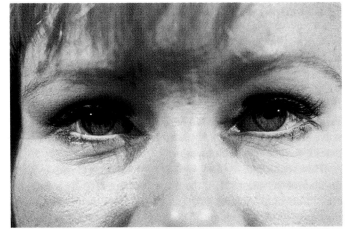

Figure 43-23d

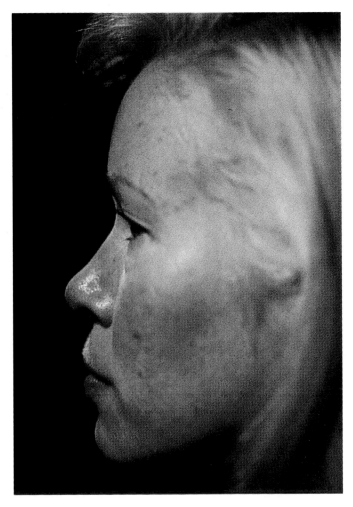

Figure 43-23e

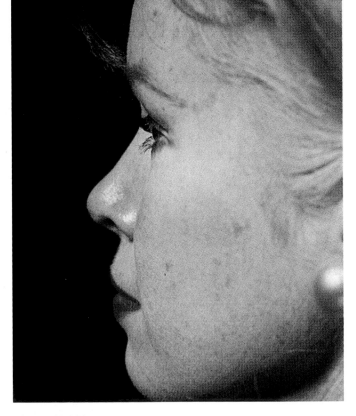

Figure 43-23f

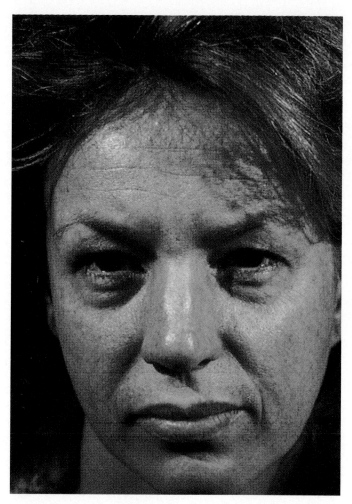

Figure 43-24a (a–f) A 48-year-old patient demonstrating six weeks postoperative result of standard upper lid blepharoplasty, and skin muscle flap lower lid blepharoplasty. Transcutaneous approach was selected to allow conservative excision of hypertrophic lower lid orbicularis muscle. Lower lid incision is barely visible even at this early postoperative stage.

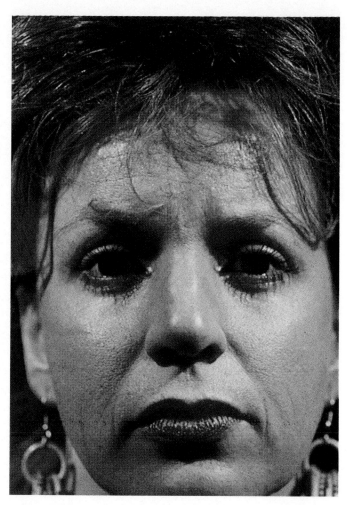

Figure 43-24b

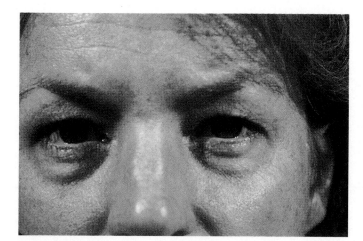

Figure 43-24c

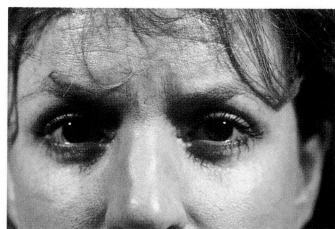

Figure 43-24d

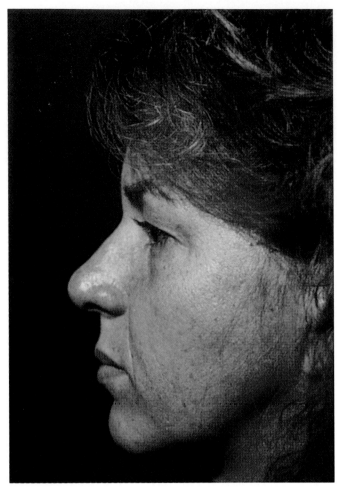

Figure 43-24e

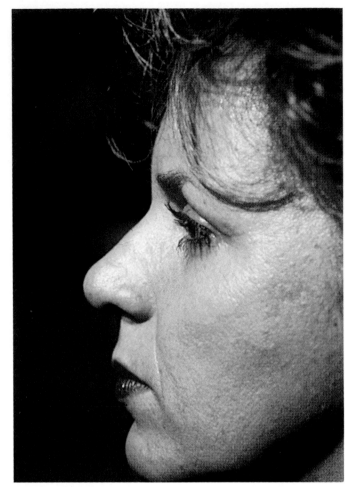

Figure 43-24f

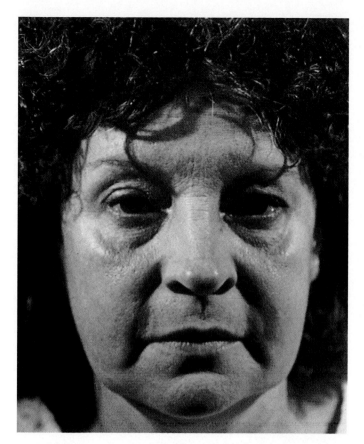

Figure 43-25a   (a–f) A 57-year-old patient demonstrating six weeks postoperative result of upper lid blepharoplasty with aggressive excision of skin, muscle and fat, and skin muscle flap lower lid blepharoplasty. The patient also underwent middle and lower face lift, without any forehead lift. Restoration or creation of a high set upper lid crease combined with sufficient skin excision over the lateral canthus to the orbital rim, is often sufficient to yield good results even in the presence of moderate brow ptosis. This patient also demonstrates malar "bags" which are not affected by lower lid blepharoplasty and should be pointed out to the patient preoperatively.

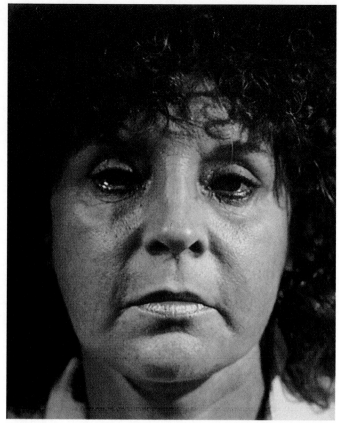

Figure 43-25b

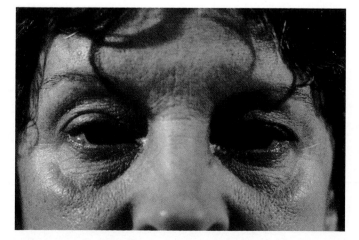

Figure 43-25c

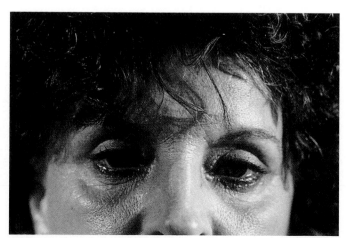

Figure 43-25d

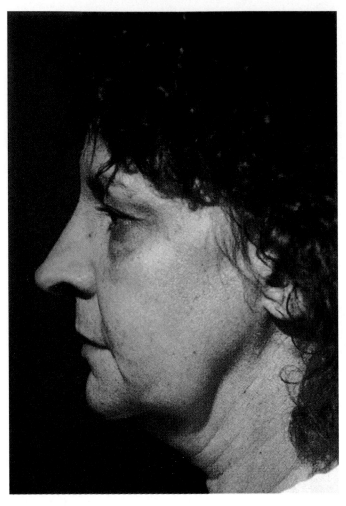

Figure 43-25*e*

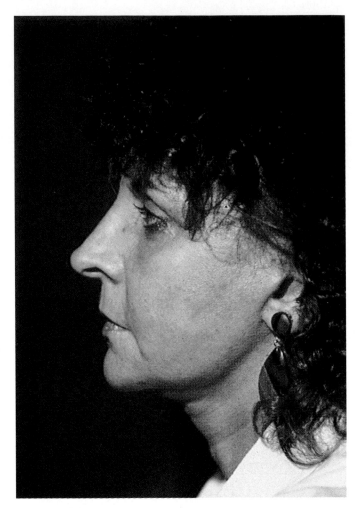

Figure 43-25*f*

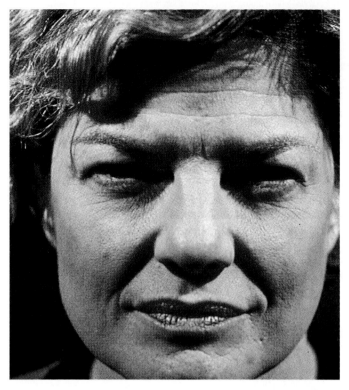

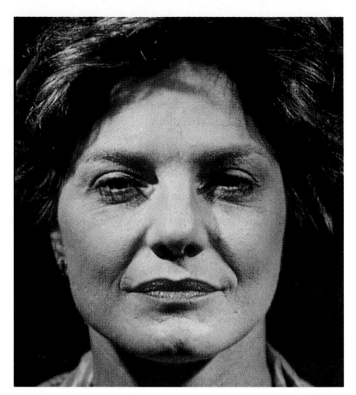

Figure 43-26a (*a–d*) A 46-year-old patient demonstrating six months postoperative results of upper (coronal brow lift), middle, and lower face lift. Upper lid blepharoplasty alone would be counter indicated in the presence of such severe brow ptosis. While many surgeons choose to perform upper lid blepharoplasty at the same time as the brow lift, the author prefers to wait 6–12 months after the brow lift, which assures better accuracy of the upper lid skin excision.

Figure 43-26b

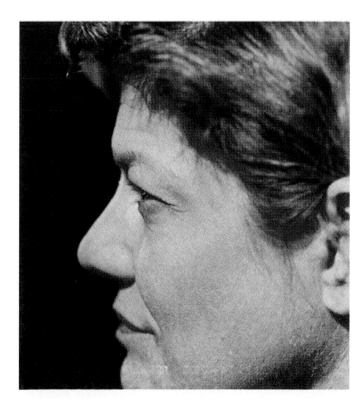

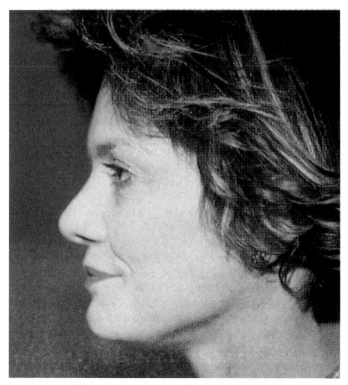

Figure 43-26c

Figure 43-26d

Epidermis

In the epidermis, minimal tissue changes occur.[21] At the light microscopic level, there is no decrease in epidermal thickness,[27] although the epidermal surface area increases. At the electron microscopic level, the basal lamina and the basal surfaces of basal epidermal cells show a more undulated appearance. Within the cytoplasm of basal and prickle cells, there are larger bundles of tonofilaments, forming tonofibrils which are scattered throughout the cell. The intercellular spaces throughout all layers of the epidermis become reduced, measuring 50 to 100 Å.[28] Increased epidermal mitotic activity during tissue expansion may be the cause of the decreased intercellular space as well as the undulation of the basal lamina.[21] The combination of a lack of epidermal thinning along with increased epidermal mitosis during expansion supports the idea of a net gain in epidermal tissue as opposed to just tissue "loan."[1]

Dermis

In contrast to the epidermis, the dermis undergoes significant change during tissue expansion in animal models.[27,28] There is a notable decrease in the thickness as seen by light microscopy. This decrease in thickness is most rapid in the first few weeks of expansion, further decreasing at a slower rate thereafter.[27] At the electron microscopic level, fibroblasts are found in increased numbers and show pronounced rough endoplasmic reticulum. This signifies increased metabolic activity, as compared to normal skin. Myofibroblasts develop in the deeper dermis,[28] and elastic tissue becomes thicker and compact, forming clusters. The papillary and reticular dermis become filled with thick bundles of collagen fibers.[21] The tension during chronic tissue expansion increases collagen synthesis in both the dermis and the fibrous capsule surrounding the implant.[29] The collagen fibers also have more biaxial orientation and are stronger and stiffer than collagen synthesized in normal wound healing.[30] The large bundles of compacted collagen fibers show cross-banding of normal periodicity.[2]

Appendages

Skin appendages such as hair follicles and glands continue activity and become further spaced apart but quantitatively remain unchanged.[21] The hair becomes imperceptibly less dense, sweat glands become compacted but remain open and continue to function, and small dermal blood vessels show not alterations. In chronic expansion, the expanded dermis is free of inflammatory cells.[28]

Muscle

Muscle shows a marked decrease in thickness and mass during chronic tissue expansion; however, no functional loss in muscle strength is observed clinically.[21] With electron microscopy, a large amount of sarcoplasm is noted in relation to the number of myofibrils,[28] and the sarcoplasmic reticulum enlarges. Also, the number and size of mitochondria increase.[21]

Fat

Fat is the most intolerant to chronic tissue expansion. There is a decrease in the thickness of fat layers and the number of fat cells.[21,29] Although this loss is permanent, fat necrosis can be avoided with judicious expansion.[21]

Capsule Formation

With chronic tissue expansion, a dense fibrous capsule will form within days after implantation.[21,29] This capsule is composed of elongated fibroblasts and occasional myofibroblasts which lie between collagen bundles oriented parallel to the implant surface.[28] The fibroblasts within the capsule show highly active rough endoplasmic reticulum with prominent cisternae and collagen fibers with a typical periodicity.[28,29] At the junction of the capsule and host tissue, a rapid proliferation of blood vessels occurs. This neovasculature contributes to the increased viability of the flap.[5,21]

ISLE Technique

In rapid tissue expansion with the ISLE technique, a study via light microscopy showed there are no significant changes seen in the epidermis, dermis, dermal appendages, adipose tissue, or muscle. Special staining of collagen and elastin revealed a slight degree of alignment, with no evidence of microfragmentation. Increased duration of expansion, larger volumes at each interval of expansion, and shorter periods between expansion caused increased inflammatory responses and ecchymotic changes.[25]

COMPLICATIONS

The complications of tissue expansion vary widely depending on a multitude of factors, such as the experience of the surgeon, patient selection or indications, the involved anatomic site, and the level of difficulty of a particular case. In chronic tissue expansion, the lower extremities have the highest complication rate, while the chest, trunk, and back of the hands have lower rates.[21,31–35]

Infection

Infection rates are less than 1 percent with the use of sterile tissue expanders and sterile technique. When infection does occur, it is usually secondary to a local wound infection or to an infection elsewhere in the body.[21] Prophylactic measures such as perioperative intravenous antibiotics should be employed, but long-term antibiotics are not recommended.[21,31-35] Treatment modalities used in infection control include irrigation, drainage, and antibiotic therapy. If therapy is unsuccessful, the implant must be removed until the infection is resolved.[17]

Hematoma

Hematoma formation predisposes a patient to flap necrosis, capsule formation, and infection. Hematomas can also increase the tension of tissues already undergoing expansion. Treatment consists of the immediate removal of the expander, evacuation of the hematoma, and establishment of hemostasis. The occurrence of hematomas can be minimized by meticulous hemostasis and, if necessary, suction drains.[21,31-35]

Pain

Pain may be elicited during the active inflation period of the tissue expander. The severity of pain coincides with the tenseness of the expanded skin, and it also seems to signal the attainment of the skin's inflation limit, as determined by skin color and decreased capillary refill. Pain can immediately be relieved by withdrawal of only a few milliliters of saline.[31,34] This pain is also temporary, decreasing within 4 to 6 h as the expanded tissue becomes less tense. In general, pain varies with anatomic site of expansion. For example, scalp and breast expansion are associated with little pain, while expansion of the flank, back, temporal areas, and feet are associated with greater pain.[21]

Ischemia

Tissue expansion may create some degree of hypoxia. As the overlying tissue becomes compressed, blood flow decreases. Overly vigorous or prolonged inflation of an expander may result in tissue ischemia or necrosis; however the onset of pain usually prevents this. Adequate capillary refill is regained by removing a sufficient amount of saline from the expander.[31] Necrosis is also prone to develop in areas with a predisposition to decreased blood supply, as in previous radiation therapy or burns.[21,31-33]

In chronic expansion, implant exposure may follow wound dehiscence, pressure necrosis over a persistent fold in the expander, erosion through an inadequate tissue cover, or manipulation by a psychotic patient.[21,31,33,35] The cheek and neck have been found to be particularly susceptible to focal pressure necrosis and implant exposure. This is secondary to the effects of gravity, which cause the implants to slip downward. The most common cause of incisional dehiscence is the formation of an insufficient pocket that places the implant in contact with the suture line.[21] To prevent exposure, inflation of the implant should be delayed until 2 weeks after the initial procedure.[21,31] Envelope folds can be avoided by slow expansion or emptying the expander if folds occur and then refilling it while manipulating the overlying skin. Therapy for implant exposure includes antibiotic coverage while expansion progresses.

Implant failure

Implant failures rarely occur.[21,31-35] Manufacturing errors, such as an injection port that lacks a solid back to stop needle exit, are uncommon. Implant deflation, valve leakage, and perforation are also rare occurrences.[31] The device is usually removed following deflation, with resumption of expansion after 1 to 2 weeks for chronic expansion. Implant leakage does not always require replacement, depending upon the amount of leakage.[33]

Neurapraxia

Neurapraxia is a rare complication. Traction over a peripheral nerve or direct mechanical force may lead to compression by the implant. Slight deflation can quickly resolve neurapraxia if it is recognized and treated early, before the onset of focal demyelination.[17]

STAR Technique

When the STAR technique is used, it is necessary to monitor visually for signs of blanching, cyanosis, ischemia, irritation, infection, or hematoma, just as with any other surgical device. Excessive tightening or prolonged attachment to the skin surface will cause the same complications seen in overtightening of a traditional suture ligature or prolonged presence of any suture material in the skin.[16]

ISLE Technique

With use of the ISLE technique, distal flap or marginal ischemia can occur, causing flap loss, wound separation, infection, and mixed pigmentation. It is mandatory to assess adequate dermal bleeding closely during surgery to avoid the complications of decreased flap perfusion. The surgeon should immediately lower tension on the expanded flap until satisfactory dermal bleeding is noted.[25]

In addition to the risk of ischemia resulting from the ISLE procedure, small hematomas can sometimes occur and are preventable. Also, it is recommended that intraoperative antibiotics are used to minimize the risk of infection.[25]

INDICATIONS

Specific applications of tissue expansion in dermatologic surgery are almost limitless as long as there is sufficient normal skin adjacent to the defect. Expansion can provide tissue that will match the recipient site in color, texture, and hair-bearing characteristics while simultaneously minimizing the donor site deformity. Either rapid or chronic expansion can be used as an adjunct in wound closures. Since chronic tissue expansion is at least a two-staged procedure, it is usually reserved for closing larger lesions that would have customarily required staged excisions or complicated closures involving skin grafts or flaps.[24]

Although tissue expansion was initially adapted by Radovan in 1978[9,10] for reconstructive use in the postmastectomy patient, a multitude of applications now exist. For instance, in head and neck reconstruction, although the conventional use of distant flaps may provide the quantity of tissue needed for function and symmetry, the aesthetic quality may be compromised.[32] Thus, it is preferable to use local tissue which can be made available through tissue expansion. Expansion in the head and neck is challenging, however, because careful planning is required to match expanded skin with the variable characteristics of facial skin, such as specific skin tone, hair-bearing qualities, sebaceous gland content, and thickness of skin (Fig. 44-3a–d).[31,32,36] Tissue expansion is a useful adjunct for the reconstructive therapy of scalp skin in which unique hair-bearing characteristics and relative lack of mobility have made other methods inadequate or difficult (Fig. 44-4a–e). Hair follicles are not increased but become uniformly separated from one another,[24,37] and hair growth is not

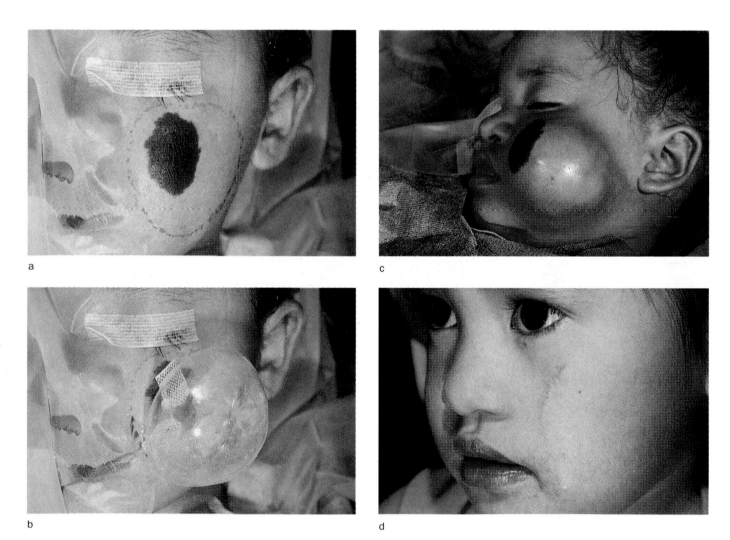

a

b

c

d

Figure 44-3   (a) This 14-month-old patient presented with an intermediate sized congenital pigmented nevus to the left cheek. The nevus measured 2.5 × 3.5 cm in dimensions. (b) In May 1992, the patient underwent the first stage of reconstruction with the insertion of a 20-cc round expander with a remote valve system. The expander was inserted through a 1.5 cm incision behind the ear lobule in the subcutaneous fat plane. The expander was positioned under the nevus and into the adjacent normal tissue. (c) After six weeks of serial expansion, the implant was filled gradually to 40 cc without significant distortion to the nose or lower lid. (d) The patient is shown two years after the nevus was removed and the defect resurfaced with the expanded skin in a vertical line of closure. The scar has healed without pigmentation or hypertrophy. Sensation has returned to the normal level. No lower lid ectropion was present. All facial muscles were functioning symmetrically in the post-operative period.

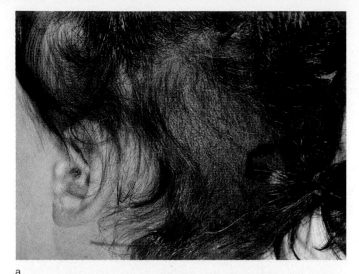

a

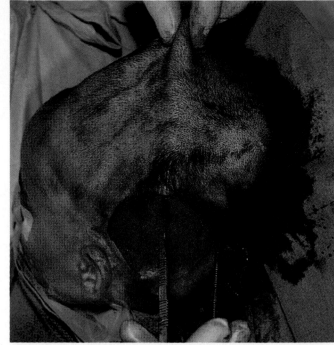

d

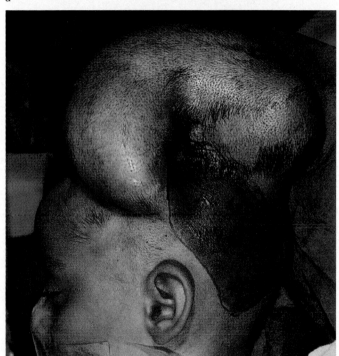

b

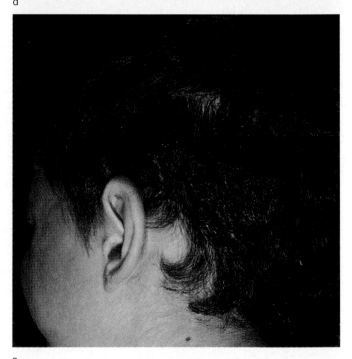

e

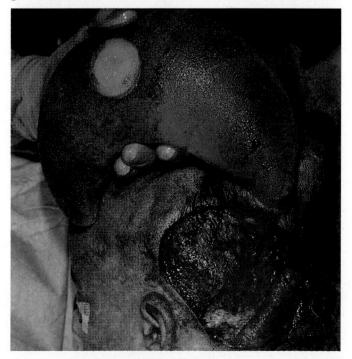

c

Figure 44-4 (*a*) This 4-year-old patient presented with a 5 × 7 cm cresent-shaped congenital large nevus to the left temporo-parietal and occipital area of his scalp. The patient was indicated for the removal and resurfacing with expanded scalp tissue on the basis of potential malignant changes in the future. (*b*) On December 1993, an endoscopic-assisted insertion of a 600 cc cresent-shaped expander was inserted through a 2.5 cm incision along the right temporoparietal area of his scalp. The expander had an incorporated valve. Over a period of four months, the expander was slowly inflated by serial filling up to 630 cc, creating a hemispheric mound of 18 cm across. (*c*) The entire nevus was excised down to the galea aponeurosis and temporoparietalis fascia after intra-operative expansion of up to 730 cc was performed for five minutes. (*d*) After capsulectomy and base capsulotomy, the expanded flap was able to be advanced with complete coverage and minimal dog-ear presence. (*e*)The patient is shown one and a half years after surgery. There was minimal scar alopecia of less than 5 mm across the length of the scar. Normal sensation recurred after a year with almost-normal density of hair.

interrupted. Conversely, significant hair growth occurs.[21] Scalp defects due to congenital deformities, localized radiation therapy, stabilized male pattern baldness, and cicatricial alopecia caused by trauma or inflammation can be corrected.[37]

Lesions on the trunk or extremities sufficiently large enough to require serial excisions or grafting should instead be considered for tissue expansion. Expansion may also be used for the removal of tattoos, giant cerebriform nevi, or large congenital nevi on any location, particularly the extremities.

Also, expansion can be used subsequently to below knee amputations, for covering the stump before fitting prostheses.[31,38] Additionally, expansion in the extremities can augment the cutaneous territory of fasciocutaneous or musculocutaneous flaps or improve extremity donor defects.[31,32,39]

Tissue expansion can be an instrumental adjunct in reconstructive surgery after removal of a malignancy,[31] particularly basal cell carcinomas removed through Mohs' surgery (Fig. 44-5a–f). Because basal cell carcinomas grow slowly, chronic

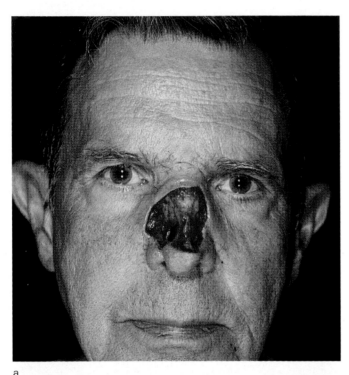

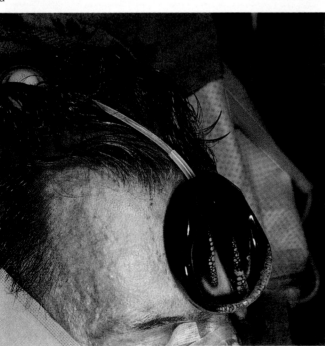

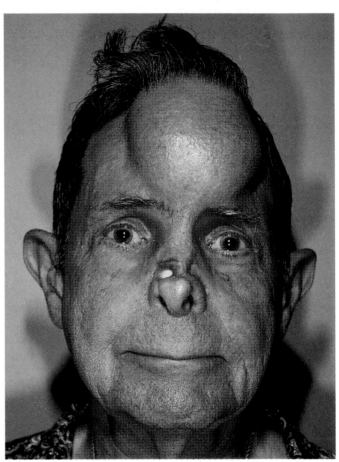

Figure 44-5   (a) This 68-year-old patient underwent Mohs chemosurgery to the nose for a sclerotic and invasive basal cell multifocal cancer with removal of skin, cartilage, and lining. The right upper lateral and cephalic portions of the alar cartilage were excised two days prior to his planned reconstruction consisting of turned down flaps for mucosal lining and insertion of a 100-cc round expander. (b) The expander was positioned under the galea of the forehead through a 1.5 cm incision behind the precapillary line. The expander was partially filled with methylene blue to determine any leak of the system during its insertion. The expander was filled to tissue tolerance at surgery to decrease the incidence of hematoma formation and maintenance of pocket size. (c) After 12 weeks of slow serial expansion, the expander contained about 125 cc of saline. The hemispheric flap measured about 16 cm across. During the time for chronic expansion, the defect underwent cicatrization and secondary contraction.

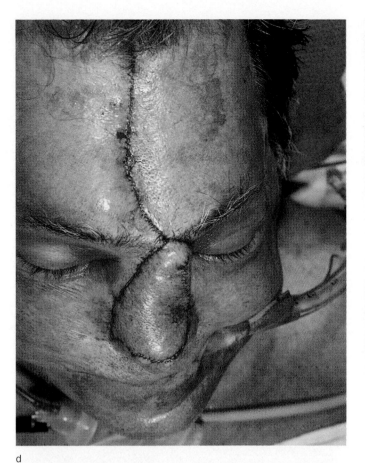

d

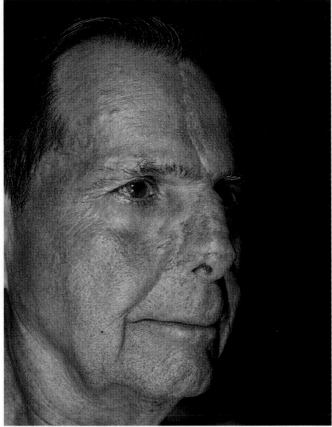

f

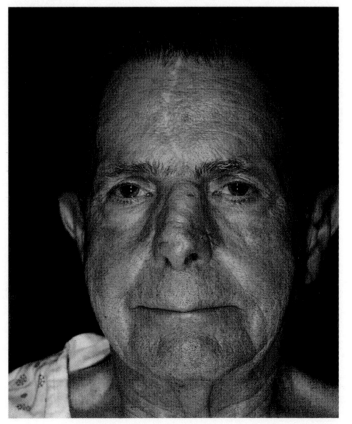

e

Figure 44-5 (*d*) Intraoperative expansion was performed at the second stage to gain more potential tissue. The recipient site was prepared by recreating the defect, positioning a left conchal cartilage graft to replace the upper lateral and alar cartilage lobular defect, and transposing the expanded glabellar flap over the reconstructive site. The glabellar flap measured about 9 cm across to permit side-to-side coverage of the nasal lobule. The donor forehead site was approximated in a single vertical line closure without crowding the brow heads. (*e–f*) After three months, the flap was inset and divided at its neurovascular pedicle. Further refinements to the alar folds were added. The flap subsequently underwent two defattening procedures with insertion of a spreader graft and septal relocation.

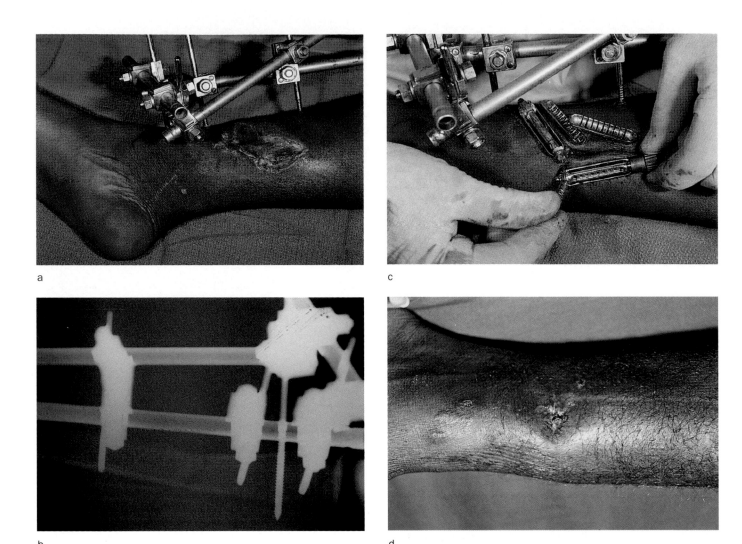

a

b

c

d

Figure 44-6   (*a–b*) This 17-year-old male was involved in a motor vehicle accident sustaining facial lacerations and a type III-A injury to his left lower extremity. The distal tibia was fractured
with bone exposure, temporary nerve damage, and vascular contusion. The skin defect measured
2.5 × 6 cm in dimensions. External fixation was performed to align the fracture site. After two de-
bridements and irrigation, and delayed skin closure was planned. (*c*) Three weeks after the injury,
a delayed skin closure was obtained by the application of two suture tension assisted reel (STAR)
devices. The skin was advanced every two days by tightening the suture reel. In four days, the skin
edges were approximated as edema was reduced and the skin stretched. (*d*) Eight days after application of the STAR devices, the skin was primarily closed without need of a muscle pedicle or free
flap. Six months later, primary bone healing was noted with skin healing.

expansion can be done prior to surgery so that repair of the
defect can be executed simultaneously with tumor excision.

The STAR technique can be employed for various clinical
situations.[16] It can effectively stretch skin either preoperatively,
as in cycled presuturing, or intraoperatively, as in excision,
flap, and scalp reduction surgery (Fig. 44-6*a–d*). It may prove
valuable in improving cicatrization and cosmesis of surgical
skin closures.

Besides its use in planned intraoperative procedures, the
STAR technique may also be used for unexpected intraoperative conditions. For instance, if the width of a defect or the

size of a flap is larger than anticipated, or if attaining frozen
sections necessitates making a larger defect than originally
estimated, the skin can be expanded to adapt to these unfore-
seen circumstances. In addition, if excessive bleeding or oozing occurs and extensive undermining might be further detrimental, the STAR device may be extemporaneously attached
to expand tissue as an alternative to continued surgery.

Clinical experience with ISLE indicates that this procedure
can be used for reconstruction of almost any body surface
area with defects less than 4.5 cm in diameter (Fig. 44-7*a–d*).[25]
When ISLE is used as the sole mode of expansion, up to

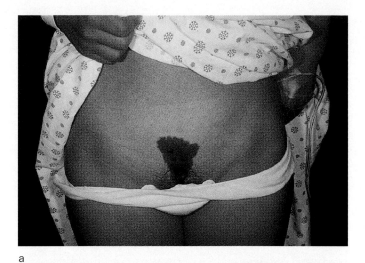

a

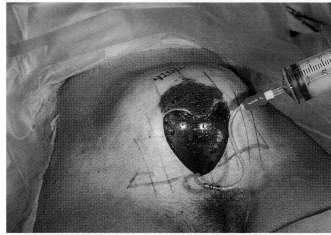

c

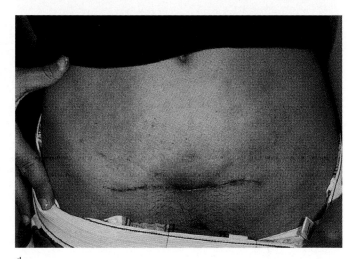

b

d

Figure 44-7 (*a*) This 13-year-old patient presented with a 4 × 5 cm congenital nevus to the suprapubic area. The patient desired to have the nevus removed by intraoperative expansion technique rather than by chronic expansion method. (*b*) A 320-cc intraoperative expander was planned to be inserted in the subcutaneous fat through an intralesional incisional. (*c*) Intraoperative expansion was serially done by filling the expander to its limits for three minutes, deflation for three minutes, and reexpansion twice more. Additional tissue was recruited enabling the nevus to be removed with primary closure. (*d*) The patient is shown about three months after completion of her procedure. There was minimal distortion of the umbilicus without elevation of the suprapubic hairline. Sensation is slowly returning to normal.

2.5 cm of tissue can be gained from use of each intraoperative expander, depending on the anatomic site. Even more tissue can be generated to approximate large defects with use of multiple expanders. When used in conjunction with conventional long-term expansion as the final step before reconstruction, rapid intraoperative expansion can gain an additional 1 to 3 cm of tissue prior to flap advancement. This depends on the site of expansion, age of the patient, and local tissue factors.

Regarding the future role of tissue expansion in facial dermatologic surgery, expanding skin to make primary closures would be a critical advantage. Specifically in locations of limited tissue mobility, such as the nasal tip or upper lip, the possibility of having a single linear closure as opposed to a complicated, distant flap would greatly improve the final cosmetic result. It would also decrease postoperative complications, compared to larger reconstructive procedures.[17]

There are unique advantages and disadvantages involved with the use of each type of tissue expansion. With immediate tissue expansion, tissue may be expanded either linearly (i.e., STAR device) or spherically. Immediate expansion takes advantage of the skin's ability to creep mechanically. Although immediate expansion is rapid and effective, the maximal expansion achieved is self-limited and relatively modest. In distinction, chronic tissue expansion is based on the skin's ability to creep biologically. Although chronic tissue expansion takes weeks and is more technically demanding, it results in the generation of significantly more tissue. Both immediate and chronic tissue expansion present a valuable alternative to the more traditional methods of surgical reconstruction (i.e., flaps and grafts).

CONCLUSION

Tissue expansion serves as a highly useful complement to surgical reconstruction of skin defects. It offers significant aesthetic as well as functional advantages to concealing both large and small defects. Concealing defects is accomplished through using adjacent tissue of similar color, texture, and hair-bearing characteristics, all of which are especially essential in reconstructing cosmetically important areas such as the face, scalp, and hands. In addition, the expanded soft tissue permits production of a broad-based rotation or advancement flap from the neighboring normal skin or hair-bearing scalp that can be manipulated without tension.

REFERENCES

1. Austad ED et al: Tissue expansion: Dividend or loan? *Plast Reconstr Surg* **78**:63–67, 1986
2. Mustoe TA et al: Physical, biomechanical, histologic, and biochemical effects of rapid versus conventional tissue expansion. *Plast Reconstr Surg* **83**:687–691, 1989
3. Gibson T et al: The mobile microarchitecture of dermal collagen: A bioengineering study. *Br J Surg* **522**:764–770, 1965
4. Gibson T: The physical properties of skin, in *Reconstructive Plastic Surgery,* edited by JM Converse. Philadelphia, Saunders, pp 69–77, 1977
5. Liang MD et al: Presuturing: A new technique for closing skin defects: Clinical and experimental studies. *Plast Reconstr Surg* **83**:681–686, 1989
6. Burnett W: Yank meets native. *National Geographic* **88**:105–128, 1945
7. Weeks GS: Into the heart of Africa. *National Geographic* **110**:257–263, 1956
8. Neumann CG: The expansion of an area of skin by progressive

9. Radovan C: Reconstruction of the breast after radical mastectomy using temporary expander (letter). *Plast Surg Forum* **1**:41, 1980
10. Radovan C: Breast reconstruction after mastectomy using the temporary expander. *Plast Reconstr Surg* **69**:195–206, 1982
11. Hirshowitz B et al: Reconstruction of the tip of the nose and ala by load cycling of the nasal skin and harnessing of extra skin. *Plast Reconstr Surg* **77**:316–319, 1986
12. Sasaki GH: Intraoperative expansion as an immediate reconstructive technique. *Facial Plastic Surgery* **5**:362–378, 1988
13. Johnson T et al: Immediate intraoperative tissue expansion. *J Am Acad Dermatol* **22**:283–287, 1990
14. Gibson T: Discussion: Reconstruction of the tip of the nose and ala by load cycling of the nasal skin and harnessing of extra skin. *Plast Reconstr Surg* **77**:320–321, 1986
15. Liang MD et al: Presuturing: A new technique for closing large skin defects: Clinical and experimental studies. *Plast Reconstr Surg* **81**:694–702, 1988
16. Cohen BH, Cosmetto AJ: The suture tension adjustment reel: A new device for the management of skin closure. *J Dermatol Surg Oncol* **18**:112–123, 1992
17. Marcus J et al: Tissue expansion: Past, present, and future. *J Am Acad Dermatol* **23**:813–825, 1990
18. van Rappard JHAA et al: Surface area increase in tissue expansion. *Plast Reconstr Surg* **82**:833–837, 1988
19. Brobman GF, Huber J: Effects of different-shaped tissue expanders on transluminal pressure, oxygen tension, histopathologic changes, and skin expansion in pigs. *Plast Reconstr Surg* **76**:731–736, 1985
20. Swanson NA, Argenta LC: Tissue expansion, in, *Dermatologic Surgery: Principles and Practice,* edited by RK Roenigk, HH Roenigk Jr. New York, Marcel Dekker, pp 347–354, 1989
21. Argenta LC et al: Advances in tissue expansion. *Clin Plast Surg* **12**:159–171, 1985
22. Garner WL et al: Effects of rate of tissue expansion on the creation of new tissue. *Surgical Forum of Plastic Surgery* **38**:591–593, 1987
23. Marks MW et al: Rapid expansion: Experimental and clinical experience. *Clin Plast Surg* **14**:455–463, 1987
24. Roenigk RK, Wheeland RG: Tissue expansion in cicatricial alopecia. *Arch Dermatol* **123**:641–646, 1987
25. Sasaki GH: Intraoperative sustained limited expansion (ISLE) as an immediate reconstructive technique. *Clin Plast Surg* **14**:563–573, 1987
26. Moy RL et al: Decrease in skin closing tension intraoperatively with suture tension adjustment reel, balloon expansion and undermining. *J Dermatol Surg Oncol* **20**:368–371, 1994
27. Austad ED, Rose GL: A self-inflating tissue expander. *Plast Reconstr Surg* **70**:588–593, 1982
28. Pasyk KA et al: Electron microscopic evaluation of guinea pig

skin and soft tissues "expanded" with a self-inflating silicone implant. *Plast Reconstr Surg* **70:**37–45, 1982

29. Pasyk KA et al: Intracellular collagen fibers in the capsule around silicone expanders in guinea pigs. *J Surg Res* **36:**125–133, 1984

30. Langrana NA et al: Effects of mechanical load in wound healing. *Ann Plast Surg* **10:**200, 1983

31. Manders EK et al: Soft-tissue expanders: Concepts and complications. *Plast Reconstr Surg* **74:**493–507, 1984

32. Radovan C: Tissue expansion in soft-tissue reconstruction. *Plast Reconstr Surg* **74:**482–490, 1984

33. Austad ED: Complications in tissue expansion. *Clin Plast Surg* **14:**549–450, 1987

34. Dickson WA et al: Experience with an external valve in small volume tissue expanders. *Br J Plast Surg* **41:**373–377, 1988

35. Antonyshyn O et al: Complications of soft tissue expansion. *Br J Plast Surg* **41:**239–249, 1988

36. Argenta LC et al: Selective use of serial expansion in breast reconstruction. *Ann Plast Surg* **11:**188–195, 1983

37. Manders EK et al: Skin expansion to eliminate scalp defects. *Ann Plast Surg* **12:**305–312, 1984

38. Rees RS et al: Tissue expansion: Its role in traumatic below-knee amputations. *Plast Reconstr Surg* **77:**133–137, 1986

39. Hallock GG: Tissue expansion. *Contemporary Surgery* **29:**34–39, 1986

Index

Page numbers in *italics* refer to illustrations; page numbers followed by t refer to tables.

Abnormal surface scar(s), treatment of, 131–133
Abreaction, 139
Absorbable suture(s), 78–79, 79t
Acetone, as prepeel agent, 508–509
Acinetobacter, 57
ACLS (advanced cardiac life support), 113
Acne, chemical peels for, 512–513, *513*
  dermabrasion for, 496–497, *496*
Acne flare(s), 501
Acne scar(s), revision of, 260–261
Acquired digital fibrokeratoma, 279, *279*
Acquired immunodeficiency virus (AIDS), 497–498. See also *Human immunodeficiency virus (HIV)*
Acrochordons, 224
Actinic cheilitis, laser treatment for, 449–450
Actinic keratoses, chemical peels for, 512
  dermabrasion for, *497*
Adenosquamous carcinoma, 108
Adhesive bandage(s), 25–26
Adhesive tape(s), 25
Adipose, 352
Adnexal neoplasm, benign, 107
Adnexal tumors, malignant, 242–243, *243*
Adson forceps, 92, *92*, *93*, 95
Advanced cardiac life support (ACLS), 113
Advancement flap, for forehead reconstruction, 354–355, *354–356*
  for lip reconstruction, 334, *335*, 336, *337*, 341, *342*
  for nasal reconstruction, 387
  method of, 310–317, *311–317*
AFX. See *Atypical fibroxanthoma (AFX)*
Age spot(s), 226
Aggressive-growth basal cell carcinoma, 107
Aging skin, dermabrasion for, *497*, 498, *498*
AHAs (alpha hydroxy acids), as peeling agent, 505, 506–507
AIDS, 497–498
Ala, reconstruction of, 398
Alar groove tumors, Mohs micrographic surgery for, 575–576, *575*
Alcohol(s), as skin preparation agent, 57–58
Alexandrite laser. See *Q-switched alexandrite laser*
Alginate(s). See *Calcium alginate(s)*
Algosteril, 29
Allergic reaction(s), 117–118
Allograft(s), definition of, 297

Alopecia, cicatricial, complication from browlift, 596
Alopecia reduction(s) (ARs), 471, *471*, 487
Alpha hydroxy acid(s) (AHAs), as peeling agent, 505, 506–507, 507t
Anaphylaxis, 117–118
Anatomy, browlift, *594*, 595
  ear, 37, 363, *364*
  eyelid, 583–585, *583–585*
  face, 35–43, *36*, *72*, *73*
  facial nerve, 40–42, *41*, *42*, 45, 109, *109*
  forehead, 349–353, *350–353*
  lips, 36–37, 329–331, *330*, *331*
  lymphatics of head, 40, *40*
  mouth, 36–37
  nail, 266–268, *266*, *267*
  neck, 43–45, *44*, *45*
  nose, 37, 381–382, *381*, *382*
  parotid gland and duct, 40, *41*, 110
  periorbital region, 37
  resting/relaxed skin tension lines (RSTLs), 38, *38*, 201, 202, *202*, 211, 253, *253*
  sclerotherapy, 405, *406*
  skin, 495–496
  Superficial Musculoaponeurotic System (SMAS), 38, 211, 212, *213*, 350–352, *350–352*, 357–359, *358*, 595
  temple, 356–359, *356–359*
Anesthesia. See *General anesthesia; Local anesthesia*
Angiofibroma(s), 230–231
Angiogenesis, 11
Angiolipoma(s), 229
Angiosarcoma, 244
Angled iris scissors, 94, *94*
Angular artery, 39, *39*
Angular vein, 39, *39*
Ankle(s), nerve block for, *73*, 74
  sclerotherapy for, 409
Anterior triangle of neck, 44, *44*
Antibacterial ointment(s), 24, 24t
Antibiotic prophylaxis, 60–61, 127, 532–533
Anticoagulant(s), 102
Antihistamine(s), 117–118
Anti-inflammatory drug(s), 102
Apical angle, 187–188, *189*
Appendages, histologic changes in, following tissue expansion, 608
Appose, 82
Arbitration versus litigation, 141
Argon laser, background of, 451
  complications and contraindications for, 452

indications for, 451–452, 451t
  mode and wavelengths of, 446t, 451
  technique of, 452
Argon pumped continuous wave tunable dye laser, background of, 456–457
  complications and contraindications for, 457
  indications for, 457
  mode and wavelengths of, 446t, 456
  technique of, 457
Arteriovenous fistula, as complication of hair replacement, 492
Asian blepharoplasty, 585, 588, *589*
Aspirin, 102
A-to-L plasty, 334, *335*
A-to-T flap, 312, 355, *356*
A-to-T plasty, 334, *336*
Atropine, for cardiac arrest, 120, 121
Atypical fibroxanthoma (AFX), 243
Auricular nerve, *109*, 110
Auriculotemporal nerve, 358, *358*
Australian punch, 89–90, *90*
Autograft(s), definition of, 297
Autoimmune disease, injectable bovine collagen and, 423
Autologous fat grafting. See *Microlipoinjection*
Autologous punch grafting, for stable leukoderma, 286, 288
Avulsion. See *Nail avulsion*
Axial pattern flap(s), 310

Baker phenol chemical peel solution, 505, 506
Baker-Gordon phenol peel, 507–508, 507t, 510, 512
Baldness, classification of, *544*. See also *Hair replacement; Scalp reduction*
Balloon expansion, 606–607, *606*, *607*
Bandage scissors, 96–97, *96*
Band-Aid strip, 25–26
Banner flap, for ear reconstruction, *368–369*, 369
  for nasal reconstruction, 389
  method of, *322*, 323, *323*
Bard-Parker scalpel(s), 85–86, *86*, 522
Basal cell carcinoma (BCC), age of patient, 108
  aggressive-growth basal cell carcinoma, 107
  clinical presentation of, 235
  cryosurgery for, 157–158, *157*, 157t, *158*, 237
  duration of, 105
  electrodesiccation and curettage for, 236–237

Basal cell carcinoma (BCC) (*continued*)
excision for, 237
growth pattern of, 106, 107
high-risk locations of, 236, *236*
histology of, 106, 107, 235–236
imitators of, 107–108
incidence of, 105, 235
infiltrative basal cell carcinoma,
106–107, *106*
lip reconstruction, *343*
locations of, 105, 236, *236*
metastatic basal cell carcinoma, 238
metatypical basal cell carcinoma, 107
micronodular basal cell carcinoma,
106–107, *107*
Mohs micrographic surgery for, 107,
236, 237–238, *237*, 568, 569t
morpheic (morpheaform) basal cell carcinoma, *23*, 107, *107*, 236
nail unit excision, 278
nodular basal cell carcinoma, 106, *106*,
237
perineural spread of, 107
recurrent basal cell carcinoma,
105–106
size of, 105
subclinical extension, 105
superficial basal cell carcinoma, 106,
106
surgical treatment of, 235–238
Base of flap, definition of, 309
Basic life support (BLS), 113
Basting suture(s), buried basting suture,
182, *182*
full-thickness skin graft, 305
interrupted basting suture, 181–182,
182
running basting suture, 182
upper dermal running stitch, 182
BCC. See *Basal cell carcinoma (BCC)*
Beaver scalpel, 86–87, *87*
Benign adnexal neoplasm, 107
Benign cutaneous lesion(s), acrochordons,
224
cryosurgery for, 155t, 156
cysts, 226–232
angiofibromas, 230–231
dermatofibromas, 230, *230*
digital mucoid cysts, 228–229
epidermoid cysts, 227–228, *227*
hidrocystoma, 229
lipomas, 229–230
milia, 229
pilar cysts, 228
sebaceous hyperplasia, 231
steatocystoma multiplex, 228
syringomas, 231, *231*
trichoepithelioma, 231–232
xanthelasma, 232
dermabrasion for, 499
dermatosis papulosa nigra, 225
electrosurgery for, 148–149, *149*, *150*
laser treatment for, 447t, 448, 449t
lentigines, 226
melanocytic nevi, 225–226, *226*
proximal nail fold lesions, 273, *273*

seborrheic keratoses, 224–225
verrucae, 221–224
condylomata acuminata, 223–224
plantar warts, 223
verrucae planae, 222–223
verrucae vulgaris, 222
Benign nail unit tumor(s), acquired digital
fibrokeratoma, 279, *279*
giant cell tumors of the tendon sheath,
279–280
glomus tumors, 279
pterygium, 280, *280*
Benzalkonium chloride, as skin preparation agent, 58
Benzocaine, 66
Beta-blocker(s), 102
Bilateral occipitoparietal flap (BOP flap),
491, 492, 551
Bilobed flap, for nasal reconstruction, 392,
392, *393*
method of, 325–326, *326*, *327*
Biobrane, 29
Biological creep, 605
Biopsy, for malignant melanoma, 241
for nails, 270–271, *270*, *271*
Bipolar forceps, 95, *95*
Birhombic flap, for ear reconstruction,
363, *366–367*
Bi-rhomboid flap, for posterior ear, 379,
380
Birtcher hyfrecator, 95, *95*
Bisected graft, in hair replacement, 471
Bishop-Harmon forceps, *92*, 93
Bitemporal flap (BT flap), *491*, 492, 551,
552
Biterminal modality, 147
Bleeding. See *Postoperative bleeding*
Bleomycin, plantar warts, 223
verrucae vulgaris, 222
Blepharoplasty, anatomy of eyelid,
583–585, *583–585*
before and after photos of, *589*,
597–603
browlift combined with, 594–595
history of, 583
lower lid blepharoplasty, 590–593
anesthesia, 590
before and after photos of, *597–600*
carbon dioxide laser, 593
complications, 593
goals, 590, *590*
operation, 590–593, *590–593*
postoperative care, 593
procedures for operation, 590–593,
591–593
skin markings, 590, *590*
transconjunctival blepharoplasty,
592–593, *593*
patient evaluation, 585
upper lid blepharoplasty, 585–589
anesthesia, 586
Asian blepharoplasty, 585, 588, *589*
before and after photos of, *597–602*
female blepharoplasty, 585
goals of, 585
male blepharoplasty, 585, 588

operation, *585–589*, *586–588*
procedures for operation, *585–589*,
586–588
skin markings, *585*, 586
supratarsal fixation, 588
Blindness, as complication of lower lid
blepharoplasty, 593
Blister formation, and cryosurgery, 161,
161
Blood supply, to face, 39, *39*, 108–109,
109
to nails, 267–268, *267*
to neck, 45
BLS (basic life support), 113
BOP flap, *491*, 492, 551
Bovie electrosurgical unit, 95, 96
Bovine collagen. See *Injectable bovine collagen*
Bowen's disease, 158, *159*, 240
Braided suture(s), 77
Breast augmentation, 431
Bretylium, for cardiac arrest, 121
Browlift, anatomy of, *594*, 595
complications, 596
endoscopic browlift, 597
independent operation versus combina-
tion with face-lift and/or blepharo-
plasty, 594–595
operation, *594*, 595–596, *595*
patient evaluation, 595
planning, *594*
postoperative care, 596
Brown dermatome, 90, *91*, 523–524
Brown-Adson forceps, 92, *92*, 93
BT flap, *491*, 492, 551, *552*
Buccinator muscle, 37
"Bulk" dog-ear(s), 194
Bupivacaine (Marcaine/Sensorcaine), 67t,
68, 476
Buried basting suture, 182, *182*
Buried dermal suture, 177, *177*
Buried horizontal mattress suture, 178,
178
Buried vertical mattress suture, 178–179,
178
Burns(s), as electrosurgery danger,
147–148
Burow's flap, for dog-ear avoidance and
correction, 196, *196*
Burow's graft, for lip reconstruction, 332,
333
for nasal reconstruction, 384, *385*, 386
method of, 306–307, *306–307*
Burow's triangle, for dog-ear avoidance
and correction, 196–197, *197*
for lip reconstruction, 334, *335*, *337*
for nasal reconstruction, 389, *389*, *390*
Burow's wedge advancement flap, 312,
314, *315*
Buttocks, sclerotherapy for, 409

Café au lait macule(s), 461, *461*
Calcium alginate(s), 17, 29, 29t
Cancer. See *Malignant lesion(s); Mohs mi-
crographic surgery*

Candida infection, as complication of dermabrasion, 501
Capsule formation, histologic changes in, following tissue expansion, 608
Carbocaine. See *Mepivacaine (Carbocaine)*
Carbon dioxide laser, background on, 449
  complications and contraindications, 450–451
  for angiofibromas, 231
  for basal cell carcinoma, 238
  for Bowen's disease, 240
  for condylomata acuminata, 224
  for lower lid blepharoplasty, 593
  for matricectomy, 272
  for nail warts, 281
  for plantar warts, 223
  for scalp reduction, 558
  for sebaceous hyperplasia, 231
  for trichoepithelioma, 232
  for verrucae vulgaris, 222
  for xanthelasma, 232
  indications for, 449–450, 449t
  mode and wavelengths of, 446t, 449
  technique of, 450
Carcinoma, adenosquamous carcinoma, 108
  basal cell carcinoma, 105–108, 235–238, *236, 237,* 278
  Merkel's cell carcinoma, 244
  microcystic adnexal carcinoma, 242
  nail unit excision, 278–279, *279*
  sebaceous carcinoma, 242–243, *243*
  squamous cell carcinoma, 108, 238–239, *238,* 278–279, *279*
  verrucous carinoma, 240, *240*
Cardiac disease, 103
Cardiopulmonary resuscitation (CPR), 113, 118–119, *119*
Carotid triangle of neck, 44, *44*
Cartilage, dog-ear formation, 198–199
  nasal cartilage reconstruction, 399
  necrosis of, following cryosurgery, *162,* 163
Cartilage graft, for nasal reconstruction, 386
Castoviejo blade breaker and holder, 86, *86, 87*
Castoviejo needle-holder, 94, *94*
Catacaine, 66
Catgut suture, 78, 79t
Cellulo adipose, 352
Cerebrovascular accident (CVA), 115–116
Cervical nerve(s), *109,* 110
Cervical plexus, 44, 45
Chalazion clamp, 93, *93,* 571–572, *573*
Channeling, 148
Cheek bulk muscle, 37
Chemical disinfection, of instruments, 98
Chemical peel(s), complications of, 514–516
  deep peels, 505–506
  definition of, 505
  depths of, 505–506
  documentation of peeling process, 508

histology of, 506
history of, 505
indications for, 505, 506t, 511–514
  acne, 512–513, *513*
  actinic keratoses, 512
  lentigines, 513–514
  melasma, 513, *514, 515*
  wrinkles, 511–512, *512*
medium peels, 505–506
peeling agents, 505–516
  alpha hydroxy acids (AHAs), 505, 506–507, 507t
  combination peels, 510–511
  factors affecting efficacy of, 508t
  glycolic acid, 505t, 506–507, 509, 512–516
  Jessners' solution, 505t, 510–511, 512, 514
  phenol, 505, 506, 507–508, 510
  popular superficial peeling agents, 505t
  resorcin, 505, 505t, 510t, 511
  retinoic acid, 505t, 510, 512
  salicylic acid, 505
  trichloroacetic acid (TCA), 505, 505t, 506, 507, 509–510, 512–516
planning before procedure, 508
postpeel, 511
superficial peels, 505, 506t, 511–514
  indications for, 505, 506t, 511–514
  popular peeling agents for, 505t
technique, 508–511
  applying glycolic acid peel, 509
  applying Jessner's solution, 511
  applying phenol peel, 510
  applying resorcin, 511
  applying TCA peel, 509–510
  combination peels, 510–511
  planning the peel, 508
  skin preparation, 508–509
Chemiclave, 50t, 51
Chemotherapy, Bowen's disease, 240
Chloral hydrate, 110
Chlorhexidine, as prepeel agent, 508–509
  as skin preparation agent, 58
Chloroprocaine (Nesacaine), 67t, 68
Chondroitin sulfate, 6
Chromic gut suture, 78, 79t
Chronic balloon expansion, 606–607, *606*
Cicatricial alopecia, as complication from browlift, 596
Cigarette smoking, 104
Circumferential excision, *207,* 208
Circumferential scalp reduction, 558
Citanest. See *Prilocaine (Citanest)*
Clamp(s), towel, 96, *96*
Clark's nevus, 225
ClearSite, 28, 28t
Closure(s). See also *Suturing technique(s)*
  cold steel surgery, 167–169, *168, 169*
  combination closures, 184
  forces generated by, 190–191, *190*
  stainless steel staple closure, 183, *183*
  three-dimensional considerations and role of contour, 192–193, *192, 193*

vertical dynamics of, 193, *193*
  wound closure tapes, 183–184, *184*
Closure material(s), suture materials, 77–80
  absorbable sutures, 78–79, 79t
  catgut, 78, 79t
  characteristics of, 77–78
  cotton, 80
  future trends in, 80
  natural versus synthetic, 78
  nonabsorbable sutures, 78, 80, 80t
  nylon, 80, 80t
  polybutester, 80, 80t
  polydioxanone, 78–79, 79t
  polyester, 80, 80t
  polyglactin 910, 78–79, 79t
  polyglycolic acid, 78–79, *79,* 79t
  polyglyconate, 78–79, 79t
  polypropylene, 80, 80t
  silk, 80, 80t
  size of, 78
  stainless steel, 80
  suture needles, 80–81, *81*
  sutureless materials, 81–83
    cyanoacrylate glues, 82
    fibrin glues, 82
    staples, 82–83
    tissue glues, 81–82
    wound closure tapes, 82
Cloth packing, for instruments, 49
Clothing, for health-care personnel, 60
CO_2 laser. See *Carbon dioxide laser*
Cocaine, 66, 67t, 68
Cold steel surgery, closure, 167–169, *168, 169*
  closure of skin surface, 168–169, *169*
  commencing the closure, 168, *168*
  ellipse used in, 165–166, *165, 166,* 166t
  patient communication and, 169–170
  surgical method, 166–167, *167*
  undermining, 167, *167*
Cold sterilization, 50t, 51
Collagen. See also *Injectable bovine collagen*
  flexibility of, 212
  Gly-X-Y sequence in, 1
  origin of term, 1
  production of, 2, *2*
  Type I collagen, 2, *2, 3,* 8, 212
  Type III collagen, 2, 4, 212
  Type IV collagen, 2–4, *3,* 8
  Type V collagen, 4
  Type VI collagen, 4
  Type VII collagen, 4, *4*
  Type XII collagen, 4
  Type XIV collagen, 4
  Type XVII collagen, 4
Columella, reconstruction of, 398
Combination closure(s), 184
Combination peel(s), 510–511
Come-and-go vessel(s), 409
Comparative negligence, 139–140
Complaint, 141
Complementary flap, for torn earlobes, 580, *580*

Composite graft, definition of, 297
for nasal reconstruction, 386
Compression hosiery, for sclerotherapy, 414
Concha, reconstruction of, 374, *374–376*
Condylomata acuminata, 223–224
Condylox, 223–224
Cone(s), 132, 189–190, *189, 190, 197, 198,* 203
Conjunctival edema, as complication of lower lid blepharoplasty, 593
Contact dermatitis, treatment of, 130, *130*
Contaminating flora, 57
Contour line(s), 209–210, *210,* 219
Contractual relationship, between physician and patient, 138
Contributory negligence, 139–140
Copper vapor laser (CVL), background of, 455–456
complications and contraindications for, 456
indications for, 456
mode and wavelength of, 446t, 455
technique of, 456
Coronal browlift. See *Browlift*
Corrugator supercilii muscle, 37, *350, 351, 351*
Corticosteroid(s), 103, 117–118
Corynebacterium, 57
Cotton suture, 80
Coverstrip, 82
CPR (cardiopulmonary resuscitation), 113, 118–119, *119*
Cranial nerve(s), 109–110, *109*
Crescentic ellipse, 204–205, *204–205*
Critical margin, 564, *565*
Crus of helix, reconstruction of, 369, *370–371*
Cryoanesthesia, 65–66, 65t
Cryosurgery, advantages, side-effects, and disadvantages of, 161–163, *161, 162*
dipstick method, 155–156
equipment for, 155–156, *157*
for basal cell carcinoma, 157–158, *157,* 157t, *158,* 237
for benign lesions, 155t, 156
for condylomata acuminata, 223
for digital mucoid cysts, 229
for ingrown nail, 276, *276*
for lentigines, 226
for lentigo maligna and lentigo maligna melanoma, 160, *160*
for malignant lesions, 156–161, *157–161,* 157t
for nail warts, 280
for sebaceous hyperplasia, 231
for seborrheic keratoses, 225
for squamous cell carcinoma, 158, *159,* 160, *161,* 239
for verrucae planae, 223
for verrucae vulgaris, 222
for verrucous carcinoma, 240
indications for, 154t, 155t, 157t
mechanism of damage due to cold injury, 153–155

methods of, 155–156
palliation, 160–161
spot freeze technique, 156
Curettage. See also *Electrodesiccation and curettage (ED&C)*
for dermatosis papulosa nigra, 225
for sebaceous hyperplasia, 231
for seborrheic keratoses, 224–225
for trichoepithelioma, 232
Curette(s), 90, *90*
Cutaneous forehead, 349
Cutaneous squamous cell carcinoma, 108
Cutinova Plus, 27
Cutting instrument(s). See *Instrumentation and equipment*
Cutting needle(s), 81
CVA (cerebrovascular accident), 115–116
CVL. See *Copper vapor laser (CVL)*
Cyanoacrylate glue(s), 82
Cyst(s), angiofibromas, 230–231
complication of full-thickness skin graft, 307
dermatofibromas, 230, *230*
digital mucoid cysts, 228–229
epidermoid cysts, 227–228, *227*
hidrocystoma, 229
lipomas, 229–230
milia, 229
myxoid cysts, 273–274, *274*
pilar cysts, 228
sebaceous hyperplasia, 231
steatocystoma multiplex, 228
syringomas, 231, *231*
trichoepithelioma, 231–232
xanthelasma, 232
Cytokine(s), clinical trials of growth factors in wound healing, 12t, 13
cytokine modulation of cell proliferation and migration, 11
effects of cytokines on extracellular matrix gene expression, 9, 10t
mechanistic interactions between growth factor, 10
modulation of degradative events by, 10
pathway of normal wound repair, 9
regulation of angiogenesis by, 11
release of, due to platelet aggregation, 8
relevance of in vitro observation to wound healing in vivo, 11–12, 11t
Cytotoxic agent(s), 103

Dana's procedure, for epidermoid cysts, 228
Davidson Marking System, in Mohs micrographic surgery, 563–564
Davol dermatome, for split-thickness skin graft (STSG), 523
Davol-Simon dermatome, 90–91, *91*
Debulking excision, in Mohs micrographic surgery, 562
Decorin, 4, 6
Deep galae aponeurotica, 352, *352*
Deep peel(s). See *Chemical peel(s)*
Deep subcutaneous suture, 177–178, *177*
Deep temporal fascia, 359

Defibrillation, 119–120, *120*
Dehiscence, treatment of, 131, *131*
Delayed grafting, 305–306
Delayed primary closure, Mohs micrographic surgery, 567
Delayed wound healing, 13–14, 14t
Depressed scar(s), 132
Depressor anguli oris muscle, 36
Depressor labii inferioris muscle, 36
Depressor septi muscle, 37
Dermabrasion, acquired immunodeficiency virus and, 497–498
anatomy and healing in dermatology, 495–496
anesthesia, 500–501
before and after photos, *496–502*
complications, 501
for angiofibromas, 231
for sebaceous hyperplasia, 231
instrumentation for, 53, 97, *97,* 499–500
occlusive dressings used in, 495–496
patient selection and indications for, 495t, 496–499
technique of, 500–503
tretinoin applied preoperatively, 495, *496*
Dermal dendrocyte(s), 9
Dermal extracellular matrix, collagen, 1–4, *2–4*
cytokine effects on, 9, 10t
elastic fibers, 4–6, *5–6*
extracellular matrix deposition, 7
fibronectin, 7
glycosaminoglycans, 6–7, *7*
proteoglycans, 6–7, *7*
Derma-Prep, 25t
Dermatitis, contact, 130, *130*
Dermatofibroma(s), 230, *230*
Dermatofibrosarcoma protuberans (DFSP), 230, 242, *242*
Dermatoheliosis, 127–128
Dermatology, anatomy and healing in, 495–496
liposuction and, 530
Dermatome(s), 90–91, *91,* 523–524, *524*
Dermatosis papulosa nigra, 225
Dermis, histologic changes in, following tissue expansion, 608
Dermistik, 25, 25t
Dexon suture, 78–79, *79,* 79t
DFSP (dermatofibrosarcoma protuberans), 230, 242, *242*
Diabetes mellitus, 104
Diazepam, 110
Digit(s), pressure dressings for, 32
Digital mucoid cyst(s), 228–229
Dipstick method, of cryosurgery, 155–156
Discoloration of graft(s), as complication of hair replacement, 490
Discovery rule, 140
Disinfection of instruments, 98
Displacement force(s), in wound closure, 190–192, *190–192*
Distal nail tip excision, 275, *275*

Distant flap(s), 309
Ditigal nerve block, 72
Dog-ear(s), "bulk" dog-ears, 194
  Burow's flap for avoidance and correction of, 196, *196*
  Burow's triangle and multiple excisions for avoidance and correction of, 196–197, *197*
  complex wounds, 197–199
    cartilage, 198–199
    rotation flap, 197, *197*
    S-shaped wounds, 198
    transposition flap, 197, *197*
  corrective action for, 197–198, 199
  ellipse excision, 203
  formed by elliptical closure, 165, *165*
  geometric classification of, 189–190, *189, 190*
  geometry of wound in horizontal plane, 187–189, *188, 189*
  M-plasty for avoidance and correction of, 195–196
  "rubber duck" technique for avoidance and correction of, 196–197, *197*
  surgical technique, 193–195
    preoperative planning, 194
    suturing technique, 194–195, *195*
    tension and tension avoidance, 193–194
    undermining, 194
    wound depth, 194, *194*
  three-dimensional considerations and role of contour, 192–193, *192, 193*
  tissue dynamics and, 190–192, *190–192*
  treatment of, 132
  wound design and, 188–189
Doppler examination, 414
Dorsal nasal flap, 387, *388*
Dorsum, reconstruction of, 397–398
Double rotation flap, 319, *321*
Drain(s), 127, 128, *129*
Drapes, 59
Dressing(s), adhesive bandages, 25–26
  antibacterial ointments for, 24, 24t
  biobrane, 29
  characteristics of ideal dressing, 24, 24t
  composite dressing, 24–25
  growth dressings, 30
  history of, 23
  occlusive dressings, 14–17, 23, 26–29
    calcium alginates, 17, 29, 29t
    characteristics of, 26, 26t
    gels and hydrogels, 15–16, 28, 28t
    hydrocolloid dressings, 16–17, 28–29, 28t
    polymer films, 15, 26–27, 26t, 27t
    polymer foams, 15, 26t, 27–28
    tissue repair and, 17
    topical agents and, 17
    trade names of dressings, 16t
    wound bacteriology and, 17
  pressure dressings, 30–32
    digits, 32
    ear, 31, *32*

eyelids, 32
  nose, 31–32, *32*
  scalp, 30–31, *31*
  scrotum, 32
surgical adhesive tapes for, 25
tactifiers, 25, 25t
techniques of, 30
trade names of, 16t
Drug reaction(s), in medical history, 101, 113–114
Drug toxicity. See *Toxicity*
Dry eye, as complication of lower lid blepharoplasty, 593
Dry heat sterilization, 50t, 51, 98
Dry technique of liposuction, 535
DuoDERM, 28, 28t, 29
Duplex scanning, 414
Duranest. See *Etidocaine (Duranest)*
Dysplastic nevi, 225

Ear(s), anatomy of, 37, 363, *364*
  muscle of, 37
  pressure dressings for, 31, *32*
Ear piercing, 579–580
Ear reconstruction, anatomy of ear, 363, *364*
  combined defects, 374, *376–379*, 377–378
  concha, 374, *374–376*
  lobule, *368–370*, 369
  lower antihelix, *373*, 374
  posterior ear, 379, *379–380*
  posterior-middle helical rim, 363, 365, *367–368*, 369
  scaphoid fossa and triangular fossa of antihelix, 369, *371–373*, 374
  superior helical rim, 363, *364–367*
  tragus and crus of helix, 369, *370–371*
Ear tumor(s), Mohs micrographic surgery for, 572, *574–575*, 575
Earlobe repair
  absence of earlobe, 580–581, *581*
  completely torn earlobes, 580
  earlobe augmentation, 582, *582*
  enlarged holes, 580
  island-flap method, 581–582, *582*
  postauricular flap, 581
  preauricular flap for, 580, *580*, *582*
  reverse-contoured flap, 581
  U-flap, 581, *581*
ED&C. See *Electrodesiccation and curettage (ED&C)*
Edema, as complication of hair replacement, 490
  as complication of lower lid blepharoplasty, 593
  as complication of scalp reduction, 559
  cryosurgery, 161
  microlipoinjection and, 442
EGF (epidermal growth factor), 8
Elastic fiber(s), 4–6, *5–6*, 212
Elastic force(s), in wound closure, *190*, 191
Elastic support garment(s), after tumescent liposuction, 539

Elasticity, definition of, 212
  in wound closure, 192
Elastin, 5, *5*
Elaunin fiber(s), 5
Elective incision line(s). See *Coutour line(s); Skin tension line(s) (STLs)*
Electric dermatome(s), for split-thickness skin graft (STSG), 523–524, *524*
Electrocautery, 145–146, 167
Electrocoagulation device(s), 95–96, *95, 96*
Electrocution, as electrosurgery danger, 148
Electrode(s), for electrosurgery, 52, *52*
Electrodesiccation, for acrochordons, 224
  for seborrheic keratoses, 225
  for verrucae planae, 223
Electrodesiccation and curettage (ED&C), for basal cell carcinoma, 236–237
  for Bowen's disease, 240
  for squamous cell carcinoma, 239
  for verrucae vulgaris, 222
Electrolysis, 145
Electron microscopy, 405, 407
Electrosurgery, characteristics of high-frequency electrosurgery, 146t
  clinical applications, 148–151
    benign lesions, 148–149, *149, 150*
    hemostasis, 149, *150*, 151
    malignant lesions, 151
  dangers with high-frequency electrosurgery, 147–148
    burns and ignition, 147–148
    electrocution, 148
    pacemakers, 148
  electrocautery, 145–146, 167
  equipment for, 52–53, *52, 53*
  for hidrocystoma, 229
  for matricectomy, 272
  for nail warts, 281
  galvanic surgery, 145
  physics of high-frequency electrosurgery, 146–147, 146t
  techniques of high-frequency electrosurgery, 147
Ellipse, in cold steel surgery, 165–166, *165, 166*, 166t
  standard ellipse, 202–203, *203*
Ellipse excision, circumferential excision, 207, 208
  crescentic ellipse, 204–205, *204–205*
  M-plasty, *206–207*, 207–208
  S-plasty, 205, *206*, 207
  standard ellipse, 202–203, *203*
Emergency(ies). See *Perioperative emergency(ies)*
Emergency medications, 122, 122t
EMLA (eutectic mixture of local anesthetics), 66, 110
EMPD (extramammary Paget's disease), 243–244, *243*
Endoscopic browlift, 597
Endotracheal intubatin, 119
Enucleation, epidermoid cysts, 227–228, *227*
Epidermal growth factor (EGF), 8

Epidermis, histologic changes in, following tissue expansion, 608
Epidermoid cyst(s), 227–228, *227*
Epigard, 27
Epinephrine, allergic reactions treated by, 117
  cardiac arrest treated by, 120, 121
  concentration of, in mixing with local anesthetic, 68
  contraindications for, 70, 117
  hair replacement, 476
  lip reconstruction, 330
  midline scalp reduction, 546
  punch graft, 288
  recipe for tumescent liposuction anesthetic solution, 533, 533t
  scalp reduction, 546, 549, 550, 552, 554
  toxicity of, 60–61, 117
Epithelialized tunnel(s) or sinuses, excision of, 286, *287, 293,* 294
Epithelioma adenoides cysticum, 231
Equipment. See *Instrumentation and equipment*
Eruptive hidradenoma of Darier en Jaquet, 231, *231*
Eruptive syringoma(s), 231, *231*
Erythema, as complication of chemical peels, 514–516
  as complication of dermabrasion, 501
  cryosurgery, 161
Erythroplasia of Queyrat, 158, *159*
Etidocaine (Duranest), 67t, 68
Eutectic mixture of local anesthetics (EMLA), 66, 110
Evaluation of patients. See *Preoperative patient evaluation*
Excess tissue. See *Dog-ear(s)*
Excision. See also *Fusiform excision and variations*
  distal nail tip excision, 275, *275*
  epithelialized tunnels or sinuses, 286, *287, 293,* 294
  for acrochordons, 224
  for angiofibromas, 230–231
  for basal cell carcinoma, 237
  for Bowen's disease, 240
  for condylomata acuminata, 223
  for digital mucoid cysts, 229
  for epidermoid cysts, 227–228, *227*
  for hidrocystoma, 229
  for ice-pick scar, 286, *287,* 289
  for lipomas, 229–230
  for melanocytic nevi, 225–226
  for nails, 270–272, *270, 271,* 278–279, *279*
  for sebaceous hyperplasia, 231
  for seborrheic keratoses, *224,* 225
  for verrucous carcinoma, 240
  for xanthelasma, 232
  in Mohs micrographic surgery, 561–562
  lateral nail fold excision, 274–275, *275*
  nail unit excision and carcinoma, 278–279, *279*

partial nail unit excision, 271–272, *271*
punch excision with full-thickness autologous punch graft replacement, 284–288, 285t, *286, 287*
punch excision without autografting, 284, 284t
shave excision, *224,* 225
Excision from a distance, for lipomas, 230
Exostosis, 277
Extended glabellar flap, nasal reconstruction, 387, *388*
Extensibility, definition of, 212
Extensive scalp-lifting, *545,* 551, *552*
Extracellular matrix. See *Dermal extracellular matrix*
Extraction, of milia, 229
Extramammary Paget's disease (EMPD), 243–244, *243*
Extravasation ulcer(s), as complication of sclerotherapy, 412
Eye protection, for health-care personnel, 60
Eyebrow(s), 349, *350,* 351, *351*
Eyebrow fat pad, 352, *352*
Eyelid(s). See also *Lower eyelid(s); Upper eyelid(s)*
  anatomy of, 583–585, *583–585*
  pressure dressings for, 32
Eyelid surgery. See *Blepharoplasty*
Eyelid tumor(s), excision of, at free margin, 218, *219*
  Mohs micrographic surgery for, 571–572, *571, 573*

Face. See also *Ear(s); Eyebrow(s); Eyelid(s); Forehead; Nose*
  anatomy of, 35–43, *36,* 72, 73
  blood supply of, 39, *39,* 108–109, *109*
  local anesthesia for, 72–73, *72*
  lymphatics of, 40, *40*
  muscles of, 36–37, *36,* 213, *213, 214, 215*
  nerves of, 40–43, *41–43,* 72–73, *72,* 109, 109–110, *109*
  sclerotherapy for, 409
  surface anatomy of, 35, *36*
Facial artery, 39, *39*
Facial edema, as complication of scalp reduction, 559
Facial nerve, 40–42, *41, 42,* 45, 109, *109*
Facial vein, 39, *39*
Fast Absorbing Gut, 78
Fat, eyebrow fat pad, 352, *352*
  histologic changes in, following tissue expansion, 608
Fat grafting. See *Microlipoinjection*
"Feeders gone, spiders remain" (FGSR) phenomenon, 414, *415*
Feet. See *Foot (feet)*
Female blepharoplasty, 585
FGSR. See *"Feeders gone, spiders remain" (FGSR) phenomenon*
Fibrel, indications for, 424–425
  product and its mechanisms, 424, *425*

  side effects and complications, 426–427
  technique, 425–426
Fibrillin(s), 5–6, *5*
Fibrin, 8
Fibrin foam, 424
Fibrin glue(s), 82
Fibroblast(s), 8, 10
Fibroepithelial polyps, 224
Fibronectin, 7, 8
Fibroxanthoma, atypical, 243
Field block, 71–72
Fitzpatrick skin type, and chemical peels, 505, 508, 577/585
  pulsed dye laser, 446t, 452–455
Flap(s). See *specific types of flap*
Flap surgery, advancement flaps, 310–317, *311–317*
  checklist for selection of flap closure, 327–328
  classification of flaps, 309–310
  definitions concerning, 309
  lip reconstruction for partial-thickness wounds, 331–341, *332–342*
  rotation flaps, 310, 317–319, *317–321*
  selection of flap closure, 326–328
  transposition flaps, 310, 319, 322–326, *322–327*
Flash sterilization, 98
Flat wart(s), 222–223
5–Fluorouracil, for actinic kratoses, 512
Follow-up visits, 127
Foot (feet), nerves of, 74, *74*
  sclerotherapy for, 409
Force vectors, in wound closure, *190, 191, 191*
Forceps, 92–93, *92, 93, 95, 95*
Forehead, anatomy of, 349–353, *350–353*
  corrugator supercilii muscle of, *350, 351, 351*
  cutaneous forehead and eyebrow, 349
  deep galae aponeurotica, 352, *352*
  eyebrow fat pad, 352, *352*
  frontalis muscle of, *350, 351, 351*
  muscular layer of, 351, *351*
  orbicularis oculi muscle of, *350,* 351, *351*
  pericranium, 353
  procerus muscle of, *350, 351, 351*
  relaxed skin tension lines of, 357, *357*
  subcutaneous forehead and eyebrow, 349, *350*
  subgaleal space, 352–353, *352, 353*
  superficial galea aponeurotica, 351
  superficial musculoaponeurotic system of, 350–352, *350–352*
Forehead flap, for nasal reconstruction, 395, *395–396,* 397
Forehead reconstruction, advancement flaps for, 354–355, *354–356*
  anatomy of forehead, 349–353, *350–353*
  island pedicle flaps for, 355, *356*
  primary fusiform closure for, 354, *354*
  rotation flaps for, 355
  secondary intention, 355–356, *357*

skin grafts for, 356
tissue expansion for, 355
transposition flaps for, 355
Foreign body reaction, as complication of scalp reduction, 559
Fox currette, 90, 90
Fragile vein syndrome, 415–416
Fraise(s), for dermabrasion, 53, 97, 97
Frazier hook, 92
Free cartilage graft, for nasal reconstruction, 386
Free flap(s), 309–310
Freeze-thaw cycle (FTC), 156
Frontalis muscle, 350, 351, 351
Frontonasal flap, 387, 388
Fruit acid(s). See Alpha hydroxy acid(s) (AHAs); Glycolic acid
FTC (freeze-thaw cycle), 156
FTSG. See Full-thickness skin graft (FTSG)
Full-thickness flap (FTP), for scaphoid fossa and triangular fossa of antihelix, 369, 371–373, 374
Full-thickness graft (FTG)
    for concha, 374, 374–375
    for lower antihelix, 373, 374
Full-thickness lip defect(s), 341, 343, 343–346
Full-thickness skin graft (FTSG), advantages and disadvantages of, 298
    basting sutures for, 305
    Burow's grafts, 306–307, 306–307
    complications of, 307
    definition of, 297
    delayed grafting, 305–306
    donor site selection, 298
    failure of, 307
    for lip reconstruction, 332, 333–334
    for nasal reconstruction, 383–386, 384, 385, 385t
    indications for, 298
    perioperative management, 304–305
    physiology of, 297–298
    surgical technique, 298–300, 300–304
Fusiform closure, for forehead reconstruction, 354, 354
    for lip reconstruction, 334
    for temple reconstruction, 359, 361
Fusiform excision and variations, circumferential excision, 207, 208
    crescentic ellipse, 204–205, 204–205
    ellipse excision, 202–208, 203
    M-plasty, 206–207, 207–208 preoperative evaluation, 201–202
    relaxed skin tension lines (RSTLs), 201, 202, 202
    S-plasty, 205, 206, 207

Galeotomy, 558
Gallium-arsenide laser, 446t, 464
Galvanic surgery, 145
GAP repair technique, 424
Gas sterilization, 50t, 51, 98
Gel(s), for occlusive dressings, 15–16, 28, 28t

General anesthesia, versus local anesthesia for tumescent liposuction, 530–531, 535–536
Geometric broken line, 260, 260
Geometric classification, of dog-ears, 189–190, 189, 190
Giant cell tumor(s) of the tendon sheath, 279–280
Glabellar rotation flap, for nasal reconstruction, 387, 388
Glabellar turn-down flap, 323, 323
Glomus tumor(s), 279
Glove(s), 59
Glue(s), cyanoacrylate glues, 82
    fibrin glues, 82
    tissue glues, 81–82
Glycolic acid, applying, in chemical peel, 509
    as peeling agent, 505t, 506–507
    for acne, 512–513
    for actinic keratoses, 512
    for lentigines, 514
    for melasma, 513
    for wrinkles, 512
Glycosaminoglycan(s), 6–7, 7
Gly-X-Y sequence, 1
Gold vapor laser, background of, 458
    complications and contraindications for, 458–459
    indications for, 458
    mode and wavelength of, 446t, 458
    technique of, 458
Gradle scissors, 88, 88, 94
Graefe forceps, 93
Graft elevation, as complication of hair replacement, 490
Grafting. See Full-thickness skin graft (FTSG); air replacement; Microlipoinjection; Punch graft; Split-thickness skin graft (STSG)
Granuloma, and liquid silicone, 431, 432
Growth dressing(s), 30
Gut suture, 78, 79t
Guthrie hook, 92, 92

Hair follical damage, by cryosurgery, 162, 163
Hair removal, for infection control, 59
Hair replacement, age and, 476
    alopecia reductions (ARs), 471, 471, 487
    anesthesia for, 476
    bandages used in, 489, 489, 490
    before and after photographs, 473–475, 482–485, 588
    blond hair, 471, 473
    cleaning and insertion of grafts, 489–490, 489, 490
    coarse, dark and/or dense hair, 485–488
    donor site for, 476–483, 477, 478, 480, 481
    early transplanting, 472, 474
    female patients, 474, 475, 476

fine-textured and less dense hair, 482–484, 483–485
hairpieces used after, 476
minigrafting, 470–471, 471
    micrografting, 470
    round minigrafting, 470, 488–489
    slit grafting, 470–471, 487–489
Negroid-type hair, 471, 474
planning of, 471–476, 472–475
postoperative complications, 490–492
    arteriovenous fistula, 492
    cicatricial alopecia, 491, 492
    discoloration of grafts, 490
    edema, 490
    graft elevation, 490
    hematoma, 491
    hypertrophic scarring, 492
    hypoesthesia, 490–491
    infection, 492
    keloidal healing, 492
    mild pruritus, 490
    osteomyelitis, 492
    postoperative bleeding, 492
preoperative instructions for, 476
"prone pillow" for, 471, 471
recipient area, 482–486, 483–489, 488
scalp reducation before or after, 545
schematic drawing of typical density distribution, 486–487, 486
standard round grafting, 469, 470
straight Caucasian hair, 471, 474
U-shaped recipient area in, 469, 470
white and salt-and-pepper hair, 471, 473
Hairpiece(s), after hair replacement, 476
Half-buried horizontal mattress suture, 176, 176
Halsted hemostat, 95, 95
Hand washing, in operating room, 58–59
HBV (hepatitis B virus), 54, 60, 82, 86, 98, 104–105
HCD (hydrocolloids), 16–17, 28–29, 28t
Head. See Ear(s); Eyebrow(s); Eyelid(s); Forehead; Face; Nose
Healing. See Wound healing
Health maintenance organization(s) (HMOs), 141
Helical rim advancement flap, 363, 365, 367–368, 369
Helium-neon laser, 446t, 464
Hemangioma, argon laser treatment for, 451–452
    pulsed dye laser treatment for, 454
Hematoma, as complication of browlift, 596
    as complication of hair replacement, 491–492
    as complication of liposuction, 540
    as complication of scalp reduction, 559
    as complication of split-thickness skin graft (STSG), 527
    as complication of tissue expansion, 609
    subungual hematoma, 272
    treatment of, 129, 129
Hemorrhage, 114–115

Hemostasis, electrosurgery for, 149, *150*, 151
  Mohs micrographic surgery, 562
  punch graft, 292
Hemostat(s), 95, *95*
Hemostatic instrument(s), electrocoagulation devices, 95–96, *95, 96*
  hemostats, 95, *95*
Hepatitis B virus (HBV), 54, 60, 82, 86, 98, 104–105
Herpes simplex, as complication of chemical peels, 514–516
  as complication of dermabrasion, 501
  as complication of injectable bovine collagen, 422
Hexachlorophene, as skin preparation agent, 58
Hidrocystoma, 229
High-frequency. See *Electrosurgery*
Hip(s), sclerotherapy for, 409
Histiocytoma, 243
Histology, of chemical peels, 506
HIV (human immunodeficiency virus), 54, 60, 82, 86, 98, 104–105, 142
HMO(s) (health maintenance organizations), 141
Horizontal mattress suture, 175–176, *175, 176*
H-plasty, 312, *314*
HPV (human papilloma virus), 221–222
Human immunodeficiency virus (HIV), 54, 60, 82, 86, 98, 104–105, 142. See also *Acquired immunodeficiency virus (AIDS)*
Human papilloma virus (HPV), 221–222
Hyaluronic acid, 6
Hydrocolloid(s) (HCD), 16–17, 28–29, 28t
Hydrocortisone sodium succinate, 118
Hydrogel(s), 15–16, 28, 28t
Hydroquinone, 226
Hydroxypolyethoxydodecane, as sclerosant, 410
Hyperpigmentation, as complication from pigmented lesion dye laser, 462
  as complication of chemical peels, 514–516
  as complication of dermabrasion, 501
  as complication of pulsed dye laser, 455
  as complication of Q-switched ruby laser, 460
  cryosurgery and, 163
Hypertonic saline, as sclerosant, 410
Hypertrophic scarring, as complication of carbon dioxide laser, 450–451
  as complication of chemical peels, 514–516
  as complication of hair replacement, 492
  treatment of, 133, 261, *263*
Hypertrophy, as complication of full-thickness skin graft, 307
Hypesthesia, as disadvantage of scalp-lift, 551

Hypnotic(s), 64, 64t
Hypoesthesia, as complication of hair replacement, 490–491
Hypopigmentation, as complication from pigmented lesion dye laser, 462
  as complication of Q-switched ruby laser, 460
  cryosurgery and, 163, *163*
Hysensitivity reaction, complication of injectable bovine collagen, 422–423

Ice-pick scar, excision of, 286, *287, 289*
Ignition, 147–148
Immediate balloon expansion, 607, *607*
Immunosuppressive agent(s), 103
Infection, as complication of dermabrasion, 501
  as complication of hair replacement, 492
  as complication of injectable bovine collagen, 422
  as complication of tissue expansion, 608–609
  as complications after split-thickness skin graft (STSG), 527
  treatment of, 129–130, *130*
Infection control, drapes, 59
  gloves, 59
  hair removal, 59
  operating room protocols, 61, 61t
  prophylactic antibiotics, 60–61
  skin preparation, 57
  skin preparation agents, 57–58
    alcohols, 57–58
    benzalkonium chloride, 58
    chlorhexidine, 58
    hexachlorophene, 58
    iodine and iodophor, 58
  surgical scrubbing, 58–59
  universal precautions, 60
Infectious disease(s), in medical history, 104–105
Infiltrative basal cell carcinoma, 106–107, *106*
Informed consent, 138–139
Infraorbital nerve, 73
Ingrown nail, 276, *276*
Inhalant(s), 64–64, *64*
Injectable anesthetics. See *Local anesthesia*
Injectable bovine collagen, adverse treatment responses, 422–423
  formulations, 419–420
  injectable collagen implant and autoimmune disease, 423
  maintenance of correction and fate of implant, 421–422
  patient selection and skin testing, 420
  technique of injection, 420–421, *420–422*
Injectable tissue augmentation, 419
Inner knee, sclerotherapy for, 407, 409
Instrument tie, 171, *172*

Instrumentation and equipment. See also *Sterilization of equipment; and specific instruments*
  bandage scissors, 96–97, *96*
  care of instruments, 97–98
  chemical disinfection of, 98
  cleaning of surgical instruments, 48, *48*, 98
  construction of surgical instruments, 47–48, *48*
  cryosurgery, 155–156, *157*
  cutting instruments, 85–91
    curettes, 90, *90*
    dermatomes, 90–91, *91*
    punches, 89–90, *89, 90*
    scalpels, 85–88, *86, 87*
    tissue-cutting scissors, 88–89, *88, 89*
  dermabrasion, 53, 97, *97*, 499–500
  electrocautery, 146
  electrosurgery, 52–53, *52, 53*
  hemostatic instruments
    electrocoagulation devices, 95–96, *95, 96*
    hemostats, 95, *95*
  instrument packing, 48–50, *49, 50*
  laser equipment, 53
  ligation/cauterization of occipital arteries, 552
  local anesthesia, 70–71, *71*, 71t
  lubrication of joints of instruments, 98
  luster or satin finish for instruments, 47
  midline scalp reduction, 546
  Mohs micrographic surgery, 571–572, *573, 576*
  nail surgery, 268–269, *269*
  needles, 70–71, 71t
  paramedian or lateral scalp reduction pattern, 550
  perioperative emergencies, 121–122, 121t, 122t
  periosteal elevators, 97, *97*
  punch graft, 288
  scalp lift technique, 554
  split-thickness skin graft (STSG), 522
  storage of instruments, 51
  surgical tray setup, 51–52
  suturing instruments, 93–95
    needle-holders, 47, *48*, 93–94, *94*
    staplers, 94–95, *94*
    suture-cutting scissors, 94, *94*
  syringes, 70, *71*
  tissue-holding instruments, 92–93
    chalazion clamp, 93, *93*
    forceps, 92–93, *92, 93*
    skin hooks, 92, *92*
  towel clamps, 96, *96*
  undermining instruments, 91–92, *91*
  Y or Mercedes scalp reduction pattern, 549
Internal carotid system, 109
Interrupted basting suture, 181–182, *182*
Interrupted subcutaneous suture, 176–179, *177, 178*
Interrupted suture(s), buried dermal suture, 177, *177*

buried horizontal mattress suture, 178, *178*

buried vertical mattress suture, 178–179, *178*

deep subcutaneous suture, 177–178, *177*

half-buried horizontal mattress suture, 176, *176*

horizontal mattress suture, 175–176, *175, 176*

interrupted subcutaneous suture, 176–179, *177, 178*

simple interrupted suture, 173, *173*

vertical mattress suture, 173–175, *174*

Intertemporal-fascial plane, 359

Intraoperative sustained limited expansion (ISLE), 607, *607*, 608, 609, 614–615

Inverted cone(s), 189–190, *189, 190*

Iodine, as skin preparation agent, 58

Iodophor, as skin preparation agent, 58

Iontophoresis, 66, 145

Iris scissors, 88, *88*, 94, *94*

Ischemia, as complication of tissue expansion, 609

Island graft, 306–307, *306–307*

Island pedicle flap, for earlobe repair, 581–582, *582*

   for forehead reconstruction, 355, *356*

   for nasal reconstruction, 392, 395

   for skin reconstruction, 336, 339, *339*, 341, *342*

   method of, 312, *316*, 317, *317*

   skin flaps, 392, 395

ISLE (intraoperative sustained limited expansion), 607, *607*, 608, 609, 614–615

Isthmus catagen cyst(s), 228

JC-5 Tape Adherent, 25t

Jessners' solution, as peeling agent, 505t, 511

   as prepeel agent, 508, 508t

   for lentigines, 514

   for wrinkles, 512

   in combination peels, 510–511, 512

   preparation of, 508t

Jeweler's forceps, *92*, 93, 95

Karapandzic flap, 343, *345*

Kaye scissors, 91–92, *91*

Keloid(s), treatment of, 133

Keloidal healing, as complication of hair replacement, 492

Keratinocyte migration, 7–8

Keratoacanthoma, 240, *240*

Keratoses simplex, 514

Key suture, definition of, 309

Keyes punch, 89

Knee, sclerotherapy for inner knee, 407, 409

Knot security, of suture, 77–78

Laboratory procedures, in Mohs micrographic surgery, 564–565, *565, 566*, 576

   in sclerotherapy, 414

Laceration(s), of nails, 280, *280*

Lagophthalmos, as complication of lower lid blepharoplasty, 593

Lalonde forceps, 92

Laminin, 8

Langer's line(s). See *Skin tension line(s)*

Lap-joint principle, for torn earlobes, 580, *580*

Laser(s). See also *Carbon dioxide laser*

   acronym meaning, 445

   argon laser, 446t, 451–452, 451t

   argon pumped continuous wave tunable dye laser, 446t, 456–457

   carbon dioxide laser, 446t, 449–451

   copper vapor laser, 446t, 455–456

   equipment, 53

   for sclerotherapy, 409

   future of, in dermatology, 464

   gallium-arsenide laser, 446t, 464

   gold vapor laser, 446t, 458–459

   helium-neon laser, 446t, 464

   history of, 445

   laser-tissue interactions, 445–446

   lesions treatable by laser, 446–449

     benign lesions, 447t, 448, 449t

     malignant and premalignant lesions, 447t, 448–449, 449t

     pigmented lesions, 447–448, 447t, 449t, 451t

     vascular lesions, 446–447, 447t, 449t, 451t

   low-energy laser systems, 464

   neodymium:yttrium-aluminum-garnet laser, 446t, 462–463, *463*

   photodynamic therapy with tunable dye laser, 457–458

   properties of, 445

   pulsed dye laser, 446t, 452–455

   pulsed (dye) pigmented laser, 446t, 460–462, *461*

   Q-switched Alexandrite laser, 446t, 460–462, *461*

   Q-switched ruby laser, 446t, 459–450, *459, 460*

   tunable dye laser, 456–458

   types of, used in dermatology, 446t, 449–464

Lateral nail fold excision, 274–275, *275*

Lateral scalp reduction pattern, anesthesia for, 550

   instrumentation for, 550

   preoperative considerations for, 550

   technique of, 550–551

Lateral thigh, sclerotherapy for, 407

Lawsuit(s), 141

Legal issue(s). See *Medicolegal issues*

Lentigines, 226, 513–514

Lentigo maligna (LM), 160, 226, 242

Lentigo maligna melanoma, 160, *160*

Lentigo simplex, 226

Lesion(s). See *Benign cutaneous lesion(s); Malignant lesion(s)*

Leukoderma, 286, 288

Levator anguli oris muscle, 37

Levator labii superioris alaeque nasi muscle, 36–37

Levator labii superioris muscle, 36

Levator muscle, *584*

Lidocaine (Xylocaine), bactericidal properties of, 532

   characteristics of, 67t, 68

   for cardiac arrest, 120, 121

   for hair replacement, 476

   for lip reconstruction, 330–331

   for nail surgery, 265–266, *266*

   for punch graft, 288

   for scalp reduction, 546, 549, 550, 552, 554

   for tumescent liposuction, 69t, 533–535, 533t

   pharmacokinetics of, 533–534

   recipe for tumescent liposuction anesthetic solution, 69t, 533, 533t

   safe dose of, 534

   topical lidocaine, 66

   toxicity of, 69, 70t, 534–535, 535t

Ligation/cauterization of occipital arteries, anesthesia for, 552

   instrumentation for, 552

   preoperative considerations for, 552, *552*

   technique of, 552–553, *553*

Line(s). See *Contour line(s); Minimum skin tension line(s) (MSTLs); Relaxed skin tension line(s) (RSTLs); Skin tension line(s)*

Lip(s), anatomy of, 36–37, 329–331, *330, 331*

   motor innervation of, 330

   muscles of, 36–37

   relaxed skin tension lines of, 329, *330*

   sensory innervation of, 330

   vascular supply to, 331

Lip proper muscle, 37

Lip reconstruction, anatomy of lips, 329–331, *330, 331*

   anesthesia for, 330–331

   full-thickness wounds, 341, 343, *343–346*

   partial-thickness wounds, 331–341, *332–342*

     advancement flaps, 334, *335*, 336, *337*, 341, *342*

     basic principles for, 331

     full-thickness skin graft, 332, *333–334*

     local flaps, 332, 334

     mucosal advancement flaps, 341, *342*

     rotation flaps, 336, *338*

     second intention wound healing, 332, *332*

     skin graft, 332, *333–334*

     transposition flaps, 339, *340, 341*

   postoperative considerations, 343, 346

   preoperative considerations, 329–331, *330, 331*

Lip tumor(s), Mohs micrographic surgery for, 575

Lipoma(s), 229–230
Liposuction, areas treated by, 529
  complications after, 540
  differences between plastic surgery and
      dermatology for, 530
  dry technique of, 535
  for lipomas, 230
  French experience of, 438
  good candidates for, 530
  local versus general anesthesia for,
      530–531, 535–536
  tumescent liposuction with local anesthe-
      sia, 529–540
  wet technique of, 535–536
Liquid nitrogen. See Cryosurgery
Liquid silicone, animal studies, 427
  clinical experience, 427, 428–430
  complications, 428, 431–432, 432, 433
  current status of, 432, 437
  for breast augmentation, 431
  for granulomas, 431, 432
  illegality of, 432
  literature review, 427–428, 431–432
  nodularity beading, 431–432
  overcorrection, 431–432, 432, 433
  physical characteristics, 427
  volume of, 428, 431
Lister bandage scissors, 96–97, 96
Litigation versus arbitration, 141
Liver spots, 226
LM (lentigo maligna), 160, 226, 242
LMM (lentigo maligna melanoma), 160,
      160
Lobule "rim advancement" flap, 369, 370
Local anesthesia, adverse reactions to,
      69–70, 70t, 117–118
  cryoanesthesia, 65–66, 65t
  equipment for, 70–71, 71, 71t
  for cryosurgery, 161
  for dermabrasion, 500–501
  for hair replacement, 476
  for ligation/cauterization of occipital ar-
      teries, 552
  for lip reconstruction, 330–331
  for lower lid blepharoplasty, 590
  for microlipoinjection, 439, 439t
  for midline scalp reduction, 546
  for Mohs micrographic surgery,
      561–562
  for nail surgery, 265–266, 266
  for paramedian or lateral scalp reduc-
      tion pattern, 550
  for punch graft, 288
  for scalp lift technique, 554
  for split-thickness skin graft (STSG),
      521
  for tumescent liposuction, 533–535
  for upper lid blepharoplasty, 586
  for Y or Mercedes scalp reduction pat-
      tern, 549
  improved safety with, 530
  inhalants, 64–64, 64
  injectable anesthetics
    addition of vasoconstriction and neu-
        tralizing agents, 68–69
    mechanism of action, 66–67

structure and classifcation o, 67–68,
      67, 67t
    technique of injection, 71–74, 72–74
  iontophoresis, 66
  opthalmic anesthetics, 66
  preoperative medications, 63–64, 64t,
      110–111
  surface anesthesia, 65
  topical anesthetics, 66
  toxicity of, 69–70, 70t, 116–117,
      534–535
  versus general anesthesia for tumescent
      liposuction, 530–531, 535–536
Local flap(s), definition of, 309
  for lip reconstruction, 332, 334
Longitudinal melanonychia, 277
Low-energy laser system(s), 464
Lower antihelix, reconstruction of, 373,
      374
Lower eyelid(s), anatomy of, 583–585,
      583–585
Lower eyelid tumor(s), Mohs micro-
      graphic surgery for, 571–572, 571,
      573
Lower lid blepharoplasty, anesthesia for,
      590
  carbon dioxide laser in, 593
  complications of, 593
  goals of, 590, 590
  postoperative care for, 593
  procedures for operation, 590–593,
      591–593
  skin markings for, 590, 590
  transconjunctival blepharoplasty,
      592–593, 593
Lower lip tumor(s), Mohs micrographic
      surgery for, 575
Low-flow hemangioma, argon laser treat-
      ment for, 452
Lubrication, of joints of instruments, 98
Luster finish for instruments, 47
Lying cone(s), 189, 189, 198
Lymphatics, of head, 40, 40
Lyofoam, 27

Macronychia, 265
Macrophage(s), 9
Male blepharoplasty, 585, 588
Malignant adnexal tumors, 242–243
Malignant and premalignant lesion(s), la-
      ser treatment for, 447t, 448–449,
      449t
Malignant fibrous histiocytoma (MFH),
      243
Malignant lesion(s), angiosarcoma, 244
  atypical fibroxanthoma, 243
  basal cell carcinoma, 105–108,
      235–238, 236, 237, 278
  Bowen's disease, 240
  carbon dioxide laser treatment for, 450
  cryosurgery for, 156–161, 157–161,
      157t
  dermatofibrosarcoma protuberans, 242
  electrosurgery for, 151

extramammary Paget's disease,
      243–244, 243
  keratoacanthoma, 240, 240
  lentigo maligna, 242
  lesion, 105–108, 106, 107, 108
  malignant adnexal tumors, 242–243
  malignant fibrous histiocytoma, 243
  malignant melanoma, 108, 241–242,
      241
  Marjolin's ulcer, 239–240
  melanocytic nevi, 108
  Merkel's cell carcinoma (MCC), 244
  microcystic adnexal carcinoma, 242
  Mohs micrographic surgery for,
      568–570, 569t, 570t
  nails, 278–279, 279
  sebaceous carcinoma, 242–243, 243
  split-thickness skin graft (STSG) used
      in removal of, 519–520
  squamous cell carcinoma, 108,
      238–239, 278–279, 279
  verrucous carcinoma, 240, 240
Malignant melanoma, description of, 108,
      241–242, 241
  Mohs micrographic surgery for, 569,
      569t
Malpractice, 139–141, 413–414
Mandibular division, of trigeminal nerve,
      42–43, 43, 72, 73
Mapping, in Mohs micrographic surgery,
      562–565, 563–565
Marcaine. See Bupivacaine (Marcaine/Sen-
      sorcaine)
Marjolin's ulcer, 239–240
Mask(s), 60
Mast cell(s), 8–9, 8
Mastisol, 25, 25t
Matricectomy, carbon dioxide laser tech-
      nique, 272
  chemical technique, 272
  electrosurgery technique, 272
  phenol matricectomy, 272
  scalpel technique, 272
Matrix metalloproteinase(s) (MMPs), 9,
      10
Maxillary division, of trigeminal nerve,
      42, 43, 72, 73
Maxon suture, 79, 79t
Mayo scissors, 91, 91
MCC. See Merkel's cell carcinoma
      (MCC)
Mechanical creep, 605
Medical history, cardiac disease, 103
  cigarette smoking, 104
  diabetes mellitus, 104
  drug reactions, 101
  for preoperative patient evaluation,
      101–105
  infectious diseases, 104–105
  medications affecting surgery, 101–103
  nutritional factors, 104
  pregnancy, 104
  vascular disease, 103
Medical malpractice, 139–141, 413–414
Medical record(s), 140–141

Medication(s), affecting surgery, 101–103
  anticoagulants, 102
  aspirin, 102
  beta-blockers, 102
  drug reactions recorded in medical history, 101, 113–114
  drug toxicity, 116–117
  emergency medications, 122, 122t
  immunosuppressive agents, 103
  neuroleptic agents, 103
  nonsteroidal anti-inflammatory drugs (NSAIDs), 102
  preoperative medications, 63–64, 64t, 110–111
Medicolegal issue(s), consent to treatment, 138–139
  contractual relationship between physician and patient, 138
  establishing physician-patient relationship, 137–138
  human immunodeficiency virus (HIV) infection, 142
  medical malpractice, 139–141, 413–414
  terminating physician-patient relationship, 138
Medium peel(s). See *Chemical peel(s)*
Melanocytic nevi, 108, 225–226, *226*
Melanoma, lentigo maligna melanoma, 160, *160*
  malignant melanoma, 108, 241–242, *241*
  Mohs micrographic surgery for malignant melanoma, 569, 569t
Melasma, chemical peels for, 513, *514*, *515*
Memory, of suture, 77
Mental nerve, 73
Mentalis muscle, 36
Meperidine hydrochloride, 110
Mepivacaine (Carbocaine), 67t, 68
Mercedes scalp reduction pattern, anesthesia for, 549
  instrumentation for, 549
  preoperative considerations for, 549
  technique of, 549, *550*
Merkel's cell carcinoma (MCC), 244
Metastatic basal cell carcinoma, 238
Metatypical basal cell carcinoma, 107
Methoxyflurane (Pentrane), 64–65, *64*
Metzenbaum scissors, 91, *91*
MFH. See *Malignant fibrous histiocytoma (MFH)*
Microcystic adnexal carcinoma, 242
Micrografting, in hair replacement, 470
Micrographic surgery. See *Mohs micrographic surgery*
Microlipoinjection, anesthesia for, 439, 439t
  animal models and basic research, 438
  clinical results and evaluation, 440–441, *440*, *441*
  complications of, 441–442
  cosmetic surgical experience, 438
  current cross-specialty experience, 438

historical attempts at grafting fat, 437–438
injectable substances for soft-tissue augmentation, 437
liposuction and the French experience, 438
proposed research areas, 442
techniques, 438–440
Micronodular basal cell carcinoma, 106–107, *107*
Microscopic examination, in Mohs micrographic surgery, 565–566
Midline scalp reduction, anesthesia for, 546
  instrumentation for, 546
  preoperative considerations, 546
  technique of, 547–548, *547*, *548*
Milia, as complication of dermabrasion, 501
  as complication of full-thickness skin graft, 307
  as complication of lower lid blepharoplasty, 593
  management of, 229
  treatment of, 133
Minigrafting, in hair replacement, 470–471, *471*
Minimum skin tension line(s) (MSTLs), 165, *166*, 166t
MMP(s), (matrix metalloproteinases), 9, 10
MMS. See *Mohs micrographic surgery*
Mmunigrafts, in hair replacement, 470
Mohs micrographic surgery, facilities for, 576
  fixed tissue technique, 570–571
  for alar groove and nasolabial groove tumors, 575–576, *575*
  for basal cell carcinoma, 107, 236, 237–238, *237*
  for Bowen's disease, 240
  for ear tumors, 572, 574–575, *575*
  for lower eyelid tumors, 571–572, *571*, *573*
  for lower lip tumors, 575
  for squamous cell carcinoma, 238, 568–569
  for verrucous carcinoma, 240
  fresh tissue technique
    advantages of, 570, 570t
    basal cell carcinoma, 568, 569t
    debulking excision, 562
    disadvantages of, 570
    excision, 561–562
    hemostasis, 562
    indications for, 569–570, 570t
    laboratory processing, 564–565, *565*, *566*
    local anesthesia, 561–562
    location of cancer, 569
    malignant melanoma, 569, 569t
    mapping, 562–565, *563–565*
    microscopic examination, 565–566
    multidisciplinary approach, 567–568
    orientation, 562–563
    primary versus recurrent cancers, 569

results, 568–569, 569t
    saucerizing excision, 562
    squamous cell carcinoma, 568–569
    tissue marking, 563–564, *564*
    wound management, 566–567, *568*
  future of, 576
  histopathology laboratory for, 564–565, *565*, *566*, 576
  history of, 561
  instrumentation for, 571–572, *573*, 576
Monofilament suture(s), 78
Monoterminal modality, 147
Morpheic (morpheaform) basal cell carcinoma, *23*, 107, *107*, 236
Morphine sulfate, 110
Mosquito hemostat, 95, *95*
Motor nerve(s), 109–110, *109*
Mouth, muscles of, 36–37. See also *Lip(s)*
Mouth-to-mask ventilation, 119, *119*
M-plasty, for dog-ear avoidance and correction, 195–196
  for lip reconstruction, 334
  variation of ellipse excision, *206–207*, 207–208
MSTL(s) (minimum skin tension lines), 165, *166*, 166t
Mucosal advancement flap, for lip reconstruction, 341, *342*
Multifilament suture(s), 77
Muscle(s), ear, 37
  facial muscles, 36–37, *36*, 213, *213*, *214*, *215*
  forehead, *350*, 351, *351*
  histologic changes in, following tissue expansion, 608
  lips, 36–37
  mouth, 36–37
  neck, 44–45, *44*
  nose, 37
  periorbital, 37
  scalp, 37
  temple, 359, *359*
Myocardial infarction, 118
Myxoid cyst(s), 273–274, *274*

Nail(s), anatomy of, 266–268, *266*, *267*
  anesthesia for, 265–266, *266*
  benign nail unit tumors, 279–280
    acquired digital fibrokeratoma, 279, *279*
    giant cell tumors of the tendon sheath, 279–280
    glomus tumors, 279
    pteryglum, 280, *280*
  biopsy and small excisions, 270–271
    nail matrix, 271, *271*
    nail plate and nail bed, 270–271, *270*, *271*
  blood and nerve supply to, 267–268, *267*
  carcinoma and nail unit excision, 278–279, *279*
  chronic paronychia, 272–273, *273*
  clinical terminology on, 265

Nail(s) (*continued*)
  distal nail tip excision, 275, *275*
  exostosis, 277
  ingrown nail, 276, *276*
  instrumentation for, 268–269, *269*
  lateral nail fold excisions, 274–275, *275*
  longitudinal melanonychia, 277
  matricectomy, 272
  minor lacerations, 280, *280*
  myxoid cysts, 273–274, *274*
  nail avulsion, 269–270, *270*
  nail plate debridement, 278
  onychogryposis, 277–278
  onychoschizia, 278
  partial nail unit excision, 271–272, *271*
  pincer nail deformities, 276, *276*
  postoperative status, 269, *269*
  pre-operative status of, 265
  preparing the field, 268, *268*
  proximal nail fold lesions, 273, *273*
  proximal nail fold re-creation, 273
  racqet thumbnail, 278, *278*
  split nail deformities, 277, *277*
  split-thickness graft nail bed reconstruction, 280
  subungual hematoma, 272
  warts, 280–281
Nail avulsion, 269–270, *270*, 280–281
Nail plate debridement, 278
Nail unit excision, 278–279, *279*
Naloxone hydrochloride, 110
Narcotic preanesthesia, 64, 64t, 110
Nasal ala, reconstruction of, 398
Nasal anatomy, 381–382, *381*, *382*
Nasal bone, reconstruction of, 399
Nasal cartilage, reconstruction of, 399
Nasal lining, reconstruction of, 399
Nasal reconstruction, anatomy of nose, 381–382, *381*, *382*
  approaches to, 383
  cosmetic subunit and aesthetic aspects, 382, *382*
  major nasal reconstruction, 399
  physiology of nose, 382–383
  primary closure, 383
  prosthetics, 397
  regional approach to, 397–398
    ala, 398
    columella, 398
    dorsum, 397–398
    nasal root/glabella, 397
    nasal sidewall, 398
    tip and supratip, 398
  secondary intention healing, 383 secondary procedures and scar revision, 397
  skin flaps
    advancement flaps, 387
    biloped flap, 392, *392*, *393*
    forehead flap, 395, *395–396*, 397
    general features, 386–387
    nasalis myocutaneous flap, *394*, 395
    nasolabial flap, 389–392, *389–391*
    pedicle flap, 392, *394*, 395
    rhombic flap, 387, *389*

  rotation flaps, 387, *388*
  subcutaneous island pedicle flap, 392, 395
  transposition flaps, 387
  skin grafts, 383–386
    composite grafts, 386
    free cartilage grafts, 386
    full-thickness skin grafts, 383–386, *384*, *385*, 385t
    split-thickness skin grafts, 383
Nasal root/glabella, reconstruction of, 397
Nasal sidewall, reconstruction of, 398
Nasal tip and supratip, reconstruction of, 398
Nasalis muscle, 37
Nasalis myocutaneous flap, *394*, 395
Nasolabial flap, for nasal reconstruction, 389–392, *389–391*
Nasolabial fold flap, 323, *323*
Nasolabial groove tumors, Mohs micrographic surgery for, 575–576, *575*
Natural suture(s), 78
Nd:YAG laser. See *Neodymium:yttrium-aluminum-garnet laser*
Neck, anatomy of, 43–45, *44*, *45*
  blood supply of, 45
  muscles of, 44–45, *44*
  nerves of, 45
  triangles of, 44, *44*
Necrosis, as complication of injectable bovine collagen, 422
  as complication of scalp reduction, 551, 559
  partial necrosis, 128, *128*
  treatment of, 131, *132*, 413, *413*
Needle(s), cutting needles, 81
  injection of local anesthetics, 70–71, 71t
  measurements defining size of, 81, *81*
  points of, 81, *81*
  pop-offs, 81
  reverse cutting needles, 81
  suturing, 80–81, *81*
Needle-holder(s), 47, *48*, 93–94, *94*
Needle-stick(s), 60
Negative dog-ear(s), 189–190, *189*, *190*
Negligence, 139–140
Neodymium:yttrium-aluminum-garnet laser, background of, 462
  complications and contraindications for, 463
  indications for, 462
  mode and wavelength of, 446t, 462
  technique of, 462–463
Neoplasm(s), benign adnexal neoplasms, 107
Neo-Synephrine. See *Phenylephrine (Neo-Synephrine)*
Neovascular vessels, as complication of sclerotherapy, 411–412, *411*, 416
Nerve(s), face, 40–43, *41–43*, 72–73, *72*, 109, 109–110, *109*
  feet, *74*, 75
  lips, 330
  motor nerves, 109–110, *109*

  nails, 267–268, *267*
  neck, 45
  scalp, 42–43, *43*
  sensory nerves, 42–43, *43*, *109*, 110
  temple, 358, *358*
Nerve block, 72–74, *73*
Nerve damage, as complication of liposuction, 540
Nesacaine. See *Chloroprocaine (Nesacaine)*
Neural structure(s). See *Nerve(s)*
Neurapraxia, as complication of tissue expansion, 609
Neuroleptic agent(s), 103
Nevi, melanocytic, 225–226, *226*
Nevocytic, 225
Nevus of Ota, laser treatment for, 459, *460*
Nitrogen. See *Cryosurgery*
Nitroglycerin, 118
Nitrous oxide, 64, 65
Nodular basal cell carcinoma, 106, *106*, *237*
Nodularity beading, 431–432
Nonabsorbable suture(s), 78, 80, 80t
Nonextravasation ulcer(s), 412–413, *412*
Nonsteroidal anti-inflammatory drug(s) (NSAIDs), 102
Nonsurgical scar revision, 261, *263*
Normal flora, 57
Norwood classification of male pattern baldness, *544*
Nose. See also *Nasal reconstruction*
  anatomy of, 381–382, *381*, *382*
  muscles of, 37
  physiology of, 382–383
  pressure dressings for, 31–32, *32*
Novafil, 80
Novocaine. See *Procaine (Novocaine)*
NSAID(s) (nonsteroidal anti-inflammatory drugs), 102
Nu-Derm, 27
Nurolon, 80
Nutritional factors, in medical history, 104
Nylon suture, 80, 80t

Occipital arteries, injury to, 559
  ligation/cauterization of, in scalp reduction, 552–553, *552*, *553*, 559
Occipitofrontalis muscle, 37
Occlusive dressing(s), calcium alginates, 17, 29, 29t
  characteristics of, 26, 26t
  gels and hydrogels, 15–16, 28, 28t
  history of, 23
  hydrocolloids, 16–17, 28–29, 28t
  polymer films, 15, 26–27, 26t, 27t
  polymer foams, 15, 26t, 27–28
  tissue repair and, 17
  topical agents and, 17
  trade names of, 16t
  wound bacteriology and, 17
Ointment(s), antibacterial, 24, 24t
Omiderm, 27, 27t

Ongoing care. See *Postoperative and ongoing care*
Onychauxis, 265
Onychogryposis, 265, 277–278
Onychomadesis, 265
Onychomycosis, 265
Onychorrhexis, 265
Onychoschizia, 265, 278
Onythocryptosis, 265
Operating room protocols, 61, 61t
Ophthalmic division, of trigeminal nerve, 42, *43*, *72*, 73
OpSite, 26, 27t, 28
Op-Site Wound Closure, 82
Opthalmic anesthetics, 66
Orbicularis oculi muscle, 37, *350*, 351, *351*
Orbicularis oris muscle, 37
Oriental blepharoplasty, 585, 588, *589*
Osteomyelitis, complication of hair replacement, 492
O-T advancement flap, 312, *314*, *316*
O-to-Z double rotation flap, 319, *321*
Overcorrection, and liquid silicone, 431–432, *432*, *433*

Pacemakers, as electrosurgery danger, 148
Padgett dermatome, for split-thickness skin graft (STSG), 523–524
Pain, as complication of tissue expansion, 609
Pain management, 111, 127
Palliation, cryosurgery for, 160–161
Panniculitis, postliposuction, 540
Paper packing, for instruments, 49
Paper/transparent pouches, for instruments, 49, *49*, *50*
Paramedian scalp reduction pattern, anesthesia for, 550
  instrumentation for, 550
  preoperative considerations for, 550
  technique of, 550–551
Paronychia, chronic, 272–273, *273*
Parotid gland and duct, 40, *41*, 110
Partial closure, in Mohs micrographic surgery, 567
Partial nail unit excision, 271–272, *271*
Partial-thickness lip defect(s), 331–341, *332–342*
Patient evaluation. See *Preoperative patient evaluation*
Patient-physician relationship, consent to treatment, 138–139
  contractual nature of, 138
  establishing, 137–138
  human immunodeficiency virus (HIV) infection, 142
  malpractice and, 139–141, 413–414
  terminating, 138
PDGF (platelet-derived groth factor), 8
PDL. See *Pulsed dye laser (PDL)*
PDS suture, 79, 79t
Pedicle, definition of, 309
Pedicle flap, for combined ear defects, 374, *376–379*, *377–378*

for nasal reconstruction, 392, *394*, 395
for scaphoid fossa and triangular fossa of antihelix, 369, *371–373*, 374
method of, 310
Pedi-Pre-Tape, 25t
Pedi-Skin adherent, 25t
Peel(s). See *Chemical peel(s)*
Pentrane. See *Methoxyflurane (Pentrane)*
Pericranium, 353
Perioperative emergency(ies), allergic reactions, 117–118
  anaphylaxis, 117–118
  cardiac arrest, 118–121, *119*, *120*, 120t
  cerebrovascular accident, 115–116
  drug reactions and, 113–114
  drug toxicity, 116–117
  equipment and medications, 121–122, 121t, 122t
  hemorrhage, 114–115
  myocardial infarction, 118
  prevention of, 113–114
  seizures, 115
  training and preparation for, 113
  vasovagal syncope, 114
Periorbital region, muscles of, 37
Periosteal elevators, 97, *97*
Peripheral nerve block, 72, 74
Periungual verrucae, 280–281
Peroneal nerve, 74, *74*
Phenol, applying, in chemical peel, 510
  as peeling agent, 505, 506, 507–508
  Baker phenol chemical peel solution, 505, 506
  Baker-Gordon phenol peel, 507–508, 507t, 510, 512
  toxicity of, 505
Phenol matricectomy, 272
Phenylephrine (Neo-Synephrine), 66
Photodynamic therapy with tunable dye laser, background of, 457
  complications and contraindications for, 458
  indications for, 457–458
  technique of, 458
Physician-patient relationship, consent to treatment, 138–139
  contractual nature of, 138
  establishing, 137–138
  human immunodeficiency virus (HIV) infection, 142
  malpractice and, 139–141, 413–414
  terminating, 138
Piezosurgery, for epidermoid cysts, 227
Pigmentary abnormality(ies), 132–133
Pigmentation, as complication of sclerotherapy, 412. See also *Hyperpigmentation; Hypopigmentation*
Pigmented lesion(s), laser treatment for, 447–448, 447t, 449t, 451t
  Q-switched ruby laser treatment for, 459, *460*
Pigmented lesion dye laser (PLDL), 460–462, *461*
Pilar cyst(s), 228
Pincer nail deformity(ies), 276, *276*

Pinch graft(s), for split-thickness skin graft (STSG), 522–523, *523*
"Pinch test," 165, *166*
Pitcher-lip deformity(ies), *189*, 190, *190*
Pityrosporum, 57
Plantar wart(s), 223
Plastic surgery, and liposuction, 530
Platelet-derived groth factor (PDGF), 8
PLDL. See *Pigmented lesion dye laser (PLDL)*
PM/DM (polymyositis/dermatomyositis), 423
Podophyllin, 223
Poikiloderma of Civatte, 454, *454*
Polidocanol, as sclerosant, 410, *410*
Polybutester suture, 80, 80t
Polydioxanone (PDS) suture, 79, 79t
Polyester suture, 80, 80t
Polyglactin 910 (Vicryl) suture, 79, 79t
Polyglycolic acid (Dexon) suture, 78–79, 79, 79t
Polyglyconate (Maxon) suture, 79, 79t
Polymer film(s), 15, 26–27, 26t, 27t
Polymer foam(s), 15, 26t, 27–28
Polymyositis/dermatomyositis (PM/DM), 423
Polypropylene suture, 80, 80t
Pontocaine. See *Tetracaine (Pontocaine)*
Pop-off(s), 81
Port-wine hemangioma, laser treatment for, 451–452, 453, *453*, *454*
Postauricular flap, for earlobe repair, 581
Post-auricular transposition flap, 363, *364–367*
Posterior ear, reconstruction of, 379, *379–380*
Posterior tibial nerve, 74, *74*
Posterior triangle of neck, 44, *44*
Posterior-middle helical rim, reconstruction of, 363, 365, *367–368*, 369
Postliposuction panniculitis, 540
Postoperative analgesia, 111, 127
Postoperative and ongoing care, complications, 128–133
  abnormal surface scar, 131–133
  bleeding, 128, *129*
  contact dermatitis, 130, *130*
  dehiscence, 131, *131*
  hematoma, 129, *129*
  infection, 129–130, *130*
  miscellaneous complications, 133
  necrosis, 128, *128*, 131, *132*
  prevention of, 128
  suture reactions, 130, *130*
  for blepharoplasty, 593
  for browlift, 596
  for hair replacement, 490–492
  for lip reconstruction, 343, 346
  for punch graft, 292–294
  for split-thickness skin graft, 526–528
  for tumescent liposuction, 537–540
  routine care
    antibiotic prophylaxis, 127
    drains, 127
    follow-up visits, 127

Postoperative and ongoing care, complications, (*continued*)
  instructions to patients, 111, 126–127, *126*
  ongoing care, 127–128
  pain management, 111, 127
  suture removal, 127
  wound care principles, 125–126, 126t
Postoperative bleeding, treatment of, 128, *129*
  with cryosurgery, 163
  with full-thickness skin graft, 307
  with hair replacement, 492
  with scalp reduction, 559
Pox scar(s), revision of, 260
Preanesthesia, 63–64, 64t, 110–111
Preauricular flap, for earlobe repair, 580, *580, 582*
Pre-auricular transposition flap, 363, *364–367*
Pregnancy, as contraindication for epinephrine, 70
  in medical history, 104
  sclerotherapy and, 403, *404*, 409
Premalignant lesion(s), laser treatment for, 447t, 448–449, 449t
Preoperative patient evaluation and considerations, anatomic considerations, 108–110, *109*
  motor nerves, 109–110, *109*
  neural structures, 109–110, *109*
  parotid gland, 110
  sensory nerves, *109*, 110
  vascular structures, 108–109, *109*
  day of surgery, 110–111
  dog-ears and, 194
  for fusiform excision, 201–202
  for hair replacement, 550
  for ligation/cauterization of occipital arteries, 552, *552*
  for lip reconstruction, 329–331, *330, 331*
  lesion, 105–108
    basal cell carcinoma, 105–108, *106, 107*
    malignant melanoma, 108
    melanocytic nevi, 108
    squamous cell carcinoma, 108
  medical history, 101–105, 102t
    cardiac disease, 103
    cigarette smoking, 104
    diabetes mellitus, 104
    drug reactions, 101
    general factors, 102t
    infectious diseases, 104–105
    medications affecting surgery, 101–103
    nutritional factors, 104
    pregnancy, 104
    vascular disease, 103
  postoperative instructions, 111
  preoperative sedation, 110–111
  scalp lift technique, 553–554
  scalp reduction, 546, 549, 550, 552–554, *552*

tumescent liposuction, 531–533, *531, 534*
Preoperative sedation, 63–64, 64t, 110–111
Pressure dressing(s), digits, 32
  ear, 31, *32*
  eyelids, 32
  nose, 31–32, *32*
  scalp, 30–31, *31*
  scrotum, 32
Prilocaine (Citanest), 66, 67t
Primary cancer, Mohs micrographic surgery for, 569
Primary closure, for lower antihelix, *373, 374*
  for nasal reconstruction, 383
  for tragus and crus of helix, 369, *370–371*
  in Mohs micrographic surgery, 566–567
Primary contraction, 298
Primary defect(s), definition of, 309
Primary fusiform closure, for forehead reconstruction, 354, *354*
  for temple reconstruction, *359*, 361
Primary motion, definition of, 309
Procaine (Novocaine), 67t, 68
Procerus muscle, 37, *350*, 351, *351*
Prolene, 80
"Prone pillow," 471, *471*
Prophylactic antibiotics, 60–61, 127, 532–533
Propionibacterium, 57
Propranolol, 117
Prosthetics, and nasal reconstruction, 397
Proteoglycan(s), 6–7, *7*
Protrusion(s). See *Dog-ear(s)*
Proximal nail fold lesions, 273, *273*
Proximal nail fold re-creation, 273
Proximate II stapler, 95
Proxi-Strip, 82
Pruritus, as complication of hair replacement, 490
  treatment of, 133
Pterygium, 280, *280*
Ptosis, as complication of lower lid blepharoplasty, 593
Pulmonary emboli, as complication of sclerotherapy, 412
Pulsed dye laser (PDL), background of, 453
  complications and contraindications for, 455
  indications for, 453–454, *453, 454*
  mode and wavelengths of, 446t, 452–453
  technique of, 455
Pulsed (dye) pigmented laser, background of, 461
  complications and contraindications for, 462
  indications for, 461–462, *461*
  mode and wavelength of, 446t, 460
  technique of, 461–462
Punch(es), 89–90, *89, 90*

Punch elevation, 284, *285*
Punch excision with full-thickness autologous punch graft replacement, 284–288, 285t, *286, 287*
Punch excision with suturing, for acne scars and pox scars, 260
Punch graft, autologous punch grafting for stable leukoderma, 286, 288
  donor and recipient sites, *291*
  donor-recipient punch choices, 290t
  excision of epithelialized tunnels or sinuses, 286, *287, 293*, 294
  history of, 283
  instruments and supplies for, 288
  postoperative considerations for, 292–294
  preoperative instructions for, 288
  procedure for punch grafting, 288–294, *289*, 290t, *291*, 292t, *293*
  punch elevation, 284, *285*
  punch excision with full-thickness autologous punch graft replacement, 284–288, 285t, *286, 287*
  punch excision without autografting, 284, 284t
  sequelae, 292t
  success of, 283–284
  technique of, 288–294
Purpura, as complication from pigmented lesion dye laser, 462

Q-switched alexandrite laser, background of, 460–461
  complications and contraindications for, 462
  indications for, 461, *461*
  mode and wavelength of, 446t, 460–461
  technique of, 461–462
Q-switched ruby laser, background of, 459
  complications and contraindications for, 460
  indications for, 459, *459, 460*
  mode and wavelength of, 446t, 459
  technique of, 459–460
Quarter grafting, in hair replacement, 471

Racqet thumbnail, 278, *278*
Radiation therapy, for basal cell carcinoma, 238
  for Marjolin's ulcer, 240
  for squamous cell carcinoma, 239
  for verrucous carcinoma, 240
Rake(s), 92, *92*
Random pattern plap(s), 310
Razor blade, 86, *86, 87*, 522
Reactive forces, in wound closure, *190*, 191
Recurrent basal cell carcinoma, 105–106
Recurrent cancer, Mohs micrographic surgery for, 569
Relaxed skin tension line(s) (RSTLs), 38, *38*, 201, 202, *202*, 211, 253, *253*
Resident cells of the dermis, 8–9, *9*

Resident flora, 57

Resorcin, as peeling agent, 505, 505t, 510t, 511
preparation of, 510t

Resting skin tension line(s) (RSTLs), 38, 38, 201, 202, 202, 211, 253, 253

Retinoic acid, as peeling agent, 505t
for actinic keratoses, 512
in combination peels, 510

Reverse cutting needle(s), 81

Reverse-contoured flap, for earlobe repair, 581

Revision, of Mohs surgery defects, 567

"Revolving door" island flap, 374, 375–376

Rh-123 (rhodamine-123), 452

Rhinophyma, carbon dioxide laser treatment for, 450
dermabrasion for, 499, 502

Rhodamine-123 (Rh-123), 452

Rhombic flap, for nasal reconstruction, 387, 389
for tragus and crus of helix, 369, 370–371
method of, 322, 324–325, 324

Rieger's flap, for nasal reconstruction, 387, 388

Ring block, 71–72

Risorius muscle, 36

Rotation flap, definition of, 310
dog-ear formation and, 197, 197
for forehead reconstruction, 355
for lip reconstruction, 336, 338
for nasal reconstruction, 387, 388
for temple reconstruction, 360, 361
method of, 317–319, 317–321

Round grafting, in hair replacement, 469, 470, 477, 477, 478, 479–481

Round minigrafting, in hair replacement, 470, 488–489

RSTL(s) (relaxed skin tension lines), 38, 38, 201, 202, 202, 211, 253, 253

"Rubber duck" technique, 196–197, 197

Running basting suture, 182

Running horizontal mattress suture, 180, 180

Running locked suture, 179–180, 179

Running subcutaneous suture, 181, 181

Running subcuticular suture, 180–181, 181

Running suture(s), running horizontal mattress suture, 180, 180
running locked suture, 179–180, 179
running subcutaneous suture, 181, 181
running subcuticular suture, 180–181, 181
simple running suture, 179, 179

Salicylic acid, as peeling agent, 505

Saphenous nerve, 73, 74, 74

Satellite cyst(s), 228

Satin finish for instruments, 47

Saucerizing excision, in Mohs micrographic surgery, 562

Scalp, lymphatics of, 40, 40
muscles of, 37
nerves of, 42–43, 43
pressure dressings for, 30–31, 31

Scalp extenders, 558

Scalp lift technique, anesthesia for, 554
complications of, 551, 559
extensive scalp-lifting, 545, 551, 552
instrumentation for, 554
preoperative considerations for, 553–554
technique of, 554–558, 555–557

Scalp reduction, adjuncts to, 558
carbon dioxide laser, 558
galeotomy, 558
scalp extenders, 558
before or after hair replacement, 545
circumferential reduction, 558
complications, 559
extensive scalp-lifting, 545, 551, 552
history of, 543–544
indications for, 543
ligation/cauterization of occipital arteries, 552–553, 552, 553
anesthesia, 552
instrumentation, 552
preoperative considerations, 552, 552
technique, 552–553, 553
midline reduction, 545–548, 545
anesthesia, 546
instrumentation, 546
preoperative considerations, 546
technique, 547–548, 547, 548
Norwood classification of male pattern baldness, 544
paramedian or lateral pattern, 545, 549–551
anesthesia, 550
instrumentation, 550
preoperative considerations, 550
technique, 550–551
patient selection, 544–545
scalp lift technique, 553–558, 555–557
anesthesia, 554
instrumentation, 554
preoperative considerations, 553–554
technique, 554–558, 555–557
stretch-back following, 559
types of, 545–558
Y or Mercedes pattern, 545, 548–549
anesthesia, 549
instrumentation, 549
preoperative considerations, 549
technique, 549, 550

Scalpel(s), 85–88, 86, 87

Scaphoid fossa, reconstruction of, 369, 371–373, 374

Scar revision, basic principles of, 250–251
excision of ice-pick scar, 286, 287, 289
functional and cosmetic concerns, 249–250
methods
geometric broken line, 260, 260
punch excision with suturing, 260
shave abrasion, 261
specialized techniques, 260–261, 262
W-plasty, 260, 260
Z-plasty, 253, 255, 258, 258, 259, 260
nasal reconstruction, 397
nonsurgical scar revision, 261, 263
scar analysis, 251, 253–255, 253–257
sequential healing and ability of skin to heal, 250–251, 250–252

Scarring, abnormal surface scar, 131–133
as complication of chemical peels, 514–516
dermabrasion for, 498–499, 499–501
measures of, 14, 16t

SCC. See Squamous cell carcinoma (SCC)

Scissors, bandage scissors, 96–97, 96
blunt-tipped scissors for undermining, 91–92, 91
suture-cutting scissors, 94, 94
tissue-cutting scissors, 88–89, 88, 89
tungsten-carbide inserts for, 47, 48, 88, 89

Sclerotherapy, anatomy and, 405, 406
basic principles of, 403
clinical profiles, 414–416
complications, 411–413
extravasation ulcers, 412
neovascular vessels, 411–412, 411, 416
nonextravasaton ulcers, 412–413, 412
pigmentation, 412
pulmonary emboli, 412
thrombophlebitis, 412
thrombosis, 412
compression hosiery, 414
controversies on, 414
Doppler examination, 414
duplex scanning, 414
electron microscopy and, 405, 407
fragile vein syndrome, 415–416
gender considerations, 403, 404
injecting feeder veins, 414, 415
insurance for, 413
laboratory procedures, 414
laser for resistant vessels, 409
location, 407, 409
ankle/feet, 409
buttocks, 409
face, 409
hips, 409
inner knee, 407, 409
lateral thigh, 407
patient evaluation, 404–405, 405, 406
photography to document, 414
posttraumatic vessels, 407
pre- and posttreatment vessel populations, 407, 408
pregnancy, 403, 404, 409
public misperception and malpractice, 413–414
resistant vessels, 409
responses to, 404, 407, 408
sclerosant interaction in clinical setting, 407

Sclerotherapy, anatomy and (continued)
  sclerosants, 409–411
    choice of, 410
    equivalent concentrations of, 410
    general rules, 409
    high concentrations of, 411
    hypertonic saline, 410
    low concentrations of, 411
    polidocanol, 410, 410
    selection of sclerosant concentrations,
        410–411, 410
    sotradecol, 410
  sclerotherapeutic crudity, 404
  spectrum of posttreatment response, 404
  treatment for extravasation/impending
      tissue necrosis, 413, 413
  unpredictable fragility of veins, 405,
      406
  varicosity and, 405, 405, 406
  vascular growth dynamics, 403–404
    etiology/taxonomy, 404
    proliferation and quiescence,
        403–404
  vessel size and color, 407
  wider uses of, 416
Scrotum, pressure dressings for, 32
Scrubbing, surgical, 58–59
Sebaceous carcinoma, 242–243, 243
Sebaceous cyst(s), 228
Sebaceous hyperplasia, 231
Seborrheic keratoses, 224–225
Secondary contraction, 298
Secondary defect(s), definition of, 309
Secondary intention, forehead reconstruc-
      tion, 355–356, 357
  lip reconstruction, 332, 332
  Mohs micrographic surgery, 567, 568
  nasal reconstruction, 383
  temple reconstruction, 361
  typical course of, 13
Secondary motion, definition of, 309
Sedation, preoperative, 110–111
Seizure(s), 115
Sensorcaine. See Bupivacaine (Marcaine/
      Sensorcaine)
Sensory nerve(s), 42–43, 43, 109, 110
Seroma, as complication of liposuction,
      540
  as complication of split-thickness skin
      graft (STSG), 527
Shave abrasion, scar revision, 261
Shave excision, 224, 225–226
Shaw scalpel(s), 87–88, 87, 146
Side/length ratio of wounds, 187, 188
Side/side ratio of wounds, 187, 188
Silicone gel sheeting, and hypertrophic
      scarring, 261, 263
Silk suture, 80, 80t
Simple closure, in Mohs micrographic sur-
      gery, 566–567
Simple interrupted suture, 173, 173
Simple lentigines, 226
Simple running suture, 179, 179
Single-arm (Burow's wedge) advancement
      flap, 312, 314, 315
Skin, anatomy of, 495

biological or mechanical creep of, 605
contaminating or transient flora of, 57
elasticity of, 192
layers of, 13
normal or resident flora of, 57
preparation of, for infection control,
      57–58
Skin cancer. See Malignant lesion(s)
Skin flap(s). See specific types of flap
Skin graft. See also Full-thickness skin
      graft (FTSG); Split-thickness skin
      graft (STSG)
  contraction of, 298
  definition of, 297–298
  for forehead reconstruction, 356
  for lip reconstruction, 332, 333–334
  physiology of, 297–298
Skin hook(s), 92, 92
Skin reconstruction, 336, 339, 339
Skin tag(s), 224
Skin tension line(s) (STLs). See also Mini-
      mum skin tension line(s) (MSTLs);
      Relaxed skin tension line(s)
      (RSTLs)
  determining direction of, 216–218,
      216–219
  diagrams of, 166, 210–211, 211
  direction of, 214–216, 214, 215
  extrinsic factors in development of,
      212, 213
  facial muscles and, 213, 213
  factors in development of, 212, 213
  historical aspects of, 211–212
  intrinsic factors in development of, 212
  sleep lines, 214
  terminology for, 210
  variability in direction of, 213–219,
      213–219
SkinPrep, 25, 25t
Sleep line(s), 214
Slit grafting, in hair replacement,
      470–471, 487–489
Slot deformity, as complication of scalp re-
      duction, 559
SMAS (Superficial Musculoaponeurotic
      System), 38, 211, 212, 213,
      350–352, 350–352, 357–359,
      358, 595
Soft-tissue augmentation, fibrel, 423–427,
      437
  indications for, 424–425
  product and its mechanisms, 424, 425
  side effects and complications,
      426–427, 437
  technique, 425–426
  ideal filler, 423–424
  injectable bovine collagen, 419–423,
      437
    adverse treatment responses,
        422–423
    formulations, 419–420, 437
    injectable collagen implant and auto-
        immune disease, 423
    maintenance of correction and fate of
        implant, 421–422
    patient selection and skin testing, 420

technique of injection, 420–421,
      420–422
  injectable tissue augmentation, 419
  liquid silicone, 427–433, 437
    animal studies, 427
    breast augmentation, 431
    clinical experience, 427, 428–430
    complications, 428, 431–432, 432,
        433
    current status of, 432, 437
    granulomas, 431, 432
    illegality of, 432
    literature review, 427–428, 431–432
    nodularity beading, 431–432
    overcorrection, 431–432, 432, 433
    physical characteristics, 427
    volume of, 428, 431
Solar lentigines, 226
Sorbsan Topical Wound Dressing, 29
Sotradecol, as sclerosant, 410
Spencer suture scissors, 94, 94
Spinal accessory nerve, 44, 45, 109–110,
      109
S-plasty, variation of ellipse excision, 205,
      206, 207
Splicing, 2, 2
Split nail deformity(ies), 277, 277
Split-thickness graft nail bed reconstruc-
      tion, 280
Split-thickness skin graft (STSG), anesthe-
      sia for, 521
  classification of, 519, 520
  definition of, 297, 519
  donor sites for, 520–521
  for forehead reconstruction, 356
  for nasal reconstruction, 383
  indications for, 519–520
  postoperative expectations and complica-
      tions, 526–528
    cosmetic considerations, 528
    functional complications, 527–528
    hematomas and seromas, 527
    infection, 527
    movement, 527
    technical considerations, 527
  sterile technique, 521
  surgical dressings, 526, 526
  surgical techniques, 521–526
    electric dermatomes, 523–524, 524
    instrumentation, 522
    pinch grafts, 522–523, 523
    preparations for surgery, 521–522
    securing the graft, 524–526, 525
Spot freeze technique, of cryosurgery, 156
Spread scar(s), 132
Squamous cell carcinoma (SCC), adeno-
      squamous carcinoma, 108
  clinical appearance of, 238, 238
  cryosurgery for, 158, 159, 160, 161
  cutaneous squamous cell carcinoma,
      108
  incidence of, 238
  Mohs micrographic surgery for, 238,
      568–569
  nail unit excision, 278–279, 279
  surgical treatment of, 238–239

S-shaped wound(s), dog-ear formation, 198
Staged flap(s), 310
Stainless steel staple closure, 183, *183*
Stainless steel suture, 80
Standard round grafting, in hair replacement, 469, *470, 477, 477, 478, 479–481*
Standing cone(s), 189, *189, 197, 198,* 203
Staphylococcus infection, 57, 61, 501
Staple(s), 82–83
Stapler(s), 94–95, *94*
Staple-remover, 94, *94*
STAR technique, 607, 614
Statute of limitations, 140
Statutes of repose, 140
Steam autoclave, 50–51, 50t, 98
Steatocystoma multiplex, 228
Stein-Abbe-Estlander flap, 343
Sterilization of equipment, dermabrasion equipment, 53
 dermabrasion fraises and brushes, 53
 dermabrasion handpieces, 53
 equipment maintenance, 53
 electrosurgical equipment, 52–53, *52, 53*
  electrosurgical electrodes, 52, *52*
  electrosurgical handles and cords, 52–53, *52–53*
 human immunodeficiency virus and hepatitis B virus cross-contamination risks, 54, *54*
 laser equipment, 53
 methods
  chemiclave, 50t, 51
  cold sterilization, 50t, 51
  dry heat sterilization, 50t, 51, 98
  flash sterilization, 98
  gas sterilization, 50t, 51, 98
  steam autoclave, 50–51, 50t, 98
 surgical instruments
  cleaning of, 48, *48,* 98
  construction of, 47–48
  nonpacked instruments, 48–49
  packing of, 48–49, *48, 49*
  sterilization methods, 50–51, 50t, 97–98
  storage of, 51
  surgical tray setup, 51–52
Steri-Srip, 82
Steroid(s), 228–229
Stevens tenotomy scissors, 88, *88,* 91
STL(s). See *Skin tension line(s) (STLs)*
Stress relaxation, 606
Stretch-back, following scalp reduction, 559
Strip harvesting, in hair replacement, 478–481
Stroke, 115–116
STSG. See *Split-thickness skin graft (STSG)*
Subcutaneous forehead, 349, *350*
Subcutaneous island pedicle flap, for nasal reconstruction, 392, 395
Subcutaneous suture(s), in cold steel surgery, 168–169, *168*

Subgaleal space, 352–353, *352, 353*
Submandibular triangle of neck, 44, *44*
Submental triangle of neck, 44, *44*
Submuscular fibroadipose layer, of eyebrow, 352
Subungual hematoma, 272
Subungual verrucae, 281
Sun-damaged facial skin, laser treatment for, 450
Superficial anatomy. See *Anatomy*
Superficial basal cell carcinoma, 106, *106*
Superficial galea aponeurotica, 351
Superficial Musculoaponeurotic System (SMAS), 38, 211, 212, *213,* 350–352, *350–352,* 357–359, *358,* 595
Superficial peel(s). See *Chemical peel(s)*
Superficial peroneal nerve, 74, *74*
Superficial temporal artery, 39, *39,* 108–109, *109,* 358, *358*
Superficial temporal fascia, 357–358
Superficial temporal vein, 39, *39*
Superior auricular muscle, 37
Superior helical rim, reconstruction of, 363, *364–367*
Supraorbital nerve, 73, *109,* 110
Supratarsal fixation, 588
Supratrochlear nerve, 73, *109,* 110
Sural nerve, 74, *74*
Surface anesthesia, 65
Surface scar(s), abnormal, 131–133
Surgery. See *specific surgical techniques*
Surgical gut suture, 78, 79t
Surgical instrument(s). See *Instrumentation and equipment; Sterilization of equipment*
Surgical scar(s), dermabrasion for, 498–499, *499*
Surgical scrubbing, 58–59
Surgical tray setup, 51–52
Surgical wound dressing(s). See *Dressing(s)*
Suture(s), absorbable sutures, 78–79, 79t
 catgut, 78, 79t
 polydioxanone (Ethicon), 79, 79t
 polyglactin 910 (Vicryl), 79, 79t
 polyglycolic acid (Dexon), 78–79, *79,* 79t
 polyglyconate (Maxon), 79, 79t
 characteristics of, 77–78
 knot security of, 77–78
 memory of, 77
 natural sutures, 78
 nonabsorbable sutures, 78, 80, 80t
  cotton, 80
  nylon, 80, 80t
  polybutester, 80, 80t
  polyester, 80, 80t
  polypropylene, 80, 80t
  silk, 80, 80t
  stainless steel, 80
 size of, 78
 synthetic sutures, 78
Suture reaction(s), treatment of, 130, *130*
Suture Strip Plus, 82

Suture tension adjustment reel, 606
Suture-cutting scissors, 94, *94*
Suturing instruments, needle-holders, 47, *48,* 93–94, *94*
 staplers, 94–95, *94*
 suture-cutting scissors, 94, *94*
Suturing technique(s). See also *Closure(s)*
 basting suture, 181–182
  buried basting suture, 182, *182*
  for full-thickness skin graft, 305
  interrupted basting suture, 181–182, *182*
  running basting suture, 182
  upper dermal running stitch, 182
 combination closures, 184
 dog-ear formation and, 194–195, *195*
 instrument tie, 171, *172*
 interrupted suture, 173–179
  buried dermal suture, 177, *177*
  buried horizontal mattress suture, 178, *178*
  buried vertical mattress suture, 178–179, *178*
  deep subcutaneous suture, 177–178, *177*
  half-buried horizontal mattress suture, 176, *176*
  half-buried vertical mattress suture, 174–175, *174*
  horizontal mattress suture, 175–176, *175, 176*
  interrupted subcutaneous suture, 176–179, *177, 178*
  simple interrupted suture, 173, *173*
  vertical mattress suture, 173–175, *174*
 key suture, 309
 needles, 80–81, *81*
 running suture, 179–181
  running horizontal mattress suture, 180, *180*
  running locked suture, 179–180, *179*
  running subcutaneous suture, 181, *181*
  running subcuticular suture, 180–181, *181*
  simple running suture, 179, *179*
 stainless steel staple closure, 183, *183*
 subcutaneous sutures in cold steel surgery, 168–169, *168*
 suture materials, 77–80, 79t, 80t
 suture removal, 127, 182–183, *183*
 wound closure tapes, 183–184, *184*
Synthetic suture(s), 78
Syringe(s), 70, *71*
Syringoma(s), 231, *231*

TAC. See *Triamcinolone (TAC)*
Tachycardia, after liposuction, 540
Tactifier(s), 25, 25t
Tape(s), composite bandages, 25
 wound closure tapes, 82, 183–184, *184*
Tarsorrhaphy, 593

Tattoo(s), alexandrite laser treatment for, 461
  argon laser treatment for, 452
  carbon dioxide laser treatment for, 450
  neodymium:yttrium-aluminum-garnet laser treatment for, 462–463, *463*
  pigmented lesion dye laser treatment for, 461
  Q-switched ruby laser treatment for, 459, *459*
  removal of, 499
TCA. See *Trichloroacetic acid (TCA)*
Tegaderm Plus, 26–27, 27t
Telangiectasia, argon laser treatment for, 451, 452
  pulsed dye laser treatment for, 453
Telogen effluvium, as complication of scalp reduction, 559
Temple, adherence of superficial fascia and skin to, 358–359
  anatomy of, 356–359, *356–359*
  cutaneous innervation of, 357
  deep temporal fascia of, 359
  intertemporal-fascial plane, 359
  relaxed skin tension lines of, 357, *357*
  superficial musculoaponeurotic system of, 357–359, *358*
  superficial temporal artery and auriculotemporal nerve of, 358, *358*
  superficial temporal fascia of, 357–358
  temporalis muscle of, 359, *359*
Temple reconstruction, anatomy of temple, 356–359, *356–359*
  preparation for, 361
  primary fusiform closure, 359, 361
  rotation flaps for, *360*, 361
  secondary intention, 361
  transposition flaps for, 361
Temporal artery, 358, *358*
Temporalis muscle, 359, *359*
Tennis headband, 30–31, *31*
Tension, definition of, 212
  dog-ears and, 193–194
Termination of physician-patient relationship, 138
Tetracaine (Pontocaine), 66, 67t, 68
Thigh, sclerotherapy for, 407
30–degree-angle flap, 324, 325, *325*, *326*
Thrombophlebitis, as complication of sclerotherapy, 412
Thrombosis, as complication of sclerotherapy, 412
Tibial nerve, 74, *74*
Tincture of benzoin, 25, 25t
Tissue compression and reactive expansion, in wound closure, *190*, 191, *192*
Tissue expansion, advantages and disadvantages of, 616
  complications, 608–609
    hematoma, 609
    implant failure, 609
    infection, 608–609
    ischemia, 609
    ISLE technique, 609

neurapraxia, 609
  pain, 609
  for forehead reconstruction, 355
  future role of, 615–616
  histologic changes, 607–608
    appendages, 608
    capsule formation, 608
    dermis, 608
    epidermis, 608
    fat, 608
    muscle, 608
  history of, 605–606
  indications for, 609–616, *610–615*
  technique, 606–607, *606*, *607*
    chronic balloon expansion, 606–607, *606*
    immediate balloon expansion, 607, *607*
    STAR technique, 607, 614
Tissue glue(s), 81–82
Tissue marking, in Mohs micrographic surgery, 563–564, *564*
Tissue-holding instruments. See *Instrumentation and equipment*
Topical agent(s), for condylomata acuminata, 223
  for lentigines, 226
  for plantar warts, 223
  for verrucae planae, 223
  for verrucae vulgaris, 222
  occlusive dressings and, 17
Topical anesthetics, 66
Tort law of negligence, 139
Towel clamps, 96, *96*
Toxicity, of local anesthetics, 69–70, 70t, 116–117, 534–535
Trachyonychia, 265
Track marks, 255
Tragus and crus of helix, reconstruction of, 369, *370–371*
Tranquilizer(s), 64, 64t
Transconjunctival blepharoplasty, 592–593, *593*
Transient flora, 57
Transplanting hair. See *Hair replacement*
Transposition flap, banner flap, *322*, 323, *323*, *368–369*, 369
  definition of, 310
  dog-ear formation and, 197, *197*
  for forehead reconstruction, 355
  for lip reconstruction, 339, *340*, *341*
  for nasal reconstruction, 387
  for posterior ear, 379, *379–380*
  for temple reconstruction, 361
  helical rim advancement flap, 363, 365, *367–368*, 369
  lobule "rim advancement" flap, 369, *370*
  method of, 319, 322–326, *322–327*
  pre- or post-auricular transposition flap, 363, *364–367*
  rhombic flap, *322*, 324–325, *324*, 369, *370–371*
Tretinoin, in dermabrasion, 495, *496*
  lentigines, 226
  verrucae planae, 223

Triamcinolone, 228–229
Triamcinolone (TAC), 261
Triangles of neck, 44, *44*
Triangular fossa of antihelix, reconstruction of, 369, *371–373*, 374
Trichilemmal cyst(s), 228
Trichloroacetic acid (TCA), applying, in chemical peel, 509–510
  as peeling agent, 505, 505t, 506, 507
  for acne, 512–513
  for actinic keratoses, 512
  for lentigines, 226, 514
  for melasma, 513
  for verrucae planae, 223
  for wrinkles, 512
  for xanthelasma, 232
  in combination peels, 510–511
Trichoepithelioma, 107–108, 231–232
Trigeminal nerve, 42–43, *43*, *72*, 73, *109*, 110
Trilobed flap, for nasal reconstruction, 392
Tumescent liposuction, areas treated by, 529
  before and after photographs, *531*, *534*, *535*, *538*
  complications of, 540
  differences between plastic surgery and dermatology for, 530
  disadvantages of, 540
  general anesthesia for, 530–531, 535–536
  good candidates for, 530
  improved safety with local anesthesia, 530
  intraoperative considerations
    anesthetic solution formulation, 533, 533t
    hemostasis, 535–536
    infiltration technique, 536–537, 536t
    intravascular fluid status, 536
    lidocaine pharmacokinetics, 533–534
    liposuction cannulas, 537
    liposuction technique, 537
    patient's modesty, anxiety, and physical comfort, 533
    safe lidocaine dose, 534
    toxicity of local anesthetic, 534–535, 535t
  local anesthesia for, 69t, 529–540, 533t
  mechanical advantages of, 531
  postoperative considerations, 537–540
    bruising, 537
    drainage, 538–539
    elastic support garments, 539
    immediate postoperative recovery, 538
    inflammation, 539–540
    instructions for care after liposuction, 532t, 538
    physical activity, 539
    reduced pain, 537–538
    wound care and bathing, 539
  preoperative considerations, 531–533, *531*, *534*
    diet, 531–532

instructions for care before liposuction, 532t
prophylactic antibiotics, 532–533
technique, 529
Tumor(s). See *Benign cutaneous lesion(s); Benign nail unit tumor(s); Malignant lesion(s)*
Tunable dye laser, 456–458
Tungsten-carbide inserts, for instruments, 47, *48*, 88, *89*, 93, *94*
Tyrell hook, 92, *92*

U-flap, for earlobe repair, 581, *581*
Ulcer(s), extravasation ulcers, 412
nonextravasation ulcers, 412–413, *412*
Undermining, 167, *167*, 194
Undermining instrument(s), 91–92
Ungraft(s), in hair replacement, 470
Universal precautions, 60
Upper cervical nerve(s), *109*, 110
Upper dermal running stitch, 182
Upper eyelqid(s), anatomy of, 583–584, *583–585*
crease formation for, *584*
Upper lid blepharoplasty, anesthesia for, 586
Asian blepharoplasty, 585, 588, *589*
female blepharoplasty, 585
goals of, 585
male blepharoplasty, 585, 588
procedures for operation, *585–589*, 586–588
skin markings for, *585*, 586
supratarsal fixation, 588

Varicose veins, 405, *405*, *406*
Vascular disease, 103
Vascular lesion(s), laser treatment for, 446–447, 447t, 449t, 451t
Vascular structure(s). See *Blood supply*
Vasoconstrictor(s), 68
Vasodepressor syncope, 114
Vasovagal syncope, 114
Ventricular fibrillation (VF), 120, 120t
Ventricular tachycardia (VT), 120, 120t
Verrucae, carbon dioxide laser treatment for, 449
condylomata acuminata, 223–224
human papilloma virus (HPV) causing, 221–222
nails, 280–281
periungual verrucae, 280–281
plantar warts, 223
subungual verrucae, 281
verrucae planae, 222–223
verrucae vulgaris, 222
Verrucae planae, 222–223
Verrucae vulgaris, 222
Verrucous carcinoma, 240, *240*
Versican, 6–7, *7*
Vertical mattress suture, 173–175, *174*
VF (ventricular fibrillation), 120, 120t

Vicryl suture, 79, 79t
Vigilon, 28, 28t
Vision loss, as complication of injectable bovine collagen, 422
Voluntary binding arbitration, 141
VT (ventricular tachycardia), 120, 120t
V-Y advancement flap, nasal reconstruction, 387

Wart(s). See *Verrucae*
Web formation, 218, *219*
Webster needle-holder, 93–94, *94*
Weck knife, for split-thickness skin graft (STSG), 522
Wen(s), 228
Westcott scissors, 88, *88*
Wet technique of liposuction, 535–536
Wire brush(es), for dermabrasion, 53, 97, *97*
Wound(s). See also *Closure(s); Closure material(s); Dressing(s); Infection; Infection control; Wound healing*
apical angle of, 187–188, *189*
bacteriology of, 17
depth of, 13, *13*
depth of, and dog-ears, 194, *194*
geometry of, in horizontal plane, 187–189, *188*, *189*
side/length ratio of, 187, *188*
side/side ratio of, 187, *188*
Wound closure(s). See *Closure(s); Closure material(s)*
Wound closure tape(s), 82, 183–184, *184*
Wound dressing(s). See *Dressing(s)*
Wound healing. See also *Closure(s); Closure material(s); Dressing(s); Infection; Infection control*
biochemistry and physiology of, 14, 15t
cytokines, 9–13
clinical trials of growth factors in wound healing, 12t, 13
cytokine modulation of cell proliferation and migration, 11
effects of cytokines on extracellular matrix gene expression, 9, 10t
mechanistic interactions between growth factor, 10
modulation of degradative events by cytokines, 10
pathway of normal wound repair, 9
regulation of angiogenesis by cytokines, 11
relevance of in vitro observation to wound healing in vivo, 11–12, 11t
delayed wound healing, 13–14, 14t
dermal extracellular matrix, 1–7
collagen, 1–4, *2–4*
elastic fibers, 4–6, *5–6*
extracellular matrix deposition, 7
fibronectin, 7
glycosaminoglycans, 6–7, *7*
proteoglycans, 6–7, *7*
dynamics of, 190–192, *190–192*

factors hindering normal healing, 126t
in Mohs micrographic surgery, 566–567
instructions to patients, 111, 126–127, *126*
integrated healing response
biochemistry and physiology of wound healing, 14, 15t
delayed wound healing, 13–14, 14t
measures of healing and scarring, 14, 16t
wound healing process, 13–14, *13*, 14t
keratinocyte migration, 7–8
measures of healing and scarring, 14, 16t
pathway of normal wound repair, 9
principles of wound care, 125–126, 126t
process of, 13–14, *13*, 14t
resident cells of the dermis, 8–9, *9*
three-dimensional considerations and role of contour, 192–193, *192*, *193*
vertical dynamics of, 193, *193*
Wound infection. See *Infection*
W-plasty, 217, 260, *260*
Wrinkle(s). See also *Skin tension line(s)*
chemical peels for, 511–512, *512*
dermabrasion for, *497*, 498, *498*
Wrist block, 74

Xanthelasma, 232
Xenograft(s), definition of, 297
Xylocaine. See *Lidocaine (Xylocaine)*

Y scalp reduction pattern, anesthesia for, 549
instrumentation for, 549
preoperative considerations for, 549
technique of, 549, *550*

ZC. See *Zyderm collagen (ZC)*
ZI. See *Zyderm I (ZI) collagen*
Zimmer dermatome, for split-thickness skin graft (STSG), 523–524
ZP. See *Zyplast (ZP)*
Z-plasty, for lip reconstruction, 341, *342*
for redirection of incision along STLs, 217, *218*
for torn earlobes, 580, *580*
method of, *253*, 255, 258, *258*, *259*, 260
Zyderm collagen (ZC), 419–423, 437
Zyderm I (ZI) collagen, 419–423
Zygomaticus major and minor muscle(s), 36
Zyplast (ZP), 419–423

ISBN 0-07-036471-0

90000>

9 780070 364714

LASK:PRIN&TECH US